P9-DGB-738

STAYING WELL INFORMED CAN BE AN IMPORTANT PART OF STAYING WELL

Compiled by a team of leading medical educators working with the nation's foremost medical publisher, this invaluable sourcebook can help you help yourself to better health, by providing complete, current information on every significant medical issue.

Especially adapted from a standard reference for health professionals, *Mosby's Medical, Nursing, and Allied Health Dictionary,* this fully revised and updated guide features in-depth entries, charts, tables, and drawings to aid you in making faster, better-informed decisions about your health.

Praise for *Mosby's Medical, Nursing, and Allied Health Dictionary*

"SUPERB!"
—Episcopal Hospital School of Nursing, Philadelphia

"THE BEST! VERY COMPREHENSIVE AND EASY TO READ." —University of Wisconsin

"EXCELLENT! The longer definitions go happily beyond the usual medical dictionary."
—Loyola University, Chicago, Illinois

THE

MOSBY

MEDICAL

ENCYCLOPEDIA

REVISED EDITION

WALTER D. GLANZE
Managing editor

KENNETH N. ANDERSON
Editor and medical writer

LOIS E. ANDERSON
Consulting editor and writer

Ⓟ

A PLUME BOOK

The ideas, procedures, and suggestions contained in this encyclopedia are not intended as a substitute for consulting with your physician. All matters regarding your health require medical supervision.

PLUME
Published by the Penguin Group
Penguin Books USA Inc., 375 Hudson Street, New York, New York 10014, U.S.A.
Penguin Books Ltd, 27 Wrights Lane, London W8 5TZ, England
Penguin Books Australia Ltd, Ringwood, Victoria, Australia
Penguin Books Canada Ltd, 10 Alcorn Avenue, Toronto, Ontario, Canada M4V 3B2
Penguin Books (N.Z.) Ltd, 182-190 Wairau Road, Auckland 10, New Zealand

Penguin Books Ltd, Registered Offices: Harmondsworth, Middlesex, England

Published by Plume, an imprint of Dutton Signet, a division of Penguin Books USA Inc.
Published by arrangement with the Mosby Company. For information address the
Mosby Company, 11830 Westline Industrial Drive, St. Louis, Missouri 63146.

First Plume Printing, November, 1985
First Plume Printing (Revised Edition), June, 1992

            15   17   19   20   18   16   14

Copyright © 1985, 1992 by the C. V. Mosby Company
All rights reserved

 REGISTERED TRADEMARK—MARCA REGISTRADA

ISBN 0-452-26672-6

Printed in the United States of America

Without limiting the rights under copyright reserved above, no part of this publication
may be reproduced, stored in or introduced into a retrieval system, or transmitted, in any
form, or by any means (electronic, mechanical, photocopying, recording, or otherwise),
without the prior written permission of both the copyright owner and the above publisher
of this book.

BOOKS ARE AVAILABLE AT QUANTITY DISCOUNTS WHEN USED TO PROMOTE PRODUCTS OR
SERVICES. FOR INFORMATION PLEASE WRITE TO PREMIUM MARKETING DIVISION, PENGUIN
BOOKS USA INC., 375 HUDSON STREET, NEW YORK, NEW YORK 10014.

CONTENTS

EDITORS' FOREWORD

THIS MAJOR NEW REFERENCE WORK contains 22,000 entries providing complete current information about pregnancy and child care, in addition to signs and symptoms of the major diseases and the recommended treatments for them. It is based on the traditional *Mosby's Medical Nursing and Allied Health Dictionary,* used by hundreds of thousands of physicians, nurses, and allied health personnel in their education and health care practices. It is a valuable encyclopedia of medical knowledge for both the professional and nonprofessional and should be in every home and office library.

All too often, the words we want most to understand are the words that describe our bodies and their normal or abnormal conditions. And the language of health seems hopelessly difficult. It's little wonder that doctors have been accused of creating a secret language to deliberately baffle patients and prevent them from learning the true condition of their health and the nature of the medications prescribed.

Actually, doctors have been striving for centuries to create a reasonable language that even they can understand. Most medical terms are derived from Greek or Latin words; some are combinations of Greek and Latin words. One advantage of this system is that doctors in all parts of the world, by using the same medical term for the same body part or health condition, will speak and write in an international language regardless of their native tongues. Thus, the word "acroparesthesia" means a tingling or numbness in the hands or feet to a doctor in France, India, Japan, or Mexico, as well as to a doctor in one of the English-speaking nations. The doctor also knows immediately what medical condition is being described, since part of the term, "acro," refers to an extremity of the body. Another part, "para," can mean near or beyond, and "esthesia" is translated as sensation or feeling. The three parts of the medical term are derived form Greek words, and in addition to having a universal meaning, a term such as "acroparesthesia" offers an economy of wordage to the doctor since it often saves time and space to say or write the 15-letter medical term rather than using the nine words, "a tingling or numbness in the hands or feet." The reading will find throughout this encyclopedia examples of "combining forms," which help in understanding the use of many Greek or Latin prefixes or suffixes commonly found in medical terms.

Adding to the confusion of medical terms for many persons is the practice of naming diseases, injuries, instruments, and even units of matter and energy for people. In some instances, however, there is an advantage. For example, it is probably easier even for doctors to remember a term like "Reiter's syndrome" than the more exact medical description of "arthritis associated with nonbacterial urethritis and conjunctivitis." And it seems less confusing to some medical people to use the term "Parkinson's disease" than the older "paralysis agitans," which suggests a contradiction of paralysis the excessive movement. In this encyclopedia, the editors have included the alternative terms where a disease or condition is commonly known by more than one name.

Like diseases, medicines are likely to have more than one name. In fact, there are some drugs with as many as 80 different brand names. This encyclopedia has been carefully screened to make sure that brand-name drugs listed on the following pages are identified also by their generic names. A further effort has been made to ensure that the drugs listed in this encyclopedia are those currently prescribed by physicians in the United States. Particularly valuable for readers who take prescription or nonprescription drugs is the "Guide to Common Drug Interactions," which describes adverse reactions of various classes of drugs, such as antihistamines, diuretics, and oral contraceptives.

A unique feature of this medical encyclopedia is its combination of easy-to-understand readability and up-to-date medical accuracy. Each definition has been reviewed by a team of English-language experts to ensure that it can be easily understood by a person without the special education or training usually needed to comprehend complex medical terms. Each definition also was reviewed by a qualified health professional after final editing as a further guarantee of reliability.

Among the entries on disease, drugs, and procedures, there are many that have paragraphs with separate headings; the information given there is of special importance to the nurse and the patient. Examples of such subheadings are "diagnosis," "treatment," "patient care," "caution," "adverse effects," "method," and "outcome." Twenty-two tables, more than 100 illustrations, and 9 appendixes are valuable sources of information and complement the encyclopedia entries.

The pronunciation system developed for this encyclopedia is basically a system that most readers are familiar with because of its use in most popular English-language dictionaries, including many common desk dictionaries.

The editors

GUIDE TO THE ENCYCLOPEDIA

ALPHABETIC ORDER

The entries are alphabetized in dictionary style, that is, letter by letter, disregarding spaces or hyphens between words. For example:

analgesic	artificial lung
anal membrane	artificially acquired immunity
analog	artificial pacemaker

The alphabetic order is alphanumeric, that is, numbers are placed as though they were spelled-out numerals, and words and numbers form a single list (with few exceptions). For example:

Nilstat
90-90 traction
ninth nerve

NATURAL HEADWORDS

Entry "headwords" of more than one word are given according to usage, in their natural order. For example: **abdominal surgery,** not **surgery, abdominal,** and **achondroplastic dwarf,** not **dwarf, achondroplastic.**

The second word (**surgery** and **dwarf**) is usually listed at its own alphabetic place, with a reference to the other entry.

NUMBERED DEFINITIONS

If a headword has more than one meaning, the meanings are numbered, and often they are given with the field of the meaning. For example: **"fractionation, 1.** (in neurology) . . . **2.** (in chemistry) . . . **3.** (in bacteriology) . . ."

Words that are spelled alike but have quite different meanings and origins are usually given as separate entries, with small raised numbers. For example: "**aural[1],** of or pertaining to the ear or hearing . . ." followed by the entry "**aural[2],** of or pertaining to an aura."

THE BOLDFACE WORDS OF AN ENTRY

Besides the headword itself, an entry may include several types of boldface words (in the following order):

1. *A headword abbreviation.* For example: **central nervous system (CNS)**

2. *Plurals (or the singular) of the headword.* For example: "**carcinoma,** *pl.* **carcinomas, carcinomata**" (and "**data,** *sing.* **datum**")

3. *Hidden entries.* These are expressions that can best be explained inside a more general entry. For example, the entry **equine encephalitis** continues as follows: "... **Eastern equine encephalitis (EEE)** is a severe form of the infection . . . **western equine encephalitis (WEE),** which occurs . . . **Venezuelan equine encephalitis (VEE),** which is common in . . ."

4. *Indirect cross-references.* These are implied references to other defined entries, usually beginning with the phrase "Kinds of . . ." For example: **"dwarf,** . . . Kinds of dwarfs include **achondroplastic dwarf, Amsterdam dwarf,** and **thanatophoric dwarf."**

5. *Synonyms.* These are terms with the same or a very closely related meaning. They are identified with the phrase "Also called" or "Also spelled" (or, for verbs and adjectives, the word "Also"). For example: **abducens nerve,** . . . Also called **sixth nerve."**

6. *Cross-references.* These are direct cross-references to another entry for additional information. They begin with "See also" or "Compare." For Example: **abdominal aorta,** . . . See also **descending aorta.**

7. *Parts of speech.* These are forms that are closely related to the headword. They are shown as run-on entries that do not need their own definition. For example: **"abalienation,** . . . **—abalienate,** *v.,* **abalienated,** *adj."*

REFERENCE ENTRIES

A reference entry is an undefined entry that refers to a defined entry for information. There, the term usually appears in boldface—see above. A reference entry says "See . . ."

Some reference entries refer indirectly to a lightface term in the defined entry. For example: **"air sickness:** See **motion sickness."** and **"motion sickness,** . . . Examples are . . . air sickness . . ."

A reference entry may also appear in the form of a numbered sense of a defined entry. For example: **"hyperalimentation, 1.** overfeeding or the . . . **2.** See **total parenteral nutrition."** (The entry **total parenteral nutrition** shows the synonym **hyperalimentation.)**

A reference entry that would be derived from a boldface term in an immediately neighboring entry is not listed again as a headword. For example: **"acardius amorphus,** . . . Also called **acardius anceps."** But **acardius anceps** is not listed again as a reference entry because it would immediately follow the entry (the next entry is **acariasis**). Therefore:

If a term is not listed as an entry at the expected place, the reader might find it among the boldface terms of the immediately preceding or the immediately following entry.

OTHER KINDS OF ENTRIES

1. *Abbreviation entries.* These entries give the full form in boldface if it is listed, in turn, as a defined entry. For example: **"ABC,** abbreviation for **aspiration biopsy cytology"** or **"H,** symbol for **hydrogen."** If the full form is not listed as an entry, it is given in italics. For example: **"CBF,** abbreviation for *cerebral blood flow."*

2. *Combining forms.* See the definition of the entry **combining form** in this encyclopedia. Combining forms are helpful in understanding many terms in which they appear—even many terms that are not in a dictionary.

3. *Entries with special paragraphs.* Among the entries on diseases, drugs, and procedures, there are many that have paragraphs with separate headings. The information given there is especially meaningful to the nurse and the patient. Examples of such headings are "diagnosis," "treatment," "patient care," "caution," "adverse effects," "method," and "outcome."

PRONUNCIATION

The pronunciation system of this dictionary is basically a system that most readers know from their use of popular English dictionaries, especially the major college or desk dictionaries. All symbols for English sounds are ordinary letters of the alphabet with few changes, and with the exception of the schwa, /ə/ (the neutral vowel). See the Pronunciation Key.

1. *Accents.* Pronunciation is given with heavy and light accents, and with a raised dot that shows that two neighboring symbols are pronounced separately. For example:

anoopsia /an′ō·op′sē·ə/
cecoileostomy /sē′kō·il′ē·os′təmē/
methemoglobin /met′hēməglō′bin, met·hē′məglō′bin/

2. *Truncation.* Sometimes the pronunciation is shortened (truncated), especially for alternative or derived words. For example:

defibirillate /difī′brilāt, difib′-/
bacteriophage /baktir′ē·əfāj′, ...—**bacteriophage** -of′əjē/, *n.*

3. *Letterword or acronym.* In an acronym, each letter stands for something but the acronym is pronounced as a word. In a letterword, each letter is pronounced as itself. If the pronunciation of an abbreviation is not shown, the abbreviation is usually a letterword. For example:

ABO blood groups [read /ā′bē′ō′/, not /ā′bō/]

If the abbreviation is an acronym, this is indicated by pronunciation:

AWOL /ā′wôl/

4. *Foreign sounds.* See the Pronunciation Key. Certain foreign words and proper names are given in English approximations. Examples are **Müller** /mil′ər/, which is closer to German than would be /mY′lər/, or **jamais vu,** for which three acceptable

pronunciations are given: /zhämävY′/ (near-French) and the approximations /zhämävē′/ and (farthest removed from French but popular) /zhämävoo͞′/.

At any rate, the English speaker should not hesitate to follow whatever is usage in his or her working or social environment.

Many of the numerous *Latin* terms in this dictionary are not given with pronunciation, mainly because there are different ways (all of them understood) in which Latin is pronounced by the English speaker.

5. *Latin and Greek plurals.* The spelling of Latin and Greek plurals is shown in most cases. However, when the plural is regular according to Latin and Greek rules, the pronunciation is usually not included.

PRONUNCIATION KEY

Vowels

SYMBOLS	KEY WORDS
/a/	hat
/ä/	father
/ā/	fate
/e/	flesh
/ē/	she
/er/	air, ferry
/i/	sit
/ī/	eye
/ir/	ear
/o/	proper
/ō/	nose
/ô/	saw
/oi/	boy
/o͞o/	move
/o͝o/	book
/ou/	out
/u/	cup, love
/ur/	fur, first
/ə/	(the neutral vowel, always unstressed, as in) ago, focus
/ər/	teacher, doctor

Consonants

SYMBOLS	KEY WORDS
/b/	book
/ch/	chew
/d/	day
/f/	fast
/g/	good
/h/	happy
/j/	gem
/k/	keep
/l/	late
/m/	make
/n/	no
/ng/	sing drink
/ng·g/	finger
/p/	pair
/r/	ring
/s/	set
/sh/	shoe, lotion
/t/	tone
/th/	thin
/*th*/	than
/v/	very
/w/	work
/y/	yes
/z/	zeal
/zh/	azure, vision

Foreign sounds

/œ/ as in (French) **feu**/foe/, **Europe**/œrôp′/; (German) **schön** /shœn/, **Goethe** /gœ′tə/

/Y/ as in (French) **tu**/tY/, **déjà vu** /dāzhävY′/; (German) **grün** /grYn/, **Walküre** /vulkY′rə/

/kh/ as in (Scottish) **loch**/lokh/, (German) **Rorschach** /rôr′shokh/; **Bach** /bokh, bäkh/

/*kh*/ as in (German) **ich** /i*kh*/, **Reich** /rī*kh*/; (which is similar to the sound in the English word **fish**: /ish/, /rīsh/)

/N/ This symbol does not represent a sound but indicates that the preceding vowel is a nasal, as in French **bon** /bôN/, **en face** /äNfäs′/, or **international** /aNternäsyōnäl′/.

CREDITS

Appreciation is expressed to the following Mosby-Year Book authors whose titles provided a valuable resource toward the compilation of this encyclopedia.

Austrin, M.G.: Young's learning medical terminology, ed. 6, 1987.

Ballinger, P.W.: Merrill's atlas of radiographic positions and radiologic procedures, ed. 6, 1986.

Barnard, K.E., and Erickson, M.L.: Teaching children with developmental problems: a family care approach, ed. 2. 1976.

Bauer, J.D., Ackermann, P.G., and Toro, G.: Clinical laboratory methods, ed. 9, 1982.

Beck C.M., Rawlins, R.P., and Williams, S.R.: Mental health — psychiatric nursing, 1984.

Beck, E.W.: Mosby's atlas of functional human anatomy, 1982.

Billings, D.M., and Stokes, L.G.: Medical-surgical nursing: common health problems of adults and children across the life span, ed. 2, 1987.

Bower, F.L., and Bevis, E.O.: Fundamentals of nursing practice: concepts, roles, and functions, 1979.

Brooks, S.M., and Paynton-Brooks, N.: The human body: structure and function in health and disease, ed. 2, 1980.

Budassi, S. A., and Barber, J.M.: Mosby's manual of emergency care: practices and procedures, ed. 2, 1984

Burrell, L.O., and Burrell, Z.L., Jr.: Critical care, 1982

Bushong, S.C.: Radiologic science for technologists, ed. 3, 1984.

Butler, R.N., and Lewis, M.I.: Aging and mental health, ed. 3, 1982.

Campbell, J.M., and Campbell, J.B.: Laboratory mathematics: medical and biological applications, ed. 3, 1984.

Conover, M.B.: Understanding electrocardiography: physiological and interpretive concepts, ed. 4, 1984.

Daily, E.K., and Schroeder, J.S.: Techniques in bedside hemodynamic monitoring, ed. 3, 1984.

DeYoung, L.: Dynamics of nursing, ed. 5, 1985.

Fogel, C.I., and Woods, N.F.: Health care of women: a nursing perspective, 1981.

Goth, A.: Medical pharmacology: principles and concepts, ed. 11, 1984.

Gould, J.A., and Davies, G.J.: Orthopaedic and sports physical therapy, 1985.

Groër, M.W., and Shekleton, M.E.: Basic pathophysiology: a conceptual approach, ed. 2, 1983.

Hahn, A.B., Barkin, R.L., and Oestreich, S.J.K.: Pharmacology in nursing, ed. 16, 1986.

Hilt, N.E., and Cogburn, S.B.: Manual of orthopedics, 1980.

Hood, G.H., and Dincher, J.R.: Total patient care, ed. 6, 1984.

Ingalls, A.J., and Salerno, M.C.: Maternal and child health nursing, ed. 6, 1987.

Iorio, J.: Childbirth: family centered nursing, ed. 3, 1975.

Irwin, S., and Tecklin, J.S.: Cardiopulmonary physical therapy, 1985.

Jensen, M.D., and Bobak, I.M.: Maternity and gynecologic care: the nurse and the family, ed. 3, 1985.

Kaye, D., and Rose, L.F., editors: Fundamentals of internal medicine, 1983.

Kim, M.J., McFarland, G.K., and McLane, A.M.: Pocket guide to nursing diagnoses, ed. 2, 1987.

Lawrence, R.A.: Breastfeeding: a guide for the medical profession, ed. 2, 1985.

Malasanos, L., et al.: Health assessment, ed. 2, 1981.

McLane, A.M.: Classification of nursing diagnoses, 1987.

McClintic, J.R.: Human anatomy, 1982.

McPherson, S.P., and Spearman, C.B.: Respiratory therapy equipment, ed. 3, 1985.

Pagliaro, A.M., and Pagliaro, L.A.: Pharmacologic aspects of nursing, 1986.

Parcel, G.S.: Basic emergency care of the sick and injured. ed. 3, 1986.

Pasquali, E.A., et al.: Mental health nursing: a holistic approach, ed. 2, 1985.

Perry, A.G., and Potter, P.A.: Clinical nursing skills and techniques, 1986.

Phibbs, B.: The human heart: a consumer's guide to cardiac care, 1982.

Phillips, C.R.: Family-centered maternity/newborn care, ed. 2, 1987.

Phipps, W.D., Long, B.C., and Woods, N.F.: Medical-surgical nursing: concepts and clinical practice, ed. 3, 1987.

Pierog, S.H., and Ferrara, A.: Medical care of the sick newborn, ed. 2, 1976.

Potter, P.A., and Perry, A.G.: Basic nursing: theory and practice, 1987.

Quaal, S.J.: Comprehensive intra-aortic balloon pumping, 1984.

Rosen, P., et al.: Emergency medicine: concepts and clinical practice, ed. 2, 1987.

Saxton, D., Pelikan, P., Nugent, P., and Needleman, S.: Mosby's Assesstest, 1987.

Schottelius, B.A., and Schottelius, D.D.: Textbook of physiology, ed. 18, 1978.

Seidel, H.M., Ball, J.W., Dains, J.E., and Benedict, G.W.: Mosby's guide to physical examination, 1987.

Slonim, N.B., and Hamilton, L.H.: Respiratory physiology, ed. 5, 1987.

Smith, A.L.: Microbiology and pathology, ed. 12, 1980.

Spearman, C.B., and Sheldon, R.L.: Egan's fundamentals of respiratory therapy, ed. 4, 1982.

Stanhope, M., and Lancaster, J.: Community health nursing, 1984.

Stuart, G.W., and Sundeen, S.J.: Principles and practice of psychiatric nursing, ed. 3, 1987.

Taylor, C.M.: Mereness' essentials of psychiatric nursing, ed. 12, 1986.

Thibodeau, G.A.: Textbook of anatomy and physiology, ed. 12, 1987.

Tucker, S.M., et al.: Patient care standards, ed. 3, 1983.

U.C.S.F.: Mosby's manual of clinical nursing procedures, 1981.

Umphred, D.A.: Neurological rehabilitation, 1985.

Warner, C.G.: Emergency care: assessment and intervention, ed. 3, 1983.

Whaley, L.F., and Wong, D.L.: Nursing care of infants and children, ed. 1, 2, and 3, 1979, 1983, 1987.

Whaley, L.F., and Wong, D.L.: Essentials of pediatric nursing, ed. 2, 1985.

Wilkins, R.L., Sheldon, R.L., and Krider, S.J.: Clinical assessment in respiratory care, 1985.

Williams, S.R.: Nutrition and diet therapy, ed. 5, 1985.

Zschoche, D.A.: Mosby's comprehensive review of critical care, ed. 3, 1986.

Artists

Ernest W. Beck, B.S., M.A., Medical Illustrator
Glenna Deutsch
John Hagen
David Mascaro
Karen Waldo
Marcia Williams, Marcia Williams Medical Illustrations
Donald O'Connor

THE
MOSBY
MEDICAL
ENCYCLOPEDIA

A

A68, symbol for a protein found in the brains of patients with Alzheimer's disease. It is also found in the normal brains of fetuses and infants but begins to disappear by the age of 2 years.

āa, āā, ĀĀ, (in prescriptions) abbreviation for **ana,** meaning equal amounts of each ingredient.

AA, 1. abbreviation for **achievement age. 2.** abbreviation for **Alcoholics Anonymous.**

Aaron's sign, pain and soreness between the navel and the right hip bone during an attack of appendicitis.

abacterial /ab′aktē′rē·əl/, any place free of bacteria.

abactio, abortion or labor started by drugs or surgery.

Abadie's sign, a twitch of the eyelid that can occur with a too-active thyroid gland. It can occur when no disease is present.

abaissement /äbāsmäN′/, a falling, lowering, or depressing.

abalienation /əbāl′yənā′shən/, a state of physical decline or mental illness.

abarticular /ab′ärtik′yōōlər/, not having a joint.

abarticulation, dislocation of a joint.

abasia /əbā′zhə/, inability to walk.

Abbe-Estlander operation /ab′ē-est′-/, a type of skin graft on the mouth. A flap of skin from the healthy lip is attached to the injured lip. Inside the skin flap is a small artery that sends blood to the graft. After the graft "takes," the flap is removed.

Abbokinase, a trademark for a drug used to dissolve blood clots in deep veins (urokinase).

Abbot pump /ab′ət/, a small pump that allows exact amounts of a drug to go through an intravenous (IV) tube.

Abbott's method, a way to correct a crooked spine (scoliosis). The patient is placed in a plaster jacket that helps straighten the spine.

abdomen /ab′dəmən, abdō′mən/, the part of the body between the chest and the hips. Also called (*informal*) **belly.** See also **abdominal cavity.**

abdominal actinomycosis. See **actinomycosis.**

abdominal aorta, the large artery (aorta) that passes through the belly. It supplies blood to many different parts of the body, as the testicles, ovaries, kidneys, stomach, and the legs. See also **descending aorta.** Compare **thoracic aorta.**

abdominal aortography, the process of taking an x-ray of the abdominal aorta. A substance that blocks x-rays is used to outline the interior of the blood vessel.

abdominal bandage, a broad bandage often used after stomach surgery. It gives support to the belly.

abdominal binder, a bandage or elastic band that is wrapped around the stomach area. A binder is sometimes used after stomach surgery for support and to lessen pain. A kind of abdominal binder is the **Scultetus binder.**

abdominal breathing, a breathing technique in which the diaphragm and stomach muscles do most of the work. It is sometimes used with patients who have breathing difficulties. Patients learn to contract the stomach muscles to push the diaphragm upward and empty the lungs.

abdominal cavity, the space in the body that holds part of the esophagus, stomach, small intestines, liver, gallbladder, pancreas, spleen, kidneys, and tubes that deliver urine from the kidneys to the bladder (ureters).

abdominal delivery, the birth of a child through a surgical cut through the skin of the abdomen. This is also called **cesarean section.**

abdominal-diaphragmatic breathing, breathing in which the stomach moves out and the diaphragm moves downward when breathing in.

abdominal fistula, an abnormal opening from an organ to the outside of the body. For example, a colostomy is an opening from the bowel to the surface of the stomach area. This is done by surgery to unblock the bowels or when part of the bowel is removed.

abdominal hernia, a loop of bowel that bulges through the muscles of the abdomen. This can happen at an old surgical scar. Also called **ventral hernia.** See also **hernia.**

abdominal hysterectomy, removing the uterus through the abdomen.

abdominal inguinal ring, a part of the muscles in the groin. It is naturally weak, and hernias may occur here.

abdominal pain, pain in the belly that can be sudden or long-term, local or general. It can be an important symptom because surgery or medical treatment may be needed. The most common causes of severe pain are infection, a tear in the abdominal contents, and blockage of the bloodstream, intestine, or kidney. Conditions causing pain that may need surgery include appendicitis, pouches in the intestines (diverticulitis), gallbladder problems, pancreas infection, a bleeding peptic ulcer, blocked intestines, pouches in an artery wall (abdominal aortic aneurysms), and damage to an organ. Other causes of pain that may require surgery include serious pelvic inflammatory disease, a break in an ovarian lump (cyst), and pregnan-

1

cies outside the uterus. Pain during pregnancy may be caused by the weight of the fetus, or squeezing or moving the bowels. In addition, contractions during premature labor may cause severe pain. Some diseases that can cause pain include systemic lupus erythematosus, lead poisoning, hypercalcemia, sickle cell anemia, diabetic acidosis, porphyria, tabes dorsalis, and black widow spider poisoning.

abdominal pregnancy, a pregnancy in which the fetus develops outside of the uterus. This can occur because of a defect in the fallopian tube or uterus. This is rare. Diagnosis is made by ultrasound or x-ray films. The placenta and fetus must be removed.

abdominal pulse, the pulse of the large artery (abdominal aorta) that carries blood to the organs and legs.

abdominal quadrant, any one of the four areas of the belly divided by two imaginary lines, one vertical and the other horizontal. They intersect at the belly button. They are labeled: left (meaning patient's left) upper quadrant (LUQ), left lower quadrant (LLQ), right upper quadrant (RUQ), and right lower quadrant (RLQ).

abdominal reflex, a reflex caused by firmly stroking the skin of the belly. The muscles contract and the navel moves toward the side stroked. See also **superficial reflex.**

abdominal regions, nine parts of the belly, made by four imaginary lines, in a tic-tac-toe pattern.

abdominal splinting, a rigid contraction of the muscles of the stomach wall. It is usually an unconscious reaction to pain caused by a stomach disorder or following surgery. Abdominal splinting may hamper adequate breathing and cause respiratory problems.

abdominal surgery, any operation on the belly, usually done with general anesthesia. Before surgery, blood and urine tests are done. Often an enema is given. The skin is shaved and cleaned. A drug is often given at bedtime to aid sleep. Eating and drinking are not allowed after midnight before surgery. Shortly before surgery a calming drug is usually given, along with a drug to reduce saliva and respiratory secretions. After surgery the patient is checked to be sure all intravenous (IV) tubes and catheters are working. The dressing is checked for bleeding or drainage. The patient is turned from side to side and is helped to cough and breathe deeply. Drugs are given as needed for pain. Some kinds of abdominal surgery are **appendectomy, cholecystectomy, colostomy, gastrectomy, herniorrhaphy, laparotomy.** See also **acute abdomen.**

abdominocentesis. See **paracentesis.**

abdominocyesis /abdom′inōsĭ·ē′sis/, a pregnancy outside the womb in the abdomen.

abdominoscopy /abdom′inos′kəpē/, a way to examine the abdominal cavity. A tool like a small telescope with a light is used. This method is used for diagnosis. It has the advantage of needing only a small cut, rather than the larger ones necessary for exploratory surgery. See also **endoscopy, laparoscopy, peritinoscopy.**

abducens nerve /abdoō′sənz/, the sixth cranial nerve, which starts in the brain and goes to the muscle that turns the eye out. Also called **abducent nerve, nervus abducens.**

abduction, movement of an arm or leg away from the body. Compare **adduction.**

abduction boots, a set of casts for the legs, with a bar joining the casts at ankle level to keep the toes pointed out. This prevents the end of the thigh bone (femur) from moving inside the hip socket. These casts are often used after hip surgery to allow the bone to heal.

abductor, a muscle that allows a body part to move away from the middle of the body or to move one part away from another. For example, the triceps muscle that straightens the arm is an abductor muscle. Compare **adductor.**

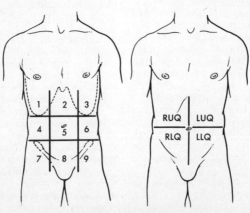

Abdominal regions

abenteric, about organs or body parts other than the intestine.

Abernathy's sarcoma /ab'ərna'thēz/, a tumor, usually cancerous, made up of fat cells. Occurs on the trunk.

aberrant /aber'ənt/, **1.** not found in the usual or expected course, as a blood vessel that appears in an unusual place. **2.** describing an abnormal individual.

aberrant goiter, a large extra thyroid gland or one not located in the normal position. Normally the thyroid gland is located behind the Adam's apple.

aberrant ventricular conduction (AVC), the brief abnormal electric signal of the heart found with some types of irregular heart beats. This can be caused by scar tissue or by an overdose of digitalis, a drug given for heart failure. Also called **aberrancy, ventricular aberration.**

aberratio humorum, any body fluid, as blood, that flows in the wrong direction.

aberration, **1.** any change from the normal course or condition. **2.** abnormal growth. **3.** a thought or belief lacking reason. **4.** change in the number or structure of genes. **5.** bad image caused by unequal bending of light rays through a lens.

aberratio testis, a testicle that does not move down correctly.

abetalipoproteinemia /əbā'təlip'ōprō'tinē'mē·ə/, a rare inherited disorder in which fat is not correctly used. The patient has bad red blood cells, low or no betalipoproteins (which carry cholesterol in the bloodstream), and no cholesterol. Also called **Bassen-Kornzweig syndrome** /-kôrn'zwīg/.

abient /ab'ē·ənt/, moving away from a stimulus. Compare **adient.** –**abience,** *n.*

ability, able to act in a certain way because of having the right skills and mental or physical fitness.

abiochemistry. See **inorganic chemistry.**

abiology, the study of inanimate things.

abiosis /ab'ē·ō'sis/, a lifeless condition or one that is not compatible with life.

abiotrophy /ab'ē·ot'rəfē/, an early loss of energy or the breakdown of certain parts of the body, usually because of a lack of certain foods. –**abiotrophic** /ab'ē·ətrō'fik/, *adj.*

abirritant, a drug or substance that relieves irritation.

ablation /ablā'shən/, the act of cutting off any part of the body, or removal of a growth or damaged tissue.

ablatio placentae. See **abruptio placentae.**

ablatio retinae. See **retinal detachment.**

ablepsia /əblep'sē·ə/, blindness. Also called **ablepsy.**

abnerval current, an electric current that passes from a nerve to and through muscle.

abnormal behavior, acts that deviate from normal. These may range from short-term inability to deal with a stress to total withdrawal from the realities of everyday life. See also **behavior disorder.**

abnormal psychology, the study of mental and emotional problems, including neuroses and psychoses. It also includes normal things that are not fully understood, as dreams and other states of consciousness.

ABO blood groups, the main system for labeling blood based on properties of the red blood cell. The four blood types in this group are A, B, AB, and O. See also **blood group, Rh factor, transfusion.**

aboiement /ä'bô·ämäN'/, uncontrolled animal-like sounds, as barking. Aboiement maybe a symptom of Gilles de Tourette's syndrome.

aborted systole, a heart beat that is too early and may be so weak that a pulse is not felt in the wrist.

abort, **1.** to birth a fetus before it can survive. See also **spontaneous abortion. 2.** to end a pregnancy before the fetus is able to live. See also **induced abortion. 3.** to end anything in the early stages, as to stop the course of a disease, to stop growth, or to halt a project.

abortifacient /əbôr'tifā'shənt/, a drug or substance that causes abortion.

abortion, a spontaneous or deliberate ending of pregnancy before the fetus can be expected to live. Kinds of abortion include **habitual abortion, infected abortion, septic abortion, threatened abortion, voluntary abortion.**

abortion-on-demand, the right of a pregnant woman to have an abortion done at her request.

abortus, a fetus weighing less than 600 g (about 1⅓ pounds) at time of abortion.

abortus fever, a form of brucellosis. This infection is caused by *Brucella abortus,* bacterium that causes abortion in cows. Infection in humans results from drinking milk from infected cows, from handling infected meat, or from skin contact with the wastes of infected animals. Symptoms include chills, fever, aches, pains, and diarrhea. Also called **Rio Grande fever.** See also **brucellosis.**

abouchement /ä'bōōshmäN'/, the joining of a small and a large blood vessel.

aboulia. See **abulia.**

abrachia /əbrā'kē·ə/, the lack of arms. –**abrachial,** *adj.*

abrade, /əbrād/, to remove the top layer or other layers of skin, usually by scraping or rubbing.

abrasion, a scraping or rubbing away of a surface. It may be the result of trauma, as a skinned knee. Compare **laceration.**

abreaction, an emotional release from recalling a painful past event. See also **catharsis.**

abrosia /əbrō′zhə/, a state of fasting or not eating food. See also **anorexia.**

abruptio placentae, parting of the placenta from the uterus before birth. It occurs about once in 200 births. Because it often results in severe bleeding, it is serious. If it is not at the end of the pregnancy, the mother rests in bed and is watched carefully. If the pregnancy is close to the end (usually 7 months or more) the baby is often delivered by cesarean section. Also called **ablatio placentae.** Compare **placenta previa.** See also **Couvelaire uterus.**

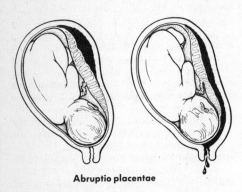

Abruptio placentae

abscess, a hole filled with pus and surrounded by swollen tissue. It forms as a result of a local infection. Healing usually occurs after it drains or is opened.

absence seizure. See **petit mal seizure.**

absenteeism, absence from work, presumably for health-related reasons. Absenteeism varies according to job assignments. The most common medical causes are the flu and job-related skin diseases.

absent without leave (AWOL), a patient who leaves the institution to which he or she is admitted without permission.

absolute discharge, a final and complete end to the patient's relationship with a hospital.

absolute growth, total increase in size from birth to being full-grown.

absolute humidity, the actual amount of water in a given volume of air, usually described in grams per cubic meter or pounds per cubic foot or cubic yard.

absolute temperature, temperature that is measured from a base of absolute zero using either the Kelvin or Rankine scale.

absolute zero, the temperature at which molecules stop moving. Absolute zero is −273°C on the Kelvin scale or −460°F on the Rankine scale.

absorb, 1. taking up of substances, as when the intestines absorb fluids. 2. the energy moved to tissues by radiation, as an absorbed dose of radioactivity.

absorbable gauze, a gauzelike material that can be taken up by the body. It is put on a wound to stop the flow of blood.

absorbance, the amount of light or other radiant energy absorbed by an object or person.

absorbent dressing, a dressing placed on a wound or cut to absorb fluid or other drainage.

absorbent gauze, a gauze for soaking up fluids.

absorbifacient /absôr′bifā′shənt/, anything that aids absorption.

absorption, 1. taking one substance into another, as dissolving a gas in a liquid or removing a liquid with a sponge. 2. substances passing into tissues, as digested food being absorbed into intestinal walls. 3. the absorbing of energy rays by living or nonliving matter, as pavement holding warmth from the sun.

absorption rate constant, a value that describes how much drug is taken up by the body in a set amount of time.

abstinence, choosing to avoid some thing or activity, as no food during a religious day.

abstract /ab′strakt, abstrakt′/, a short version of an article or speech.

abstract thinking, the last stage in the growth of the thought processes. During this phase, the child can begin to change thoughts with ease. The child can use general concepts. Problem solving is done by using logic. This type of thinking appears from about 12 to 15 years of age, in most cases after some schooling. Compare **concrete thinking, syncretic thinking.**

abtraction, a defect in which the jaw or teeth are too low.

abulia /əboō′lē-ə/, a loss of the ability to act on one's free will or to make decisions. Also spelled **aboulia.**

abuse, 1. wrong use of equipment, a substance, or a service (as a drug) either on purpose or not. See also **drug abuse.** 2. to attack or injure, as in **child abuse.**

ABVD, an anticancer drug composed of doxorubicin, bleomycin, vinblastine, and dacarbazine.

-ac, a combining form referring to an agent derived from acetic acid that reduces inflammation.

a.c., short for *ante cibum,* a Latin phrase meaning 'before meals.'

abutment, a tooth, root, or implant to support dentures or a bridge.

abutment tooth, a tooth that supports a dental bridge.

AC, short for **alternating current.**

acalculia /a′kalkoō′li-ə/, the inability to solve simple mathematic problems.

acampsia /əkamp′sē-ə/, a defect in which a joint becomes rigid. See also **ankylosis.**

acantha /əkan'thə/, a spine, as the spinelike projection of a backbone (vertebra).

acanthiomeatal line, /əkan'thē·ō'mē·ā'təl/, an imaginary line that extends from the outside of the ear canal to the center of the base of the front nasal spine. A full upper denture is constructed so that the teeth close parallel to this line.

acanthion, a point at the center of the base of the front nasal spine.

acantho-, a prefix meaning 'thorny or spiky.'

acanthocyte /əkan'thəsīt'/, an abnormal red blood cell with spurlike projections giving it a thorny look.

acanthocytosis /akan'thōsītō'sis/, the presence of acanthocytes in the blood.

acanthoma /ak'anthō'mə/, any harmless or malignant tumor of the skin.

acanthoma adenoides cysticum. See **trichoepithelioma.**

acanthoma verrucosa seborrheica. See **seborrheic keratosis.**

acanthosis /ak'ənthō'sis/, a thickening of the skin, as in eczema and psoriasis.

acanthosis nigricans /nē'grikanz'/, a skin disease marked by dark colored, wartlike areas in the armpit or other body folds like the genital area. See also **acanthosis.**

acapnia /akap'nē·ə/, a lack of carbon dioxide in the blood, usually caused by hyperventilation.

acarbia /akär'bē·ə/, a decrease in the bicarbonate level in the blood.

acardia /akär'dē·ə/, a rare birth defect in which the heart is absent.

acariasis /ak'ərī'əsis/, any disease caused by an acarid mite, as scrub typhus.

acarid /ak'ərid/, one of the many mites that are members of the order Acarina. Several types can infect humans. See also **chiggers, scabies.**

accelerated hypertension. See **malignant hypertension.**

accelerated idiojunctional rhythm /id'ē·ō-/, a heart rhythm that is faster than the normal rate. If the heart is otherwise normal, this condition is not a problem.

accelerated idioventricular rhythm (AIVR), a condition in which the heart beats faster than the normal rate but slower than 100 beats per minute (50 to 100 per minute).

acceleration, an increase in the speed of an object. Compare **deceleration. –accelerator,** n.

acceleration phase, (in birth) the first part of active labor. The cervix opens more quickly during this time.

acceptable daily intake (ADI), the most of anything that can be safely taken. Taking more than the ADI may cause problems.

acceptor, a person who receives living tissue from another person or organism, as a blood transfusion. Compare **donor.**

access cavity, a hole made in a tooth for cleaning, shaping, and filling the pulp space.

accessory, a structure that serves one of the main systems of the body. For example, the hair, the nails, and the sweat glands are accessories of the skin.

accessory diaphragm, a birth defect in which a second diaphragm or part of one develops in the chest. It may be separated from the true diaphragm by part of the lung.

accessory movements, joint movements that are necessary for total mobility but not controlled directly and voluntarily. Examples include rotations and gliding motions.

accessory muscle, a muscle that is an exact copy of another. It is usually noticed as a swelling under the skin. Treatment is not necessary if the accessory muscle does not interfere with normal function.

accessory nerve, either of a pair of nerves in the head needed for speech, for swallowing, and for certain movements of the head and shoulders. Each nerve has a cranial and a spinal part, connects with certain nerves in the neck, and connects to the brain. Also called **eleventh cranial nerve, nervus accessorius, spinal accessory nerve.**

accessory pancreatic duct, a small opening into the pancreatic duct or the first section of the small intestine (duodenum).

accessory pathway, an extra muscle tract in the heart. It may become a life-threatening problem when combined with a condition in which the heart rate rises to more than 400 beats a minute (atrial fibrillation).

accessory root canal, a branching to the side of the pulp canal in a tooth.

accessory phrenic nerve, the nerve that joins the nerve at the base of the neck (phrenic) or in the chest.

accessory sinus of the nose. See **paranasal sinus.**

accessory tooth, an extra tooth that does not look like a normal tooth in size, shape, or position.

accident, any unexpected or unplanned event that results in death, injury, property damage, or a combination of serious effects.

acclimate /əklī'mit, ak'līmāt/, to adjust to a different climate, especially to changes in altitude and in weather. Also **acclimatize** /əklī'mətīz'/. –**acclimation, acclimatization,** n.

accommodation (A, acc, Acc), 1. the state of adapting to something. 2. the ongoing process of a person to adjust to his or her surroundings, both physically and mentally. 3. the adjustment of the muscles and lens of the eye to distances. See also **accommodation reflex.**

accommodation reflex, a change by the eyes for close vision. It includes the pupils getting smaller, the eyes moving together, and focusing. Also called **ciliary reflex.** See also **light reflex.**

accomplishment quotient, a person's achievement age compared with mental age. The value is given as a ratio multiplied by 100. See also **achievement quotient, intelligence quotient.**

accretio cordis /əkrē'shē·ō/, a state in which there is scarlike tissue of the sack covering the heart (pericardium) that has grown to a structure around the heart.

accretion /əkrē'shən/, 1. growth or increase by adding to something. 2. the growing together of parts that are normally separated. 3. the gathering of foreign material, especially within a hole. –accrete, v., accretive, adj.

accumulated dose equivalent, an estimate of the maximum safe dose of radiation over a lifetime. It is used for persons working with radioactive materials or x-rays.

accurate empathy, a communication technique used by nurses to convey an understanding of the patient's feelings and experiences.

Accurbron, a trademark for a drug to treat bronchial asthma (theophylline).

Accutane, a trademark for a drug to treat acne (isotretinoin).

acebutolol, a drug given for high blood pressure, chest pain (angina), and irregular heart beats. Also called **butanamide.**
★CAUTION: This drug is not given to patients with asthma, heart failure, or blood vessel disease.
★ADVERSE EFFECTS: The side effects of this drug include slow heart beat, gas, leg pains, nausea, headache, skin rashes, dizziness, and drowsiness.

acedia /əsē'dē·ə/, a state of tiredness and a type of depression, marked by not caring and slow thinking.

acentric /āsen'trik/, having no center or being away from the center.

acephalobrachia /asef'əlōbrā'kē·ə/, a birth defect in which a fetus lacks both arms and a head.

acephaly /əsef'əlē/, a birth defect in which the head is absent or not properly formed.

acetabulum /as'ətab'yələm/, pl. **acetabula,** the large, cup-shaped, hip socket holding the ball-shaped head of the thigh bone (femur).

acetaldehyde, a colorless liquid with a strong odor. In the body, acetaldehyde is made in the liver. It is also made commercially to make various aromas and flavors. Exposure to high levels of this liquid can cause headache, eye injury, runny nose, and lung problems.

acetaminophen /əset'əmin'əfin/, a pain-relieving and fever-reducing drug used in many over-the-counter drugs.
★CAUTION: Known allergy to this drug prohibits its use.
★ADVERSE EFFECTS: Among the most serious side effects are severe allergy and severe anemia. Overdose can result in fatal liver failure.

acetanilide, a pain relieving drug that reduces fever and joint swelling in arthritis. Because acetanilide has caused a blood problem, it has been replaced by acetaminophen in most cases. See **acetaminophen.**

acetazolamide /as'ətəzō'ləmīd/, a drug used for treating water buildup (edema), pressure buildup in the eye (glaucoma), and epilepsy (primarily petit mal).

Acetest /as'ətest/, a trademark for tablets used to test urine for abnormal amounts of acetone. Patients with diabetes mellitus or other metabolic problems can have high levels of this substance in the urine. This test allows patients with diabetes to check their acetone level at home.

acetoacetic acid /as'ətō·əsē'tik, əsē'tō-/, a colorless compound that is in normal urine in small amounts and in large amounts in the urine of patients with diabetes mellitus, especially in an acid buildup (ketoacidosis). Also called **acetone carboxylic acid, acetylacetic acid, diacetic acid.**

acetohexamide, a drug taken by mouth to treat diabetes mellitus when insulin is not required.

acetone /as'ətōn/, a colorless, sweet-smelling liquid found in small amounts in normal urine and in larger amounts in the urine of patients with diabetes.

acetone bodies. See **ketone bodies.**

acetone carboxylic acid. See **acetoacetic acid.**

acetonide grouping, a chemical combination similar to acetone, commonly found in some steroid drugs, such as flucinolone acetonide.

acetophenetidin. See **phenacetin.**

acetylacetic acid. See **acetoacetic acid.**

acetylcarbromal. See **acecarbromal.**

acetylcholine, a substance in the body that allows messages to travel from one nerve to another. For example, a person who decides to pick up a pen can act on the thought only when the hand receives the message from the brain. This process in normal persons occurs in a fraction of a second. See also **acetylcholinesterase, atropine.**

acetylcholinesterase, an enzyme that stops acetylcholine. It reduces or prevents the movement of nerve signals.

acetylcysteine, a drug used for treating many lung problems.
★CAUTION: Known allergies to this drug prohibit its use.
★ADVERSE EFFECTS: Among the most serious side effects are sore mouth, nausea, runny nose, and asthmalike problems.

acetylsalicylic acid. See **aspirin.**

achalasia /ak'əlā'zhə/, the inability of a muscle to relax.

Achard-Thiers syndrome /ash'ärtērz'/, a hormonal disorder seen in women after menopause who have diabetes. The syndrome causes growth of body hair in a male pattern. See also **hirsutism, hypertrichosis.**

ache, 1. a pain that is steady, dull, and not too strong. An ache may be local, as a stomach ache, headache, or bone ache. It may be general, as the ache of the flu. **2.** to suffer from a dull, steady pain.

achievement age, the level of a person's educational growth. It is measured by a test and compared with the normal score for persons the same age.

achievement quotient (AQ), a number score of a person's achievement age. It is the scores from achievement tests, divided by the person's actual age and multiplied by 100.

achievement test, a standard test that measures a person's knowledge in many fields of study.

Achilles tendon /əkil′ēz/, the tendon of the calf muscles. It is the thickest and strongest tendon in the body. It begins near the middle of the back of the leg and connects to the heel bone. Also called **calcaneal tendon, tendo calcaneus, tendon of Achilles.**

Achilles-tendon reflex, the response to a sharp tap given to the tendon at the back of the ankle causing the foot to move up. This does not happen in patients with nerve damage in the legs. Patients with an underactive thyroid often have a slow reflex. A very quick reflex may be caused by an overactive thyroid or by a disease of the brain. Also called **ankle reflex, calcaneal tendon reflex.** See also **deep tendon reflex.**

achlorhydria /ā′klôrhī′drē·ə/, a state in which hydrochloric acid is missing from the gastric juice in the stomach. Digestion of protein (as meat) is hard for patients with this problem, but otherwise digestion is close to normal. See also **achylia, pernicious anemia. –achlorhydric,** *adj.*

acholia, 1. the absence or decrease of bile fluids. **2.** any thing that stops the flow of bile from the liver into the small intestine. **–acholic,** *adj.*

acholuria, the lack of bile colors in the urine, indicating a possible liver problem.

achondrogenesis, /ākon′drōjen′əsis/, a form of dwarfism characterized by very short arms and legs and excess fluid in the tissues of the head and trunk. It is transmitted genetically.

achondroplasia /ākon′drōplā′zhə/, a problem with the growth of cartilage in the growth plates of the long bones and skull. The bones fuse too soon. Growth stops and dwarfism results. One type, called familial achondroplasia, is inherited.

achondroplastic dwarf, this most common type of dwarf has short limbs, a normal-sized trunk, large head with a sunken nose and small face, stubby hands, and a sway back. This results from an inherited defect of the bones, and there are often other physical defects. Usually these people have normal intelligence. See also **achondroplasia.**

achromatic vision. See **color blindness.**

achromia, the absence or loss of normal skin coloring. It may be present at birth, such as albinism, or the result of a disease, such as psoriasis.

achromocyte /ākrō′məsīt/, a red blood cell shaped like a new moon that is pale in color. It does not indicate disease. Occasionally these blood cells are found in healthy people. Also called **achromatocyte** /ā′krōmat′əsīt/.

Achromycin V, a trademark for an antibiotic (tetracycline hydrochloride).

achylia /ākī′lē·ə/, a lack of or not enough hydrochloric acid and pepsinogen, chemicals needed for digesting food in the stomach.

achylous /əkī′ləs/, **1.** describes a lack of gastric or other digestive juices. **2.** referring to a lack of chyle, a milky fluid made in the intestines during digestion.

acid, 1. a substance that turns blue litmus paper red, has a sour taste, and reacts with bases to form salts. See also **alkali. 2.** *slang.* lysergic acid diethylamide (LSD). See **lysergide.**

acid-base balance, a normal condition in which the body makes acids and bases at the same rate they are removed. See also **acid, base.**

acid-base metabolism, the acts that maintain the balance of acids and bases in the body. When this balance is upset, either too much acid is present (acidosis) or the opposite (alkalosis). Acidosis may be caused by diarrhea, vomiting, kidney disease (uremia), uncontrolled diabetes mellitus, and some drugs. Alkalosis may be caused by too much of an alkaline drug (antacids), vomiting, and some drugs that increase urine production (diuretics). See also **acid-base balance, acidosis, alkalosis, pH.**

acid bath, a bath taken in water with a mineral acid. It helps reduce excess sweating.

acid burn, damage to the body caused by a strong acid. The type of burn depends on the kind of acid and the length of time and amount of tissue exposed. Emergency treatment includes washing the area with large amounts of water. Compare **alkali burn.**

acid dust, highly acid bits of dust that collect in the air. This is the reason for much of the smog over towns and cities. High levels can be dangerous for patients with lung problems. See also **acid rain.**

acidify, 1. to make a substance acid. **2.** to become acid. Compare **alkalize.**

acidophilic adenoma, a tumor of the pituitary. These can cause the pituitary to make too much growth hormone, causing abnormal growth of the body (gigantism) or enlarged bones in the arms and legs (acromegaly). Also called **eosinophilic adenoma.**

acidophilus milk /as′idof′ələs/, milk that has *Lactobacillus acidophilus* added. It is used with some bowel problems to change the bacteria in the stomach and intestines.

acidosis, an abnormal increase in hydrogen in the body from too much acid or the loss of base. The many forms of acidosis are named for the cause. For example, renal tubular acidosis results when the kidney fails to get rid of hydrogen or collect bicarbonate. Compare **alkalosis.**

acid-perfusion test, a test of the response of the esophagus to acid. Sensitivity to acid may be caused by stomach acid moving into the esophagus (reflux esophagitis). Also called **Bernstein test.**

acid phosphatase, an enzyme found in the kidneys, blood serum, semen, and prostate. It is higher in serum of patients with cancer of the prostate and in trauma victims. See also **alkaline phosphatase.**

acid poisoning, a condition caused by swallowing a toxic acid as hydrochloric, nitric, phosphoric, or sulfuric acids. Emergency treatment includes giving large amounts of water or milk to weaken the acid. Vomiting should not be brought on. The victim must be taken quickly to the hospital. Compare **alkali poisoning.**

acid rain, rain with high acid content caused by air pollution from industry, motor vehicles, and other sources. Acid rain is blamed for many health problems, fish kills, and the ruin of timber. Also called **acid precipitation, acid snow.**

acid rebound, a condition in which stomach acid is produced in greater amounts than normal. It may occur after the initial effects of an antacid wear off.

acid salt, a salt having some degree of acidity, as sodium bicarbonate.

acid therapy, a way of taking off warts. Plaster patches with a mild acid are placed on the warts.

acidulous /əsid′yələs/, slightly acidic or sour.

aciduria, the presence of acid in the urine.

acinar adenocarcinoma. See **acinic cell adenocarcinoma.**

acinic cell adenocarcinoma, an uncommon cancer that grows in certain glands, especially the salivary glands. Also called **acinar adenocarcinoma, acinous adenocarcinoma.**

acinitis, any swelling of the tiny, grape-shaped portions of certain glands.

acinous adenocarcinoma. See **acinic cell adenocarcinoma.**

acinus /as′inəs/, pl. **acini, 1.** any small saclike structure, as one found in a gland. Also called **alveolus. 2.** a part of the lung.

Aclovate, a trademark for a topical corticosteroid (alclometasone dipropionate).

acmesthesia /ak′misthē′zhə/, the feeling of a pinprick or a sharp point touching the skin.

acne /ak′nē/, a breakout of pimples. It usually occurs in or near the oil glands on the face, neck, shoulders, and upper back. Its cause is not known but involves bacteria that bother the skin. Treatment includes antibiotics, topical vitamin A, benzyl benzoate, and dermabrasion. See also **comedo.**

acne artificialis, an eruption in the skin caused by an external irritation as tar. It can also be caused by swallowing some irritating substance.

acne cachecticorum, a breakout of the skin that may occur in patients who are very weak. It is marked by soft pus-filled pimples.

acne conglobata /kong′glōbā′tə/, a severe form of acne with abscesses, lumps (cysts), scars, and thick, raised scars (keloids).

acneform /ak′nifôrm′/, like acne. Also **acneiform** /aknē′əfôrm/.

acneform drug eruption, an acnelike skin response to a drug.

acnegenic /ak′nijen′ik/, causing or making acne.

acne indurata, skin condition with many pimples that often make severe scars. Also called **chronic acne vulgaris.**

acne keratosa, a skin problem with hard cone-shaped plugs that appear at the corners of the mouth and affect the surrounding skin.

acne necrotica miliaris, a rare, long-term skin problem. Pus forms around the hair roots on the forehead and scalp. It occurs mostly in adults.

acne neonatorum, a skin problem in infants caused by large oil glands. Small pimples and lumps (cysts) show on the nose, cheeks, and forehead.

acne papulosa, small pimples that usually do not get infected.

acne rosacea. See **rosacea.**

acne vulgaris, a common form of acne seen in teenagers and young adults. It is probably caused by male sex hormones working on the oil glands. Bacteria, which live around the hair root, become more active and pimples are formed.

acognosia /ak′og·nō′zhə/, a knowledge of cures.

acoria /akôr′ē·ə/, a state of always being hungry even when the desire for food is small.

acorn-tipped catheter, a flexible hollow tube with an acorn-shaped tip. It is used often in urology.

acou-, acu-, a prefix meaning hearing.

acousma /əkōōz′mə/, pl. **acousmas, acousmata,** hearing strange sounds that are not there.

acoustic, referring to sound or hearing. Also **acoustical.**

acoustic cavitation, a potential biologic effect of ultrasonography. It is marked by broad-ranging vibrations of microscopic gas bubbles. As normally used, ultrasound does not cause this condition in human tissues.

acoustic impedance, the effect of an object on sound waves passing through it. Sound waves include those used in ultrasonography. Acoustic impedance is affected by the speed of the sound wave and the density of the object in its path. The acoustic impedance of bone may be nearly five times as great as that of blood.

acoustic nerve, a pair of nerves in the skull (cranial) important to hearing. The nerves connect the inner ears with three areas in the brain. Also called **eighth cranial nerve.**

acoustic neuroma, a benign tumor of the acoustic (eighth cranial) nerve that grows in the ear canal. The symptoms depend on the place and size of the tumor. Symptoms are ringing in the ear (tinnitus), loss of hearing, headache, facial numbness, swelling in the eye (papilledema), dizziness, and an unsteady walk. Also called **acoustic neurilemmoma, acoustic neurinoma, acoustic neurofibroma.**

acoustic shadow, an image produced by ultrasonography. It indicates the presence of dense material in soft tissue. It is often used to detect gallstones.

acoustic trauma, a slow loss of hearing. This can be caused by loud noise over a long time. A sudden loss of hearing may be caused by an explosion, a blow to the head, or other accident. Hearing loss may be for a short time or permanent, partial or total.

acquired, referring to a feature, state, or disease that happens after birth. It is not inherited but is a response to the environment. Compare **congenital, familial, hereditary.**

acquired immune deficiency syndrome (AIDS) /ādz/, a disease of the system that fights infection. The problem is found mostly in gay men and intravenous (IV) drug users. AIDS can also occur in women who have sex with bisexual men and in children whose parents have the disease. The cause is thought to be a virus called HTLV-3. This virus is thought to be spread through exchange of body fluids, as in sex. The first symptoms are extreme fatigue, fever, night sweats, chills, swollen lymph glands, swollen spleen, loss of appetite with weight loss, severe diarrhea, and depression. As the disease goes on, the patient may become weaker because of many infections. A form of pneumonia (*Pneumocystis carinii*) often occurs, as does swelling of the cover of the spine (meningitis) or swelling of the brain (encephalitis). Most patients get cancer, especially Kaposi's sarcoma, Burkitt's lymphoma, and non-Hodgkin's lymphoma. Treatment is mainly with chemotherapy. Drugs have been used, with little success. The death rate is 90% for patients who have had the disease more than 2 years. See **HTLV, retrovirus.**

acquired immunity, any form of protection from infection that is gotten after birth. It may be natural or not. With **naturally acquired immunity** the body is able to fight off infections successfully after having the disease. Immunity can come from the mother during pregnancy. The mother can also pass this immunity to a baby through her milk. **Artificially acquired** immunity is gotten by vaccination. Compare **natural immunity.** See also **active immunity, passive immunity.**

acquired reflex. See **conditioned reflex.**

acrid, sharp, bitter, and unpleasant to the smell or taste.

acro-, a prefix meaning arms and legs.

acrocephalosyndactylism. See **Apert's syndrome.**

acrocephaly. See **oxycephaly.**

acrochordon /ak′rōkôr′don/, a harmless skin tag growing on the eyelids or neck or in the armpit or groin.

acrocyanosis /ak′rōsī′ənō′sis/, a problem of the hands and feet, more often the hands. The symptoms are a blue color, coldness, and sweating of the hands and feet. It is caused by a spasm of the blood vessels and is usually started by cold or by mental stress. Also called **Raynaud's phenomenon, Raynaud's sign.**

acrodermatitis, any breaking out of the skin of the hands and feet caused by a parasitic mite.

acrodermatitis enteropathica /en′tərōpath′ikə/, a rare, long-term disease of infants. The symptoms are blisters on the skin and mucous membranes, hair loss, diarrhea, and failure to thrive. It may cause death if not treated.

acrodynia /ak′rōdin′ē-ə/, a disease in infants and young children. The signs are itching, swelling from water, pink or red skin rash on the arms, legs, and face, sweating, stomach upsets, problems with light, crabby times or no energy. Also called **pink disease, Swift's disease.**

acromegalic eunuchoidism, a problem in men with a disease that makes the bones in the arms and legs get larger. The signs are wasting of the genitals and breast growth. It is caused by a benign tumor (adenoma) in the pituitary. Also called **retrograde infantilism.**

acromegaly /ak′rəmeg′əlē/, a long-term problem in which bones of the face, jaw, arms, and legs get larger. It occurs in middle-aged patients. It is caused by too much growth hormone. It is treated by x-rays to shrink the pituitary, or part of the pituitary gland is removed. Also called **acromegalia.** Compare **gigantism.** See also **adenohypophysis, growth hormone.**

acromicria, /ăk′rəmik′rē-ə/, an abnormality characterized by unusually small hands and feet. The person may also have extremely small facial features, such as nose and ears.

acromioclavicular articulation, the joint between the collarbone and shoulder blade.

acromion /əkrō′mē-ən/, the outer part of the shoulder blade. It forms the highest point of the shoulder and connects with the collarbone. Also called **acromion process.**

acronym, a word formed by the first letters of a name or phase. For instance, *CAT* is the acronym for *C*omputerized *A*xial *T*omography.

acroosteolysis, an occupation disease that mainly affects people who work with polyvinylchloride (PVC) plastic materials. It is characterized by decreased blood supply to the hands and feet, loss of bone tissue in the hands, and sensitivity to the cold. A form of the disease found in people who do not work with plastics is thought to be inherited.

acroparesthesia /ak'rōpar'isthē'zhə/, very sensitive arms or legs. It is often caused by pressure or irritation of the nerves. The signs are tingling, numbness, and stiffness in the fingers, the hands, and the forearms.

acrophobia, a fear of high places that does not make sense and causes one to be very nervous. See also **obsession, phobia.**

acrotic /əkrot'ik/, **1.** referring to the surface or to the skin glands. **2.** referring to the lack of or a weak pulse.

acrylic resin base, a base for a set of false teeth made of this resin. Compare **denture base.**

acrylic resin dental cement, a cement for fixing broken teeth.

ACTH, short for **adrenocorticotropic hormone.**

Acthar, a trademark for a drug used to treat kinds of arthritis and allergies (corticotropin).

Actidil, a trademark for a drug used to treat allergies (triprolidine hydrochloride).

Actifed, a trademark for a drug used to treat allergies and hay fever (pseudoephedrine hydrochloride and triprolidine hydrochloride).

actin, a protein found in muscles that helps them get tight and relax. Also called **actinin.** See also **myosin.**

acting out, to show mental pain in acts that are usually slightly crazy and uptight. Acting out may be destructive or harmful. See also **transference.**

actinic /aktin'ik/, referring to sending rays, as sunlight or x-rays.

actinic dermatitis, a skin swelling or rash caused by sun, x-rays, or atomic radiation. It can cause skin cancer.

actinic keratosis, a thickening of the skin. It happens slowly and usually affects a small spot. This problem is caused by too much time in the sun. Also called **senile keratosis, senile wart, solar keratosis.**

Actinomyces /ak'tinōmī'sēz/, a genus of bacteria. Many species that may cause disease in humans, as *Actinomyces israelii,* normally live in the mouth and throat. See also **actinomycosis.**

actinomycin D. See **dactinomycin.**

actinomycosis /ak'tinōmīkō'sis/, a long-term problem that causes deep, lumpy holes with a thin, grainy pus. It is seen most often in patients who live in the country. It is caused by *Actinomyces israelii,* a bacterium that normally lives in the bowel and mouth. There are four main types of actinomycosis. **Cervicofacial actinomycosis** occurs when the bacteria spreads into the mouth, throat, and neck, after a tooth or tonsil infection. **Thoracic actinomycosis** may be a problem if the holes with pus spread down the throat. It may result from breathing the bacteria into the lungs. **Abdominal actinomycosis** may occur after appendicitis, pouches (diverticulum) of the large bowel, or a hole in the stomach. A case may happen after an intrauterine device (IUD), a method of birth control, is put in place. **Generalized actinomycosis** may involve the skin, brain, liver, and urogenital system.

action current. See **action potential.**

action potential, an electric signal sent across a nerve and across a muscle cell. Also called **action current.**

Activase, a trademark for a commercial form of a synthetic clot-dissolving substance.

activated charcoal, a general-purpose antidote used to treat poisoning and to control intestinal gas.
    ★CAUTION: There are no known reasons for not using it, but activated charcoal does not work for poisoning caused by a strong acid or base or by cyanide.
    ★ADVERSE EFFECTS: There are no known serious side effects.

activated 7-dehydrocholesterol. See **vitamin D₃.**

activated partial thromboplastin time (APTT), a timed blood test for the speed of clotting. This test is used to learn about clotting problems.

activation factor. See **factor XII,** found in the blood.

activator, 1. a substance, force, or device that prompts activity of something. **2.** a device worn in the mouth that works on the muscles around the mouth.

active algolagnia. See **sadism.**

active assisted exercise, moving the body or part of the body mostly through one's own efforts. A therapist or some other device, as an exercise machine, assists. See also **exercise, passive exercise.**

active euthanasia. See **euthanasia.**

active exercise, repeated movement of a part of the body by contracting and relaxing the muscles. Compare **passive exercise.** See also **aerobic exercise, anaerobic exercise.**

active immunity, a form of long-term, gained immunity. It protects the body from new infection. Compare **passive immunity.** See also **immune response.**

active movement, moving the muscles and joints without outside help. Compare **passive movement.**

active play, playing, not watching. Compare **passive play.**

active resistance exercise, moving the body against a checking force. See also **progressive resistance exercise.**

active resistance training (ART), a conditioning or rehabilitation program designed to improve a patient's muscle strength and endurance. The program uses progressive resistance exercises and muscle overloading.

active specific immunotherapy, a treatment for cancer in which the patient is injected with irradiated tumor cells. The injected cells promote the making of antibodies that kill the tumor cells.

active treatment. See **treatment.**

activities of daily living (ADL), normal, everyday actions, as eating, dressing, washing, or brushing the teeth. Accidents or illnesses may make it hard to do these.

activity intolerance, a condition of general weakness, sitting much of the time, oxygen imbalance, or bed rest. The patient may have weakness, fast heart rate, blood pressure changes, and shortness of breath when activity is tried.

activity tolerance, the type and amount of exercise a patient may be able to perform without undue exertion or possible injury.

actual cautery, the applying of heat to destroy tissue.

actual charge, the amount charged by a medical person for a service. This may not be the same as that paid by an insurance plan.

acu-, **1.** a prefix referring to a needle. **2.** a prefix referring to hearing.

acuity, the clearness or sharpness of one of the senses, as visual acuity.

acuminate wart. See **condyloma acuminatum.**

acupressure /ak'yəpresh'ər/, a therapy of putting pressure on set points of the body. It is used to relieve pain, make anesthesia, or control a body function.

acupuncture /ak'yəpunk'chər/, a therapy for relieving pain or changing a function of the body. Fine, wire-thin needles are put into the skin at set places along a series of lines called meridians. The needles are twirled, given a slight electric charge, or warmed. See also **moxibustion.** –**acupuncturist,** *n.*

acupuncture point, a point on the skin along the meridians, or lines, of the body.

acute, **1.** begins quickly and is intense or sharp, then slowing after a short time. **2.** sharp or severe. Compare **chronic.**

acute abdomen, the quick onset of severe pain in the belly. It should be examined right away, because surgery may be needed. Facts about the start, length of time, type of pain, location, and other symptoms are needed so that a correct diagnosis can be made. The nurse or doctor will ask questions about changes in bowel habits, weight loss, bloody stool, diarrhea, color of stool, and what makes the pain better or worse. Constant, increasing pain is often caused by appendicitis or a pouch in the intestines (diverticulitis). However, pain that starts and stops can mean a blockage of the bowel, kidney stones, or gallstones. Also called **surgical abdomen.** See also **abdominal pain.**

acute air trapping, a condition in which small tubes in the breathing system collapse without warning. The patient is unable to either inhale or exhale and may panic. The episode can usually be treated by a series of sharp, forceful squeezes to the sides of the chest, causing the lungs to empty. People prone to episodes of acute air trapping often learn to control their breathing with pursed-lip breathing.

acute alcoholism, being drunk from too much alcohol. Symptoms are tremors, daze, loss of good movement, and often nausea, loss of water, and headache. Compare **chronic alcoholism.** See also **alcoholism.**

acute bacterial arthritis. See **septic arthritis.**

acute care, treatment for a serious illness, for an accident, or after surgery. It is usually given in a hospital by trained persons. It may also involve intensive care. This kind of care is usually for only a short time. Compare **chronic care.**

acute cervicitis. See **cervicitis.**

acute childhood leukemia, cancer of the blood-forming tissues. It is the most common cancer in children, particularly those between 2 and 5 years of age.

★DIAGNOSIS: The two major types of serious leukemia are **acute lymphoid leukemia (ALL)** and **acute myelocytic or monocytic (nonlymphoid) leukemia (AML).** ALL is usually a disease of children, whereas AML occurs in all age groups. The exact cause of the disease is not known, although many things are possible, as hereditary problems, inability to fight infection, viruses, and cancer-causing environment, as radiation. In acute leukemia, large, not-fully-formed white blood cells build up quickly and enter other tissues of the body. This causes a decrease in red blood cells. Patients get infections and bleed more easily. Their bones may weaken and break. Symptoms include fever, pale color, fatigue, loss of appetite, infections, bone and joint pain, bleeding under the skin, and bigger spleen, liver, and lymph nodes. Start may be sudden or not. The diagnosis is made by testing bone marrow.

★TREATMENT: Treatment of leukemia is a three-stage process of chemotherapy and radiation. In the first stage, all leukemic cells are destroyed within a 4- to 6-week period with drugs and therapy. The main drugs used in ALL are steroids. In children with AML the main drugs are 6-thioguanine, daunomycin, cytosine arabinoside, 5-azacytidine, vincristine, and prednisone. The child is usually put in the hospital because of the side effects of the drugs and the high risk of problems. The second stage is to prevent leukemia cells from entering the nervous system. This therapy usually consists of high doses of radiation to the head and doses of methotrexate put into the spinal cord. In some cases only the drug is given. In small children the radiation is limited to the skull to prevent stunted growth, but older children may have radiation to the skull and spine. The purpose of the third stage is to maintain remission. It usually begins after the child has left the hospital. It uses many sets of drugs. Complete blood counts are done weekly or monthly, and bone-marrow tests are done every 3 to 4 months. Maintenance therapy is stopped after 2 to 3 years if there is no sign of the disease. Treatment past 3 years is not done because the side effects of the drugs get worse with long use. Relapse occurs in about 20% of the cases. If it does, the child begins the treatment cycle again, usually with prednisone, vincristine, and a set of other drugs not tried before. Other treatments for prolonging remission include BCG vaccine or bone-marrow transplant.

★PATIENT CARE: Care for the child involves much physical and mental support. The child and parents should be prepared for the many procedures, including intravenous (IV) tubes, having bone marrow and spinal fluid samples taken, and x-ray treatment. Most of the drugs used may cause problems, as infection, bleeding, and iron-poor blood. Infection is a main problem and one of the most frequent causes of death. It is important that both the child and parents avoid all known sources of infection. Prevention can also help to decrease bleeding under the skin. Attention is given to skin and mouth care and cleanliness of the genital and anal areas. Activities that could result in an accident should be watched. Although corticosteroid drugs (as prednisone) usually cause hunger and produce a sense of well-being, they also cause moon face. This side effect goes away when steroid therapy is stopped. See also **acute lymphocytic leukemia, acute myelocytic leukemia, leukemia.**

acute cholecystitis. See **cholecystitis.**

acute circulatory failure, a drop in heart output that results in tissues receiving inadequate oxygen. The cause may not be related to the heart. It usually happens so rapidly that the body does not have time to adjust to the changes. If not controlled immediately, the condition usually progresses to shock syndrome.

acute confusional state, a central nervous system problem caused by interference with essential biochemical processes. Symptoms may include difficulties with thinking, awareness, memory, and orientation. These may be accompanied by restlessness, apprehension, irritability, and apathy. The condition may be associated with delirium, toxic psychosis, or acute brain syndrome.

acute delirium, mental problem that is quick, severe, and short-lived. See also **delirium.**

acute disease, a disease with symptoms that are usually severe but last only a short time. One either gets better, moves into long-term phase, or dies. See also **chronic disease.**

acute epiglottitis, a severe bacterial infection of the upper breathing system that occurs in young children, usually between 2 and 7 years of age. The symptoms are sore throat, barking high-pitched breathing, and swelling of tissue that keeps food from going in the lungs. Sudden blockage can occur and be fatal. The infection is generally caused by the bacterium *Hemophilus influenzae,* type B, although sometimes strep may be the cause. Infection occurs from air particles or direct contact. Compare **croup.**

★DIAGNOSIS: The infection begins suddenly and moves quickly. The first signs—sore throat, hoarseness, fever, and difficult swallowing—may be followed by an inability to swallow, drooling, shortness of breath, high-pitched breathing, crabbiness, and fear. The child who is not getting enough oxygen appears frightened and anxious. The color of the skin can be pale to blue. The diagnosis is made by testing mucus from the nose, throat, or blood for bacteria. Pushing down the tongue shows a swollen, cherry-red epiglottis.

★TREATMENT: The airway is opened by placing a tube in the mouth and throat or by putting a tube through a cut in the throat. Moisture and oxygen are given, and mucus is removed. Fluids given in the vein are usually required, and antibiotics are started right away. Penicillin, ampicillin, or chloramphenicol is most often given.

★PATIENT CARE: A child will receive intensive care. One must change cloths and bed sheets often to prevent chilling. The worst phase passes within 24 to 48 hours. Airway tubes are not usually needed after 3 to 4 days. As the child gets better, breathing gets easier. There is usually quick recovery so that bed rest and quiet activity to relieve boredom become the main concerns. The infection may spread, causing ear infections, pneumonia, and bronchitis. Also called **acute epiglottiditis.**

acute febrile polyneuritis. See **Guillain-Barré syndrome.**

acute gastritis. See **gastritis.**

acute glaucoma. See **glaucoma.**

acute glomerulonephritis. See **postinfectious glomerulonephritis.**

acute hallucinatory paranoia, paranoia in which one sees and hears things that are not there and believes things that are not true. Also called **paranoia hallucinatoria.**

acute hallucinosis. See **alcoholic hallucinosis.**

acute hemorrhagic conjunctivitis, an eye disease that is easy to get and is usually caused by enterovirus type 70. This virus is found mostly in humid areas with many people. Symptoms are eye pain, itching, redness, sensitivity to light, swelling of the eyelid, and lots of watery discharge. It is treated by keeping the eye clean and by using drugs.

acute hemorrhagic leukoencephalitis. See **acute necrotizing hemorrhagic encephalopathy.**

acute hypoxia, a sudden or rapid loss of available oxygen. It may result from suffocation, blockage of the airway, heavy internal bleeding, or sudden failure of the cardiorespiratory system. Symptoms may include abnormal breathing, headache, confusion, and loss of consciousness.

acute idiopathic polyneuritis. See **Guillain-Barré syndrome.**

acute idiopathic thrombocytopenic purpura. See **idiopathic thrombocytopenic purpura.**

acute illness, any illness in which the person experiences severe symptoms that do not last for long but interfere with normal functioning.

acute intermittent porphyria (AIP), a birth defect in the chemistry of food breakdown (metabolic disorder). It involves sudden attacks of pain from the nerves. Women are affected more often and attacks often are started by hormone changes of menstruation, pregnancy, and during puberty. Other factors that can start an attack are starvation or crash dieting, infections, and a wide range of drugs. Any part of the nervous system can be affected. A common effect is belly pain. Other effects can include nerve damage, inadequate salt, seizures, coma, hallucinations, and difficult breathing. A high-carbohydrate diet may reduce the attacks. See also **porphyria.**

acute interstitial nephritis. See **interstitial nephritis.**

acute laryngotracheobronchitis. See **croup.**

acute lymphoblastic leukemia. See **acute lymphocytic leukemia.**

acute lymphocytic leukemia (ALL), a blood cancer marked by many not-fully-formed white blood cells that collect in the bone marrow, the blood, the lymph nodes, the spleen, the liver, and other organs. The number of normal blood cells is reduced. About 80% of the 2,250 cases a year in the United States occur in children, most of whom are between 2 and 5 years of age. See also **acute childhood leukemia.**

acute mastitis. See **mastitis.**

acute mountain sickness. See **altitude sickness.**

acute myelocytic leukemia (AML), a cancer of blood-forming tissues marked by rapid growth of not-fully-formed granular leukocytes, a type of white blood cell. The symptoms may begin quickly. The typical ones are spongy bleeding gums, iron-poor blood, fatigue, fever, shortness of breath, large spleen, joint and bone pains, and many infections. Greenish tumors (chloromas) may develop in bone or soft tissue. AML may occur at any age, but it usually affects young adults. The diagnosis is made by blood and bone tests. Chemotherapy with various drugs is the main form of treatment. Also called **acute granulocytic leukemia (AGL), acute nonlymphocytic leukemia (ANLL), acute myeloge-** nous leukemia, myeloid leukemia, splenomedullary leukemia, splenomyelogenous leukemia. See also **acute childhood leukemia, chronic myelocytic leukemia.**

acute necrotizing gingivitis, an infection of the gums and throat. It causes bad-smelling sores, fever, and swollen lymph nodes in the neck. It is usually seen with poor cleaning of the mouth. It is most common in patients who live in crowded areas and who do not have enough of the right food to eat. Other causes are hormone changes (as at puberty and during pregnancy), diabetes mellitus, leukemia, or other severe disease. Treatment is scraping the gums (scaling) and antibiotics. Daily use of dental floss and toothbrushing, and routine teeth cleaning every 6 months can keep the mouth healthy. Also called **trench mouth, Vincent's angina, Vincent's infection.**

acute necrotizing hemorrhagic encephalopathy, a disease of the brain that gets worse over time. Typical signs are severe headache, fever, and vomiting. Convulsions may occur, and the patient may rapidly lose consciousness. Treatment consists of removing spinal fluid to ease pressure on the brain and giving large doses of steroids. Also called **acute hemorrhagic leukoencephalitis.**

acute necrotizing ulcerative gingivitis (ANUG), a gum disease that mainly affects the triangular pad of gum (gingiva) between the teeth, causing decay and sores. Treatment and prevention is the same as above.

acute nonlymphocytic leukemia. See **acute myelocytic leukemia.**

acute pain, severe pain, as may follow surgery, trauma, occur with heart attacks, or other diseases. Serious pain in patients with skeletal problems is caused by the covering over the bones (periosteum), the joint surfaces, and the artery walls. Muscle pain after bone surgery results from lack of blood to the muscle. Serious belly pain often causes the patient to lie on one side and draw up the legs in the fetal position. Compare **chronic pain.** See also **pain intervention.**

acute paranoid disorder, the psychological condition of false beliefs of being persecuted. The disorder begins and develops quickly, and usually lasts less than 6 months. It is most commonly seen in persons who have seen big changes in their environment, such as immigrants, refugees, prisoners, military inductees, and, in a less severe form, those leaving home for the first time.

acute promyelocytic leukemia, a cancer of the blood-forming tissues. It causes severe bleeding, bruises, a low blood-clotting factor (fibrinogen) level and blood platelet count. See also **leukemia.**

acute psychosis, a psychological disorder in which the ability to process facts is lessened. It sometimes has a known physical cause. Delirium and acute brain syndrome are associated with known physical disorders of the brain. These cause disorientation, loss of memory, and lapses in consciousness.

acute pyelonephritis. See **pyelonephritis.**

acute pyogenic arthritis, a bacterial infection of one or more joints. It is caused by trauma or a stab wound and occurs most often in children. Typical symptoms are pain, redness, and swelling in the joint, muscle spasms, chills, fever, sweating, and more white blood cells. Treatment is mainly with antibiotics, although in some cases the fluid in the joint is removed. Therapy is sometimes needed after the injury heals.

acute radial nerve palsy, damage to the radial nerve of the arm, causing a weakening of the muscles of the forearm. It may be caused by too much pressure on the radial nerve.

acute radiation exposure, exposure for a short time to much radiation. It will cause death.

acute respiratory distress syndrome (ARDS), an emergency caused by failure of the lungs to work. This may follow heart and lung bypass surgery, severe infection, blood transfusions, too much oxygen, trauma, pneumonia, or other lung infections. It may also occur in Guillain-Barré syndrome, muscular dystrophy, myasthenia gravis, emphysema, asthma, or polio. Also called **adult respiratory distress syndrome, congestive atelectasis, pump lung, shock lung, wet lung.** See also **chronic obstructive pulmonary disease.**
★DIAGNOSIS: The symptoms include shortness of breath and quick breathing. Tests of the blood show low amounts of oxygen and more carbon dioxide in the blood. The changes that occur within the lungs may include damage to the very small blood vessels, bleeding, and swelling.
★TREATMENT: The patient usually requires mechanical assistance with breathing. Oxygen, mist, and respiratory therapy are also used.
★PATIENT CARE: The patient requires constant and careful care. Confusion, the skin getting red, and changes in actions may be caused by too much carbon dioxide. Oxygen levels that are too high can cause the heart to race and the blood pressure to rise. Breathing failure brings falling blood pressure and a blue tinge to the skin, caused by lack of oxygen (cyanosis). The patient is weighed often, x-ray films of the chest are taken, and secretions are checked.

acute rheumatic arthritis, arthritis that occurs during rheumatic fever.

acute rhinitis. See **rhinitis.**

acute schizophrenia, the sudden onset of identity crisis. The symptoms include confusion, emotional turmoil, fear, depression, and strange behavior. Also called **undifferentiated schizophrenia.** See also **schizophrenia, schizophreniform disorder.**

acute toxicity, the harmful effect of a poison that acts in seconds, minutes, hours, or days after entering the body.

acute transverse myelitis, a serious condition marked by swelling of the spinal cord. It is the worst form and can develop quickly. Nerve problems often last after improvement. It may develop from many causes, as multiple sclerosis, measles, pneumonia, and exposure to poisons, as carbon monoxide, lead, and arsenic. Some poisons can destroy a whole part of the spine and can cause bleeding.
★DIAGNOSIS: Acute transverse myelitis starts very quickly with nerve damage below the spinal cord damage. Pain and numbness below this part of the spine usually occur. Within 2 days, one or both legs may be unable to move. The severe spinal cord damage may cause shock with low blood pressure and low body heat. Loss of bowel control and reflexes are common.
★TREATMENT: There is no good treatment and chance of complete recovery is poor. Any other infection is treated.
★PATIENT CARE: Care of the patient involves watching for any signs of spinal shock, as low blood pressure and much sweating. Tubes for draining urine are used. Good skin care is needed to prevent infections and bed sores. Physical therapy, bowel and bladder training, instruction, and good cheer are important throughout the healing process.

ACVD, short for *atherosclerotic cardiovascular disease.*

acyanotic congenital defect, /āsī′ənot′ik/, a heart defect present at birth that does not produce a bluish skin discoloration under normal circumstances. However, the condition does increase the work of breathing, and physical activity may cause problems with blood flow.

acyclovir, an antiviral drug used to treat herpes, including genital herpes (acycloguanosine). It is an ointment for treating herpes of the eye (herpes simplex keratitis) and other types of herpes. Acyclovir does not work on other viral infections.
★CAUTION: Known allergy to this drug prohibits its use.
★ADVERSE EFFECTS: The ointment may cause itching. The form taken by mouth may cause too much sweating, headache, and nausea.

acyesis /a′sī-ē′sis/, **1.** the lack of pregnancy. **2.** sterility in women.

ad-, a prefix meaning 'to, toward, addition to, or making more intense.'

A/D, short for **analog-to-digital.**

ADA, **1.** short for **American Dental Association. 2.** short for **American Diabetes Association. 3.** short for **American Dietetic Association.**

adactyly /ādak'tilē/, a birth defect in which one or more fingers or toes are missing.

adamantinoma. See **ameloblastoma.**

adamantoblastoma. See **ameloblastoma.**

ADAMHA, abbreviation for United States *Alcohol, Drug Abuse, and Mental Health Administration.*

Adam's apple, *informal.* the bulge at the front of the neck made by the thyroid cartilage of the voice box. Also called **laryngeal prominence.**

Adams-Stokes syndrome, a state of sudden fainting. It is caused by incomplete heart block. Seizures may also happen. Also called **Stokes-Adams syndrome.** See also **infranodal block.**

adaptation, a change or response to stress of any kind.

adaptation syndrome. See **general adaptation syndrome.**

adaptive response, an appropriate reaction to an environmental demand.

adaptor RNA. See **transfer RNA.**

addiction, a great need for something. Stopping is very hard, and there is usually a severe response. Compare **habituation.**

addictive personality, a personality marked by traits of compulsive and habitual use of a substance or practice to cope with emotional pain caused by conflict and anxiety.

Addisonian anemia. See **pernicious anemia.**

Addisonian crisis, Addison's crisis. See **adrenal crisis.**

Addison's disease, a life-threatening disease caused by partial or complete failure of the adrenal gland. This gland makes many hormones that control many body functions. Causes include autoimmune diseases, infection, tumor, or bleeding in the adrenal gland. Also called **Addisonism, Addison's syndrome.** See also **adrenal crisis, hypoadrenalism.** ★DIAGNOSIS: This is marked by weakness, loss of strength, darkening of the skin, loss of hunger, loss of water, weight loss, and stomach and intestine problems. Other symptoms are restlessness, depression, and sensitivity to cold. The onset is usually gradual, over a period of weeks or months. ★TREATMENT: Treatment includes replacing the natural hormones with glucocorticoid and mineralocorticoid drugs, drinking more fluids, controlling salt and potassium intake, and eating foods high in carbohydrate and protein. The patient's need for glucocorticoid, mineralocorticoid, and salt is made larger by stress, as in infection, trauma, and surgery. After release from the hospital, sugar in the blood or urine must be checked, the urine checked for acetone, and corticoid drugs must be continued. ★PATIENT CARE: The patient's ability to fight infection, to work, and to feel good must be maintained. Weight and fluid are checked. Good eating is a must. The patient should learn to avoid stress after leaving the hospital.

Addison's keloid. See **morphea.**

Addison's syndrome. See **Addison's disease.**

adduction, movement of a limb toward the body. Compare **abduction.**

adductor /əduk'tər/, a muscle that acts to draw a part toward the midline of the body. Compare **abductor, tensor.**

adductor brevis, a triangular muscle in the thigh. It acts to pull and turn the thigh to the center of the body and to bend the leg. Compare **adductor longus, adductor magnus, gracilis, pectineus.**

adductor canal, a triangular channel in the thigh under the sartorius muscle and between the adductor longus and vastus medialis muscles. Blood vessels and a large nerve pass through the adductor canal. Also called **Hunter's canal.**

adductor longus, the top-most of the three adductor muscles of the thigh. It pulls the thigh. Compare **adductor brevis, adductor magnus, gracilis, pectineus.**

adductor magnus, the long, heavy, triangular muscle of the middle of the thigh. It turns the thigh to the center of the body and bends it on the hip. The lower section straightens the thigh and turns it to the side.

adenalgia /ad'ənal'jə/, a state marked by pain in any of the glands. Also called **adenodynia** /ad'ənōdin'ē·ə/.

adenectomy /ad'ənek'təmē/, the removal by surgery of any gland.

Aden fever. See **dengue fever.**

adenitis /ad'əni'tis/, a swelling of a lymph node or gland. Serious adenitis of the nodes in the neck causes a sore throat and stiff neck, looking like mumps if severe. Swelling of the nodes in the belly is often painful and may cause symptoms like appendicitis. See also **lymphadenitis.** Compare **acinitis.**

adeno-, aden-, a prefix meaning gland.

adenoacanthoma /ad'ənō·ak'anthō'mə/, a tumor that may be cancerous or harmless, made from gland tissue.

adenoameloblastoma /ad'ənō·am'əblastō'mə/, *pl.* **adenoameloblastomas, adenoameloblastomata,** a harmless tumor of the upper jaw bone (maxilla). It grows in tissue that normally makes teeth, and it is most often seen in young people.

adenocarcinoma /ad'ənōkärsinō'mə/, *pl.* **adenocarcinomas, adenocarcinomata,** any one of a large group of cancerous tumors of the glands. The types of tumors are named for the tissue. For example, cancer of the uterine cervix is marked by tumor cells looking like the cells of the cervix. –**adenocarcinomatous,** *adj.*

adenocarcinoma in situ, a growth of abnormal gland tissue that may become cancerous. It is most common in the lining of the uterus (endometrium) and in the large intestine.

adenocarcinoma of the kidney. See **renal cell carcinoma.**

adenocele /ad′ənōsēl′/, a cystlike tumor of a gland.

adenochondroma /ad′ənōkondrō′mə/, *pl.* **adenochondromas, adenochondromata,** a tumor containing tissue from glands and cartilage, as a tumor of the salivary glands. Also called **chondroadenoma.**

adenocyst /ad′ənōsist′/, a harmless tumor in which the cells form glandlike lumps (cysts). Also called **adenosystoma.** A kind of adenocystoma is **papillary adenocystoma lymphomatosum.**

adenocystic carcinoma, a cancerous tumor that occurs most often in the salivary glands, breast, and mucous glands of the upper and lower breathing tract. Also called **adenoid cystic carcinoma, adenomyoepithelioma, cribriform carcinoma, cylindroma, cylindromatous carcinoma.**

adenodynia. See **adenalgia.**

adenoepithelioma /ad′ənō·ep′ithē′lē·ō′mə/, a tumor made of cells from glands and the covering of the body's surfaces (epithelium).

adenofibroma /ad′ənōfībrō′mə/, a tumor of the connective tissues that contains glandlike parts. Connective tissue is the material that binds the body together and supports it, as bone, cartilage, and mucus.

adenofibroma edematodes, a tumor made of glandlike parts and connective tissue in which there is marked swelling, as in a pouchlike growth in the nasal passage (nasal polyp).

adenohypophysis /ad′ənōhīpof′isis/, the front (anterior) lobe of the pituitary gland, which is at the base of the brain. It gives off many hormones, including growth hormone. Hormones from the hypothalamus gland control the adenohypophysis. The hormones of the adenohypophysis control the thyroid, gonads, adrenal cortex, breast, and other endocrine glands. Also called **anterior pituitary.**

adenoid /ad′ənoid/, **1.** having a glandlike look. **2.** adenoids, a growing larger of the spongy (lymphoid) tissue in the space above the soft roof of the mouth (nasopharynx). See **pharyngeal tonsil.** –**adenoidal,** *adj.*

adenoidal speech, a muted, nasal way of speaking caused by larger adenoids. This usually occurs in children. It is fixed by removal.

adenoid cystic carcinoma. See **adenocystic carcinoma.**

adenoidectomy /ad′ənoidek′təmē/, removal of the adenoids. Surgery is done because the adenoids are large, cause blockage, or are infected. Normal adenoids may be removed with the tonsils. Before surgery blood tests are done to check blood clotting. A sickle cell test is done for black patients. A general anesthesia is used in children, but local anesthesia may be used in adults. See also **tonsillectomy.**

adenoid hyperplasia, a state in which large adenoids cause partial breathing blockage, especially in children.

adenoleiomyofibroma /ad′ənōlī′ōmī′ōfibrō′mə/, a glandlike tumor with parts of smooth muscle, connective tissue and covering of the surfaces of the body (epithelium).

adenolipoma /ad′ənōlipō′mə/, a tumor of gland and fat.

adenolipomatosis /ad′ənōlipōmətō′sis/, a state marked by the growth of many adenolipomas in the groin, armpits, and neck.

adenolymphoma. See **papillary adenocystoma lymphomatosum.**

adenoma /ad′ənō′mə/, a tumor in which the cells are glandlike. They often grow on glands and may cause them to secrete a great deal.

adenoma sebaceum /sebā′sē·əm/, a condition in which the skin consists of many, wart-like, yellowish-red, small waxy bumps (papules) on the face. They are not true adenomas but tumors made of fully-grown connective tissue (fibromas). This is part of a problem called tuberous sclerosis. See also **tuberous sclerosis.**

adenomatoid /ad′ənō′mətoid/, looking like a glandlike tumor.

adenomatosis /ad′ənōmətō′sis/, a state in which two or more glands are large or grow tumors. The most common glands are the thyroid, adrenals, and pituitary.

adenomatous goiter /ad′ənō′mətəs/, a large thyroid because of a tumor or many jellolike bumps (colloid nodules).

adenomyoepithelioma. See **adenocystic carcinoma.**

adenomyofibroma /ad′ənōmī′ōfibrō′mə/, a fibrous tumor that has gland and muscle tissue.

adenomyoma /ad′ənōmī·ō′mə/, a tumor of the lining (endometrium) of the womb. It usually causes menstrual cramps (dysmenorrhea).

adenomyomatosis /ad′ənōmī′ōmətō′sis/, harmless lumps (nodules) that resemble adenomyomas found in or beside the womb.

adenomyosarcoma /ad′ənōmī′ōsärkō′mə/, a cancerous tumor that grows in soft tissue and has gland and muscle tissue. A kind of adenomyosarcoma is **Wilms' tumor.**

adenomyosis /ad′ənōmī·ō′sis/, **1.** a state marked by harmless tumors made of gland tissue and muscle cells. **2.** a cancerous state marked by tumors in the wall of the womb or the ducts from the ovary to the womb (oviducts).

adenopathy /ad′ənop′əthē/, a growth of any gland, especially a lymph gland. –**adenopathic,** *adj.*

adenosarcoma /ad′ənōsärkō′mə/, a cancerous glandlike tumor of the soft tissues of the body.

adenosarcorhabdomyoma /ad′ənōsär′kōrab′-dōmī·ō′mə/, a tumor composed of gland muscle and connective tissue.

adenosis /ad′ənō′sis/, **1.** a disease in any gland,

especially a lymph gland. **2.** an abnormal growth of a gland.

adenovirus /ad'ənōvī'rəs/, a virus that causes problems with upper lung infection, or stomach and intestine infection.

adenylate cyclase, an enzyme that begins the conversion of adenosine triphosphate (ATP) to cyclic adenosine monophosphate (cAMP), a controller of many activities that take place in a cell.

adermia /ədur'mē·ə/, defect in or lack of skin. This state may be a birth defect or it may be gotten.

ADH, short for **antidiuretic hormone.**

adhere, the act of two things sticking to each other.

adherence, the state of clinging or being closely attached.

adhesion /adhē'zhən/, a band of scar tissue that binds two surfaces normally apart from each other. They are most commonly found in the belly after surgery, swelling, or injury. More surgery may be needed to pull apart the tissues. See also **adhesiotomy, intestinal obstruction.**

adhesiotomy /adhē'sē·ot'əmē/, separating scar tissue by surgery that binds. This is often done to open an intestinal blockage. See also **abdominal surgery.**

adhesive absorbent dressing, a spongelike dressing with a sticky back.

adhesive pericarditis, scar tissue the binds the layers of the sack around the heart (pericardium) or the pericardium and the partition between the lungs (mediastinum), diaphragm, or chest wall. It may interfere with the normal movements of the heart.

adhesive peritonitis, a problem of the membrane lining the belly cavity (peritoneum). It is marked by scar tissue between two surfaces. There may be oozing of serum and pus, belly pain and tenderness, vomiting, constipation, and fever.

adhesive plaster, a strong fabric covered on one side with a sticky matter. Often able to repel water, it may be used to hold bandages and dressings in place, to hold still a part, or to put pressure on a wound. Also called **adhesive tape.**

adhesive pleurisy, inflammation of the covering of the lungs (pleura) with oozing of fluid. This makes the layers of the pleura fuse together. The main symptom is pain when breathing in or moving.

adhesive skin traction, a type of traction in which the weights are applied to the skin with sticky straps. This can be used to set broken bones. Compare **nonadhesive skin traction.**

adiathermance /a'dī·əthur'məns/, the state of not being affected by radiated heat.

adient /ad'ē·ənt/, tending to move toward rather than away from stimuli. Compare **abient. –adience,** *n.*

Adie's pupil /ā'dēz/, a state of the eyes in which one pupil reacts much more slowly to light or focusing than the other. Also called **tonic pupil.**

Adie's syndrome, the state of Adie's pupil and slowed or no tendon reflexes. Also called **Adie-Holmes syndrome, Weill's syndrome.** See **Adie's pupil.**

adipectomy. See **lipectomy.**

adiphenine hydrochloride /ədif'ənin/, a drug that relaxes smooth muscles, which are in most organs. It is used for treating spasms of the intestines and urinary tract. Side effects include widening of the pupils and dry mouth.

adipo-, adip-, a prefix meaning fat.

adipocele /ad'ipōsēl'/, a loop of an organ or tissue through an opening and holding fat or fatty tissue. Also called **lipocele.**

adipocyte /ad'ipōsīt'/, a fat cell.

adipofibroma /ad'ipōfībrō'mə/, a fiber tumor with fatty part. It grows on connective tissue, as cartilage.

adiponecrosis /ad'ipōnikrō'sis/, breaking down of fatty tissue in the body. **–adiponecrotic,** *adj.*

adiponecrosis subcutanea neonatorum, skin of newborns with patchy spots of hard fatty tissue and bluish-red bruises. It is often a result of delivery, and it clears up in a few days. Also called **pseudosclerema, subcutaneous fat necrosis.**

adipose /ad'ipōs/, fatty. Adipose tissue is made of fat cells arranged in lobes. See also **fat, fatty acid, lipoma.**

adipose tumor. See **lipoma.**

adiposogenital dystrophy /ad'ipō'sōjen'itəl/, a problem of young boys in which the genitals are small and female qualities grow, including the distribution of fat. It is caused by hypothalamic gland problem or by a tumor in the front pituitary gland. Treatment may include giving testosterone, starting a weight-loss program, and removing the tumor either by surgery or x-ray therapy. Also called **adiposogenital syndrome, Fröhlich's syndrome.**

adiposogenital syndrome. See **adiposogenital dystrophy.**

adipsia, lack of thirst.

aditus /ad'itəs/, an approach or entry.

adjunctive psychotherapy, a form of therapy that works on improving a person's outlook without trying to solve basic emotional problems. Some kinds are **music therapy, occupational therapy, physical therapy, recreational therapy.**

adjunct to anesthesia, any drug given before or during surgery that aids the patient's comfort and safety. Drugs may be given before surgery to reduce fear, calm the patient, reduce mouth watering, and secretions of the lungs, and prevent slowed heart beat. During surgery hypnotic and pain-killing drugs are given to help the effects of other drugs. Drugs are given to relax the muscles during surgery. Drugs that excite the nerves (analeptics) are given after surgery to reverse the effects of the anesthetic. Carbon dioxide and oxygen are given to maintain normal breathing.

adjustable orthodontic band, a thin metal ring that is fitted to a tooth to allow braces or other devices to be attached. It is usually made of stainless steel and has an adjusting screw to change the size.

adjusted death rate. See **standardized death rate.**

adjustment reaction, a sudden, short-term response to great stress in people who have no mental illness. It may occur at any age and can be mild or severe. Symptoms include worry, withdrawal, depression, brooding, temper outbursts, crying spells, acting out to get attention, bed wetting, loss of appetite, aches, pains, and muscle spasms. It can result from taking an infant from its mother, the birth of a brother or sister, loss or change of a job, death of a loved one, or forced retirement. See also **neurotic disorder.**

adjuvant chemotherapy /ad'jəvənt/, the use of anticancer drugs after a cancer has apparently been removed, but when there is a significant risk that undetectable cancer cells may still be present. Adjuvant chemotherapy is most commonly used in treating breast cancer.

adjuvant therapy /ad'jəvənt/, the treatment of a disease with substances that help the action of drugs. The term is used to describe drugs that help the body produce antibodies.

ADL, short for **activities of daily living.**

ad lib, short for the Latin *ad libitum,* meaning to be taken as wanted. The term is sometimes used in drug prescriptions.

administration of parenteral fluids, giving intravenous (IV) solutions to maintain the right amount of fluids in the body, increase the amount of blood, replace lost electrolytes (such as potassium or sodium), or provide some nutrition. See **parenteral.**
★METHOD: Fluid is given through a vein, usually in the patient's arm or leg. A needle is put into a vein and taped in place. A tube connects the needle to a bottle of germ-free solution. The fluid is made to run into the vein slowly.
★PATIENT CARE: While the fluid is given, the entire IV system is kept closed so that it stays sterile. The flow rate and amount of solution is watched closely, and the area where the needle is put in is checked often. Infants, aged patients with blood-flow problems or kidney disease, and burn patients need special attention.

adnexa, *sing.* **adnexus,** tissue or structures in the body that are next to or near another structure. The ovaries and the uterine tubes are adnexa of the uterus, for example.

adnexitis, a swelling of the adnexal organs of the uterus, as the ovaries or the fallopian tubes.

-adol, a combining form referring to a drug that relieves pain (analgesic).

adolescence, the time in growth between the onset of sexual maturity (puberty) and adulthood. It usually begins between 11 and 13 years of age, when breast growth, beard growth, pubic hair growth, and other related changes occur (secondary sex characteristics). It spans the teen years, and ends at 18 to 20 years of age when the person has a fully developed adult body. During this time the person undergoes great physical, psychologic, emotional, and personality changes. See also **postpuberty, prepuberty, psychosexual development, psychosocial development, pubarche.**

adolescent, referring to or typical of adolescence.

adolescent vertebral epiphysitis. See **Scheuermann's disease.**

adrenal cortex, the outer part of the adrenal or suprarenal gland. The adrenal cortex makes three kinds of hormones that are vital to the body. See **adrenal gland.**

adrenal cortical carcinoma, a cancerous tumor of the adrenal cortex that may cause adrenogenital syndrome or Cushing's syndrome. Such tumors vary in size, occur at any age, and are more common in females than in males. The cancer often spreads to the lungs, liver, and other organs. See also **adrenogenital syndrome, Cushing's syndrome.**

adrenal crisis, a sudden, life-threatening lack of a hormone made by the adrenal cortex. There is a lack of the hormone glucocorticoid, a drop in fluids, as blood, urine, and saliva, and high potassium levels in the blood (hyperkalemia). Also called **Addisonian crisis, adrenergic crisis.** See also **Addison's disease, adrenal cortex.**
★DIAGNOSIS: The patient seems to be in shock or coma with a low blood pressure and loss of pulses. The patient may have had Addison's disease in the past. Laboratory tests show hyperkalemia and decreased salt (hyponatremia).
★TREATMENT: An intravenous (IV) solution of sodium chloride with the hormone glucocorticoid is given right away. Drugs may be needed to correct the low blood pressure. If the patient is vomiting, a stomach tube is passed through the nose to the stomach. The patient must rest in bed. Blood pressure, temperature, and other vital signs must be watched. After the first crucial hours the patient is treated for Addison's disease and the steroid is given at lower doses. The reason for the adrenal crisis is not known. Infection and a failure to increase the steroid dose is a common cause of crisis in patients who have Addison's disease.
★PATIENT CARE: The patient's room is kept

quiet and dark. The patient is not moved unless it cannot be avoided and is not allowed to do self-care. If the condition is seen and treated right away, recovery is good. When the patient is discharged from the hospital he or she must seek medical aid in any stressful instance, both physical and emotional, to prevent the crisis from occurring again.

adrenalectomy /ədrē′nəlek′təmē/, removal of one or both adrenal glands, or part of the gland. This lowers the excess secretion of adrenal hormones when there is an adrenal tumor or a cancer of the breast or prostate. Steroids are given by mouth for a few days after surgery. The dosage is later cut down. When both glands are taken out, the steroids are given for life. Stress and fatigue must be avoided. See also **Addison's disease, Cushing's syndrome.**

adrenal gland, the organ that sits on top of each kidney. The gland has two parts: the cortex and the medulla. The adrenal cortex secretes the hormones corticosteroids and androgens. The adrenal medulla makes epinephrine and norepinephrine.

Adrenalin, a trademark for a drug used to treat severe allergies, spasms of the large air channels of the lungs (bronchial spasms), and a clogged nose and throat (epinephrine).

adrenaline. See **epinephrine.**

adrenalize /ədrē′nəlīz/, to stimulate or excite.

adrenal medulla, the inner part of the adrenal gland. The adrenal medulla secretes epinephrine and norepinephrine. These regulate blood pressure and heart rate. See **adrenal cortex.**

adrenal virilism, the growth of male secondary sexual characteristics in a female. This state is due to too much androgenic hormones or by tumors of the ovary. See also **virilization.**

adrenarche /ad′rinär′kē/, the very busy action of the adrenal cortex that occurs at about 8 years of age. Larger amounts of various hormones, especially androgens, are made as the body prepares for puberty.

adrenergic /ad′rinur′jik/, referring to nerves that secrete epinephrine or epinephrinelike substances. Compare **cholinergic.** See also **sympathomimetic.**

adrenergic blocking agent. See **antiadrenergic.**

adrenergic drug. See **sympathomimetic.**

adrenergic fibers, nerve fibers of the self-controlling nerves, the part of the nervous system that controls the heart, smooth muscles, and glands (autonomic nervous system). These fibers give off the hormones norepinephrine and, in some areas, dopamine. Norepinephrine raises blood pressure and speeds up the heart. Dopamine is a chemical needed for the nervous system to work.

adrenocorticotropic /ədrē′nōkôr′tikōtrop′ik/, referring to excitement of the adrenal cortex.

adrenocorticotropic hormone (ACTH), a hormone made by the front pituitary gland. It excites the growth of the adrenal gland cortex and its secretion of corticosteroids. ACTH secretion is controlled by the hypothalamus gland. ACTH increases when a patient has stress, fever, sudden low blood sugar, and major surgery. ACTH is also made commercially and is used to treat rheumatoid arthritis, acquired hemolytic anemia, severe allergy, skin diseases, and many other defects. Also called **adrenocorticotrophic hormone, corticotropin.**

adrenodoxin /ədrē′nōdok′sin/, a protein, made by the adrenal glands, that is needed to make steroids.

adrenogenital syndrome /ədrē′nōjen′itəl/, a state in which too many androgens are made by the adrenal glands. This may be caused by an adrenal tumor, large, inherited adrenal gland, or an inborn defect. Girls born with this syndrome may have a very large clitoris and labia that have grown together. More than usual growth of body hair, low pitched voice, acne, and lack of a menstrual period occur at puberty. Male hair growth and muscle size may also occur at puberty. Boys with this syndrome have early growth of the penis and prostate and of hair in the pubic and armpit areas. However, their testicles stay small and not fully formed. Children with the defect are quite tall, but the growth plates of their bones (epiphyses) close too soon, and as adults they are very short. See also **adrenal virilism, pseudohermaphroditism.**

adrenoleukodystrophy (ALD), a rare, inherited childhood defect of the body's food chemistry. It affects only boys. It is known by wasting of the adrenal glands and widespread loss of a cell structure in the brain (cerebral demyelination). The result is progressive mental decay, loss of speech or understanding (aphasia), loss of ability to function (apraxia), and, in the end, blindness.

Adriamycin. See **doxorubicin hydrochloride.**

adromia /ədrō′mē·ə/, a state in which a nerve that serves a muscle becomes unable to function.

Adrucil, a trademark for an agent that controls or kills cancer cells (fluoracil).

ADRV, abbreviation for **adult rotavirus.**

adult, 1. one who is fully physically mature and who has reached the mental potential and the emotional growth typical of a mature person. **2.** a person who has reached full legal age. Compare **child.**

adult celiac disease. See **celiac disease.**

adult day care center, a place for the supervised care of older adults. These centers provide services as meals and company during set day hours. The people go to their homes each night.

adulteration, the lowered quality or watered-down state of the purity of any substance, process, or act.

adult hemoglobin. See **hemoglobin A.**

adulthood, the phase of growth known by physical and mental maturity.

adult onset diabetes. See **non-insulin-dependent diabetes.**

adult polycystic disease. See **polycystic kidney disease.**

adult respiratory distress syndrome (ARDS). See **acute respiratory distress syndrome.**

adult rickets, a disease that affects adults and looks like rickets. See also **osteomalacia, rickets.**

adult rotavirus (ADRV), a form of rotavirus that causes severe diarrhea in adults. It resembles the usual rotavirus but does not react against rotavirus antibodies. ADRV antibodies have been found in adults in China and Australia. See also **rotavirus.**

advanced life support. See **Emergency Medical Technician Advanced Life Support.**

adventitious /ad′ventish′əs/, referring to a state that is brought on by accident or to a random action.

adventitious bursa, a defect of the liquid sacs in a joint that is due to rubbing or pressure.

adventitious crisis, an accidental, uncommon, and unexpected tragedy that may affect an entire community or population. Examples include earthquakes, floods, and airplane crashes. In addition to injuries, deaths, and property damage, an adventitious crisis often results in emotional problems that require long-term counseling.

adventitious sounds, breath sounds that are not normally heard. They may be heard along with normal breath sounds.

adverse drug effect, a harmful side effect of a drug given in normal amounts.

adverse reaction, any harmful or unintended effect of a medication, diagnostic test, or therapeutic intervention.

advocacy, 1. a process whereby a nurse provides a patient with the information to make certain decisions. 2. a method by which patients, their families, attorneys, health professionals, and citizen groups can work together to develop programs that ensure the availability of high-quality health care for a community.

adynamia /ad′inā′mē·ə/, physical and mental fatigue caused by a disease.

adynamia episodica hereditaria, a rare inherited defect seen in infants. The patient may suffer from attacks of muscle weakness and be unable to move. The drug acetazolamide is often given to prevent the attacks. Also called **hyperkalemic periodic paralysis.**

adynamic fever, a high fever with a weak pulse, nervous depression, and cool, moist skin. Also called **asthenic fever.**

adynamic ileus. See **ileus.**

Aedes /ā·ē′dēz/, a type of mosquito, found in hot, wet regions. Many species can give diseases to humans, including dengue fever, equine encephalitis, St. Louis encephalitis, tularemia, and yellow fever.

aerate /er′āt/, to add air, carbon dioxide, or oxygen to a substance.

aero-, aer-, a combining form referring to air or to gas.

Aerobacter aerogenes. See *Enterobacter cloacae.*

aerobe /er′ōb/, a tiny organism that needs oxygen to live and grow. Kinds of aerobes are **facultative aerobe, obligate aerobe.** Compare **anaerobe.**

aerobic /erō′bik/, 1. referring to the presence or need of air or oxygen. 2. referring to aerobic exercise.

aerobic exercise, any physical exercise that makes the heart and lungs work harder to meet the muscles' need for oxygen. The exercise causes harder breathing than light exercise and improves the heart and lungs. Running, bicycling, swimming, and cross-country skiing are types of aerobic exercise. Also called **aerobics.** See also **active exercise, passive exercise.**

aerobic glycolysis. See **glycolysis.**

aerobics. See **aerobic exercise.**

aerodontalgia /er′ōdontal′jə/, a pain in the teeth caused by air trapped in the teeth when the air pressure changes, as may occur at high altitudes.

aeroembolism. See **embolism.**

aerophagy /erof′əjē/, swallowing air, often leading to belching, stomach upset, and gas. Also called **aerophagia** /er′ōfā′jə/.

aerosinusitis /er′ōsī′nəsī′tis/, soreness, swelling, or bleeding of the sinuses. It is caused when air expands in the sinuses. This occurs when air pressure goes down. Also called **barosinusitis.**

aerosol /er′əsol′/, 1. small particles in a gas or air. 2. a gas under pressure that contains a drug which is breathed in. Drugs for asthma attacks and problems in the canals of the nose are often given in aerosols.

Aerosporin, a trademark for an antibiotic used to treat meningitis, liver infection, blood poisoning due to bacteria (septicemia), and infections of the ear, lungs, urinary tract, and joints (polymyxin B sulfate).

aerotitis /er′ətī′tis/, an inflamed ear that is due to changes in air pressure. Also called **barotitis.**

aerotitis media, soreness or bleeding in the middle ear. It is caused by a difference between the air pressure in the middle ear and the air outside. This can occur with quick changes in altitude, in diving, or in pressure chambers.

Symptoms are pain, ringing in the ear (tinnitus), trouble hearing, and dizziness (vertigo). Also called **barotitis media.**

Æsculapius /es′kyo͞olā′pē·əs/, the ancient Greek god of medicine. His symbol in modern medicine is a staff with a snake wrapped around it.

afebrile /āfē′bril, āfeb′ril/, without fever.

affect, the way in which a person's feelings are shown. **–affective,** *adj.*

affective disorder. See **major affective disorder.**

affective learning, learning behaviors that express feelings in attitudes, appreciations, and values.

affective melancholia. See **depression.**

affective psychosis, a psychotic reaction in which the primary symptom is a severe problem in mood or emotions.

affect memory, a feeling that returns when a certain time is recalled.

afferent /af′ərənt/, moving toward the center of an organ or system. This usually refers to blood vessels, lymph channels, and nerves. Compare **efferent.**

affiliated hospital, a hospital that works with a medical school or health program.

afibrinogenemia /afi′brinōjenē′mē·ə/, a rare blood disorder known by a low or absent clotting factor in the blood (fibrinogen).

aflatoxins, a group of cancer-causing, poisonous factors made by *Aspergillus flavus* food molds. These poisons cause liver death (necrosis) and liver cancer in test animals. Aflatoxins are thought to be the cause of the high rate of liver cancer in people in regions of Africa and Asia, who may eat moldy grains, peanuts, or other *Aspergillus* infected foods. See *Aspergillus.*

AFP, short for **alpha fetoprotein.**

African lymphoma. See **Burkitt's lymphoma.**

African sleeping sickness. See **African trypanosomiasis.**

African tick fever. See **relapsing fever.**

African tick typhus, an infection transmitted by ixodial ticks, characterized by fever, rash, and swollen lymph nodes. At the onset of the infection a buttonlike skin irritation with a black center appears. The rash usually begins on the forearms and spreads over the rest of the body. The fever may last as long as two weeks, but death or complications are rare.

African trypanosomiasis, a disease caused by the parasites *Trypanosoma brucei,* which are given to humans in the bite of the tsetse fly. African trypanosomiasis occurs only in the tropical areas of Africa, where tsetse flies are found. Kinds of African trypanosomiasis are **Gambian trypanosomiasis, Rhodesian trypanosomiasis.** Also called **African sleeping sickness, sleeping sickness.** See also **trypanosomiasis, tsetse fly.**

Afrin, a trademark for a drug that clears the nose and decreases stuffiness for easy breathing (oxymetazoline hydrochloride).

afterbirth, the material expelled from the womb after a baby is born.

aftercare, health care after release from a hospital. A patient may need care for a health problem that no longer requires hospital care.

afterdepolarization, the space after a heart beat when there is no electric activity in the heart. (depolarization). It is thought to be the time that parts of the heart beat at random when the patient has had too much digitalis.

afterload, the pressure against which the left lower chamber of the heart (ventricle) must eject the blood during a beat. The pressure is made by the amount of blood that is already flowing and the vessel walls themselves. About 90% of the oxygen needed by the heart is used in the afterload effort.

afterpains, cramps that often occur in the first days after giving birth.

Ag, symbol for **silver.**

AGA, short for **appropriate for gestational age.**

agalactia, inability of the mother to make enough milk to breast feed an infant after birth.

agammaglobulinemia /agam′əglob′yo͞olinē′mē·ə/, a rare defect, in which there is not enough gamma globulin in the blood. This increases the chances of infection. See also **Bruton's agammaglobulinemia, immune gamma globulin.**

aganglionic megacolon. See **Hirschsprung's disease.**

ageism, /ā′jizəm/, an attitude that discriminates, separates, stigmatizes, or otherwise disadvantages older adults on the basis of age.

agenesia corticalis, the failure of some of the brain cells to grow in the embryo. It causes loss of motor function in the brain of the infant (infantile cerebral paralysis), and severe mental retardation.

agenesis /ājen′əsis/, **1.** born without an organ or part. **2.** the state of being unable to reproduce (sterility) or maintain an erection (impotence). Also called **agenesia** /ā′jinē′zhə/. Compare **dysgenesis. –agenic,** *adj.*

agenetic fracture, a bone break caused by faulty bone growth.

ageniocephaly /ājen′ē-ōsef′əlē/, faulty skull growth in which the brain, skull, and sense organs are normal but the lower jaw is malformed.

agenitalism /ājen′itəliz′əm/, the absence of the ovaries or testicles or problems of function. It is caused by lack of sex hormones.

agenosomia /əjen′əsō′mē·ə/, a birth defect in which the genitals are defective or missing, and the intestines stick out through the abdominal wall.

agenosomus /əjen′əsō′məs/, a fetus with agenosomia.

Agent Orange, a U.S. military code name for a mixture of two chemicals, 2,4-D and 2,4,5-T, used to kill crops in Southeast Asia during the war in Vietnam. The chemical mix contained the highly poisonous chemical dioxin. This chemical causes cancer and birth defects in animals and chloracne and slight or severe long-term scarring (porphyria cutanea tarda) in humans. See **dioxin.**

agglutination /əgl$\overline{oo}$'tinā'shən/, the clumping together of cells as a result of their contact with certain antibodies. See also **agglutinin, blood typing, precipitin.**

agglutination inhibition test, a way to test the blood for foreign invadors (antigens). One type of pregnancy test is based on agglutination inhibition.

agglutinin /əgl$\overline{oo}$'tinin/, a kind of defender cell (antibody) that interacts with foreign invaders (antigens) by agglutination. Compare **precipitin.** See also **agglutination, blood typing, hemagglutination.**

agglutinin absorption, removing antibodies from immune blood.

agglutinogen /ag'l$\overline{oo}$tin'əjin/, an antigen that causes agglutination.

aggregate anaphylaxis, a severe allergy caused by injecting a foreign substance (antigen).

aggression, physical, verbal, or symbolic act or attitude that is carried out with force and assertion of the self.

aggressive personality, type of person who is quick to anger, has tantrums, is destructive or violent when frustrated.

aggressive-radical therapy, (in psychiatry) a form of therapy that introduces the political and social viewpoints of the therapist into the therapeutic process. Supporters of this technique believe that by making all values explicit, the patient will view the solution of an emotional conflict and the raising of political consciousness as one and the same.

aging, the process of growing old, caused in part by a failure of body cells to work normally or to make new cells to replace those that are dead or defective. Normal cells may be lost through infection, poor nutrition, contact with health hazards, or gene problems. See also **assessment of the aging patient, senile.**

agitated, being in a state of physical and mental excitement known by restless actions that have no purpose.

agitated depression, a form of depression known by severe worry and restlessness. See also **depression.**

agitation, a state of continuous restlessness, usually characterized by voluntary movements to express emotional tension.

agitographia /aj'itōgraf'ē·ə/, too-rapid writing in which words or parts of words are left out by mistake.

agitolalia. See **agitophasia.**

agitophasia /aj'itōfā'zhə/, too-rapid speech in which words, sounds, or parts of words are left

out, slurred, or distorted. Also called **agitolalia.**

agnathia /ag·nath'ē·ə/, a birth defect in which the lower jaw is missing totally or in part. The ears may be either joined or close together. Also called **agnathy** /ag'nəthē/. Compare **synotia.** See also **otocephaly.** –**agnathous,** *adj.*

agnathocephalus /ag·nath'əsef'ələs/, a baby before birth with agnathocephaly.

agnathocephaly /ag·nath'əsef'əlē/, a birth defect in which the lower jaw is missing, the mouth is defective, the eyes are low on the face, and the cheeks and ears are joined.

agnathus /ag·nath'əs/, a fetus with agnathia.

agnathy. See **agnathia.**

agnogenic myeloid metaplasia. See **myeloid metaplasia.**

agnosia /ag·nō'zhə/, total or partial loss of the ability to know familiar objects or persons. It is due to brain damage. The state may affect any of the senses and is therefore noted as hearing (auditory), sight (visual), smell (olfactory), taste (gustatory), or touch (tackle) agnosia. Also called **agnosis.** See also **autotopagnosia.**

agonal respiration, a type of breathing pattern of gasping, followed by no breathing. It often means the onset of lung failure.

agonal thrombus /ag'ənəl/, a clot made of blood platelets, clotting factors, and cells that forms in the heart in the process of dying.

agonist /ag'ənist/, **1.** a contracting muscle that is opposed by another muscle (an antagonist). **2.** a drug or other substance that causes a response that can be known in advance.

agoraphobia /ag'ərə-/, mental defect in which the patient is afraid to be alone in an open, crowded, or public place, as a field, tunnel, bridge, busy street, or store, where escape may be hard or help may not be at hand. The disorder can sometimes be treated with success through psychiatric help.

agranular endoplasmic reticulum. See **endoplasmic reticulum.**

agranulocyte /āgran'y$\overline{oo}$lōsīt'/, any white blood cell (leukocyte) that does not have cytoplasmic granules, as a monocyte or lymphocyte. Compare **granulocyte.** See also **leukocyte.**

agranulocytosis /āgran'y$\overline{oo}$lōsītō'sis/, a sudden condition of the blood in which there is a severe decrease in the number of granulocytes, (a type of white blood cell). This results in fever, severe fatigue and bleeding sores of the rectum, mouth, and vagina. It can occur as a side effect to a drug or be the result of radiation therapy.

agraphia /āgraf'ē·ə/, a nerve defect in which the person can no longer write. This can be due to injury to the language center in the brain. Compare **dysgraphia.**

A:G ratio, the ratio of protein albumin to globulin in the blood serum.

agrypnia. See **insomnia.**

agrypnotic /ag'ripnot'ik/, a drug or other substance that prevents sleep.

agyria /əjī'rē-ə/, **1.** an abnormal condition caused by excessive absorption and storing of silver salts in tissues. It is marked by a slate-gray coloration of the skin and mucous membranes. **2.** a cerebral cortex abnormality in which the ridges (gyri) are poorly developed.

AHA, abbreviation for **American Hospital Association.**

"aha" reaction /ähä'/, (in psychology) a sudden idea that occurs, especially during deep thought. Some psychologists link great discoveries and works of art with this reaction. It is not linked to intelligence.

AHF, short for **antihemophilic factor.**

Ahumada-del Castillo syndrome, an absence of menstruation in non-pregnant females that may be associated with a pituitary gland tumor. It also is characterized by the presence of breast milk.

AID, short for **artificial insemination donor.**

AIDS /ādz/, short for **acquired immune deficiency syndrome.**

AIH, short for **artificial insemination husband.**

air, the clear gas with no odor that surrounds the earth. It is made of 78% nitrogen, 21% oxygen, almost 1% argon, small amounts of carbon dioxide, hydrogen, and ozone, traces of helium, krypton, neon, and xenon, and amounts of water vapor that vary.

air bath, exposing the body to warm air to aid in restoring health. Also called **balneum pneumaticum** /bal'nē-əm nōōmat'ikəm/.

airborne contaminants, materials in the air that can affect people's health. Inhaled contaminants may cause tissue damage, tissue reaction, disease, or physical blockage. Contaminants may affect the respiratory system or be absorbed into the bloodstream and damage other organs or the blood itself.

air cells of the nose. See **nasal sinus.**

air conditioner lung. See **humidifier lung.**

air embolism, the presence of air in the blood that blocks the flow of blood through a vessel. Air can enter a vessel by needle, during surgery, or through a puncture wound. See also **decompression sickness, embolus, gas embolism.**

air encephalography. See **encephalography.**

air fluidization, the process of blowing warm air through a collection of tiny beads to create a fluidlike environment. The technique is used in special mattresses designed to reduce pressure against a patient's skin. See also **air-fluidized bed.**

air-fluidized bed, a bed with body support provided by thousands of tiny soda-lime glass beads suspended by pressurized warm air. The patient rests on a polyester filter sheet that covers the beads. The special bed is designed for use by patients with pressure sores or grafts on their backs, burns, or donor areas.

airplane splint, a splint used to prevent a broken arm from moving while it heals. The splint holds the arm up at shoulder level, with the elbow bent.

air pump, a pump that forces air in or out of a cavity or chamber.

air sickness. See **motion sickness.**

air thermometer, a thermometer that uses air instead of mercury. See also **thermometer.**

airway, any tube that allows air to move into and out of the lungs. Examples are tubes on an anesthesia machine, a tube used for mouth-to-mouth resuscitation, and the nose, mouth, and throat.

airway obstruction, anything that blocks the wind pipe and will not let oxygen enter or be absorbed by the lungs. It can be caused by bronchospasm, choking, croup, chronic obstructive lung disease, goiter, tumor, or pneumothorax.

★DIAGNOSIS: If the blockage is minor, as in sinusitis or pharyngitis, the patient is able to breathe, but not normally. If the blockage is severe, the patient may grasp the neck, gasp, become blue (cyanotic) and faint.

★TREATMENT: Severe airway obstruction is a life-threatening emergency. Food, mucus, or a foreign object may be removed by hand, by suction, or with the Heimlich maneuver. Blockage of the airway that is due to swelling or allergies may be treated with drugs to open the passages, with steroids, by inserting a tube to open the airway, and by giving oxygen. Inserting a tube through a cut in the throat (tra-

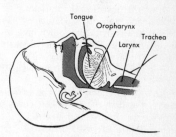

Airway obstruction by tongue

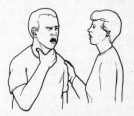

Airway obstruction: Victim gives international choking sign; rescuer asks if victim can speak

cheotomy) may be needed if the blockage cannot be cleared within a few minutes.

★PATIENT CARE: The patient is usually very scared and may resist care out of panic. The patient should be reassured, but treatment must not be delayed. See also **aspiration, cardiopulmonary resuscitation, Heimlich maneuver.**

akathisia /ak´əthē´zhə/, an abnormal state in which the person is restless and agitated, as muscles of the neck and face jerk over and over, a side effect of long-term doses of antipsychotic drugs (in tardive dyskinesia).

akinesia /ā´kinē´zhə, ā´kīnē´zhə/, an abnormal state of physical and mental inactivity or inability to move the muscles.

akinetic apraxia, the inability to make a quick move without thinking. See also **apraxia.**

akinetic mutism, a state in which a person is not able or will not move or make sounds.

akinetic seizure, a type of seizure disorder observed in children. It is a brief, generalized seizure in which the child suddenly falls to the ground.

Akineton, a trademark for a drug (biperiden hydrochloride or biperiden lactate) used to treat a problem that gets worse with time and is known by the muscles not moving (parkinsonism).

Al, symbol for **aluminum.**

ala /ā´lə/, *pl.* **alae, 1.** any winglike structure. **2.** the axilla, or armpit.

ALA, abbreviation for **aminolevulinic acid.**

ala auris, the outside, visible part of the ear (auricle).

ala cerebelli /ser´əbel´ī/, the winglike portion of the central lobe of the cerebellum, the part of the brain that instructs the muscles.

ala cinerea /sinir´ē·ə/, the spot shaped like a triangle on the floor of the fourth hollow chamber of the brain. The vagus nerve starts here.

alactasia. See **lactase deficiency.**

ala nasi /nā´sī/, the outer flaring wall of each nostril.

alanine (Ala), an amino acid found in many proteins in the body. It is broken down by the liver. See also **amino acid, protein.**

alanine aminotransferase (ALT), an enzyme normally present in the clear liquid part of the blood (serum) and tissues of the body, specially the tissues of the liver. It is let into the serum with an injury. The level may grow in patients with severe liver damage. Also called **glutamic-pyruvic transaminase.** Compare **aspartate aminotransferase.**

Al-Anon, a worldwide group. They give help and guidance to people who have alcoholics in their lives (families, friends, coworkers). See also **Alcoholics Anonymous.**

ala of the ethmoid, a small piece on the ethmoid bone, which is a small bone lying between the eyesockets and at the root of the nose.

ala of the ilium, the upper flaring part of the hip (iliac) bone.

ala of the sacrum, the flat bone on each side of the sacrum, which is the lower part of the backbone.

alar ligament, one of a pair of ligaments that joins the axis to the occipital bone at the base of the skull and limits turning of the head. Also called **check ligament, odontoid ligament.** Compare **membrana tectoria.**

alarm reaction, the first stage of adapting. One uses the many defenses of the body or the mind to cope with a stress. See also **stress.**

alastrim /al´əstrim/, a mild form of smallpox, thought to be caused by a weak strain of *Poxvirus variolae.* Also called **Cuban itch, milkpox, variola minor.** See also **smallpox.**

Alateen, a world-wide group. They give help and guidance to the children of alcoholics. See also **Alcoholics Anonymous.**

ala vomeris /vō´məris/, a piece of bone on each side of the upper border of the vomer (part of the nose).

alba /al´bə/, a Latin term for "white," as in linea alba.

Albers-Schönberg disease. See **osteopetrosis.**

Albert's disease, an inflammation of the fluid-filled sac that lies between the Achilles tendon and the heel bone. It is most frequently caused by injury, but may also result from wearing poorly fitted shoes, increased strain on the tendon, or rheumatoid arthritis. If treatment is delayed, the inflammation may cause erosion of the heel bone. Also called **anterior Achilles bursitis.**

albinism /al´biniz´əm/, a birth defect marked by partial or total lack of pigment in the body. Total albinos have pale skin that does not tan, white hair, pink eyes, rapid, eye movement they cannot control (nystagmus), uneven eye curvature (astigmatism), and a response to light (photophobia). Compare **piebald, vitiligo.**

Albright's syndrome /ôl´brīts/, a state in which parts of the bone act like tumors, brown spots form on the skin, and hormones do not work right. It causes very early puberty in girls but not in boys. Also called **Albright-McCune-Sternberg syndrome, osteitis fibrosa disseminata.**

albumin /albyōō´min/, a protein found in almost all animal tissues and in many plant tissues. Amounts and types of albumin in urine, blood, and other body tissues form the basis of many laboratory tests.

albumin A, a blood serum substance that gathers in cancer cells but does not circulate in cancer patients.

albumin (human), a substance that expands the volume of blood and is used for treating hypoproteinemia, hyperbilirubinemia, and hypovolemic shock.

★CAUTION: Severe iron-poor blood (anemia) or heart failure prohibits its use.

★ADVERSE EFFECTS: Among the most serious are chills, low blood pressure, fever, and itching.

-albuminuria, a suffix meaning too many serum proteins in the urine.

albuterol, a drug used to treat spasms in the windpipe in patients with obstructive airway disease.

★CAUTION: Known allergy to this drug prohibits its use.

★ADVERSE EFFECTS: Among the most serious are rapid heart beat, inability to sleep (insomnia), dizziness, and high blood pressure.

alcalase, a protein enzyme found in certain laundry detergents. It is a cause of enzymatic detergent asthma.

alclometasone dipropionate, a topical steroid. It is prescribed for the relief of symptoms of inflammation and itching of certain skin disorders.

★CAUTION: children may absorb proportionally greater amounts of the drug and should be treated with the smallest amount needed.

★ADVERSE EFFECTS: among adverse reactions reported are burning, stinging, and itching.

Alcock's canal, a canal formed by the muscles in the pelvis (obturator internus muscle and the obturator fascia). The nerve and vessels effecting the outer sex organs (pudendal) pass through the canal. Also called **pudendal canal.**

alcohol, 1. (*USP*) a liquid that contains between 92.3% and 93.8% ethyl alcohol. It is used as a skin cleaner and to break down other things. 2. a clear, colorless liquid that is made by brewing sugar with yeast. Examples are beer and whiskey. 3. a compound derived from a hydrocarbon. Some kinds are rubbing, sugar, and unsaturated.

alcohol bath, a way to lower a high body temperature. Alcohol is mixed with an equal amount of warm water. The patient is sponged on the arms and legs, then on the trunk. The patient is turned only once, from the back to the front and then back. A hot-water bottle can be placed at the feet and a cold cloth on the head to speed up heat loss, to make the patient feel better, and to reduce the heat of the blood flowing to the brain.

alcoholic cirrhosis. See **cirrhosis.**

alcoholic fermentation, the changing of simple sugar to alcohol.

alcoholic hallucinosis, a mental disorder caused by alcohol. The symptoms are mainly hearing things that are not there, fear, and false feelings of being punished. It is seen with serious alcoholism right after stopping or reducing drinking. Also called **acute hallucinosis.** See also **alcoholic psychosis, hallucinosis.**

alcoholic hepatitis, liver injury caused by too much alcohol.

alcoholic ketoacidosis, the fall in the acid in the blood, as seen in alcoholics.

alcoholic-nutritional cerebellar degeneration, a sudden loss of ability to move the legs together, as seen in poorly nourished alcoholics. The patient walks, if at all, with the legs far apart. Treatment consists of good food, stopping drinking, and physical therapy. Also called **cerebellar cortical degeneration.** See also **alcoholism.**

alcoholic paranoia, unfounded fears as seen with long-term alcoholism.

alcoholic psychosis, any severe mental disorder, as delirium tremens, Korsakoff's psychosis, and acute hallucinosis. Each is caused by brain damage that comes from the too much alcohol.

Alcoholics Anonymous (AA), a worldwide nonprofit group, founded in 1935, whose members are alcoholics who no longer drink. The purpose of AA is to help others stop drinking and stay sober.

alcoholic trance, a state of being active while not being aware because of too much alcohol.

alcoholism, the extreme dependence on alcohol that is marked by bad behaviors. It is a long-term illness that starts slowly and may occur at any age. The most frequent medical problems are mental changes and breakdown (cirrhosis) of the liver. The problems are worse when not enough food has been eaten. Patients may suffer from belly problems (gastritis), nerve damage, hearing things that are not there, and heart problems. Suddenly not drinking causes weakness, sweating, and very quick reflexes. The severe form of quitting is called delirium tremens. Caution must be used in giving drugs to the patient, because interactions with alcohol are common. The treatment of alcoholism consists of mental therapy (especially group therapy, as in Alcoholics Anonymous), electroshock treatments, or drugs, as disulfiram, that cause one to not want any alcohol. See also **acute alcoholism, chronic alcoholism, delirium tremens.**

alcohol poisoning, poisoning caused by drinking alcohol, as ethyl, isopropyl, or methyl. Ethyl alcohol (grain alcohol) is in whiskies, brandy, gin, and other drinks. In most cases, it is lethal only if large amounts are drunk in a short time. Isopropyl alcohol, found in cosmetics and solvents, is more poisonous, and drinking 8 ounces may cause breathing or heart failure. Methyl alcohol (wood alcohol) is very poisonous. It may cause nausea, vomiting, belly pain, and blindness. Death may come after drinking only 2 ounces. Treatment includes pumping the belly, giving baking soda and sugar through the veins, and, if necessary, blood dialysis (hemodialysis).

alcohol withdrawal syndrome, the symptoms that come with suddenly not drinking alcohol.

These may include tremor, seeing and hearing things that are not there, nervous system problems, and seizures.

ALD, short for **adrenoleukodystrophy.**

Aldactazide, a trademark for a drug that causes one to empty the bladder. It has two diuretics (hydrochlorothiazide and spironolactone). It is used for treating high blood pressure and to reduce fluids.

Aldactone, a trademark for a diuretic (spironolactone).

Aldoclor, a trademark for an antihypertensive drug with specific amounts of both clorothiazide and methyldopa.

aldolase /al'dəlās/, an enzyme in muscle tissue that is necessary for storing energy in the cells. See also **glycolysis.**

Aldomet, a trademark for a drug used for treating high blood pressure (methyldopa).

Aldoril, a trademark for a drug that is used to treat too much fluid in the body (diuretic hydroclorothiazide) and high blood pressure (antihypertensive-methyldopa).

aldosterone /al'dōstərōn', aldos'tərōn/, a steroid hormone made by the adrenal cortex that controls sodium and potassium in the blood.

aldosteronism /al'dōstərō'nizəm, aldos'-/, a state in which too much aldosterone is made. This can occur from a disease of the adrenal cortex or, more often, as a second problem caused by another disease. Too much aldosterone causes the body to keep salt and get rid of potassium. The symptoms are increased blood pressure, too much base in the pH of the blood, muscular weakness, muscle contractions (tetany), numbness (paresthesias), kidney disease (nephropathy), and heart failure. Also called **hyperaldosteronism.**

aldosteronoma /al'dōstir'ənō'mə/, an aldosterone-secreting tumor (adenoma) of the adrenal cortex that causes too much aldosterone in the system with holding salt, increased blood volume, and high blood pressure.

-aldrate, a combining form referring to an antacid aluminum salt.

Aleppo boil. See **oriental sore.**

aleukemic leukemia /ā'o͞okē'mik/, a type of leukemia in which the white blood cell (leukocyte) count is normal and few abnormal leukocytes are found in the blood. Also called **subleukemic leukemia.** See also **leukemia.**

aleukemic myelosis. See **myeloid metaplasia.**

aleukia /ālo͞o'kē-ə/, a marked decrease or total lack of white blood cells or blood platelets. Compare **leukopenia, thrombocytopenia.** See also **aplastic anemia.**

Alexander technique, a mental-health therapy introduced by Frederick Alexander. It focuses on individual variations in body musculature, posture, the breathing process and the correction of defects to avoid stress, tension, and possible loss of function.

alexia /əlek'sē-ə/, a nervous system defect, in which the person cannot understand written words. Compare **dyslexia.** **–alexic,** *adj.*

alexithymia /əlek'sithī'mē-ə, -thim'ē-ə/, an inability to consciously experience and communicate feelings.

alga /al'gə/, *pl.* **algae** /al'jī/, any of a large group of water plants with chlorophyll. Many types of algae can be found worldwide in fresh-water, saltwater, and on land. All belong to the phylum Thallophyta. **–algal,** *adj.*

algesi-, alg-, alge-, algo-, a combining form referring to pain.

algid malaria, a form of malaria caused by the protozoan *Plasmodium falciparum.* Symptoms of this disease are cold skin, extreme weakness, and severe diarrhea. See also **falciparum malaria, malaria.**

algodystrophy /al'gōdis'trəfē/, a painful wasting of the muscles of the hands, often accompanied by tenderness and a loss of bone calcium. The condition may begin in the hand or in the shoulder and spread over the entire limb, causing contractures, swelling, and a bluish skin tone. It may be associated with injury, heart disease, stroke, or a viral infection.

algolagnia /al'gōlag'nē-ə/, a term that is used to describe the sexual preference for sadism or masochism. See also **sadism, sadomasochism.**

algologist, **1.** a person who studies or treats pain. **2.** a person who studies algae. Also called **phycologist.**

algology, **1.** the branch of medicine that is concerned with the study of pain. **2.** the branch of science that is concerned with algae. Also called **phycology.**

algophobia, a mental defect in which there is too much fear of feeling pain or of seeing pain in others.

algor mortis, the drop in body temperature and accompanying loss of skin tone that occur after death. Also called **death chill.**

alienation, the act or state of being separated from others or isolated. See also **depersonalization.**

alimentary bolus. See **bolus,** def. 1.

alimentary canal. See **digestive tube.**

alimentation, nourishment. See also **feeding.**

alkalemia, increased pH of the blood, so that it is too alkaline.

alkali /al'kəlī/, a compound with the chemical qualities of a base. Alkalis join with fatty acids to make soaps, turn red litmus paper blue, and enter into chemical reactions. See also **acid, base.** **–alkaline,** *adj.* **alkalinity,** *n.*

alkali burn, tissue damage caused by an alkaline compound, as lye. Treatment includes flushing with water to wash off the chemical. Then vinegar or another mildly acidic substance mixed with water is put on the burn to make neutral any alkali that is left and to lessen the pain.

The patient should be taken right away to a hospital or other treatment center if the damage is severe. Compare **acid burn**.

alkaline-ash, substance in the urine that has a pH higher than 7.

alkaline-ash producing foods, foods that are eaten to make an alkaline pH in the urine, reducing the chance of acidic stones (urinary calculi) forming in the kidney. Some of the foods that result in alkaline ash are milk, cream, buttermilk, fruit (except prunes, plums, and cranberries), vegetables (except corn and lentils), almonds, chestnuts, coconuts, and olives.

alkaline bath, a bath in which sodium bicarbonate is mixed in the water. This is used for skin problems.

alkaline phosphatase, an enzyme in bone, the kidneys, the intestine, blood plasma, and teeth. It may be present in the blood serum in high levels in some diseases of the bone, liver, and in some other illnesses.

alkalinize /al'kəlinīz/, **1.** to make a substance alkaline by adding a base. **2.** to become alkaline. Also **alkalize** /al'kəlīz/. Compare **acidify**.

alkali poisoning, a poisoning caused by swallowing an alkaline agent, as ammonia, lye, and some soap powders. Emergency treatment includes giving large amounts of water or milk to water down the alkali. The patient must not vomit and mild acids should not be given. The patient is taken without delay to the hospital to watch for any damage to the esophagus or any food chemistry defects, and for flushing out the stomach. Compare **acid poisoning**.

alkaloid /al'kəloid/, any of a large group of organic compounds made by plants or made synthetically. Examples include many drugs, as atropine, caffeine, cocaine, morphine, nicotine, and quinine. The term also may be applied to some synthetic chemicals, as procaine.

alkalosis /al'kəlō'sis/, a disorder of body fluids in which the pH level is greater than 7.44. Alkalosis of the lungs may be caused by too much air coming into the lungs (hyperventilation). Treatment of alkalosis restores the normal acid-base balance. Compare **acidosis**.

alkaptonuria /alkap'tōnŏŏr'ē·ə/, a rare inherited defect in which tyrosine, an amino acid, is not fully used. Large amounts of glycosuric acid are given off, staining the urine dark. Usually, the defect does not cause symptoms until middle age, at which point ochronosis, a type of arthritis, may develop. See also **ochronosis**. –**alkaptonuric,** adj.

Alkeran, a trademark for a drug used to treat cancer (melphalan).

alkylating agent /al'kilā'ting/, a drug that causes a chemical process to disrupt cell division, especially in fast-growing tissue. Such drugs are very useful in the treatment of cancer. The types of alkylating agents used in medicine are the alkyl sulfonates, the ethylenimines, the nitrogen mustards, the nitrosoureas, and the triagenes. The most widely used agent is cyclophosphamide.

ALL, abbreviation for **acute lymphocytic leukemia**. See also **acute childhood leukemia**.

allantoidoangiopagus /al'əntoidō·an'jē·op'əgəs/, twin fetuses from one egg that are two different sizes, which are joined by the vessels of the umbilical cord. Also called **omphaloangiopagus**. See also **omphalosite**. –**allantoidoangiopagous,** adj.

allantoin /əlan'tō·in/, a white crystal-forming substance found in many plants, allantoic and amniotic fluids, and fetal urine.

allantois /əlan'tois/, a tube that comes out of the yolk sac in the embryo and includes the allantoic vessels. In human embryos, allantoic vessels become the umbilical vessels. See also **body stalk, umbilical cord.** –**allantoic** /al'əntō'ik/, adj.

allele /əlēl'/, **1.** one of two or more possible forms of a gene on the chromosomes. **2.** also called **allelomorph** /əlē'ləmôrf/. One of two or more contrasting qualities carried by alternative genes.

Allen test, a method to test the function of the artery on the thumb side of the wrist (radial artery). A catheter is put in the artery. The patient then makes a fist while a nurse presses the middle (ulnar) artery of the wrist. This causes the hand to become pale. Pressure is continued while the fist is opened. If the flow of blood through the radial artery is good, the hand should flush and get its color back.

allergen /al'ərjin/, a foreign substance that can cause an allergic response in the body but is only harmful to some people. Some common allergens (also called antigens) are pollen, animal dander, house dust, feathers, and varied foods. About one of every six Americans is allergic to one or more allergens. Normal people are immune to allergens, but in others the immune system may be too sensitive to foreign substances and even to substances made by the body. The body normally protects itself against allergens by the complex chemical workings of the immune system. Skin tests are the most common way to find the allergens. Desensitization treatments often help people who react to allergens. See also **antigen**. –**allergic,** adj.

allergenic extract, an extract of the protein of a substance to which a person may be sensitive. The extract can be used for diagnosis or for desensitization therapy.

allergic, pertaining to allergy.

allergic alveolitis. See **diffuse hypersensitivity pneumonia**.

allergic asthma, a form of asthma caused by breathing in a airborne substance. This allergen causes antibodies to form in the cells of the lung sacs. Histamine is then released, which causes the bronchial muscles to contract. This causes the coughing and wheezing of asthma. Mental factors may cause asthma attacks in patients whose bronchi are already infected with allergic material. Treatments are more effective for pollen sensitivity than for house dust, animal hair, molds, and insects. Often, a daily pattern of histamine release is seen, causing many degrees of attacks at different times of the day. Also called **extrinsic asthma.** Compare **intrinsic asthma.** See also **asthma, asthma in children, asthmatic eosinophilia, status asthmaticus.**

allergic bronchopulmonary aspergillosis, a form of asthma that occurs when the fungus *Aspergillus fumigatus* grows in the bronchial tube, causing an allergic reaction. The symptoms are like those of asthma, including breathing difficulty and wheezing. Blood tests usually reveal antibodies to *A. fumigatus.* Treatment is with steroid drugs and antiasthma drugs. Compare **aspergillosis.**

allergic conjunctivitis, an abnormal condition of excess blood in the membrane lining of the eye (conjunctiva) because of an allergy. Common allergens that cause this condition are pollen, grass, skin medications, air pollutants, and smoke.

★DIAGNOSIS: The common signs of allergic conjunctivitis are tearing and pain, a yellow discharge, and redness of the conjunctiva. Diagnosis is commonly based on allergy tests to identify the allergen.

★TREATMENT: Treatment of allergic conjunctivitis commonly includes eyedrops to reduce blood flow into the eye, cold compresses to relieve itching, and an oral histamine to reduce swelling and tearing.

allergic coryza, stuffy nose caused by an allergen to which the patient is allergic.

allergic interstitial pneumonitis. See **diffuse hypersensitivity pneumonia.**

allergic reaction, an allergic response to an allergen to which a patient has been exposed before and has developed antibodies against. Exposure causes the release of histamine and many symptoms, as itching, skin rash (eczema), breathing difficulty, diarrhea, nasal irritation, sinusitis, and throat spasm (laryngospasm).

allergic rhinitis, a swelling of the nasal passages, usually with watery nasal discharge and itching of the nose and eyes. This is caused by an allergic reaction to house dust, animal dander, or pollen. The condition may be seasonal, as in hay fever, or not, as in allergy to dust or animals. Treatment includes taking antihistamines, avoiding the antigen, and by injecting the antigen in gradually increasing amounts.

allergic vasculitis, a swelling of the blood vessels that is caused by an allergen. Swelling sometimes occurs in patients treated with drugs, as iodides, penicillin, sulfonamides, and thiourea.

Symptoms are itching, a slight fever, and pimples, blisters, rashes, or small ulcers on the skin.

allergy, a reaction to generally harmless antigens. More than 20 million Americans have allergic reactions to cigarette smoke, house dust, and pollens. Nasal irritation (allergic rhinitis), which is caused by allergens in the air, affects mostly young children and adolescents but occurs in all age groups. Allergies are labeled according to how the body's cells react to the allergen. Allergies are also divided into those that cause responses right away and those that cause delayed responses. Those allergic reactions that occur right away release substances into the blood flow, as histamine. Delayed allergic reactions, as skin rash or poison ivy, may take many days to show up. Some common symptoms of allergy are lung congestion, allergic eye swelling, fluid buildup, fever, itching, and vomiting. Severe allergic reactions can cause shock and death. Symptoms that last a short time, as those of hay fever, bee stings, and itching, can be treated with steroid drugs. When allergic reactions are life-threatening, steroids may be given in the vein. For milder diseases, as hay fever, antihistamines are usually given. See also **allergy testing, immunoglobulins.**

allergy testing, any one of the many tests used to name the allergens that cause the allergy. Such tests are helpful to know which treatment will stop allergies or reduce their severity. Skin tests are used most often for allergy testing. Small amounts of the test allergens are placed on or under the skin. If the patient is sensitive to the allergen, the skin will turn red in the test area, often in 20 minutes.

alligator forceps, a tonglike device with heavy teeth and a double clamp. These forceps are used in surgery on the bone structure.

alloeroticism, alloerotism. See **heteroeroticism.**

alloesthesia /al′ō·esthē′zhə/, a referred pain or other sensation. It may be felt on the same or the opposite side of the body but not at the site stimulated.

allogamy. See **cross fertilization.**

allogenic /al′ōjen′ik/, **1.** referring to a being or cell that is from the same species but looks distinct due to different genes. **2.** tissues that are transplanted from the same species but have distinct genes.

allograft, the transfer of tissue between two beings with unlike genes, as an organ transplant between two humans who are not identical twins. Also called **homograft.** Compare **autograft, isograft, xenograft.** See also **graft.**

allometric growth, the increase in size of different organs or parts of an organism at many rates.

allometry /əlom′itrē/, the study of the changes of the many parts of an organism as they relate to its growth. See also **allometric growth. –allo-metric**, *adj.*

allopathic physician /al'ōpath'ik/, a doctor who treats disease and injury with active treatments, as medicine and surgery. The treatment is meant to have the opposite effect from that which is caused by the disease or injury. Almost all doctors in the United States are allopathic. Compare **chiropractic, homeopathy.**

allopathy /əlop'əthē/, a system of treatment in which a disease is treated by creating a state in which it cannot thrive. For example, an antibiotic that kills a certain bacterium is given for an infection.

alloplastic maneuver, a process that is part of adaptive change, in which the outer setting is changed. Compare **autoplastic maneuver.**

allopurinol /al'əpyōŏr'ənôl/, a drug used to prevent gout attacks and kidney stones caused by uric acid.

★CAUTION: It is not prescribed for children (except those with too much uric acid in the blood from cancer), for nursing mothers, or for patients with a sudden, short-term attack of gout. Known allergy to this drug prohibits its use.

★ADVERSE EFFECTS: Among the most serious side effects to this drug are blood defects, rashes, and other allergies. Stomach upset and problems with vision also may occur.

allorhythmia /al'ōrith'mē·ə/, any problem heart rhythm that tends to be repeated.

allowable dose. See **maximum permissible dose.**

alloxan, a substance that is found in the intestine in diarrhea. Because it can kill the cells of the pancreas that secrete insulin, alloxan may cause diabetes.

alloy /al'oi/, a mixture of two or more metals. A number of alloys have medical uses, as those used for false limbs (prostheses) and in tooth fillings. See also **amalgam.**

aloe /al'ō/, the juice of the varied species of *Aloe* plants. Once used to empty the bowels, the practice has been stopped because it often causes severe cramps. The most common use of aloe today is for mild skin burns and rash.

alopecia /al'əpē'shē·ə/, partial or complete loss of hair that results from aging, hormone defects, drug allergy, anticancer treatment, or skin disease. See also **baldness.**

alopecia areata /er'ē·ā'tə/, a disease in which there are well-defined bald patches, often round or oval in shape, on the head and other hairy parts of the body. The cause is not known. The state usually clears up within 6 to 12 months without treatment. It is common for alopecia areata to recur. Compare **alopecia totalis, alopecia universalis.**

alopecia totalis, an uncommon defect in which all the hair on the scalp is lost. The cause is not

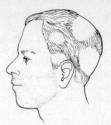

Alopecia areata

known, and the baldness is not reversible. No treatment is known. Compare **alopecia areata, alopecia universalis.**

alopecia universalis, a total loss of hair on all parts of the body, sometimes as an extension of alopecia areata. Compare **alopecia areata, alopecia totalis.**

alpha (α), the first letter of the Greek alphabet, often used in chemistry to denote one type of a chemical compound from others.

alpha-adrenergic blocking agent. See **antiadrenergic.**

alpha-adrenergic receptor. See **alpha receptor.**

alpha alcoholism, a mild form of alcoholism in which the dependence is emotional instead of physical. The person may drink excessive amounts of alcohol to relieve physical pain or mental distress. The person usually retains control and is able to voluntarily stop drinking.

alpha-antitrypsin. See **antitrypsin.**

alpha fetoprotein (AFP), a protein normally produced by the liver, yolk sac, and stomach tract of a human fetus. High levels may be found in the blood of adults who have certain diseases. AFP is measured in amniotic fluid to check for fetal defects, as incomplete growth of the spine (spina bifida). High levels may be present in adults with liver breakdown (cirrhosis), some types of hepatitis, and some cancers. AFP levels are used to check the results of surgery and chemotherapy for cancerous tumors.

alpha$_2$-interferon /in'tərfir'on/, a protein molecule that has been found effective in controlling the spread of common colds caused by rhinoviruses. It is administered as a nasal spray.

alpha receptor, the receptor cells that certain hormones of the adrenal gland (norepinephrine) and certain drugs attach to. When attached in this way, the receptors cause the blood vessel to get smaller, the pupils of the eye to get bigger, and some skin muscles to contract. Also called **alpha-adrenergic receptor.** Compare **beta receptor.**

alpha redistribution phase, a period after intravenous administration of a drug when the amount of drug in the blood begins to fall from its peak. It is caused primarily by the drug spreading throughout the body.

alpha rhythm. See **alpha wave.**

alpha state, a waking state that is relaxed and peaceful. It can be known by the alpha rhythm of the brain waves. These can be recorded on a machine that graphs brain impulses (electroencephalograph). In the alpha state there are tranquil feelings and a lack of tension. Biofeedback training and meditation techniques are ways of reaching the state.

alpha-tocopherol. See **vitamin E.**

alphavirus, any of a group of very small viruses made of a single molecule. Many alphaviruses live in the cells of insects and are given to humans through insect bites.

alpha wave, one of the four types of brain waves. Alpha waves, the "relaxed waves" of the brain, are the main waves recorded by electroencephalograms. Blinking the eyes affects the patterns of the alpha waves. Also called **alpha rhythm.** Compare **beta wave, delta wave, theta wave.**

alprostadil, a proprietary form of prostaglandin E_1 used to keep the ductus arteriosis open in certain newborns. It is recommended for newborns awaiting surgery to correct heart defects present at birth.

★CAUTION: None

★ADVERSE EFFECTS: The most common adverse effects include an absence of automatic breathing, fever, seizures, bleeding in the brain, and flushing.

ALS, 1. short for **antilymphocyte serum. 2.** short for **advanced life support. 3.** short for **amyotrophic lateral sclerosis.**

alseroxylon, a combination of reserpine and other alkaloids extracted from *Rauwolfia serpentina.* It is used in oral sedatives and medications that lower blood pressure.

Älstrom's syndrome, an inherited disease in which several organs are resistant to hormones. It can cause childhood blindness, diabetes insipidus, and gout.

altered state of consciousness (ASC), any state of awareness that differs from the normal aware state. Altered states of consciousness have been achieved, especially in Eastern cultures, by many persons by using techniques, as not eating, deep breathing, whirling, and chanting. Western science now knows that such techniques can affect the chemistry of the body and help to bring on the desired state. Most people are able to enter altered states of consciousness. These states can be used to improve health and help fight disease.

alternobaric vertigo, a condition in which the sense of balance is impaired. It is caused by unequal pressure in the middle ear, as may be experienced by divers during ascent.

alt.h., abbreviation for the Latin prescription term *alternis horis,* meaning every other hour.

altitude, any location on earth with reference to a fixed surface point, which is usually sea level. Several types of health problems are associated with altitude extremes, including increased exposure to ultraviolet radiation. Many effects are related to lowered oxygen pressure at higher altitudes. See also **altitude sickness**.

altitude sickness, a sickness linked with the low oxygen in the air at high altitudes. The sickness is often brought on by mountain climbing or travel in unpressurized aircraft. Persons with altitude sickness may feel dizzy, crabby, breathless, blissful, or have a headache. Older people and those with lung or heart disorders may suffer breathing problems, heart failure, or fainting, needing emergency treatment. A long-term form of altitude sickness causes a higher red blood cell count, which results in blood that is thick and does not move easily through the blood vessels. Also called **acute mountain sickness. See polycythemia.**

altruism /al'trōō·iz'əm/, a sense of concern for the welfare of others. It may be expressed by individuals or social systems.

alum, a substance that causes the skin cells to contract (astringent). It is used mainly in lotions and douches.

alum bath, a bath taken in water and alum, used mainly for skin defects.

aluminum (Al), a widely used metal and the third most abundant of all the elements. Its atomic number is 13; its atomic weight is 26.97. It is light and strong and used in aircraft parts, false limbs, and dental work. It is also found in many antacids, antiseptics, astringents, and styptics. Aluminum salts, as aluminum hydroxychloride, can cause allergies in some patients. Aluminum hydroxychloride is the most often used agent in antiperspirants and also works well as a deodorant.

Alupent, a trademark for a drug used to treat breathing defects, as bronchial asthma, bronchitis, and emphysema (metaproterenol sulfate).

alveolar air, the respiratory gases in an air sac of the lung. Alveolar air can be analyzed by collecting the last portion of air expelled by maximum exhalation.

alveolar canal, any of the canals of the upper jaw through which the blood vessels and the nerves to the upper teeth pass. Also called **dental canal.**

alveolar cell carcinoma, a cancerous tumor of the lung. This form of lung cancer is less common than others. It is known by a bad cough and a large amount of spit. Also called **bronchiolar carcinoma.**

alveolar dead space. See **dead space.**

alveolar distending pressure, the pressure difference between the air sac of the lung and the space between the membranes surrounding the lungs (intrapleural space).

alveolar duct, any of the air passages in the lung that branch out from the air sacs (bronchioles).

alveolar fistula. See **dental fistula.**

alveolar gas, the gas mixture located in the area of the lungs where gas exchange takes place.

alveolar gas volume, the total amount of gas in the area of the lungs where respiratory gas exchange occurs. It is indicated by the symbol V_A.

alveolar macrophages, defense cells within the lungs that act by surrounding and digesting foreign substances that may be inhaled.

alveolar pressure (P_A), the pressure in the air sacs of the lungs.

alveolar process, the part of the jaw that forms the dental arch and serves as a bony structure to hold the teeth. See also **alveolar ridge.**

alveolar proteinosis, a disorder in which various blood components accumulate in the air sacs of the lungs. The disease usually affects previously healthy young adults, more males than females. The cause is unknown and symptoms vary, but only the lungs are affected. The condition may be treated by washing out the lungs and air passages. Other infections may also occur.

alveolar ridge, the bony ridge of the jaw that contains the tooth sockets. See also **alveolar process.**

alveolectomy, removal of part of the dental alveolar process to take out a tooth, change the line of the jaw after tooth removal, or prepare the mouth for false teeth.

alveoli, small pockets that stick out along the walls of alveolar sacs in the lung. This is where carbon dioxide leaves the blood and oxygen is taken on by the blood.

alveolitis /al′vē·əli′tis/, an allergic lung reaction caused by breathing in a foreign body (antigen). Symptoms are breathing problems, cough, sweating, fever, weakness, and pain in the joints and muscles lasting from 12 to 18 hours. If it recurs often, it may lead to long-term lung disease with weight loss, and worse breathing problems. X-ray films of the lungs will show the defect. Kinds of alveolitis include **bagassosis, farmer's lung, pigeon breeder's disease.**

alveolus /alvē′ələs/, *pl.* **alveoli,** a small saclike structure. The word is often used in place of **acinus.** See also **dental alveolus, pulmonary alveolus. –alveolar,** *adj.*

alymphocytosis /alim′fōsītō′sis/, an abnormal decrease in the number of white cells (lymphocytes) in the blood.

Alzheimer's disease /älts′hīmərz/, a form of brain disease. It can lead to confusion, memory loss, restlessness, problems with perception, speech trouble, trouble moving, and fearing things that are not there. The patient may become too excited, refuse food, and lose bowel or bladder control. The disease often starts in later middle life with slight defects in memory and behavior. Alzheimer's disease occurs as often in men as it does in women. The exact cause is not known, but real breakdown of the cells of the brain does occur. There is no treatment, but good nutrition may slow the progress of the disease, which lasts about 7 years in most people who have it. Also called **senile dementia-Alzheimer type (SDAT).**

Am, symbol for **americium.**

AMA, short for **American Medical Association.**

amalgam /əmal′gəm/, **1.** a mixture or combination. In dentistry the substances used to fill cavities, often a mix of silver and another substance. **2.** a mix of mercury and another metal or metals.

amalgam carrier, a dental device that holds plastic amalgam for putting into a prepared tooth cavity or mold.

amalgam carver, a dental device for shaping plastic amalgams used in some tooth fillings.

amalgam condenser, a dental device used for compacting plastic amalgam in filling teeth.

Amanita, a genus of mushrooms. Some species, as *Amanita phalloides,* are poisonous if eaten, causing images to appear that are not real, stomach upset, and pain. Liver, kidney, and nervous system damage can result.

amantadine hydrochloride /əman′tədēn/, a drug used to prevent and treat the flu virus A_2, and for relief of symptoms of Parkinson's disease. ★CAUTION: It is used with caution in patients with heart failure and during pregnancy and breast feeding. Known allergy to this drug prohibits its use.

★ADVERSE EFFECTS: Among the most serious side effects are confusion, mood changes, and skin blotches. Nervousness, blurred sight, and slurred speech also may occur.

amasesis /am′əsē′sis/, a defect in which the person is not able to chew food. This may be caused by failure of the chewing muscles to work, crowded teeth, poorly-fitted false teeth, or a mental problem.

amastia /əmas′tē·ə/, lack of breasts in women. This may be caused by an inherited defect, or a growth problem. Also called **amazia.**

amaurosis /am′ôrō′sis/, blindness caused by something outside the eye itself. For example, amaurosis can be caused by a disease of the optic nerve or brain, diabetes, kidney disease, or poisoning from alcoholism. Amaurosis of one or both eyes may come after an emotional shock and may last for days or months. Amaurosis may be present with the sudden onset of certain stomach upset. One kind of amaurosis is inherited. **–amaurotic** /am′ərot′ik/, *adj.*

amaurosis congenita of Leber. See **Leber's congenital amaurosis.**

amaurosis fugax /foo'gaks/, short-term blindness. Compare **amaurosis.**

amaurosis partialis fugax, short-term partial blindness, often caused by lack of blood to parts of the eye as a result of a blood vessel disease.

amaurotic familial idiocy. See **Tay-Sachs disease.**

Ambenyl, a trademark for a drug use to treat coughs from colds or allergies (codeine sulfate, bromodiphenhydramine hydrochloride and diphenhydramine hydrochloride, potassium guaiacolsulfonate).

ambi-, a combining form meaning 'on both sides.'

ambient air standard, the highest amount allowed of any air pollutant, as lead, nitrogen dioxide, sodium hydroxide, or sulfuric dioxide. Federal authorities in the United States have said that the air in some cities is dangerous to breathe. Research has shown a strong link between many diseases and poisonous chemicals. Little is known about the exact effects and movement of air pollutants.

ambient pressure, the atmospheric pressure, or pressure in the environment or surrounding area.

ambiguous genitalia, outer genitals that are not normal or typical of either sex, as occurs in pseudohermaphroditism.

ambivalence /ambiv'ələns/, **1.** a state in which a person has conflicting feelings, attitudes, drives, or desires, as love and hate, tenderness and cruelty, pleasure and pain. To some degree, ambivalence is normal. **2.** the state of being uncertain or unable to choose between opposites. **–ambivalent** /ambiv'ələnt/, *adj.*

ambivert /am'bivurt'/, a person who can be very withdrawn and antisocial at some times and very outgoing and social at other times.

amblyopia /am'blē·ō'pē·ə/, reduced vision in an eye that appears to be normal. Kinds of amblyopia are **alcoholic amblyopia, suppression amblyopia, tobacco amblyopia, toxic amblyopia.**

ambo-, amb-, a combining form meaning 'both or on both sides.'

Ambu-bag, a trademark for a breathing bag used to aid patients' breathing in an emergency.

ambulance, an emergency vehicle used to take patients to a hospital or other treatment center in cases of accident, trauma, or severe illness.

ambulatory, able to walk, hence referring to a patient who is not confined to bed.

ambulatory automatism, moving about without aim or performing acts without knowing it. See also **fugue, poriomania.**

ambulatory care, health services given to those who come to a hospital or other health care center and who leave after treatment on the same day.

ambulatory schizophrenia, a mild form of schizophrenia, characterized mainly by a tendency to respond to questions with vague and irrelevant answers. The person also may seem somewhat eccentric and wander aimlessly.

ambulatory surgery center, a health care center that deals with relatively minor surgeries, which do not need overnight hospitalization. For example, cataracts, hernia repair, and some knee surgeries are types of surgery done in these centers.

AM care, routine hygiene care that is given patients before breakfast or early in the morning.

amcinonide, a steroid ointment and cream used to treat skin trouble.

★CAUTION: Viral and fungal diseases of the skin, blood-flow problems, or known allergy to steroids prohibits its use.

★ADVERSE REACTIONS: Among the most serious side effects are skin allergies. These side effects may occur from long-term use or from covering the area with dressings.

amdinocillin, a drug derived from penicillin that is used as an antibiotic but is not taken orally. It is prescribed for treatment of certain types of urinary infections.

★CAUTION: Known allergy to penicillin prohibits its use.

★ADVERSE EFFECTS: Among the most serious adverse effects reported are: an increase in the number of two-lobed white blood cells (eosinophilia), inflammation of a vein, elevated serum aspartate aminotransferase and serum alkaline phosphatase, skin rash, an abnormal increase in the number of platelets in the blood, diarrhea, nausea, dizziness, and various blood disorders.

ameba /əmē'bə/, a microscopic, single-celled organism. Several species may live in humans, including *Entamoeba coli* and *E. histolytica.* Also spelled **amoeba.** See also **amebiasis.** **–amebic,** *adj.*

amebiasis /am'ēbī'əsis/, an infection of the intestine or liver by an ameba, often *Entamoeba histolytica.* The amebae are present in food or water that has had contact with infected feces. Mild amebiasis may not have symptoms. Severe infection may cause diarrhea, belly pain, jaundice, loss of appetite, and weight loss. It is dangerous in infants, the aged, and disabled patients. Also spelled **amoebiasis.** See also **ameba, amebic abscess, amebic dysentery, hepatic amebiasis.**

amebic abscess, a collection of pus formed by dead tissue, usually in the liver, caused by *Entamoeba histolytica.* The amebae enter the body in food or water that has had contact with feces. They pass along the stomach tract into the intestine and then invade the liver, causing pus to collect. Symptoms are nausea, vomiting, belly pain, and severe diarrhea. See also **amebiasis.**

amebic dysentery, an inflammation of the intestine caused by *Entamoeba histolytica*. Symptoms are frequent, loose stools flecked with blood and mucus. Amebic dysentery is often accompanied by an amebic abscess. Also called **intestinal amebiasis**. See also **amebiasis, hepatic amebiasis**.

amebicide, a drug or other agent that is destructive to amebas.

amelanic melanoma /am′ilan′ik/, a tumor that lacks color.

amelanotic /am′ilənot′ik/, referring to tissue that has no color because it lacks the substance that makes color (melanin).

amelia /əmē′lē·ə/, a birth defect, marked by the lack of one or more limbs. The term may be changed to refer to the exact number of legs or arms missing at birth, as **tetramelia** for the lack of all four limbs.

ameloblast /am′iloblast′/, a cell from which tooth enamel is made. –**ameloblastic** /-blas′tik/, *adj*.

ameloblastic fibroma, a dental tumor in which there is a growth of connective and other tissues but no growth of dentin or enamel.

ameloblastic hemangioma, a tumor that grows on cells that cover the tooth bud of the fetus. See also **hemangioma**.

ameloblastic sarcoma, a cancerous tumor of the tooth, in which soft tissue grows but dentin or enamel does not.

ameloblastoma /am′əlōblastō′mə/, a highly destructive, cancerous, fast-growing tumor of the jaw. Also called **adamantinoma, adamantoblastoma, epithelioma adamantinum**.

amelodentinal /am′əlōden′tinəl/, referring to both the enamel and dentin of the teeth.

amelogenesis /am′əlōjen′əsis/, the forming of the enamel of the teeth. –**amelogenic**, *adj*.

amelogenesis imperfecta, an inherited defect in which the teeth are brown in color. The cause can be either severe lack of calcium or poor growth of the enamel. The state is classed by its severity. In agenesis there is complete lack of enamel. In enamel hypoplasia, there is not enough enamel. In enamel hypocalcification, there is a normal amount of enamel, but it is soft and lacks calcium. Also called **hereditary brown enamel, hereditary enamel hypoplasia**. Compare **dentinogenesis imperfecta**. See also **enamel hypocalcification, enamel hypoplasia**.

amenorrhea /ā′menərē′ə/, the absence of the monthly flow of blood and discharge of mucous tissues from the uterus through the vagina (menstruation). Amenorrhea is normal before sexual maturity, during pregnancy, after menopause, and in other phases of the menstrual cycle. Abnormal amenorrhea is caused by malfunction of the hypothalamus gland, pituitary gland, ovary, or uterus. It can be caused by drugs, or by removal of both ovaries or the uterus. A woman born without a uterus will not menstruate. **Primary amenorrhea** is the failure of menstrual cycles to begin. **Secondary amenorrhea** is the stopping of menstrual cycles once they have begun to occur. See also **hypothalamic amenorrhea, postpill amenorrhea**. –**amenorrheic**, *adj*.

amentia /āmen′shə/, 1. a term no longer used for mental retardation. See **mental retardation**. 2. also called **confusional insanity**. Lack of interest, and confusion, close to stupor, as in Stearns' alcoholic amentia.

American Academy of Allergy and Immunology (AAAI), a national organization of doctors who treat allergies and immune system defects.

American Academy of Nursing (AAN), the honor society of the American Nurses' Association.

American Academy of Physical Medicine and Rehabilitation (AAPMR), a national association of professional health care workers who are concerned with physical disability and techniques and devices to make the body work better.

American Academy of Physicians' Assistants (AAPA), a national organization of physicians' assistants or associates.

American Association for Respiratory Therapy (AART), a national organization of nurses and other health workers who work with respiratory therapy.

American Association of Colleges of Nursing (AACN), a society of nursing schools.

American Association of Critical Care Nurses (AACN), a society of nurses who work in critical care units.

American Association of Industrial Nurses (AAIN), a society of nurses working in industry and dealing with issues of health in the workplace.

American Association of Medical Colleges (AAMC), a society of teachers and deans of medical schools.

American Association of Nephrology Nurses and Technicians (AANNT), a society of nurses and other persons working with dialysis and kidney diseases.

American Association of Neurological Nurses (AANN), a society of nurses working with patients who have diseases of the nervous system.

American Association of of Neuroscience Nurses (AANN), a society of nurses working with patients with nerve problems. The group works with the American Association of Neurological Surgeons.

American Association of Nurse Anesthetists (AANA), a society of certified registered nurse anesthetists.

American Association of Oral and Maxillofacial Surgeons (AAOMS), a society of oral surgeons who work with the jaws, mouth, and teeth.

American Association of Pathologists and Bacteriologists (AAPB), a society of specialists in pathology and bacteriology.

American College of Obstetricians and Gynecologists (ACOG), the society of obstetricians and gynecologists.

American College of Physicians (ACP), a society of physicians.

American College of Prosthodontists, a society of dentists who work in rebuilding teeth or the mouth.

American College of Radiologists (ACR), a society of doctors who work in radiology.

American College of Surgeons (ACS), a society of doctors who work in surgery.

American Hospital Association (AHA), a society of persons, institutions, and groups that works to better the health care of all people. The AHA publishes many journals and newsletters.

American leishmaniasis, a group of infections caused by many types of very small, one-celled animals (protozoan), *Leishmania.* The disease causes ugly sores of the nose, mouth, and throat. The diseases are seen in the forests of southern Mexico and in Central and South America. Illness may be for a long time, making it easy for a patient to get other infections. Kinds of American leishmaniasis are **chiclero's ulcer, espundia, forest yaws, uta.** Also called **mucocutaneous leishmaniasis, New World leishmaniasis.** See also **leishmaniasis.**

American Medical Association (AMA), a society made up of licensed doctors in the United States. The AMA keeps lists of all qualified doctors (including those who are not members) in the United States, and publishes many journals. See also **British Medical Association (BMA).**

American mountain fever. See **Colorado tick fever.**

American Nurses' Association (ANA), the society of registered nurses in the United States. The ANA publishes the *American Nurse* and *The American Journal of Nursing.*

American Psychiatric Association (APA), a society of psychiatrists. It publishes the *Diagnostic and Statistical Manual of Mental Disorders.*

American Red Cross, a national organization that helps people with many health, safety, and disaster relief programs. It is connected with the International Committee of the Red Cross. The Red Cross was begun at the Geneva Convention of 1864. The American Red Cross has more than 130 million members in about 3,100 chapters. It depends largely on volunteers to make the programs work. They collect and give more blood than any other agency in the United States. American Red Cross nursing and health programs have courses at home on being a parent, care before and after birth, and first aid. The mark for the American Red Cross is a red cross on a field of white.

American Registry of Radiologic Technologists (ARRT), a society of persons working in radiology.

American Society of Parenteral and Enteral Nutrition, an organization that provides education, support, and accreditation to persons who specialize in nutrition that is provided through intravenous, enteral, or related types of feeding.

American Speech, Language, and Hearing Association (ASHA), the professional association that certifies audiologists and speech-language pathologists.

American trypanosomiasis. See **Chagas' disease.**

American Type Culture Collection (ATCC), a group that saves samples of cellular and microbiologic cultures. It can send the cultures to research centers and laboratories.

Ameslan /am'islan/, short for American Sign Language, a way of talking with the deaf. Words and letters are made with the hands and fingers.

Ames test, a way of testing if something causes cancer. A strain of *Salmonella* bacteria is mixed with a sample of the item to be tested. It is then checked for genetic mutations. Also called **mutagenicity test.**

ametropia /am'itrō'pē·ə/, an eye problem. The image made on the back of the eyeball is wrong because of how light is bent when it enters the eye. Astigmatism, farsightedness (hyperopia), and nearsightedness (myopia) are types of ametropia. **–ametropic,** *adj.*

Amicar, a trademark for a drug used to treat bleeding that may happen after surgery or in severe illness (aminocaproic acid).

amide-compound local anesthetic, a compound that causes a loss of feeling in an area. Some kinds are **bupivacaine, dibucaine, etiodocaine, lidocaine, mepivacaine, prilocaine.**

Amigo, a trademark for a battery-operated scooterlike vehicle used to get around by some patients who cannot walk.

amikacin sulfate, an antibiotic used to treat various severe infections.

★CAUTION: This drug must not be used with diuretics. Known allergy to this or other similar antibiotics prohibits its use. The drug is used with caution in patients who have poor kidneys or myasthenia gravis.

★ADVERSE EFFECTS: The more serious side effects are kidney damage, hearing and balance problems, and nerve and muscle problems. Stomach and intestinal upsets, pain at the site of the shot, and allergic reactions may occur.

Amikin, a trademark for an antibiotic (amikacin sulfate).

amiloride hydrochloride, a drug used to treat heart failure or high blood pressure. It is often given with something to increase the release of urine (diuretic).

★CAUTION: This drug must not be used with potassium-conserving drugs. Too much potassium in the blood, poor kidney function, or known allergy to this drug prohibits its use.

★ADVERSE EFFECTS: Among the most serious side effects are headache, diarrhea, nausea and vomiting, loss of hunger, too much calcium in the blood, dizziness, brain disease, problems with sex, muscle cramps, irregular heart beats, confusion, and numbness.

amine pump, *informal.* a system in some nerve endings that absorbs epinephrine, a chemical of the nervous system. Bad reactions to some drugs, as antidepressants, block this. This causes a large amount of another chemical, norepinephrine, in heart tissue, resulting in heart rhythm disorders. See also **monoamine oxidase inhibitor.**

amino acid, an organic compound necessary for forming peptides, a piece of protein, and proteins. Digestion releases the individual amino acids from food. More than 100 are found in nature, but only 22 occur in animals. In humans eight are essential for life: isoleucine, leucine, lysine, methionine, phenylalanine, threonine, tryptophan, and valine. Arginine and histidine are essential in infants.

aminoaciduria /amē′nō·as′idoŏr′ē·ə/, the abnormal presence of amino acids in the urine. It usually indicates an inborn chemical defect, as in cystinuria.

aminocaproic acid /əmē′nōkəprō′ik, am′inō-/, a drug given to stop bleeding.

★CAUTION: Active blood clotting within blood vessels prohibits its use.

★ADVERSE EFFECTS: Among the most serious side affects are blood clots and low blood pressure. A man may be unable to ejaculate. Nasal congestion, diarrhea, and allergic reactions may occur.

aminolevulinic acid (ALA) /am′inōlev′ōōlin′ik/, the substance that gives rise to the oxygen-carrying portion of red blood cells. It may be detected in the urine of some patients with porphyria, liver disease, and lead poisoning.

aminophylline /am′ənōfil′in, əmē′nō-/, a drug that opens the bronchus. It is used for treating bronchial asthma, emphysema, and bronchitis.

★CAUTION: Known allergies to this or a similar drug prohibits its use. It is used with caution in patients who have peptic ulcer and those in whom heart stimulation would be harmful.

★ADVERSE EFFECTS: Among the more serious side effects are stomach and intestinal upsets, uneven or rapid heart beat, and nervousness.

aminosuccinic acid. See **aspartic acid.**

aminotransferase, an enzyme that helps move an amino group from one chemical compound to another. Aspartate amino transferase (AST) is present in blood and many tissues, specially the heart and liver. It is given off by cells that have been damaged. A high blood level of AST can occur with a heart attack or liver disease. Also called **transaminase.**

amiodarone hydrochloride, an oral drug that prevents, eases, or corrects an abnormal heart rhythm. It is prescribed for life-threatening, recurrent abnormal heart rhythms that do not respond to other drugs.

★CAUTION: This drug should not be given to patients with certain heart rhythm problems unless used along with a pacemaker.

★ADVERSE EFFECTS: Among the most serious adverse effects reported are pulmonary toxicity, liver dysfunction, nausea, vomiting, constipation, loss of appetite, weakness, fatigue, tremor, involuntary movements, visual disorders, abnormally slow heart rate, and congestive heart failure.

amitosis /am′ətō′sis/, a simple type of cell division. The nucleus and cytoplasm split in two. –**amitotic,** *adj.*

amitriptyline, a drug used to treat depression.

AML, short for **acute myelocytic leukemia.**

ammonia, a pungent, colorless gas made of nitrogen and hydrogen. It is made when organic matter containing nitrogen breaks down. It is used as a stimulant, a detergent, and an emulsifier.

ammonium ion, an ion formed by the reaction of ammonia with a hydrogen ion. It dissolves in water but does not pass easily through cell membranes.

amnesia, a loss of memory caused by brain damage or by severe emotional trauma. Some types are **anterograde amnesia, hysteric amnesia, posttraumatic amnesia, retrograde amnesia.**

amnestic apraxia, inability to do an act when asked because of not remembering the request. See also **apraxia.**

amniocentesis /am′nē·ōsentē′sis/, removing a small amount of the fluid (amniotic) that is in the womb during pregnancy. It is usually done between the sixteenth and twentieth weeks. Testing the fluid can check for fetal abnormalities, as Down's syndrome, spina bifida, and Tay-Sachs disease. The sex of the fetus can also be learned. Later in pregnancy it may be done to learn the age of the fetus.

★METHOD: Using ultrasound scanning, the position of the fetus and the location of the placenta can be learned. The skin on the woman's belly is cleaned. A local anesthetic is given. A needle attached to a syringe is put into a part of the womb where there is the least chance of touching the placenta or the fetus. Less than 1 ounce of fluid is removed. In testing for birth defects, 3 or more weeks are usually needed before a diagnosis can be made. This waiting period can be stressful. The woman is warned to report any signs of infection or labor.

★PATIENT CARE: The woman must sign an informed-consent form, which explains the procedure and possible adverse effects.

★ADVERSE REACTIONS: Problems are rare.

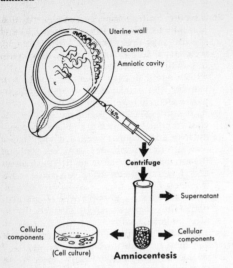

Uterine wall
Placenta
Amniotic cavity

Centrifuge

Supernatant

Cellular
components

Cellular
components

(Cell culture)   **Amniocentesis**

Miscarriage occurs in approximately 1% of the
women. Putting a hole in the placenta or a
blood vessel in the umbilical cord may cause
bleeding and blood disease of the fetus. This
could be fatal. Infections in the mother or fetus may occur, but they are rare.

amnion /am'nē·on/, the membrane that covers
the fetal side of the placenta. It contains the
amniotic fluid. Compare **chorion.**

amniotic fluid /am'nē·ot'ik/, a liquid made by the
amnion and the fetus. It usually totals about
1,500 ml (a little more than 1½ quarts) at 9
months. It surrounds the fetus during pregnancy, providing it with protection. It is swallowed, processed, and excreted as fetal urine
at a rate of 50 ml (more than 2 ounces) every
hour. Amniotic fluid is clear, though cells and
fat give it a cloudy look.

amniotic sac, a thin-walled bag that contains the
fetus and fluid during pregnancy. The wall of
the sac extends from the edge of the placenta
and surrounds the fetus.

amobarbital, a barbiturate given to relieve nervousness and to help one sleep. It is also given
to prevent tremors.

amoeba. See **ameba.**

amorph /ā'môrf, əmôrf'/, a gene that does not
effect a trait.

amorphous crystals, ill-defined crystals without
shape, usually phosphates.

amoxapine, a drug used to treat depression.

amoxicillin, a type of penicillin taken by mouth.
It is used to treat different infections.
★CAUTION: Known allergy to any penicillin
prohibits its use.
★ADVERSE EFFECTS: Among the most serious
side effects are allergic reactions, nausea, and
diarrhea. Many allergic reactions and rashes
are common.

Amoxil, a trademark for an antibiotic (amoxicillin).

AMP, short for **adenosine monophosphate.**

amphetamines, a group of drugs that works on
the nervous system. These include amphetamine dextroamphetamine and methamphetamine. These drugs are abused by some people
because they cause one to stay awake and feel
great. Abuse causes the user to act driven, feel
fearful, hear and see things that are not there,
and consider suicide. They have street names,
as **black beauties, lid poppers, pep pills,** and
speed. See also **amphetamine sulfate, dextroamphetamine sulfate, methamphetamine sulfate.**

amphiarthrosis. See **cartilaginous joint.**

amphigenetic /am'fig·net'ik/, **1.** made by the
union of reproductive cells from both sexes. **2.**
bisexual, or having tissue from both ovaries
and testicles.

amphigonadism /am'fig·ō'nədiz'əm/, true hermaphroditism; having tissue from both testicles and ovaries. –**amphigonadic,** adj.

amphigonous inheritance, having traits from
both parents. Also called **biparental inheritance, duplex inheritance.**

amphoric breath sound, an abnormal, hollow
blowing sound from the chest heard with a
stethoscope. It is caused by a hollow place
opening into the bronchus, or by air in the
chest (pneumothorax).

amphotericin B /am'fəter'əsin/, a drug used to
treat fungus infections.
★CAUTION: Known allergy to this drug prohibits its use.
★ADVERSE EFFECTS: Among the most serious
side effects are blood clots, blood defects, kidney problems, nausea, and fever. When used
on the skin, allergic reactions can occur.

ampicillin /am'pəsil'in/, a penicillin used to treat
many infections caused by a broad range of
organisms.

amplitude, width or breadth of range or extent.

amplitude of accommodation (AA), the range of
the eye for near and distant vision.

amplitude of convergence, the amount of increase in the power needed to turn the eyes
from distant vision to close vision. Also called
fusional amplitude, vergence ability.

ampule /am'pyo͞ol/, a small, sterile glass or plastic container. It holds a dose of a drug to be
given in the vein or in the muscle. Also spelled
ampoule.

ampulla /ampo͞o'lə/, a rounded, saclike opening
of a duct, canal, or tube, as the tear duct,
fallopian tube, or rectum.

ampullary tubal pregnancy /ampo͞o'ərē,
am'pəler'ē/, a kind of pregnancy that occurs
in the openings of one of the fallopian tubes.
See also **tubal pregnancy.**

amputation, the removal of a part of the body,
often a leg, arm, finger, or toe. Amputations

are done in cases of severe infections or gangrene, to remove cancerous tumors, and in severe injury. A general anesthesia is used. The part is removed and a flap is cut from muscle, skin, and connective tissue to cover the end of the bone. A section is left open for drainage if there is an infection. The patient may begin to learn to use the affected limb within 1 to 2 days after surgery. Kinds of amputation include **closed amputation, congenital amputation, open amputation, primary amputation, secondary amputation.**

amputee, a patient who has had one or more arms or legs removed. See also **congenital amputation.**

amrinone lactate, a drug that increases the force of the contraction of the heart wall. It is administered intravenously and prescribed in the short-term management of congestive heart failure in patients who do not respond to other drugs.
★CAUTION: The drug may interact with other heart medications. Any combination therapy should be closely monitored.
★ADVERSE EFFECTS: Among more serious adverse reactions are reduction in platelets, abnormal heart rhythm, low blood pressure, nausea, vomiting, liver problems, and allergic reactions.

Amsler grid, a device for looking at the eyes. The grid has a checkerboard pattern of dark lines with one dark spot in the middle. To check for a defect in the field of vision, the person covers or closes one eye and looks at the spot with the other eye. If the person sees a defect, blank, or other fault in the grid, there is a problem with the field of vision of the eye.

Amsterdam dwarf, a person with de Lange's syndrome. The person will be short and suffer severe mental retardation as well as many other defects.

amu, abbreviation for **atomic mass unit.**

amusia, loss of ability to recognize melodies. The condition may follow a stroke or other types of brain damage.

amygdalin /əmig′dəlin/, a chemical that is found in bitter almonds and apricot pits. It is thought by some to be a potential cure for cancer. It is sold under the trademark of Laetrile. Also called **vitamin B$_{17}$.**

amylase /am′ilās/, an enzyme that aids the breakdown of starch in digestion. Alpha-amylase is found in saliva, juice of the pancreas, malt, certain bacteria, and molds. It helps to convert starches to sugars. Beta-amylase is found in grains, vegetables, and malt. It helps to convert starch to a form of sugar. See also **enzyme.**

amylene hydrate, a clear, liquid that smells like camphor. It can be mixed with alcohol, chloroform, ether, or glycerin and is used as a solvent and as a calming drug (sedative).

amyl nitrite, a drug that opens up blood vessels. It is used to relieve smothering chest pain and spasms (angina pectoris).
★CAUTION: Known allergy to this drug or to other nitrites prohibits its use.
★ADVERSE EFFECTS: Among the more serious side effects are low blood pressure, allergies, nausea, headache, and dizziness.

amylo-, amyl-, a combining form referring to starch.

amyloidosis /am′iloidō′sis/, a disease in which a waxy, starchlike, protein (amyloid) builds up in tissues and organs. There are two main forms of the defect. **Primary amyloidosis** often occurs with a bone tumor. Patients with **secondary amyloidosis** usually suffer from another long-term disease, as tuberculosis, osteomyelitis, rheumatoid arthritis, or Crohn's disease. The cause of both types of amyloidosis is not known. Almost all organs are affected, and their function is impaired. There is no known cure for amyloidosis. Patients with kidney amyloidosis are treated with kidney dialysis. When possible, kidney transplant is done.

amylopectinosis. See **Andersen's disease.**

amyoplasia congenita. See **arthogryposis multiplex congenita.**

amyotonia /ā′ī·ōtō′nē·ə/, a defect of the muscles. The muscles lose tone, become weak, and waste. It is usually due to disease of the nerves that supply the muscles (motor neurons). **–amyotonic,** adj.

amyotonia congenita. See **Oppenheim's disease.**

amyotrophic lateral sclerosis (ALS) /ā′mī·ōtrof′ik/, a disease of the nerves that supply the muscles (motor neurons). The symptoms are wasting of the muscles of the hands, forearms, and legs. It can spread to most of the body. It results from a breaking down of the nerves that supply the muscles where they begin, in the brain and spinal cord. ALS usually starts in middle age and quickly gets worse, causing death within 2 to 5 years. There is no known treatment. Also called **Lou Gehrig's disease.** See also **Aran-Duchenne muscular atrophy.**

an-, ana-, 1. a combining form meaning 'not.'

ANA, short for **American Nurses' Association.**

anabolic steroid, any one of many drug compounds that are taken from a male hormone (testosterone), or prepared synthetically. Anabolic steroids aid body growth, counter the effects of a female hormone (estrogen), and cause physical features to become more male. Anabolic steroids are used to treat severe anemias and leukemia, and breast cancer.

anabolism /ənab′əliz′əm/, any process that produces energy in which simple substances are converted into more complex matter. It is a process that occurs in living matter. Compare **catabolism. –anabolic** /an′əbol′ik/, adj.

anaclisis /an′əkli′sis/, **1.** a state in which a person is mentally dependent on other people. This is normal in childhood but not in adulthood. **2.** a state in which a person chooses a love object because he or she is like the mother, father, or other caretaker in infancy. The person may or may not be aware of why he or she chose that love object. **–anaclitic** /an′əklit′ik/, *adj.*

anaclitic depression, a syndrome in infants that occurs after sudden separation from the mother figure. Symptoms include tension, fear, withdrawal, constant crying, refusal to eat, and sleep problems. After a while, stupor sets in, which can lead to severe impairment of the infant's physical, social, and mental growth. If the mother figure returns or is replaced in 1 to 3 months, the infant recovers quickly with no long-term effects. See also **hospitalism.**

anacusis /an′əkoo̅′sis/, a total loss of hearing.

anadipsia /an′ədip′sē·ə/, extreme thirst. It often occurs in the manic phase of manic-depressive psychosis. The state is the result of lack of body fluids due to too much sweating, frequent urination, and constant motion.

Anadrol-50, a trademark for hormones that is used as an anabolic steroid (oxymetholone).

anaerobe /aner′ōb/, a microorganism that grows and lives without oxygen. An example is *Clostridium botulinum,* which causes botulism. Anaerobes are found throughout nature and in the body. See also **anaerobic infection.**

anaerobic /an′ərō′bik/, **1.** referring to the absence of air or oxygen. **2.** able to grow and live without air or oxygen.

anaerobic exercise, a type of exercise that does not need extra oxygen. The exercise uses up the food stored in the muscles quickly, often within 3 or 4 minutes. Lactic acid builds up in the tissues, which makes muscles feel sore. Examples of anaerobic exercise are weight lifting, wrestling, and sprinting. Compare **aerobic exercise.** See also **active exercise, passive exercise.**

anaerobic infection, an infection caused by an anaerobic organism. It usually occurs in deep puncture wounds. Tissue that has little oxygen because of injury, cell death, or too much bacteria may also be infected with anaerobes.

anaerobic myositis. See **gas gangrene.**

anal /ā′nəl/, referring to the anus.

anal canal, the end of the intestinal tract, about 4 cm (about 1½ inches) long, that ends at the anus.

anal character, a kind of personality with patterns of behavior that begin in the anal stage of infancy. Anal behavior can include extreme neatness, stubborness, too much concern with being perfect, clean or prompt, and stinginess. It can also include the extreme opposites of these behaviors. See also **anal eroticism, anal stage, psychosexual development.**

anal crypt, the place in the wall of the rectum that holds networks of veins. This place can become sore and swollen, which is then called hemorrhoids.

analeptic. See **central nervous system stimulant.**

anal fissure, a bleeding sore or cut in the skin of the anus.

anal fistula, an open sore on the skin surface near the anus, usually as a result of an infection of the anal crypt.

analgesia /an′əljē′zē·ə/, pain relief that does not cause the patient to fall asleep.

analgesic /an′əljē′zik/, a drug that relieves pain. There are two kinds. One causes a stupor and is habit-forming (narcotic). The other lacks these side effects. Narcotics are usually given for severe pain. Compare **anodyne.** See also **pain intervention.**

analgesic cocktail, *informal.* a tailored mix of drugs used for pain relief in certain diseases. For example, cancer patients may be given a mix of alcohol and morphine. See also **lytic cocktail.**

analog /an′əlog/, **1.** something that is similar in appearance or function to another object. However, the source or final product differ. For example, the eye of a fly and the eye of a human are analogs. **2.** a drug or other compound that acts like another substance but has different effects. Also spelled **analogue.** Compare **homolog.**

anal reflex, a nerve reflex caused by stroking the skin around the anus. This should result in a contraction of the anal muscle (sphincter). This reflex may be lost in a nerve (neurological) disease.

anal stage, the period in development, occurring between 1 and 3 years of age, when bowel functions and the sensations of the anus are the major source of physical pleasure. It is thought to be important in deciding personality type. Adult patterns of behavior linked with fixation on this stage can include too much concern with being neat, clean, perfect, and on time. They can also include their extreme opposites. Also called **anal phase.** See also **anal character, psychosexual development.**

anal stenosis. See **imperforate anus.**

analysand /ənal′isand′/, a patient who is undergoing psychoanalysis.

analysis, 1. the act of breaking down substances into their parts. It is done so that the nature and qualities of these parts may be understood. **Qualitative analysis** is naming the elements in a substance; **quantitative analysis** is the measurement of each element in a substance. **2.** *informal.* psychoanalysis. **–analytic,** *adj.* **analyze,** *v.*

analyst, 1. a psychoanalyst. **2.** a person who analyzes the chemical, physical, or other properties of a substance.

analytic psychology, **1.** the system in which sensations and feelings are analyzed and listed by type. Compare **experimental psychology. 2.** a way to analyze the psyche that follows the concepts of Carl Gustav Jung. It stresses a group unconscious and a mystical factor in the growth of the personal unconscious. It is unlike the system of Sigmund Freud. Analytic psychology does not stress the importance of sexual factors on early mental growth. Also called **Jungian psychology.**

anamnesis /an'amnē'sis/, **1.** memory of the past. **2.** all the facts that will be used to analyze the state of a patient. These can include family, memories, past feelings or responses, and environment. Compare **catamnesis.**

anaphase /an'əfāz/, a stage in division of a cell's nucleus. See also **interphase, meiosis, metaphase, mitosis, prophase, telophase.**

anaphia /anā'fē·ə/, the loss of the ability to feel something touching the skin.

anaphylactic hypersensitivity /an'əfilak'tik/, an allergic response to a foreign substance (antigen). A skin test causes raised, red skin and swelling within 30 minutes. Substances are released from cells that cause the arteries to get bigger and the muscles to contract. Many allergies, hay fever, and insect sting reactions are anaphylactic hypersensitivity reactions. See also **anaphylactic shock, immunoglobulins.**

anaphylactic shock, a severe and sometimes fatal allergic response to a foreign substance, (allergen), as a drug, vaccine, certain food, insect venom, or chemical. It can occur within seconds from the time of contact with the substance. It is commonly marked by trouble breathing and extremely low blood pressure. The more quickly any reaction occurs in a person after contact, the more severe the shock is likely to be.
★DIAGNOSIS: Anaphylactic shock can occur within seconds or minutes after contact with an allergen. The first symptoms are intense worry, weakness, sweating, and shortness of breath. Other symptoms may include falling blood pressure, shock, uneven heart beat, wheezing, trouble in swallowing, nausea, and diarrhea.
★PATIENT CARE: The patient should be rushed to an emergency care center. A shot is given in the muscle or vein to treat the shock.

anaphylactoid purpura. See **Henoch-Schönlein purpura.**

anaphylaxis /an'əfilak'sis/, a severe allergic response to a foreign substance (antigen) that the patient has had contact with before. The response causes the release of substances that affect muscle. The response may be redness and swelling, itching, and water build-up. In severe cases there may be extremely low blood pressure, spasm of the lungs, and shock. The severity of symptoms depends on the amount of the foreign substance and how it got into the body. Anaphylaxis can be caused by insect stings, iodide-containing fluids used for x-ray testing, aspirin, and antitoxins from animal serum. Substances used to test and treat patients with allergies can also cause this type of shock. Allergy to penicillin is the most common cause of anaphylactic shock. Kinds of anaphylaxis are **aggregate anaphylaxis, antiserum anaphylaxis, cutaneous anaphylaxis, cytotoxic anaphylaxis, indirect anaphylaxis, inverse anaphylaxis.** –**anaphylactic, anaphylactoid,** adj.

anaplasia /an'əplā'zhə/, a breakdown in the structure of cells and in their relation to each other. Anaplasia occurs in cancer. Compare **metastasis.** –**anaplastic,** adj.

anaplastic astrocytoma. See **glioblastoma multiforme.**

anarthria /anär'thrē·ə/, the loss of control of the muscles of speech. It results in the patient being unable to say words. The defect is usually caused by damage to a nerve.

anasarca /an'əsär'kə/, general, massive fluid build up (edema). Anasarca is often seen in kidney disease when fluid retention is a problem that goes on for a long period of time. See also **edema.** –**anasarcous,** adj.

anastomosis /ənas'tōmō'sis/, pl. **anastomoses,** joining two parts as blood vessels to allow flow from one to the other. It may be done to bypass a bulging of an artery wall (aneurysm) or a blocked artery. Using general anesthesia, a length of the patient's vein or a piece of Dacron, Teflon, or Orlon is grafted to the prepared vessels. The blood flow through the graft must be kept up. If the blood does not flow, the graft may close. This is a major problem that requires surgery and sometimes amputation. Kinds of anastomoses are **end-to-end anastomosis, side-to-side anastomosis.** See also **aneurysm, bypass.**

anastomosis at elbow joint, the natural meeting of blood vessels at the elbow joint.

anatomic crown, the part of a tooth covered by dental enamel. Compare **artificial crown, clinical crown, complete crown, dowel crown, partial crown.**

anatomic curve, a normal curve of the segments of the spinal column. When looking at the spine from the side, the neck (cervical) curve looks like it curves inward. The upper back (thoracic) curve looks like it curves outward. The lower (lumbar) curve looks like it curves inward.

anatomic dead space, an area in the throat and air passages that contain air that does not reach the air sacs during breathing. Certain lung defects, as emphysema, increase the amount of anatomic dead space. Compare **physiologic dead space.**

anatomic impotence. See **impotence.**

anatomic position, a position of the body in which a person stands erect, facing directly forward, feet pointed forward and slightly apart, arms hanging down at the sides with palms facing forward. This is the standard neutral position referred to in medical texts. It is used to describe sites or motions of parts of the body.

anatomic snuffbox, a small, cuplike low space on the back of the hand near the wrist where the thumb and index finger tendons form a "v." It is formed by moving the thumb outward, the wrist upward, and stretching the fingers apart.

anatomic zero joint position, the beginning point of the natural range of movement of a joint.

anatomy, 1. the study of structures and organs of the body. Kinds of anatomy are **applied anatomy, comparative anatomy, descriptive anatomy, gross anatomy, microscopic anatomy, surface anatomy.** 2. the structure of an organism. 3. a text on anatomy. Compare **physiology.** 4. *archaic.* dissection of a body.

Anavar, a trademark for a hormone (androgen) used as a growth-promoting (anabolic) drug (oxandrolone).

Ancobon, a trademark for a drug used to treat fungus infections (flucytosine).

anconeus, a muscle of the forearm. It works to straighten the forearm.

ancrod /ang'krod/, the poison of the Malayan pit viper, a snake. It prevents clotting of the blood. It is used to treat certain clotting defects.

Ancylostoma /ang'kilos'təmə/, a tiny worm (nematode) that lives in the intestines and causes hookworm disease. See also *Necator.*

ancylostomiasis /an'səlos'təmī'əsis/, hookworm disease caused by *Ancylostoma.* Infection by *Ancylostoma* is harmful and hard to treat. It is less common than *Necator americanus,* which is the hookworm most often found in the southern United States. Treatment for hookworm infection is drugs to rid the body of the worms. Blood or iron may be given if the patient is anemic. Infection may be prevented by keeping soil free of fecal matter and by wearing shoes. See also **hookworm.**

Andersen's disease, a rare disease caused by an inherited lack of an enzyme. It causes the animal starch glycogen to collect in an abnormal manner. Infants with the disease are normal at birth but fail to thrive. They soon show an enlarged liver and spleen, and weak muscles. They develop liver or heart failure. Also called **amylopectinosis, glycogen storage disease type IV.**

-andr-, a combining form that refers to any steroid hormone that increases growth of male physical qualities.

andro-, andr-, a combining form referring to man or to the male.

androgen /an'drəjin/, any steroid hormone that increases growth of male physical qualities. Natural hormones, as testosterone, are used as therapy during the male change of life. Androsterone is also an androgen. Androgens may be given orally or in the vein. **–androgenic,** *adj.*

androgynous /androj'inəs/, 1. having some qualities of both sexes. Social role, behavior, personality, and appearance are not due to the physical sex of the person. 2. hermaphroditic. Compare **gynandrous. –androgyny,** *n.*

android pelvis, a type of pelvis in which the structure is typical of the male. It is common in women. The bones are thick and heavy. The opening is heart-shaped. Childbirth may be hard unless the android pelvis is large and the baby is small.

andropause /an'drəpôs/, a change of life for males. It may be expressed through a career change, divorce, or reordering of life. It is associated with a lowering of the levels of male hormones that occurs in men during their late 40's or early 50's. See also *menopause.*

androsterone /andros'tərōn/, one of the male sex hormones (androgens). It is seldom used in therapy. See also **testosterone.**

anecdotal, referring to medical knowledge based on observations and not yet confirmed by scientific studies.

anechoic /an'ekō'ik/, (in ultrasonography) free of echoes or without echoes.

Anectine, a trademark for a muscle relaxant used with anesthesia (succinylcholine chloride).

anemia, a decrease in red cells in the blood. The ability to carry oxygen is reduced. Anemia is noted by the hemoglobin content of the red cells and by red cell size. See also **hemolytic anemia, hypoplastic anemia, iron deficiency anemia, iron metabolism.**

★DIAGNOSIS: Depending on its severity, anemia may cause one or more symptoms. These include fatigue, difficult breathing during activity, dizziness, headache, insomnia, and pale skin and mucous membranes. Loss of hunger, unsettled stomach, irregular heart beats and murmurs also occur. Iron deficiency is the most common cause. Blood tests are done to find the type of anemia and the cause.

★TREATMENT: The treatment of anemia depends on the cause. Severe anemia may call for blood transfusion. Treatment also includes giving vitamins to replace what the blood lacks, as iron for iron deficiency anemia.

★PATIENT CARE: It is important that the patient is on a balanced diet to supply the food the blood needs. An anemic patient must also get a lot of rest. The patient must be aware of signs of increasing anemia or blood loss.

anemia of pregnancy, a state of pregnancy in which there is a decrease of red cells in the blood. This decrease can occur because the amount of blood plasma expands more than the number of red blood cells. This anemia may also be caused by a problem in the making of red cells (erythrocytes). It can also be caused by a loss of red blood cells through bleeding. This type of anemia is common in about one half of all pregnancies. It may result from a lack of iron, folic acid, or vitamin B$_{12}$. Too much loss of red blood cells through bleeding may result from abortion, bleeding hemorrhoids, intestinal parasites, defects of the placenta, or weakness of the uterus.

anemic anoxia, a state in which there is lack of oxygen in body tissues. The cause is a decrease in the number of red blood cells.

anencephaly /an'ensef'əlē/, a birth defect in which there is no brain or spinal cord, the skull does not close, and the spinal canal remains a groove. Carried on the genes, it can be found early in pregnancy by looking at the amniotic fluid (amniocentesis). See also **neural tube defect.**

anergic stupor, a kind of mental defect in which the person is quiet, listless, and nonresistant.

anergy, **1.** lack of activity. **2.** an immune defect in which the body does not fight off foreign substances well enough. This state may be seen in advanced tuberculosis and other serious infections, in AIDS, and in some cancers. **–anergic,** *adj.*

Anestacon, a trademark for an anesthetic put into the urethra before surgery or tests on that part of the body (2% lidocaine hydrochloride).

anesthesia, the lack of normal sensation, especially awareness of pain. It is brought on by an anesthetic drug or by hypnosis. It can also occur with damage to nerve tissue. Anesthesia for medical purposes may be used on the skin (topical) or in part or all of the body. See also **general anesthesia, Guedel's signs, local anesthesia, regional anesthesia, topical anesthesia, and specific anesthetic agents.**

anesthesia dolorosa, a bad pain in an anesthetized area. Also called **analgesia algera.**

anesthesia machine, a machine for giving anesthetics that are breathed in. It is the source of the gas used and has a meter to measure the flow of gas; containers to mix the anesthetic and the carrier gas; and a system for bringing the gas to the patient.

anesthesia patients, classification of, the system by which the American Society of Anesthesiologists lists anesthesia patients in five categories. Class I includes patients who are generally healthy, without serious physical or mental problems. For these patients anesthesia is needed only for a local problem, as a hernia or fibroid uterus. Class II includes patients who have mild to moderate health problems, as anemia, mild diabetes, high blood pressure, too much fat, or long-term bronchitis. Class III includes patients who have severe health prob-

lems or disease, as severe diabetes. Class IV includes patients who have a life-threatening problem, as kidney disease. Class V includes patients who have little chance of survival, as a person in shock with a massive lung clot (pulmonary embolus). The letter E is added to the roman numeral to indicate an emergency.

anesthesia screen, a metal upside down U-shaped frame that is put on the sides of an operating table, 12 to 18 inches above a patient's upper chest. It is covered with a sheet to protect the sterile area from breathing by the patient or the anesthetist.

anesthesiologist /an'əsthē'zē·ol'əjist/, a doctor trained to give anesthetics and to support lungs, heart, and blood-flow systems during surgery. Compare **nurse anesthetist.**

anesthesiology, the branch of medicine that deals with the control of sensations of pain and with giving drugs to relieve pain during surgery. See also **anesthesiologist, nurse anesthetist.**

anesthetist /ənes'thətist/, **1.** a person who gives anesthesia. **2.** an anesthesiologist. See also **nurse anesthetist.**

aneuploidy /an'yōōploi'dē/, any difference in the number of chromosomes that has to do with individual chromosomes rather than whole sets. There may be fewer chromosomes, as in Turner's syndrome, or more chromosomes, as in Down's syndrome. Compare **euploidy.** See also **monosomy, trisomy.**

aneurysm /an'yōōriz'əm/, a bulging of the wall of a blood vessel, usually caused by hardening of the arteries (atherosclerosis) and high blood pressure (hypertension). It is sometimes caused by injury, infection, or an inherited weakness in the vessel wall. Aneurysms are most dangerous in the large artery of the heart (aorta). They also occur in smaller vessels and are common in the legs of older patients. A sign of an arterial aneurysm is a pulsating swelling. It makes a blowing murmur that can be heard with a stethoscope. An aneurysm may break open and cause bleeding, or clots may form in the pouch and block smaller vessels. Kinds of aneurysms include **aortic aneurysm, bacterial aneurysm, berry aneurysm, cerebral**

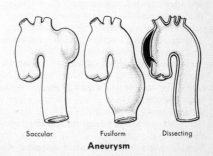

Saccular Fusiform Dissecting

Aneurysm

aneurysm, compound aneurysm, dissecting aneurysm, fusiform aneurysm, mycotic aneurysm, racemose aneurysm, Rasmussen's aneurysm, saccular aneurysm, varicose aneurysm, ventricular aneurysm.　–aneurysmal, *adj.*

aneurysmal bone cyst,　a saclike bone tumor that usually develops in long bones but may occur in any bone, including the spine. It causes pain and swelling and tends to increase gradually in size. It usually is removed surgically, but radiation may be used when the tumor cannot be easily reached.

aneurysm needle,　a needle that has a handle, used to repair aneurysms.

angel dust.　See **phencyclidine hydrochloride (PCP)**.

anger,　a feeling of displeasure, rage, upset, or hostility.

angiitis /anjē·ī'tis/,　an inflamed state of a blood or lymph vessel. A kind of angiitis is **consecutive angiitis**. See also **vasculitis**.

angina /anji'nə, an'jinə/,　**1.** a cramping chest pain and choking feeling caused by lack of oxygen to the heart muscle (angina pectoris). **2.** a symptom of some diseases that is known by a feeling of choking, suffocation, or crushing pressure and pain. Kinds of angina are **intestinal angina, Ludwig's angina, Prinzmetal's angina, streptococcal angina.**　–anginal, *adj.*

angina decubitus,　a state in which attacks of angina pectoris occur when the patient is lying down.

angina dyspeptica,　a painful state caused by gas swelling of the stomach. It causes the same symptoms as angina pectoris.

angina epiglottidea,　a painful state caused when the top of the windpipe (epiglottis) becomes inflamed.

angina pectoris,　a cramping pain in the chest. It is caused most often by a shortage of oxygen to the heart (myocardial anoxia). It is often linked with hardening of the arteries (atherosclerosis) of the heart. The pain usually travels down the inside of the left arm. It often occurs with a feeling of suffocation and impending death. Attacks of angina pectoris are often related to exertion, emotional stress, and contact with intense cold. The pain may be relieved by rest and drugs, as nitroglycerin.

angio-, angei-, angi-,　a combining form referring to a vessel, usually a blood vessel.

angioblastic meningioma /an'jē·ōblas'tik/,　a tumor of the blood vessels in the membranes that cover the spinal cord or the brain.

angioblastoma /an'jē·ōblastō'mə/,　a tumor of blood vessels in the brain. Kinds of angioblastomas are **angioblastic meningioma, cerebellar angioblastoma**.

angiocardiogram /an'jē·ōkär'dē·ōgram'/,　an x-ray film (radiograph) of the heart and the vessels of the heart. A fluid that can be seen on x-ray films (radiopaque) is put into a vein that goes

directly to the heart. X-rays films are taken as the radiopaque substance passes through the heart and its vessels.

angiocatheter /an'jē·ōkath'ətər/,　a hollow, flexible tube put into a blood vessel to take blood or give fluids.

angiochondroma /an'jē·ōkondrō'mə/,　a tumor made up of cartilage that forms too many blood vessels.

angioedema.　See **angioneurotic edema**.

angiofibroma /an'jē·ōfībrō'mə/,　an angioma that has fiberlike tissue. Also called **fibroangioma**.

angiogenesis /an'jē·ōjen'əsis/,　the ability to grow blood vessels. It is a common feature of cancerous tissue. Angiogenesis in breast tissue is thought of as a sign that breast cancer may follow.

angiography /an'jē·og'rəfē/,　the x-ray study of the inside of the heart and blood vessels. It is done after a dye is injected. It is used to test for heart attacks (myocardial infarction), blocked vessels (vascular occlusion), hardened deposits in the arteries, stroke, high blood pressure, kidney tumors, lung clots, and lung vessel problems.　–angiographic, *adj.*

angiohemophilia.　See **von Willebrand's disease**.

angiokeratoma /an'jē·ōker'ətō'mə/,　a horny tumor on the skin. It appears as clumps of swollen blood vessels, clusters of warts, and thickened skin, especially in the scrotum and the fingers and toes.

angiokeratoma circumscriptum,　a rare skin defect in which pimples and bumps appear in small patches on the legs or on the trunk.

angiokeratoma corporis diffusum,　a somewhat rare disease that runs in families. Certain fats are stored in many parts of the body. This causes blood vessel, urinary, and skin problems, and, in some cases, muscle defects. Symptoms of the disease are water retention, high blood pressure, enlarged heart, and skin bumps. Albumin and blood cells show up in the urine. Also called **Fabry's disease, Fabry's syndrome**.

angiolipoma /an'jē·ōlipō'mə/,　a harmless tumor that has blood vessels and tissue.

angioma /an'jē·ō'mə/,　any harmless tumor made up mainly of blood vessels (hemangioma) or lymph vessels (lymphangioma). Most angiomas are present at birth.

angioma arteriale racemosum /ärtē'ri·ā'lē ras'-əmō'səm/,　a tumor that contains a network of many small, newly made, dilated blood vessels. Later, normal blood vessels become affected.

angioma cutis,　a wartlike tumor made of a network of dilated blood vessels.

angioma lymphaticum.　See **lymphangioma**.

angioma serpiginosum,　a skin disease that shows up as rings of tiny red dots. Also called **Hutchinson's disease**.

angiomatosis /an'jē·ōmətō'sis/,　a state in which

the patient has many blood vessel tumors.

angiomyoma, *pl.* **angiomyomas, angiomyomata,** a tumor made of blood vessels and muscle tissue.

angiomyosarcoma /an'jē·ōmī'ōsärkō'mə/, a tumor made of blood vessels, muscles, and connective tissue.

angioneuroma. See **glomangioma.**

angioneurotic anuria, a defect in which the patient produces almost no urine. It is caused when tissue in the kidney is destroyed.

angioneurotic edema, a sudden, painless, swelling lasting a short time. It affects the face, neck, lips, throat, hands, feet, genitals, or abdominal organs. It may be caused by a food or drug allergy, infection, or mental stress, or it can be inherited. For severe forms, shots of a hormone may be given (epinephrine). A tube may be put in through the nose or through a cut in the throat to allow breathing (tracheotomy). Also called **angioedema** /an'jē·ōdē'mə/. See also **anaphylaxis, serum sickness, urticaria.**

angiosarcoma /an'jē·ōsärkō'mə/, a rare, cancerous tumor made of tissue that grows around blood vessels. This condition occurs most often in older patients. It is also linked to contact with vinyl chloride and arsenic. Also called **hemangiosarcoma, malignant hemangioendothelioma.** Compare **angioma.**

angiospasm, a sudden, short-term spasm of a blood vessel. Also called **vasospasm.** See also **vasoconstriction.**

angiotensin /an'jē·ōten'sin/, a substance in the blood that causes blood vessels to constrict. This raises blood pressure. It causes the hormone aldosterone to be released from the adrenal cortex. Angiotensin increases right after the egg is released (ovulation) during the menstrual cycle. It may be the cause of the higher levels of aldosterone during that time.

angiotensin sensitivity test (AST), a test to determine sensitivity to a substance (angiotensin II) in the blood that raises blood pressure.

angle, the geometric relationships between the surfaces of the body.

angle board, a device used in dentistry. It is used to find the angles between a patient's head, the x-ray beam, and the x-ray film.

angle-closure glaucoma. See **glaucoma.**

angle of incidence, the angle at which an ultrasound beam hits the point where two different types of tissues, such as bone and muscle, meet.

angle of Treitz /trīts/, a sharp curve or bend at the point where the upper section of the small intestine meets the middle section.

Angle's classification, a system of classes in dentistry of the varied types of poor bite (malocclusion). The system was set up by Edward Angle, American orthodontist. Classes are based on the relation of teeth in the upper and lower jaws.

angular movement, one of the four basic kinds of movement by the joints of the body. For example, the angle between the forearm and upper arm gets smaller when the arm is bent and gets larger when the arm is extended. Compare **circumduction, gliding, rotation.**

angular stomatitis, soreness and swelling at the corner of the mouth.

angulated fracture, a break in which the fragments of bone are angled.

angulation, an angled shape. See also **horizontal angulation, vertical angulation.**

anhedonia /an'hēdō'nē·ə/, a state in which a person is not able to feel pleasure or happiness when such feelings would be normal. **–anhedonic,** *adj.*

anhidrosis /an'hidrō'sis, an'hī-/, an abnormal lack of sweating.

anhydride, a chemical compound made when water is taken out of a substance. **–anhydrous,** *adj.*

anicteric /an'ikter'ik/, referring to the absence of a yellow discoloring of the skin and eyes (jaundice).

anicteric hepatitis /an'ikter'ik/, a mild form of hepatitis in which there is no jaundice (icterus). It is mostly seen in infants and young children. Symptoms include loss of appetite, stomach upset, and slight fever. The infection may be mistaken for flu or go unnoticed. Compare **hepatitis.** See also **jaundice.**

anideus /anid'ē·əs/, incomplete growth of an early fetus (embryo) made up of a simple rounded mass. Few body parts can be seen.

aniline /an'ilēn/, an oily, colorless, poisonous liquid with a strong odor and burning taste. It is now used in making certain dyes. Workers who come in contact with aniline are at risk of getting blood diseases.

anima /an'imə/, 1. the soul or life. 2. the active substance in a drug. 3. a person's true, inner being, as distinct from outward personality (persona). 4. the female part of the male persona. Compare **animus.**

animal starch. See **glycogen.**

animus /an'iməs/, 1. the active or rational soul; the active agent of life. 2. the male part of the female persona. 3. a deep resentment that is under control but may break out under stress. Compare **anima.**

anion /an'ī·ən/, 1. an ion with a negative charge that is drawn to the positive electrode (anode) in electrolysis. 2. an atom, molecule, or radical with a negative charge. Compare **cation.**

anise /an'is/, the fruit of the *Pimpinella anisum* plant. Extract of anise is used in drugs that relieve gas (carminatives) and loosen mucus in the lungs (expectorants).

aniseikonia /an'īsīkō'nē·ə/, a defect in which

each eye sees the same image differently.

aniso-, a combining form meaning 'unequal or dissimilar.'

anisocytosis /anī′sōsītō′sis/, a defect of the blood in which the red blood cells differ in size.

anisogamete, a sperm or egg germ cell (gamete) that differs a great deal in size and structure from the one with which it unites. Compare **heterogamete, isogamete. –anisogametic,** *adj.*

anisogamy /an′īsog′əmē/, sexual uniting of gametes that are of unequal size and structure. Compare **heterogamy, isogamy. –anisogamous,** *adj.*

anisognathic, referring to a defect in which the upper (maxillary) and the lower (mandibular) jaws differ greatly in size.

anisokaryosis /anī′sōker′ē-ō′sis/, great difference in the size of the nucleus of cells that are the same type.

anisomastia /anī′sōmas′tē-ə/, a condition in which one female breast is much larger than the other.

anisometropia /anī′sōmetrō′pē-ə/, a defect in which each eye refracts light with a different strength.

anisopia /an′īsō′pē-ə/, a condition in which the vision in one eye is better than in the other.

anisopoikilocytosis /anī′sōpoi′kilōsītō′sis/, a defect of the blood. The red blood cells differ in size and shape.

anisotropine methybromide, a drug used for treating peptic ulcer.

★CAUTION: Glaucoma, blockage of the urinary system or the digestive tract, blocked intestines, heart defects, severe ulcerative colitis, or myasthenia gravis prohibits its use.

★ADVERSE EFFECTS: Among the most serious side effects are blurred vision, rapid heart beat, dilation of the pupils and other eye problems, impotence, confusion, trouble in urinating, constipation, allergies, and itching.

ankle, 1. the joint of the three bones of the foot at the leg (tibia, talus, fibula). 2. the part of the leg where it joins the foot.

ankle bandage, a figure-of-eight bandage that is looped under the sole of the foot and around the ankle. The heel may be covered or left bare, although it is better to cover it.

ankle bone. See **talus.**

ankle clonus, an involuntary reflex in the tendon that makes the foot move up and down repeatedly. It may be caused by pressure on the foot or a central nervous system disease.

ankle reflex. See **Achilles tendon reflex.**

ankyloglossia, a defect of the mouth in which the membrane under the tongue is too short (lingual frenulum). It limits the movement of the tongue and impairs the speech. It may be corrected. Also called **tongue-tie.**

ankylosing spondylitis /ang′kilō′sing/, a long-term swelling disease of unknown cause. It first affects the spine and nearby structures. It of-

ten progresses to a joining together (ankylosis) of the bones of the spinal column. In extreme cases the patient stoops forward, which is called a "poker spine" or "bamboo spine." The disease affects mostly men under 30 years of age. There is a strong chance that it can be inherited. As well as the spine, the joints of the hip, shoulder, neck, ribs, and jaw are often involved. When the joints where the ribs join the spine are involved, it may be hard for the patient to expand the rib cage while breathing. Many patients with the disease also have bowel disease that involves swelling, heat, redness, and pain. The aim of treatment is to relieve pain and swelling in the joints, usually with drugs. Physical therapy aids in keeping the spine as erect as possible. In advanced cases surgery may be done to straighten a badly bent spine. Compare **rheumatoid arthritis.** See also **ankylosis.** Also called **Marie-Strümpell disease.**

ankylosis /ang′kilō′sis/, 1. "freezing" of a joint, often in a position that is not normal. It is due to destruction of cartilage and bone, as occurs in rheumatoid arthritis. 2. also called **arthrodesis, fusion.** Fixing a joint through surgery to relieve pain or give support.

anlage /on′lägə/, the layer of cells from which an organ or structure grows. See also **blastema.**

ANLL. short for **acute nonlymphocytic leukemia.** See **acute myelocytic leukemia.**

annihilation, the changing of matter into energy.

anodic stripping voltametry /anod′ik/, a chemical process used to detect trace metals.

anodontia /an′ōdon′tē-ə/, an inherited defect in which some or all of the teeth are missing.

anodyne /an′ədīn/, a drug that relieves or lessens pain. Compare **analgesic.**

anomalo-, a combining form meaning 'uneven or irregular.'

anomaly /ənom′əlē/, 1. change from what is regarded as normal. 2. inherited problem with growth of a structure, as the lack of a limb or the presence of an extra finger. – **anomalous,** *adj.*

anomia /ənō′mē-ə/, a form of memory loss (aphasia) in which the patient cannot name objects. It is caused by an injury to a part of the brain.

anomie /an′əmē/, a state of not caring, feeling apart from others, and feeling worried, confused, and upset. It is due to the loss of social norms and goals that were valued at another point in time. Also spelled **anomy.**

anoopsia /an′ō·op′sē-ə/, a defect in which one or both eyes are fixed in an upward position. Also called **hypertropia.**

Anopheles /ənof′əlēz/, a genus of mosquito that gives malaria-causing parasites to humans. See also **malaria,** *Plasmodium.*

anoplasty, an operation to restore function of the anus.

anorchia, inherited lack of one or both testicles. Also called **anorchism.**

anorectal /an'ōrek'təl, ā'nō-/, referring to the anal and rectal portions of the large intestine.

anorectic /an'ōrek'tik/, **1.** referring to appetite loss. **2.** causing a loss of appetite, as an anorexiant drug.

anorexia /an'ōrek'sē·ə/, a loss of appetite that results in the patient not being able to eat. The state may be caused by unpleasant food, illness, or surroundings. It may also have a mental cause. Compare **pseudoanorexia.** See also **anorexia nervosa. –anorexic,** *adj.*

anorexia nervosa, a mental problem in which there is a long-term refusal to eat. It causes wasting, lack of menstrual cycle, mental problem with body image, and a fear of becoming fat. The state is seen mainly in teenagers, mostly girls. It is often linked with mental stress or conflict, as worry, anger, and fear. This stress may be due to a big change in the patient's life. Treatment consists of improving health, followed by therapy to get over the emotional conflicts.

anorexiant, drug or other substance that causes loss of appetite. Examples include amphetamine, diethylpropion, fenfluramine, and mazindol.

anorthopia /an'ôrthō'pē·ə/, a visual problem in which straight lines appear to be curved or angular. The person may also have difficulty seeing that objects are symmetrical.

anosigmoidoscopy /an'ōsig'moidos'kəpē/, a procedure in which a device with a light (endoscope) is used to look at the lining of the anus, rectum, and colon.

anosmia /anoz'mē·ə/, loss or impairment of the sense of smell. This is often a short-term state caused by a head cold or lung infection. Swelling or blockage of the nasal passages keeps odors from getting to the region that senses smells (olfactory region). It can get to be a permanent state when any part of the olfactory nerve is destroyed. This may happen with a brain injury, tumor, or disease, as can occur in chronic rhinitis. In some cases, the state may be caused by mental factors, as fear linked with a certain smell. Also called **olfactory anesthesia.** Compare **hyperosmia. –anosmatic, anosmic,** *adj.*

anosmia gustatoria, a state in which the patient is not able to smell foods.

anosognosia /an'əsognō'zə/, a condition in which the patient is not able to tell when there has been an injury to the body. It may be caused by an injury in the brain.

anovular menstruation, menstrual bleeding that occurs even though an egg has not been released from the ovary (ovulation). The egg (ovum) either stays in the follicle and breaks down, or in rare cases is fertilized. This causes an ovarian pregnancy.

anovulation /an'ovyōōlā'shən/, failure of the ovaries to produce, mature, or release eggs. The cause can be ovaries that have not matured, old ovaries, pregnancy, breast feeding, or disturbance of the hypothalamus, pituitary gland, and ovary from stress or disease. Anovulation may be a side effect of drugs given for other defects. **–anovulatory** /anov'yōōlətôrē/, *adj.*

anoxemia, a lack of sufficient oxygen in the blood.

anoxia /anok'sē·ə/, a lack of oxygen. Anoxia may occur in a small space or affect the whole body. It can be the result of poor supply of oxygen to the lungs. It can also occur when the blood is not able to carry oxygen to the tissues, or the tissues are not able to absorb the oxygen from the blood. Kinds of anoxia include **cerebral anoxia, stagnant anoxia. –anoxic,** *adj.* See also **hypoxemia, hypoxia.**

ansa /an'sə/, *pl.* **ansae,** a looplike structure that looks like a curved handle of a vase.

ansa cervicalis, a loop of nerves in the nerve network near the top of the spinal cord.

Antabuse, a trademark for a drug used to treat alcohol abuse (disulfiram).

antacid /antas'id/, **1.** opposing acidity. **2.** a drug or substance in the diet that buffers, makes neutral, or absorbs hydrochloric acid in the stomach. Antacids that contain aluminum and calcium may cause constipation; those with magnesium have a laxative effect.

antagonist, 1. one against or opposed to another. **2.** anything, as a drug or muscle, that has an opposite action or competes for the same thing. Kinds of antagonists include **antimetabolite, associated antagonist, direct antagonist, narcotic antagonist.** Compare **agonist. 3.** a tooth in the upper jaw that comes in contact during chewing or biting with a tooth in the lower jaw.

ante-, a combining form meaning 'before in time or in place.'

antecubital, at the bend of the elbow on the inside of the arm.

anteflexion, a position of an organ in which it is tilted forward, folded over on itself. This is not a normal state.

antegonial notch, a depression or low place that is present at the corner of the lower jaw.

antenatal. See **prenatal.**

antenatal diagnosis. See **prenatal diagnosis.**

antepartal care, care of a pregnant woman throughout the maternity cycle. It begins with conception and ends when labor starts. A complete health history and background is taken. Diseases in the family and infectious illness are noted. A physical exam is done to assess the skin, thyroid gland, heart, breasts, abdomen, lungs, and pelvic organs. The vaginal part of the pelvic exam may include a pap smear and tests for gonorrhea, yeast infection, and *Trichomonas.* Monthly tests look at blood pressure, weight, and urine content. Tests for syphilis, *Chlamydia,* genital herpes, or other viral infections are done. The heart of the fetus is measured and listened to. Blood tests are done. Sometimes fluid is withdrawn from the embryonic sac (amniocentesis) if certain defects in the fetus are suspected.

★PATIENT CARE: The mother is urged to discuss her concerns about the pregnancy, to learn about the processes, to report changes in the baby's movement, to take a class to prepare for labor, and to plan for the infant's needs.
See also **intrapartal care, prenatal nutrition, postpartal care.**

anterior (A), the front of a structure or a part facing toward the front. Compare **posterior.** See also **ventral.**

anterior Achilles bursitis. See **Albert's disease.**

anterior atlantoaxial ligament, one of five ligaments connecting the bones (atlas and axis) at the top of the spinal column.

anterior atlantooccipital membrane, one of two broad, close-woven fiberlike sheets that form part of the joint between the spine and the skull (atlantoccipital joint). Compare **posterior atlantooccipital membrane.**

anterior cardiac vein, one of many small blood vessels that return blood to the heart when it is out of oxygen. See also **coronary sinus.**

anterior crural nerve. See **femoral nerve.**

anterior cutaneous nerve, one of a pair of branches of the network of nerves near the top of the spine (cervical plexus). It arises from the second and the third nerves in the neck, and branches to the skin of the neck and upper chest.

anterior determinants of cusp, the shapes of the front teeth that decide the "hills and valleys" of the back teeth. They are important in restoring the back teeth.

anterior fontanel, a diamond-shaped area just above the baby's forehead. See also **fontanel.**

anterior longitudinal ligament, the broad, strong ligament attached to the front surfaces of the backbones (vertebrae). It goes from the skull to the lower back.

anterior mediastinal node, a lymph node in one of the three groups of chest (thoracic) nodes of the lymph system. This node drains lymph from nodes of the thymus, heart area, and breastbone (sternum).

anterior mediastinum, a space between the flat bone in the center of the chest (sternum), the fourth through the seventh ribs, and the sac around the heart (pericardium). It goes downward as far as the diaphragm.

anterior nares, the ends of the nostrils that open into the nasal space and allow breathing in and out. Each is an oval opening that measures about 1.5 cm (about ¾ inch) in length and about 1 cm (less than ½ inch) across. Also called **nostrils.** Compare **posterior nares.**

anterior neuropore, the opening of the spine in the early fetus (embryonic neural tube) in the front part of the forebrain. Compare **posterior neuropore.** See also **horizon.**

anterior pituitary. See **adenohypophysis.**

anterior tibial artery, one of the two branches of the major leg (popliteal) artery. The anterior tibial artery starts in back of the knee, splits into six branches, and supplies the muscles of the leg and foot.

anterior tibial node, one of the small lymph glands of the leg. Compare **inguinal node, popliteal node.**

anterior tooth, any one of the teeth in the front of the mouth (incisors and canine teeth). Compare **posterior tooth.**

anterocclusion /an'tərōkloo'shən/, faulty bite (malocclusion) in which the lower teeth are in front of the teeth in the upper jaw. Compare **anteversion.**

anterograde amnesia, the loss of memory of the events that occur after an injury. Compare **anterograde memory, retrograde amnesia.**

anterograde memory, the memory of events of long ago but not of those that happen recently. Compare **anterograde amnesia.** Also called **senile memory.**

anteroposterior /an'tərōpostir'ē·ər/, from the front to the back of the body. The term is often used to describe the direction of an x-ray beam.

anteversion, 1. the condition of an organ that is abnormally tilted forward. **2.** the forward tilting of teeth. Compare **anterocclusion. 3.** the angle between the neck and shaft of the thigh bone. The normal angle is between 15 and 20 degrees.

anthelmintic /ant'helmin'tik/, referring to a drug that destroys or prevents infection caused by parasitic worms, as filariae, flukes, hookworms, pinworms, roundworms, schistosomes, tapeworms, trichinae, and whipworms.

anthracosis /an'thrəkō'sis/, a long-term lung disease of coal miners. It is caused by coal dust in the lungs. It forms black bumps on the bronchioles that result in emphysema. The condition is made worse by cigarette smoking. There is no real treatment. The progress of the disease may be halted by staying away from coal dust. Also called **black lung, coalworker's pneumoconiosis, miner's pneumoconiosis.** See also **inorganic dust.**

anthracosis linguae. See **parasitic glossitis.**

anthralin /an'thrəlin/, a drug that is put on the skin. It is used to treat psoriasis and long-term swelling of the skin.
★CAUTION: Kidney disease or known allergy to this drug prohibits its use. It is not put on broken skin or near the eyes.

★ADVERSE EFFECTS: The most serious side effect is kidney failure.

anthrax /an'thraks/, a disease that affects mostly farm animals (cattle, goats, pigs, sheep, and horses), and is caused by the bacterium *Bacillus anthracis.* Anthrax in animals is usually fatal. Humans most often get it through a break in the skin when in direct contact with infected animals and their hides. They may also get anthrax of the lungs by breathing in the bacterium. The type that infects the skin begins with a reddish-brown sore that breaks open and then forms a dark scab. The symptoms that follow include internal bleeding, muscle pain, headache, fever, nausea, and vomiting. The lung form, called woolsorter's disease, is often fatal unless treated early. Treatment for both forms is penicillin G or tetracycline. A vaccine is available for people for whom anthrax is a work hazard. Also called **malignant pustule.**

anthropo-, a combining form referring to a human being.

anthropoid pelvis, a type of pelvis in which the opening is oval; the front-to-back (anteroposterior) diameter is much greater than the side-to-side (transverse). If the pelvis is large, normal childbirth is possible. This type of pelvis is present in 40% of nonwhite women and in more than 25% of white women.

anthropometry /an'thrəpom'itrē/, the science of measuring the human body for height, weight, and size of different parts. This includes measuring skinfolds. Also called **anthropometric measurement.** –**anthropometric,** *adj.*

anti-, ant-, a combining form meaning 'against.'

antiadrenergic /an'ti·ad'drənur'jik/, 1. referring to blocking signals sent by the nerves that release the chemical norepinephrine. These kinds of nerves are called adrenergic nerves and have two types of receivers called alpha and beta. 2. an antiadrenergic drug. These are drugs that block the response to norepinephrine by alpha-adrenergic receptors. They cause blood flow to increase and blood pressure to decrease. Drugs that block beta-adrenergic receptors slow the heart beat. Also called **sympatholytic.** Compare **adrenergic.**

antianabolic, referring to drugs or other agents that prevent or slow processes in which simple substances are converted into more complex matter.

antianemic, 1. referring to a substance or method that corrects or prevents a shortage of red blood cells. 2. a drug used to treat or to prevent a shortage of red blood cells (anemia). Whole blood transfusions are given to treat anemia from sudden blood loss. Packed red cells are usually given when the shortage is due to constant blood loss. Transfusions of parts of the blood are used to treat aplastic anemia. Iron deficiency anemia, the most common form of anemia, is treated with doses of iron

ferrous sulfate, fumerate, or gluconate taken by mouth. Iron is given by vein to patients who are not able to absorb iron from the digestive tract. It is also given by vein to those who get nausea and diarrhea when taking iron by mouth. Vitamin B_{12} (cyanocobalamin) is injected for pernicious anemia. Folic acid is given to correct a shortage of that vitamin. It is given for anemia due to poor nutrition. It is also given for liver disease due to alcohol abuse.

antianginal drug, any drug that enlarges the arteries of the heart, thereby improving blood flow. This will prevent symptoms of angina pectoris.

antiantibody, an antibody formed by the blood to fight off a foreign antibody that can cause an allergic response. See also **antibody, immune gamma globulin.**

antiarrhythmic, 1. referring to a treatment or drug that prevents, relieves, or corrects a heart rhythm problem. 2. an agent used to treat an uneven heart beat (arrhythmia). A device that gives an electric shock is often used to restore a normal rhythm in patients with rapid, uneven heart beats. A pacemaker can be surgically placed in a patient with a very slow heart rate or other heart beat problems. The electrode tube (catheter) of an external pacemaker may be threaded through a vein to the heart in cases of complete heart block. Drugs may be given to restore normal heart rate. See also **arrhythmia.**

antibacterial /an'tibaktir'ē·əl/, 1. referring to a substance that kills bacteria or prevents their growth. 2. an antibacterial (antibiotic drug).

antiberiberi factor. See **thiamine.**

antibiotic, referring to the ability to kill or prevent the growth of a living organism. Antibiotics are also called antibacterial or antimicrobial drugs. They can be made from cultures of microorganisms. They can also be made artificially. Side effects to antibiotics can include rash, fever, spasm of the bronchial tubes, inflamed blood vessels, kidney and ear problems, stomach upset, vomiting, fatigue, and lack of sleep. They are used to treat infections.

antibiotic anticancer agents, drugs that may act against infection (antibiotics) as well as cancer (anticancer). Examples include bleomycin, dactinomycin, daunorubicin, and mitomycin.

antibiotic sensitivity tests, a type of test to find out what antibiotic will work to get rid of a certain bacteria. After the organism has been found in a sample of mucus, blood, or other body tissue, it is grown in the laboratory. A number of antibiotic drugs are tested on the bacterium. If the growth is stopped by the drug, the bacterium is said to be sensitive to that antibiotic. If it keeps growing in spite of the antibiotic, it is said to be resistant to that drug.

antibody (Ab), a molecule made by lymph tissue. It defends the body against bacteria, viruses, or other foreign bodies (antigens). Each antibody reacts to a certain foreign body. Antibodies are also called immunoglobulins. See also **antiantibody, antigen determinant, plasma protein, T cell.**

antibody instructive theory, a theory that each contact with an antigen causes the body to make a new antibody.

antibody specific theory, a theory about the growth of antibodies. It states that at birth a person's cells are able to make antibodies to fight off a small number of foreign bodies. The theory holds that the body has a large number of lymph cells. Each is able to make a different antibody. This theory explains why many people have allergies to certain foreign bodies, as pollen. Also called **clonal selection theory.** See also **autoimmunity.**

antibromic. See **deodorant.**

anticancer diet, a diet designed to reduce the kinds of eating habits that may be associated with cancer. It is based on recommendations of the American Cancer Society, National Cancer Institute, and National Academy of Sciences. It includes a reduction in fatty foods, adequate amounts of high-fiber foods, foods rich in vitamins A and C, and vegetables such as broccoli, cabbage, and cauliflower. The diet limits alcohol and salt-cured, smoked, or nitrate-cured foods. It also recommends that obesity be avoided.

anticholinergic, **1.** referring to a blocking of certain receivers on the nerve. This causes the body to stay in a "fight or flight" state, with high blood pressure, rapid breathing, and dry mouth. **2.** an anticholinergic drug that lessens muscle spasms in the bladder, lung, and intestine. It also relaxes the iris muscles of the eye; decreases substances released by the stomach, lung, and mouth; decreases sweating; and speeds up the heart. Many anticholinergic drugs reduce symptoms like those in Parkinson's disease. Also **parasympatholytic.** Compare **cholinergic.**

anticholinergic agent. See **anticholinergic.**

anticholinesterase /an'tikol'ənes'tərās/, a drug that stops the action of a chemical that sends nerve signals (acetylcholine). Anticholinesterase drugs are used to treat sudden, local muscle fatigue (myasthenia gravis).

anticipatory adaptation /antis'əpətôr'ē/, the process in which a person prepares to deal with a situation that may be distressing. An example would be a student trying to relax before learning the results of an important test.

anticipatory guidance /antis'əpətôr'ē/, the help given to a person who is afraid of an event that is about to occur. One example is preparing a child for surgery by explaining what will happen.

anticoagulant, **1.** referring to a substance that prevents or delays blood clots (coagulation). **2.** an anticoagulant drug.

anticonvulsant, referring to a drug or treatment that prevents seizures. It may also make the seizure less severe. One type of seizure treated is convulsive, as epilepsy. Many of these drugs may cause birth defects when given to pregnant women.

antideformity positioning and splinting, the use of splints, braces, or similar devices to prevent or control deformities of the bones and muscles that may result from disuse, burns, or other injuries.

antidepressant, referring to a drug or a treatment that prevents or relieves depression. See also **antipsychotic.**

antidiarrheal, a drug or other agent that relieves the symptoms of diarrhea.

antidiuretic, referring to a drug or treatment that keeps the body from making urine. Antidiuretic hormone (vasopressin), made in the hypothalamus, decreases the amount of urine formed in the body. **–antidiuresis,** *n.*

antidiuretic hormone (ADH), a hormone that decreases the making of urine. It does this by causing water to be soaked up by the kidneys. ADH is given off by the hypothalamus and stored in the pituitary gland. ADH is released when the blood volume falls, when a large amount of salt shows up in blood, or when pain, stress, or certain drugs are present. Nicotine, and large doses of certain drugs cause ADH to be released. Alcohol slows the making of the hormone. Artificial ADH is used to treat a type of diabetes. Also called **vasopressin.**

antidote /an'tidōt/, a drug or other substance that stops the action of a poison. An antidote may coat the stomach. This will keep the poison from being soaked up. It may also work to oppose the action of the poison, as giving a relaxing drug to a patient who has taken a large amount of a stimulant.

antidromic conduction /an'tidrom'ik/, the sending of a nerve signal backward. It is not normal but has been done in experiments. Compare **orthodromic conduction.**

antiembolism hose, elastic stockings worn to prevent clots (emboli). They are often worn after surgery or when the patient is restricted to bed. They help the return flow of the blood to the heart. This keeps the blood from pooling in the veins. This helps avoid varicose veins and clotting (thromboembolic) defects.

antiemetic, referring to a drug or treatment that prevents or relieves nausea and vomiting.

antiestrogen drug, a hormone-based drug used primarily in cancer chemotherapy. The group of drugs includes tamoxifen. They are used mainly in treating tumors that depend on the presence of estrogen, such as those found in breast cancer.

antifebrile. See **antipyretic.**

antifungal, referring to a substance that kills fungi or prevents their growth.

antigalactic, referring to a drug or other agent that prevents or reduces the flow of breast milk in some mothers of newborns.

anti-GBM disease, a kidney disorder related to an immune reaction. It involves the glomular basement membrane (GBM), which is damaged in the reaction. The kidney itself may be the cause of the reaction.

antigen /an'tijən/, a substance foreign to the body, often a protein. It causes the body to form an antibody that responds only to that antigen. Antigens can cause allergic reactions in some people.

antigen-antibody reaction, a process of the immune system in which certain white blood cells (lymphocytes) respond to a foreign body (antigen). The cells then make antibodies to protect the body from infection. The poison antigens are made harmless when they are bound to antibodies. The antigen-antibody reaction may start right away with antigen contact, or it may start as much as 48 hours later. Antigen-antibody reactions are normal to the immune response of the body. Some people have a too-responsive antigen-antibody reaction. This causes the immune system to fight off healthy cells of the body. There are many theories about why this happens. See also **serum sickness.**

antigen determinant, a small spot on the surface of an antigen that fits onto a certain part of an antibody, much like a lock and key. When an antibody binds to an antigen, an antigen-antibody complex is formed. Also called **epitope.** See also **antibody.**

antigenicity /an'tijənis'ətē/, causing antibodies to be made. The degree of antigenicity depends on the kind and amount of the foreign substance (antigen). It also depends on how sensitive a person is to the antigen.

antigerminal pole. See **vegetal pole.**

antiglobulin /an'tiglob'yoolin/, an antibody against a certain type of human protein (globulin). It can occur normally or be made in laboratory animals. Antiglobulins are used to find antibodies, as in blood typing. See also **precipitin.**

antiglobulin test, a test to find antibodies that coat and damage red blood cells as a result of disease. It is used to check for a number of blood defects. Also called **Coombs' test.** See also **autoimmune disease, erythroblastosis fetalis.**

antigravity muscles, the muscles that keep joints or other body parts in proper position by opposing the effects of gravity on the body. Examples include the muscles of the jaw that automatically keep the jaw up and the mouth closed.

antihemophilic C factor. See **factor XI.**

antihemophilic factor (AHF), blood clotting factor VIII. It is a substance that stops bleeding. It is used to treat a lack of factor VIII (hemophilia A).
★ADVERSE EFFECTS: The most serious side effect is hepatitis. This can happen when the blood plasma used to treat the patient is infected. Allergic reactions may also occur.

antihemorrhagic, any drug or other agent used to prevent or control bleeding.

antihistamine, a substance that reduces the effects of histamine. Histamine is a chemical made by the body as a response to a foreign substance (allergen). It can cause itching, breathing trouble, and increased heart beat in allergic reactions. Many antihistamine drugs can be gotten over the counter to treat allergies, as hay fever and itching. Antihistamines should not be overused. The drugs should not be left in reach of children who could swallow them. The misuse of these drugs can cause death. Side effects of prescribed use can include fatigue, nausea, constipation, and dryness of the throat and breathing tract. About 25% of the people who use antihistamines feel some side effect. **–antihistaminic,** adj.

antihypercholesterolemic, a drug that prevents or controls an increase of cholesterol in the blood. Examples include clofibrate and colestipol.

antihypertensive, referring to a drug or treatment that reduces high blood pressure. Certain drugs that increase the making of urine (diuretics) lower the blood pressure. They do this by decreasing blood volume.

antiinflammatory, referring to a drug or treatment that reduces inflammation or swelling.

antiinitiator, a substance that may cause cancer but may also protect cells against cancer if given before exposure to a carcinogen. An anti-initiator given after exposure to a substance that causes cancer may also promote and encourage cancer development instead of block it.

antileprotic, a drug or other agent used to treat leprosy.

antilipidemic /antilip'idē'mik/, referring to a diet or drug that reduces the amount of fats (lipids) in the blood. Antilipidemic diets and drugs are prescribed to reduce the risk of disease of the blood vessels and heart muscle (atherosclerotic cardiovascular disease, or ACVD). In ACVD, fat collects in the vessel or heart that has cholesterol in it. Groups of people who eat low-fat diets have lower cholesterol levels and less heart disease. A low-fat diet is thought to help to prevent heart disease, in the view of many heart specialists. A number of drugs are used to reduce fats in the blood stream, but it is not certain how these affect ACVD. Side effects of these drugs may include gallstones, uneven heart beat, blood clots, and the loss of vitamins. See also **hyperlipidemia.**

Antilirium, a trademark for a drug that is used to reverse the effects of anesthesia (physostigmine salicylate).

antilymphocyte serum (ALS), a serum given to help the body accept the new tissue in an organ transplant. It is also used with chemotherapy for cancerous tumors. ALS has had good results in some cases of leukemia and in kidney transplant. The side effects include serious serum sickness, infection, severe allergy, and kidney failure.

antimalarial, 1. referring to a drug that kills or stops the growth of malaria organisms (plasmodia). Antimalarial also refers to a way to kill mosquitos that carry the disease, as spraying insecticides or draining swamps. **2.** an antimalarial drug that kills or prevents the growth of plasmodia in humans. See also **malaria.**

antimetabolite, a drug similar to a chemical that is needed to make DNA in the body. An antimetabolite interferes with the making of DNA. Antimetabolites are used as anticancer drugs.

antimicrobial, referring to a substance that kills microorganisms or stops their growth.

Antiminth, a trademark for a drug used to treat infection from worms (pyrantel pamoate).

antimitochondrial antibody, an antibody that acts against mitochondria. Mitochondria are structures in the body's cells that make the cell's energy. These antibodies are not normally present in the blood of healthy people. A test to find these antibodies in the blood is helpful in finding liver disease. Low levels may occur in long-term hepatitis, liver disease caused by drugs, and other diseases. High levels are found in severe liver disease, as primary biliary cirrhosis.

antimitotic, referring to the prevention of cell division.

antimony /an'təmōnē/, a chemical element that occurs in nature, both free and as a salt. Its symbol is sb. Its atomic number is 51; its atomic weight is 121.8. Antimony is a bluish metal that has a crystal structure. Antimony compounds are used to treat parasite infections, as filariasis, leishmaniasis, schistosomiasis, and trypanosomiasis. It is also used to bring on vomiting in cases of poisoning.

antimony poisoning, poisoning caused by swallowing or breathing antimony or antimony compounds. The symptoms are vomiting, sweating, diarrhea, and a metallic taste in the mouth. Irritation of the skin or mucous membrane may result from contact. Severe poisoning will look like arsenic poisoning. Dimercaprol is used to treat antimony poisoning. Antimony is common in many substances used in medicine and industry.

antimony potassium tartrate, a drug used to treat infection caused by the parasite *Schistosoma japonicum.*

★CAUTION: Low red blood cell level (anemia), severe liver, kidney, or heart problems, or known allergy to this drug prohibits its use.

★ADVERSE EFFECTS: Among the most serious side effects are collapse of the blood flow system from too rapid injection, and coughing and vomiting during and after injection. Sometimes serious allergic reactions and blood problems occur. Also called **tartar emetic.**

antimuscarinic, a drug that causes the "flight or fight" response, with raised blood pressure, fast heart beat, and dry mouth.

antimutagen /an'timyōō'təjən/, **1.** any substance that lowers the rate of changes in cell structure (mutation), or protects the body against a mutagen. **2.** any method that protects cells against drugs that cause cell mutations. **–antimutagenic,** *adj.*

antimycotic. See **antifungal.**

antineoplastic, a drug that controls or kills cancer cells. See also **alkylating agent, antimetabolite.**

antineoplastic antibiotic, a drug made from a microorganism or by artificial means. It is used to treat cancer. Antineoplastic antibiotics slow down bone marrow function and often cause nausea and vomiting. Many types also cause hair loss.

antineoplastic hormone, a chemical made by the body or by artificial means. It is used to control some cancers. Hormone treatment slows the growth of the tumor. Hormones are used with other methods to treat cancer of the prostate, and breast cancer.

antineuritic vitamin. See **thiamine.**

antinuclear antibody, an antibody that works on the nucleus of a cell. Antinuclear antibodies are found in patients with various diseases, as systemic lupus erythematosus (SLE).

antioxidant, a chemical or other agent that prevents or reduces the process in which the oxygen content of a substance is increased (oxidation). Antioxidants may be added to foods containing fats or oils to prevent spoiling.

antiparasitic, 1. referring to a drug or treatment that kills parasites or stops their growth. **2.** an antiparasitic drug, including amebicides, anthelmintics, antimalarials, schistosomicides, trichomonacides, and trypanosomicides.

antiparkinsonian, referring to a drug or treatment used to treat parkinsonism. Drugs for this nervous system defect are of two kinds. One kind makes up for the lack of a chemical in the brain tissues (dopamine). Another kind will balance the effects of too much of another chemical (acetylcholine) in the brain. Levodopa is given to patients to reduce the stiffness, slowness, drooling, and lack of balance that is typical of the disease. The drug does not stop the course of the disease or condition. Other drugs may help to relieve tremors and rigidity and make movement easier. See also **tardive dyskinesia.**

antiperistaltic, 1. referring to a substance that reduces the movement of the intestines (peristalsis). **2.** an antiperistaltic drug. Narcotics, as paregoric, diphenoxylate, and loperamide hydrochloride, are antiperistaltic drugs used to give relief in diarrhea. Anticholinergic drugs reduce spasms of the muscles of the intestines.

antipernicious anemia factor. See **cyanocobalamin.**

antiprotoplasmatic, referring to agents that damage the living substance of a cell (protoplasm).

antipruritic, 1. referring to a drug or treatment that helps relieve or prevent itching. **2.** an antipruritic drug. Anesthetics that are put on the skin (topical), corticosteroids, and antihistamines are used as antipruritic agents.

antipsychotic, 1. referring to a drug or treatment that lessens the symptoms of a severe mental illness (psychosis). **2.** an antipsychotic drug. Phenothiazine drugs are given most often to treat schizophrenia and other psychotic defects. Common side effects of this type of drug are a dry mouth, blurred vision, and parkinsonian symptoms. See also **antidepressant, neuroleptic, tranquilizer.**

antipyretic, 1. referring to a drug or treatment that reduces fever. **2.** an antipyretic drug. The most widely used are acetaminophen, given by mouth or through the rectum, aspirin, and other salicylates. A lukewarm alcohol sponge or tub bath may decrease a high fever. A cooling blanket is sometimes used for patients with a prolonged, high fever. Also called **antifebrile, antithermic, febrifuge.**

antipyretic bath, a bath with lukewarm water to reduce a fever.

antirachitic, referring to an agent used to treat rickets.

antiscorbutic vitamin. See **ascorbic acid.**

antiseborrheic, referring to a drug or other agent that is applied to the skin to control a condition in which the production of too much grease causes very oily skin or dry scales (seborrhea).

antiseptic, 1. tending to stop the growth of microorganisms. **2.** a substance that stops the growth of microorganisms.

antiseptic dressing, a dressing treated with a germ or bacteria killing drug. It is placed on a wound or an incision to prevent or treat infection.

antiseptic gauze, gauze soaked in an antiseptic fluid. It is sometimes packaged in separate, sealed packets.

antiserum, the straw-colored fluid of the blood (serum) of an animal or human that contains antibodies against a certain disease. Antiserum is used to transfer immunity against that disease. Antiserum does not cause the patient to produce his or her own antibodies. There are two types of antiserum, antitoxin and antimicrobial serum. Antitoxin destroys the poison (toxin) made by the bacteria, but it does not kill the bacteria itself. Antimicrobial serum destroys bacteria. An antiserum that acts on more than one strain of bacteria is called polyvalent. A univalent antiserum acts on only one type of bacteria. Also called **immune serum.** Compare **vaccine.**

antiserum anaphylaxis, an extreme allergic reaction in a normal person. It is caused by injecting serum from a person with that allergy. Also called **passive anaphylaxis.**

antisialogogue, a drug that reduces saliva secretion.

antisocial personality, a person who displays attitudes and behavior that run against the customs, standards, and morals accepted by society. Also called **psychopathic personality, sociopathic personality.** See also **antisocial personality disorder.**

antisocial personality disorder, repeated behavior patterns that lack morals and ethics. These patterns bring a person into conflict with society. A person with this defect may be aggressive, impulsive, irresponsible, hostile, and immature and show poor judgment.

antisocial reaction. See **antisocial personality disorder.**

antispasmodic, a drug or other agent that prevents muscle spasms in certain muscles, including muscles in the uterus, digestive system, or urinary tract.

antistreptolysin-O test (ASOT, ASLT) /an'tis-trep'təli'sinō'/, a test to find and measure antibodies in the blood to streptolysin-O. This is a poison that is made by certain types of the bacteria streptococci. The test is often used to help diagnose rheumatic fever. High levels may mean the patient has had a recent infection. See also **Lancefield's classification.**

antithermic. See **antipyretic.**

antithyroid drug, any one of many drugs that can lower the level of thyroid hormones. These drugs are often used to treat an overactive thyroid (hyperthyroidism). The main antithyroid drugs are thioamides. These drugs are often given to control hyperthyroidism before the thyroid is removed. These drugs should not be taken during pregnancy. They can cause low levels of thyroid hormones (hypothyroidism) and goiter in the baby. Mothers who breast feed their children should not take these drugs.

antitoxin, an antiserum that is often made from the serum of horses that have immunity against a certain organism. Examples of antitoxins are botulism antitoxin given to patients who have a type of food poisoning (botulism), and tetanus and diphtheria antitoxins which are given to prevent those infections.

antitrypsin, a protein produced in the liver that blocks the action of certain enzymes, including trypsin. A lack of adequate antitrypsin is associated with emphysema. Also called alpha-antitrypsin.

antitubercular, any of a group of drugs used to treat tuberculosis. At least two drugs, and usually three, are used in various combinations in treating tuberculosis.

antitussive /an'titus'iv/, **1.** against a cough. **2.** any of a large group of habit-forming and non-habit-forming (narcotic and nonnarcotic) drugs that act on the nervous system to reduce the action of the cough reflex. Because the cough reflex is needed to clear the upper breathing tract of released fluids, antitussives should not be used with a cough that produces sputum. Codeine and hydrocodone are strong narcotic antitussives. Dextromethorphan works just as well and is not habit-forming. Antitussives are given by mouth, often in a syrup with a substance to help bring up the mucus (expectorant), and alcohol. They may also be given in a capsule with an antihistamine and a mild painkiller.

antivenin /an'tiven'in/, a substance with antibodies that cause venom to become harmless. It is made from the serum of immunized horses. Antivenin transfers this immunity and is given in first aid for snake and insect bites.

Antivert, a trademark for an antihistamine drug (meclizine hydrochloride).

antiviral, destructive to viruses.

antivitamin, a substance that stops the action of a vitamin.

antixerophthalmic vitamin. See **vitamin A.**

Anton's syndrome, a form of a condition (anasognosia) in which the patient is not able to tell when there has been an injury to the body. In this form of the condition a person with partial or total blindness refuses to admit to any visual problem, even though medical evidence shows that there is a problem. The patient usually makes excuses for being unable to see, suggesting, for example, that the light is inadequate.

antral gastritis, a defect in which the lower part (antrum) of the stomach near the opening to the duodenum (pyloris) becomes too narrow. It is not a true inflamed stomach lining (gastritis), but is either a sore in the stomach lining, or tumor.

antrum cardiacum, a small passage where the esophagus joins the stomach.

antrum of Highmore. See **maxillary sinus.**

Anturane, a trademark for a drug used to treat gout (sulfinpyrazone).

anular, describing a ring-shaped sore around a clear, normal, unaffected disk of skin.

anular ligament, a ligament that goes around the end of the bone on the thumb side of the forearm (radius).

anuria /əno̅o̅r'ē·ə/, the state of being unable to urinate, the failure to produce urine, or urinating less than about 3½ ounces a day. Anuria may be caused by kidney failure, a severe decline in blood pressure, or blockage of the urinary tract. A fast decline in urinary output occurs in sudden kidney failure. Although patients can live up to 2 weeks with anuria, death may occur within 24 hours after complete loss of urinary function. Poisoning from holding urine (uremia) occurs in anuria as the waste products build up in the bloodstream. Treatment of anuria includes limiting potassium and protein in the diet, drugs to help get rid of potassium, limiting fluid intake, and running blood tests often. It may also be treated by removing waste with a machine (dialysis). The patient must be protected from infection and injury. Also called **anuresis** /an'yoo̅re̅'sis/ anuric, anuretic, *adj.* Compare **oliguria.**

anus /ā'nəs/, the opening at the end of the anal canal.

anxietas /angzī'ətas/, a state of anxiety, nervousness, fear, or worry. Anxietas often goes along with a feeling of pressure in the stomach. Kinds of anxietas are **anxietas presenilis, restless legs syndrome.**

anxietas presenilis, a state of extreme anxiety linked with the change of life.

anxietas tibiarum. See **restless legs syndrome.**

anxiety, a feeling of worry, upset, uncertainty, and fear that comes from thinking about some threat or danger. Anxiety is often mental, rather than a response to real events. The cause of the problem is complex and may involve a mental conflict about values and goals of life. It can also be due to a change in health, income, role, home life, or friendships.

anxiety attack, a sudden response of intense anxiety and panic. Symptoms depend on the person and how severe the attack is. Often the symptoms include fast heart beat, shortness of breath, dizziness, faintness, sweating, paleness, stomach upset, and a vague feeling of doom. Attacks often occur suddenly, and last from a few seconds to 1 hour or longer. They may come as often as many times a day or once a month. Treatment may include giving drugs, if needed, and psychotherapy to help to understand the stresses. See also **anxiety, anxiety neurosis.**

anxiety complex. See **castration anxiety.**

anxiety dream, a dream that occurs during rapid-eye-movement (REM) sleep and is accompanied by restlessness and a gradual increase in pulse rate. Anxiety dreams tend to occur in children, who usually recall the content clearly.

Signs of anxiety

Appearance

↑ Muscle tension (rigidity)
Skin blanches, pales
↑ Perspiration, clammy skin
Fatigue
↑ Small motor activity (e.g., restlessness, tremor)

Behavior

↓ Attention span
↓ Ability to follow directions
↑ Acting out
↑ Somatizing
↑ Immobility

Conversation

↑ Number of questions
Constant seeking of reassurance
Frequent shifting of topics of conversation
Describes fears with sense of helplessness
Avoids focusing on feelings
Focuses on equipment or procedures

Physiological signs mediated through autonomic nervous system

↑ Heart rate
↑ Rate or depth of respirations
Rapid extreme shifts in body temperature, blood pressure, menstrual flow
Diarrhea
Urinary urgency
Dryness of mouth
↓ Appetite
↑ Perspiration
Dilation of pupils

Signs of anxiety are dependent on the degree of anxiety. Mild anxiety heightens the use of capacities, whereas severe and panic states severely paralyze or overwork capacities.

anxiety hierarchy, a list of various situations or conditions that cause anxiety, listed in order according to the amount of anxiety they cause.

anxiety neurosis, a mental conflict or problem in which anxiety lasts for a long time. The patient may feel mildly tense, worried, afraid, tired, unable to make a decision, restless, or easy to anger. In more severe cases, the symptoms may be more hostile towards others. In extreme cases, the mental upset may lead to physical problems, as tremors, muscle tension, rapid heart beat, breathing problems, high blood pressure, and sweating. Other physical signs include changes in skin color, nausea, vomiting, diarrhea, restlessness, lack of sleep, and changes in appetite. The symptoms of anxiety may be helped with drugs, but psychotherapy is the better treatment. Also called **anxiety reaction, anxiety state.** See also **anxiety, anxiety attack.**

anxiolytic /angk'sē·ōlit'ik/, a sedative or minor tranquilizer used primarily to treat episodes of anxiety. Kinds of anxiolytics include barbiturates, benzodiazepines, chlormezanone, hydroxyzine, meprobamate, and tybamate.

AORN, abbreviation for **Association of Operating Room Nurses.**

aorta /ā·ôr'tə/, the main artery of the heart. It starts at the opening of the heart's lower left chamber (ventricle). In the belly, it narrows and branches into the two common iliac arteries that supply blood to the legs.

aortic aneurysm, a bulge in the wall of the aorta caused by deposits of cholesterol (atherosclerosis), high blood pressure, or syphilis. Syphilitic aneurysms almost always occur in the chest portion of the aorta (thoracic aorta). They often involve the aortic arch. More common atherosclerotic aneurysms are in the belly (abdominal) section. A bulging abdominal aortic aneurysm may get in the way of the urinary tract, spine, or other structure, and cause pain. In many cases the first sign is life-threatening bleeding that is caused by the breaking open of the lesion. An aneurysm that is still intact can be found by x-ray films of the belly, by another type of film of the blood vessels (angiogram), or by using special sound waves (ultrasound). Treatment of small aneurysms includes drugs to reduce the blood pressure, relieve pain, and reduce the force of the heart beats. Large aneurysms are removed, and the part of the aorta is replaced with a plastic tube. See also **dissecting aneurysm.**

aortic arch. See **arch of the aorta.**

aortic arch syndrome, a blockage of the part of the aorta that forms an arch. Conditions as atherosclerosis, inflamed arteries (arteritis), and syphilis may cause aortic arch syndrome. The symptoms include fainting, short-term blindness, loss of use of part of the body, and memory loss.

aortic body reflex, a normal chemical reaction in the body. It is caused by a decrease in oxygen in the blood. This causes faster breathing to build up oxygen supplies. See also **carotid body reflex.**

aortic regurgitation, the reverse flow of blood from the aorta back into the left lower heart chamber (ventricle). Also called **aortic insufficiency.**

aortic stenosis, a defect in which the aortic valve in the heart is more narrow than is normal. It can be caused by a birth defect or rheumatic fever. Aortic stenosis blocks the flow of blood from the left lower heart chamber (ventricle) into the aorta. This causes a lower output of blood from the heart and lung congestion. Symptoms include faint pulses, problems with exercise, chest pain, and a heart murmur. Diagnosis is made by putting a tube into the heart (cardiac catheterization) and graphing the sounds of the heart (echocardiography). Surgery is often done to correct the defect. See also **congenital cardiac anomaly, valvular disease, valvular heart disease.**

aortic valve, a valve in the heart between the left lower heart chamber (ventricle) and the aorta. It has three leaves that close when the heart beats to prevent blood from flowing back into the heart from the aorta. Compare **mitral valve, pulmonary valve, tricuspid valve.**

aortitis /ā′ôrtī′tis/, an inflammation of the aorta. It can occur in syphilis and sometimes in rheumatic fever.

aortography /ā-ôrtog′rəfé/, a method to diagnose heart diseases. The aorta and its branches are injected with a fluid that will show on x-ray films. –**aortographic,** *adj.*

aortopulmonary fenestration, a birth defect in which there is an abnormal opening between the ascending aorta and the main artery to the lungs (pulmonary artery). This allows blood with oxygen and blood without oxygen to mix. As a result, there is less oxygen available to the body.

APA, 1. short for **American Psychiatric Association. 2.** short for **American Psychological Association.**

apareunia /ā′pərōō′nē-ə/, an inability to perform sexual intercourse because of a physical or emotional problem.

apathetic hyperthyroidism, a form of excess thyroid production that tends to affect mainly older adults, who have stereotyped "senile" physical features and are apathetic and inactive rather than overactive in behavior. Medical treatment not only restores normal behavioral activity but also results in a loss of wrinkles and a younger physical appearance. Untreated, the patient is likely to succumb to the effects of stress or acute illness.

apathy /ap′əthē/, a lack of emotion, feeling, concern, or passion; a lack of care for things that are normally exciting or moving. The state is often seen in patients with certain types of mental illness, as neurasthenical neurosis and schizophrenia. –**apathetic,** *adj.*

apatite, a mineral made of calcium and phosphate that is found in the bones and teeth.

APC, short for **aspirin, phenacetin, caffeine.**

aperient /əpir′ē-ənt/, a mild laxative.

aperitive /əper′itiv/, a stimulant of the appetite.

Apert's syndrome /operz′/, a rare defect in which the head and face are deformed and the fingers and toes are fused together. The exact cause of Apert's syndrome is not known, but it seems to be a genetic defect. Symptoms of Apert's syndrome are a long, pointed head,

wide-set and bulging eyes, and defects of the jaws. The treatment of Apert's syndrome usually includes surgery of the skull bones to prevent pressure on the brain. The fingers and toes can also be corrected. Also called **acrocephalosyndactylism.**

aperture, an opening in an object or structure.

aperture of frontal sinus, the opening between the sinus in the forehead (frontal sinus) and the nasal cavity.

aperture of larynx, the opening between the two sections of the windpipe (pharynx and larynx).

aperture of sphenoid sinus, a round opening between the sinus behind the eye (sphenoid sinus) and the nasal cavity.

apex /ā′peks/, *pl.* **apices** /ā′pisēz/, the top, the end, or the tip of a structure, as the apex of the heart, the apices of the teeth.

apex beat, a pulsation of the left lower chamber (ventricle) of the heart. It can sometimes be seen on the skin of the chest.

apex cordis, the pointed lower border of the heart.

apexification, the process of closing the root of a tooth with hard tissue.

apexigraph /āpek′sigraf′/, a dental device used to find the position of the apex of a tooth root.

apex pulmonis /pəlmō′nis/, the rounded upper border of each lung that rises above the collar bone into the root of the neck.

Apgar score /ap′gär/, a test to determine a newborn baby's physical health. It is done 1 minute and 5 minutes after birth. Scoring is based on a rating of five factors that refer to how well the infant is able to adjust to life outside the womb. A doctor, Virginia Apgar, MD, created the system to tell quickly which infants require treatment right away or transfer to an intensive care nursery.

★METHOD: The infant's heart rate, breathing, muscle tone, reflexes, and color are scored from a low value of 0 to a normal value of 2. The five scores are combined, and the totals at 1 minute and 5 minutes are written. For example, Apgar 9/10 is a score of 9 at 1 minute and 10 at 5 minutes.

★NURSING CARE: A low 1-minute score requires on-the-spot treatment, oxygen is given, the nose and throat are cleared of mucus, and the infant may be transferred to an intensive

Infant evaluation at birth – Apgar scoring system

	0	1	2
Heart rate	Absent	Slow (below 100 beats/minute)	Over 100 beats/min
Respiratory effort	Absent	Slow or irregular	Good crying
Muscle tone	Limp	Some flexion of extremities	Active motion
Response to catheter in nostril (tested after oropharynx is clear)	No response	Grimace	Cough or sneeze
Color	Blue or pale	Body pink, extremities blue	Completely pink

care nursery. A baby with a low score after 5 minutes needs expert care. This may include assisted breathing, putting in a catheter, heart massage, or drugs.

★OUTCOME: A score of 0 to 3 is given to infants with severe distress, a score of 4 to 7 means moderate distress, and a score of 7 to 10 is normal. About 50% of infants with 5-minute scores of 0 to 1 die, and infants that survive have three times as many defects at 1 year of age as at birth.

APHA, short for **American Public Health Association.**

aphagia /əfā′j·ə/, loss of the ability to swallow, either from disease or mental causes. See also **dysphagia.**

aphagia algera, the refusal to eat or swallow due to pain caused by swallowing.

aphakia /əfā′kē·ə/, a state in which part or all of the lens of the eye is missing. This is usually because it has been removed, as in the treatment of cataracts.

aphasia /əfā′zhə/, a nerve defect in which there are problems with speaking or speech is lost. It is due to an injury to certain areas of the brain. There are many forms and degrees of aphasia. For example, a patient with aphasia may be able to speak but not to form words that can be understood. The patient may be able to understand speech and writing and form thoughts but not be able to speak. Aphasia may be the result of a severe head injury, lack of oxygen, or stroke. It is sometimes short term, as when a swelling in the brain goes down and language returns. Constant hard work and practice by the patient and the patient's family have helped to restore normal speaking ability. See also **Broca's area.**

aphemia /əfē′mē·ə/, a loss of the ability to speak. It can be caused by physical or emotional problems.

apheresis, a procedure in which blood is removed from a patient, one or more elements are removed, and the rest of the blood is returned to the patient. Apheresis is used to treat certain diseases. It is also used to get blood elements to treat other patients or for research purposes. Also called **pheresis.** See also **leukapheresis, plasmapheresis, plateletpheresis.**

aphonia /āfō′nē·ə/, a defect in which the patient is not able to make normal speech sounds. Aphonia is caused by overuse of the vocal cords, disease, or mental upset, as hysteria. See also **speech dysfunction. –aphonic, aphonous,** adj.

aphonia clericorum, loss of the voice from overuse.

aphonia paralytica /par′əlit′ikə/, loss of the voice caused by paralysis or disease of the nerves in the throat.

aphonia paranoica, a loss of speech functions that has no physical cause. This defect is common in some forms of mental illness.

aphonic speech /āfon′ik/, a speech defect in which everything is whispered.

aphoria /əfôr′ē·ə/, a condition in which physical weakness is not improved by exercise.

aphrasia /əfā′zhə/, a form of a nerve defect (aphasia) in which there are problems with speaking. A person may be able to speak or understand single words but not communicate in meaningful phrases or sentences.

-aphrodisia, a combining form meaning a state of sexual arousal.

aphronia /əfrō′nē·ə/, a state in which the patient is not able to make common sense decisions. **–aphronic,** n., adj.

aphthous fever. See **foot-and-mouth disease.**

aphthous stomatitis /af′thəs/, a condition that happens over and over again in which there are painful canker sores on the mucous membranes of the mouth. The cause is unknown, but aphthous stomatitis may be an immune response. See also **canker sore.**

apical /ap′ikəl, ā′pi-/, 1. referring to the top or apex. 2. referring to the end of a tooth root.

apical curettage, the surgical removal of the top (apex) of a tooth root. Also called **root amputation, root resection.** Compare **root curettage, subgingival curettage.**

apical fiber, any one of the many fibers of the ligament in the gum tissue around the teeth (periodontal ligament). They go from tooth to bone.

apical lordotic view, an x-ray made by positioning the patient leaning backward at an angle of about 45 degrees.

apical odontoid ligament, a ligament that connects the spine to the skull.

apical pulse, the heart beat as heard with a stethoscope placed over the top (apex), or pointed lower part, of the heart.

apicectomy /ap′isek′təmē/, the surgical removal of the top part of the root of a tooth. It is usually done along with root canal therapy. Also called root amputation, root resection.

aplasia /əplā′zhə/, 1. a defect in the growth of the fetus that causes a missing organ or tissue. 2. a failure of the normal process of blood cell production and growth. See also **aplastic anemia, hyperplasia.**

aplasia cutis congenita, absence at birth of a small area of skin. The defect occurs mainly on the scalp but sometimes on the limbs and trunk. The area may be covered by a thin membrane or scar tissue, or it may be raw and covered with sores. The defect is inherited.

aplastic, referring to the absence or defective growth of a tissue or organ.

aplastic anemia, a blood defect in which the bone marrow can no longer make blood cells.

It may be caused by cancer of the bone marrow, or by contact with poisonous chemicals, radiation, or antibiotics or other drugs. Compare **alymphocytosis, hemolytic anemia, hypoplastic anemia.** See also **aleukia, leukopenia.**

apnea /apnē′ə, ap′nē·ə/, an absence of automatic breathing. Kinds of apnea include **cardiac apnea, central sleep apnea, deglutition apnea, periodic apnea of the newborn, primary apnea, reflex apnea, secondary apnea.** –**apneic,** *adj.*

apneustic breathing, a pattern of breathing in which the person breathes in for a long time and then fails to breathe out. The rate of apneustic breathing is usually around 1.5 cycles per minute.

apocrine gland, one of the large, deep glands that are in the armpit, anal, genital, and breast areas of the body. The apocrine glands become active only after puberty, and they release sweat that has a strong, easy to identify odor. Compare **eccrine gland.** See also **exocrine gland.**

apodial symmelia. See **sirenomelia.**

apoenzyme, an enzyme without any or with less than the entire amount of cofactors.

apolipoprotein, the protein part of lipoprotein complexes.

aponeurosis /ap′ōnŏōrō′sis/, *pl.* **aponeuroses,** a strong sheet of fiberlike tissue that attaches muscles to bone (tendon) or holds muscles together (fascia).

aponeurosis of the obliquus externus abdominis, the strong membrane that covers the entire surface of the belly. It lies on top of the rectus abdominis muscles.

apophyseal /ap′əfiz′ē·əl/, referring to the part near the end of a long bone that is enlarged and somewhat uneven.

apophyseal fracture /ap′əfiz′ē·əl/, a break that separates an outgrowth (apophysis) of a bone from the main bone tissue at a point where a tendon attaches.

apophysis /əpof′i·sis/, any small projection or outgrowth, usually on a bone.

apophysitis /əpof′əsī′tis/, a state in which the outgrowth (apophysis) of a bone becomes inflamed.

apoplexy /ap′əplek′sē/, *obsolete.* a stroke that results in paralysis.

apothecaries' measure /əpoth′əker′ēz/, a system of liquid measurements. It was first based on the minim, equal to one drop of water. It has now been set at 0.06 ml. The measures are 60 minims equal 1 fluid dram, 8 fluid drams equal 1 fluid ounce, 16 fluid ounces equal 1 pint, 2 pints equal 1 quart, 4 quarts equal 1 gallon. See also **apothecaries' weight, metric system.**

apothecaries' weight, a system of weights. The system was based on the weight of a plump grain of wheat. It is now set at 65 mg. The weights are 20 grains equal 1 scruple, 3 scruples equal 1 dram, 8 drams equal 1 ounce, 12 ounces equal 1 pound. Compare **avoirdupois weight.** See also **apothecaries' measure, metric system.**

apparatus, a device or a system made of different parts that act as one to do a special function.

apparent death. See **death.**

appendage, an extra piece that is attached to a part or organ. Also called **appendix.**

appendectomy /ap′əndek′təmē/, removal of the appendix through a cut in the right lower part of the belly. It is done in acute appendicitis to take out a swollen appendix before it breaks open. Often it is done with other surgery of the belly region. Unless the appendix has burst and infection has set in, care of the patient is routine. If the appendix has burst, a drain may be left in the cut, dressings are changed more often, and drugs are given. The pain may be severe. Fluids through the vein, sedatives, and narcotic painkillers are given. See also **abdominal surgery, peritonitis.**

appendicitis /əpen′disī′tis/, inflammation of the appendix, usually severe, which if not dealt with leads to a break and infection (peritonitis). The most common symptom is constant pain in the right lower part of the belly. To help the pain, the patient keeps the knees bent. Symptoms are vomiting, a low-grade fever of 99° to 102° F, tenderness, a rigid belly, and fewer or no bowel sounds. The problem is caused by a blockage at the opening of the appendix, disease of the bowel wall, an adhesion, or a parasite. Treatment involves taking out the appendix within 24 to 48 hours of the first symptoms. Delay usually results in break and infection as feces can get in the belly. The fever rises when infection begins. The patient may have sudden relief from pain followed by more, widespread pain. Appendicitis occurs most often in young adults and more often in males. A kind of appendicitis is **chronic appendicitis.** See also **peritonitis.**

appendix dyspepsia, trouble with digestion caused by long-term appendicitis. See also **dyspepsia.**

appendix epididymidis, a lump (cyst) sometimes found on the tube for sperm (epididymis) near the testicles.

appendix epiploica, *pl.* **appendices epiploicae,** one of the fat pads, ¾ to 4 inches (2 to 10 cm long), found in the membrane lining the belly (peritoneum), along the large intestine, and at the upper part of the rectum.

appendix vermiformis. See **vermiform appendix.**

apperception, a way of learning based on a person's experiences. –**apperceptive,** *adj.*

appliance, something made for a set purpose, as a dental device.

applied anatomy, the study of the structure of the organs of the body as it relates to disease. Also called **practical anatomy.** Types are pathologic anatomy, radiologic anatomy, surgical anatomy. See also comparative anatomy.

applied chemistry, the practical use of the study of chemical elements and compounds.

applied psychology, a practical use of psychology, as clinical psychology, child psychology, industrial psychology, educational psychology.

apposition, the placing of objects very close together, as in the layering of tissue cells.

appositional growth, an increase in size caused by new tissue at the edge of a part or structure, as in new layers in bone. Compare interstitial growth.

approach-approach conflict, a conflict caused by the need to choose between two or more things that are wanted.

approach-avoidance conflict, a conflict caused by something that is both wanted and not wanted.

appropriate for gestational age (AGA) infant, a newborn whose size and growth are normal for the pregnancy.

approximation, (in psychiatry) the movement of one individual toward another in the development of a relationship.

approximator, a medical instrument used to pull together the edges of tissues that have been separated, as in closing a wound or repairing a fractured rib.

apraxia /əprak′sē·ə/, loss of the ability to do simple or routine acts. This involves the nervous system. It occurs in many forms. Ideational apraxia is a failure to understand the use of an object. Motor apraxia is an inability to use an object or perform a task needing a certain arm or leg muscle. Amnestic apraxia is an inability to do something because of forgetting the command. Apraxia of speech is caused by brain damage. The person is unable to control the speech muscles and cannot speak understandably. –apraxic, adj.

Apresoline Hydrochloride, a trademark for a drug used to treat high blood pressure (hydralazine hydrochloride).

aprosody /āpros′odē/, a speech defect. There are no normal changes in pitch, sound, and rhythm.

aprosopia /āprəsō′pē·ə/, a birth defect. Part or all of the face is missing. There are usually other defects.

aptitude, a natural talent to learn or know a skill.

aptitude test, any standard test to check a person's ability to learn certain skills. Compare achievement test, intelligence test, personality test, psychologic test.

AQ, short for achievement quotient.

aqua amnii. See amniotic fluid.

AquaMEPHYTON, a trademark for vitamin K. It is used to treat blood clotting and other blood problems (phytonadione).

aqueduct, any canal, channel, or passage through or between body parts.

aqueous /ā′kwē·əs, ak′wē·əs/, 1. watery or waterlike. 2. a drug made with water. See also aqueous humor.

aqueous humor, the clear, watery fluid that moves in the eyeball.

Ar, symbol for argon.

Ara-A. See vidarabine.

arabinosylcytosine. See cytarabine.

arachidonic acid /ar′əkidon′ik/, an essential fatty acid in lecithin. It is a building block of some prostaglandins.

arachnodactyly /ərak′nōdak′tilē/, a birth defect. One has long, thin, spiderlike fingers and toes. It is seen in Marfan's syndrome.

arachnoid /ərak′noid/, a fiberlike structure like a spiderweb, as the arachnoid membrane. – arachnoidal, adj.

arachnoidea spinalis, the arachnoid membrane of the brain that covers the spinal cord to its base. It also has branches that cover the nerves as they pass through the holes between the back bones. Also called arachnoid of the spinal cord, spinal arachnoid.

arachnoid membrane, one of the three thin membranes covering the brain and the spinal cord. Also called arachnoid.

arachnoid of the spinal cord. See arachnoidea spinalis.

Aramine, a trademark for a drug used for severe, life-threatening high blood pressure (metaraminol bitartrate).

Aran-Duchenne muscular atrophy /aran′dōōshen′/, a form of breakdown of the nerves in the muscles (amyotrophic lateral sclerosis). It affects the hands, arms, shoulders, and legs in the beginning. It later spreads throughout the body. Also called progressive spinal muscular atrophy.

arbitrary interference, a faulty thought process in which a judgment based on insufficient evidence leads to an incorrect conclusion.

arbitrator, an impartial person who must settle a disagreement between people.

arborization test. See ferning test.

arbovirus /är′bōvī′rəs/, any one of more than 300 viruses carried by insects. These viruses cause infections. The infections are marked by two or more of the following: fever, rash, brain swelling, and bleeding into the internal organs or skin. Yellow fever, and swelling of the brain and spinal cord are two common arboviral infections. There are vaccines that prevent infection from some arboviruses.

ARC, abbreviation for AIDS-related complex.

arch, any structure that is curved or has a bow-like appearance. Also called arcus.

arch bar, any one of many types of wires, bars or splints that are shaped like the arch of the teeth. They are used to treat broken jaws and to make stable injured teeth.

archenteric canal. See **neurenteric canal.**

archenteron, *pl.* **archentera,** the simple digestive cavity formed in the early fetus (embryo) of many animals.

archetype /är′kətīp′/, **1.** an original model or pattern from which something is made. **2.** a Jungian mental concept of an inherited idea or way of thinking that comes from the experiences of the human race. It is present in the unconscious of a person in the form of drives, moods, and concepts. See also **anima.**

archinephric canal. See **pronephric duct.**

archinephron. See **pronephros.**

architectural barriers, structural features of homes and public buildings that prevent or limit disabled persons from entering or moving around inside. For example, a person in a wheelchair needs a ramp, doorways at least 32 inches wide, a space at least 60 inches by 60 inches for wheelchair turns, and counters no more than 26.5 inches above floor level.

arch length, the length of the arch of the teeth. This is usually measured through the points of contact between joining teeth.

arch length deficiency, the difference in a dental arch between the length needed to allow room for all of the natural teeth and the actual space available.

arch of the aorta, one of the four parts of the large artery of the heart (aorta). Also called **aortic arch.**

arch width, the width of a dental arch. It is determined by measuring between the canine teeth, the first molars, and the second premolars.

arch wire, a wire fastened to two or more teeth through fixed attachments. It is used to guide tooth movement.

arcing spring contraceptive diaphragm /är′king/, a kind of flexible disk for birth control that fits against the lower end of the uterus (cervix). It has a flexible metal spring that forms the rim. The spring is a combination of a flexible coil spring and a flat band spring of stainless steel. This kind of diaphragm is given for a patient whose vagina muscles are relaxed and will not afford strong support. This is a common problem in patients whose bladder or rectum pushes through the vagina (cystocele and rectocele). It is also a common problem in patients whose uterus has sagged into the vagina (uterine prolapse). If the uterus is in an abnormal position, the arcing spring may offer better protection than the coil or flat spring. It is stronger and better able to hold the diaphragm in place. It is less likely to slip out of position in the vagina, thereby leaving the narrow lower end of the uterus (cervix) exposed. Many women who have had a vaginal childbirth are fitted with an arcing spring diaphragm. The reason is that some loss of vaginal muscle strength commonly occurs. An unusually long or short vagina or a vagina of unusual form is often best fitted with an arcing spring diaphragm. Compare **coil spring contraceptive diaphragm, flat spring contraceptive diaphragm.** See also **contraceptive diaphragm fitting.**

arcuate scotoma /är′kyo͞o·at/, a blind area in the shape of an arc that may develop in the field of vision of a person with glaucoma. It is caused by damage to nerve fibers in the retina.

arcus senilis, a dull-looking ring, gray to white in color, that surrounds the edges of the cornea in the eye. The condition is caused by deposits of fat in the cornea or by breakdown of tissue. It occurs mainly in older persons. Also called **gerontoxon.**

ARDS, 1. abbreviation for **adult respiratory distress syndrome. 2.** abbreviation for **acute respiratory distress syndrome.**

area, a space that contains a specific structure of the body or within which certain functions take place. For example, the aortic area is the space around the large heart artery.

area under the concentration curve (AUC), a method of measurement of the amount of a drug available to the target tissue based on a plot of blood concentrations sampled at frequent intervals. It is directly proportional to the total amount of unaltered drug in the patient's blood.

areflexia /ā′rēflek′sē·ə/, a condition of the nervous system in which the reflexes are missing.

Arenavirus /ar′inəvī′rəs/, a genus of viruses usually carried to humans by mouth or skin contact with the waste matter of wild rodents. Individual arenaviruses are linked to geographic areas, where they occur. For example, **Bolivian hemorrhagic fever** occurs in one river valley in Bolivia. **Lassa fever** occurs in Nigeria, Liberia, and Sierra Leone. **Argentine hemorrhagic fever** is limited to two farm provinces in Argentina. The symptoms are fever, muscle pain, rash, bleeding, mental confusion, low blood pressure, and ulcers of the mouth. There is no specific drug or vaccine.

areola /arē′ōlə/, *pl.* **areolae, 1.** a small space or a cavity within a tissue. **2.** a circular area of a different color surrounding a feature, as the discolored skin around a lesion with pus (pustule). **3.** the part of the iris around the pupil.

areola mammae /mam′ē/, the colored, circular area around the nipple of each breast. Also called **areola papillaris.**

areolar gland /arē′ələr/, one of the large oil glands in the parts (areolae) around the nipples on the breasts of women. The areolar glands give off an oily fluid that protects the nipple during nursing. They have bundles of muscles that cause the nipples to become erect when aroused. Also called **gland of Montgomery.**

Arfonad, a trademark for a drug used to control high blood pressure (trimethaphan camsylate).

Arg, abbreviation for **arginine.**

argentaffin cell /är'jentaf'in/, a cell that gives off serotonin. Serotonin is a chemical that narrows blood vessels. These cells occur in most parts of the stomach and intestines. Also called **enterochromaffin cell, Kulchitsky's cell.** See also **carcinoid, carcinoid syndrome.**

argentaffinoma /är'jentaf'inō'mə/, a cancerlike tumor growing from argentaffin cells in the stomach and intestines. The tumor occurs chiefly in middle-aged or elderly patients. It may begin as a small raised area in the early stage, surrounding the bowel later.

Argentine hemorrhagic fever, an infectious disease. It is caused by an arenavirus carried to humans through the feces of rodents. The early symptoms are chills, fever, headache, aching muscles, loss of appetite, nausea, vomiting, and weakness. As the disease continues, the patient may get high fever, loss of body fluids, falling blood pressure, and flushed skin. Abnormally slow heart beat, bleeding from the gums and internal tissues, and blood in the urine may also occur. Nervous system disorders, shock, and fluid in the lungs may occur as well. There is no specific treatment for the disease other than fluids, rest, warmth, and a balanced diet. See also **arenavirus, Bolivian hemorrhagic fever, Lassa fever.**

arginine (Arg), an amino acid made by the digestion of proteins. It can also be made artificially. Certain compounds made from arginine, especially arginine glutamate and arginine hydrochloride, are used to treat excess ammonia in the blood because of liver disease. See also **urea cycle.**

argininemia /är'jininē'mē·ə/, an inherited disorder with an increased amount of arginine in the blood. It is caused by a lack of an enzyme (arginase). Without arginase, ammonia cannot be changed into urea. Partial lack may result in ammonia in the blood, convulsions, a large liver, mental retardation, and growth failure. Complete absence of arginase causes death.

argininosuccinic acidemia, an inherited metabolism disorder. Symptoms include seizures and mental retardation. Treatment involves mainly a low-protein diet containing essential amino acids or amino acid analogs.

argon (Ar), a colorless, odorless, chemically inactive gas. It is one of the six rare gases in the atmosphere. Its atomic weight is 39.95; its atomic number is 18.

Argyll-Robertson pupil, a pupil of the eye that narrows when focused for near vision but not in response to light. It is most often seen with syphilis, which affects the nervous system.

ariboflavinosis /ārī'bōflā'vinō'sis/, a condition caused by lack of vitamin B_2 in the diet. The symptoms are sores at the corners of the mouth, on the lips, and around the nose and eyes. Other symptoms are scaling of the skin (seborrheic dermatitis) and many vision disorders. See also **riboflavin.**

Arica therapy, a mental-health treatment that focuses on altered states of consciousness. Its goal is to increase the powers of the mind.

Aristocort, a trademark for a steroid drug (triamcinolone). The tablets, syrup, and injections are used for severe allergies, rheumatic diseases, and other severe diseases. The cream and ointment are used for swelling of the skin (dermatitis).

–arit-, a combining form referring to a drug used to treat any of the many swelling conditions (rheumatism) of the bursae, joints, ligaments, or muscles.

arithmetic/logic unit (ALU), the part of a computer that calculates, compares, and performs logical operations.

arithmetic mean. See **mean,** def. 2.

Arlidin, a trademark for a drug that widens blood vessels. It is used for diseases of the circulation (nylidrin hydrochloride).

arm, 1. the part of the upper limb of the body between shoulder and elbow. The bone of the arm is the humerus. The muscles of the arm are the coracobrachialis, the biceps brachii, the brachialis, and the triceps brachii. The nerves are the ulnar nerve and the radial nerve. Blood is supplied by many arteries, as the brachial artery and the radial collateral artery. **2.** *nontechnical.* the arm and the forearm.

arm bone. See **humerus.**

arm cylinder cast, a cast made of plaster of Paris or fiberglass. It is used for keeping rigid the arm from the wrist to above the elbow. It is most often applied to aid the healing of a dislocated elbow or to correct a defect of the elbow.

armpit. See **axilla.**

Arnold-Chiari malformation /är'nəldkē·är'ē/, an inborn bulging (herniation) of the brain stem and lower lobe of the brain (cerebellum) through the base of the skull into the spinal canal. This defect often occurs with brain and spine disorders (meningocele and spina bifida). See also **neural tube defect.**

–arol, a combining form referring to a certain type of drug (anticoagulant) used to prevent blood from clotting.

aroma, any agreeable odor, especially of food, drink, spices, or flavored drug.

aromatic bath, a bath with drugs in which aromatic substances or needed oils are added to the water.

array processor, a part of a computer system that organizes huge amounts of data so that it can be handled more easily by the host computer. They are contained in computerized tomography (CT) equipment to reduce the time needed to complete an image.

arrest, to inhibit, restrain, or stop. For example, to arrest the course of a disease. See also **cardiac arrest.**

arrested dental caries, dental decay (caries) that has stopped developing. The demineralized area in the tooth remains as a cavity.

arrested development, fetal development that stops. This results in birth defects. Also called **developmental arrest.**

arrheno-, a combining form meaning "male."

arrhenoblastoma /ərē′nōblastō′mə/, a tumor of the ovary whose cells release male sex hormone. This causes a woman to develop male characteristics, as deep voice and body hair. Also called **andreioma, andreoblastoma, androma, arrhenoma, Sertoli-Leydig cell tumor.**

arrhenogenic /arē′nōjen′ik/, making only male offspring.

arrhenokaryon /arē′nōkar′ē·on/, an organism that is made from an egg that has chromosomes only from the father.

arrhythmia /ərith′mē·ə, ərith′mē·ə/, any change in the normal pattern of the heart beat. Kinds of arrhythmias include **atrial fibrillation, atrial flutter, heart block, premature atrial contraction, sinus arrhythmia.** Also spelled **arhythmia.** Compare **dysrhythmia.** See also **antiarrhythmia.** –**arrhythmic, arrhythmical,** *adj*.

ARRT, abbreviation for **American Registry of Radiologic Technologists.**

arsenic (As) /är′sənik/, an element that occurs throughout the earth's crust in metal arsenides, arsenious sulfides, and arsenious oxides. Its atomic number is 33; its atomic weight is 74.91. This element has been used for centuries as a drug and as a poison. It continues to have limited use in some drugs used to treat tropical disease (trypanosomiasis), as melarsoprol and tryparsamide. The introduction of drugs without arsenic that have less dangerous side effects has greatly reduced its use. The large amount of arsenic in the world places it in the food chain. Many compounds with arsenic are used as dyes, pesticides, herbicides, and feed additives for poultry and livestock. Fruit, vegetables, fish, and shellfish have significant concentrations of arsenic. The average daily human consumption of this element is about 900 micrograms. Most is consumed in food and water. The average concentration in the human adult is about 20 mg. It is stored mainly in the liver, the kidney, the stomach and intestines, and the lungs. Small amounts are found in the muscles and nerves. Long-term exposure to inorganic arsenic may cause severe damage to the lining of the stomach and intestines, kidneys, nervous system, bone marrow, liver, and blood system. Small doses of inorganic arsenic cause mild widening of the blood vessels. Larger doses lead to widening of the blood capillaries, heart disorders, and smaller blood volume. Studies show a strong link between the amount and length of time of arsenic exposure and lung cancer in metal workers. Federal laws on arsenic levels in food and industry have greatly lessened the number of arsenic poisonings. –**arsenic** /ärsen′ik/, **arsenical,** *adj*.

arsenical stomatitis, a mouth condition linked to arsenic poisoning. The symptoms are dry, red, and painful mucous membrane in the mouth, ulcers, bleeding gums, and loose teeth. Compare **Atabrine stomatitis, bismuth stomatitis.** See also **arsenic poisoning.**

arsenic poisoning, poisoning caused by eating or breathing arsenic. Small amounts absorbed over a period of time may result in long-term poisoning. Nausea, headache, coloring and scaling of the skin, thickened skin, loss of desire for food, and white lines across the fingernails are symptoms of long-term poisoning. Consuming large amounts of arsenic results in severe stomach and intestine pain, diarrhea, vomiting, and swelling of the feet and hands. Kidney failure and shock may occur. Death may result. Diagnosis is confirmed when arsenic is found in the urine, hair, or fingernails. Treatment includes flushing the stomach with water and giving the drug dimercaprol. Fluids given in the veins and other treatment as needed for anemia, kidney failure, or shock, are also given.

ART, abbreviation for **active resistance training.**

Artane, a trademark for a drug used to treat parkinsonism (trihexyphenidyl hydrochloride).

arteria alveolaris inferior. See **inferior alveolar artery.**

arterial, referring to an artery.

arterial blood gas, the oxygen and carbon dioxide in the blood of arteries. This is measured by many methods to see whether oxygen intake and distribution is normal and whether the acid-base status (pH) is adequate. The oxygen content of arterial blood becomes less in lifelong obstructive lung disease, chest deformities, and some muscle diseases. Overweight, breathing diseases have the same effect. Abnormal oxygen pressures are seen in excess red blood cells (polycythemia), hyperventilation, anemias, heart failure, long-term obstructive lung disease, and certain muscle disorders. The carbon dioxide content is increased in shortness of breath (emphysema), excess aldosterone (aldosteronism), and severe vomiting. It is decreased in starvation, acute kidney failure, acid pooling caused by diabetes (diabetic acidosis), and severe diarrhea. The normal pH of arterial blood is 7.40.

arterial circle of Willis, a group of arteries at the base of the brain. It is formed by the front and back brain arteries and branches of the inner carotid and the basilar arteries. These three arterial trunks supply the two lobes of the brain.

arterial insufficiency, lack of enough blood flow in arteries. It is caused by cholesterol deposits (atherosclerosis) or clots (emboli), and by damaged, diseased, or weak vessels. Other causes are an abnormal connection between an artery and a vein (fistula), bulging artery walls (aneurysms), clotting problems, or heavy use of tobacco. Signs of arterial insufficiency include pale, bluish, or spotted skin over the affected area. Numbness, tingling, loss of a sense of temperature, muscle pains, and reduced or absent pulses are also seen. In advanced disease, weakness of muscles of the arms or legs occurs. The disorder may be diagnosed by checking pulses, by x-ray tests of blood vessels (angiography), by ultrasound, by blood studies, and by skin temperature tests. Normally placing an arm in hot water increases the skin temperature of the opposite arm. This usually does not occur in arterial disease. Placing the patient's hand in ice water raises the blood pressure greatly. In the normal individual the blood pressure increases only slightly. Treatment of arterial insufficiency may include a diet low in saturated fats, moderate exercise, and sleeping on a firm mattress. Surgery and the use of drugs to widen the blood vessels are two additional treatments.

arterial pressure, the stress placed on the walls of the arteries by the flow of blood. The amount of arterial pressure is the product of how much blood the heart pumps and the resistance in the blood vessels. Arterial blood pressure is commonly measured with a blood pressure cuff (sphygmomanometer) and stethoscope. Stress, high blood volume, low blood volume, and many drugs may alter the arterial pressure. See also **afterload blood pressure.**

arterial wall, the fiberlike wall of the vessels that move blood with oxygen from the heart to structures throughout the body. The arteries, like the veins, are cylindric tubes. They are enclosed by three layers of tissue: the inner layer (tunica intima), the middle layer (tunica media), which makes up most of the arterial wall, and the outer layer (tunica adventitia). The middle layer in smaller arteries is almost entirely muscular. It is more elastic in larger arteries. The thickness of the outer layer changes with the location of the artery. In protected areas, as the stomach and skull, the outer layer of the arteries is very thin. In more exposed locations, as in the limbs, it is much thicker. Larger arteries have a thick inner layer. In older patients the layer may have deposits of cholesterol and calcium salts or other deposits. See also **artery.**

arteriogram /ärtir′ē·əgram′/, an x-ray film of an artery that has been injected with a dye. See also **angiography.** –**arteriographic,** *adj.*

arteriole /ärtir′ē·ōl/, any one of the tiny vessels of the arterial circulation. Blood flowing from the heart is pumped through the arteries to the arterioles, which form part of the capillaries. The blood flows from the capillaries into the veins and returns to the heart. The muscular wall of the arterioles narrows and widens in response to chemicals made by the nerves. Thus, arterioles play an important role in blood vessel resistance and in controlling blood pressure. See also **artery.**

arteriosclerosis, a common disorder of the arteries. It is marked by thickening, loss of elasticity, and hardening of the walls through calcium. This results in less blood supply, especially to the brain and legs. The condition often develops with aging. It also often occurs with high blood pressure, kidney disease, hardening of the connective tissues (scleroderma), diabetes, and excess of lipids in the blood (hyperlipidemia). Symptoms include leg cramps when walking (intermittent claudication), changes in skin temperature and color, altered pulses, headache, dizziness, and memory defects. Drugs to widen the blood vessels and exercise to stimulate circulation may relieve symptoms of arteriosclerosis. However, there is no specific treatment for the disorder. Kinds of arteriosclerosis are **atherosclerosis, Mönckeberg's arteriosclerosis.**

arteriovenous /ärtir′ē·ōvē′nəs/, referring to arteries and veins.

arteriovenous angioma of the brain, an inborn tumor. It is made up of a tangle of coiled, usually widened arteries and veins, and areas of hardened brain tissue. The tumor may grow deeply into the brain, causing seizures and paralysis.

arteriovenous fistula, an abnormal communication between an artery and vein. It can occur from a birth defect, injury, infection, bulge in an artery wall (aneurysm), or a cancer. An arteriovenous fistula is often made by surgery. It gives access to the bloodstream of patients receiving dialysis.

arteriovenous oxygen (a-vo₂) difference, the amount of oxygen in the arteries minus the amount of oxygen in the central veins.

arteritis /är′tərī′tis/, a swelling condition of the walls of one or more arteries. It may occur as a disease in itself. It also may go together with another disorder, as rheumatoid arthritis and rheumatic fever.

arteritis obliterans. See **Friedländer's disease.**

arteritis umbilicalis, a swelling of the umbilical artery in newborn infants. It is usually caused by the bacteria *Clostridium tetani.*

artery, any one of the large blood vessels carrying blood with oxygen from the heart to the rest of the body. The artery is a hollow tube enclosed by three layers of tissue. Most of the arteries in the body are about ³⁄₁₆ inch (4 mm) in diameter. The muscle walls of arteries keep the blood moving away from the heart and nerves that supply the arteries direct the flow of blood. See also **arteriole, arterial wall.**

artery forceps, any tongs (forceps) used for grasping, pressing together, and holding the end of an artery during surgery. Generally self-locking, its handles are scissorlike. Also called **hemostatic forceps.**

arthr-, arthro-, a combining form referring to a joint.

arthralgia /ärthral'jē·ə/, any pain that affects a joint. **–arthralgic,** *adj.*

arthritis /ärthrī'tis/, any swelling of the joints, marked by pain and swelling. See also **osteoarthritis, rheumatoid arthritis.**

arthritis deformans. See **rheumatoid arthritis.**

arthrocentesis /är'thrōsintē'sis/, puncturing a joint with a needle and withdrawing fluid (synovial fluid) from the joint. Arthrocentesis is done to get samples of synovial fluid for diag-

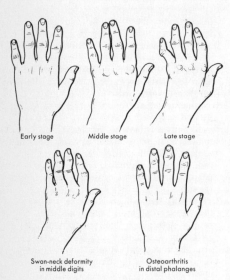

Early stage   Middle stage   Late stage

Swan-neck deformity   Osteoarthritis
in middle digits   in distal phalanges

Arthritic deformities

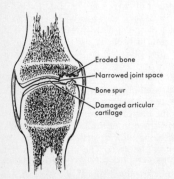

Eroded bone
Narrowed joint space
Bone spur
Damaged articular cartilage

Arthritis: joint changes

nosis. A local anesthetic is usually given first. Normal synovial fluid is a clear, straw-colored, slightly thick liquid. If swelling is present, as in rheumatoid arthritis, the fluid is watery and cloudy. Synovial fluid samples are also cultured. Examination with a microscope then is done to diagnose an infection of the joints.

arthrodesis. See **ankylosis,** def. 2.

arthrodia. See **gliding joint.**

arthrogram /är'thrəgram/, an x-ray film of a joint after the injection of a dye that illuminates inner structures.

arthrogryposis multiplex congenita, stiffness of one or more joints that is present at birth. It is often linked to incomplete growth of the muscles that move the joints. It is also linked to the breakdown of the nerves that supply those muscles. Physical therapy to loosen the joints is the only treatment.

arthrokinematic /är'thrəkin'əmat'ik/, referring to the movement of joint surfaces.

arthron /är'thron/, a joint, including all of its parts and the muscles next to it.

arthropathy /ärthrop'əthē/, any disease or abnormal condition affecting a joint.

arthroplasty /är'thrəplast'ē/, the surgical reconstruction or replacement of a painful, broken-down joint. Arthroplasty gives again movement to a joint in joint disease (osteoarthritis and rheumatoid arthritis). It can correct an inborn defect. Two basic types of arthroplasty are: (1) The bones of the joint are reshaped and soft tissue or a metal disk is placed between the reshaped ends. (2) All or part of the joint is replaced with a metal or plastic joint. See also **osteoarthritis.**

arthropod /är'thrəpod'/, a member of the Arthropoda, a large major group of animal life that includes crabs and lobsters, mites, ticks, spiders, and insects. Arthropods generally have a jointed shell (exoskeleton) and paired, jointed legs. They bite, sting, and cause allergic reactions. They carry viruses and other disease-causing organisms.

arthroscopy /ärthros'kəpē/, examination of the interior of a joint. It is done by putting a specially designed microscope-like device (endoscope) through a small cut. The procedure is used chiefly in knee problems. Arthroscopy permits removal of cartilage or fluid from the joint (synovial fluid), the diagnosis of a torn meniscus, and the removal of loose bodies in the joint space. **–arthroscopic,** *adj.*

Arthus reaction /är'tōōs/, a rare, severe, direct allergic reaction to injection of a foreign substance (allergen). The allergen usually is not harmful. However, in certain individuals it causes a reaction. A sudden local swelling reaction with bleeding, and tissue death occurs at the site of injection. See also **serum sickness.**

articul-, a combining form referring to a joint.

articular capsule, an envelope of tissue that surrounds a joint. It is made up of an outer layer of white fiberlike tissue and an inner synovial membrane. See also **fibrous capsule.**

articular disk, the platelike end of certain bones in movable joints. It is sometimes closely linked to surrounding muscles or with cartilage.

articular fracture, a broken bone involving the articular surfaces of a joint.

articulatio cubiti. See **elbow joint.**

articulatio ellipsoidea. See **condyloid joint.**

articulatio genus. See **knee joint.**

articulation. See **joint.**

articulation of the pelvis, any one of the connections between the bones of the pelvis.

articulatio plana. See **gliding joint.**

articulatio sellaris. See **saddle joint.**

articulator, a dental device used to make and test dentures. It represents the jaw hinge (temperomandibular joints). Upper jaw (maxillary) and lower jaw (mandibular) casts may be attached to it. Some articulators are adjustable. They allow movement of attached casts in many relationships.

artifact, anything irrelevant or unwanted, as a substance, structure, or piece of information. In x-ray films electronic signals may appear as an artifact on an image, thereby confusing the results of any examination.

artificial airway, a plastic or rubber device that can be inserted into the breathing (respiratory) tract to promote breathing or to remove substances (secretions).

artificial blood. See **perfluorocarbons.**

artificial classification cavity, any tooth decay (cavity) that may be classified in one of six groups. Class 1: cavities linked to structural tooth defects, as pits and fissures. Class 2: cavities in the sides of premolars and molars. Class 3: cavities in the sides of the canines and incisors that do not interfere with the edge of the tooth. Class 4: cavities in the sides of canines and molars that require restoring the edge of the tooth. Class 5: cavities, except pit cavities, near the gum. Class 6: cavities on the edges and cusp tips of the teeth.

artificial crown, a dental device (prosthesis) that restores part or all of the crown part of a natural tooth.

artificial fever, a higher body temperature caused by artificial means. Injecting malarial parasites, a vaccine that causes fever, or applying heat to the body will produce this condition. An artificial fever may be given to a patient to stop a disease that is sensitive to higher body temperatures. Also called **fever therapy.**

artificial heart, a mechanical device of molded polyurethane. It is made up of two chambers implanted in the body and powered by an air compressor outside the body. Mechanical hearts have been tested on animals since 1957. The first artificial heart for humans was implanted in December 1982. The patient was a retired dentist at the University of Utah Medical Center in Salt Lake City. The mechanical heart was attached to the upper chambers (atria) and major blood vessels of the patient's normal heart with Dacron fittings. The first artificial heart for humans kept the patient alive for 112 days. Also called **Jarvik-7.**

artificial impregnation. See **artificial insemination.**

artificial insemination, putting semen into the vagina or uterus by mechanical means rather than by sexual intercourse. This is planned along with the expected time of the discharge of the egg (ovum) from the ovary. Thus fertilization can occur. Kinds of artificial insemination are **artificial insemination-donor, artificial insemination-husband.** Also called **artificial impregnation.** See also **menstrual cycle.**

artificial insemination donor (AID), artificial insemination in which the semen is given by an unknown donor. It is used mainly in cases where the husband is sterile. Also called **heterologous insemination.** Compare **artificial insemination husband.**

artificial insemination husband (AIH), artificial insemination in which the semen is given by the husband. It is used mainly in cases of impotency or when the husband is incapable of sexual intercourse because of some physical disability. Also called **homologous insemination.** Compare **artificial insemination-donor.**

artificial kidney, a device used to rid the blood of substances that are usually released in urine. It usually is made up of a set of tubes for passing the blood between the patient and a dialysis machine. Also called **kidney machine.** See also **hemodialysis, peritoneal dialysis.**

artificial limb. See **prosthesis.**

artificial lung. See **Drinker respirator.**

artificially acquired immunity. See **acquired immunity.**

artificial pacemaker. See **pacemaker.**

artificial respiration, the process of continuing breathing by the hands and mouth of another person or mechanical means when normal breathing has stopped. Breathing may stop because of swelling, a foreign body, mucus, nerve disorders, and severe asthma. Other causes are exhaustion, drug overdose, or trauma to the chest wall. Before trying to give artificial respiration, the airway is checked. Any obstruction is removed. See also **cardiopulmonary resuscitation (CPR), resuscitation, ventilator.** (See illustration on p. 64).

artificial stone, a material similar to but stronger than plaster of Paris. It is used for making dental casts.

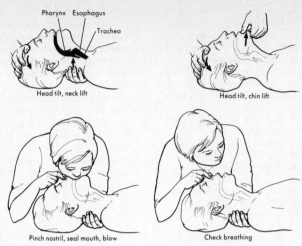

Pharynx Esophagus

Trachea

Head tilt, neck lift

Head tilt, chin lift

Pinch nostril, seal mouth, blow

Check breathing

Artificial respiration

art therapy, a type of mental-health treatment in which the patient is encouraged to express his or her feelings through various forms of artwork.

aryepiglottic folds /er′ē·ep′iglot′ik/, folds of mucous membranes that extend around the edges of the voicebox from the point where it meets the lid (epiglottis). They serve to close off the voicebox while the person is swallowing.

aryl hydrocarbon hydroxylase (AHH), an enzyme that changes cancer-causing chemicals in tobacco smoke and in polluted air into active cancer-causing agents within the lungs.

As, symbol for **arsenic.**

ASA, 1. abbreviation for **American Society of Anesthesiologists. 2.** abbreviation for **aspirin** (acetylsalicylic acid).

asbestosis, a life-long lung disease. It is caused by breathing asbestos fibers. It results in lung disorders, as pleural fibrosis. Asbestos miners and workers are most often affected. The disease sometimes occurs in other people who have been exposed to asbestos building materials. The disease gets worse. Shortness of breath develops eventually into failing to breathe. See also **chronic obstructive pulmonary disease, inorganic dust.**

ascariasis /as′kərī′əsis/, an infection caused by a parasitic worm, *Ascaris lumbricoides.* The eggs are passed in human feces. This infects the soil and allows that the infection is carried on to others through hands, water, or food. After hatching in the small intestine, the larvae travel through the wall of the intestine. Then they are carried by the lymph system and bloodstream to the lungs. Early breathing symptoms are coughing, wheezing, and fever. The larvae then go to the throat. They are swallowed, they mature in the intestine where

they release eggs, and the cycle is repeated.

Ascaris /as′kəris/, a genus of large parasitic intestinal roundworms, as *Ascaris lumbricoides.* They cause serious infection (ascariasis). It is found throughout temperate and tropical regions.

ascending aorta, one of the four main sections of the large artery of the heart (aorta). It branches into the right and left coronary arteries.

ascending colon, the part of the large intestine (colon) that extends upward from the first part of the colon (cecum) in the lower right side of the stomach to where the colon turns (the transverse colon) and crosses the stomach about the level of the navel.

ascending oblique muscle. See **obliquus internus abdominis.**

ascending pharyngeal artery, one of the smallest arteries that branch from the outer carotid artery, deep in the neck. It takes blood to many organs and muscles of the head.

ascending urography. See **urography.**

asceticism, (in psychiatry) a defense mechanism that involves rejecting all impulses based on instinct. The concept comes from the ancient religious belief that material things are evil and only spiritual things are good.

ascites /əsī′tēz/, an abnormal pooling of fluid in the abdominal cavity containing large amounts of protein and other cells. Ascites is usually noticed when more than one pint (500 ml) of fluid has collected. The condition may lead to general abdominal swelling, dilution of the blood, or less urinary output. The most common cause is liver disease (cirrhosis). However, ascites can be caused by cancer, kidney disease, congestive heart failure, or other diseases. The fluid can be removed with a needle (paracentesis). This relieves pain and improves breathing and organ function. See also **paracentesis**. −ascitic, *adj.*

ascites adiposus. See **chylous ascites.**

ascorbemia /as′kôrbē′mē·ə/, the presence of vitamin C (ascorbic acid) in the blood in larger-than-normal amounts. It usually means an excess of ascorbic acid in the diet.

ascorbic acid /əskôr′bik/, a water-soluble, white crystalline vitamin (vitamin C). It is in citrus fruits, tomatoes, berries, and potatoes. Fresh, green, leafy vegetables, as broccoli, brussels sprouts, collards, turnip greens, parsley, sweet peppers, and cabbage also contain vitamin C. It is needed by the body to form collagen and fiber for teeth, bone, cartilage, connective tissue, skin, and capillary walls. It also helps in fighting bacterial infections. Symptoms of its lack are bleeding gums, tendency to bruising, swollen or painful joints, and nosebleeds. Anemia, lowered resistance to infections, and slow healing of wounds and fractures are other symptoms. Severe lack results in scurvy. An excess of ascorbic acid may cause a burning sensation during urination, diarrhea, skin rash, and nausea. It may disturb the absorption and processing of vitamin B_{12}. Also called **antiscorbutic vitamin, cevitamic acid, vitamin C.** See also **ascorbemia, bioflavonoid, citric acid, infantile scurvy, scurvy.**

ascorburia /as′kôrbyŏŏr′ē·ə/, ascorbic acid in the urine in larger amounts than normal.

ascribed role, an assigned role in society, based on age, sex, or other factors about which the individual has no choice. See also **assumed role.**

Asendin, a trademark for a drug used to relieve depression (amoxapine).

asepsis /āsep′sis/, the absence of germs. **Medical asepsis** is the removal of disease organisms or infected material. **Surgical asepsis** is protection against infection before, during, or after surgery by using sterile technique. −aseptic, *adj.*

aseptic bone necrosis, a type of bone and joint damage that may occur in workers who are repeatedly exposed to compressed-air environments, as in diving or tunneling occupations. It apparently results from blocking of small arteries in the bones by nitrogen bubbles, followed by death of the bone from decreased blood supply. There may be no symptoms or the person may experience severe pain and the joint may collapse.

aseptic fever, a fever that is not caused by infection. Mechanical trauma, as a crushing injury, can cause fever even when no organism is present.

aseptic gauze, 1. sterile gauze prepared and packed for surgical use. 2. any gauze that is free of microorganisms.

aseptic meningitis, a swelling of the brain and spine (cerebrospinal) membranes (meninges). It can be caused by a number of viruses, including coxsackieviruses, nonparalytic polio viruses, echoviruses, and mumps. The disease is especially common in children during the late summer and early fall. In about one third of the children, no organism can be found. The fluid of the brain and spinal cord shows white blood cells but no bacteria. Symptoms vary depending on the cause. They may include fever, headache, stiff neck and back, nausea, and skin rash. No specific treatment is available. Complete recovery, without complication or lasting problems, is usual.

aseptic technique, any health-care procedure in which added precautions are used to prevent contamination of a person, object, or area.

Asepto syringe, a trademark for a blunt-tipped syringe fitted with a bulb at the top. It is used mainly for flushing out wounds.

asexual /āsek′shŏŏ·əl/, 1. referring to an organism that has no sexual organs. 2. referring to a process that is not sexual. −asexuality, *n.*

asexual dwarf, an adult dwarf whose sex organs are not well developed.

asexualization /āsek′shŏŏ·əlīzā′shən/, the process of making one unable to reproduce. This may be by castration, vasectomy, taking the ovaries away, tying the tubes, or other means.

asexual reproduction, a type of reproduction found in plants and lower animals. Offspring are formed without male-female union. Examples are budding, fission, and spore formation. Compare **sexual generation.**

ASHA, abbreviation for **American Speech, Language, and Hearing Association.**

Asherman syndrome, lack of menstruation (amenorrhea) in a woman with normal hormones. It may be caused by scar tissue (adhesions) that form as a result of surgical scraping (curettage) or infection. It is treated by curettage to remove adhesions. It is followed by placing a device in the uterus to prevent adhesions from re-forming during healing.

asialorrhea. See **hyposalivation.**

Asian flu. See **influenza.**

asiderosis, a lack of sufficient iron and a cause of a decrease in red cells in the blood (anemia).

ASLT, abbreviation for **antistreptolysin-O test.**

Asn, abbreviation for **asparagine.**

ASOT, abbreviation for **antistreptolysin-O test.**

asparagine (Asn) /aspar′əjin/, an amino acid found in many proteins in the body. It is termed "nonessential" because it can be made by the body and need not be included in the diet. It acts as a drug that promotes the release of urine. See also **amino acid, protein.**

aspartame, a white, almost odorless crystalline powder with an intensely sweet taste. It is used as an artificial sweetener. It is about 180 times as sweet as the same amount of sugar. It is used to give a better flavor to cold or uncooked foods. Aspartame tends to lose its sweetness in the presence of heat and moisture. Excess use of aspartame should be avoided by patients with phenylketonuria (PKU).

aspartate aminotransferase (AST) /aspär'tāt/, an enzyme normally present in blood serum and in the heart and liver. AST is released into the blood after injury and as a result of heart attack and liver damage. Also called **glutamicoxaloacetic transaminase, serum glutamicoxaloacetic transaminase.** Compare **alanine aminotransferase.**

aspartic acid (Asp) /aspär'tik/, an amino acid in sugar cane, beet molasses, and the breakdown products of many proteins. It is termed "nonessential" because it can be made by the body and need not be included in the diet. Aspartic acid is used in culture media, dietary supplements, and detergents. It is also used in drugs that kill funguses and germs. Also called **aminosuccinic acid.** See also **amino acid, protein.**

ASPEN, abbreviation for **American Society of Parenteral and Enteral Nutrition.**

aspergillic acid /as'pərjil'ik/, an antibiotic substance that grows on *Aspergillus.*

aspergillosis /as'pərjilō'sis/, an infection caused by the fungus *Aspergillus.* It usually affects the ear but is capable of infecting any organ. The infection is relatively uncommon. It typically occurs in a patient already weakened by some other disorder. Treatment of skin infections is with fungicides. Amphotericin B is used to treat systemic aspergillosis, especially if it has spread to the lungs. Compare **allergic bronchopulmonary aspergillosis.**

Aspergillus /as'pərjil'əs/, a genus of fungi that commonly infects the laboratory and causes hospital infection. Infection from breathing in spores is rare.

aspermia /āspur'mē·ə/, a state of not producing or releasing semen.

asphyxia /asfik'sē·ə/, severe oxygen lack. It leads to blood with low oxygen content, loss of consciousness, and, if not corrected, death. Some of the more common causes of asphyxia are drowning, electric shock, breathing vomit, and a foreign body stuck in the breathing tract. Breathing toxic gas or smoke, and poisoning are other causes. Artificial respiration and oxygen are promptly given to avoid damage to the brain. See **artificial respiration.** –**asphyxiate,** *v.,* **asphyxiated,** *adj.*

aspirant, the fluid, gas, or solid particles that are removed from the body using a suction device (aspiration).

aspirant maneuver, a procedure used in making x-ray films of part of the throat (laryngopharyngeal area). The patient breathes out completely, then slowly breathes in while making a harsh, high-pitched sound. This is done so that the cavity (ventricle) of the voicebox can be clearly seen in the x-ray.

aspirating needle, a long hollow needle used to take fluid from a cavity, vessel, or structure of the body.

aspiration, 1. the act of taking a breath, inhaling. 2. the act of withdrawing fluid, as mucus or blood, from the body by a suction device. See also **aspiration pneumonia.** –**aspirate,** *n.*

aspiration biopsy, taking living tissue away with a fine needle attached to a syringe. The purpose is to examine the tissue under a microscope. See also **cytology, needle biopsy.**

aspiration biopsy cytology (ABC), a microscopic examination of cells taken directly from living body tissue with a fine needle. It is used mainly for diagnosis. Compare **exfoliative cytology.**

aspiration drug abuse, inhaling certain chemicals for purposes unrelated to illness. Examples include glue sniffing and cocaine snorting.

aspiration of vomitus, breathing vomit into the lungs. See also **aspiration pneumonia.**

aspiration pneumonia, an inflammatory condition of the lungs and bronchial tubes. It is caused by taking foreign material or vomit into the lungs. Compare **bronchopneumonia.** See also **pneumonia.**

★DIAGNOSIS : Aspiration pneumonia most often occurs when a patient vomits during or after surgery while under anesthesia. It also occurs when a patient is intoxicated or otherwise unconscious and vomits.

★TREATMENT: Treatment involves suctioning the vomit from the lungs and giving oxygen. Artificial respiration may be needed. Steroids are usually given to treat the swelling. The vomitted matter (sputum) is checked for bacteria. Any infection is treated with antibiotics.

aspirator, any instrument that takes a substance away from body cavities by suction, as a bulb syringe, pump, or hypodermic needle.

aspirin, a pain-killing, fever-reducing, and inflammation-relieving drug. It is used to reduce fever and to relieve pain and swelling.

★CAUTION: Bleeding disorders, peptic ulcer, pregnancy, the use of anticlotting drugs, or known allergy prohibits its use.

★ADVERSE EFFECTS: Among the most serious adverse reactions are stomach and intestinal problems (ulcers, bleeding). Use of large doses over a long time can cause blood clotting defects, and liver and kidney damage. Reye's syndrome in children may be caused by aspirin. Some asthmalike and other allergic reactions are seen occasionally. Ringing in the ears (tinnitus) and stomach discomfort (dyspepsia) are the most common side effects.

aspirin poisoning. See **salicylate poisoning.**

Assam fever. See **kala-azar.**

assertiveness, a form of behavior that is designed to claim one's own rights without denying the rights of others.

assertive training, a technique used in behavior therapy to help people become more self-assertive and self-confident in their relationships. It teaches direct, honest statement of feelings and beliefs. Also called **assertion training.**

assessment, 1. an evaluation of a condition. 2. an examiner's evaluation of the disease or condition based on the patient's report of the symptoms and the examiner's findings. It includes data gotten through laboratory tests, physical examination, and medical history.

assessment of the aging patient, an evaluation of the changes brought about by advancing years in an elderly patient.
★METHOD: The patient is measured, weighed, examined, observed, and questioned about physical and behavioral changes. Height normally diminishes 0.5 inch with aging. Weight steadily decreases in men over 65 years of age but increases in women. The skin is examined for dryness, wrinkles, sagging, thinning over the back of the hands, areas of pigment changes, warts, skin tags, and widened capillaries. The hair is examined for greying, lack of luster, and thinning on the scalp and in the armpit and the pubic areas. Observations are made of enlargement of the nose and ears relative to face size. The eyes are checked for dryness, discoloration of the whites and iris, a ring near the edge of the cornea. Decreased size of the pupil, and loss of peripheral vision are also noted. Tests are taken to see if there is hearing loss, especially of high-frequency tones. The lungs are examined for decreased breath volume. The patient is evaluated for heart problems and inadequate circulation. Examination of the mouth may show receding gums, loss of teeth and taste, and lessened salivation. The elderly patient may have muscle wasting, broken-down joints, shortened finger muscles, bone disease (osteoporosis), stand with the legs apart for balance, and move slowly. The sense of position, of smell, and of touch and the sensitivity to heat and cold may be less. Reflexes may be decreased. Signs of aging often found in women are pendulous, flaccid breasts. Vaginal narrowing and shortening, and lessened lubrication, causing painful intercourse are other common signs. Women who take estrogen for a long time may have uterine bleeding, breast pain, weight gain, fluid retention, and high blood pressure. Signs of aging in men include decrease in the size and firmness of the testicles and in the amount of semen. Increased diameter of the penis, and enlargement of the prostate gland are other signs. Sexual desire and a sense of satisfaction usually do not become less.
★OUTCOME: Aging does not develop at a uni-

form rate. Its effects may vary widely from one patient to the next. In many cases, changes considered normal in elderly patients are actually diseases that may respond to treatment.

assimilation, 1. the process of incorporating nutrition into living tissue. 2. the incorporation of new experiences into a person's consciousness.

assisted breech, a technique in which a baby being born feet or buttocks first is permitted to be born spontaneously as far as its navel. The infant is then helped the rest of the way by the physician or midwife. Also called **partial breech extraction.** Compare **breech extraction.**

assisted ventilation, the use of mechanical or other types of devices to help maintain breathing. It usually uses pressure to push air or oxygen into the lungs. See also **IPPB.**

associate degree in nursing, an academic degree awarded on satisfactory completion of a two-year course of study. It is usually offered at a community or junior college.

associated antagonist, one of a pair of muscles or group of muscles that pull in opposite directions. Their combined action results in moving a part in one direction.

association, 1. a connection, union, joining, or combination of things. 2. connecting feelings, emotions, sensations, or thoughts with particular persons, things, or ideas.

association area, any part of the main portion of the brain (cerebrum) involved in integrating sensory information, as vision. Also called **association cortex.**

association of ideas, a mental connection made between similar or concurring ideas, feelings, or perceptions.

association test, a technique used in psychiatry and in educational and psychological evaluation. A person is asked to respond to a word with the first thing that comes to mind. The time taken to respond and the associations made are compared to pretested responses. They are classified for diagnosis. Also called **word association test.**

associationist model of learning, a theory that defines learning as a change in behavior caused by reinforced practice.

associative looseness, a type of thought disorder in which relationships among ideas are rooted in fantasy rather than reality.

associative play, a form of play in which a group of children do similar or identical activities without direction, or a definite goal. The children may borrow or lend toys or pieces of play equipment. They may do like others in the group. However, each child acts independently, as on a playground or among a group riding tricycles or bicycles. Compare **cooperative play.** See also **parallel play, solitary play.**

assumed role, a role in life that a person intentionally chooses or achieves. Examples include roles such as wife and dentist. See also **ascribed role**.

astasia, a problem with nerves involved with moving (motor nerves) in which the patient cannot stand without assistance.

astatine (At), a very unstable, radioactive element. It occurs naturally in very small amounts. Its atomic number is 85; its atomic weight is 210.

asteatosis /as′tē·ətō′sis/, a dry skin condition that results when insufficient oil is produced by the glands in the skin. The dryness may cause scales or cracks. The condition is treated with creams and ointments that replace the missing skin oils.

-aster, a combining form meaning "star-shaped."

astereognosis /əstir′ē·ognō′sis/, a nervous system disorder. It is marked by an inability to recognize objects by touch.

asterixis /as′tərik′sis/, a hand-flapping tremor. It often goes together with processing (metabolic) disorders. The tremor is usually seen when the arm is extended and the wrist is flexed backwards. Asterixis is seen often in patients in a coma from liver disease. Also called **flapping tremor, liver flap.**

asteroid body, an irregular, star-shaped structure that develops in certain cells. It is seen in some diseases.

asthenia /asthē′nē·ə/, **1.** the lack or loss of strength or energy; weakness; debility. **2.** lack of dynamic force in the personality. Kinds of asthenia include **asthenia gravis hypophyseogenea, myalgic asthenia, neurocirculatory asthenia, tropical anhidrotic asthenia.** See also **adynamia. –asthenic,** *adj.*

asthenic habitus, a body with a slender build with long limbs, an angular profile, and prominent muscles or bones. Compare **athletic habitus, pyknic.** See also **ectomorph.**

asthenic personality, a personality with low energy, lack of enthusiasm, and oversensitivity to physical and emotional strain. A person who has this kind of personality may be easily tired and self-pitying. He or she may blame others for any physical and emotional problems.

asthenopia, a condition in which the eyes tire easily because of weakness of the eye muscles. Symptoms include pain in or around the eyes, headache, dimness of vision, dizziness, and slight nausea.

asthma /az′mə/, a lung disorder marked by attacks of breathing difficulty, wheezing, coughing, and thick mucus coming from the lungs. The episodes may be started by breathing foreign substances (allergens) or pollutants, infection, vigorous exercise, or emotional stress. Treatment includes getting rid of the cause if possible. Sprays or wideners of the bronchi

taken by mouth, and steroid drugs are also used. Certain drugs must not be used by persons with asthma (for example, some of the drugs for treating circulatory disease [beta-adrenergic drugs], barbiturates, and narcotics). Repeated attacks often result in shortness of breath (emphysema) and permanent obstructive lung disease. Also called **bronchial asthma.** See also **allergic asthma, asthma in children, intrinsic asthma, organic dust, status asthmaticus.**

asthma crystal. See **Charcot-Leyden crystal.**

asthma in children, a condition of attacks of breathing distress, wheezing, prolonged breathing out, and a cough. It usually begins between 3 and 8 years of age. Asthmatic attacks are caused by a narrowing of the airways. This results from muscle spasm in the lungs, swelling of the bronchial tubes, or excess mucus. Asthma in children is usually caused by an allergy to a foreign substance (allergen), as pollen, mold, house dust, certain foods, animal hair and skin, feathers, insects, smoke, and various chemicals or drugs. In infants, especially those born into a family with a history of allergic reactions, food allergy is a common cause. In some instances, the attacks are caused by other events, as infection or swelling, obstruction by a foreign body, physical stress resulting from weakness, exposure to cold air, or psychological stress. Such cases are classified as nonallergic, or intrinsic, asthma. There is a strong hereditary factor associated with the disease. As many as 75% of children with asthma have a family history of the disorder. The child usually has other allergic symptoms, as hay fever, eczema, or skin eruptions (urticaria). The disease occurs twice as often in boys as in girls before puberty. Both boys and girls are affected equally during adolescence.

★DIAGNOSIS: The condition is often confused with breathing tract infections, obstruction of the bronchial tubes or throat, and cystic fibrosis. Diagnosis is by examining the sputum and taking long function tests. Asthma attacks vary greatly in frequency, how long they last, and the symptoms. The attacks can range from occasional periods of wheezing, mild coughing, and slight breathlessness to severe attacks that can lead to airway obstruction and total inability to breathe. An attack may begin slowly or abruptly. It is often preceded by an upper respiratory infection. In general, episodes caused by infection have a slow beginning and last longer. Attacks caused by allergens are sudden and subside quickly if the cause is removed. Typically, an attack begins with shortness of breath, wheezing, and a hacking cough. As secretions increase, breathing out becomes longer. The cough gets deeper and more rattling, and a large quantity of thick sputum is made as the attack becomes less. The child appears afraid and speaks in a panting manner. He or she may assume a bent-over position to breath easier. A sudden increase in the rate of breathing, repeated hacking, and coughing without sputum mean a lack of air. This is a medical emergency. Children with life-long asthma develop a barrel chest from the continuous hyperventilated state. They usually carry their shoulders high to make better use of the muscles of breathing. ★TREATMENT: A sudden asthmatic attack is a medical emergency. It needs direct relief with drugs that widen the bronchi and removal of excess bronchial releases. The major drugs used to relieve bronchospasm are the beta-adrenergic agents, the methylxanthines, steroids, expectorants, and sedatives. Antibiotics are used when infection is the cause of an attack. Failure to stop the attack results in status asthmaticus. This is a serious prolonged state needing hospitalization. The child has usually lost too much water. Thus hospital care includes intravenous fluids and humidified oxygen. Bronchodilators to relieve bronchospasm and antibiotics to reduce risk of infection are also given. Children with mild, infrequent attacks are treated with bronchodilators in aerosol sprays. They give quick relief and are effective in controlling an attack when it begins. The drug is usually given by mouth in younger children. Those with persistent asthma get daily doses of a bronchodilator by mouth, often theophylline, usually in combination with an expectorant and steroids. Sometimes the home environment can be changed to lessen contact with the allergen. Making the patient less sensitive (hyposensitization) is advised when an allergen is known and cannot be avoided. Physical exercise and play activities are important aspects of therapy, especially those that promote proper breathing techniques. Children with emotional problems need special attention. Psychological stresses often trigger asthmatic attacks. For this reason psychotherapy or behavior therapy is often required. Prognosis for children with asthma varies considerably. Many children lose their symptoms at puberty. Much depends on the number and severity of symptoms, emotional factors, and the family history of allergy.

asthmatic eosinophilia, a form of pneumonia. It is marked by allergic spasm of the tubes of the bronchi, by coughing up tissue, and by cough and fever. The condition usually occurs in the fourth or fifth decade of life. It is twice as common in women as in men. It is a result of allergy to *Aspergillus fumigatus* or *Candida albicans*. Untreated, the condition may result in swelling of the sac around the heart (pericarditis) or of the brain (encephalitis), pooling of fluid, a large liver, and breathing failure. De-

sensitization to the allergen is usually not effective. See also **allergic asthma, eosinophilic pneumonia.**

astigmatism /əstig'mətiz'əm/, an abnormal condition of the eye in which the curve of the cornea is unequal. As a result, light rays cannot be focused clearly. Vision is blurred. The eyes tire easily. The condition usually can be corrected with contact lenses or with eyeglasses.

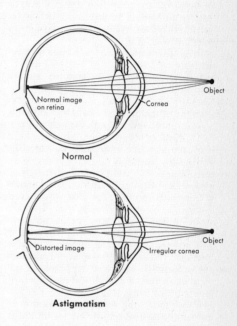

Normal image on retina — Cornea — Object

Normal

Distorted image — Irregular cornea — Object

Astigmatism

–astine, a combining form referring to an antihistamine.

astragalus. See **talus.**

astringent /əstrin'jənt/, a substance that causes tissues to contract. It is usually used on the skin. Alum and tannic acid are common astringents.

astringent bath, a bath in which an astringent is added to the water.

astro-, a combining form referring to a star, or star-shaped.

astroblastoma /as'trōblastō'mə/, *pl.* **astroblastomas, astroblastomata,** a cancerous tumor of the brain and spinal cord. Cells of an astroblastoma lie around blood vessels or, in some cases, around connective tissue.

astrocyte /as'trōsīt'/, a large, star-shaped cell found in certain tissues of the nervous system.

astrocytoma /as'trōsītō'mə/, *pl.* **astrocytomas, astrocytomata,** a tumor of the brain composed of astrocytes. It is marked by slow growth, lump (cyst) formation, and invasion of surrounding structures. Often, a highly cancerous tumor called glioblastoma grows within the tumor.

Complete removal of an astrocytoma by surgery may be possible early in the growth of the tumor. Also called **astrocytic glioma.**

astrocytosis /as'trōsītō'sis/, an increase in the supporting structure of nerve tissue (neuroglial cells). This is often seen in brain abscesses, certain brain tumors, and brain softening (encephalomalacia). Astrocytosis is actually a process of repair.

asymmetrical /āsimet'rikəl, asimet'-/, parts of the body that are unequal in size or shape, or that are different in arrangement. Also **asymmetric.** Compare **symmetrical.** –**asymmetry** /āsim'itrē, asim'-/, n.

asymmetric tonic neck reflex. See **tonic neck reflex.**

asymptomatic diabetes. See **impaired glucose tolerance.**

asynclitism /āsing'klitiz'əm/, during labor, a presentation of the top of the baby's head that is not in proper alignment with the mother's pelvis for birth. In normal labor, the baby's head is usually asynclitic at some time, especially during early labor.

asynergy /āsin'ərjē/, faulty coordination among groups of organs or muscles that normally function well together. See also **ataxia, cerebellum.**

asyntaxia /ā'sintak'sē·ə/, any interference with the proper order of growth of the fetus during development. Asyntaxia results in one or more birth defects. See also **developmental anomaly.**

asyntaxia dorsalis, failure of the primative spinal cord (neural tube) to close during the early growth of the fetus.

asystole /āsis'təlē/, the absence of a heart beat. Cardiotoxic asystole is a brief period of cardiac arrest. It is caused by speeding up of the heart rate. Asystole requires immediate cardiopulmonary resuscitation with cardiac massage. If these measures fail to start heart contractions, a defibrillator may be used to shock the heart into working again. Also called **cardiac arrest, cardiac standstill.**

At, symbol for **astatine.**

Atabrine Hydrochloride, a trademark for a drug used to treat malaria (quinacrine hydrochloride).

Atabrine stomatitis, an abnormal mouth condition. It may be caused by the drug Atabrine. The symptoms are similar to those of a skin disease (lichen planus). Compare **arsenical stomatitis, bismuth stomatitis.**

Atarax, a trademark for a drug used to treat distress and itching from allergies (hydroxyzine hydrochloride).

atavism /at'əviz'əm/, traits or characteristics in a person that are more like those of a grandparent or earlier ancestor than like the parents. Atavistic data may offer hints of genetic or family health factors to a physician. –**atavistic,** adj.

ataxia /ətak'sē·ə/, a blocked ability to coordinate movements. A staggering walk and poor balance may be caused by damage to the spinal cord or brain. This can be the result of birth trauma, inborn disorder, infection, tumor, poison, or head injury. See also **hereditary ataxia.**

ataxia-telangiectasia, a rare genetic disease involving an immune system that works poorly. It begins in childhood. It develops slowly with brain breakdown and frequent breathing infections. Widened capillaries are clearly visible on the ears, face, and the membranes lining the eye. Also called **Louis-Bar syndrome.**

ataxic breathing, a type of breathing linked to an injury in the breathing centers of the brain. The symptoms are poorly coordinated breathing in and out.

ataxic speech, abnormal speech marked by faulty formation of the sounds. The cause is a disorder of the nerves to the muscles.

atelectasis /at'ilek'təsis/, an abnormal condition marked by the collapse of lung tissue. This prevents the breathing exchange of carbon dioxide and oxygen by the blood. Symptoms include lessened breath sounds, fever, and more difficulty in breathing. The condition may be caused by obstruction of the major airways and bronchioles. It may also be caused by pressure on the lung from fluid or air in the area around the lungs (pleural space), or by pressure from a tumor outside the lung. Loss of lung tissue may cause increased heart rate, higher blood pressure, and faster breathing.

atelectatic rale /at'iləktat'ik/, an abnormal intermittent crackling sound heard when listening to the chest with a stethoscope. It usually disappears after the patient being examined coughs or breathes deeply several times.

ateliotic dwarf /at'əlē·ot'ik/, a dwarf whose skeleton is incompletely formed during bone development.

atelo-, a combining form meaning imperfect or incomplete.

atenolol, a drug used to treat high blood pressure.

★CAUTION: Abnormally slow heart beat or heart failure prohibits its use.

★ADVERSE EFFECTS: Among the more serious side effects are slow heart beat, dizziness, and nausea.

atherectomy catheter /ath'ərek'təmē/, a specially designed hollow, flexible tube (catheter) for cutting away deposits from the lining of an artery.

atheroembolic renal disease /ath'ərō·embol'ik/, a condition in which the kidneys gradually or rapidly fail because the arteries that serve them are blocked. It is associated with disorders of the arteries (atherosclerosis) and high blood pressure. It occurs most frequently in persons over 60 years of age.

atheroma /ath'ərō'mə/, an abnormal mass of fat,

as in an oil gland (sebaceous), lump (cyst) or in deposits in an artery wall.

atheromatosis /ath'ərōmətō'sis/, the development of many atheromas.

atherosclerosis /ath'ərōsklərō'sis/, a common disorder of the arteries. Yellowish plaques of cholesterol, fats, and other remains are deposited in the walls of large and medium-sized arteries. The vessel walls become thick and hardened. The vessel narrows. This lessens circulation to organs and other areas normally supplied by the artery. These plaques (atheromas) are major causes of heart disease, chest pain (angina pectoris), heart attacks, and other disorders of the circulation. How atherosclerosis develops is not clear. It may begin with injury to the artery or with an increase of muscle in vessel walls. Excess saturated fats in the diet, faulty carbohydrate processing, or a genetic defect may be other causes. Atherosclerosis usually occurs with aging. It is often linked to overweight, high blood pressure, and diabetes. See also **arteriosclerosis.**

athetosis /ath'ətō'sis/, a condition of the nerves supplying the muscles. It is marked by slow, twisting, continuous, and involuntary movement of the arms and legs. It is seen in some forms of brain disorders (cerebral palsy). It is also seen in disorders resulting from injury to the nerves.

athiaminosis /əthī'əminō'sis/, a condition resulting from lack of thiamine (vitamin B_1) in the diet. See also **beriberi, thiamine.**

athlete's foot. See **tinea pedis.**

athlete's heart, the typical, normal but large heart of an athlete trained for endurance. It is marked by slow heart beats, and an increased pumping capacity. It also is marked by greater-than-average ability to carry oxygen to skeletal muscles. Also called **athletic heart syndrome (AHS).**

athletic habitus, a well-proportioned, muscular body with broad shoulders, thick neck, deep chest, and flat stomach. Compare **asthenic habitus, pyknic.** See also **mesomorph.**

athletic heart syndrome. See **athlete's heart.**

Ativan, a trademark for a drug used in tablet form to treat anxiety. Injections are given before surgery to deepen the anesthesia (lorazepam).

atlantooccipital joint /-oksip'itəl/, one of a pair of joints formed where the atlas of the vertebral column meets the occipital bone of the skull.

atlas, the first backbone in the neck (cervical vertebra), which connects with the occipital bone of the skull and the second backbone (axis).

atman, (in psychiatry) a concept based on Eastern Indian philosophy that the highest value is to know one's true self. The atman represents the innermost spirit and the highest controlling power of a person.

atmosphere, 1. the natural air, composed of about 20% oxygen, 78% nitrogen, and 2% carbon dioxide and other gases, that covers the surface of the earth. **2.** an envelope of gas, which may or may not be identical to the natural atmosphere, in chemical components. **–atmospheric,** *adj.*

atmospheric pressure, the pressure of the weight of the atmosphere. The atmospheric pressure at sea level is approximately 14.7 pounds per square inch. With increasing altitude the pressure becomes less. At 30,000 feet, the air pressure is 4.3 pounds per square inch. Also called **barometric pressure.**

atomic mass unit (amu), the mass of a neutral (uncharged) atom of an element.

atomizer, a device for spraying a liquid as a fine mist or vapor.

atonia /ātō'nē·ə/, an abnormal lack of muscle tone.

atonia constipation, constipation caused by failure of the large intestine (colon) to respond to normal prompting for bowel movement. It may occur in elderly or bedridden patients. It may also happen after long use of laxatives. To prevent fecal material from hardening in the colon and rectum, a laxative taken by mouth or a mild suppository may be given. Patients are told to develop regular, unhurried bowel habits. A diet rich in fruits, whole grains, and vegetables can help correct or avoid constipation. Also called **colon stasis, lazy colon.** See also **fecalith, inactive colon.**

atonic /əton'ik/, **1.** weak, or lacking normal tone, as a muscle that is soft. **2.** lacking vigor, as an atonic ulcer, which heals slowly.

atonic bladder. See **flaccid bladder.**

atonic impotence. See **impotence.**

atopic /ātop'ik/, referring to a hereditary tendency to develop immediate allergic reactions, as asthma, allergic skin disease (atopic dermatitis), or hay fever. Atopic reactions are caused by an antibody in the skin and sometimes the bloodstream. **–atopy,** *n.*

atopic dermatitis, an intensely itching swelling of the skin. It is commonly found on the face, knees, and elbows of allergy-prone patients. It is most common in infants. It often clears completely by 18 months of age. The foreign substance (allergen) causing the dermatitis should be detected by allergy testing so it can be avoided. Treatment includes steroids, tar ointments, antihistamines, and wet compresses of Burow's solution. Also called **atopic eczema, infantile eczema.** Compare **contact dermatitis.** See also **atopic.**

atopic eczema. See **atopic dermatitis.**

atopognosia /ātop'əgnō'zhə/, a disorder in which a person cannot properly locate a sensation.

ATP, abbreviation for **adenosine triphosphate.**

ATPase, abbreviation for **adenosine triphosphatase.**

atransferrinemic anemia /ā'transfer'inē'mik/, a disease in which iron fails to move from the liver or other locations where it is stored to tissues in which red blood cells develop. In addition to a decrease in the number of red blood cells in the blood (anemia), the patient usually suffers from an increased deposit of iron in a variety of tissues (hemosiderosis).

atresia /ətrē'zhə/, the absence of a normal body opening, duct, or canal, as the anus, vagina, or ear canal.

atresic teratism /ətrē'sik/, a birth defect in which any of the normal openings of the body, as the mouth, nostrils, anus, or vagina, fail to form.

atrial failure /ā'trē·əl/, an abnormal condition marked by the failure of one of the upper heart chambers (atrium) to fill completely with blood. The atria normally provide a pumping function for the heart. In normal persons or in patients with mild heart disease, loss of atrial pumping may not change the amount of blood pumped at rest. However, the amount of blood may decrease during exercise. Heart failure caused by atrial failure may begin with irregular contractions of the upper heart chambers (atrial fibrillation) in patients who have heart disease.

atrial fibrillation, a heart condition marked by rapid, unsystematic contractions of the upper heart chambers (atria). This causes the lower chambers (ventricles) to beat irregularly at the rate of 130 to 150 a minute. The atria may discharge more than 350 electric impulses a minute. The lower chambers cannot contract in response to all these impulses and the contractions become disordered. Atrial fibrillation occurs most often in heart diseases, as mitral stenosis and atrial infarction. The rapid pulsations result in a decreased amount of blood pumped to the body. The disorganized contractions of the atria can cause blood clots to form in the atria.

atrial flutter, a condition marked by rapid, regular contractions of the upper heart chambers (atria), about 300 beats per minute. The lower chambers of the heart (ventricles) cannot respond to this. They contract at a lower rate, usually about 150 beats per minute. Compare **atrial fibrillation.**

atrial gallop, an abnormal heart rhythm in which a low-pitched, extra sound is heard when listening to the heart with a stethoscope. It is often heard in heart disease caused by high blood pressure. See also **gallop, heart sound.**

atrial myxoma, a benign, gelatinlike tumor that grows in the wall dividing the upper chambers (atria) of the heart. It may cause irregular heart beats, nerve swelling, nausea, weight loss, weakness, breathlessness, fever. It may occasionally lead to fainting caused by obstruction of the flow of blood through the heart.

atrial septal defect (ASD), a birth defect of the heart in which there is an abnormal opening in the wall (septum) between the two upper heart chambers (atria). The severity of the condition depends on the size and location of the hole. Atrial septal defects cause an increased flow of blood containing oxygen into the right side of the heart. Surgery can close the hole in most cases. Unless the defect is severe, it is usually not done until later childhood to prevent problems. Also called **atrioseptal defect.** See also **endocardial cushion defect.**

atrioseptal defect. See **atrial septal defect.**

atrioventricular (AV) block /ā'trē·ōventrik'yələr/, the slowed electric impulse of the heart. It occurs at the atrioventricular node, bundle of His, or its branches. An overdose of digitalis, heart disease, or severe heart attack may cause the condition. AV block is a common reason a cardiac pacemaker is inserted. See also **heart block, intraatrial block, intraventricular heart block, sinoatrial block.**

atrioventricular (AV) node, an area of specialized heart muscle that receives the electric impulse of the heart from the sinoatrial (SA) node. The impulse then travels to the atrioventricular bundle of His, which carries it to the ventricles. The AV node is located in the septal wall of the right atrium.

atrioventricular septum, a small portion of wall that separates the upper heart chambers (atria) from the lower heart chambers (ventricles) of the heart.

atrioventricular valve, a valve in the heart through which blood flows from the upper heart chambers (atria) to the lower heart chambers (ventricles). The valve between the left atrium and left ventricle is called the mitral valve. The right valve is called the tricuspid valve. Also called **cuspid valve.**

at risk, referring to a person or population who is vulnerable to a particular disease or injury. The factors determining risk may be environmental or physical. An example of an environmental factor is exposure to toxic wastes. An example of a physical factor is genetic tendency to develop a disease.

atrium /ā'trē·əm/, *pl.* **atria,** a chamber or cavity, as the right and left atria of the heart or the nasal cavity.

atrium of the heart, one of the two upper chambers of the heart. Blood lacking oxygen returns from the body to the right atrium. The left atrium receives blood with oxygen from the veins in the lungs. Blood is emptied into the lower heart chambers (ventricles) from the atria.

-atrophia, -trophy, 1. a combining form meaning a 'condition of malnutrition.' 2. a combining form meaning a 'continuous decline of a body part.'

atrophic catarrh, an abnormal condition marked by swelling and discharge from the nose. It goes together with the loss of mucous membranes. Compare **hypertrophic catarrh.** See also **catarrh.**

atrophic fracture, a spontaneous fracture caused by wasting away (atrophy). This sometimes occurs in elderly patients.

atrophic gastritis, a long-term inflammation of the stomach, with the breakdown of the mucous membranes of the stomach. This is sometimes seen in elderly patients. It is also seen in patients with dangerous (pernicious) anemia. Atrophic gastritis may cause pain just below the breastbone.

atrophoderma, the wasting away or decrease in size of the skin. It may affect the entire body surface or only small areas.

atrophy /at′rəfē/, a wasting or loss of size of a part of the body because of disease or other influences. A muscle may atrophy because of lack of physical exercise. Nervous system or muscle disease are other causes. Cells of the brain and nervous system may atrophy in old age because of restricted blood flow to those areas. See also **aging.** –**atrophic,** *adj.*

atropine sulfate, a drug used to treat irritability of the stomach and intestines, swelling of the eye, irregular heart beats, neurological disorders (parkinsonism), certain kinds of poisoning, and as a boost to anesthesia.

★CAUTION: Obstruction of the stomach and intestines, certain eye diseases (glaucoma), swelling of the liver (hepatitis), kidney disease, or known allergy to this or similar drugs prohibits its use.

★ADVERSE EFFECTS: Among the more serious side effects are rapid heart beat, chest pain, loss of taste, nausea, diarrhea, skin rash, blurred vision, and eye pain. Dry mouth and constipation are common effects.

attachment, 1. the state or quality of being attached. 2. a mode of behavior in which one person relates in a dependent manner to another; a feeling of affection or loyalty that binds one person to another. See also **bonding.** 3. any device, as a retainer or artificial crown, used to secure a partial denture to a natural tooth in the mouth.

attachment apparatus, the combination of tissues that support the teeth.

attending physician, the physician who is responsible for a particular patient.

attention, the mental process in which a person concentrates on a specific issue, object, or activity.

attention deficit disorder, a syndrome affecting children, adolescents, and, rarely, adults. It is marked by learning and behavior disabilities. The symptoms may be mild or severe. They are caused by nervous system disorders. Usually there are no other nervous system problems or psychiatric problems. The patients with the disease are usually of normal or above-average intelligence. Symptoms include blocked vision, language, memory, and motor skills. Other symptoms are short attention span, impulsiveness, emotional instability, and sometimes overactivity. The condition is 10 times more common in boys than in girls. It may result from genetic factors, chemical imbalance, or injury or disease at or after birth. Also called **hyperactivity, hyperkinesis, minimal brain dysfunction.** See also **learning disability.**

attenuation, the process of reduction, as the weakening of a disease organism.

Attenuvax, a trademark for a vaccine against measles virus.

attitudinal reflex, any reflex triggered by a change in position of the head.

attraction, a tendency of the teeth or other jaw structures to grow above their normal position.

attrition, the process of wearing away or wearing down by friction.

atypical measles syndrome (AMS), a form of measles (rubeola) that tends to infect people who were immunized by a vaccine that was not stored properly. Symptoms, a bit different from those seen with typical measles, begin with a sudden high fever, headache, stomach pain, and coughing. The measles rash may appear only 1 or 2 days later. It usually starts on the hands and feet rather than on the head and neck. The infection may be complicated by swelling of the hands and feet, and pneumonia.

atypical somatoform disorder, an abnormal condition in which physical symptoms and complaints appear to be related to the person's excessive concern with an imagined defect in appearance or ability.

Au, symbol for **gold.**

audioanalgesia, the use of music to relax and to distract a patient's mind from pain, as during dentistry. The procedure has also been tried during labor.

audiogram /ô′dē·əgram′/, a chart showing the sharpness of hearing as shown by a person's ability to hear sounds and to distinguish different speech sounds. See also **audiometry.**

audiology, the study of hearing, especially impaired hearing that cannot be corrected.

audiometer /ô′dē·om′ətər/, an electric device for testing the hearing and for measuring the conduction of sound through bone and air. Earphones are placed over the ears. The ear not being tested gets a masking noise from the machine. The ear being tested is aroused by a series of tones, from very low to very high frequencies at various decibels. The patient signals when a tone is heard. The results are noted on an audiogram.

audiometry /ō'dē·om'itrē/, testing the sense of hearing. Pure tone audiometry determines the patient's ability to hear frequencies, usually ranging from 125 to 8,000 hertz (Hz). It can determine if a hearing loss is caused by a middle-ear problem or by one in the inner ear or the auditory nerve. In this test the patient sits in a soundproof booth. The operator slowly increases the decibel level. The patient signals when sounds are first heard through the earphones. Speech audiometry tests the ability to repeat certain words. Impedance audiometry is a method of testing the middle ear by measuring muscle responses to sound with a probe inserted in the ear canal. Cortical audiometry measures the response of the brain to pure tones. Localization audiometry is a method for measuring a patient's ability to locate the source of a sound.

audit, a review and evaluation of health-care procedures.

auditory canal, one of two passageways for sound to pass through the ear. One leads from the outer ear to the eardrum. The other, located within the skull, contains the nerve that sends signals from the inner ear to the brain (auditory nerve). Compare **eustachian tube (auditory tube).**

auditory nerve, either of the pair of nerves in the inner ear that send impulses to the brain regarding hearing and balance. Also called **acoustic nerve, eighth cranial nerve.**

auditory ossicles, the small bones in the middle ear (incus, malleus, and stapes) that connect with each other and the ear drum (tympanic membrane). Sound waves are carried through these bones as the tympanic membrane vibrates.

auditory system assessment, an evaluation of the patient's ears and hearing. It includes searching for present and past diseases or conditions that may be responsible for a hearing loss. ★METHOD: The patient is asked if he or she has any of the following: earaches, reduced or no hearing in one or both ears, dizziness (vertigo), a feeling of fullness, itching, or the heart pulsating in the ears. The patient is asked if there is a ringing or buzzing in the ears or a popping noise when yawning or swallowing. Other questions are if the voice echoes, if the ears drain a clear, yellow, red, or dark substance, and if oils, cotton swabs, or other objects are used to clean the ears. Examination includes blood pressure, pulse, temperature, and breathing, the ability to hear or to lipread or use a hearing aid. The patient's startle reflex, tolerance of loud sounds, allergies, use of drugs, especially of eardrops, are carefully noted. The presence of ear infection or other ear disorders are observed. Heart disease, high blood pressure, brain tumor, head injury, or skull fracture are some other diseases that are investigated. Diagnosis may be made by an audiogram, audiometric test, a mastoid x-ray film, or by an ear examination. Rinne and Weber tuning-fork tests, and tests for any ear drainage are also used for diagnosis.

auditory tube. See **eustachian tube.**

Auer rod /ou'ər/, abnormal, needle-shaped or round bodies in the white blood cells of a patient with leukemia. The finding of Auer rods in the blood may help to keep different types of leukemia apart. Also called **Auer body.**

aura /ôr'ə/, *pl.* **aurae** /ôr'ē/, a sensation of light or warmth that may be noted before an attack of migraine headache or an epileptic seizure.

aural /ôr'əl/, referring to the ear or hearing. **–aurally,** *adv.*

aural forceps, a dressing forceps with fine, bent tips, used in aural surgery.

auramine, a yellow dye used in paints, textiles, and rubber products. It has been found to cause bladder cancer in humans. Also called **dimethyl aniline.**

auranofin, an oral drug prescribed for the treatment of rheumatoid arthritis. ★CAUTION: It should not be given to patients who have health problems that are caused or aggravated by medicines containing gold. ★ADVERSE EFFECTS: Among the most severe adverse reactions reported are diarrhea, stomach pain, nausea, vomiting, rash, itching, inflammation of the mouth, blood and urine abnormalities, and increased liver enzymes.

Aureomycin, a trademark for a tetracycline antibiotic (chlortetracycline hydrochloride).

auricle /ôr'ikəl/, **1.** the external ear. Also called **pinna. 2.** the left or right upper heart chamber (atrium), so named because of its earlike shape.

auricularis anterior, one of three outer muscles of the ear. Some people can voluntarily contract the auricularis anterior to move the ears. Compare **auricularis posterior, auricularis superior.**

auricularis posterior, one of three outer muscles of the ear. It serves to draw the auricula backward. Compare **auricularis anterior, auricularis superior.**

auricularis superior, a thin, fan-shaped muscle that is one of three outer muscles of the ear. It acts to draw the auricula upward. Compare **auricularis anterior, auricularis posterior.**

auriculin, a hormonelike substance made in the upper chambers (atria) of the heart. It promotes the release of urine.

auriculoventriculostomy /ôrik'yoŏlōventrik'yoŏlos'təmē/, a surgical procedure that directs brain and spine (cerebrospinal) fluid into the blood circulation. It treats water on the brain (hydrocephalus). This is usually done in the newborn. A hole is drilled through the side of the skull. A polyethylene tube is inserted. The tube is passed into the jugular vein in the neck. Thus the cerebrospinal fluid drains into the bloodstream. Also called **ventriculoatrial shunt, ventriculoatriostomy.**

auriosis. See **chrysiasis.**

aurothioglucose /ôr′ōthī′ōglo͞o′kōs/, gold used to treat adult and juvenile rheumatoid arthritis. ★CAUTION: Severe uncontrolled diabetes, kidney or liver disease, a history of infectious swelling of the liver (hepatitis), high blood pressure, and heart failure prohibits its use. Pregnancy or known allergy to this drug also prohibits its use. ★ADVERSE EFFECTS: Among the most serious side effects are kidney damage and many allergic reactions. Skin disease (dermatitis) and ulcers of the mucous membranes are common.

auscultation /ôskəltā′shən/, the act of listening for sounds within the body to evaluate the condition of the heart, lungs, intestines, or other organs or to hear the fetal heart beat. Auscultation may be done with the ear alone. However, usually a stethoscope is used. The frequency, intensity, duration, and quality of the sounds are noted. During auscultation of the chest, the patient usually sits upright. He or she breathes slowly and deeply through the mouth. The front and back of the chest are auscultated from top to bottom. The sounds of the right and left sides are compared. The heart and stomach may be auscultated with the patient lying down or sitting upright. –**auscultate,** v.

Australia antigen, hepatitis B surface antigen (HBsAG). It is found in the blood serum of a patient who has serum hepatitis or who is a carrier for that virus. Blood banks routinely examine blood for Australia antigen. The purpose is to avoid passing on a liver disease (hepatitis) infection to a patient receiving a transfusion. See also **hepatitis.**

Australian lift, a type of shoulder lift used to move patients who are unable to sit upright by themselves.

autacoid /ô′təkloid/, any of a group of substances, as hormones, that are made in one organ and are transported by blood or lymph to another part of the body.

authenticity, (in psychiatry) being open in feelings and actions; a quality of being genuine and trustworthy.

authoritarian personality, the characteristics of a person who believes in obedience and acting strictly according to the rules.

authority, a relationship between two or more persons or groups in which one influences the other(s) through ideas, commands, suggestions, or instructions.

authority figure, a person who influences others by virtue of status, strength, knowledge, or other recognized superiority.

autism, a mental disorder. It is marked by extreme withdrawal into fantasy. Autism goes together with delusion, hallucination, and an inability to talk or to otherwise relate to people. Schizophrenic children are often autistic. See also **infantile autism. –autistic,** adj.

autistic phase, a normal period of development that lasts from birth to around 1 month. Children then realize that they cannot satisfy their body needs by themselves.

autistic thought, a form of thinking in which ideas have a private meaning to the individual. In autistic thinking, fantasy life may be interpreted as reality.

auto-, a combining form referring to self.

autoantibody /ô′tō·an′tibod′ē/, an antibody that reacts against the patient's own body. Normally antibodies attack foreign invaders (antigens). There are several mechanisms that may lead to the making of autoantibodies. For example, antibodies made against certain streptococcal bacteria during infection may react with heart tissue. This causes rheumatic heart disease. Another mechanism is that normal body proteins may be changed to antigens by chemicals, infection, or drugs.

autoantigen /ô′tō·an′tijin/, a normal body substance that causes an abnormal production of autoantibody. This results in a reaction of the body against tissues in the body (autoimmune reaction). See also **autoantibody.**

autochthonous idea /ôtok′thənəs/, an idea that begins in the unconscious and arises spontaneously in the mind, independent of any conscious train of thought.

autodiploid /ô′tōdip′loid/, referring to a person, organism, or cell containing two genetically identical or nearly identical chromosome sets.

autoeroticism, 1. sensual, usually sexual, satisfaction of the self. It is usually done through stimulating one's own body without the participation of another person. Satisfaction comes from stroking, masturbation, fantasy, or from other oral, anal, or visual sources. 2. sexual feeling or desire occurring without any outer stimulus. 3. (in Freudian psychoanalytic theory) an early phase of psychosexual development. It occurs in the oral and the anal stages. Also called **autoerotism.** Compare **heteroeroticism. –autoerotic,** adj.

autoerythrocyte sensitization /ô′tō·ərith′rəsīt/, an unusual disorder marked by the spontaneous appearance of painful bleeding under the skin on the front areas of the arms and legs. The cause is allergy to the patient's own red blood cells.

autogenic therapy, a mental-health therapy based on the concept that natural forces in the brain are able to remove disturbing influences. It involves biofeedback exercises.

autogenous /ôtoj′ənəs/, 1. self-creating. 2. originating from within the organism, as a poison or vaccine.

autograft, transplantation by surgery of any tissue from one part of the body to another part in the same patient. Autografts are commonly used to replace skin lost in severe burns. Compare **allograft, isograft, xenograft.** See also **graft.**

autographism. See **dermatographia.**

autoimmune, referring to the development of an immune response to one's own tissues.

autoimmune disease, one of a large group of diseases marked by a change of the immune system of the body. Normally, the immune system controls the body's defenses against infection. Sometimes these defenses are turned against the body itself. This leads to chronic and often deadly diseases. The cause of autoimmune disease is not known. However, many researchers believe that in some cases a virus infection may "retrain" the body's defense cells (T cells) to attack the wrong tissues. There are two general categories of autoimmune diseases. The first are the collagen diseases. The second are the autoimmune blood destroying (hemolytic) disorders. Treatment includes steroid, antiswelling, and immunosuppressive drugs. The symptoms are treated as needed. For example, a transfusion for bleeding, pain relievers, and physical therapy for preventing crippling. Diet may be regulated, as iron might be given to treat anemia in a patient with a certain blood disease (thrombocytopenic purpura). Calories might be reduced in a weight-loss diet for a patient with rheumatoid arthritis. Surgery is some times done to correct or prevent further complications. Many of these diseases have periods of crisis and periods of no symptoms. During a crisis, the patient may be hospitalized and need extensive treatment.

autoimmunity, an abnormal condition in which the body reacts against its own tissues. Autoimmunity may result in allergy and autoimmune disease. Although there are several theories to explain autoimmunity, it is not yet fully understood. See also **antibody specific theory, autoimmune disease.**

autolet, a small, sharp instrument used to obtain certian blood samples from capillaries.

autologous transfusion /ôtol'əgəs/, a procedure in which blood is removed from a person, stored for a period of time, and then returned to the person's own circulation.

automatic bladder. See **spastic bladder.**

automatic infiltration detector, a device that sounds an alarm and automatically stops intravenous fluids when the fluid leaks out of the vein. The device detects any cooling of the skin where the intravenous needle is inserted, a common sign of infiltration.

automaticity, a property of specialized excitable tissue that allows it to create electrical impulses that can travel across cell membranes, as in the pacemaker cells of the heart.

automatic speech, speech containing words or phrases spoken without thinking. It often consists of expletives, profanities, and greetings.

automation, use of a machine made to follow repeatedly and automatically a set order of operations.

automatism /ôtom'ətiz'əm/, **1.** involuntary function of an organ system. It can be independent of outer stimulation, as beating of the heart, or dependent on outer stimulation but not consciously controlled, as the dilation of the pupil of the eye. **2.** mechanical, repetitive, and undirected behavior that is not consciously controlled, as in brain disorder (psychomotor epilepsy), hysteric states, and sleepwalking.

autonomic /ô'tənom'ik/, **1.** having the ability to function independently without outside influence. **2.** referring to the autonomic nervous system.

autonomic drug, any of a large group of drugs that copy or change the function of the autonomic nervous system.

autonomic dysreflexia, reflexes that are confused as the result of blocked function of the autonomic nervous system. It is caused by simultaneous sympathetic and parasympathetic activity. It occurs in patients paralyzed from the neck down (quadriplegics) and some paralyzed from the waist down (paraplegics). The symptoms are paleness below and flushing above the spinal cord injury, high blood pressure, slowed heart beat, and convulsions.

autonomic nervous system, the part of the nervous system that regulates vital functions of the body that are not consciously controlled (involuntary). It includes the activity of the heart, the smooth muscles (as digestive muscles), and the glands. It has two divisions: the **sympathetic nervous system** speeds up heart rate, narrows blood vessels, and raises blood pressure; the **parasympathetic nervous system** slows heart rate, increases intestinal and gland activity, and relaxes ringlike muscles that close passages (sphincters).

autonomic neuropathy, damage to nerves of the autonomic nervous system. This type of neuropathy can cause extreme drops in blood pressure when standing up (orthostatic hypotension), for example.

autonomic reflex, any of a large number of normal reflexes that regulate the functions of the body's organs. Autonomic reflexes control activities as blood pressure, heart rate, intestinal activity, sweating, and urination.

autonomous bladder. See **flaccid bladder.**

autonomy /ôton'əmē/, the quality of having the ability to live independently. **–autonomous,** *adj.*

autonomy drive, a type of behavior in which the person attempts to control the environment to serve the individual's own purposes.

autopagnosia, an inability to recognize and identify the parts of one's own body. It is linked generally to disease of the brain. It is diagnosed when a patient is unable to perform a task, as touching the right ear with the left thumb.

autoplastic maneuver, a process that is part of adaptation, involving an adjustment within the self. Compare **alloplastic maneuver.**

autoplasty /ô'təplas'tē/, a plastic surgery procedure in which parts of the patient's own tissues are used to replace or repair body areas damaged by disease or injury.

autopolyploid /ô'tōpol'iploid/, referring to an individual, organism, or cell that has more than two genetically identical or nearly identical sets of chromosomes.

autopsy /ô'topsē/, an examination after death that is done to determine the cause of death. Also called **necropsy, thanotopsy.**

autopsy pathology, the study of disease by a pathologist's examination of the body after death. This includes looking at tissues under a microscope and doing laboratory tests.

autoserous treatment /ô'təsir'əs/, treatment of an infectious disease by injecting the patient with his or her own serum.

autosite /ô'təsīt/, the larger, more normally formed member of unequal-sized joined twins. The other smaller fetus is dependent on the autosite for various functions and for nutrition and growth. Compare **parasitic fetus. –autositic,** *adj.*

autosomal /ô'təsō'məl/, **1.** referring to or characteristic of a non-sex determining chromosome (autosome). **2.** referring to any condition carried by an autosome.

autosomal dominant inheritance, a pattern of inheritance in which a dominant gene on a non-sex determining chromosome (autosome) makes a certain characteristic. Males and females are affected in equal numbers. Affected individuals usually have an affected parent. Normal children of an affected parent do not carry the trait.

autosomal inheritance, a pattern of inheritance in which traits depend on the presence or absence of certain genes on the non-sex determining chromosomes (autosomes). The pattern may be dominant or non-dominant (recessive), and males and females are affected in equal numbers. Most hereditary disorders are the result of a defective gene on an autosome.

autosomal recessive inheritance, a pattern of inheritance in which a non-dominant (recessive) gene on a non-sex determining chromosome (autosome) results in a person being either a carrier of a trait or being affected. Males and females are affected with equal frequency. There is usually no family history of the trait. Instead, it is manifested when two unaffected parents who are both carriers of a particular recessive gene have a child. Cystic fibrosis, phenylketonuria, and galactosemia are examples of autosomal recessive inheritance. Compare **autosomal dominant inheritance.** See also **recessive.**

autosome /ô'təsōm/, any chromosome that is not a sex chromosome and that appears as an identical (homologous) pair. Humans have 22 pairs of autosomes, which carry all genetic traits other than those that are sex-linked. Also called **euchromosome.** Compare **sex chromosome.**

autosplenectomy /ô'tōsplinek'təmē/, a continuous shrinking of the spleen. It may occur in sickle-cell anemia. The spleen is replaced by fiberlike tissue. It becomes nonfunctional.

autosuggestion, an idea, thought, attitude, or belief suggested to oneself, often as a formula or chant, as a means of controlling one's behavior. Compare **suggestion.**

autotopagnosia /ô'tōtop'əg·nō'zhə/, the inability to recognize or locate the various parts of the body because of organic brain damage. It is generally associated with brain tumors and strokes. It is also characterized by the patient's inability to distinguish right from left. Retraining involves touching parts of the patient's body and asking the patient to name the area touched, and by having the patient put together human figure puzzles. Also called **body-image agnosia, body-scheme disorder.** See also **agnosia, proprioception.**

autotransfusion, a procedure in which blood is collected from an active bleeding site, cleansed, and returned to the body. It may be used in cases of major trauma or in major surgery.

autumn fever. See **leptospirosis.**

auxanology /ôks'ənol'əjē/, the scientific study of growth and development. **–auxanologic, auxanological,** *adj.*

auxesis /ôksē'sis/, *pl.* **auxeses,** an increase in size or amount caused by the cells growing larger. This is the opposite of most growth, which is caused by an increase in the number of cells. Also called **auxetic growth.** Compare **merisis.**

available arch length, the length or space in a dental arch that is available for all the natural teeth.

avantin. See **isopropyl alcohol.**

avascular /āvas'kyōōlər/, referring to an area not receiving a sufficient supply of blood. The reduced flow may be the result of blockage by a blood clot. It may also be from stopping the blood flow during surgery or when controlling bleeding.

aversion therapy, a form of behavior therapy in which punishment, unpleasant, or painful stimulation are used to stop undesirable behavior. Electric shock and drugs that cause nausea are examples of aversion therapy. The therapy is used in treating conditions as drug abuse, alcoholism, gambling, overeating, smoking, and various sexual abnormalities. Also called **aversive conditioning.** See also **behavior therapy.**

aversive stimulus, a stimulus, as electric shock, that causes emotional or physical pain. See also **aversion therapy.**

avidin, a protein in raw egg white that reacts with part of the B complex vitamins (biotin).

avitaminosis /āvī'təminō'sis/, a lack of one or more essential vitamins. It may result from lack of vitamins in the diet. It may also be the result of the inability to use the vitamins because of disease. Also called **hypovitaminosis.**

AV nicking, a blood vessel abnormality on the retina of the eye that is visible on examination, It is caused when a vein is pressed together by an artery (AV) crossing it. The vein appears "nicked" because of narrowing or spasm. It is a sign of high blood pressure, hardening of the arteries (arteriosclerosis), and other disorders of the blood vessels.

avoidance, a conscious or unconscious defense mechanism, physical or psychological in nature. A person tries to avoid or escape from something unpleasant, conflicts, or feelings, as anxiety, fear, pain, or danger.

avoidance-avoidance conflict, a conflict resulting from the confrontation of two or more events that are equally undesirable. Also called **double-avoidant conflict.** See also **conflict.**

avoidance conditioning, the establishment of certain patterns of behavior to avoid unpleasant or painful stimulation.

avoidant personality, a personality disorder in which the individual is overly sensitive to rejection and is reluctant to start a relationship because of a fear of not being accepted without criticism. The person has a strong desire for affection and acceptance and may be distressed by not being able to relate to others comfortably.

avoirdupois weight /av'ərdəpoiz'/, the English system of weights in which there are 7,000 grains, 256 drams, or 16 ounces to 1 pound. One ounce in this system equals 28.35 grams. 1 pound equals 453.59 grams. Compare **apothecaries' weight.** See also **metric system.**

avulsed teeth /əvulst/, teeth that have been forcibly displaced from their normal position.

avulsion, the separation, by tearing, of any part of a structure, as an avulsion fracture.

avulsion fracture, a bone fracture caused when a strong ligament or tendon forcibly pulls a fragment of bone away.

awake anesthesia, a treatment in which painkillers and anesthesia are used without loss of consciousness. Dental treatments, surgery on a limb, and certain kinds of head surgery are commonly done using awake anesthesia. Also called **conscious sedation.**

awareness context of death, the awareness by a terminally ill patient that he or she is dying and the awareness by those caring for the person that he or she knows that death is imminent. See also **emotional care of the dying patient, stages of dying.**

axial (A), 1. referring to or situated on the center (axis) of a structure or part of the body. 2. (in dentistry) relating to the long axis (root to tip) of a tooth.

axial current, the central part of the bloodstream as it flows through a vessel.

axial gradient, the variation in the chemical processes (metabolic rate) in different parts of the body.

axial spillway, a groove that crosses a rounded projection (cusp) or a marginal ridge and extends onto an axial surface of a tooth.

axilla /aksil'ə/, pl. **axillae,** a pyramid-shaped space forming the underside of the shoulder between the upper part of the arm and the side of the chest. Also called **armpit.**

axillary artery /ak'sələr'ē/, the artery that supplies each arm. Called the subclavian artery at the collar bone, it becomes the axillary at the shoulder. Where it crosses the bicep it becomes the brachial artery.

axillary nerve, the nerve that runs through the armpit (axilla), winds around the bone in the upper arm (humerus), and supplies part of the shoulder muscles (deltoid) and the shoulder joint.

axillary node, one of the lymph glands of the armpit (axilla) that help to fight infections in the chest, armpit, neck, and arm. They also drain lymph from those areas. The 20 to 30 axillary nodes are divided into the following groups: The lateral group is the lymph vessels that drain the whole arm. The anterior group is the vessels that drain the chest muscles. The posterior group is the vessels that drain the muscles of the back of the neck and the muscles of the chest wall. The central group is the vessels that drain the lymph from the nodes of the three groups just named. The medial group drains lymph from the breast and carries the lymph away. See also **lymphatic system, lymph node.**

axillary vein, one of a pair of veins of the arm that begins at the top of the arm near the bicep and becomes the subclavian vein near the collar bone. It receives oxygen-poor blood from certain veins.

axis, pl. **axes** /ak'sēz/, 1. an imaginary line that passes through the center of the body, or a part of the body. 2. the second backbone located in the neck (cervical vertebra). The first backbone in the neck (atlas) rotates around the axis, allowing the head to turn, extend, and flex. Also called **epistropheus, odontoid verte-bra.**

axis artery, one of a pair of extensions of the subclavian arteries. It runs into the upper arm and continues into the forearm as the palmar interosseous artery.

axis traction, 1. during childbirth, the process of pulling a baby's head with forceps in a direction of least resistance through the mother's birth canal. 2. *informal.* any mechanical device attached to forceps to aid in pulling in the proper direction.

axoaxonic synapse /ak′sō·akson′ik/, a type of neuron link (synapse) in which the extension (axon) of one neuron comes in contact with the axon of another neuron. See **axon.**

axodendritic synapse /ak′sōdendrit′ik/, a type of neuron link (synapse) in which the extension (axon) of one neuron comes in contact with the threadlike extensions (dendrites) of another neuron.

axodendrosomatic synapse /ak′sōden′drōsōmat′ik/, a type of neuron link (synapse) in which the extension (axon) of one neuron comes in contact with both the threadlike extensions (dendrites) and the cell body of another neuron.

axon /ak′son/, the cylinderlike extension of a nerve (neuron) cell that conducts electric impulses (synapses) away from the neuron. Also called **axis cylinder.** Compare **dendrite.**

axon flare, widening of the blood vessels, reddening, and increased sensitivity of skin surrounding an injured area. It is caused by nerve damage. Injury or stroking of the skin results in local reddening. Histamine or a histamine-like substance is released, and raised skin (wheal formation) occurs. A pin prick in the involved area causes intense pain.

axonotmesis /ak′sənotmē′sis/, a break in the transmitting portion of a nerve cell (axon) with subsequent breakdown of the end portion. Connective tissue of the nerve, including the protective cells surrounding the nerves, may remain intact.

axoplasmic flow /ak′sōplaz′mik/, the continuous pulsing movement of the cytoplasm between the cell body of a neuron and the fiber of the extension of the nerve cell (axon). The cytoplasm supplies the axon with substances vital for activity and for repair. The nerve fiber is totally dependent on the cell body for nutrition. Any interruption in the axoplasmic flow

caused by disease or injury results in the breakdown of the axon.

axosomatic synapse /ak′sōsōmat′ik/, a type of neuron link (synapse) in which the extension (axon) of one neuron comes in contact with another neuron.

azathioprine, an immunosuppressive drug used to prevent organ rejection after organ transplantation. It is also used to treat systemic inflammatory diseases.

–azepam, a combining form referring to a drug similar to diazepam, which is used to treat anxiety.

azidothymidine (AZT) /az′ədōthī′midēn/, See **zidovudine.**

Azlin, a trademark for an antibiotic (azlocillin).

azlocillin sodium, a penicillin antibiotic used to treat infections of the lower respiratory tract, urinary tract, skin, bone, joints, and blood poisoning (septicemia).

★CAUTION: Allergy to any of the penicillins prohibits its use.

★ADVERSE EFFECTS: The most serious side effects are reactions caused by a foreign protein (anaphylaxis), convulsive seizures, pain near the breastbone, blood disorders, and kidney and liver problems.

azo dye /ā′zō/, a chemical substance used in commercial coloring materials. Some forms may cause cancer.

–azoline, a combining form referring to a substance that reduces allergic responses (antihistamine) or narrows blood vessels.

azoospermia /āzō′əspur′mē·ə/, lack of sperm in the semen. It may be caused by dysfunction of the testicles or by blockage of the tubes in which sperm is stored (epididymis). It may also be caused by vasectomy. Infertility but not impotence is linked to azoospermia. Compare **oligospermia.**

–azosin, a combining form referring to a type of drug used to treat high blood pressure.

azotemia /az′ōtē′mē·ə/, excess amounts of nitrogen compounds in the blood. This poisonous condition is caused by failure of the kidneys to remove urea from the blood. It is characteristic of uremia. See also **uremia.** **–azotemic,** *adj.*

AZT, abbreviation for **azidothymidine.**

azygous /az′əgəs/, occurring as a single being or part, as any unpaired physical structure (for example, the mouth). Also **azygos.** **–azygos** /az′əgos′/, *n.*

azygous vein, one of the seven veins of the chest.

B

B, symbol for **boron.**

Ba, symbol for **barium.**

B.A., abbreviation for **Bachelor of Arts.**

babbling, a stage of speech development in which a series of sounds is produced.

Babcock's operation, removal of a varicosed saphenous vein by inserting an acorn-tipped rod, tying the vein to the rod and drawing it out. Also called **subcutaneous stripping.**

babesiosis /bəbē′sē·ō′sis/, an infection caused by the protozoa *Babesia.* The organism enters the body through the bite of ticks. Symptoms include headache, fever, nausea and vomiting, aching, and blood disorders. Also called **babesiasis.**

Babinski's reflex /bəbin′skēz/, extending the big toe upward and fanning the other toes when the sole of the foot is stroked. The reflex is normal in newborn infants. It is abnormal in children and adults in whom it may indicate a brain injury. Also called **Babinski's sign.**

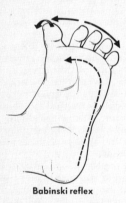

Babinski reflex

baby, **1.** an infant or young child, especially one who is not yet able to walk or talk. **2.** to treat gently or with special care.

Baby Jane Doe regulations, rules established in 1984 by the United States Health and Human Services Department. State governments are required to investigate complaints about parental decisions involving the treatment of handicapped infants. The rules also allowed the federal government to have access to children's medical records. Hospitals are required to post notices urging doctors and nurses to report any suspected cases of infants denied proper medical care. Also called **Baby Doe rules.**

baby talk, **1.** the speech patterns and sounds of young children learning to talk. It is character-ized by mispronunciation, repetition, and speech modifications, as lisping or stuttering. See also **lallation. 2.** the intentionally oversimplified manner of speech that imitates young children learning to talk. It is often used by adults in addressing children or pets. **3.** the speech patterns that occur in some mental disorders, especially schizophrenia.

bacampicillin hydrochloride, a penicillin used to treat respiratory tract, urinary tract, skin, and gonococcal infections.

★CAUTION: Known sensitivity to this drug or other penicillins prohibits its use.

★ADVERSE EFFECTS: Among the most serious side effects are allergic reactions, gastritis, enterocolitis, and transient blood disorders.

bacill-, a combining form referring to any rod-shaped bacteria.

Bacillaceae /bas′əlā′si·ē/, a family of *Schizomycetes* bacteria of the order *Eubacteriales,* consisting of rod-shaped cells. These bacteria commonly appear in soil. Some are parasitic on insects and animals and can cause disease. The family includes the genus *Bacillus,* which needs air (aerobic) and the genus *Clostridium,* which can live without air (anaerobic).

bacillary dysentery. See **shigellosis.**

bacille Calmette-Guérin (BCG) /kalmet′gāraN′/, a weakened strain of tubercle bacilli, used in many countries as a vaccine against tuberculosis. It appears to prevent the more serious forms of tuberculosis and to give some protection to persons living in areas where tuberculosis is common. BCG is also given to stimulate the immune system in patients who have certain kinds of cancer. See also **tuberculin test, tuberculosis.**

bacilliform /bəsil′ifôrm/, rod-shaped in form, like a bacillus.

bacilluria /bas′əloo͞or′ē·ə/, the presence of bacilli in the urine.

Bacillus, a genus of air-consuming (aerobic), spore-producing bacteria in the family Bacillaceae. There are 33 species, three of which cause disease. See also **Bacillaceae.**

Bacillus anthracis, a species of nonair-consuming (anaerobic) bacteria that causes anthrax. The spores of this organism, if inhaled, can cause a pulmonary form of anthrax. The spores can live for many years in animal products, as hides and wool, and in soil. See also **anthrax, woolsorter's disease.**

bacillus Calmette-Guérin vaccine. See **BCG vaccine.**

bacitracin /bas′itrā′sin/, an antibacterial used to treat some skin infections.

★CAUTION: Known allergy to this drug prohibits its use.

★ADVERSE EFFECTS: Among the more serious side effects are kidney damage and skin rash.

back, the back part of the trunk between the neck and the pelvis. The back is divided by a furrow created by the spine. The skeletal portion of the back includes the chest (thoracic) and lower (lumbar) backbones (vertebrae) and both shoulder blades (scapulas).

backache, pain in the spine or muscles of the back. Causes may include muscle strain or other muscular disorders, pressure on the root of a nerve, or a ruptured vertebral disk. Treatment may include heat, ultrasound, and devices to provide support, bed rest, surgery, pain relievers, and muscle relaxers.

back-action condenser, a dental instrument for compacting filling material (amalgams).

background radiation, naturally occurring radiation given off by materials in the soil, ground waters, and building material. Radioactive substances in the body, especially potassium 40 (40K), and cosmic rays from outer space also give off background radiation. The average person is exposed each year to 44 millirad (mrad) of cosmic radiation, 44 mrad from the environment, and 18 mrad from naturally occurring internal radioactive sources.

back pressure, pressure that builds in a blood vessel or a cavity as fluid accumulates. The pressure increases and extends backward if the normal passageway for the fluid is not opened. See also **backward failure.**

backtracking, a communication technique in which the patient and the therapist review what they have discussed previously to regain focus.

backward failure, heart failure that develops when the lower heart chamber (ventricle) cannot empty. Blood backs up in the pulmonary veins and the lungs, causing fluid accumulation (pulmonary edema).

baclofen, a muscle relaxant used to treat spasticity in multiple sclerosis.

★CAUTION: Known allergy to this drug prohibits its use.

★ADVERSE EFFECTS: Among the more serious side effects are confusion, low blood pressure, shortness of breath, impotence, nausea, and temporary drowsiness.

bacteremia /bak′tirē′mē·ə/, the presence of bacteria in the blood. Bacteremia is diagnosed by growing organisms from a blood sample. Treatment is antibiotics. Compare **septicemia.** See also **septic shock.** —**bacteremic,** adj.

bacteremic shock. See **septic shock.**

bacteria /baktir′ē·ə/, sing. **bacterium,** the small one-celled microorganisms of the class Schizomycetes. Some are round (cocci), rod-shaped (bacilli), spiral (spirochetes), or comma-shaped (vibrios). The nature, severity, and outcome of any infection caused by a bacterium depend on the species.

bacterial aneurysm, a dilation in a small area of the wall of a blood vessel caused by the growth of bacteria. This condition often follows septicemia or bacteremia. See also **mycotic aneurysm.**

bacterial endocarditis, a bacterial infection of the lining of the heart (endocardium) or the heart valves or both. The symptoms are a heart murmur, prolonged fever, bacteremia, enlarged spleen, and blood clot. Prompt treatment with antibiotics is essential to prevent destruction of the valves and heart failure. See also **endocarditis, subacute bacterial endocarditis.**

bacterial food poisoning, illness from eating food contaminated by certain bacteria. Acute infectious gastroenteritis caused by various species of salmonella is characterized by fever, chills, nausea, vomiting, diarrhea, and general discomfort beginning 8 to 48 hours after the contaminated food is eaten and continuing for several days. Similar symptoms caused by staphylococcus appear much sooner and rarely last more than a few hours. Food poisoning caused by the organism *Clostridium botulinum* produces stomach and intestinal symptoms, disturbances of vision, weakness or paralysis of muscles, and, in severe cases, respiratory failure. See also **botulism.**

bacterial meningitis. See **meningitis.**

bacterial plaque, a film made up of microorganisms that cling to the teeth and often cause tooth decay and infections of the gums. Mucin secreted by the salivary glands is also a component of plaque. Also called **dental plaque.**

bacterial protein, a protein produced by a bacterium.

bacterial resistance, the ability of certain types of bacteria to develop a resistance to the effects of specific antibiotics.

bactericidal /baktir′isī′dəl/, destructive to bacteria. Compare **bacteriostatic.**

bacterio-, bacter-, a combining form referring to any bacteria.

bacteriologic sputum examination, a laboratory procedure to determine the presence or absence of bacteria in a sample of material (sputum) coughed up from a patient's lungs.

bacteriology, the scientific study of bacteria. —**bacteriological, bacteriologic,** adj.

bacteriolysin /baktir′ē·əli′sin/, an antibody that breaks down a particular species of bacteria.

bacteriolysis /baktir′ē·ol′əsis/, the breakdown (lysis) of bacteria.

bacteriophage /baktir′ē·əfāj′/, any virus that causes bacteria to disintegrate. —**bacteriophagic,** adj., **bacteriophagy** /-of′əjē, n/.

bacteriophage typing, the process of identifying a species of bacteria according to the type of virus that attacks it.

bacteriostatic /baktir′ē·əstat′ik/, tending to restrain the development of bacteria. Compare **bacteriocidal.**

bacteriuria /baktir′ēyŏŏr′ē·ə/, the presence of bacteria in the urine. More than 100,000 bacteria per ml of urine usually means a urinary tract infection is present. See also **urinary tract infection.**

bacteroid /bak′təroid/, referring to or resembling bacteria.

Bacteroides /bak′təroi′dēz/, a genus of bacilli that can live without air (anaerobic). They are normally found in the large intestine, mouth, genital tract, and upper respiratory system. Severe infection may result when a break occurs in the mucous membranes and the bacillus enters the circulation, causing clots and bacteremia.

Bactrim, a trademark for a drug containing two antibacterials (sulfamethoxazole and trimethoprim).

baffling, the process of removing large water particles from the mist in a jet atomizer. It is done to ensure that the mist that enters the patient's breathing passages is therapeutic.

bag, a flexible pouch designed to contain gas, fluid, or semisolid material, as crushed ice. A breathing bag (Ambu-bag) is used to control the flow of gases entering the lungs of a patient. Several types of bags are used to widen the anus, vagina, or other body openings.

bagasse /bəgas′/, the crushed fibers and residue left after syrup is extracted from sugar cane.

bagassosis /bag′əsō′sis/, a lung disease caused by an allergic reaction to bagasse. The symptoms are shortness of breath, fever, and malaise. Treatment may include steroid drugs. To prevent a recurrence of the condition, bagasse should be avoided. See also **diffuse hypersensitivity pneumonia, organic dust.**

bagging, *informal.* artificial respiration performed with a respirator bag, as an Ambu-bag or Hope resuscitator. The bag is squeezed to force air into the patient's lungs as the mask is held over the mouth. During surgery, the anesthetist may also use this technique to correct the breathing pattern of an unconscious patient.

bag of waters, the membrane sac of amniotic fluid surrounding the fetus during pregnancy. See **amnion.**

Bainbridge reflex, a heart reflex consisting of an increased pulse rate, resulting from stimulation of the wall of the left upper heart chamber (atrium). It may be produced by large amounts of intravenous fluids.

Baker's cyst, a sac (cyst) in or under the skin filled with fluid or semi-solid materials that forms at the back of the knee. It is often associated with rheumatoid arthritis and may appear only when the leg is straightened.

BAL, abbreviation for **British antilewisite.** See **dimercaprol.**

balance, 1. an instrument for weighing. **2.** a normal state of physical equilibrium. **3.** a state of mental or emotional equilibrium.

balanced anesthesia, *informal.* a type of technique for general anesthesia in which more than one anesthetic is used. A mixture of anesthetics is given according to the needs of a particular patient for a particular operation.

balanced articulation, the simultaneous contacting of the upper and lower teeth as they glide over each other.

balanced diet, a diet containing all of the essential nutrients in adequate amounts needed by the body for growth, energy, repair, and maintenance of normal health.

balanced occlusion, 1. a closure (occlusion) of the teeth in which all the surfaces are in harmony. **2.** the upper and lower teeth on both sides make contact together.

balanced suspension, a system of splints, ropes, slings, pulleys, and weights for suspending the legs. It is used as an aid to healing of fractures or after surgical operations.

balanced traction, a system of balanced suspension that supplements traction for treating fractures of the legs or after various operations on the lower parts of the body.

balancing factors, events that contribute to the cause and results of a crisis.

balancing side, the side of the mouth opposite the chewing side.

balanic /bəlan′ik/, referring to the penis or the clitoris.

balanitis /bal′əni′tis/, inflammation of the penis.

balanitis xerotica obliterans /zirot′ikə-oblit′ərans/, a long-term skin disease of the penis, characterized by white, hardened tissue surrounding the opening (meatus).

balano-, a combining form referring to the penis.

balanoplasty /bal′ənōplas′tē/, an operation involving plastic surgery of the penis.

balanoposthitis /bal′ənōposthi′tis/, a generalized inflammation of the penis and foreskin. The symptoms are soreness, irritation, and discharge, occurring as a complication of bacterial or fungal infection. The cause is often a common venereal disease, in which case it is treated with antibiotics. Circumcision may be considered in severe cases.

balanopreputial /bal′ənōpripyŏŏ′shəl/, referring to the penis and the foreskin.

balanorrhagia /bal′ənōrā′jē·ə/, balanitis with an excessive amount of pus.

balantidiasis /bal′əntidī′əsis/, an infection caused by swallowing the cysts of the protozoan *Balantidium coli.* In some cases the organism is a harmless inhabitant of the large intestine, but infection with *B. coli* usually causes diarrhea. Occasionally, the protozoan invades the intestinal wall and produces ulcers or abcesses, which may cause dysentery and death.

Balantidium coli /bal'əntid'ē·əm/,　the largest and the only protozoan species with hairlike projections (cilia) that can produce disease in humans, as balantidiasis. It is a normal inhabitant of the domestic hog and is transmitted to humans by swallowing the cysts excreted by the hog.

baldness,　absence of hair, especially from the scalp. See also **alopecia.**

BAL in Oil,　a trademark for a drug used to treat poisoning with arsenic, gold, mercury, and lead (dimercaprol).

Balkan frame,　an overhead, rectangular frame, fixed to the bed for attaching splints, for suspending immobilized limbs, and for traction weights and pulleys.

Balkan tubulointerstitial nephritis /tōō'byəlō·in'tərstish'əl/,　a chronic kidney disorder marked by reduced kidney function, large amounts of protein in the urine, death of tissue, and anemia. It develops gradually, but end-stage disease occurs within 5 years after the first signs. About one-third of the patients also suffer from cancer of the urinary tract. The disease is common in the Balkans but is not hereditary.

ball-and-socket joint,　a synovial joint in which the round head of one bone is held in the cuplike cavity of another bone. This allows a limb to move in many directions. The hip and shoulder joints are ball-and-socket joints. Also called **enarthrosis, spheroidea.** Compare **condyloid joint, pivot joint, saddle joint.**

ballismus,　an abnormal condition characterized by violently flinging the arms about and, occasionally, the head. The cause is a brain injury. **Hemiballismus** is a form of the condition that involves only one side of the body. Also called **ballism.**

ballistic movement,　an extremely rapid movement, such as a tennis serve or boxing punch. It requires a high level of coordination.

ballistocardiogram /bəlis'tōkär'dē·əgram'/,　a recording of the body vibrations that are caused by the beating of the heart. When the blood is pumped into the large heart artery (aorta) and the pulmonary arteries, it causes a vibration beginning at the head and traveling to the feet. The patient is placed on a special table, a ballistocardiograph, that is so delicately balanced that body vibrations can be recorded by a machine attached to the table. It is used to determine how elastic the aorta is and the amount of blood the heart is able to handle.

ball of the foot,　includes the part of the foot where the toe bones and foot bones meet and the pad of tissue that surrounds it.

balloon septostomy.　See **Rashkind procedure.**

balloon-tip catheter,　a tube (catheter) with an inflatable sac around one end. After the catheter is inserted, the sac is inflated with air or sterile water. The inflated sac secures the catheter in the correct position. Kinds of balloon-

tip catheters include **Foley catheter** for inserting into the urinary bladder and **Swan-Ganz catheter** for measuring the pressure in the pulmonary artery.

ballottable head,　a fetal head that has not descended very far into the birth canal.

ballottement /bä'lôtmäN', bəlot'ment/,　a technique of feeling (palpating) an organ or structure by bouncing it gently and feeling it rebound. In late pregnancy, a fetal head that can be ballotted is said to be **floating** or **unengaged.** This is in contrast to a fixed or an engaged head, which cannot be easily dislodged from the pelvis.

ball thrombus,　a relatively round blood clot containing platelets, fibrin, and cell fragments. It can block a blood vessel or a valve of the heart.

ball-valve action,　the opening and closing of a hole by a buoyant, ball-shaped mass that acts as a valve. Some kinds of objects that may act in this manner are kidney stones, gallstones, and blood clots.

balm,　**1.** also called **balsam.** a healing or a soothing substance, as a medicinal ointment. **2.** an aromatic plant of the genus *Melissa* that is steeped in water and taken to relieve pain.

balneology /bal'nē·ol'əjē/,　a field of medicine that deals with the healing characteristics of various mineral waters, especially in baths. **–balneologic,** *adj.*

balneotherapy /bal'nē·ōther'əpē/,　use of baths in the treatment of many diseases and conditions.

balneum pneumaticum.　See **air bath.**

balsam,　any of a variety of resinous saps, generally from evergreens.

bamboo spine,　the typically rigid spine of advanced ankylosing spondylitis. Also called **poker spine.** See also **ankylosing spondylitis.**

band,　**1.** a bundle of fibers that encircles a structure or binds one part of the body to another. **2.** a strip of metal that fits around a tooth and serves as an attachment for orthodontic appliances.

band adapter,　an instrument for fitting an orthodontic band to a tooth.

bandage,　a strip of cloth that is wound around a part of the body in a variety of ways. It is used to hold a dressing, put pressure over a compress, or immobilize a limb or other part of the body.

bandage shears,　a sturdy pair of scissors used to cut through bandages. The blades of most bandage shears are angled, and the lower blade has a rounded blunt tip to avoid harming the skin when the scissors are inserted under the bandage.

band cell,　any one of the granular white blood cells that has a curved or indented nucleus.

band pusher,　an instrument used for adapting metal orthodontic bands to the teeth.

band remover,　an instrument used for removing orthodontic bands from the teeth.

bank blood, unclotted (anticoagulated) preserved blood collected from donors in pints (500 ml) and refrigerated for future use. Bank blood is used after it is matched to the recipient's blood. See also **packed cells, pooled plasma, whole blood.**

Banthine, a trademark for a drug used to treat peptic ulcer and irritable bowels (methantheline bromide).

Banti's syndrome /ban'tēz/, a serious disorder involving several organ systems. The blood vessels that lie between the intestines and the liver are obstructed, leading to congestion of the veins, an enlarged spleen, stomach and intestinal tract bleeding, cirrhosis of the liver, and destruction of red and white blood cells. Early symptoms are weakness, fatigue, and anemia. The spleen is sometimes removed, and a passage between the portal vein and the vena cava (portacaval shunt) is created to improve circulation to the liver. Also called **Banti's disease.** See also **cirrhosis, portacaval shunt, portal hypertension.**

bar, a measure of air pressure, equal to about 1 standard atmosphere (1 atm).

Bárány's syndrome. See **caloric test.**

-barb, a combining form referring to a substance derived from barbituric acid.

barber's itch. See **sycosis barbae.**

barbiturate /bärbich'ŏŏrāt, -ərit/, a class of drugs that acts as a sedative or induces sleep. These drugs depress the respiratory rate, blood pressure, temperature, and nervous system. They are addictive. Among the more common barbiturates are amobarbital, butabarbital, pentobarbital, phenobarbital, secobarbital, and thiopental.

barbiturism /bärbich'əriz'əm/, **1.** sudden or long-term poisoning by any of the barbiturates. Excessive amounts of these drugs may be fatal or may produce physical and psychological changes, as depressed respiration, lack of oxygen, disorientation, and coma. **2.** addiction to a barbiturate.

Bard-Pic syndrome /bärd'pik'/, a condition characterized by progressive jaundice, enlarged gallbladder, and deterioration associated with advanced pancreatic cancer.

Bard's sign, the increased movements of the eyeball in uncontrolled rapid eye movement (nystagmus) when the patient tries to follow a target moved from side to side.

bariatrics /ber'ē·at'riks/, the field of medicine that focuses on the treatment and control of obesity and diseases associated with obesity.

baritosis, a benign disease caused by an accumulation of barium dust in the lungs. The condition is most likely to affect persons who are involved with the mining and processing of barite, a product used in the manufacture of paint.

barium (Ba) /ber'ē·əm/, a pale yellow, metallic element classified with the alkaline earths. Its atomic number is 56; its atomic weight is 137.36. Fine, milky barium sulfate is given to patients before x-ray films are taken of the digestive tract.

barium enema, an enema of barium sulfate given before x-ray films are taken of the lower intestinal tract. The x-rays cannot pass through the barium, so abnormalities can be seen on the x-ray film. This is used for diagnosing obstruction, tumors, or disorders as ulcerative colitis. The patient takes only liquids the night before and has no breakfast before the examination. After the x-ray films are taken, the barium is removed by a cleansing enema. Also called **contrast enema.**

barium meal, swallowing barium sulfate before x-ray films are taken of the esophagus, stomach, and intestinal tract. It is used to diagnose conditions as inability to eat (dysphagia), peptic ulcer, and other disorders. The movement of the barium through the stomach and intestinal tract is followed by fluoroscopy, x-ray films, or both. Before the test, the patient receives nothing by mouth for at least 8 hours. Also called **barium swallow.** See also **G.I. series.**

barium swallow. See **barium meal.**

Barlow's disease. See **infantile scurvy.**

Barlow's syndrome, an abnormal heart condition characterized by a murmur and a click. These symptoms are associated with back flow of blood caused by prolapse of the mitral valve located between the upper and lower heart chambers. Also called **electrocardiographic-auscultatory syndrome.**

baro-, bar-, a combining form referring to pressure.

barognosis, pl. **barognoses,** the ability to evaluate weight, especially that held in the hand.

barograph /ber'əgraf'/, an instrument that continuously monitors atmospheric (barometric) pressure and provides a record on paper of pressure changes.

barometer /bərom'ətər/, an instrument for measuring atmospheric pressure. It usually consists of a slender tube filled with mercury, sealed at one end, and inverted into a reservoir of mercury. At sea level the normal height of mercury in the tube is 760 mm. **–barometric,** adj.

barometric pressure. See **atmospheric pressure.**

baroreceptor /ber'ōrisep'tər/, one of the pressure-sensitive nerve endings in the walls of the upper chambers (atria) of the heart and in the large blood vessels (the vena cava, the aortic arch, and the carotid sinus). Baroreceptors stimulate reflex mechanisms that allow the body to adapt to changes in blood pressure by dilating or constricting the blood vessels.

barosinusitis. See **aerosinusitis.**

barotitis. See **aerotitis.**

barotitis media. See **aerotitis media.**

barotrauma /ber'ōtrô'mə, -trou'mə/, physical injury sustained as a result of exposure to increased environmental pressure. For example, barotitis media or rupture of the lungs or sinuses may occur among deep-sea divers. Compare **decompression sickness.**

Barr body. See **sex chromatin.**

barrel chest, a large, rounded chest, considered normal in some stocky people and others who live in high-altitude areas and consequently develop larger lung capacities. Barrel chest, however, may also be a sign of emphysema.

Barré's pyramidal sign /bärāz'/, the inability of a patient who is paralyzed on one side to remain in a flexed position. This occurs only on the paralyzed side when lying down with the lower legs flexed 90 degrees at the knees. The leg on the paralyzed side straightens.

Barrett's esophagus. See **Barrett's syndrome.**

Barrett's syndrome, a harmless ulcerlike area in the esophagus. It is caused most often by long-term irritation of the esophagus from digestive juices flowing back into the esophagus. Also called **Barrett's esophagus.**

barrier, **1.** a wall or other obstacle that can block the passage of substances. Barrier methods of contraception, as the condom or diaphragm, prevent sperm from entering the uterus. Membranes of the body act as screenlike barriers to permit water or certain other molecules to move from one side to the other, while preventing the passage of other substances. **2.** something nonphysical that obstructs, as barriers to communication.

barrier creams, ointments, lotions and similar preparations that are applied to the skin to protect it from various substances that may cause allergic reactions, irritation, or cancer. A sunscreen used to protect against skin cancer is an example of a barrier cream.

barrier nursing, nursing care of a patient in isolation to prevent the spread of infection. Gown, mask, and gloves are worn by staff and visitors entering the room. The number of staff entering the room is kept to a minimum, and visitors are limited. Contaminated substances are handled according to strict guidelines.

bartholinitis /bär'təlini'tis/, an inflammatory condition of one or both Bartholin's glands, caused by bacterial infection. Usually, the microorganism is either *Streptococcus* or *Staphylococcus.* Gonorrhea can also cause the infection. The condition is characterized by swelling of one or both glands, pain, and abscess. A passageway (fistula) may develop between the gland and the vagina, anus, or anywhere in the area.

Bartholin's cyst /bär'təlinz/, a cyst that grows from one of the Bartholin glands or from its ducts and fills with clear fluid.

Bartholin's duct, the major duct of the sublingual gland beneath the tongue.

Bartholin's gland, one of two small glands located on the wall near the opening of the vagina. These glands help lubricate the vagina. Also called **greater vestibular glands.**

Bartonella /bär'tənel'ə/, a genus of small round bacilli. These are parasites that infect red blood cells and the lymph nodes, liver, and spleen. They are transmitted by the bite of a sandfly of the genus *Phlebotomus.*

bartonellosis /bär'tənəlō'sis/, a sudden infection caused by *Bartonella,* which is transmitted by the bite of a sandfly. It is characterized by fever, severe anemia, and bone pain. Several weeks after the first symptoms, many warty-looking areas appear on the skin. The disease is common in the valleys of the Andes in Peru, Colombia, and Ecuador.

Barton forceps. See **obstetric forceps.**

Barton's fracture, a fracture of the forearm involving the bone on the thumb side of the arm (radius) near the wrist. It is often accompanied by dislocation of the wrist onto the radius.

Bartter's syndrome /bär'tərz/, a rare hereditary disorder, characterized by kidney enlargement and overactive adrenal glands. Early signs in childhood are abnormal physical growth and mental retardation.

barye /ber'ē/, a measure of atmospheric pressure equal to 1/1,000th of a millibar.

basal, referring to the fundamental or the basic. For example, "basal metabolic rate" means the lowest rate at which chemical activity (metabolism) occurs in the body.

basal acid output (BAO), the minimum amount of digestive juice produced in a given period of time. This measurement is used in the diagnosis of various diseases of the stomach and intestines.

basal anesthesia, **1.** a state of unconsciousness just short of complete surgical anesthesia in depth. The patient does not respond to words but still reacts to pinprick or other unpleasant sensation. **2.** also called **narcoanesthesia,** any form of anesthesia in which the patient is completely unconscious, in contrast to awake anesthesia.

basal body temperature, the temperature of the body taken in the morning, orally or rectally, after at least 8 hours of sleep. It is taken before doing anything else, including getting out of bed, moving around, talking, eating, or drinking.

basal body temperature method of family planning, a natural method of family planning that relies on identifying the fertile period during a woman's menstrual cycle. The basal body temperature rises 0.5° to 1.0° F during ovulation. The rate and pattern of the increase varies greatly from woman to woman, and somewhat from cycle to cycle in any one woman. Several cycles (six is recommended) are observed, and the woman keeps careful records of her temperature at the same time every morning before getting out of bed. It may be taken orally or rectally but should be done the same way every day. Many factors may change the reading, including infection, stress, a bad night's sleep, medication, or environmental temperature. If any of these factors are present the woman notes them on her record. The fertile period is considered to continue until the temperature is above the baseline for 5 days. The rise can happen slowly over 5 days or it can increase rapidly, reaching a plateau for 3 or 4 days. For birth control, the days following that period are considered "safe" unfertile days. Abstinence is required from 6 days before the earliest day that ovulation was noted to occur until the fifth day after the rise in temperature in the current cycle. Compare **calendar method of family planning, ovulation method of family planning.**

basal bone, 1. the bone of the upper and lower jaw, which provides support for artificial dentures. 2. the fixed bone structure that limits the movement of teeth.

basal cell, any one of the cells in the base layer of epithelium. Epithelium is the lining of the internal and external surfaces of the body, including organs, blood vessels, and skin (epidermis).

basal cell acanthoma. See **basal cell papilloma.**

basal cell carcinoma, a malignant tumor of the epithelium that begins as a small bump and enlarges to the side. It develops a central crater that erodes, crusts, and bleeds. The tumor rarely spreads to other organs (metastasis), but surrounding tissue is destroyed. In 90% of cases, the tumor grows between the hairline and the upper lip. The main cause of the cancer is excessive exposure to the sun or to x-rays. Treatment is surgical removal or x-ray therapy. Also called **basal cell epithelioma, basaloma, carcinoma basocellulare, hair matrix carcinoma.** See also **rodent ulcer.**

basal cell papilloma, a benign skin tumor characterized by numerous yellow or brown raised oval areas. These tumors usually develop in middle age. Also called **basal cell acanthoma, seborrheic keratosis, seborrheic wart.**

basal ganglia, the islands of gray matter within each one of the lobes of the brain (cerebrum). They are involved in posture and coordination.

basal lamina, a thin substance lying just under the epithelium. Also called **basement lamina.**

basal membrane, a sheet of tissue that lies just under the pigmented layer of the retina in the eye.

basal metabolic rate (BMR), the amount of energy used in a certain amount of time by a person. The test is done after the person fasts for 14 to 18 hours and is awake and resting in a comfortable, warm environment. The rate is the amount of oxygen used, which is expressed in calories consumed per hour per square meter of body surface area or per kilogram of body weight. This test was used to determine how well the thyroid gland functioned. It is seldom used now, however, because much more accurate tests have been developed.

basal metabolism, the amount of energy needed to maintain essential body functions, as respiration, circulation, temperature, intestinal activity, and muscle tone.

basaloid carcinoma, a rare, malignant tumor of the anal canal. These tumors contain areas that resemble basal cell carcinoma of the skin. The tumor may spread to the skin of the genital area.

basaloma. See **basal cell carcinoma.**

basal seat, the oral tissues and structures that support a denture.

basal temperature. See **basal body temperature.**

basal tidal volume, the amount of air inhaled and exhaled by a healthy person at complete rest. It varies according to age, weight, and sex.

base, 1. a chemical compound that combines with an acid to form a salt. Compare **alkali.** 2. a molecule that takes up protons. 3. the major ingredient of a compounded material, particularly one that is used as a drug. Petroleum jelly is frequently used as a base for ointments.

Basedow's goiter /bä′sədōz/, an enlarged thyroid gland, characterized by oversecretion of thyroid hormone. It occurs after iodine therapy.

base-forming food, a food that makes urine less acid. Base-forming foods include mainly fruits, vegetables, and dairy products.

baseline fetal heart rate, the fetal heart rate pattern during labor between contractions of the uterus. An electronic fetal monitor is used to detect very fast or slow rates (less than 120 or more than 160 per minute). These abnormalities sometimes mean the baby's oxygen supply is interrupted.

basement lamina. See **basal lamina.**

basement membrane, the fragile, deepest layer of tissue that secures the layers of epithelium.

base of the heart, the portion of the heart opposite the tip. The base is tilted to the right side of the body. It forms the upper border of the heart and lies just below the second rib.

base of the skull, the floor of the skull to which the spine attaches.

baseplate, a temporary form that represents the base of a denture. It is used for making records of the jaw relationships, arranging artificial teeth, or for trial placement in the mouth to assure a precise fit of a denture.

bas-fond /bäfôN′/, the bottom or base of any structure, especially the urinary bladder.

basi-, basio-, a combining form referring to a foundation or a base.

basic health services, the minimum amount of health care considered necessary to maintain health and protection from disease.

basifacial, referring to the lower portion of the face.

basilar, referring to a base.

basilar artery, the single artery at the base of the skull that is formed by the junction of the two vertebral arteries. It supplies blood to the internal ear and parts of the brain.

basilar artery insufficiency syndrome, insufficient blood flow through the basilar artery; can be caused by a blockage. Symptoms of this syndrome are dizziness, blindness, numbness, depression, speech problems, difficulty swallowing, and weakness on one side of the body.

basilar artery occlusion, a blockage of the artery at the base of skull (basilar artery). It causes many serious problems, ranging from blindness to paralysis.

basilar membrane, the cell structure that forms the floor of the duct of the cochlea, which is the spiral tube inside the ear and the main organ of hearing.

basilar plexus, the network of interlaced veins between the layers of the membrane that protects the brain (dura mater) over the base of the skull.

basilic vein /bəsil′ik/, one of the four veins of the arm near the surface. It runs along the inside of the forearm.

basiloma /bas′ilō′mə/, *pl.* **basilomas, basilomata,** a cancer composed of basal cells. A kind of basiloma is **basiloma terebrans.** Also called **basaloma.**

basiloma terebrans /ter′əbrənz/, a basal cell cancer that invades surrounding tissue.

basioccipital, referring to the base of the back of the skull (occipital bone).

basis pedunculi cerebri. See **crus cerebri.**

basket cell, a degenerated white blood cell.

basophil /bā′səfil/, a white blood cell with a nucleus that contains granules. Basophils represent 1% or less of the total white blood cell count. The number of basophils increases in bone marrow (myeloproliferative) diseases and decreases in severe allergic reactions. Compare **eosinophil, neutrophil.** See also **agranulocyte, differential white blood cell count, granulocyte, leukocyte, polymorphonuclear leukocyte.**

basophilic adenoma, a tumor of the pituitary gland. Cushing's syndrome is often caused by a basophilic adenoma. Compare **acidophilic adenoma, chromophobic adenoma.**

basophilic leukemia, a cancer of blood-forming tissues, characterized by large numbers of immature basophils. See also **acute myelocytic leukemia.**

basophilic stippling, the abnormal presence of spotted basophils in the red blood cells. Stippling is characteristic of lead poisoning. See also **basophil, lead poisoning.**

basosquamous cell carcinoma /bā′sōskwā′məs/, a malignant skin tumor composed of basal and squamous cells.

Bassen-Kornzweig syndrome. See **abetalipoproteinemia.**

bath, a cleansing routine performed daily by or for almost all hospitalized patients. A daily bath helps prevent infection, preserves the unbroken condition of the skin, stimulates circulation, promotes oxygen intake, maintains muscle tone and joint mobility, and provides comfort.

bath blanket, a thin, lightweight blanket used to cover a patient during a bath. It absorbs moisture while keeping the patient warm. See also **blanket bath.**

bathesthesia /bath′əsthē′zhə/, a sensitivity of internal parts of the body. It is associated with organs or structures beneath the surface, as muscles and joints.

bathy-, batho-, a combining form referring to depth, deep.

bathycardia /bath′əkär′dē·ə/, an unusually low position of the heart in the chest. It usually does not cause any problems with functioning.

Batten's disease, a progressive brain disease (encephalopathy) of children with disturbed metabolism of polyunsaturated fatty acids.

battered woman syndrome (BWS), repeated episodes of physical assault on a woman by the man with whom she lives, often resulting in serious physical and emotional damage to the woman. Such violence tends to follow a predictable pattern. The violent episodes usually follow verbal argument and are accompanied by verbal abuse. Almost any subject—housekeeping, money, childrearing—may begin the episode. Often the violent episodes become more frequent and severe over time—once a month becomes once a week; a shove becomes a punch. Studies show that the longer the woman stays in the relationship, the more likely she is to be seriously injured. Less and less provocation seems to be enough to trigger an attack once the syndrome has begun. The use of alcohol increases the severity of the assault; a man who usually shoves or slaps his partner is more likely to punch or kick her if he is drunk. Other drugs do not have this effect; the man is more likely to be abusive as the drug is wearing off. Battering occurs in cycles of violence. The first phase is characterized by the man acting increasingly irritable, edgy, and tense. Verbal abuse, insults, and criticism increase, and shoves or slaps begin. The second phase is the violent activity. As the tension mounts, the woman becomes unable to calm the man, and she may argue or defend herself. The man uses this as the justification for his anger and assaults her, often saying that he is "teaching her a lesson." The third stage is characterized by apology and remorse on the part of the man, with promises of change. The calm continues until tension builds again. The battered woman syndrome occurs at all socioeconomic levels. It is estimated that in the United States between 1 million and 2 million women a year are beaten by their husbands or lovers. Men who grew up in homes in which the father abused the mother are more likely to beat their wives than are men who lived in nonviolent homes. Personal and cultural attitudes also affect the incidence of wife battering. Aggressive behavior is a normal part of male socialization in most cultures; physical aggression may be condoned as a means of resolving a conflict. The battered woman syndrome is much better recognized now than a decade ago, and several different agencies can assist and protect the woman. In many communities the police have programs to remove the man and to refer the woman to help. Social service departments, battered women's shelters, and counseling services' hotlines can provide both emergency services and long-term help.

battery, 1. two or more electrolytic cells connected together to form a single source providing direct current or voltage. 2. a series of tests to determine the cause of a particular illness or the degree of skill in an area. 3. the unlawful use of force on a person. See **assault.**

Battey bacillus /bat′ē/, any of a group of mycobacteria that cause a long-term lung disease resembling tuberculosis. These organisms are resistant to most of the common antibiotic drugs. Surgical removal of involved lung tissue may be necessary and may improve the outcome in serious cases.

battledore placenta /bat′əldôr′/, a placenta to which the umbilical cord is attached at the edge.

Battle's sign, a small area of bleeding under the skin behind the ear. It may indicate a fracture of a bone of the lower skull.

Baudelocque's diameter. See **external conjugate.**

Baudelocque's method, turning the baby from a face-first position to a crown-first position just before delivery.

Baynton's bandage /bān′tənz/, a spiral adhesive wrap applied to the leg over a dressing. It is used to treat ulcers of the leg.

bayonet condenser, a dental instrument for compacting filling material.

BBB, abbreviation for **blood-brain barrier.**

B cell, a type of white blood cell (lymphocyte) that comes from the bone marrow. It is one of the two lymphocytes that play a major role in the body's immune response. Compare **T cell.** See also **plasma cell.**

BCG, abbreviation for **bacille Calmette-Guérin.**

BCG vaccine, an immunizing vaccine against tuberculosis.

★CAUTION: Loss of gammaglobulins, immune system suppression, or use of steroids or isoniazid prohibits its use. It is not given after vaccination for smallpox, nor is it given to patients with a positive tuberculin reaction or a burn.

★ADVERSE EFFECTS: Among the most serious side effects are severe allergic reactions and development of tuberculosis. Pain, inflammation, and nodules may develop at the site of injection.

BCNU. See **carmustine.**

B complex vitamins, a large group of water-soluble substances that includes **vitamin B$_1$ (thiamine), vitamin B$_2$ (riboflavin), vitamin B$_3$ (niacin), vitamin B$_6$ (pyridoxine), vitamin B$_{12}$ (cyanocobalamin), biotin, choline, carnitine, folic acid, inositol,** and **para-aminobenzoic acid.** The B complex vitamins are essential in breaking down carbohydrates into glucose to provide energy, for breaking down fats and proteins, for normal functioning of the nervous system, for maintenance of muscle tone in the stomach and intestinal tract, and for the health of skin, hair, eyes, mouth, and liver. They are found in brewer's yeast, liver, whole-grain cereals, nuts, eggs, meats, fish, and vegetables and are produced by the intestinal bacteria. Maintaining milk-free diets or taking antibiotics may destroy these bacteria. Symptoms of vitamin B deficiency include nervousness, depression, insomnia, nerve problems, anemia, hair loss, acne or other skin disorders, and excessive cholesterol in the blood. See also specific vitamins.

Be, symbol for **beryllium.**

beaded, resembling a row of beads.

beaker cell. See **goblet cell.**

beam, a bedframe fitting for pulleys and weights, used for patients requiring weight traction. See **Balkan frame.**

BE amputation, an amputation of the arm below the elbow.

bean, the pod-enclosed flattened seed of numerous legumes. Some beans are used in preparing drugs.

beat, the force of contraction of the heart muscle. It is felt and recorded as the pulse.

Becker's muscular dystrophy, a degenerative disease of the muscles causing progressive weakness. It occurs in childhood between 8 and 20 years of age. The disease is inherited. Also called **benign pseudohypertrophic muscular dystrophy.** Compare **Duchenne's muscular dystrophy.**

Beck operation, a type of surgery that provides additional circulation to the heart. It is performed when the vessels of the heart are diseased and supply inadequate amounts of blood to the heart. The surgery is sometimes done in two stages, usually about 3 weeks apart.

Beck's Diagnostic Inventory (BDI), a system of classifying criteria for depression. It was developed by A.T. Beck in the 1970s as a diagnostic and therapeutic tool for the treatment of childhood mental disorders. Also called **Beck depression inventory (BDI).** See also **DSM-III.**

Beck's triad, a combination of three symptoms that characterize compression of the heart: high pressure in the veins, low pressure in the arteries, and a small, quiet heart.

Beckwith's syndrome, a hereditary disorder in infants of low blood sugar (hypoglycemia) and overproduction of insulin.

Beckwith-Wiedemann syndrome. See **EMG syndrome.**

beclomethasone dipropionate, a type of steroid (glucocorticoid) used in an inhaler in the treatment of bronchial asthma.

★CAUTION: Status asthmaticus, severe asthma attack, or known allergy to this drug prohibits its use.

★ADVERSE EFFECTS: Among the more serious side effects are the symptoms of adrenal insufficiency. Hoarseness, sore throat, and fungal infections of the throat may occur.

bed, a supporting tissue, as the nail beds of specialized skin over which the fingernails and the toenails move as they grow.

bedbug, a bloodsucking arthropod of the species *Cimex* that feeds on humans and other animals. The bedbug can be removed after covering it with petrolatum. The bite causes itching, pain, and redness.

Bedford finger stall, a removable finger splint that holds the injured finger in a brace or cast, along with the adjacent finger. It can be worn for prolonged periods of time.

Bednar's aphthae /bed′närz/, small, yellowish, slightly elevated ulcerated patches that occur on the roof of the mouth in infants who place infected objects in their mouths. It is also associated with marasmus, which is a type of malnutrition. Compare **Epstein's pearls, thrush.**

bedside manner, the behavior of a nurse or doctor as perceived by a patient.

bedsore. See **decubitus ulcer.**

bedwetting. See **enuresis.**

Bee-cell pessary. See **pessary.**

beef tapeworm. See *Taenia saginata.*

beef tapeworm infection, an infection caused by the tapeworm *Taenia saginata,* transmitted to humans when they eat contaminated beef. The adult worm can live for years in the intestines without causing any symptoms. See also **tapeworm infection.**

bee sting, an injury caused by the venom of bees, usually accompanied by pain and swelling. The stinger of the honeybee usually remains implanted and should be removed carefully. Pain

may be relieved by applying an ice pack or a paste of sodium bicarbonate and water. Allergic individuals are encouraged to carry emergency kits with them when the possibility of bee sting exists. Compare **wasp.**

behavior, **1.** the manner in which a person acts or performs. **2.** any or all of the activities of a person, including physical and mental activity. Kinds of behavior include **abnormal behavior, automatic behavior, invariable behavior, variable behavior.**

behavioral reflex. See **conditioned response.**

behavioral science, any of the disciplines that observe and study human activity, including psychological and emotional development, relationships, values, and mores. Psychiatry, psychology, sociology, and anthropology are all behavioral sciences.

behavior disorder, any of a group of antisocial behavior patterns occurring primarily in children and adolescents. The behavior disorders include overaggressiveness, overactivity, destructiveness, cruelty, truancy, lying, disobedience, perverse sexual activity, criminality, alcoholism, and drug addiction. The most common reason for such behavior is hostility, which may be obvious. It is started by a disturbed relationship between the child and the parents, an unstable home situation, and, in some cases, by organic brain dysfunction. See also **antisocial personality disorder.**

behaviorism, a school of psychology founded by John B. Watson that studies and interprets behavior by observing people's responses to things. Behaviorism is not concerned with consciousness, mental states, or ideas and emotions. See also **neobehaviorism.**

behavior modification. See **behavior therapy.**

behavior systems model, a theory describing factors that may affect the stability of a person's behavior. The model examines systems of behavior, not the behavior of an individual at any particular time.

behavior therapy, a kind of psychotherapy that attempts to modify patterns of behavior by substituting a new response to a given stimulus. Some "quit smoking" programs use this technique successfully. Also called **behavior modification.** See also **biofeedback.**

Behçet's disease, a rare and severe illness of unknown cause, mostly affecting young males and characterized by eye inflammation and atrophy. Ulcers appear on the mouth and the genitals. Also called **Behçet's syndrome.**

Behla's bodies. See **Plimmer's bodies.**

BEIR-III Report, a report, *"The Biological Effects of Low Doses of Ionizing Radiation,"* by the National Academy of Sciences; it estimates the risk of cancer deaths from exposure to radiation at various dose levels.

bejel /bej′əl/, a nonvenereal form of syphilis common among children in the Middle East and North Africa. It is transmitted by person-to-person contact and by sharing drinking and eating utensils. The main sore is usually on or near the mouth and is followed by the development of pimplelike sores on the trunk, arms, and legs.

Békésy audiometry /bek′əsē/, a method of testing hearing. The patient presses a signal button while listening to a pure tone that is progressively diminished in intensity. When the sound is no longer heard, the patient releases the button.

bel, a unit that expresses intensity of sound. An increase of 1 bel approximately doubles the intensity or loudness of most sounds.

belching. See **eructation.**

belladonna, the dried leaves, roots, and flowering or fruiting tops of *Atropa belladonna,* a common perennial called deadly nightshade. It contains hyoscyamine, which is a source of atropine.

Bell's law, an axiom stating that the nerves at the internal part of the spinal cord control the muscles and those at the outer part control the senses. Also called **Bell-Magendie law, Magendie's law.**

Bell's palsy, a paralysis of the facial nerve. It is caused by injury to the nerve, compression of the nerve by a tumor, or, possibly, from an unknown infection. Any or all branches of the nerve may be affected. The patient may not be able to open an eye or close the mouth. The condition may be on one side or both, temporary or permanent.

Bell's phenomenon, a sign of facial paralysis, manifested by the upward and outward rolling of the eyeball when the patient tries to close the eyelid.

belly. See **abdomen.**

belly button. See **umbilicus.**

belonephobia /bel′ənəfō′bē·ə/, a morbid fear of sharp-pointed objects, especially needles and pins.

Benadryl, a trademark for an antihistamine used to treat allergic reactions (diphenhydramine hydrochloride).

Bence Jones protein /bens/, a protein found almost exclusively in the urine of patients with multiple myeloma. See also **multiple myeloma, protein.**

bench research, *informal.* any research done in a controlled laboratory setting using other than human subjects.

bending fracture, a fracture indirectly caused by bending an extremity, as the foot or the big toe.

bendroflumethiazide /ben′drōflo͞o′məthī′əzīd/, a diuretic and antihypertensive drug used to treat high blood pressure and water retention.

★CAUTION: Kidney dysfunction or known allergy to this drug, to other thiazide drugs, or to sulfonamides prohibits its use.

★ADVERSE EFFECTS: Among the more serious side effects are loss of potassium, high blood sugar, excess uric acid in the blood, and various allergic reactions.

bends. See **decompression sickness.**

Benedict's qualitative test, a test for sugar in the urine. A mixture of urine and Benedict's solution is heated in boiling water for 5 minutes and then cooled. A substance will form that is rated by color: orange or red means more than 2% sugar (called 4+), yellow means 1% to 2% sugar (called 3+), olive green means 0.5% to 1% sugar (called 2+), and green means less than 0.5% sugar (called 1+). Also called **Benedict's method.**

Benemid, a trademark for a drug used to treat gout (probenecid).

benign, not cancerous and therefore not an immediate threat, even though treatment of a benign tumor eventually may be required for health or cosmetic reasons. See **benign neoplasm.** Compare **malignant.**

benign hypertension, a misnomer implying an innocent form of high blood pressure. Any hypertension can be dangerous. See also **essential hypertension.**

benign intracranial hypertension. See **pseudotumor cerebri.**

benign juvenile melanoma, a benign, pink or fuchsia raised area on the skin with a scaly surface, usually on a cheek. It occurs most commonly in children between 9 and 13 years of age. It may be mistaken for a malignant melanoma. Also called **compound melanocytoma, spindle cell nevus, Spitz nevus.**

benign mesenchymoma, a benign tumor made of meshlike connective tissue.

benign neoplasm, a tumor (neoplasm) that has a fiber capsule and a regular shape. It does not grow very fast nor become widespread. A benign neoplasm does not invade surrounding tissue or spread to distant sites. It causes harm only by pressure and does not usually return after removal. Some kinds of benign neoplasms are **adenoma, fibroma, hemangioma, lipoma.** See also **malignant neoplasm.**

benign nephrosclerosis, a kidney problem in which arteries in the kidney thicken, stiffen, and harden. It is associated with high blood pressure.

benign prostatic hypertrophy, enlargement of the prostate gland, common among men after 50 years of age. The condition is not malignant or inflammatory, but may lead to obstruction of the urethra, interfering with the flow of urine. This can increase frequency of urination, the need to urinate during the night, pain, and urinary tract infections. Treatment consists of regular sexual release, hot baths, massage of the prostate, avoiding alcohol and drinking excessive fluids, and urinating as soon as the urge occurs. Surgery is sometimes necessary. Compare **prostatitis.** See also **prostatectomy.**

benign pseudohypertrophic muscular dystrophy. See **Becker's muscular dystrophy.**

benign stupor, a state of apathy or lethargy, as occurs in severe depression.

benign suicide, (in psychology) indirect self-destructive behavior. It is most likely to occur in older persons who find it impossible to deal with the loss of a loved one and refuse to eat, take medications, or take care of other needs. Also called **subintentional suicide.**

benign thrombocytosis. See **thrombocytosis.**

benign tumor. See **benign.**

Bennet's small corpuscle. See **Drysdale's corpuscle.**

Bennet hand tool test, a test used in occupational therapy and job-aptitude testing to measure hand function, coordination, and speed of performance.

Bennett's fracture, a fracture of the hand that runs through the base of the thumb and into the wrist. Bennett's fracture may be caused by the thumb being forced backward or by being dislocated.

Benoquin, a trademark for a cream that corrects the abnormal pigmentation of skin in vitiligo (monobenzone).

bent fracture, a fracture caused by the bone being forcibly bent. The actual fracture may be some distance from the area that was bent.

bentonite, colloidal, hydrated aluminum silicate, which, when added to water, swells to approximately 12 times its dry size. It is used as a bulk laxative and as a base for skin-care preparations.

bentonite test, a blood test for the presence of rheumatoid factor.

Bentyl, a trademark for a drug used to treat intestinal irritability and spasms (dicyclomine hydrochloride).

benzalkonium chloride, a disinfectant and fungicide prepared in water that comes in various strengths.

benzathine penicillin G. See **penicillin G benzathine.**

Benzedrex, a trademark for a drug used to treat low blood pressure (propylhexedrine).

benzene poisoning, poisoning caused by swallowing benzene, inhaling benzene fumes, or exposure to benzene-related products, as toluene or xylene. The symptoms are nausea, headache, dizziness, and incoordination. In severe cases, respiratory failure or extremely rapid heart beat may cause death. Long-term exposure may result in aplastic anemia or a form of leukemia. Benzene poisoning by inhalation is treated with breathing assistance and oxygen. Poisoning from swallowing benzene is treated by flushing the stomach with water. See also **nitrobenzene poisoning.**

benzethonium chloride /ben′zəthō′nē·əm/, a disinfectant for the skin and for treating some infections of the eye, nose, and throat. It is also used as a preservative in some drugs.

benzo(a)pyrene dihydrodial epoxide (BPDE-I), a substance associated with tobacco smoke that causes cancer.

benzocaine, an anesthetic for the skin used in many over-the-counter compounds for itching and pain. Although not poisonous, some people become sensitive to it over prolonged or frequent use. Use of benzocaine may cause a blood disorder (methemoglobinemia) in infants and small children. A minimum of 5% benzocaine is required in a compound to be effective.

benzodiazepine   derivative /ben′zōdī·az′əpin/, one of a group of drugs used to relieve anxiety or insomnia. The tranquilizers include chlordiazepoxide, diazepam, oxazepam, and chlorazepate. The hypnotics are flurazepam and nitrazepam. Diazepam is also used to relieve spasm of the muscles and to prevent seizures. Tolerance and physical dependence occur with prolonged high doses. Withdrawal symptoms, including seizures and serious psychosis, may occur if the drug is abruptly discontinued. Adverse reactions to the benzodiazepines include drowsiness, muscle incoordination, and increased aggression and hostility. However, these reactions are not commonly seen in patients who take only the usual recommended dose.

benzoic acid /benzō′ik/, a substance usually used with salicylic acid as an ointment for treating athlete's foot and ringworm of the scalp. Mild irritation may occur at the site of application.

benzonatate /benzō′ənāt/, a drug used to suppress coughing. It is not a narcotic.
★CAUTION: Known allergy to this drug prohibits its use.
★ADVERSE EFFECTS: A serious reaction may be convulsions. Vertigo, headache, constipation, and allergic reactions, usually mild, sometimes occur.

benzoyl peroxide, an antibacterial drying agent used to treat acne.
★CAUTION: Known allergy to this drug prohibits its use. It is not used in the eye, on inflamed skin, or on mucous membranes.
★ADVERSE EFFECTS: Among the more serious side effects are excess drying of the skin and allergic contact dermatitis.

benzphetamine   hydrochloride, a drug that causes loss of appetite and is used to treat obesity.
★CAUTION: Arteriosclerosis, cardiovascular disease, high blood pressure, glaucoma, overactive thyroid gland, or known allergy to this or other similar drugs prohibits its use.
★ADVERSE EFFECTS: Among the more serious side effects are restlessness, insomnia, rapid

heart beat, increased blood pressure, and dry mouth.

benzthiazide, a drug used to treat high blood pressure and water retention.

benztropine mesylate, a drug used to treat parkinsonism. It is used in combination with other drugs, as levodopa.

★CAUTION: Known allergy to this drug prohibits its use. It is not given to children under 3 years of age.

★ADVERSE EFFECTS: Among the most serious side effects are blurred vision, dry mouth, nausea and vomiting, constipation, depression, and skin rash.

benzyl alcohol, a clear, colorless, oily liquid derived from certain balsams. It is used as an anesthetic on the skin and to prevent bacteria from growing in solutions for injection. Also called **phenyl carbinol, phenyl methanol.**

benzyl benzoate, a clear, oily liquid with a pleasant, aromatic odor. It is used to destroy lice and scabies, as a solvent, and as a flavor for gum.

benzylpenicillin. See **penicillin G.**

bereavement, a form of depression with symptoms of anxiety; a common reaction to the loss of a loved one.

Berger's disease, a kidney disorder in which the urine periodically contains abnormal substances, such as blood and excess protein. The condition may progress to kidney failure over a period of many years. The disease usually begins in children or young adults. Males are affected twice as often as females. Treatment is similar to that of other kidney diseases. Also called **mesangial IgA nephropathy** /mesan′-jē-əl/.

Bergonié-Tréboneau law /ber′gônē′trā′bônō′/, a rule in x-ray therapy stating that the sensitivity of tissue depends on the number of cells, their activity, and the length of time they are actively reproducing.

beriberi /ber′ēber′ē/, a disease of the nerves of the arms and legs caused by a deficiency of thiamine. It is usually caused by a diet limited to polished white rice and is common in eastern and southern Asia. Rare cases in the United States are associated with stressful conditions, as underactive thyroid gland, infections, pregnancy, breast feeding, and alcoholism. Symptoms are fatigue, diarrhea, appetite and weight loss, disturbed nerve function causing paralysis and wasting of limbs, water retention, and heart failure. Also called **athiaminosis, kakke disease.** See also **thiamine.**

berkelium (Bk), an artificial radioactive element. Its atomic number is 97; its atomic weight is 247.

Berlock dermatitis, an abnormal skin condition caused by a reaction to oil of bergamot (psoralens), which is commonly used in perfumes, colognes, and pomades. Dark patches and sores appear on the skin. This condition affects mostly women and children and may result from using products that contain psoralens and exposure to ultraviolet light. Although only about 5% of the radiation of the sun is ultraviolet light and much of that is absorbed by oxygen and ozone, the level of ultraviolet radiation reaching the earth, especially on a sunny day, is sufficient to cause the condition to appear. Also called **Berloque dermatitis.**

Bernard-Soulier syndrome /bernär′soolyā/, a blood-clotting disorder caused by lack of an essential glycoprotein in the platelets.

Bernstein test. See **acid perfusion test.**

berry aneurysm, a small, saclike dilation of the wall of an artery in the brain. It occurs most frequently where several arteries join at the base of the brain. A berry aneurysm may be the result of a congenital defect and may rupture without warning, causing bleeding into the brain.

berylliosis /bəril′ē·ō′sis/, poisoning that results from inhaling dusts or vapors that contain beryllium.

beryllium (Be), a steel-gray, light-weight metallic element. Its atomic number is 4; its atomic weight is 9.012. Beryllium occurs naturally as beryl and is used in metallic alloys and in fluorescent powders.

bestiality, 1. a brutal or animal-like character or nature. 2. conduct or behavior characterized by beastlike appetites or instincts. 3. also called **zooerastia** /zōō·əras′tē·ə/, sexual relations between a human being and an animal. 4. sodomy. See also **zoophilia.**

beta (β), the second letter of the Greek alphabet, used as a combining form with chemical names to distinguish one of two or more forms or to show the position of substituted atoms in certain compounds. Compare **alpha.**

beta-adrenergic blocking agent. See **antiadrenergic.**

beta-adrenergic receptor. See **beta receptor.**

beta-adrenergic stimulating agent. See **adrenergic.**

beta-alaninemia /-al′əninē′mē·ə/, an inherited metabolic disorder in which the person lacks the enzyme, beta-alanine-alpha-ketoglutarate amino transferase. Symptoms include seizures, drowsiness, and, if uncorrected, death. The condition is sometimes treated with pryidoxine.

beta-carotene, an ultraviolet screening agent used to reduce sensitivity to the sun in patients with erythropoetic protoporphyria.

★CAUTION: It is used with caution in patients with impaired kidney or liver function. Known allergy to this drug prohibits its use.

★ADVERSE EFFECTS: No serious side effects have been observed. The skin may turn slightly yellow while taking this drug. Diarrhea may occur.

beta cells, 1. cells that produce insulin. They are located in the islands of Langerhans in the pancreas. The insulin production by the beta cells tends to speed the movement of glucose, amino acids, and fatty acids out of the blood and into the cells. 2. the basophilic cells of the anterior lobe of the pituitary gland.

beta decay, a type of radioactivity that results in the emission of beta particles, as electrons or positrons. See also **beta particle.**

Betadine, a trademark for an antiinfective that is used on the skin (povidone-iodine).

beta fetoprotein, a protein found in fetal liver and in some adults with liver disease. It is identical with normal liver ferritin. See also **alpha fetoprotein, ferritin, fetoprotein.**

beta-galactosidase. See **lactase.**

beta-hemolytic streptococci, the disease-causing streptococci of groups A, B, C, E, F, G, H, K, L, M, and O. These organisms cause most of the acute streptococcal infections seen in humans, including rheumatic fever, scarlet fever, many cases of pneumonia and septicemia, and strep throat. Penicillin is usually prescribed to treat these infections. Untreated streptococcal infection may lead to kidney disease and rheumatic fever.

beta-hydroxyisovaleric aciduria, an inherited metabolic disease caused by the lack of an enzyme needed to process the amino acid leucine. The condition results in an unpleasant urine odor, retardation, and weakening of the muscles. See also **maple syrup urine disease.**

betamethasone, a steroid (glucocorticoid) available as an oral drug or as a lotion, cream, or ointment. The skin preparations are used to treat skin inflammation, as dermatitis. The oral form is given for severe allergy and a variety of serious diseases.
★CAUTION: Systemic fungal infections, viral and fungal infections of the skin, impaired circulation, or known allergy to this drug prohibits its use.
★ADVERSE EFFECTS: Among the more serious side effects linked to long-term use of the drug are stomach and intestinal, hormone, nerve, and fluid and electrolyte disturbances.

beta-naphthylamine, an organic compound used in aniline dyes and a cause of bladder cancer in humans.

beta-oxidation, a process in which fatty acids are used by the body as a source of energy.

beta particle, an electron or positron emitted from the nucleus of an atom during radioactive decay. Beta particles have a range of 3 feet (10 meters) in air and .04 inches (1 mm) in soft tissue. Also called **beta rays.**

beta receptor, any one of the adrenergic receptors of the nervous system that responds to epinephrine. Activation of beta receptors causes various reactions, as relaxation of the bronchial muscles, and an increase in the speed and force of the heart beat. Also called **beta-adrenergic receptor.** Compare **alpha receptor.**

beta rhythm. See **beta wave.**

betatron /bā′tətron/, a machine that produces high-energy electrons for x-ray treatment.

beta wave, one of the four types of brain waves, characterized by relatively low voltage and a frequency of more than 13 Hz. Beta waves are the "busy waves" of the brain. They can be recorded by electroencephalograph when a patient is awake and alert with eyes open. Also called **beta rhythm.** Compare **alpha wave, delta wave, theta wave.**

bethanechol chloride /bethan′əkol/, a drug used to treat urinary retention and to increase intestinal action.
★CAUTION: Uncertain strength of the bladder, obstruction of the stomach and intestinal or urinary tract, overactive thyroid gland, peptic ulcer, bronchial asthma, cardiovascular disease, epilepsy, Parkinson's disease, low blood pressure, or known allergy to this drug prohibits its use. It is not given during pregnancy.
★ADVERSE EFFECTS: Among the more serious side effects are flushing, headache, stomach and intestinal distress, diarrhea, excess salivation, sweating, and very low blood pressure.

bevel, any angle, other than a right angle, between two planes or surfaces.

bezoar /bē′zôr/, a hard ball of hair and vegetable fiber that may develop within the intestines of humans but more often is found in the stomachs of ruminants (cattle, sheep, goats, deer, and other cud-chewing animals).

bhang /bang/, an Asian Indian hallucinogenic, composed of dried leaves and the young stems of uncultivated marijuana (*Cannabis sativa*). It is usually drunk as a boiled mixture with milk, sugar, or water; produces euphoria. It also may be smoked or chewed. Also spelled **bang.** See also **cannabis.**

Bi, symbol for **bismuth.**

BIA, abbreviation for **bioelectrical impedance analysis.**

bias, 1. an oblique or a diagonal line. 2. a prejudiced or subjective attitude. 3. distortion of a statistic caused by the process of gathering information. 4. a voltage applied to an electronic device, as a vacuum tube or a transistor, to control operating limits.

biasing, a method of treating problems with nerves and muscles. A muscle is contracted against resistance. It results in the muscle tissue being more responsive and sensitive to stretching.

bibliotherapy, a type of group therapy in which books, poems, and newspaper articles are read in the group to help prompt the members to think about events in the real world and to relate to one another.

bicarbonate of soda. See **sodium bicarbonate.**

bicarbonate precursor, an injection of sodium lactate used to treat metabolic acidosis. It is changed by the body to sodium bicarbonate.

bicarbonate therapy, a procedure to increase the amount of bicarbonate stored in a patient's body. It is usually performed only in certain cases and as a stopgap measure.

bicarbonate transport, the route by which most of the carbon dioxide is carried in the bloodstream.

biceps. See **biceps brachii.**

biceps brachii, the long muscle that stretches over the bone of the upper arm (humerus). It flexes the arm and the forearm. Also called **biceps, biceps flexor cubiti.** Compare **brachialis, triceps brachii.**

biceps femoris, one of the muscles on the back of the thigh. The biceps femoris flexes the leg and rotates it to the side. Also called **hamstring muscle.**

biceps flexor cubiti. See **biceps brachii.**

biceps reflex, a contraction of a biceps muscle when the tendon is tapped. See also **deep tendon reflex.**

biCNU, a trademark for one of a group of drugs used in the chemotherapy of certain tumors (carmustine).

biconcave, curved in (concave) on both sides, a term usually applied to a lens. **–biconcavity,** *n.*

biconvex, bulging out (convex) on both sides, a term usually applied to a lens. **–biconvexity,** *n.*

bicornate, having two horns or processes.

bicornate uterus, an abnormal uterus that may be either a single or a double organ with two branches. It is associated with a high incidence of premature labor, spontaneous abortion, and infertility.

bicuspid /bīkus′pid/, **1.** having two cusps or points. **2.** also called **premolar tooth.** one of the two teeth between the molars and canines of the upper and lower jaw.

bicuspid valve. See **mitral valve.**

b.i.d., (in prescriptions) abbreviation for *bis in die* /dē′ā/, a Latin phrase meaning "twice a day." A drug prescribed this way should be taken 12 hours apart, for example at 7 AM and 7 PM.

bidactyly /bīdak′tilē/, an abnormal condition in which the second, third, and fourth fingers on the same hand are missing. Also called **lobsterclaw deformity.** **–bidactylous,** *adj.*

bidet /bidā′/, a plumbing fixture designed for use as a sitz bath. It is usually equipped with extensions for cleaning the genital and rectal areas of the body.

biduotertian fever, a form of malaria with overlapping attacks of chills, fever, and other symptoms. It is caused by infection with two strains of *Plasmodium,* each having its own cycle of symptoms, as in quartan and tertian malaria. Compare **double quartan fever.** See also **malaria.**

bifid, split into two parts.

bifocal, **1.** referring to the characteristic of having two foci. **2.** having two areas of different focal lengths in a lens.

bifurcation, a splitting into two branches, as the windpipe (trachea), which branches into the two bronchi of the lungs just below the collarbone.

Bigelow's lithotrite /big′əlōz/, a long-jawed instrument passed through the urethra to crush a stone in the bladder. See also **lithotrite.**

bigeminal pulse, an abnormal pulse in which two beats in close succession are followed by a pause during which no pulse is felt. See also **trigeminal pulse, trigeminy.**

bigeminy /bījem′inē/, **1.** an association in pairs. **2.** an irregular heart beat characterized by two beats in rapid succession followed by a pause. **–bigeminal,** *adj.*

bilabe /bī′lāb/, a narrow forceps used to remove small stones from the bladder.

bilaminar, referring to the characteristic of having two layers.

bilaminar blastoderm, the stage of development in the embyro before the middle layer (mesoderm) forms. Compare **trilaminar blastoderm.**

bilateral, **1.** having two sides. **2.** occurring or appearing on two sides. A patient with bilateral hearing loss may have partial or total deafness in both ears. **3.** having two layers.

bilateral long-leg spica cast, an orthopedic cast made of plaster of Paris, fiberglass, or other material that encases the trunk as far as the nipples and both legs as far as the toes. A horizontal crossbar to improve immobilization connects the cast at ankle level. Compare **one-and-a-half spica cast, unilateral long-leg spica cast.**

bile, a bitter, yellow-green secretion of the liver. Bile is stored in the gallbladder and is released when fat enters the first part of the small intestine (duodenum). Bile emulsifies these fats, preparing them for further digestion and absorption in the small intestine. Also called **gall.** See also **biliary obstruction, jaundice.** **–biliary,** *adj.*

bile acid, a steroid acid of the bile, produced during the breakdown of cholesterol.

bile duct. See **biliary duct.**

bile solubility test, a test used to determine whether an infection is caused by pneumococci or streptococci. Pneumococci dissolve in ox bile, resulting in a clear solution; streptococci do not dissolve, resulting in a cloudy solution.

bilharziasis. See **schistosomiasis.**

biliary /bil′ē·erē/, referring to bile or to the gallbladder and its ducts, which transport bile to the duodenum. These are often called the **biliary tract** or the **biliary system.** Also called

bilious. See also **bile, biliary calculus.**

biliary atresia, congenital absence or underdevelopment of one or more of the biliary structures. It causes jaundice and early liver damage. See also **biliary cirrhosis.**

biliary calculus, a stone formed in the biliary tract, consisting of bile pigments and calcium salts. Biliary calculi may cause jaundice, right-sided pain, obstruction, and inflammation of the gallbladder. If stones cannot pass into the duodenum, a cholangiogram will reveal their location, and they can be surgically removed. Also called **choledocholithiasis, gallstones.** See also **cholangitis, cholecystitis, cholelithiasis.**

biliary cirrhosis, an inflammatory condition in which the flow of bile through the liver is obstructed. Biliary cirrhosis most commonly affects women in their middle years, and its cause is unknown. It is characterized by abdominal pain, jaundice, clay-colored stools, and enlargement of the liver and spleen. Compare **biliary calculus, biliary obstruction.**

biliary colic, a type of pain specifically associated with the passing of stones through the bile ducts. Also called **cholecystalgia.** See also **biliary calculi.**

biliary duct, a duct through which bile passes from the liver to the duodenum.

biliary fistula, an abnormal passage from the gallbladder, a bile duct, or the liver to an internal organ or to the surface of the body. Biliary fistulae may open into the large intestine, duodenum, liver duct, or abdominal cavity.

biliary obstruction, blockage of the common or cystic bile duct, usually caused by one or more gallstones. It interferes with bile drainage and produces an inflammatory reaction. Uncommon causes of biliary obstruction include cysts or inflammation of the common bile duct, pancreatic and duodenal tumors, Crohn's disease, pancreatitis, and roundworm infection. Stones, consisting chiefly of cholesterol, bile pigment, and calcium, may form in the gallbladder and in the liver duct in patients of either sex at any age but are more common in middle-aged women. Increased amounts of cholesterol in the blood, as occurs in obesity, diabetes, underactive thyroid gland, biliary stasis, and inflammation of the biliary system promote the formation of gallstones.
★DIAGNOSIS: Biliary obstruction is characterized by severe pain near the breastbone that may radiate to the back and shoulder, nausea, vomiting, and profuse sweating. The dehydrated patient may have chills, fever, jaundice, clay-colored stools, dark, concentrated urine, and an electrolyte imbalance. There may also be a tendency to bleed because the absence of bile prevents the synthesis and absorption of vitamin K, which is necessary for clotting.
★TREATMENT: The patient is placed in bed and a tube inserted through the nose to the stomach for suctioning. Intravenous fluids with vitamins and medication for pain are given. When the tube is removed, the patient initially receives a low-fat liquid diet and progresses to a soft or normal diet. Removal of the gallbladder (cholecystectomy) is the usual treatment, but, in most cases, surgery is delayed until the patient's condition is stabilized and any clotting problems (caused by vitamin K malabsorption) are corrected.
★PATIENT CARE: If surgery is not performed, it is important that the patient stay on a low-fat diet and report any recurrence of symptoms. Cholecystectomy usually requires several days of hospitalization. See **cholecystectomy.**

biliary tract cancer, a relatively rare malignant tumor in a bile duct, occurring slightly more often in men than in women. It is characterized by progressive jaundice, itching, weight loss, and, in the later stages, by severe pain. X-ray studies (cholangiography) are done to determine the site of the tumor, and in some cases surgery can successfully remove it. In cases of an inoperable tumor, various surgical procedures may be performed to improve the flow of bile and reduce discomfort. Radiation treatments are also used.

bilingulate /bīling'gyəlit/, having two tongues or two tonguelike structures.

bilious /bil'yəs/, **1.** referring to bile, **2.** characterized by an excessive secretion of bile, **3.** characterized by a disorder affecting the bile.

bilirubin /bil'iroo'bin/, the orange-yellow pigment in bile, formed principally by the breakdown of hemoglobin in red blood cells. Bilirubin normally travels in the bloodstream to the liver, where it is converted to a water-soluble form and excreted into the bile. In a healthy person, about 0.01 ounce (250 mg) of bilirubin is produced daily, and most of that is excreted from the body in the stool. The characteristic yellow skin of jaundice is caused by bilirubin in the blood and in the tissues of the skin. See also **jaundice, van den Bergh test.**

bilirubinuria, the presence of bilirubin in urine.

biliuria /bil'iyoor'ē·ə/, the presence of bile in the urine.

Billings method, a method of estimating ovulation time by changes in the cervix mucus during the menstrual cycle.

Billroth's operation I, the surgical removal of the area (pylorus) where the stomach joins the beginning of the small intestine (duodenum). The duodenum is attached to the stomach. This surgery is performed for stomach cancer.

Billroth's operation II, the surgical removal of the pylorus and duodenum. The cut end of the stomach is joined to the small intestine.

Biltricide, a trademark for a drug used to rid the body of Schistosoma flukes (praziquantel).

bimanual palpation, the examination of a woman's pelvic organs in which the examiner places one hand on the stomach and one or two fingers of the other hand in the vagina.

bimaxillary, referring to the right and left upper jaw (maxilla).

bilobate, having two lobes.

bilobulate, having two small lobes. Also **bilobular.**

bilocular, divided into two cells.

bimanual, referring to the functioning of both hands.

binary fission /bī'nərē/, direct division of a cell or nucleus into two equal parts. It is the common form of asexual reproduction of bacteria, protozoa, and other lower forms of life. Also called **simple fission.** Compare **multiple fission.**

binaural stethoscope /bīnôr'əl/, a stethoscope having two earpieces.

bind, **1.** to bandage or wrap in a band. **2.** to join together with a band. **3.** to combine or unite molecules.

Binet age /binā'/, the mental age of a person, especially a child, as determined by the Binet-Simon tests. The tests are evaluated on the basis of tested intelligence of the "normal" person at any given age. The Binet age corresponding to "profoundly retarded" is 1 to 2 years of age; to "severely retarded," 3 to 7 years of age; and to "mildly retarded," 8 to 12 years of age.

binocular, **1.** referring to both eyes, especially regarding vision. **2.** a microscope, telescope, or field glass that can accommodate viewing by both eyes.

binocular fixation, the process of having both eyes directed at the same object at the same time. This is essential to having good depth perception.

binocular parallax /par'əlaks/, the difference in the angles formed by the sight lines to two objects situated at different distances from the eyes. Binocular parallax is a major factor in depth perception. Also called **stereoscopic parallax.**

binocular vision, the use of both eyes simultaneously so that the images perceived by each eye are combined to appear as a single image. Compare **diplopia.**

binomial, containing two names or terms.

binovular, developing from two distinct eggs, as in dizygotic twins. Also called **diovular.** Compare **uniovular.**

bio-, a combining form referring to life.

bioactive, referring to a substance that has an effect on or causes a reaction in living tissue.

bioassay /bī'ō·as'ā, -əsā'/, a laboratory test to find the amount of a drug or other substance in a sample by comparing its effect on an organism, an animal, or another tissue with that of a standard preparation. Also called **biologic assay.**

bioavailability, the amount of drug or other substance that is active in the tissues.

biochemical marker, any substance that is found in the urine, blood, or other body tissues that may indicate the presence of a disease or other abnormal condition.

biochemistry, the chemistry of living organisms and life processes. Also called **biologic chemistry, physiologic chemistry.**

bioelectrical impedance analysis (BIA), a method of measuring the fat composition of the body by its resistance to electricity. See also **total body electrical conductivity (TOBEC).**

bioelectricity, electric current that is generated by living tissues, as nerves, brain, heart, and muscles. The electric impulses of human tissues are recorded by electrocardiograph, electroencephalograph, and similar sensitive devices.

bioenergetics, a system of exercises based on the concept that natural healing is enhanced by bringing into harmony the patient's body rhythms and the natural environment.

bioequivalent /bī'ō·ikwiv'ələnt/, referring to a drug that has the same effect on the body as another drug, usually one nearly identical in its chemical structure. **–bioequivalence,** *n.*

biofeedback, a process monitoring certain functions of the body, as blood pressure, muscle tension, and brain wave activity. The patient can see or hear this information and is taught to alter these functions through relaxation. Biofeedback may be used to treat many conditions, as high blood pressure, insomnia, and migraine headache.

bioflavonoid /bī'ōflā'vənoid/, a term for any of a group of colored substances found in many fruits and essential for the absorption and processing of vitamin C (ascorbic acid). The bioflavonoids are needed to maintain collagen and capillary walls. They also may aid in protection against infection. Deficiency can result in a tendency to bleed or bruise easily. The bioflavonoids are not toxic. Also called **vitamin P.** See also **ascorbic acid.**

biogenesis /bī'ōjen'əsis/, **1.** the doctrine that living material can originate only from existing life and not from inanimate matter. Also called **biogeny** /bī·oj'ənē/, **2.** the origin of life and living organisms; ontogeny and phylogeny. **–biogenetic,** *adj.*

biogenetic law. See **recapitulation theory.**

biogenic /bī'ōjen'ik/, **1.** produced by the action of a living organism, as fermentation. **2.** essential to life and the maintenance of health, as food, water, proper rest.

biogenic amine, one of a large group of naturally occurring compounds, most of which transmit nerve impulses. The most dominant, norepinephrine, is involved in functions as emotional reactions, memory, sleep, and arousalfrom sleep. Acetylcholine and dopamine are other biogenic amines.

biologic, 1. referring to living organisms and their products. 2. any substance made from living organisms or the products of living organisms that is used in diagnosis, prevention, or treatment of disease. Kinds of biologics are **antigens, antitoxins, serums, vaccines.**

biological activity, the capacity of a substance to change the functions of a cell. The capacity is related not only to the nature of the substance, but also to its concentration and the length of time the cell is exposed to it.

biologic assay. See **bioassay.**

biologic half-life, the time required for the body to eliminate one half of a dosage of any substance by regular physical processes. Also called **metabolic half-life.** See also **effective half-life, half-life.**

biological monitoring, 1. a process of measuring the levels of various drugs or other substances within a patient during diagnosis or therapy. 2. the measurement of poisonous substances in the environment and the identification of health risks to the population. It is often done through analysis of samples of blood, hair, urine, sweat, saliva, and exhaled air.

biologic psychiatry, a school of psychiatric thought that stresses the physical, chemical, and nervous system as the causes of and treatments for mental and emotional disorders.

biology, the scientific study of plants and animals. Some branches of biology are **biometry, ecology, molecular biology,** and **paleontology.**

biome /bī′ōm/, all plants, animals, and microorganisms of a particular region.

biomechanics, the study of mechanical laws and their application to living organisms, especially the human body and its movement. **–biomechanical,** adj.

biomedical engineering, a system of techniques in which knowledge of biological processes is applied to solve practical medical problems.

bionics /bī·on′iks/, the science of applying electronic principles and devices, as computers and solid-state miniaturized circuitry, to medical problems. Artificial pacemakers used to correct abnormal heart rhythms are an example. **–bionic,** adj.

biophore /bī′əfôr′/, according to German biologist A.F.L. Weismann, the basic hereditary unit contained in the germ plasm from which all living cells develop and all inherited characteristics are transmitted. Compare **gemmule.**

biopotenitals, electrical charges produced by various tissues of the body, particularly muscle tissue during contractions. Electrocardiography, for example, measures changing potentials in heart muscle contractions.

biopsy, 1. removing a small piece of living tissue from an organ or other part of the body for microscopic examination to establish a diagnosis or follow the course of a disease. 2. the tissue removed for examination. 3. informal. to remove tissue for examination. Kinds of biopsy include **aspiration biopsy, needle biopsy, punch biopsy, surface biopsy.** **–bioptic,** adj.

bioptome tip catheter /bī·op′tōm/, a flexible, hollow tube (catheter) with a special tip designed to obtain samples of the tissue of the lining of the heart. It is used to monitor heart transplant patients for early signs of tissue rejection.

biorhythm, any cyclical, biological event, as the sleep cycle, the menstrual cycle, or the respiratory cycle. **–biorhythmic,** adj.

-biosis, a combining form meaning 'life.'

biostatistics, numeric data on births, deaths, diseases, injuries, and other factors affecting the general health and condition of human populations. Also called **vital statistics.**

biosynthesis, any of thousands of chemical reactions continually occurring throughout the body. In biosynthesis, molecules form more complex biomolecules, especially carbohydrates, fats, proteins, nucleotides, and nucleic acids.

biotaxis /bī′ōtak′sis/, the ability of living cells to develop into certain forms and arrangements. See also **cytoclesis.** **–biotactic,** adj.

biotechnology, the study of the relationships between humans or other living organisms and machinery. Examples include the health effects of word processor equipment on office workers or the industrial application of the results of biological research, particularly in fields as recombinant DNA or gene splicing.

-biotic, 1. a combining form referring to life. 2. a combining form meaning 'possessing a specified mode of life.'

biotic potential, the possible growth rate of a population of organisms under ideal conditions. These conditions include the absence of predators and the presence of unlimited nourishment and space for growth.

biotin /bī′ətin/, a colorless, crystalline, water-soluble B complex vitamin that helps produce fatty acids. It also helps the body use protein, folic acid, pantothenic acid, and vitamin B_{12}. Rich sources are egg yolk, beef liver, kidney, unpolished rice, brewer's yeast, peanuts, cauliflower, and mushrooms. Large quantities of raw egg whites in the diet can produce biotin deficiency, but this occurs only in experimental studies.

biotope, a specific biological habitat or site.

biotransformation /bī′ōtrans′fərmā′shən/, the chemical changes a substance undergoes in the body, as by the action of enzymes. See also **metabolic.**

Biot's respiration /bē·ōz′/, an abnormal respiratory pattern, characterized by irregular breathing with periods of not breathing. The breathing may be slow and deep or rapid and shallow and is often accompanied by sighing. Biot's respiration occurs in patients with meningitis or increased pressure on the brain.

biovular twins. See **dizygotic twins.**

bipara /bip'ərə/, a woman who has given birth twice in separate pregnancies.

biparental inheritance. See **amphigonous inheritance.**

biparietal /bīpərī'ətəl/, referring to the two parietal bones that form the top and sides of the head.

biparous, referring to the birth of two infants in a single pregnancy.

bipartite, having two parts.

biped, 1. having two feet. 2. any animal with only two feet.

bipenniform /bīpen'ifôrm'/, having the bilateral symmetry of a feather, as the pattern formed by the fibers of certain muscles.

biperiden, a drug used to treat Parkinson's disease and drug-caused disorders of movement and coordination (extrapyramidal symptoms).
★CAUTION: Narrow-angle glaucoma, asthma, blockage of the urinary tract or the stomach or intestines, or known allergy to this drug prohibits its use.
★ADVERSE EFFECTS: Among the more serious side effects are blurred vision, nervous system problems, rapid heart beat, dry mouth, reduced sweating, and allergic reactions.

biphasic /bīfā'zik/, having two phases, parts, or stages.

bipolar, 1. having two poles, as in certain types of electrotherapy using opposite poles (positive and negative). 2. a nerve cell that has electric signals traveling both to and away from the center (afferent and efferent).

bipolar disorder, a mental disorder characterized by periods of mania and depression. Characteristics of the manic phase are excess emotional displays, excitement, overactivity, excess joy, a high degree of energy, inability to concentrate, and reduced need for sleep, often coupled with unrealistic ideas about one's worth. In the depressive phase, apathy and underactivity are seen along with feelings of excess sadness, loneliness, guilt, and lowered sense of one's worth. Most people with this disorder respond well to the drug lithium.Also called **folie circulaire.** /fool̄e' serk̄eler'/.

bipolar lead, two electrodes for heart test (electrocardiogram) that are placed on different parts of the body.

bird breeder's lung. See **pigeon breeder's lung.**

bird-face retrognathism, an abnormal profile with an undeveloped lower jaw. It may be caused by problems in the growth of the jaw joint from injury or infection. Compare **prognathism.**

bird-headed dwarf, a person affected with Seckel's syndrome, a birth defect characterized by

shortness; a normal body shape; a small head with very small jaws, large eyes, and a beaklike nose; mental retardation; and many other skeleton, skin, and genital defects. Also called **nanocephalic dwarf.**

birth, 1. event of being born, the coming of a new person out of its mother into the world. Kinds of birth are **breech birth, live birth, stillbirth.** See also **effacement, labor.** 2. the childbearing event, the bringing forth by a mother of a baby.

birth canal, *informal.* the passage that extends from the opening in the pelvis to the vaginal opening, through which an infant passes during birth. See also **clinical pelvimetry.**

birth control. See **contraception.**

birth defect. See **congenital anomaly.**

birthing chair, a chair used in labor and birth to make the mother comfortable and to make labor easier. The chair may be specially built with many technical features or it may be a simple three-legged stool with a high, slanted back and a circular seat with a large hole in it. Birthing chairs should allow the woman to sit straight up or to lay back. The chair has a lower section that may be removed or folded out of the way. Lights, mirrors, and basins may be attached to make the birth attendant's job easier. The upright position seems to shorten the time in labor, particularly the period just before delivery, probably because of gravity and increased help by the mother. The chair is not to be used with anesthesia.

birth injury, injury to a baby while being born. Some kinds of birth injury are **Bell's palsy, cerebral palsy, Erb's palsy.**

birthmark. See **nevus.**

birth rate, the number of births during a given period in relation to the total population of a certain area. The birth rate is usually counted as the number of births per 1000 of population.

birth trauma, any physical injury to an infant during birth.

birth weight, the weight of a baby when born, usually about 3500 g (7.5 lbs). In the United States, 97%of newborns weigh between 2500 g (5.5 lbs) and 4500 g (10 lbs). Babies who are full term but weigh less than 2500 g are called **small for gestational age.** Babies who weigh more than 4500 g are called **large for gestational age** and are often infants of mothers with diabetes.

bisacodyl /bisak'ōdil/, a laxative given for constipation, to empty the bowel before or after surgery, or before x-ray studies are done.
★CAUTION: Stomach and bowel pain, nausea, vomiting, breaks in the rectum, open hemorrhoids, or known allergy to this drug prohibits its use.
★ADVERSE EFFECTS: Among the more serious side effects are cramping, stomach and bowel pain, and diarrhea.

bisect, to divide into two equal lengths or parts.

bisexual /bīsek'shoo·əl/, **1.** having sex organs of both sexes (hermaphroditic). **2.** having physical or psychological features of both sexes. **3.** engaging in both heterosexual and homosexual activity.

bisexual libido, the tendency in a person to seek sexual pleasure with people of either sex.

bisferious pulse /bisfer'ē·əs/, an arterial pulse that has two peaks that can be felt with the hand, the second being slightly stronger than the first. It may be detected when the force exerted by the blood on the walls of the arteries is decreased. Compare **dicrotic pulse.**

bis in die (b.d., b.i.d.), a Latin phrase, used in prescriptions, meaning "twice a day." It is more commonly used in its abbreviated form.

bismuth (Bi), a reddish, crystal-like metal element. Its atomic number is 83; its atomic weight is 209. It is combined with many other elements, as oxygen, to make salts used in making many drugs.

bismuth stomatitis, an abnormal mouth condition caused by using bismuth compounds over long periods. It is characterized by a blue-black line on the gum next to the teeth or darkening of the inside cheek in the mouth. Other symptoms are a sore tongue, metal taste, and a sense of burning in the mouth. Compare **arsenical stomatitis, Atabrine stomatitis.**

bite, 1. the act of cutting, tearing, holding, or gripping with the teeth. **2.** a record of the bite or relationship of the teeth to each other. Compare **closed bite, open bite.**

bitegage /bīt'gāj'/, a dental device that helps gain proper bite of the teeth in the upper and lower jaw.

biteguard splint, a device, usually made of resin, for covering the biting and chewing surfaces of the teeth. This protects them from injury during processes to keep the teeth rigid and stable. See also **Gunning's splint.**

bitemporal, referring to both temples or both bones (temporal) of the temple.

biteplane /bīt'plān/, a removable dental device for covering the biting surfaces of the teeth to prevent them from touching.

biteplate, a device used in dentistry for diagnosis or treatment. It is made of wire and plastic, worn in the palate, and may also be used to correct problems of the jaw joint.

bite reflex, a swift, involuntary biting action that may be triggered by stimulation of the mouth. The bite can be difficult to release in some cases, such as when a spoon or tongue depressor is placed in a patient's mouth.

bite-wing film, a type of dental x-ray film that has a central tab or wing on which the teeth close to keep the film position rigid while x-ray films are taken.

biting in childhood, a natural behavior and reflex in infants. It begins at about 5 to 6 months of age in response to solid foods in the diet and the beginning of teething. The activity is a step in the development of the child, because it is the first willful action the infant learns, and through it the infant learns to control the surroundings. The behavior also forces the infant into one of the first inner conflicts, because biting can have both pleasing and displeasing results. Biting during breast feeding causes the nipple to withdraw and anxiety in the mother, yet it is also a means of making teething more comfortable. Toddlers and older children often use biting to show hostility to their parents and other children, especially during play or to gain attention. Most children normally outgrow this behavior unless they have severe emotional problems. See also **psychosexual development, psychosocial development.**

Bitot's spots /bitōz'/, white or gray triangular deposits on the white of the eye next to the outer edge of the cornea. This is a sign of a lack of vitamin A. Also called **Bitot's patches.**

bitrochanteric lipodystrophy, an abnormal and excess amount of fat on the buttocks and the outer part of the upper thighs. It occurs most commonly in women. See also **lipodystrophy.**

bitterling test, a Japanese test for pregnancy in which a female bitterling fish is placed in about 1 quart (1 liter) of fresh water containing less than ½ ounce (10 ml) of the urine of the woman being tested. If the woman is pregnant, the long tube for eggs (oviduct) of the bitterling grows from its belly.

biuret test, a method for finding urea and other proteins in blood. In an alkaline solution, copper sulfate reacts with proteins to produce a purple color, which is called the biuret reaction.

bivalve cast, a cast used to keep a part of the body rigid. It is used to heal broken bones or to correct a bone defect. The cast is cut in half to watch for pressure under the cast, especially with a patient who has little or no feeling in the part of the body in the cast. If dangerous pressure areas are found, "windows" are often cut out of the cast over the pressure areas to correct the problem.

bizarre leiomyoma. See **epithelioid leiomyoma.**

Bk, symbol for **berkelium.**

black beauties, *slang.* amphetamines.

black damp. See **damp.**

Black Death, *informal.* bubonic plague, usually referring to the epidemic in the fourteenth century that killed more than 25 million people in Europe. See also **bubonic plague, plague,** *Yersinia pestis.*

Blackett-Healy method, a procedure for positioning a patient for making x-rays of the shoulder area. The patient is placed lying on the back with the affected shoulder centered to the middle of the film, with the arm away from the body and elbow bent. The opposite shoulder is raised about 15 degrees and supported with a sandbag.

black eye, a bruise on the eyelid. It is treated with ice packs for the first 24 hours to reduce swelling, then with hot compresses to aid the blood in leaving the bruise.

black fever. See **kala-azar.**

blackhead. See **comedo.**

black light. See **Wood's light.**

black lung. See **anthracosis.**

black lung disease. See **pneumoconiosis.**

blackout, *informal.* a temporary loss of vision or consciousness resulting from lack of oxygen to the brain.

black plague. See **bubonic plague.**

black spots film fault, a defect in an x-ray film, seen as dark spots thoughout the image area. It is caused by dust particles or developer on the film or by outdated film.

black tongue. See **parasitic glossitis.**

blackwater fever, a serious problem of chronic falciparum malaria. The symptoms are liver disease (jaundice), kidney failure, and dark red or black urine caused by heavy internal bleeding. See also **falciparum malaria, malaria,** *Plasmodium.*

black widow spider, a poisonous spider (arachnid) found in many parts of the world. The poison injected with its bite causes sweating, stomach cramps, nausea, headaches, and many degrees of dizziness. Small children, old people, or those with heart conditions are most severely affected.

black widow spider antivenin, a vaccinating drug used to treat a black widow spider bite.

★CAUTION: Known allergy to this drug or to horse serum prohibits its use.

★ADVERSE EFFECTS: Among the more serious side effects are allergic reactions.

bladder, 1. a sac that holds fluids. 2. the urinary bladder.

bladder cancer, the most common cancer of the urinary tract. It is characterized by one or more tumors that tend to return. Cancer of the bladder is more than twice as common in men than in women, is more common in urban than in rural areas, and may be more common in the future. The risk for developing bladder cancer is increased with cigarette smoking and exposure to cancer-causing agents (carcinogens), as aniline dyes, beta-naphthylamine, aromatic hydrocarbons, or benzidine. Other risk factors are long-term urinary tract infections, kidney stone disease, and infection with the fluke that causes schistosomiasis. Early symptoms of a bladder cancer include bloody urine, frequent or painful urination, and the growth of lumps (cystitis). Some tumors can be burned off, or part of the bladder can be removed. However, total removal of the bladder (cystectomy) may be necessary. In patients needing a cystectomy, a pathway is built to move urine to the large intestine or to an opening in the stomach area. External radiation may be given before surgery or to lessen the discomfort in patients who cannot have surgery. Small tumors on the bladder wall are sometimes treated with internal radiation. In this type of treatment, radioisotopes in a balloon or radon seeds are put directly into the bladder. See also **cystectomy.**

bladder flap, *informal.* a fold of stomach lining (peritoneum) that is cut open during a low cesarean section (a "bikini cesarean"). It allows the bladder to be separated from the uterus so that the cut can be made low on the uterus. See also **cesarean section.**

bladder stone. See **vesicle calculus.**

Blalock-Taussig procedure /blā'loktô'sig/, surgical building of an artery (shunt) as a temporary correction for an inborn heart defect, as in an infant born with tetralogy of Fallot. The artery above the collarbone (subclavian) is joined end-to-end with the artery that carries blood to the lungs. This shunt moves blood from the circulation to the lungs. Permanent correction is done later in early childhood. See also **heart surgery.**

blame placing, the process of placing responsibility for one's behavior on others.

blanch, 1. causing to become pale. 2. whitening or bleaching a surface or substance. 3. becoming white or pale, as from narrowing of the blood vessels, which happens with fear or anger.

bland, mild or having a soothing effect.

bland aerosols, gas mixtures that consist of water, salt solution, or similar substances that have no significant drug interaction. They are used primarily to provide humidity and to soften secretions to a more liquid form.

bland diet, a nonirritating diet. It is often given to treat many different stomach and bowel diseases, and after stomach or bowel surgery. The diet may include eggs, meat, poultry, fish, and enriched fine cereals; milk is usually important. A bland diet may include or exclude specific foods. Spicy or highly seasoned foods, carbonated beverages, raw fruits and vegetables, and rich desserts are avoided. See also **sippy diet.**

blanket bath, wrapping the patient in a wet pack and then in blankets.

blast cell, any immature cell, as a red blood cell (erythroblast), a white blood cell (lymphoblast), or a nerve cell (neuroblast).

blastema /blastē'mə/, *pl.* **blastemas, blastemata,** 1. any mass of living protoplasm able to grow and separate. 2. in certain animals, a group of cells able to grow back a lost or damaged part or to make a complete organism in asexual reproduction.

blastic transformation, a late stage in a cancer of the bone marrow (chronic granulocytic leukemia) in which affected blood cells grow more quickly and become more like each other but different from normal blood cells. The signs are anemia, lack of blood platelets, and more than half the blood cells in the bone marrow being too immature for use in the body. In this stage the patient has developed resistance to therapy and has entered a final stage of leukemia.

blastid, the site in the fertilized egg (ovum) where the nucleus forms. Also called **blastide.**

blastin, any substance that gives food to or helps the growth or reproduction of cells.

blasto-, a combining form referring to a very early fetus (embryo) or developing stage. In general, the first 5 weeks after conception the term "embryo" is used; after that, the term is "fetus."

blastocyte /blas′təsīt/, a very early embryonic cell before any cell layer has formed. **–blastocytic,** adj.

blastocytoma. See **blastoma.**

blastogenesis /blas′tōjen′əsis/, **1.** nonsexual reproduction by budding. **2.** the theory that hereditary traits are carried by the first cell of an organism (germ plasm). **3.** the development of the embryo during the separation and formation of the germ layers. **–blastogenetic,** adj.

blastogenic, **1.** beginning in the first cell of an organism (germ plasm). **2.** beginning the growth of tissue. **3.** relating to or characterized by blastogenesis.

blastokinin /blas′təki′nin/, a substance that is released by the uterus in many mammals. It may help an early cell (the blastocyst) become attached to the wall of the uterus. Also called **uteroglobulin.**

blastoma /blastō′mə/, pl. **blastomas, blastomata,** a tumor of embryonic tissue that develops from the early substance (blastema) of an organ or tissue. Also called **blastocytoma.** **–blastomatous,** adj.

blastomatosis /blast′tōmətō′sis/, the development of many tumors of embryonic tissue.

Blastomyces /blas′tōmī′sēz/, a genus of yeastlike fungus. The species *Blastomyces dermatitidis* causes an infectious disease (blastomycosis).

blastomycosis /blas′tōmīkō′sis/, an infectious disease caused by a yeastlike fungus, *Blastomyces dermatitidis.* It usually affects only the skin but may invade the lungs, kidneys, nervous system, and bones. The disease is most common in young men living in North America, particularly the southeastern United States, but outbreaks have occurred in Africa and Latin America. Skin infections often begin as small bumps on the hand, face, neck, or other exposed areas where there has been a cut, bruise, or other injury. These bumps spread gradually into surrounding areas. When the

lungs are involved, the patient usually has a cough, shortness of breath, chest pain, chills, and a fever with heavy sweating. Also called **Gilchrist's disease.** See also **fungus, mycosis.**

blastosphere. See **blastula.**

blastula, an early stage of the process in which a fertilized egg develops into an embryo. The blastula is the form in which the embryo becomes planted in the wall of the uterus. Also called **blastosphere.**

BLB mask, abbreviation for **Boothby-Lovelace-Bulbulian mask.**

bleb /bleb/, a gathering of fluid under the skin, forming bumps that are smaller than normal blisters.

bleed, **1.** to lose blood from the blood vessels of the body. The blood may flow out through a natural opening, or a break in the skin, or it may flow into a space, an organ, or the spaces between the tissues. **2.** to cause blood to flow from a vein or an artery.

bleeder, **1.** *informal.* a patient who has a blood clotting disease (hemophilia) or any other vessel or blood condition linked to a tendency to bleed. **2.** *informal.* a bleeding blood vessel, especially one cut during surgery.

bleeding, the release of blood from the circulation as a result of damage to one or more blood vessels. See also **blood clotting.**

bleeding diasthesis, a tendency to abnormal blood clotting.

bleeding time, the time needed for blood to stop flowing from a tiny wound. A test of bleeding time is the Ivy method, in which a blood pressure cuff on the upper arm is inflated and a small wound is made with a scalpel on the inner surface of the arm. Normal Ivy bleeding time is from 2 to 6 minutes. See also **hemostasis.**

blending inheritance, the apparent blending in the offspring of distinct and unlike traits of the parents. For example, a very tall father and very short mother may have a child of medium height. The grandchildren would then be of medium height.

blennorrhea /blen′ərē′ə/, excess release of mucus. Also called **blennorrhagia.**

Blenoxane, a trademark for an anticancer drug (bleomycin sulfate).

bleomycin sulfate, an anticancer antibiotic used to treat many cancers.

★CAUTION: Allergy to this drug prohibits its use.

★ADVERSE EFFECTS: Among the most serious side effects are lung problems (pneumonitis, pulmonary fibrosis), very high fever, and collapse of the circulation. Rashes and skin reactions commonly occur.

blepharal, referring to the eyelids.

blepharitis /blef′əri′tis/, an inflammatory, very contagious infection of the eyelash and oil glands of the eyelids. It is characterized by swelling, redness, and crusts of dried mucus on the lids. **Ulcerative blepharitis** is caused by a bacteria infection. **Nonulcerative blepharitis** may be caused by psoriasis, seborrhea, or an allergic reaction.

blepharoadenoma /blef′ərō·ad′inō′mə/, a gland-like tumor of the eyelid.

blepharoatheroma /blef′ərō·ath′ərō′mə/, a tumor of the eyelid.

blepharoplegia /blef′ərōplē′jə/, paralysis of the eyelid.

blepharospasm, a spasm of the eyelid.

blight, any disease of plants caused by a fungus.

blighted ovum, a fertilized egg (ovum) that fails to develop. On x-ray films or ultrasound it appears to be a fluid-filled lump (cyst) attached to the wall of the uterus. Many spontaneous abortions (miscarriages) in the first 3 months of pregnancy are actually a blighted ovum being released.

blind fistula, an abnormal passage with only one open end. The opening may be to the body surface or to an organ or structure. Also called **incomplete fistula.**

blindgut. See **cecum.**

blind intubation. See **intubation.**

blind loop, a part of the intestine that is blocked off from the rest of the intestines so that nothing can pass through it. Blind loops are sometimes created surgically during bowel operations.

blindness, unable to see.

blind spot, 1. a small, normal gap in sight caused when an image is focused on the optic disk of the retina. **2.** an abnormal gap in sight caused by an injury of the retina or other part of the eye. It is often sensed as light spots or flashes.

blister, a thin, rounded swelling of the skin that contains fluid. It is caused by irritation or burns. Also called **vesicle** or **bulla.**

bloat, a swelling or filling with gas, as when the stomach is distended from swallowing air or from intestinal gas.

Blocadren, a trademark for a drug used to treat high blood pressure (timolol maleate).

blockade, an agent that interferes with or prevents a specific action in an organ or tissue.

block anesthesia. See **conduction anesthesia.**

blocked communication, a situation in which communication with a patient is difficult because of contradictory or inconsistent verbal or nonverbal messages. To clear up blocked communication, therapists may record meetings with a patient on videotape to study eye contact and other clues to the patient's thinking process.

blocking, 1. preventing the sending of an electric signal impulse of the nervous system. For example, spinal anesthesia blocks the nerve signals to part of the body. **2.** interrupting some of the body's processes, as with some drugs. **3.** being unable to remember an event.

blocking antibody, an antibody that interferes with the action of other antibodies. See also **antigen-antibody reaction, hapten.**

blood, the liquid pumped by the heart through all of the arteries, veins, and capillaries. It is made up of a clear yellow fluid, called plasma, and many cells called the formed elements. The formed elements include red blood cells (erythrocytes), white blood cells (leukocytes), and platelets. The erythrocytes move oxygen and food to the cells and remove carbon dioxide and other wastes from the cells. The leukocytes defend the body against foreign invaders. The platelets function in blood clotting. Hormones and proteins are also contained in the blood. The normal adult has a total blood volume of 7% to 8% of body weight. This is equal to about 1 ounce per pound (70 ml/kg for men and 65 ml/kg for women) of body weight. It moves at a speed of about 1 foot per second (30 cm) with a complete circulation time of 20 seconds. Compare **lymph.** See also **blood cell, erythrocyte, leukocyte, plasma, platelet.**

blood agar, a substance for growing microorganisms in the laboratory.

blood bank, an organization that collects, processes, and stores blood to be used for transfusions and other purposes. See also **bank blood, component therapy, transfusion.**

blood-brain barrier (BBB), a feature of the brain thought to be made up of walls of small vessels (capillaries) that surround the membranes. The blood-brain barrier normally prevents many chemicals and disease-causing organisms in the blood from entering the nervous system.

blood buffers, a system of buffers made mostly of dissolved carbon dioxide and bicarbonate that help maintain the proper acid-base balance (pH) of the blood. See also **buffer, pH.**

blood cell, any one of the many cells (formed elements) of the blood, including red cells (erythrocytes), white cells (leukocytes), and platelets (thrombocytes). Together they normally make up about 50% of the total volume of the blood. See also **erythrocyte, leukocyte, platelet.**

blood clot, a semisolid, gelatin like mass that results from the clotting process of blood. It is mostly made up of red cells, white cells, and platelets enmeshed in a protein (fibrin) grouping. Compare **embolus, thrombus.** See also **blood clotting, fibrinogen.**

blood clotting, changing blood from a free-flowing liquid to a semisolid gel. The process usually starts with tissue damage and exposure of the blood to air. Within seconds of injury to the vessel wall, platelets clump at the site. If normal amounts of calcium, platelets, and tissue factors are present, a chain reaction of clotting factors (prothrombin, thrombin, and fibrinogen) produce a substance called fibrin. Fibrin forms a mesh over the wound in which all of the formed elements are kept rigid. Clotting can also occur in abnormal situations within the blood vessel, forming an embolus or thrombus. Also called **blood coagulation.** Compare **hemostasis.** See also **anticoagulant, coagulation,** table.

blood coagulation.   See **blood clotting.**

blood count,   See **complete blood count.**

blood donor,   anyone who donates blood to a blood bank or to another person. See also **blood bank, transfusion.**

blood doping,   a new technique that has been used by some athletes to increase their performance and endurance. It consists of giving a blood transfusion to add red blood cells to increase the oxygen-carrying ability of the blood. It is illegal in most competitions. Also called **blood boosting, blood packing.**

blood dyscrasia,   a condition in which any of the blood elements are abnormal, as in leukemia or hemophilia.

blood fluke,   a parasitic flatworm of the class Trematoda, genus *Schistosoma*. See also *Schistosoma,* **schistosomiasis.**

blood gas,   gas dissolved in the liquid part of the blood. Blood gases include oxygen, carbon dioxide, and nitrogen.

blood-gas determination,   an analysis of the acid-base balance (pH) of the blood. This includes measuring the amount and pressure of oxygen, carbon dioxide, and hydrogen in the blood. Blood-gas determination is important for evaluating heart failure, bleeding, kidney failure, drug overdose, shock, uncontrolled diabetes mellitus, or any other condition of severe stress. See also **acid-base balance, acidosis, alkalosis, oxygenation,** P_{CO_2}, **pH,** P_{O_2}.

blood-gas tension,   the partial pressure (the percentage of pressure the gas contributes to the total blood pressure) exerted by a gas in the blood. At equilibrium the partial pressure of a gas exerted in a liquid is the same as that of the partial pressure of the gas (in the gas phase) exerted over the liquid, regardless of solubility and other factors.

blood glucose.   See **blood sugar.**

blood group,   the labeling of blood based on the presence or lack of specific chemical substances on the surface of the red cell. Several different grouping systems have been described, the most common being the ABO blood group. Others include Auberger, Diego, Dombrock, Duffy, high-frequency, I, Kell, Kidd, Lewis, low-frequency, Lutheran, MNS, P, Rh, Sutter, and Xg. See also **ABO blood groups, blood typing.**

blood lactate,   lactic acid that appears in the blood as a result of metabolism without oxygen (anaerobic) when oxygen delivery to the tissues is not enough to support normal metabolism (aerobic).

blood lavage,   the removal of poisons from the blood by injecting blood into the veins.

blood level,   the amount of a drug or other substance in a measured amount of blood plasma, serum, or whole blood.

blood osmolality,   the osmotic pressure of blood. This measures the ability of blood to pass through a thin membrane. Blood osmolality values are abnormal in some diseases. The normal values in blood are 280 to 295 mOsm/L.

blood pH,   the hydrogen concentration of the blood, or a measure of its acidity or alkalinity. The normal pH values for whole blood from the arteries are 7.38 to 7.44; for whole blood from the veins the values are 7.36 to 7.41.

blood plasma,   the clear-yellow liquid portion of the blood with all of its formed elements and particles removed. Plasma makes up about 50% of the total volume of blood. It contains glucose, proteins, amino acids, and other foods, urea and other waste products, as well as hormones, enzymes, vitamins, and minerals. Compare **serum.** See also **blood, plasma protein, pooled plasma.**

blood platelet.   See **platelet.**

blood poisoning.   See **septicemia.**

blood pressure (BP),   the pressure of the circulating blood against the walls of the arteries, the veins, and the chambers of the heart. Overall blood pressure is kept by the complex interaction of the volume of the blood, the walls of the arteries and arterioles, and the force of the contraction of the heart. The pressure in the large artery of the heart (aorta) and the other large arteries of a healthy young adult is about 120 mm Hg during contraction (systole) and 70 mm Hg during relaxation (diastole) of the heart. See also **hypertension, hypotension.**
★METHOD: The blood pressure is most often measured by using a device called a sphygmomanometer, a stethoscope, and a blood pressure cuff. The cuff is placed around the upper arm and filled with air, tightening to stop the blood from flowing through the artery in the arm. The stethoscope is placed over the artery in front of the elbow and the pressure in the cuff is slowly released. No sound is heard until the cuff pressure falls below the systolic pressure in the artery; at that point a pulse is heard. As the cuff pressure continues to fall slowly, the pulse continues; first becoming louder, then dull and muffled. These sounds, called the sounds of Korotkoff, are caused by the disturbance of the blood flowing through the vessel. The cuff pressure at which the first sound is heard is the systolic blood pressure, and the cuff pressure at which the sounds stop is the diastolic blood pressure. The pressure in both arms is sometimes taken. A major differ-

ence between the two readings may mean there is a blockage of the vessels. The blood pressure may also be taken using the thigh with the stethoscope held behind the knee. A larger cuff is used when taking the blood pressure on the thigh or of an overweight person. Any factor that increases resistance of the vessels to the flow of blood or that affects the amount of blood pumped by the heart will change the blood pressure. Strong emotion, for example, tends to do both; therefore, the blood pressure reading is usually taken when the person is resting. Blood pressure increases with age, mainly because the veins do not expand as well. As a person grows older an increase in systolic pressure comes before an increase in diastolic pressure.

Classification of blood pressure

Diastolic blood pressure (mm Hg)	Category*
< 85	Normal blood pressure
85 to 89	High normal blood pressure
90 to 104	Mild hypertension
105 to 114	Moderate hypertension
≥ 115	Severe hypertension

Systolic blood pressure (mm Hg) when DBP < 90 mm Hg	Category
< 140	Normal blood pressure
140 to 159	Borderline isolated systolic hypertesion
≥ 160	Isolated systolic hypertension

*A classification of borderline isolated systolic hypertension (SBP 140 to 159 mm Hg) or isolated systolic hypertension (SBP ≥ 160 mm Hg) takes precedence over a classification of high normal blood pressure (DBP 85 to 89 mm Hg) when both occur in the same individual. A classification of high normal blood pressure (DBP 85 to 89 mm Hg) takes precedence over a classification of normal blood pressure (SBP < 140 mm Hg) when both occur in the same person.
From The 1984 Report of the Joint National Committee on Detection, Evaluation, and Treatment of High Blood Pressure, U.S. Dept. of Health and Human Services, Public Health Service, NIH Publication No. 84-1088, Bethesda, MD, June 1984, National Institutes of Health.

blood pump, 1. a pump for controlling the flow of blood into a blood vessel during a transfusion. **2.** the part of a heart-lung machine that pumps the blood through the machine to put oxygen into it and then through the other circulation system of the body. See also **oxygenation.**

blood serum. See **serum.**

bloodshot, a reddening of the inner surface of the eyelid and white of the eyeball caused by widening of the blood vessels.

blood smear, a small sample of blood that is smeared or spread onto a glass microscope slide for examination.

blood substitute, a substance used to replace circulating blood or to increase its volume. Plasma, human serum albumin, packed red cells, platelets, white cells (leukocytes), and clotting factors are often given in place of whole blood transfusions in the treatment of many disorders.

blood sugar, 1. one of a group of closely related substances, as glucose, fructose, and galactose, that are normally in the blood and are needed to process food. **2.** *nontechnical.* the amount of glucose in the blood. Also called **blood glucose.** See also **hyperglycemia, hypoglycemia.**

blood test, 1. any test that finds out something about the traits or properties of the blood. **2.** *informal.* a test for syphilis.

blood transfusion, giving whole blood or a part, as red cells, to replace blood lost through injury, surgery, or disease.

★METHOD: Blood for transfusion is gotten from one or more healthy donors whose ABO blood group and specific chemical substances match those of the patient getting the transfusion. The donor must also have an adequate hemoglobin level. Each 500 ml (about 1 pint) of blood collected from a donor is stored in a plastic bag and refrigerated for at most 3 weeks. The blood is removed from the refrigerator no more than 30 minutes before transfusion and is checked according to hospital policy. A needle is placed into a vein, usually in the arm, and a tube is connected to allow the blood to drip in slowly. During transfusion the position of the arm is checked, and the needle site is watched for redness, swelling, or leaking. It is stopped if a reaction occurs. A sudden reaction to the blood (hemolytic reaction), characterized by chills, fever, headache, back pain, reduced blood pressure, blood in the urine, and nausea, may occur if the patient's and donor's blood groups are not exactly matched. Giving too much blood may cause shortness of breath, lung filling and frothy sputum. Fever, chills, and an irregular heart rate may be caused by bacteria or a foreign body in the transfused blood. An allergic reaction to transfused blood may be characterized by itching, closing of the throat, and wheezing. The patient is watched for an hour after the transfusion to make certain that a reaction does not occur.

★OUTCOME: All possible efforts are made to prevent the reactions that occur in an estimated 2% to 3% of transfused patients. Sudden hemolytic reactions can be fatal; a delayed reaction, characterized by liver disease (jaundice) and anemia, may occur weeks or months after transfusion. Air bubbles in the blood (embolism) may occur if blood is given under air pressure. Viral diseases may be carried by transfused blood, but in most cases transfusion is without many risks.

blood typing, noting the specific chemical substances (antigens) on the surface of the red blood cell. This process is used to determine a person's blood group. It is the first step in testing donor's and patient's blood to be used in transfusion and is followed by cross matching. See also **ABO blood groups, blood group, Rh factor, transfusion reaction.**

blood urea nitrogen (BUN), the amount of nitrogen in the blood in the form of urea. It is a waste product of normal body functions. BUN is a rough sign of kidney function. It is high in kidney failure, shock, stomach and bowel bleeding, diabetes mellitus, and some tumors. BUN levels are lowered in liver disease, bad dietary situations, and normal pregnancy. See also **azotemia.**

blood vessel, any one of the group of tubes that carries blood. Kinds of blood vessels are **arteries, arterioles, capillaries, veins, venules.**

blood warming coil, a device made of coiled plastic tubing, used for warming blood before transfusions. The coil is often needed for patients who develop heavy stomach or bowel bleeding. Giving cold blood to these patients may cause them to go into shock. Compare **electric blood warmer.**

bloody show, blood-tinged mucus discharged from the vagina before or during labor.

Bloom's syndrome, a rare genetic disease occurring mainly in Ashkenazi Jews and carried as a recessive trait. It is characterized by slowed growth, large blood vessels on the face and arms, sensitivity to sunlight, and a risk of leukemia.

blow bottles, a device used in respiratory care to provide resistance to exhaled air. The bottles are partially filled with water, and the patient is encouraged to blow the water from one bottle to another, a practice that requires inhaling deeply and expanding the lungs to develop increased lung pressure.

blow-out fracture, a broken bone beneath the eyeball caused by a blow that suddenly increases the pressure within the eye.

blue baby, an infant born with bluish skin (cyanosis) caused by an inborn heart problem, as tetralogy of Fallot or incomplete expansion of the lungs (congenital atelectasis). Tetralogy of Fallot is the most common inborn cyanotic heart defect. These defects are diagnosed by certain tests (cardiac catheterization, angiography, or echocardiography) and are corrected surgically, usually in early childhood. See also **congenital cardiac anomaly, tetralogy of Fallot, transposition of the great vessels.**

blue bloater. See **chronic bronchitis.**

blue fever, *informal.* Rocky Mountain spotted fever, so named for the dark blue color of the skin after the infection begins. See also **rickettsiosis, Rocky Mountain spotted fever, typhus.**

blue nevus, a steel-blue skin bump (nodule) with a diameter between 2 and 7 mm (less than ⅓ inch). It is found on the face or arms, grows

very slowly, and lasts throughout life. Bumpy (nodular) blue nevi found on the buttocks or near the tailbone occasionally become cancerous. Any sudden change in the size of such a nodule demands surgical attention and tissue tests. Compare **melanoma.**

blue spot, 1. also called **macula cerulea.** One of a number of small grayish-blue spots that may appear near the armpits or around the groins of individuals infested with body or pubic lice. 2. one of a number of dark blue or mulberry-colored round or oval spots that may appear as a temporary birth defect on the tailbone of some small children. Also called **Mongolian spot.**

blunthook, a sturdy hook-shaped bar used for difficult breech births.

blunting, a decrease in the strength of emotional expression from the level one would normally expect as a reaction to a specific stiuation. It is the opposite of overaction and may be marked by unconcern, minimal response, or indifference.

blush, a brief reddening of the face and neck, commonly the result of the widening of small blood vessels. Blushing is a response to heat or sudden emotion.

B lymphocyte. See **B cell.**

BMA, abbreviation for **British Medical Association.**

BMD, abbreviation for Bureau of Medical Devices.

BMR, abbreviation for **basal metabolic rate.**

board certification, (in medicine) a process in which a person is tested in a medical specialty or subspecialty. Board certification is generally needed for a physician to practice in a hospital.

board certified, referring to a physician who has passed the certification examination given by a medical specialty board and has been certified as a specialist in a particular field of medicine. The physician is then called a fellow of the specialty organization.

boarder baby, an infant abandoned to a hospital because the mother is unable to care for him or her. Many boarder babies are infants born with AIDS or delivered to mothers who are drug-users.

board of health, a board acting on a city, county, state, provincial, or national level. The functions, powers, and duties of boards of health vary with their location. Each board is generally concerned with noting the health needs of the people and bringing projects and resources together to meet these needs.

Boas' test /bō′az/, a test for hydrochloric acid in the contents of the stomach. A glass rod is dipped in a specially made chemical and touched to a drop of filtered stomach liquid. A scarlet streak forms along the rod when hydrochloric acid is present. Also called **resorcinol test.**

body, **1.** the whole structure of an individual including the organs. **2.** a corpse. **3.** the largest or the main part of any organ. Also called **corpus, soma.**

body cavity, any of the spaces in the chest or stomach area that contain body organs. One major cavity, the chest (thoracic) cavity, is subdivided into a cavity around the heart and two lung cavities. The stomach (abdominal) cavity is not divided, but the lower portion is called the pelvic cavity.

body fluid, a liquid contained in the three fluid spaces of the body: the blood plasma, the fluid between the cells (interstitial), and the cell fluid within the cells. Blood plasma and interstitial fluid make up the extracellular fluid. The cell fluid is the intracellular fluid.

body image, a person's own concept of physical appearance. The mental picture, which may be realistic or unrealistic, is created from self-observation, the reactions of others, and the interaction of attitudes, emotions, memories, fantasies, and experiences.

body image agnosia. See **autotopagnosia.**

body jacket, a cast that covers the body but does not cover the neck or arms and legs. It is used to treat a crooked spine (scoliosis) and for keeping the patient rigid after spinal surgery. Compare **Risser cast.**

body language, a set of nonspeaking signals that can express many physical, mental, and emotional states. These include body movements, postures, gestures, expressions, and what one wears. See also **kinesics.**

body mechanics, the use of muscle actions and how the muscles keep the posture of the body.

body movement, motion of all or part of the body, especially at a joint. Some kinds of body movements are **abduction, adduction, extension, flexion, rotation.**

body odor, a smell linked to stale sweat. Fresh sweat is odorless, but after exposure to the air and bacteria on the surface of the skin, chemical changes occur to make the odor. Body odors also can be the result of discharges from many skin conditions, including cancer, fungus, hemorrhoids, leukemia, and ulcers. See also **bromhidrosis.**

body of Retzius /ret′sē·əs/, any one of the masses of protoplasm containing coloring at the base of a hair cell in the internal ear.

body plethysmograph, a device for studying lung volumes, airway resistance, and pressures in the small pockets in the lungs where gas exchange occurs. The patient sits or reclines in an airtight compartment and breathes normally. The pressure changes in the small pockets in the lungs cause equal pressure changes in the compartment, which are recorded automatically.

body position, posture of the body. Some kinds of body position are **anatomic position, decubitus, Fowler's position, prone, supine, Trendelenburg position.**

body righting reflex, any one of the nerve and muscle responses to restore the body to its normal upright position when it has been displaced. The righting reflexes involve complex mechanisms linked to the structures of the internal ear. Also involved in the righting mechanism are the many nerves to the inner ear, to muscles and tendons, and to the eyes. Interruption of the nerve signals linked to body-righting reflexes may disturb the sense of balance and cause nausea and vomiting.

body-scheme disorder. See **autotopagnosia.**

body stalk, the long part of the embryo that is connected to the membranes (amniotic sac). The stalk becomes part of the umbilical cord.

body systems model, a model for studying illness in relation to the systems of the body, as the circulation, nervous, stomach and bowel, and reproductive systems. The body systems model focuses on the disease rather than on the patient.

body temperature, the level of heat made by the body. Variations in body temperature are major signs of disease and other defects. Heat is created in the body through processing (metabolism) of food. Heat is lost from the body surface through radiation, convection, and evaporation of sweat. Heat production and loss are regulated by the hypothalamus and brain stem. Fever is usually caused by increased heat production. However, some abnormal conditions, as congestive heart failure, cause slight fevers because the heat-loss function is damaged. Diseases of the hypothalamus may cause below-normal body temperatures. Normal adult body temperature, as measured by mouth, is 98.6° F. Mouth temperatures ranging from 96.5° F to 99° F are consistent with good health, depending on the physical activity and the normal body temperature for that person. When the temperature is taken under the armpit, it is usually 1° F lower than the mouth temperature. Rectal temperatures may be 0.5° to 1.0° F higher than mouth readings. Body temperature appears to vary 1° to 2° F throughout the day, with lows recorded early in the morning and peaks between 6 PM and 10 PM.

body type, the general physical appearance of an individual human body. Three common body types are the thin, fragile body (ectomorph); the round, soft body (endomorph); and the muscular, athletic body of average size (mesomorph).

Boeck's sarcoid. See **sarcoidosis.**

Boerhaave's syndrome, a condition in which the canal leading from the mouth to the stomach (esophagus) breaks or tears on its own without warning, leading to swelling between the lungs and fluid filling the lungs. Emergency care is needed, with surgery and drainage, to save the patient's life.

Bohr effect, the effect of carbon dioxide (CO_2) and hydrogen ions (H^+) on the ability of hemoglobin molecules in red blood cells to bind to oxygen (O_2). Increasing the partial pressure of CO_2 and H^+ decreases the oxygen saturation of the hemoglobin, whereas decreasing concentrations have the opposite effect. The Bohr effect is particularly significant in the capillaries of working muscles, the inner muscle layer of the heart, and in the exchange vessels in the placenta between the mother and fetus.

boil. See **furuncle.**

boiling point, the temperature at which a substance passes from a liquid to a gas at a particular air pressure. For example, water boils at 212° F at sea level, but on Mt. McKinley in Alaska, water boils at about 175° F because the elevation is 20,320 feet and the air pressure is lower. See also **evaporation.**

-bol, a combining form indicating a steriod (anabolic) taken from the male hormone (testosterone).

Bolivian hemorrhagic fever, an infectious disease caused by a type of virus (arenavirus). It is generally carried from infected rodents to humans through food infected by rodent urine, though direct carrying between people has also been observed. About 1 to 2 weeks after exposure, the patient develops chills, fever, headache, muscle ache, loss of appetite, nausea, and vomiting. As the disease continues, low blood pressure, dehydration, slowed heart beat, lung problems, and internal bleeding may occur. Also called **Machupo.** See also **arenavirus, Argentine hemorrhagic fever, Lassa fever.**

bolus, **1.** also called **alimentary bolus.** a chewed, round lump of food ready to be swallowed. **2.** a large round mass of a drug for swallowing that is usually soft and not prepackaged. **3.** a dose of a drug or a drug injected all at once into the vein.

Bombay phenotype, a rare genetic trait involving the ABO blood groups. "Phenotype" is the genetic and individual trait of a person, as opposed to "genotype," which is the genetic trait only. The gene for the H antigen is recessive in persons with this trait so the A, B, and H antigens are suppressed. Cells of such people are phenotypically blood type O, even though genetically they are type AB. In such cases two Bombay phenotype parents may have children with blood type AB. The trait is named for the city in which it was first reported. See also **ABO blood groups.**

bonding, the attachment process that occurs between an infant and the parents, especially the mother. These ties of affection later influence both the physical and mental growth of the child. The process usually begins right after birth. Bonding is often started at birth when the nude infant is placed on the mother's stomach so that both the parents and child can see and touch one another and begin to interact. The newborn is alert for about 30 minutes to 1 hour after birth and cries, sucks, clings, grasps, and follows with the eyes, which in turn begins the parenting instincts. Especially important in starting bonding is eye-to-eye contact, holding the infant, soothing talk, and other behavior that creates emotional ties. Another needed element is the amount of contact that occurs between parents and the newborn, especially crucial with premature and sick infants. New concepts in normal birth procedures, especially the trend toward more natural childbirth, allowing the father to help in the birth, and involving parents in the care of premature and ill newborns help to build stronger parent-infant relationships. Certain behaviors are common for each parent during the early attachment process. Mothers are usually more concerned with touching and holding the infant. Fathers are more intent on eye contact with the child. By about the second to third week of life there is a definite pattern of interacting, involving an attention and nonattention cycle, during each time the parents and child are together. At the peak of the attention phase, the infant reaches out toward the parent and is very attentive. This is followed in a short time by loss of excitement in the infant and turning away from the parent. This nonattentive phase prevents the infant from being overcome by excess stimulation. Knowing these cycles, especially that the nonattention phase is not a form of rejection, helps both the mother and father develop good parenting qualities.

bone, **1.** the dense, hard, and slightly stretchy connective tissue that makes up the 206 bones of the human skeleton. It is made up of dense bone tissue (osseous) surrounding spongy tissue that contains many blood vessels and nerves. Covering the bone is a membrane called the periosteum. Long bones contain yellow marrow in the long spaces and red marrow in the ends near the joints. Red marrow also fills the spaces of the flat and the short bones, the backbones (vertebrae), the skull, the breastbone (sternum), and the ribs. Blood cells are made in active red marrow. **2.** any single element of the skeleton, as a rib, the sternum, or the femur. See also **connective tissue.** (See illustration on p. 108.)

bone cancer, a skeletal cancer occurring as the first tumor in an area of rapid growth or as a spreading tumor from cancer elsewhere in the body. First bone tumors are rare. The risk peaks during adolescence, then decreases, and rises again after 35 years of age. In adults bone

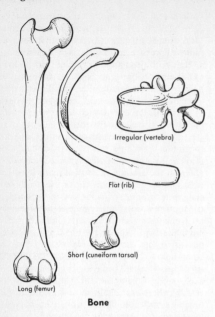

Irregular (vertebra)

Flat (rib)

Short (cuneiform tarsal)

Long (femur)

Bone

cancer is strongly linked to radiation exposure, especially in workers who apply radium paint to watch dials. Paget's disease, overactive parathyroid gland, long-term bone infection (osteomyelitis), areas where the blood supply is cut off, and fracture calluses increase the risk of bone tumors. Most bone cancers are spreading tumors found in the spine, pelvis, or other areas. Bone cancers develop rapidly but are often difficult to detect; pain that increases at night may be the only symptom. The most common bone cancers are osteosarcomas, followed by chrondrosarcomas, fibrosarcomas, and Ewing's sarcoma. Surgical treatment consists of removing slow-growing tumors or cutting off a limb if the tumor is fast-growing. X-ray therapy may be used before surgery. In tumors that are sensitive to radiation, x-ray therapy is sometimes the main treatment. Chemotherapy is often useful in curing Ewing's tumors. The use of interferon and other forms of immune therapy has been experimental.

bone graft, the moving of a piece of bone from one part of the body to another to repair a defect in the skeleton. In some cases animal bone may be transplanted in humans.

bone marrow, specialized, soft tissue filling the spaces in the cancellous part of bone shafts. Fatty, **yellow marrow** is found in the compact bone of most adult long bones, as in the arms and legs. **Red marrow** is found in many bones of infants and children and in the smaller bones, as the sternum, ribs, and backbones of adults. Red blood cells are made in red marrow.

Bonine, a trademark for a drug used to treat nausea from motion sickness (meclizine hydrochloride).

Bonnevie-Ullrich syndrome. See **Turner's syndrome.**

booster injection, giving an antigen, as a vaccine or toxoid, usually in a smaller amount than the original vaccination. A booster is given to keep the immune response at the correct level.

borate, any salt of boric acid.

borax bath, a bath in which borax and glycerin are added to the water.

borborygmus /bôr'bərig'məs/, *pl.* **borborygmi,** a stomach and bowel sound caused by overactive intestine movement (peristalsis). Borborygmi are rumbling, gurgling, and tinkling noises. Although increased intestinal movement may be noted in cases of gastroenteritis and diarrhea, true borborygmi are more intense and periodic. Borborygmi along with vomiting, bloating, and cramps may mean a blockage of the small intestine.

borderline schizophrenia. See **latent schizophrenia.**

Bordetella /bôr'ditel'ə/, a genus of coccobacilli. Some species cause infections of the breathing tract of humans. See also **parapertussis, pertussis.**

boric acid /bôr'ik/, a white, odorless powder or crystal-like substance used as a buffer. At one time boric acid was used as an antiseptic and eye wash.

Bornholm disease. See **epidemic pleurodynia.**

born out of asepsis (BOA), referring to a newborn infant that was not delivered in the usual place in a disinfected birthing unit. A BOA infant may have been born on the way to the hospital, in the hospital, on the way to the delivery room, or in a labor room.

★TREATMENT: The usual steps in caring for a newborn are carried out. The head and chest are measured, weight is taken, the baby is placed in a warmer until the temperature is normal. Vitamin K and silver nitrate are usually given, and a bath is given when the baby is warm. In many hospitals BOA infants are placed in a special nursery, isolated from other infants to prevent contagion should the BOA baby be infected.

★PATIENT CARE: Daily care for the newborn BOA is the same as that given to other newborns, but the baby is also watched for signs of infection. The parents are involved in the care of the infant as soon as is possible, and the usual instructions are given for care of the baby at home after leaving the hospital.

boron (B), a nonmetal element, similar to aluminum. Its atomic number is 5; its atomic weight is 10.8. Boron occurs in the form of dark crystals and as a greenish-yellow shapeless mass. It is the main part of boric acid, which is used mainly as a dusting powder and ointment for minor skin disorders.

Borrelia /bərel′ē-ə/, a genus of coarse, unevenly coiled spirochetes, several species of which cause tickborne and louseborne relapsing fever. Many animals are hosts for *Borrelia.*

boss, a swelling or lump on an organ, as a tumor or overgrowth of a bone surface. For example, on the forehead it is often a sign of rickets.

Boston exanthem, an epidemic disease characterized by a scattered, pale red rash on the face, chest, and back, sometimes with small ulcers on the tonsils and soft palate. The lymph glands usually do not swell, and the rash disappears by itself in 2 or 3 weeks. It is caused by echovirus 16 and needs no treatment. Compare **herpangina.**

bottle feeding, feeding an infant or young child from a bottle with a rubber nipple on the end. It is sometimes called artificial feeding because it is a substitute for or an addition to breast feeding.

★METHOD: The infant is held on one arm close to the person's body. The bottle is held at an angle to make sure that the nipple is always filled with liquid so that the infant does not swallow air while feeding. For a newborn infant, rest periods may be given every several minutes. Once or twice during feeding and again at the end the infant is helped to burp by being held upright on the person's shoulder or on its stomach on the lap. Gentle rubbing or patting on the back and pressure on the stomach often helps the infant to burp. The formula contains protein, fats, carbohydrates, vitamins, and minerals in amounts similar to those in breast milk. The formula may be warmed before feeding by placing the bottle in warm water for several minutes. This is not necessary, however. Smaller infants need larger nipple holes that need less effort. Premature or weak infants may be fed using a special, long soft nipple. Bottle feeding is used as a substitute for breast feeding when the mother is unable or chooses not to breast feed. Bottle feeding can also sometimes be substituted for breast feeding. Bottle feeding is urged if the mother has a contagious disease, a serious long-term disease, or has recently had surgery. Severe breast infection (mastitis), drug addiction, or use of drugs that are released in the breast milk usually means bottle feeding.

bottle-mouth syndrome. See **nursing-bottle caries.**

botulism /boch′əliz′əm/, an often fatal form of food poisoning caused by a poison endotoxin made by the bacillus *Clostridium botulinum.* In rare instances, the toxin may come into the human body through a wound infected by the organism, but the usual source is food. Botu-

lism differs from most other types of food poisoning in that it develops without stomach upset. Symptoms may not occur for 18 hours and up to 1 week after the infected food has been eaten. Botulism is characterized by a period of weakness followed by sight problems, as double vision, difficulty in focusing the eyes, and sensitivity to light. Muscles may become weak, and the patient often develops difficulty in swallowing. Nausea and vomiting occur in less than half of the cases. Hospitalization is necessary, and antitoxins are given. About two-thirds of the cases of botulism are fatal, usually as a result of late diagnosis and lung problems. For those who survive, recovery is slow. Most botulism occurs after eating improperly canned or cooked foods. See also *Clostridium.*

bouba. See **yaws.**

Bouchard's node /booshärz′/, an abnormal swelling of a knuckle. It usually occurs in wasting diseases of the joints, as osteoarthritis. Compare **Heberden node.**

bougie /boo′zhē, boozhē′/, a thin cylinder made of rubber, waxed silk, or other flexible material. It is put into canals of the body to widen, examine, or measure them.

boulimia. See **bulimia.**

boundary, (in psychology) an aspect of family health in which the generations are clearly defined and issues dealt with by the appropriate generation. There are also limits between the family "turf" and the larger society.

boundary lubrication, a thin layer of molecules coating each weight-bearing surface of a joint to allow a sliding action by opposing bone surfaces.

boundary maintenance mechanisms, (in psychology) behavior and practices that keep out members of some groups from the customs and values of another group.

bound carbon dioxide, carbon dioxide that passes in the bloodstream as part of a sodium bicarbonate molecule rather than as dissolved carbon dioxide or as a bicarbonate ion.

bounding pulse, a pulse that feels full and springlike when touched. A bounding pulse occurs because of increased force of the heart contraction or an increased amount of blood in the veins.

bouquet fever. See **dengue fever.**

Bourdon regulator, an adjustable device with an attached pressure gauge for controlling and measuring the contents of cylinders of oxygen and other medical gases.

boutonneuse fever /boo′tənooz′/, an infectious disease caused by *Rickettsia conorii,* which is carried to humans through the bite of a tick. The disease begins with a sore called a black spot (tache noire) at the site of the bite. A fever lasting from a few days to 2 weeks and a red rash that spreads over the body, including the palms and soles, develop. It is common in parts of Europe, Asia, Africa, and the Middle East. See also **rickettsiosis, Rocky Mountain spotted fever.**

boutonneire deformity /boo̅'tônyer'/, an abnormality of a finger marked by the fixed bending of the inner joint and the fixed straightening of the outermost joint.

Bowditch's law. See **all-or-none law.**

bowel. See **intestine.**

bowel elimination, alteration in: constipation, a condition resulting from too little food and bulk, too little physical activity, a side effect of drugs, overuse of laxatives and enemas, stomach and bowel blockage, nerve or muscle damage, weak intestinal muscles, pain on defecation, diagnostic tests, lack of privacy, pregnancy, or emotional problems. Constipation is defined as reduced times of defecation; a hard, formed stool; straining at stool; reduced bowel sounds; a feeling of stomach or rectal fullness or pressure; and nausea. Stomach and bowel pain, loss of appetite, back pain, and headache may also occur.

bowel elimination, alteration in: diarrhea, a condition caused by stress and anxiety; diet; the side effects of drugs; swelling, irritation, or faulty absorption of the bowel; or the effects of poison, infectious waste material, or radiation. The symptoms include stomach and bowel pain, cramping, increased times of defecation, increased bowel sounds, loose or liquid stools, increased need to defecate, and often a change in the color of the feces.

bowel elimination, alteration in: incontinence, a condition caused by nerve or muscle damage; depression, severe anxiety, or mental damage; life changes; not enough relaxation; little or no exercise; poor diet; work-related tensions; unmet expectations; or lacking support systems or coping methods. The symptom is the undesired passage of stool.

bowel training, a method of creating regular bowel movements by reflex conditioning. It is used to treat undesired defecation, constipation, long-term diarrhea, and patients with spinal cord injuries who develop a condition called autonomic hyperreflexia. In patients with autonomic hyperreflexia, bloating of the rectum and bladder causes high blood pressure, restlessness, chills, sweating, headache, fever, and slow heart beat.

★METHOD: The person is taught exercises to strengthen the stomach and bowel muscles, as pushing up, bearing down, and contracting the muscles. The patient is taught to note and respond promptly to signs of a full bowel, as goose pimples and sweating. The urge to defecate can be stimulated by drinking coffee, massaging the stomach, pressing the inner thigh, or stroking the anus. About 3 quarts of fluids should be drunk every day, and prune juice, orange juice, and coffee should be included.

Well-balanced meals that contain bulk and roughage are important, and constipating foods, as bananas, beans, and cabbage, are avoided. The training program may involve drinking 4 to 10 ounces of prune juice each night or 12 hours before the time set for a bowel movement. Drinking warm water, coffee, or milk 30 minutes before the set time also helps. An oiled glycerine pill may also be inserted just before the set time. No formed stools for 3 days, semiliquid feces, restlessness, and discomfort are signs of a possible severe constipation (impaction), and the condition may be treated with a laxative or with a tap water or oily enema. Patients with spinal cord injuries need to understand the importance of reporting symptoms of autonomic hyperreflexia to the physician. Emotional stress or illness may cause accidental bowel movements after the program is begun. Young persons with spinal cord injuries are able to establish a good pattern of defecation when well trained, but some elderly people may not be able to learn the program.

Bowen's disease. See **intraepidermal carcinoma.**

bowleg. See **genu varum.**

Bowman's capsule /bō'mənz/, the cup-shaped end of a renal tubule containing a glomerulus. The renal tubule is part of the filtering system in the kidneys. Also called **glomerular capsule.**

bowtie filter, (in radiology) a special bowtie-shaped filter that may be used with computerized x-ray (computed tomography) procedures to compensate for the shape of the patient's head or body. It is used with fan-shaped x-ray beams to equalize the amount of radiation reaching the film.

box bath. See **cabinet bath.**

boxer's fracture, a break of one or more of the bones in the hands (metacarpals). It usually involves the base of the fourth or fifth finger and is caused by punching a hard object.

Boyle's law, a physics law stating that the product of the volume and pressure of a gas pressed at a constant temperature remains constant.

BP, abbreviation for **blood pressure.**

BPDE-I, abbreviation for benzo(a)pyrene dihydrodoil epoxide.

Br, symbol for **bromine.**

brace, a device, sometimes jointed, to support and hold any movable part of the body in the correct position. It allows that part of the body to function, as a leg brace that permits walking and standing. Compare **splint.**

brachial /brā'kē-əl/, referring to the arm.

brachial artery, the main artery of the upper arm. It ends just below the inside bend of the elbow where it branches into the radial artery and the ulnar artery.

brachialis /brā'kē-al'is/, a muscle of the upper arm that extends from the shoulder to below the inside of the elbow. It lies under the biceps and flexes the forearm. Compare **biceps brachii, triceps brachii.**

brachial plexus, a group of nerves that branch from the upper spine and neck. The brachial plexus supplies the muscles and skin of the chest, shoulders, and arms.

brachial plexus anesthesia, an anesthetic block of the region supplied by the brachial plexus nerves. See also **regional anesthesia.**

brachial plexus paralysis. See **Erb's palsy.**

brachial pulse, the pulse of the brachial artery, felt in the space in front of the elbow.

brachiocephalic, relating to the arm and head.

brachiocephalic arteritis. See **Takayasu's arteritis.**

brachiocephalic trunk. See **innominate artery.**

brachiocephalic vein. See **innominate vein.**

brachioradialis /brā′kē·ôrā′dē·al′is/, the muscle just under the skin on the thumb (radial) side of the forearm. It flexes the forearm.

brachioradialis reflex, a reflex caused by striking the side of the forearm near the head of the radius. It is characterized by normal, slight elbow flexion and forearm rotation outward. See also **deep tendon reflex.**

brachy-, a combining form meaning 'short.'

brachycephaly /brak′isef′əlē/, a birth defect of the skull in which premature closing of the soft spot (coronal suture) results in excess growth of the head from side to side, giving it a short, broad appearance. Also called **brachycephalia, brachycephalism.** See also **craniostenosis.** –**brachycephalic, brachycephalous,** *adj.*

brachydactyly /brak′idak′təlē/, a condition of abnormally short fingers or toes.

brachytherapy, the use of radioactive materials in the treatment of cancer tumors by placing the radioactive sources in direct contact with the tissues to be treated.

Bradford frame, a rectangular frame made of pipes to which heavy movable straps of canvas are attached, running from side to side to support a patient lying on the back or the face. The straps can be removed to permit the patient to urinate or defecate while remaining rigid.

Bradford solid frame, a rectangular device of metal covered with canvas to aid in keeping patients rigid, especially children in traction. The Bradford solid frame supports the entire body and is used mostly for patients who are under 5 years of age, overactive, or mentally retarded. The main purpose of the device is to keep the patient rigid.

Bradford split frame, a rectangular device of metal covered with two separate pieces of canvas fastened at both ends of the frame. Used to keep children rigid in traction, it is divided in the middle by a large opening for defecation.

Bradley method, a method of preparing for childbirth developed by Robert Bradley, M.D.

It includes education about the physical nature of childbirth, exercise and diet during pregnancy, and ways of breathing for control and comfort during labor and birth. The father is involved in the classes and is the mother's "coach" during labor. During the early stage of labor, the woman is told to carry on her normal activities until she feels the need to focus on the contractions. During the active phase of labor, the cervix widens from about 5 cm to 10 cm (2 to 4 inches), the contractions occur every 1½ to 3 minutes and last from 40 to 90 seconds, the time between contractions tends to lessen, and the length and intensity of the contractions tend to increase. The father helps the mother by repeating reminders to relax many parts of her body, by massaging and touching her, and by arranging and rearranging pillows to support her in a "lounge chair" position. During contractions, she breathes deeply and slowly—in through the nose and out through the mouth. Her stomach lifts with each breath in and falls with each breath out. She may close her eyes and try to imagine the baby's head pressing against the cervix, causing it to widen. She is helped by the close support of the father, the midwife or obstetrician, and the nurse. When the cervix is fully widened, the contractions are strong, occurring every 1½ to 2 minutes and lasting 60 to 90 seconds. The mother, feeling the urge to bear down and push, allows her knees to fall away from each other. She breathes in and out deeply once or twice, waiting for the contraction to build in strength, then she bears down while holding her breath. She pushes as hard as necessary for 10 or 15 seconds to relieve the pressure of the contraction. The father may count seconds for her. He also checks to see that her legs and buttocks are relaxed, and he reminds her to keep her bottom relaxed, to concentrate, and to "let the baby out." As the baby is born, with the mother still in a semisitting position, the infant is placed on her stomach and then nursed as soon as it wants. The mother is given a glass of orange juice and often walks back to her room with the father and the baby. Among the advantages of the method are its simplicity, the help of the father, and the realistic approach to the efforts and discomfort of labor. Also called **husband-coached childbirth.** Compare **Lamaze method, Read method.**

brady-, a combining form meaning 'slow, dull.'

bradycardia /brad′ikär′dē·ə/, an abnormal condition in which the heart contracts steadily but at a rate of less than 60 beats a minute. The heart normally slows during sleep, and, in some physically fit people, the pulse may be quite slow. Bradycardia may be a symptom of a brain tumor, digitalis overdose, or an abnormal response of the vagus nerve (vagotonia). The blood circulating is reduced, causing faintness, dizziness, chest pain, and, eventually fainting and collapse of the circulation. Treatment may include giving atropine, implanting a pacemaker, or reducing the digitalis dose.

bradycardia-tachycardia syndrome, a heart disorder characterized by a heart rate that shifts from very slow to very fast rhythms.

bradykinesia /brad'ikinē'zhə, -kīnē'zhə/, an abnormal condition characterized by slowness of all voluntary movement and speech. This may be caused by parkinsonism, other nerve disorders, and certain tranquilizers.

bradykinin, a chemical made by the body that widens the blood vessels.

bradypnea /brad'ipnē'ə/, an abnormally slow rate of breathing.

Bragg curve, in radiation therapy, the path followed by ionizing particles. Because certain particles reach a peak of potential near the end of their path, the Bragg curve can be used to move the radiation so it reaches deep tumors while passing over normal tissues.

Braille /brāl, brä'y/, a system of printing for the blind. It is made up of patterns of raised dots or points that can be read by touch.

brain, the portion of the brain and spinal cord (central nervous system) contained within the skull. It is made up of the cerebrum, cerebellum, pons, medulla, and midbrain. Special cells in its mass of complex, soft, gray or white tissue bring together and control the functions of the central nervous system.

brain concussion, a violent jarring or shaking injury to the brain. Characteristically, after a mild concussion there may be a brief loss of consciousness followed, on awakening, by a headache. Sometimes no loss of consciousness occurs. Severe concussion may cause lengthy unconsciousness and disruption of certain vital functions of the brain stem, as breathing. The treatment for a patient recovering from a concussion is mainly watching for signs of bleeding. Because concussions can be fatal, medical attention should be sought if any of the following symptoms develops even 4 weeks after a head injury: unequally widened pupils, severe headache, confusion, loss of memory, continual drowsiness, personality changes, speech difficulties, paralysis, or loss of coordination. Also called **concussion.**

brain death, an irreversible form of unconsciousness characterized by a complete loss of brain function while the heart continues to beat. The legal definition of this condition varies from state to state. The usual medical definition of brain death includes the lack of reflexes, movements, and breathing. The pupils are widened and fixed. Because cold exposure (hypothermia), anesthesia, poisoning, or drug overdose may cause a state that resembles brain death, a diagnosis of brain death requires that the electric activity of the brain is proved to be absent.

This is proven by doing two brain tests (electroencephalograms) 12 to 24 hours apart. Also called **irreversible coma.** Compare **coma, sleep, stupor.**

brain edema. See **cerebral edema.**

brain electric activity map (BEAM), a map of the brain created by a computer that is able to respond to the brain's electric signals by a flash of light. If the wave is disordered, blocked, too small, or too large, there may be a tumor or other problem causing the abnormal pattern.

brain fever, *informal.* any swelling of the brain or lining of the brain (meninges). See also **encephalitis.**

brain scan, a painless diagnostic test using radioisotope imaging tests to identify injury, tumors, or areas where the blood supply is blocked. Radioisotopes are injected into a vein, then circulate to the brain where they gather in abnormal tissue. The radioisotopes are traced and photographed by a scanner (scintillator), and the size and location of the abnormality are found. Compare **CAT scan.** See also **isotope, radioisotope.**

brainstem, the part of the brain that includes the medulla oblongata, the pons, and the mesencephalon. It has motor, sense and reflex functions and contains the spinal tracts. The 12 pairs of nerves from the brain to the rest of the body branch off the brain stem. Compare **medulla oblongata, mesencephalon, pons.**

brain syndrome, a group of symptoms resulting from impaired function of the brain. It may be sudden and reversible or continuous and irreversible.

brain tumor, a tumor of the brain that usually does not spread beyond the brain and spinal cord. Brain tumors cause high rates of illness and death, but many are successfully treated. Brain tumors in children are usually the result of a defect during fetal growth. In adults 20% to 40% of cancers in the brain are spread from cancers in the breast, lung, stomach, intestines, kidney, or any site of a cancerous skin tumor. The cause of first brain tumors is not known, but the risk is greater for people exposed to vinyl chloride, for the brothers and sisters of cancer patients, and for patients with kidney transplants who are treated with immune supressing drugs. Symptoms of a brain tumor include headache, nausea, vomiting, swelling of the optic disk in the eye, weakness, and confusion. Many other signs also occur, as loss of sight in the eye on the side of a skull tumor. A variety of tumors may be found in the brain, but gliomas, mainly astrocytomas, are the most common cancers. Rapidly growing medulloblastomas often occur in children. Benign meningiomas are the only brain tumors more common in women than in men. Craniopharyngiomas, generally found in children and young adults, are harmless but press against important structures and are hard to get rid of. Schwannomas most often come from the eighth cranial nerve and cause deafness, but they are generally noncancerous. Surgery is the beginning treatment for most first tumors of the brain. X-ray treatment is given for tumors that cannot be operated on, medulloblastomas, tumors with many locations, and after surgery. The blood-brain barrier prevents many anticancer drugs from being effective for brain tumors.

bran bath, a bath in which bran has been boiled in the water. Bran baths are used to relieve skin irritation.

branched chain ketoaciduria. See **maple syrup urine disease.**

branchial /brang'kē·əl/, referring to the body structures of the neck and throat area, particularly the muscles.

branchial fistula, an inborn, abnormal passage from the throat to the outside surface of the neck. Also called **cervical fistula.**

brand name. See **trademark.**

brassfounder's ague. See **metal fume fever.**

brassy eye. See **chalkitis.**

Braun's canal. See **neurenteric canal.**

Braxton Hicks contraction /brak'stənhiks'/, irregular tightening of the pregnant uterus that begins during the first 3 months of pregnancy. They increase in time, length, and strength as pregnancy continues. Near the end of pregnancy, strong Braxton Hicks contractions are often hard to tell apart from the contractions of true labor. Also called **Braxton Hicks sign, false labor.**

Braxton Hicks version, one of several types of maneuvers sometimes used to turn the fetus from an undesirable position to one that promotes delivery. See also **version.**

Brazelton assessment, a system for assessing the behavior of newborns with a series of 27 reaction tests. The tests assess response to solid objects, to a pinprick, to light, and to the sound of a rattle or bell.

Brazilian trypanosomiasis. See **Chagas' disease.**

breakbone fever. See **dengue fever.**

break test, a test of a patient's muscle strength. After the patient has reached the end of a range of motion, resistance is applied in a direction opposite to the line of pull of the muscle or muscle group being tested. The resistance is released immediately if there is sign of pain or discomfort.

breakthrough bleeding, the escape of blood from the uterus between menstrual periods. This is a side effect of some women who use birth-control pills.

breast, 1. the front part of the surface of the chest. **2.** a mammary gland.

breast cancer, a cancerous tumor of breast tissue, the most common cancer in women in the United States. The rate increases between 30 to 50 years of age and reaches a second peak at 65 years of age. Risk factors include a family history of breast cancer, no children, exposure to radiation, young age when menstruation began, late menopause, being overweight, diabetes, high blood pressure, long-term cystic disease of the breast, and, possibly, hormone therapy after menopause. Women who are over 40 years of age when they bear their first child and patients with cancer in other areas also have a greater risk of getting breast cancer. Beginning symptoms, found in most cases by self-examination, include a small painless lump, thick or dimpled skin, or nipple withdrawal. As the tumor grows there may be a nipple discharge, pain, ulcers, and swollen lymph glands under the arms. The diagnosis is made by a careful physical examination, a breast scan (mammography), and examination of tumor cells. Tumors are more common in the left than in the right breast and in the upper and outer parts of the breast. Spreading through the lymph system to lymph nodes under the arm (axillary) and to bone, lung, brain, and liver is common. Surgical treatment, depending on the tumor, may be a radical, modified radical, or simple removal of the breast (mastectomy), with the removal of axillary nodes. X-ray therapy, chemotherapy, or both are usually given after surgery. If estrogen receptors are found in breast tumors, the ovaries, adrenal glands, or the pituitary gland are removed. Androgen or antiestrogen drugs may be given to reduce the amount of estrogen made by the patient and prevent the return of the cancer. Creating an artificial breast following mastectomy is becoming more common, but it is painful at first and is not approved by all physicians. Breast cancer seldom occurs in men, but those with Klinefelter's syndrome are at 60 times greater risk. See also **lumpectomy, mastectomy, scirrhous carcinoma.**

breast examination, a process in which the breasts and the surrounding structures are assessed for changes that could indicate cancer. See also **breast self-examination.**

★METHOD: The breasts are examined with the patient sitting with her arms at her sides, sitting with her arms over her head, back straight, then leaning forward, and, finally, sitting upright while contracting the pectoral muscles. The breasts are checked for identical shape and size and for surface changes, including moles or colored areas, dimpling, swelling, nipple withdrawal, unusual vein patterns showing through the skin, lumps, sores, or abnormal hair growth. The lymph nodes under the arms and around the collarbones are checked for swelling. With the patient lying on her back, each breast is shifted, and the gland area in each is felt with the flat of the fingers in circles working from the outer edges toward the nipples. The areolar areas, the nipples, and the area extending toward the armpit are then felt. Many women find it helpful to check their breasts every time they shower for the first few months after being taught how to do it to become very familiar with their own breasts.

★OUTCOME: Early diagnosis greatly improves the rate of cure in cancer of the breast. The breast examination done thoroughly is a valuable means of finding women who need further examination by tests, as xeroradiography, mammography, biopsy, or thermoradiography.

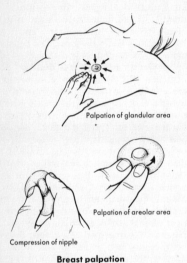

Palpation of glandular area

Palpation of areolar area

Compression of nipple

Breast palpation

breast feeding, 1. suckling or nursing, giving a baby milk from the breast. Breast feeding causes the uterus to return to its nonpregnant size. 2. taking milk from the breast. See also **breast milk, lactation.**

breast milk, human milk, the ideal food for most babies. It is easily digested, clean and warm, passes some immunities from the mother (bronchiolitis and gastroenteritis are rare in breast-fed babies), and helps the emotional bonding between mother and baby. Infants fed breast milk are less likely to become overweight or to develop a poor bite. See also **breast feeding.**

breast milk jaundice, liver disease (jaundice) and excessive bile coloring (bilirubin) in breast fed infants that occur in the first weeks of life. It is caused by a substance in the mother's milk that makes the infant unable to process and release bilirubin. The infant seems normal and healthy but the skin, the whites of the eyes, and the blood are jaundiced. If blood bilirubin is too high, breast feeding may be stopped until there is a decrease to the normal levels, usually a period of 1 to 3 days. During this

time, the infant is bottle-fed with an additional formula, and the mother uses a breast pump or empties the milk by hand.

breast pump, a device for taking milk from the breast.

breast self-examination (BSE), a method in which a woman examines her breasts and the surrounding areas for signs of change that could mean cancer. The BSE is usually done 1 week to 10 days after the first day of the menstrual cycle, when the breasts are smallest and swelling is least visible. Self-examination should be done during all phases of a woman's adult life. A woman who regularly and carefully does the examination is better able to detect small abnormalities than is a woman who is not familiar with her own breasts. The methods are similar to those of the examination of the breast done in a routine physical examination. Also called **self-breast examination.** See also **breast examination.**

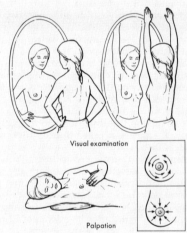

Visual examination

Palpation

Breast self-examination

breast shadows, images on chest x-rays of women. The images are caused by breast tissue but do not indicate abnormal tissue growth. The shadows enhance the underlying tissue and may cause the appearance of a disease occurring between the tissues. Breast nipples may also appear on the x-ray as coin-shaped wounds ("coin lesions"), requiring a second x-ray to be made with special markers to the nipples so the two films can be compared.

breast translumination, a method of examining the inner structures of the breast by directing light through the outer wall. See also **diaphanography.**

breath-holding, a form of voluntary stoppage of breathing that is usually, but not necessarily performed with the flap over the windpipe closed. Although breath-holding may be prolonged for several minutes, it is stopped by an involuntary break point.

breathing. See **respiration.**

breathing cycle, a cycle consisting of inhaling followed by the exhaling of a volume of gas called the tidal volume. The breathing cycle consists of inhaling once and exhaling once.

breathing frequency (f), the number of breathing cycles per a given unit of time.

breathing nomogram, a chart of scales including data for body weight, breathing frequency, and predicted volume of exhaled air, all arranged in a pattern. It allows calculation of an unknown value on one scale by drawing a line that connects known values to the two other scales.

breathing tube, a device put into the windpipe (trachea) through the mouth or nose to create an open airway for good breathing during breathing assistance. See also **extubation, intubation.**

breathing work, the energy required for breathing movements. It is a cumulative product of immediate pressure developed by the respiratory muscles and the volume of air moved during the breathing cycle.

breathlessness. See **dyspnea.**

breath odor, an odor usually produced by substances or diseases in the lungs or mouth. Certain specific odors are linked with some diseases, such as diabetes, liver failure, urea in the blood, or a pus-filled, swelled cavity in the lung. In the absence of burping, breath odors usually do not begin in the digestive tract because the throat is normally closed.

breath sound, the sound of air passing in and out of the breathing system as heard with a stethoscope. Decreased breath sounds may mean a blocked airway, collapsed lung, a lung disease (emphysema), or other long-term blocking lung disease.

breech birth, birth in which the baby comes out feet, knees, or buttocks first. Breech birth is often dangerous. The body may come out easily but the head may become trapped by an incompletely widened cervix because babies' heads are usually larger in diameter than their bodies. See also **assisted breech, breech presentation, complete breech, footling breech, frank breech, version and extraction.**

breech extraction, a birth method in which a baby being born feet or buttocks first is grabbed before any part of the trunk is born and delivered by guiding and pulling. Compare **assisted breech.**

breech presentation, a position of the fetus in which the buttocks or feet are down, rather than the head. It occurs in about 3% of births.

bregma /breg'mə/, the joining of the frontal and roof (parietal) bones on the top of the skull. **–bregmatic,** *adj.*

Brenner tumor, a noncancerous tumor of the ovary that is made up of skin (epithelial) cells covered by fiberlike connective tissue.

Brethine, a trademark for a bronchodilator drug used to treat asthma, bronchitis, and emphysema (terbutaline sulfate).

bretylium tosylate /britil'ē·əm/, a drug used to treat life-threatening irregular heart beats (ventricular arrhythmias).

★CAUTION: Known allergy to this drug prohibits its use.

★ADVERSE EFFECTS: Among the more serious side effects are low blood pressure, nausea and vomiting, chest pain (angina), and nasal stuffiness.

Bretylol, a trademark for a drug used to treat severe heart beat irregularities (bretylium tosylate).

Brevital Sodium, a trademark for a barbiturate used for anesthesia (methohexital sodium).

brewer's yeast, a preparation containing the dried cells of a yeast, used as a diet additive. It is one of the best sources of the B complex vitamins and of many minerals and amino acids.

Bricanyl, a trademark for a bronchodilator drug used to treat asthma, bronchitis, and emphysema (terbutaline sulfate).

brick dust urine, a sign of solid (precipitated) salts of uric acid in a sample of acidic urine used for testing.

bridge of Varolius. See **pons.**

bridgework, a partial denture. It may be held by clasps and be removable. It may also be fixed permanently by crowns, inlays, or other types of retainers attached to natural teeth.

bridging, positioning a patient so that bony areas of the body are free of pressure on the mattress by using pads, bolsters, or pillows.

brief psychotherapy, treatment that usually focuses on a specific problem and is limited to a specified number of sessions with the therapist. It is aimed at solving personality or behavior problems rather than trying to analyze the unconscious.

brief reactive psychosis, a short episode, usually less than 2 weeks, of abnormal behavior caused by a mental disorder (psychosis) that occurs in response to a significant psychosocial stressor.

Bright's disease, an obsolete term for a kidney disease, especially glomerulonephritis.

Brill-Symmers disease. See **giant follicular lymphoma.**

Brill-Zinsser disease /bril'zin'sər/, a mild form of typhus that returns in a patient who appears to have completely recovered from a severe case of the disease. Some rickettsiae remain in the body after the symptoms of the disease are gone, causing the symptoms to return.

brim, the edge of the upper pact on the inside of the pelvis (pelvic inlet). See also **pelvis.**

Brinnell hardness test, a means of finding out surface hardness of a material. The test is used to measure this quality in many materials used in dental treatments, as fillings, cements, and porcelains.

Briquet's syndrome. See **somatization disorder.**

Brissaud's dwarf /brisōz'/, a person affected with a dry swelling (myxedema) in infancy in which short height is linked to an underactive thyroid.

British antilewisite. See **dimercaprol.**

British Medical Association (BMA), a professional organization of physicians in the United Kingdom.

British Pharmacopoeia (BP), the official British reference work setting forth standards of strength and purity of drugs. It contains directions for making them to ensure that the same prescription written by different doctors and filled by different pharmacists will contain exactly the same ingredients in the same amounts. See also *United States Pharmacopeia (USP).*

brittle bones. See **osteogenesis imperfecta.**

brittle diabetes. See **insulin-independent diabetes mellitus.**

broad beta disease, a hereditary type of hyperlipoproteinemia in which a lipoprotein, high in cholesterol and triglycerides, gathers in the blood. The condition is characterized by yellowish nodules (xanthomas) on the elbows and knees, disease of the blood vessels, and high blood cholesterol levels. Patients with this disease are at risk of having early heart disease. See also **hyperlipidemia, hyperlipoproteinemia.**

broad ligament, a folded sheet of membrane in the abdomen (peritoneum) that is draped over the uterine tubes, the uterus, and the ovaries.

broach, a long, tapering dental instrument used for shaping and enlarging holes, particularly in removing pulp or cleaning out a root canal.

broad-spectrum antibiotic, a drug that kills and prevents the growth of a range of infectious tiny organisms.

Broca's area /brō'kəz/, the part of the brain that is involved in speech making. It is located on the front part of the brain. See also **aphasia.**

Brodie's abscess, a type of bone infection (osteomyelitis) caused by a staphylococcal infection. It usually occurs near a joint in the growth zone (metaphysis) of a long bone of a child. Also called **circumscribed abscess of bone.** See also **osteomyelitis.**

Brodmann's areas /brod'manz, brōt'monz/, the many local areas of the brain. They are linked to specific brain functions. Compare **motor area.** See also **cerebral cortex.**

brom-, bromo-, a combining form meaning 'odor, stench.'

bromhidrosis /brō'midrō'sis/, an abnormal condition in which the sweat has an unpleasant odor. The odor is usually caused by the breakdown of sweat by bacteria on the skin.

bromide /brō'mīd/, a bromine compound, especially a salt of hydrobromic acid. Bromides, once widely used as sleeping pills, are now seldom used for that purpose because they may cause serious side effects.

bromine (Br), a toxic, red-brown, liquid element of the halogen group. Its atomic number is 35; its atomic weight is 79.909. Bromine is used in photography, in making chemicals and fuels, and in drugs. Bromides are compounds of bromine that are still used in some over-the-counter drugs. Long-term use of these products may cause a toxic condition (brominism) characterized by acne, headache, loss of sexual interest, drowsiness, and weakness. See also **bromide.**

bromocriptine mesylate, a drug used to treat female infertility, Parkinson's disease, and the making of too much of the hormone prolactin. ★CAUTION: Allergy to any ergot alkaloid prohibits its use.
★ADVERSE EFFECTS: Among the more severe side effects are irregular heart rate, low blood pressure, slow heart beat, hallucinations, fainting, nausea, walking difficulty, shortness of breath, swallowing difficulty, weakness, and confusion.

bromoderma /brō'mōdur'mə/, an acnelike or nodelike skin rash. It is caused by an allergic reaction to bromides.

brompheniramine maleate /brom'fənir'əmin/, an antihistamine used to treat many allergic reactions, including nasal congestion, skin reactions, and itching.

Brompton's cocktail, a painkiller containing alcohol, morphine or heroin, cocaine, and, in some cases, a phenothiazine drug. Mixtures vary, and recently cocaine has been dropped from the mixture. The cocktail is given to help control pain in the fatally ill patient.

Bromsulphalein (BSP) test /bromsul'falin/, a trademark for a dye (sulfobromophthalein) made for use in a test that measures the ability of liver cells to remove the dye from the blood. Forty-five minutes after injection into a vein, more than 95% of the dye is cleared from the blood.

bronch-, a combining form referring to the bronchus of the lung.

bronchial asthma. See **asthma.**

bronchial breath sound, an abnormal sound heard with a stethoscope over the lungs, caused by pneumonia or pressure. Breathing in and breathing out cause loud, high-pitched sounds of equal length.

bronchial collateral flow, a network of connected capillaries in the lung tissue. In certain disease states in which there is a blockage in the artery carrying blood from the heart to the lungs, the collateral vessels may enlarge and provide a significant volume of blood to the small pouches in the lung where gas exchange occurs.

bronchial fremitus, a vibration that can be felt or heard on the chest over a bronchus clogged by fluids. It is caused by mucus rattling as the air passes during breathing.

bronchial hyperreactivity, an abnormal breathing condition characterized by spasm of the bronchus. It is a reflex response to histamine or a cholinergic drug. This is a feature of asthma and is used to tell the difference between asthma and heart disease.

bronchial secretion, a substance produced in the air passages of the lungs that consists of mucus secreted by the goblet cells and mucous glands of the air passages of the lungs, protein salts released from decaying cells, plasma fluid, and proteins (including fibrinogen) escaping the capillaries serving the lungs.

bronchial spasm, an excessive and prolonged tightening of the involuntary muscle fibers in the walls of the air passages of the lungs. The tightening may be in one area or throughout the lungs and may be caused by irritation or injury to the mucous tissues, infection, or allergies.

bronchial toilet, special care that is given to patients with a tube inserted through the neck into the windpipe (tracheostomy) and to patients with respiratory disorders, which include stimulation of coughing, deep breathing, and suctioning of the respiratory tract with a special pump.

bronchial tree, a complex of the bronchi and the bronchial tubes. The bronchi branch from the windpipe (trachea), and the bronchial tubes branch from the bronchi. The right bronchus is wider and shorter than the left bronchus. The right bronchus branches into three bronchi, one passing to each of the lobes that make up the right lung. The left bronchus is smaller in diameter but about twice as long as the right bronchus and branches into the bronchi for the upper and the lower lobes of the left lung.

bronchial venous drainage, a pattern of blood flow from the air passages, generally into the veins leading from the lungs to the heart, which otherwise carry arterial blood. Only a few air-passage veins drain to the venous system through the seven main veins of the chest or veins between the ribs.

bronchiectasis /brong′kē·ek′təsis/, an abnormal condition of the bronchial tree, characterized by irreversible widening and destruction of the bronchial walls. The condition is sometimes a birth defect, but usually it is the result of bronchial infection or of blockage by a tumor or a foreign body. Symptoms of bronchiectasis include a constant cough with excess, blood-stained sputum, a long-term sinus infection,

clubbing of the fingers, and continual moist-sounding breathing.

bronchiolar carcinoma. See **alveolar cell carcinoma.**

bronchiolar collapse, a condition in which the smallest air passages, soft-walled tubes without cartilage support, become squeezed by the pressure of surrounding structures and lack enough inhaled air to keep them open. The condition occurs in disorders such as emphysema, cystic disease, and bronchiectasis.

bronchiole /brong′kē·ōl/, a small airway of the breathing system from the bronchi to the lobes of the lung. The bronchioles allow the exchange of air and waste gases between the alveolar ducts and the bronchi. **–bronchiolar,** *adj.*

bronchiolitis /brong′kē·ōli′tis/, a viral infection of the lower breathing tract that occurs mainly in infants under 18 months of age. It causes wheezing, breathing difficulty, swelling, and blockage of the bronchioles. The most common causes are the respiratory syncytial viruses (RSV) and the parainfluenza viruses. *Mycoplasma pneumoniae,* the rhinoviruses, enteroviruses, and measles virus can also cause bronchiolitis.

★DIAGNOSIS: The condition typically begins as an upper breathing-tract infection with watery nasal discharge and, often, mild fever. Rapid breathing and a fast heart rate, cough, wheezing, and fever develop. The chest may appear barrel-shaped, and breathing becomes more shallow.

★TREATMENT: Routine treatment includes humidity and oxygen in a mist tent, vaporizer, or Croupette; giving fluids, usually through a vein; suctioning the airways to remove fluids; and rest. An airway tube is sometimes inserted. Drugs, as antibiotics, bronchodilators, steroids, cough syrups, and sleeping pills, are not used. The infection typically runs its course in 7 to 10 days, with good recovery. A major problem is bacterial infection, most commonly following long-term use of a mist tent.

bronchitis /brongki′tis/, a short-term or long-term swelling of the mucous membranes of the lungs (tracheobronchial tree). **Acute bronchitis** is characterized by a cough that releases sputum, fever, mucus-secreting structures growing larger, and back pain. Caused by the spread of viral infections to the bronchi, the swelling often occurs with childhood infections, as measles, whooping cough, diphtheria, and typhoid fever. Treatment includes bed rest, aspirin, cough drugs, and antibiotics. **Chronic bronchitis** is characterized by an excess release of mucus in the bronchi with a cough that releases sputum for at least 3 months in at least 2 years. Additional symptoms are many lung infections, blue skin from lack of oxygen, less oxygen and more carbon dioxide in the blood, and a risk to develop a heart disease (cor pulmonale) and breathing problems. Factors that may cause chronic bronchitis include cigarette smoking, air pollution, long-term infections, and abnormal growth of the bronchi. See also **chronic obstructive pulmonary disease (COPD), respiratory syncytial virus.**

bronchodilator, a drug that relaxes contractions of the bronchioles to improve breathing. Bronchodilators are given for asthma, bronchiectasis, bronchitis, and emphysema. Commonly used bronchodilators include steroids, ephedrine, isoproterenol hydrochloride, theophylline, and many related combinations of these drugs. The steroids beclomethasone dipropionate and triamcinolone can be used in aerosol form.

bronchofibroscopy. See **fiberoptic bronchoscopy.**

bronchogenic, originating in the air passages of the lungs (bronchi).

bronchogenic carcinoma, a common form of cancerous lung tumor that starts in the bronchi. Usually linked to cigarette smoking, it may cause coughing and wheezing, weakness, chest tightness, and aching joints. In the late stages, symptoms are bloody sputum, clubbing of the fingers, weight loss, and fluid around the lungs. Diagnosis is made by a range of tests. Surgery is the most effective treatment, but about 50% of cases are too far gone and not helped by surgery when first seen. Treatment to decrease the patient's discomfort includes x-ray therapy and chemotherapy.

bronchography /brongkog′rəfē/, an x-ray examination of the bronchi after they have been coated with a radiopaque substance.

bronchomotor tone, the tightness and relaxation of smooth muscle in the air-passage walls. The muscle controls the size of the airways.

bronchophony /brongkof′ənē/, an increase in strength and clearness of the voice, which may result from an increase in the thickness of lung tissue, as in cases of pneumonia when the lungs become firm and do not stretch.

bronchopneumonia, a swelling of the lungs and bronchioles, characterized by chills, fever, fast pulse and breathing, cough with bloody sputum, severe chest pain, and bloated stomach. The disease, usually a result of the spread of bacterial infection from the upper breathing tract to the lower breathing tract, caused by *Mycoplasma pneumoniae, Staphylococcus pyogenes,* or *Streptococcus pneumoniae.* Bronchopneumonia may also occur in viral and rickettsial infections. The most common cause in infants is the respiratory syncytial virus. Treatment includes an antibiotic, oxygen therapy, measures to keep the bronchi clear of fluids, and pain relievers. Compare **aspiration pneumonia, eosinophilic pneumonia, interstitial pneumonia.** See also **lobar pneumonia, respiratory syncytial virus.**

bronchopulmonary, referring to the bronchi and the lungs.

bronchoscope /brong′kəskōp′/, a curved, flexible tube for looking at the bronchi. It contains fibers that carry light down the tube and project a large image up the tube to the viewer.

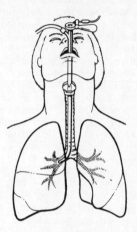

Bronchoscope

bronchoscopy /brongkos′kəpē/, an examination of the bronchial tree, using either the rigid, tubelike metal bronchoscope or the narrower, flexible fiberoptic bronchoscope. Bronchoscopy is done after the patient fasts and is given a relaxing drug. A local anesthesia is given. The test can also be used to suction, to get a tissue or fluid sample for examination, to remove foreign bodies, and to diagnose diseases.

bronchospasm, an abnormal contraction of the bronchi, resulting in narrowing and blockage of the airway. A cough with wheezing is the usual symptom. Bronchospasm is the main characteristic of asthma and bronchitis.

bronchospirometry /brong′kōspīrom′ətrē/, a technique for the study of the movement of air and gas exchange of each lung separately by inserting a tube into the main opening of either the left or the right lung. A single tube containing two smaller ones may be used to take separate samples of gas from both lungs at the same time.

bronchotomogram, an image of the upper lung area, from the windpipe to the lower air passages, produced by computerized x-ray. The procedure is used to find tumors or other causes of blockage of the lungs and windpipe.

bronchovesicular, referring to the air passages and the small pockets in the lungs where oxygen is absorbed into the blood.

bronchus /brong′kəs/, *pl.* **bronchi,** any one of several large air passages in the lungs through which inhaled air and exhaled waste gases pass. Each bronchus has a wall made up of three layers. The outer layer consists of dense fiber strengthened with cartilage. The middle layer is a grouping of smooth muscle. The inner layer is made up of mucous membrane with hairlike structures (cilia).

Bronkephrine, a trademark for a bronchodilator drug injected into the muscle. It is used to treat asthma, emphysema, and bronchitis (ethylnorepinephrine hydrochloride).

Bronkodyl, a trademark for a bronchodilator drug used to treat asthma, bronchitis, and emphysema (theophylline).

Bronkosol, a trademark for a bronchodilator drug used to treat asthma, bronchitis, and emphysema (isoetharine hydrochloride).

broth, **1.** a fluid nutrient mixture, such as a solution of milk sugar and a sulfur salt (thioglycollate), used to support the growth of bacteria for laboratory testing. **2.** a beverage or other fluid made with the juice of meat and water, as chicken bouillon.

brow, the forehead, particularly the eyebrow or ridge above the eye.

brown fat, a type of fat in newborn infants that is rarely found in adults. Brown fat is a unique source of heat energy for the infant because it makes more heat than ordinary fat.

brownian movement, a random movement of tiny particles drifting in a liquid or gas, as the continuing, irregular movement of dust particles in still water. The movement is caused when the molecules of the fluid strike the particles.

Brown-Séquard's treatment. See **organotherapy.**

Brown-Séquard syndrome /broun'säkär'/, a serious nerve disorder resulting from pressure of one side of the spinal cord at about the level of the bottom of the shoulder blades. The syndrome includes spastic paralysis on the injured side of the body, loss of a sense of posture, and loss of the senses of pain and heat on the other side of the body.

brown spider, a poisonous spider, also known as the brown recluse or violin spider, found in both North and South America. The poison from its bite usually creates a blister surrounded by white and red circles. This so-called "bull's eye" appearance is helpful in telling it apart from other spider bites. The wound usually turns into an open sore and sometimes becomes infected. Pain, nausea, fever, and chills are common, but the reaction usually goes away by itself. Steroids are sometimes given, and cleaning and applying antibiotics to the area will prevent infection. Although painful, the bite is not always a danger to adults. However, small children should get medical attention to avoid possible serious reactions.

brow presentation, a situation during birth in which the brow, or forehead, of the baby is the first part of the body to enter the birth canal. Because the size of the baby's head at this angle may be greater than the opening between the mother's hips, a cesarean section may be recommended.

Brucella abortus. See **abortus fever.**

brucellosis /brōō'səlō'sis/, a disease caused by any of several species of the coccobacillus *Brucella.* Brucellosis is most common in rural areas among farmers, veterinarians, meat packers, slaughterhouse workers, and livestock workers. Humans get brucellosis, mainly a disease of livestock, by drinking infected milk or milk products or through a break in the skin. The symptoms are fever, chills, sweating, general tiredness, and weakness. The fever often comes in waves, rising in the evening and lowering during the day, occurring at times separated by periods of no symptoms. Although brucellosis itself is rarely fatal, treatment is important because serious problems, as pneumonia, meningitis, and encephalitis, can develop. Also called **Cyprus fever, Gibraltar fever, Malta fever, Mediterranean fever, rock fever, undulant fever.** See also **abortus fever.**

Brudzinski's sign /brōōdzin'skēz/, an involuntary flexing of the arm, hip, and knee when the neck is passively flexed. This is seen in patients with meningitis.

bruise. See **contusion, ecchymosis.**

bruit /brōō'ē/, an abnormal sound heard while listening to an organ or gland, as the liver or thyroid. The specific character of the bruit, where it is, and when it occurs in a cycle of other sounds are all important in diagnosis.

Brunnstrom hemiplegia classification, a method for measuring muscle tone and voluntary control of movement in a stroke patient. Results show the patient's progress in recovering.

Brushfield's spots, pinpoint, white or light yellow spots on the iris of a child with Down's syndrome. Occasionally, they are seen in normal infants, but their lack may help to rule out Down's syndrome.

Bruton's agammaglobulinemia, an inherited condition characterized by the lack of gamma globulin in the blood. Patients with this syndrome lack antibodies to fight off foreign bodies, so they are at high risk of getting repeated infections. Compare **agammaglobulinemia.** See also **gamma globulin.**

bruxism /bruk'sizəm/, the continuous, unconscious grinding of the teeth. This occurs especially during sleep or to release tension during periods of high stress during waking hours. Also called **bruxomania.**

Bryant's traction, a device used only with infants to keep legs rigid. The device is used to treat a broken thigh (femur) or to correct an inborn dislocation of the hip. It is made up of a traction frame supporting weights, connected by ropes that run through pulleys to foot plates. Compare **Buck's traction.**

BSE, abbreviation for **breast self-examination.**

BSN, abbreviation for **Bachelor of Science in Nursing.**

BT, abbreviation for **bleeding time.**

bubble-diffusion humidifier, a device that mixes water vapor with oxygen or other gases prescribed for treatment by allowing the gas to bubble through a container of water.

bubbling rale, an abnormal chest sound characteristic of moisture moving in the lungs.

bubble oxygenator, a heart-lung device that puts oxygen in the blood while it is outside the patient's body.

bubo /byōō'bō/, *pl.* **buboes,** a very swollen lymph node usually in the armpit or groin. Buboes are linked to such diseases as chancroid, lymphogranuloma venereum, bubonic plague, and syphilis. Treatment includes antibiotics, using moist heat, and sometimes opening and drainage.

bubonic plague, the most common form of plague. The symptoms are painful swollen lymph nodes (buboes) in the armpit, groin, or neck, fever as high as 106° F, exhaustion with a high thready heart rate, low blood pressure, confusion, and bleeding into the skin from the surface blood vessels. The symptoms are caused by an endotoxin released by a bacillus, *Yersinia pestis,* usually carried by the bite of an infected rat flea. Vaccination with plague vaccine gives partial immunity; infection with the disease gives lifetime immunity. Treatment includes antibiotics and draining the buboes. Conditions that will cause a plague epidemic are when a large infected rodent population lives with a large unvaccinated human population in a damp, warm climate. Also called **Black Death, black plague.** Compare **pneumonic plague, septicemic plague.** See also **bubo.**

buccal /buk'əl/, referring to the inside of the cheek, or the gum or side of a tooth next to the cheek.

buccal administration of medication, giving a drug by mouth, usually in the form of a tablet, by placing it between the cheek and the teeth or gum until it dissolves.

buccal contour, the shape of the buccal side of a back tooth.

buccal fat pad, a fat pad in the cheek over the main muscle of the cheek (buccinator). It is very evident in infants and is often called a sucking pad.

buccal flange, the part of a denture that fits next to the cheek in the mouth.

buccal smear, a sample of cells removed from the surface of the cheeks, teeth, and gums in order to study the chromosomes to determine a person's genetic sex.

buccal splint, any material, usually plaster, placed on the cheek surfaces of fixed partial dentures to hold them in place to put them together.

buccinator /buk'sinā'tər/, the main muscle of the cheek, one of the 12 muscles of the mouth. The buccinator, served by buccal branches of the face nerve, puts pressure on the cheek, acting as an important muscle of chewing by holding food under the teeth.

buccogingival /buk'ōjinji'vəl/, referring to the structures inside the mouth, particularly the cheeks and gums.

buccolinguomasticatory triad /buk'ōling'wōmas'təkətôr'e/, a group of uncontrollable lip, tongue, jaw, and head movements seen in tardive dyskinesia.

buccopharyngeal /buk'ōfərin'jē·əl/, referring to the cheek and the throat (pharynx) or to the mouth and the pharynx.

bucket-handle tear, a tear in the knee cartilage (meniscus) that occurs lengthwise. It is a common injury in athletes and active young people. The usual cause is twisting the knee. Symptoms are pain when squatting or twisting, some swelling, and tenderness. Often the knee pops or it may lock suddenly. These tears may heal over time if the knee is supported and protected, but sometimes surgery is needed.

bucking, *informal.* **1.** gagging on an airway tube. **2.** unconsciously fighting back the air pushed into the lungs by a respirator.

buck knife, a surgical knife with a spear-shaped cutting point. It is used for cutting into the gum (gingivectomy).

Buck's traction, one of the most common bone devices for traction on the legs. Buck's traction may be used on one or both legs. It is used to line up and keep rigid the legs in the treatment of broken bones and diseases of the hip and knee. The device is usually made up of a metal bar leading from a frame at the foot of the bed and supporting traction weights connected by a rope passing through a pulley to a cast or a splint around the legs. Compare **Bryant traction.**

buclizine hydrochloride, a drug that prevents vomiting. Derived from piperazine, it also is used to treat allergies and dizziness.

Budd-Chiari syndrome /bud'kē·är'ē/, a disorder of liver circulation, characterized by blockage of the veins. This leads to a swollen liver, fluid filling the abdomen (ascites), excess growth of more blood vessels, and severe high blood pressure within the liver vessels. Also called **Chiari's syndrome, Rokitansky's disease.**

budding, a type of asexual reproduction in which the cell makes a budlike bump that eventually separates from the parent and grows into a separate organism. It is a common form of reproduction in the lower animals and plants, as sponges, yeasts, and molds.

buddy splint, a flexible splint for protecting a broken finger. It holds both the injured finger and the finger beside it so that movements of the healthy finger also force movement of the broken finger.

Buerger's disease. See **thromboangiitis obliterans.**

buffalo hump, a lump of fat on the back of the neck linked to extended use of large doses of some steriods (glucocorticoids) or the secretion of high levels of a steriod (cortisol) caused by Cushing's syndrome.

buffer, a substance or group of substances that controls the hydrogen levels in a solution. Buffer systems in the body keep the acid-base balance (pH) of the blood and the proper pH in kidney tubules. See also **blood buffers, pH.**

buffy coat transfusion. See **granulocyte transfusion.**

bulb, any rounded structure, as the eyeball and hair roots.

bulbar paralysis, a wasting nerve condition characterized by continually worsening paralysis of the lips, tongue, mouth, throat, and vocal cords.

bulbourethral gland, one of two small glands located on each side of the prostate, draining to the urethra. Bulbourethral glands release a part of semen. Also called **Cowper's gland.**

bulb syringe, a blunt-tipped, flexible syringe usually made of rubber or plastic, used mainly for flushing out openings, as the ear.

bulbus oculi. See **eye.**

bulimia /byōolim'ē-ə/, an unsatisfied desire for food, often resulting in periods of continuous eating. This is followed by periods of depression and self-denial, and in some cases, forced vomiting. Also called **boulimia.** –**bulemic,** *n.,* *adj.*

bulk. See **dietary fiber.**

bulk cathartic, a substance that softens and increases the feces in the bowel.

bulla /bŏol'ə, bul'ə/, *pl.* **bullae,** a thin-walled blister of the skin or mucous membranes containing clear fluid. Compare **vesicle.** –**bullous,** *adj.*

bulldog forceps, short, spring forceps for clamping an artery or vein during surgery.

bullet forceps, a kind of forceps made for removing a foreign object, as a bullet, from a puncture wound.

bullous disease, any disease in which blisters filled with fluid (bullae) are formed on the skin or mucous membranes. An example is pemphigus.

bullous myringitis, an inflammatory condition of the ear, characterized by fluid-filled sores on the eardrum (tympanic membrane) and severe pain in the ear. The condition often occurs with bacterial ear infection (otitis media).

Treatment includes antibiotics, pain relievers, and surgical draining of the sores. See also **otitis media.**

bumetanide, a diuretic used to treat excess fluid pooling caused by heart, liver, or kidney disease.
★CAUTION: Kidney shutdown, electrolyte loss, or known allergy to this drug prohibits its use.
★ADVERSE EFFECTS: Among the most serious side effects are loss of potassium in the blood, and excess uric acid in the blood.

Bumex, a trademark for a diuretic drug used to treat congestive heart failure and in liver and kidney disease (bumetanide).

Buminate, a trademark for a drug that expands the blood volume (human albumin).

BUN, abbreviation for **blood urea nitrogen.**

bundle branch, a part of a group of muscle fibers that carry electrical impulses within the heart.

bundle branch block, an abnormality in the conduction of the electric signal of the heart through the fibers of the bundle of His. If many fibers are affected, the heart rate is slowed.

bundle of His /his/, a band of fibers in the heart through which the electric signal is carried from the atrioventricular node to the lower chambers (ventricles). Also called **atrioventricular bundle, His bundle.**

bunion /bun'yən/, an abnormal swelling of the joint at the base of the big toe. It is caused by swelling of the bursa, usually as a result of long-term irritation and pressure from poorly fitted shoes.

Bunnell block, a small wooden block used to exercise the fingers after surgery. The exercises with the block allow each individual joint to be exercised fully while the other joints are held extended.

Bunyamwera arbovirus, one of a group of arthropod-borne viruses that infect humans. It is carried by mosquitoes from rodent hosts, causing California encephalitis, Rift Valley fever, and other diseases. The symptoms are headache, weakness, mild fever, aching, and a rash.

buphthalmos. See **congenital glaucoma.**

bupivacaine hydrochloride /byōopiv'əkān/, a local anesthetic used in caudal, epidural, peripheral, or sympathetic block.
★CAUTION: Known allergy to this drug or to any of the amide class of local anesthetics prohibits its use.
★ADVERSE EFFECTS: Among the more serious side effects are central nervous system disturbances, low blood pressure, breathing difficulties, heart attack, and allergic reactions. The side effects vary depending on the condition of the patient, the dose, and the way it is given.

buprenorphine hydrochloride, a pain-relieving drug given by injection. It is prescribed for the relief of moderate to severe pain.

★CAUTION: It is a controlled substance that is prohibited for patients who may be dependent on narcotics.

★ADVERSE EFFECTS: Among the serious side effects are reduced respiratory function, sleepiness, nausea, dizziness, headache, vomiting, shrinking of the pupils, extreme sweating, and low blood pressure.

Bureau of Medical Devices (BMD), an agency of the Food and Drug Administration organized in 1976. It provides standards for medical devices and regulates their manufacture and uses.

buret, a laboratory device used to give a range of volumes correctly. Also spelled **burette.**

Burkitt's lymphoma /bur′kits/, a cancerous tumor in the jaw or, in children, the stomach area. The tumor, which is seen mainly in Central Africa, is a gray-white, branlike mass, sometimes containing areas of bleeding and dead tissue. Central nervous system diseases often occur, and other organs may be affected. The Epstein-Barr virus may be the cause of this lymphoma. Chemotherapy usually results in complete cure of the disease. Also called **African lymphoma, Burkitt's tumor.**

burn, any injury caused by heat, electricity, chemicals, radiation, or gases. The treatment of burns includes pain relief, stopping infection, keeping fluids and electrolytes balanced, and good diet. Severe burns may cause shock. See also **chemical burn, electrocution, thermal burn.**

burn center, a health-care center that cares for patients who have been badly burned.

burning feet syndrome, a disorder of the nervous system marked by a burning feeling in the feet. The sensation is usually more severe at night than during the day. It may also involve the hands. Possible causes include injury to the long nerve stretching through the muscles of the thigh, leg, and foot (sciatic nerve), decaying of the spinal cord, and severe disorders of the outer nervous system. The condition is also linked with diabetes, kidney disease, and lack of vitamin B.

burnisher, a dental instrument with a blade or slanted end point used for smoothing out rough edges of dental work, as fillings, crowns, or dentures.

burnout, a popular term for a loss of mental or physical energy following a period of long-term, continuous job-related stress. It is sometimes characterized by physical illness.

burn therapy, the care of a patient burned by flames, a hot liquid, explosives, chemicals, or electric current. Burns are rated according to how many layers of skin are damaged. Partial-thickness burns may be first or second degree. First-degree burns involve only the top skin

		Depth of burn	Pain and pinprick sensitivity	Appearance	Healing time	End result of healing	Treatment
		Detailed classification					
	1°	Erythema only, no loss of epidermis	Hyperalgesia	Erythema		Normal skin	Allow to heal by natural processes Protect from further injury and infection
	2° Partial skin loss	Superficial, no loss of dermis	Hyperalgesia or normal		6-10 days		
		Intermediate, healing from hair follicles	Normal to hypo-algesia	Erythema to opaque, white blisters are characteristic	7-14 days	Normal to slightly pitted and/or poorly pigmented	
		Deep, healing from sweat glands	Hypoalgesia to analgesia		14-21 days	Hairless and depigmented Texture normal to pitted or flat and shiny	Elective skin grafting may save time and give better end result
	3° Whole skin loss	Deep dermal, occasionally heal from scattered epithelium	Analgesia	White opaque to charred, coagulated; subcutaneous veins may be visible	More than 21 days	Poor texture Hypertrophic Scar frequent	
		Whole skin loss, healing from edges only			Never if area is large	Hypertrophic scar and chronic granulations unless grafted	Skin grafting mandatory
	4° Deep tissue loss	Deep structure loss	May be some algesia				

Burn classification

layer (epidermis). Second-degree burns involve the epidermis and second layer of skin (corium), whereas full-thickness or third-degree burns involve all skin layers. Second-degree burns covering more than 30% of the body and third-degree burns on the face and arms and legs, or more than 10% of the body surface, are critical. In the first 48 hours of a severe burn, fluid from the vessels, salt (sodium chloride), and protein quietly pass into the burned area causing swelling, blisters, low blood pressure, and very low urine output. The body loses fluids, proteins, and salt, and the potassium level is raised. The first low fluid levels are followed by a shift of fluid in the opposite direction resulting in excess urine, high blood volume, and low blood electrolytes. Possible other problems in serious burns include collapse of the circulation, kidney damage, shutdown of the stomach and bowel system, infections, shock, pneumonia, and stress ulcer (Curling's ulcer), characterized by vomiting blood, and stomach and bowel swelling (peritonitis).
★METHOD: Fluids and electrolytes, antibiotics, tetanus vaccination, and pain drugs are given for severe burns. Often a urinary tube (catheter) and a tube through the nose to the stomach are inserted. Treatment of the burn may be by either the closed or open method. In the open method, the injured area is cleaned and exposed to air, and the patient is kept warm by a blanket or linen over a bed cradle or by a heater or lamp. In the closed method, a cream, ointment, or solution is placed on the burn, and the wound is covered with a dressing. A temporary skin graft may be used to cover the wound. This prevents loss of fluid and reduces the risk of infection, but the graft dries in 1 or 2 days and may pull and cause pain. Newly developed artificial skin holds great promise for treating severe burns. If fluids by mouth are allowed, juices and carbonated drinks are offered, but not plain water and ice chips. Fluid intake and output are measured hourly. Blood transfusions, steroid therapy, and drugs to reduce fever may be ordered, but aspirin is not given. Excess chilling and exposure to upper lung infections and wound infections are carefully avoided. Burned arms and legs are raised, and cramps are prevented by using firm supports to keep affected areas in line. This can be done by using a footboard to keep the feet at a 90 degree angle to the ankles in burns of the legs, or by having the patient grasp a ball when the back of the hand is burned. After the first important period, a high-calorie, high-protein diet is given, and the patient is offered many small meals that are high in potassium. Vitamins may be needed. The patient is helped to stand for a few minutes every hour or every

second hour and is generally able to walk in 7 to 10 days, but the recovery may take a long time. A large amount of plastic surgery and repeated skin grafts may be needed to restore function and the physical appearance of burn patients.
★OUTCOME: The outcome for the severely burned patient depends greatly on the detailed, near-constant care needed during the first phase of treatment. Scarring may cause some temporary problems, but physical therapy helps restore movement.

Burow's solution /byŏŏr′ōz/, a liquid that contains aluminum sulfate, acetic acid, solid calcium carbonate, and water. It is used as a skin cream and antiseptic for many skin disorders. Also called **aluminum acetate solution.**

burp, *informal.* **1.** to belch. **2.** a belch.

burr cell, a form of mature red blood cell (erythrocyte) in which the cells or cell fragments have tiny bumps on the surface. Compare **acanthocyte.**

bursa /bur′sə/, *pl.* **bursae, 1.** a fiber sac around the joints between some tendons and the bones under them. Lined with a membrane that releases fluid from the joint spaces (synovial fluid), the bursa acts as a small cushion that allows the tendon as it contracts and relaxes to move over the bone. **2.** a sac or closed space.

bursa of Achilles, bursa separating the tendon of Achilles and the heel.

bursitis /bursī′tis/, a swelling of the bursa, the connective tissue structure surrounding a joint. Bursitis may be caused by arthritis, infection, injury, or excess activity. The main symptom is severe pain in the joint, particularly on movement. Treatment for the pain is usually an injection of a steroid into the bursa. Other treatments are pain relievers, antiswelling drugs, cold packs, and keeping the area rigid. After the swelling has gone down, heat may be helpful. Some kinds of bursitis are **housemaid's knee, miner's elbow, weaver's bottom.** See also **rheumatism.**

bursting fracture, any broken bone that scatters bone fragments, usually at or near the end of a bone.

Buschke's disease. See **cryptococcosis.**

busulfan, a drug used to treat long-term myelocytic leukemia.
★CAUTION: Radiation, low white cells or platelets in the blood, anticancer drugs, or known allergy to this drug prohibits its use.
★ADVERSE REACTIONS: Among the more serious side effects are lung problems (busulfan lung), blood abnormalities, and severe nausea and diarrhea. It often causes menstrual periods to stop.

butabarbital sodium /byŏŏ′təbär′bitôl/, a sleeping pill used to relieve anxiety, nervous tension, and lack of sleep (insomnia).

★CAUTION: Porphyrin disturbances, seizure disorders, or known allergy to this drug prohibits its use.

★ADVERSE EFFECTS: Among the more serious side effects are liver disease (jaundice), skin rash, and excitement.

butanol. See **butyl alcohol.**

butanol extractable iodine (BEI) /byōō'tənôl/, iodine that can be separated from blood plasma proteins by a solvent, as butanol. It is used to measure thyroid function.

Butazolidin, a trademark for a drug used to treat gout, rheumatoid arthritis, osteoarthritis, and bursitis (phenylbutazone).

Butesin Picrate, a trademark for an anesthetic ointment for burns (butamben picrate).

Butisol Sodium, a trademark for a drug used to cause sleep (butabarbital sodium).

butorphanol tartrate /byōōtôr'fənôl/, a narcotic given before and during surgery. Because it gives almost immediate relief from pain when given in the vein and begins to take effect within 10 minutes when given in the muscle, it is used for moderate to severe pain after surgery. Overdose may result when butorphanol is used with other narcotic drugs.

butterfly bandage, a narrow adhesive strip with broader winglike ends used to close the edges of a surface wound and to hold the sides together as they heal. It is sometimes used instead of stitches in certain cases.

butterfly fracture, a bone break in which two cracks form a triangle.

butterfly rash, a scaling rash of both cheeks joined by a narrow band of rash across the nose. It is seen in lupus erythematosus, rosacea, and seborrheic dermatitis.

buttermilk, 1. the slightly sour-tasting liquid remaining after the solids in cream have been churned into butter. It is nearly fat free and, except for a low content of vitamin A, is comparable to whole milk. **2.** cultured milk made by adding certain organisms to fat-free milk.

buttock. See **nates.**

buttonhole, a small slitlike hole in the wall of a structure or a space of the body.

buttonhole fracture, any broken bone caused by a bullet.

buttonhook, a device designed to help patients who have lost fingers or have only limited ability to move them to button, hook, or zip clothing.

button suture, a technique in stitching (suturing) in which the ends of the suture material are passed through buttons on the surface of the skin and tied. It is used to prevent the suture from cutting through the skin.

butyl alcohol, a clear, poisonous liquid used as a solvent. Also called **butanol.**

butyr-, a combining form referring to butter.

butyric acid /byōōtir'ik/, a fatty acid occurring in rancid butter, feces, urine, sweat, and, in small amounts, in the spleen and blood. Butyric acid is used to prepare flavorings, many liquid solutions, and drugs. Also called **butanoic acid, propylformic acid.**

butyrophenone /byōō'tərōfē'nōn/, one of a small group of tranquilizers used to treat psychosis, to reduce some symptoms of Huntington's chorea and Gilles de la Tourette's syndrome, and with anesthesia. The main butyrophenones are pimozide, fluspirilene, haloperidol, and droperidol. Butyrophenones are similar to the phenothiazines.

BWS, abbreviation for **battered woman syndrome.**

bypass, any one of many types of surgery to move the flow of blood or other fluids from their normal courses. A bypass may be either temporary or permanent. Bypass surgery is often done to treat heart, stomach, and bowel disorders.

byssinosis /bis'inō'sis/, a job-related lung disease characterized by shortness of breath, cough, and wheezing. The condition is an allergic reaction to dust or fungus in cotton, flax, and hemp fibers. The symptoms are often more common on Mondays when the workers return after a weekend break. The disease is curable in the early stages. Exposure for several years results in long-term airway blockage, bronchitis, and emphysema, leading to lung failure, and high blood pressure in the lungs with heart disorders (cor pulmonale). Compare **pneumoconiosis.** See also **organic dust.**

C

c, abbreviation for **curie**.

C, **1.** symbol for **carbon**. **2.** abbreviation for **Celsius**.

Ca, symbol for **calcium**.

CA, abbreviation for **cancer, carcinoma, chronologic age**.

cabinet bath, a heated bath in which the patient is placed in a cabinet from the neck down. Also called **box bath**.

CABG, abbreviation for **coronary artery bypass graft**.

Cabot's splint, a metal support splint worn behind the thigh and leg.

cacao, 1. another spelling of cocoa. **2.** the name of the plant *Theobroma cacao*.

cacation. See **bowel movement**.

cachet /käshā'/, any wafer-shaped, flat capsule that holds a dose of a bitter-tasting drug. It is swallowed whole.

cachexia /kəkek'sē·ə/, general ill health and faulty diet. It is usually linked to a wasting disease, as tuberculosis or cancer.

cachinnation /kak'ənā'shən/, excess laughter for no reason, often part of the behavior in schizophrenia. –**cachinnate,** v.

cacodemonomania /kak'ōdē'mənōmā'nē·ə/, a confused state in which a patient claims to be possessed by the devil or an evil spirit.

cadaver, a dead body used for study.

cadmiosis, a form of a lung disease (pneumoconiosis) caused by breathing in cadmium dust.

cadmium (Cd), a metal, bluish-white element. Its atomic number is 48; its atomic weight is 112.40. Cadmium has many uses in industry. Once used in drugs, cadmium has since been replaced by less poisonous drugs. It is used in engraving, printing, and photography. Breathing the fumes during metal-plating processes can cause poisoning. Acid foods (as tomatoes and lemonade) that are prepared and stored in cadmium-lined containers can also cause poisoning.

cadmium poisoning, the side effects of swallowing cadmium, eating foods stored in cadmium cans, or breathing cadmium fumes from welding, smelting, or other industrial processes. The symptoms from breathing fumes include vomiting, difficulty in breathing, headache, exhaustion, and, possibly, years later, cancer. Cadmium causes severe stomach and bowel symptoms 30 minutes to 3 hours after swallowing. Treatment for poisoning includes fluids through the veins, special drugs and oxygen.

caduceus /kədoo'sē·əs/, the wand of the god Hermes or Mercury, shown as a staff with two serpents coiled around it. The caduceus is a medical symbol and the official symbol of the U.S. Army Medical Corps. See also **Æsculapius**.

Caesarean hysterectomy. See **cesarean hysterectomy**.

Caesarean section. See **cesarean section**.

café-au-lait spot /kaf'ā·ōlā'/, a pale tan patch of skin. It occurs in a type of bone disease (Albright's syndrome), but these spots can also occur normally. Many café-au-lait spots may develop with a tumorlike growth all over the body (neurofibromatosis). See also **Albright's syndome, neurofibromatosis**.

cafe coronary, a popular term for choking on a piece of food that gets stuck in the windpipe. Because the patient is suddenly unable to talk or breathe and collapses while eating, it is often mistaken for a heart attack. Death or brain damage can result within a few minutes if emergency treatment is not given immediately to remove the food blockage. The Heimlich maneuver is a simple and effective treatment if the person hasn't collapsed. See also **cardiopulmonary resuscitation, Heimlich maneuver**.

Cafergot, a trademark for a drug that contains caffeine and ergotamine. It is used to treat migraine headaches.

caffeine /kafēn', kaf'ē·in/, a substance found in coffee, tea, cola, and other plant products. It is used as a stimulant. Caffeine is given to treat migraine headaches, drowsiness, and mental tiredness.

★CAUTION: It is used with caution in patients with heart disease and peptic ulcer. Known allergy prohibits its use.

★ADVERSE EFFECTS: Among the most serious side effects are rapid heart beat and excess urination. Stomach and bowel distress, restlessness, and lack of sleep are common effects.

caffeinism, a poisoning condition caused by the long-term use of excess amounts of caffeine in beverages or other products. Symptoms include restlessness, anxiety, general depression, rapid heart beat, tremors, nausea, high urine output, and lack of sleep. A fatal dose is estimated to be 10 g (equal to 100 cups of coffee) for a healthy adult. See also **xanthine derivative**.

caged-ball prosthesis, an artificial heart valve made up of a plastic ball in a metal cage.

caged-lens prosthesis, an artificial heart valve made up of a plastic disk in a metal cage.

caisson disease. See **decompression sickness**.

caked breast, too much milk in the ducts of the breast following childbirth. It causes all or a part of the breast to become hard and the tissues to become filled out. Also called **lactation mastitis**.

cal, abbreviation for a positively charged calcium ion (**calcium cation**).

cal., abbreviation for **small calorie** (or **gram calorie**). See also **calorie.**

Cal., abbreviation for **large calorie** (or **kilocalorie, kilogram calorie**). See also **calorie.**

calabar swelling /kal′əbär/, an abnormal condition recognized by swollen lumps under the skin. The cause is a parasitic, filarial worm common in central and west Africa.

Caladryl, a trademark for a lotion that contains a protectant (calamine) and an antihistamine (diphenhydramine hydrochloride). It is used to relieve minor skin irritations and itching.

calamine /kal′əmīn/, a pink powder containing zinc oxide and a small amount of ferric oxide. It is used to protect and dry the skin.

Calan, a trademark for a drug used to treat chest pain (angina pectoris) (verapamil).

calc-, **1.** a combining form referring to lime or limestone. **2.** a combining form referring to the heel.

calcaneal epiphysitis, a painful disorder involving the heel where the head of the heel is separated from the bone shaft by a plate of cartilage. The condition tends to affect mainly children who are physically active and whose heel bones are still divided by a layer of cartilage. The stress of jumping and other athletic activities may break the heel bone and bone shaft from the cartilage layer where they meet. Treatment may require that the foot be put in a cast. Also called **Sever's disease.**

calcaneal spur, a painful, bony growth on the lower surface of the heel bone (calcaneus). The spur is usually caused by long-term pressure on the heel. See also **calcaneus.**

calcaneal tendon. See **Achilles tendon.**

calcaneodynia /kalkā′nē-ōdin′ē·ə/, pain in the heel.

calcaneus /kalkā′nē-əs/, the heel bone. The largest of several bones that forms the ankle. Also called **os calcis.**

calcar /kal′kär/, *pl.* **calcaria,** a spur or spurlike structure that occurs normally on many bones of the human skeleton.

calcemia, an excess level of calcium in the blood. See also **hypercalcemia, hypocalcemia.**

calcicosis, a lung disease caused by breathing marble dust.

calcifediol, a form of vitamin D used to treat bone disease and lack of blood calcium caused by long-term kidney failure. Also called **calcidol.**

★CAUTION: Calcifediol should not be given to patients with excess blood calcium, vitamin D overdose, or known allergy to this drug.

★ADVERSE EFFECTS: Among the most serious side effects are kidney poisoning, soft tissue hardening, stomach and bowel problems, brain disturbances, or excess blood levels of calcium.

calciferol /kalsif′ərôl/, a crystal-like form of vita-
min D_2. It occurs naturally in milk and fish liver oils. It is used in the diet to prevent and treat rickets, osteomalacia, and other disorders with low blood calcium. Also called **ergocalciferol, oleovitamin D_2, vitamin D_2.** See also **rickets, viosterol.**

calcific aortic disease, abnormal deposits of calcium in the large artery of the heart (aorta).

calcification, the gathering of calcium deposits in body tissues. Normally, about 99% of all the calcium in the human body is deposited in the bones and teeth. The remaining 1% is dissolved in body fluids, as the blood. Disorders that cause deposits in arteries, kidneys, lungs, and other soft tissues usually are related to parathyroid hormone activity and vitamin D levels.

Calcimar, a trademark for a thyroid hormone used to treat Paget's disease of bone and excess blood calcium (calcitonin).

calcinosis /kal′sənō′sis/, an abnormal condition recognized by deposits of calcium in the skin and muscles. The disease usually occurs in children. Also called **calcinosis universalis.**

calcitonin /kal′sitō′nin/, a hormone made in the thyroid gland. It controls the levels of calcium and phosphorus in the blood and to start the making of bones. Normally, calcitonin is released by the thyroid to lower the blood level of calcium and phosphorus and to prevent calcium from being taken in again by the bones.

calcitriol /kalsit′rē-ôl/, a hormone related to vitamin D_3, made in the kidney. It increases the absorption in the intestines of calcium and phosphorus and helps bones to reabsorb the minerals. It is used to prevent calcium loss in patients undergoing kidney dialysis.

★CAUTION: Calcitriol should not be given to patients with high blood levels of calcium, vitamin D poisoning, or an allergy to the drug.

★ADVERSE EFFECTS: Among the more serious side effects are kidney poisoning, soft tissue hardening, and stomach, bowel, and nervous system problems.

calcium (Ca), an alkaline earth metal element. Its atomic number is 20; its atomic weight is 40. It is the most common mineral and the fifth most common element in the human body, found mainly in the bones and teeth. The body needs calcium to carry nerve signals, to contract muscles, to clot blood, to help heart functions, and to work with enzymes. Calcium is absorbed mainly by the small intestine. The adult human body contains about 2.5 lbs of calcium. The daily diet amount suggested varies from 360 mg for infants to 1,200 mg for women 15 to 18 years of age. However, only about one-third of the calcium taken in by humans is absorbed, so amounts higher than the daily amounts are needed. Excess calcium in the body can cause stones (calculi) in the kidney. Too little calcium can cause rickets in children and fragile bones (osteoporosis), especially in older women.

calcium antagonist. See **calcium channel blocker.**

calcium balance, the relation between the amount of calcium absorbed by the body and the amount lost each day in urine, feces, and sweat.

calcium channel blocker, a drug that prevents calcium from entering smooth muscle cells. This causes the smooth muscles to relax and reduces muscle spasms. Calcium channel blockers are used mainly to treat heart diseases marked by spasms in the artery of the heart (angina pectoris). Also called **calcium antagonist, calcium blocker.**

calcium carbonate, a white, chalklike powder that occurs naturally in bones and shells. It is used in certain antacids. Calcium carbonate antacids are effective for short-term relief but are not suggested for constant use because they can cause excess alkaloid buildup (alkalosis) or kidney damage.

calcium chloride, a white, crystal-like powder or granules usually made into a solution. It is used to replace calcium in the blood or to control the acid-base balance. It is used to treat muscle spasms from lack of calcium (hypocalcemic tetany). Other uses include as an antidote for magnesium poisoning and in emergency treatment of heart attack.

★CAUTION: Kidney problems, irregular heart beat, excess calcium in the body, or known allergy to this drug prohibits its use. Calcium can cause a sudden drop in blood pressure and loss of consciousness.

★ADVERSE EFFECTS: Among the more serious side effects are excess calcium blood levels, nausea, vomiting, widening of the blood vessels, and heart disorders.

calcium lactate, a calcium replacer used to treat a lack of calcium, particularly in cases of muscle spasm (tetany) resulting in difficult breathing. It is given by mouth.

calcium EDTA, calcium disodium edetate, used to treat metal poisoning. See also **chelation therapy.**

calcium gluconate, a calcium salt used to treat a lack of calcium and as an antidote for fluoride or oxalic acid poisoning. It may be given in the vein or by mouth.

calcium-phosphorus ratio, the proportion of calcium to phosphorus suggested for the daily diet to keep a desired calcium balance.

calcium pump, a theoretic device for carrying calcium across a cell membrane from an area of low calcium to one of high calcium. Compare **sodium pump.**

calcium pyrophosphate dihydrate disease (CPPD), a form of pseudogout with calcium deposits in the joints. The symptoms look like arthritis or gout.

calciuria, the presence of calcium in the urine.

calculus /kal'kyələs/, pl. **calculi** /kal'kyəlī/, an abnormal stone formed in tissues when mineral salts clump together. Calculi may form anywhere in the body. The most common places are the kidneys, gallbladder, and the joints.

calculus anuria, urine that is stopped by kidney stones.

Calderol, a trademark for a drug used to treat bone disease and lack of blood calcium (calcifediol).

Caldwell-Moloy pelvic classification /kôl'dwelmәloi'/, a system for classifying the structure of the bony pelvis of the female according to shape. Categories include android, anthropoid, gynecoid, and platypelloid. Pelvic classification is done in obstetrics to predict a woman's ability to give birth normally. See also **pelvic classification.**

calefacient /kal'әfā'shәnt/, **1.** making or tending to make anything warm or hot. **2.** an agent that gives off a sense of warmth when used, as a hot-water bottle or a hot compress.

calendar method of family planning. See **rhythm method.**

calf, pl. **calves,** the fleshy mass at the back of the leg below the knee. It is made up mainly of the gastrocnemius and soleus muscles.

calf bone. See **fibula.**

caliber, the diameter of a tube or a canal, as an artery.

California encephalitis, a viral infection of the brain and spinal cord that is carried by a mosquito. The disease is named for California because it was first found in that state, but it may occur anywhere in the United States. It affects mainly children in rural or suburban areas. The symptoms are a fever that may reach 104° F, headache, stomach problems, and vomiting. See also **arbovirus, encephalitis.**

californium (Cf), an artificial chemical element. Its atomic number is 98 and its atomic weight is 251. It is a radioactive element made by hitting curium 242 with alpha particles.

caligo, dim sight, usually caused by cataracts, a cloudy cornea, or failure of the pupil to widen properly.

calipers, an instrument with two hinged, adjustable, curved legs or jaws. It is used to measure the thickness or diameter of an object. In obstetrics, calipers are used to measure a woman's pelvis.

caliper splint, a leg splint made of two metal rods extending from a band around the thigh or from a cushioned ring around the pelvis. The lower ends of the rods are attached to a metal plate under the shoe.

calisthenics, exercising the many muscles of the body according to certain routines. They may be done with or without equipment, as dumbbells. The goal of calisthenics is keeping physical health while increasing muscle strength.

callomania, an abnormal mental condition in which the patient has delusions of personal beauty.

callosity. See **callus.**

callus, 1. also called **callosity.** a common, usually painless thickening of the skin at locations of pressure or friction. Compare **corn. 2.** a bony deposit formed around the broken ends of a broken bone during healing. The bone callus is replaced by normal hard bone as the bone heals. **–callous,** *adj.*

calmodulin, a protein molecule that is necessary for many biochemical processes, including muscle contraction and the release of a chemical that carries nerve signals (norepinephrine).

calomel, a white, odorless powder that darkens when exposed to light. It is sometimes used in ointments or dusting powders. Because it irritates the bowel, calomel was once used as a laxative.

calor /kal′ôr/, heat in the body. Examples are heat caused by swelling and heat caused by the normal processes of the body.

caloric, referring to heat or calories.

caloric balance, the proportion of the number of calories taken in in food and beverages to the number of calories used during work and exercise.

caloric test, a test used to see if the inner ear is diseased or normal. The test involves flushing the ear with warm and cool water. If the ear is normal, the warm water will cause the eyes to rotate rapidly (rotatory nystagmus) toward the flushed side; cool water causes a rotatory nystagmus toward the opposite side. If the ear is damaged or diseased, nystagmus does not occur. Because the sense of balance is inside the inner ear, the difference between water and body temperature disturbs the sense of balance if the ear is normal. Also called **Barany's test.**

calorie, 1. also called **gram calorie, small calorie (cal.).** The amount of heat needed to raise 1 gram of water 1°C at 1 atmosphere pressure. **2.** also called **great calorie, kilocalorie, kilogram calorie, large calorie (Cal.).** A quantity of heat needed to raise the temperature of 1 kilogram of water 1°C at 1 air pressure. The kilocalorie unit is used by food experts when referring to the fuel or energy value of many foods. **–caloric,** *adj.*

calorigenic /kəlôr′ijen′ik/, referring to a substance or process that makes heat or energy or that increases the use of oxygen.

calorimetry /kal′ərim′ətrē/, the method of measuring heat loss or energy loss. Human body heat can be measured by putting the person in a tank of water and noting the temperature change in the water. This change is caused by the body heat. Human calorie use can also be measured in terms of the amount of oxygen breathed in and the amount of carbon dioxide breathed out during a given time. Compare **direct calorimetry, indirect calorimetry. –calorimetric,** *adj.*

calvaria /kalver′ē·ə/, the skull cap or upper, domelike part of the skull.

Calvé-Perthes disease, a bone growth problem in children that affects the upper end of the thigh bone (femur).

calvities /kalvish′i·ēz/, baldness.

calyx /kā′liks/, *pl.* **calyces** /kal′isēz, **calyxes/,** a cup-shaped structure of the body. An example is the kidney (renal) calyx, which collects urine and directs it into a tube that carries the urine to the bladder. This tube is called a ureter.

camisole, a straight jacket made from a canvas shirt with long sleeves.

camphor, a clear or white crystal-like substance with a strong odor and taste. Camphor is found in certain plants, especially *Cinnamomum camphora.* It is used as a mild irritant and antiseptic in lotions and soaps.

camphor bath, an air bath in which the air is filled with camphor vapor.

camphor salicylate, a drug made of camphor and salicylic acid. Although seldom used today, it was used in skin ointments and taken for diarrhea.

camptodactyly /kamp′tədak′təlē/, an abnormal condition in which one or more fingers become permanently bent.

camptomelia /kamp′təmē′lē·ə/, an inherited defect in which one or more limbs are bent. This causes a permanent curve of the arm or leg. See also **camptomelic syndrome. –camptomelic,** *adj.*

Campylobacter, a genus of bacteria that causes sudden infectious diarrhea in newborn infants. Symptoms may also include weight loss, vomiting, fever, poor feeding, and irritability. It is one of many highly contagious types of stomach upset in infants but may be controlled with antibiotics. Also called *Vibrio fetus.*

Canadian crutch, a wooden or a metal device that helps a disabled patient stand or walk. It is made of two uprights with a crosspiece for the hand and a crosspiece for the armpit.

Canadian Nurses' Association (CNA), the official national organization for the professional registered nurses of Canada.

canal, 1. any narrow tube or channel through an organ or between structures. An example is the **adductor canal (a canal for vessels and nerves in the thigh muscle). 2.** (in dentistry) the root and tissue canals in the teeth.

canaliculus /kan′əlik′yələs/, *pl.* **canaliculi,** a very small tube or channel, as the tiny haversian canaliculi in bone tissue.

canal of Schlemm /shlem/, a tiny vein at the corner of the eye that drains the water in the eye (aqueous humor) and funnels it into the bloodstream. A blockage of the canal can result in glaucoma. Also called **Schlemm's canal.**

canavanine /kan'əvan'in/, an agent found in alfalfa sprouts in amounts of about 15,000 ppm, or 1.5% by weight. It takes the place of arginine in proteins, causing the proteins to become inactive. In laboratory experiments, canavanine fed to monkeys produces severe poisoning syndrome similar to a continuing inflammatory disease (human lupus erythematosus).

cancellous /kan'siləs/, referring to the spongy, inner part of many bones, mainly bones that have marrow.

cancer (CA), 1. a general term for a cancerous tumor or for forms of new tissue cells that lack a controlled growth pattern. Cancer cells usually invade and destroy normal tissue cells. A cancer tends to spread to other parts of the body by releasing cells into the lymph or bloodstream. In this way cancer cells can be carried to a place in the body that may be far from the first tumor. The first site of cancer is sometimes called a primary cancer. The tumor that grows as a result of the cancer spreading is called a secondary cancer. A secondary cancer often is noticed before the primary cancer can be found. There are more than 150 different kinds of cancer and many different causes, including viruses, too much exposure to sunlight or x-rays, cigarette smoking, and chemicals in the environment. **2.** any of a large group of diseases in which malignant cells are present. The most common sites for the growth of cancerous tumors are the lung, breast, colon, uterus, mouth, and bone marrow. Many cancerous tumors or lesions are curable if found in the early stage. Warning signs for cancer may be a change in bowel or bladder habits, a nonhealing sore, unusual bleeding or discharge, a thickening or lump in the breast or elsewhere, indigestion or difficulty in swallowing, an obvious change in a wart or mole, or a nagging cough or continuing hoarseness. Treatments include surgery, radiation treatment, and chemotherapy.

cancericidal /kan'sərisi'dəl/, referring to a drug or treatment that destroys cancer cells.

cancer in situ. See **carcinoma in situ.**

cancer of the small intestine, a cancer of the upper, middle, or lower portion (duodenum, jejunum, or ileum) of the small intestine. Type of tumor may differ from site to site. Adenocarcinomas are found in the upper or middle small intestine. They form lumplike, "napkin ring" growths. Lymphomas are found in the lower small intestine. They can harm bowel function by attacking the nerves. Lymphomas

Cancer's seven warning signals

Adults	Children
Change in bowel or bladder habit	Marked change in bowel or bladder habits; nausea and vomiting for no apparent cause
Unusual bleeding or discharge	Bloody discharge of any sort: blood in urine, spontaneous nosebleed or other type hemorrhage, failure to stop bleeding in the usual time
Thickening or lump in breast or elsewhere	Swellings, lumps, or masses anywhere in the body
Obvious change in wart or mole	Any change in the size or appearance of outward growths, such as moles or birthmarks
Nagging cough or hoarseness	Unexplained stumbling in a child
A sore that does not heal	A generally run-down condition
Indigestion or difficulty in swallowing	Pains or the persistent crying of a baby or child, for which no reason can be found

From American Cancer Society: cancer facts and figures (1990), Atlanta, 1990, American Cancer Society.

can prevent the small intestine from taking in nutrients. Less common tumors of the small intestine are carcinoids, found in the lower small intestine, and sarcomas, seen in the middle and lower small intestine. Cancer of the small intestine occurs more often in men than in women.

cancer staging, a way to describe a cancer, its extent, and how far it has spread, in order to plan treatment and predict outcome.

cancer tests, certain tests always done by doctors to find early signs of cancer. They include:
1. Guaiac test for bowel cancer, which uses a stool sample from the patient. The sample is looked at for traces of blood.
2. Rectal exam, done by a doctor with a gloved finger to detect tumors in men or women and prostate cancers in men.
3. Sigmoidoscopy exam of the bowels with a lighted instrument.
4. Pelvic exam for women, done by a doctor using a gloved finger to check the female reproductive organs.
5. Pap test, done at the same time as the pelvic exam, in which cells are scraped from the surface of the cervix and looked at under a microscope.
6. Breast exam for women, for changes such as a lump or thickening of tissue. A breast exam may include an x-ray film of the breast (mammography) to find tumors before they can be felt.

cancriform /kang'krifôrm'/, referring to a tumor that looks like a cancer.

cancroid, 1. resembling a cancer. 2. a mild skin cancer.

cancrum oris, a cankerlike sore of the mouth. It can begin as a small sore of the gum and spread to the mouth and face.

Candida albicans /al′bəkanz/, a tiny, common, yeastlike fungus normally found in the mouth, digestive tract, vagina, and on the skin of healthy persons. In some situations, it may cause long-term infections of the skin, nails, scalp, mucous membranes, genitals, or internal organs. See also **candidiasis.**

Candida vaginitis. See **candidiasis.**

candidiasis /kan′didī′əsis/, any infection caused by a species of the *Candida* genus of yeastlike fungi. Many common diseases, as diaper rash, thrush, vaginitis, and dermatitis, are caused by *Candida* infestations. A warm, moist environment will aid the growth of Candida. Some drugs destroy helpful bacteria as well as harmful ones and allow the fungus to grow. Gentian violet is a drug used on the skin. Antifungal drugs, as candicidin, clotrimazole, or nystatin may be used for some infections. Also called **candidosis.**

Candiru fever /kan′diroo′/, an infection in humans caused by the bite of a sandfly. Symptoms are sudden fever, headache, and muscle aches. Recovery occurs, without treatment, in a few days. It occurs mainly in the forests of Brazil. See also **arbovirus, phlebotomus fever, sandfly fever.**

candy-striper, *informal.* a volunteer hospital helper, who wears a striped pink and white uniform.

cane, a sturdy wooden or metal walking stick used to support and allow movement to a person who can walk but is partially disabled. A cane should be of appropriate length to allow a patient with an injured leg to walk with the cane held on the side of the healthy leg. In walking, the person may rest his or her weight on the cane and the injured leg while moving the healthy leg forward. To take the next step, the weight is placed on the healthy leg while the injured leg and cane are moved forward. The cane should allow the elbow to bend at a 25° angle.

canine tooth, any one of the four teeth, two in each jaw, found on either side of the four front teeth (incisors) in the human. Canine teeth are larger and stronger than the front teeth and have deeper roots. The first set of canine teeth show around 18 months after birth. They are replaced by adult canines at 11 or 12 years of age. Canines in the upper jaw are also called **eyeteeth.**

canker, a sore, found mostly in the mouth. Causes include a food allergy, herpes infection, and emotional stress. Also called **aphthous stomatitis.**

cannabis /kan′əbis/, American or Indian hemp (Cannabis sativa) used as a source of marijuana, hashish, bhang, ganja, and other mind altering drugs. The dried flower tops of this annual contain the chemical tetrahydrocannabinols (THC) that produces the desired effects. It is mainly smoked, although it can be eaten. All parts of the plant have some mind-altering chemicals, but the highest amounts are in the flowers. Cannabis makes most people feel relaxed and happy. Some people feel panic and tension. Motor skills and sense of time are changed. It does not appear to be physically addicting. Cannabis and its products are classified as controlled substances by the U.S. government, and the trafficking of cannabis has become a large organized-crime industry. In some states, possession of a small amount (usually 1 ounce) is a misdemeanor. Cannabis is sometimes approved for cancer patients to relieve the nausea caused by chemotherapy. It is also given to patients with an increase of pressure within the eye (glaucoma) to reduce that pressure.

cannabism, the poisoning that results from too much use of cannabis.

cannula /kan′yələ/, *pl.* **cannulas, cannulae,** a flexible tube containing a pointed metal rod (trocar) that can be put in the body. When the rod is removed, fluid can drain through the tube.

cannulation, the placing of a cannula into the body, as a vein or the bladder.

cantharis /kan′thäris/, *pl.* **cantharides** /kan-ther′idēz/, the dried insects *Cantharis vesicatoria*, which contain an irritating chemical once thought to stimulate sex. Also called **Spanish fly.**

canthus /kan′thəs/, *pl.* **canthi,** each corner of the eye. The angle at which the upper and lower eyelid meet on either side of the eye.

Cantil, a trademark for an antispasm drug used to treat peptic ulcers (mepenzolate bromide).

capacitance vessels /kəpas′ətəns/, 1. the blood vessels that hold most of the body's blood volume. 2. the veins that are downstream from the smallest arteries, capillaries, and smallest veins.

Capastat, a trademark for an antibiotic drug used to treat tuberculosis (capreomycin).

capeline bandage /kap′əlin/, a caplike bandage that is wrapped to look like a cap. It is used for protecting the head, shoulder, or a stump of a limb. Also called **Hippocrates' bandage.**

capillary /kap′iler′ē/, any of the tiny blood vessels in the system that link the arteries and the veins. These tiny vessels, called arterioles and venules, are where the blood–tissue exchange occurs. The blood gives oxygen and nutrients to the cells and collects waste from the cells. The size of a capillary may be 0.008 mm, so tiny that red blood cells must pass through one at a time.

capillary fracture, any thin hairlike break.

capillary hemangioma, a birthmark caused by closely packed blood vessels near the surface of the skin. It looks like a spot of red color on the skin. It is usually found on infants and fades during childhood. Treatment is not needed unless bleeding or injury occurs. Also called **hemangioma simplex, strawberry mark.** Compare **cavernous hemangioma, nevus flammeus.**

capillary pulse. See **Quincke's pulse.**

capillary refilling, the process of blood returning to the capillaries after blood flow has been interrupted briefly. When the volume of blood pumped through the heart is reduced and the flow of blood in the fingers and toes is poor, capillary refill is slow. It is tested by pressing firmly for 5 seconds on a fingernail and measuring the speed at which blood returns after pressure is released. In a healthy person with good heart output and blood flow in the fingers and toes, capillary refilling should take less than 3 seconds. A capillary refill of more than 3 seconds is considered a sign of slow blood flow in the fingers and toes, and a time of 5 seconds is abnormal.

capillary tufting, an abnormal condition in which the capillaries in the lungs stand out as tufts, or small masses, into the small pockets in the lungs where oxygen is absorbed into the blood.

capillovenous, referring to the vein portion of the capillary beds. See also **venules.**

capillus /kəpil'əs/, *pl.* **capilli,** a body hair, especially one of the scalp hairs.

capit-, a combining form having to do with the head.

capitate bone, a large bone in the center of the wrist. Also called **os capitatum, os magnum.**

capitulum /kəpich'ələm/, *pl.* **capitula,** a small, rounded, high place on a bone where it joins another bone. The capitula of the wrist and ankle can be seen by the naked eye.

-capnia, a combining form referring to the carbon dioxide content of the blood.

capotement /käpōtmäN', kəpōt'mənt/, a splashing sound made by fluid moving in a full stomach.

caproic acid /kaprō'ik/, a fatty acid found in milk and some plant oils. It is used in the making of artificial flavors. Also called **hexanoic acid.**

capsid /kap'sid/, the layer of protein that surrounds a virus particle.

capsomere /kap'səmir/, a protein molecule that is part of the coat of a virus.

capsular pattern, A series of limitations of joint movement in different directions due to restriction of the joint capsule. It occurs in joints that are controlled by muscles and not in those joints primarily joined by ligaments.

capsule, 1. a small, oval-shaped, gelatin container that contains a powdered or liquid drug.

It is taken by mouth. Liquid drugs are usually packaged in soft gelatin capsules that are sealed to prevent leakage. Powdered drugs may be packaged in hard capsules. A capsule is coated with a substance to keep from dissolving in the stomach when the drug must be absorbed in the lower tract. Compare **tablet. 2.** a membrane or other body structure that covers an organ or part, as the capsule of the adrenal gland.

capsulectomy /kap'səlek'təmē/, the surgical removal of a capsule, usually the capsule of a joint or the capsule of the lens of the eye.

capsulotomy /kap'səlot'əmē/, a cut into a capsule.

captain-of-the-ship doctrine, the idea that the doctor is responsible for all patient care and may be held accountable.

caput /kā'pət, kap'ət/, *pl.* **capita** /cap'itə/, the head or the enlarged portion of an organ or part. The term is used with another word naming the organ part, as **caput costae,** for head of a rib, or **caput femoris,** for head of a femur.

caput epididymidis, the head of the epididymis, which is the long tube in the testicles through which sperm travel.

caput femoris, the head of the thigh bone (femur) that fits into the hip socket (acetabulum).

caput fibulae, the head of the smaller lower leg bone (fibula). It joins the shin bone (tibia) just below the knee.

caput humeri, the head of the upper arm bone (humerus). It joins the shoulder bone (scapula).

caput mallei, the head of the malleus, which is one of the bones in the inner ear.

caput mandibulae, the rounded part of the jaw hinge on the lower jaw (mandible).

caput ossis metacarpalis, the part of a bone in the hand (metacarpal) that joins to the finger bone (phalanx).

caput phalangis, the part of the first section of a finger that joins to the middle section, forming the knuckle.

caput radii, the head of one of the bones in the forearm (radius). It attaches to the upper arm bone (humerus).

caput stapedis, the head of the stapes, one of the bones in the inner ear.

caput succedaneum, a collection of fluid between the scalp and skull of a newborn. It is usually formed during labor as a result of the pressure of the cervix on the infant's head. The swelling begins to go down soon after birth. Compare **cephalhematoma, molding.**

caramiphen edisylate, a drug used to treat coughs.

★CAUTION: Known allergy to this drug prohibits its use.

★ADVERSE EFFECTS: Among the most serious side effects are dizziness, stomach upset, nausea, and lack of sleep.

carate. See **pinta.**

carb, abbreviation for a **carbonate noncarboxy-late anion.**

carbam, abbreviation for a **carbamate carboxy-late anion.**

carbamate /kär'bəmāt/, any of a group of enzymes that block the action of cholinesterase. They are used in certain medications and insecticides. Some carbamates are poisonous and may cause convulsions and death when eaten.

carbamazepine /kär'bəmaz'əpin/, a painkilling and muscle relaxing drug used to treat swollen face nerve (trigeminal neuralgia) and some kinds of seizure disorders.
★CAUTION: Carbamazepine should not be used with monoamine oxidase inhibitors or by anyone with blood problems, or known allergy to any of the tricyclic antidepressant drugs.
★ADVERSE EFFECTS: Among the more serious side effects are life-threatening blood problems, loss of sleep, dizziness, loss of balance, and nausea.

carbamide peroxide, a growth-stopping drug used to treat canker sores and other minor swellings of the gums and mouth, and to soften impacted earwax.
★CAUTION: Punctured eardrum prohibits its use in the ears.
★ADVERSE EFFECTS: The most serious side effect is local irritation, especially if the drug is put on mucous membranes.

carbamino compound, a chemical complex formed when carbon dioxide binds to proteins in the blood.

carbamino-hemoglobin, a chemical complex formed when carbon dioxide binds to hemogloblin. It accounts for nearly 25% of the carbon dioxide released in the lung.

carbenicillin disodium /kär'bənəsil'in/, a penicillin antibiotic used to treat some infections, those of burns, wounds, and the urinary tract.
★CAUTION: Known allergy to penicillin prevents its use. The drug should be used carefully by persons with allergies or kidney problems, or by persons on a low salt diet.
★ADVERSE EFFECTS: The high salt content may disturb fluid and mineral balances in patients with heart, liver, or kidney problems. Convulsions, bleeding, and blood and nerve problems can result.

carbidopa, a drug used in combination with levodopa to treat Parkinson's disease. Carbidopa allows smaller doses of levodopa to be given, with fewer side effects.
★CAUTION: Pressure within the eye (glaucoma), high blood pressure, the use of a monoamine oxidase inhibitor within the past 14 days, or known allergy to this drug prohibits its use.
★ADVERSE EFFECTS: Among the most serious side effects are stomach bleeding, uneven heartbeat, slowed muscle movements, depression, and blurred vision.

carbinoxamine maleate /kär'bənok'səmēn/, a drug used to treat many allergies, including sneezing, skin reactions, and itching.
★CAUTION: Asthma or allergy to this drug prevents its use. It is not given to newborn infants or nursing mothers.
★ADVERSE EFFECTS: Among the more serious side effects are rapid heart beat, lack of sleep, skin rash, and dry mouth.

carbo-, carbon-, a combining form meaning 'carbon, charcoal.'

Carbocaine Hydrochloride, a trademark for a local painkiller (mepivacaine hydrochloride).

carbocyclic. See **closed-chain.**

carbohydrate, a large group of sugars, starches, celluloses, and gums that all contain carbon, hydrogen, and oxygen in similar proportions. Carbohydrates are the main source of energy for all body functions and are needed to process other nutrients. They are formed by all green plants, which use the sun to combine carbon dioxide and water into simple sugar molecules. They can also be made in the body. Lack of carbohydrates can result in fatigue, depression, breakdown of body protein, and mineral imbalance.

carbohydrate loading, a diet practice of some endurance athletes. A low-carbohydrate diet is eaten for many days. Then for many days just before competing, a diet very high in carbohydrates is eaten. The theory is that the muscles will be overfull with energy for the event. See also **glycogen.**

carbohydrate metabolism, the sum of the building up (anabolic) and breaking down (catabolic) of carbohydrates in the body. This mainly involves galactose, fructose, and glucose. See also **fructose, galactose, glucose.**

carbolated camphor, a germ-preventing wound dressing made of 1.5 parts camphor and 1.0 parts each of alcohol and phenol.

carbol-fuchsin paint, a substance used to treat fungus infections on the skin. It is made of boric acid, phenol, resorcinol, fuchsin, acetone, and alcohol in water. Also called **Castellani's paint.**

carbolic acid /kärbol'ik/, a germ-preventing and germ-killing compound made from coal tar. While fairly safe in very weak solutions of about 1% for cleaning small wounds or to relieve itching, carbolic acid is a strong poison. It can be soaked up through the skin and destroy the tissue. If swallowed, it depresses the nerves and causes the lungs and blood flow to stop working. It will cause death unless emergency treatment is given promptly. Because carbolic acid has no color, it often contains a dye to warn against mistaken use. Also called **hydroxybenzene, oxybenzene, phenic acid, phenol, phenylic acid, phenylic alcohol.**

carbolic acid poisoning. See **phenol poisoning.**

carbon (C), a nonmetallic chemical element. Its atomic number is 6; its atomic weight is 12.011. Carbon occurs throughout nature as a part of all living tissue and in a vast number of carbon compounds. Carbon occurs in pure form in diamonds and coal; in impure form in charcoal, coke, and soot; and in carbon dioxide. Carbon is essential to the chemistry of the body. Carbon dioxide is important in the acid-base balance of the body and in controlling breathing. Carbon monoxide can be deadly if breathed in. Dusts with carbon in them can cause in many on-the-job lung diseases, as coal worker's pneumoconiosis, black lung disease, and byssinosis. See also **carbon 11, carbon 14.**

carbon 11, a radioisotope of carbon with a half-life of 20 minutes. Compare **carbon 14.**

carbon 14, a radioactive type of carbon with a long life. Used in research, carbon 14 is also used to find the age of very old objects. Compare **carbon 11.**

carbonate, a CO_3^{2-} anion frequently appearing in salts that don't dissolve in water, as calcium carbonate.

carbon cycle, the steps by which carbon in the form of carbon dioxide is taken from and returned to the air by living things. The process starts with plants using light to make carbohydrates. Next, carbohydrates are eaten by animals and humans. Carbon dioxide is then breathed out by animals and humans. Carbon dioxide is also released by decaying dead plants and animals. See also **Krebs' citric acid cycle.**

carbon dioxide (CO_2), a clear, odorless gas. It is found in nature, but it is also made in diverse ways. Plants and animals make carbon dioxide in breathing. Although it is mostly nonpoisonous, carbon dioxide can cause suffocation. The acid-base balance of the body is affected by the level of carbon dioxide in the blood and other tissues. Solid carbon dioxide (dry ice) is made by compressing carbon-dioxide gas at very cold temperatures. It is sometimes used to treat warts, lupus, or moles.

carbon dioxide narcosis, a condition resulting from high levels of carbon dioxide in the blood. Confusion, tremors, convulsions, and coma may occur if blood levels of carbon dioxide are too high.

carbon dioxide pressure. See **carbon dioxide tension.**

carbon dioxide retention, an increase in the body levels of carbon dioxide when it is not released at normal rates. Strangulation, slow breathing, and breath-holding are causes.

carbon dioxide stores, the amount of carbon dioxide contained the body. Under normal conditions, it remains constant.

carbon dioxide tension, a measure of the amount of carbon dioxide present in the body. Above-normal levels occur in conditions of slow blood flow, slow breathing, or increased metabolism. Below-normal levels are caused by rapid breathing or rapid blood flow. Also called **carbon dioxide pressure.** See also **carbon dioxide, hypercapnia, hypoventilation.**

carbon dioxide therapy, the inhalation of low concentrations of carbon dioxide gas to treat a medical condition. Such therapy may be used to open blood vessels, stimulate the central nervous system and areas of the brain-controlling heart rate, slow rapid breathing, assist in developing a productive cough, and control hiccups.

carbon dioxide titration curve, a line plotted on a graph showing the changes in the body's acid-base balance. These changes result from the addition or removal of carbon dioxide.

carbon fiber, a material used in radiological devices to reduce patient exposure to x-rays.

carbonic acid, an acid that is made when carbon dioxide is combined with water. Also called **seltzer, soda water.**

carbonic anhydrase inhibitor, a substance that decreases the rate of carbonic acid and hydrogen production in the kidney. This tends to increase the amount of urine produced. Some carbonic anhydrase inhibiters, as acetazolamide, are used to increase urine production (diuretics). Others are used to treat glaucoma.

carbon monoxide, a clear, odorless, poisonous gas made when carbon or other fuel is burned, as in gasoline engines. Carbon monoxide will attach to red blood cells. This prevents the blood from moving oxygen from the lungs to the body tissues.

carbon monoxide poisoning, a poisoned state in which carbon monoxide gas has been breathed and soaked up by the blood. Too much carbon monoxide limits the ability of the blood to transport oxygen. This can result in headache, loss of sleep, trouble breathing, and death. In a small enclosed space, death can occur within minutes unless emergency treatment is given. A sign of carbon monoxide poisoning in a patient is a cherry-pink skin color. It is treated by removing the patient from the source right away and giving oxygen.

carbon tetrachloride, a clear, volatile, poisonous liquid used as a solvent in dry-cleaning fluids and in fire extinguishers. Accidentally swallowing the liquid or inhaling the fumes results in headaches, nausea, depression, stomach pain, and convulsions. In poisoning by fumes, artificial respiration and oxygen may be needed. In poisoning by swallowing, the usual treatment is pumping the stomach. Carbon tetrachloride is very poisonous to the kidneys and liver, and it can cause permanent damage to these organs.

carbonuria, the presence of carbon compounds in the urine.

carboxyfluoroquinolone, any of a group of quinolone antibiotics given by mouth and effective against **Enterobacteriaceae** and **Pseudomonas.** Examples include ofloxacin and perfloxacin. The drugs differ in the amount that actually enters the bloodstream after being taken by mouth.

carboxyhemoglobin /kärbok′sēhē′məglō′bin, -hem′-/, a compound produced when carbon monoxide links with red blood cells. It is breathed into the lungs and enters the bloodstream. It blocks the sites on the cells that carry oxygen. Oxygen in the blood decreases and, when the decrease is too much, suffocation and death result. See also **carbon monoxide, oxyhemoglobin.**

carboxyl groups /kärbok′sil/, chemical units that occur in foods and tissues of living organisms. They are made of a carbon atom, a hydrogen atom, and two oxygen atoms. The workings of carboxyl groups are needed for many of the body's functions.

carbuncle /kär′bungkəl/, a group of staphylococcal sores in which pus is present in deep, connected pockets under the skin. In time, pus boils to the skin surface. Common sites for carbuncles are the back of the neck and the buttocks. Treatment includes antibiotics, hot compresses, and drainage. See also **furuncle.**

carbunculosis, a state in which a group of carbuncles is present. The problem is a form of folliculitis, in which the infecting bacteria invade the skin through hair follicles. Carbunculosis can occur with diabetes mellitus.

carcin-, a combining form referring to cancer.

carcinectomy /kär′sinek′təmē/, the removal of a cancerous tumor.

carcinoembryonic antigen (CEA), a substance sometimes measured in searching for tumors. It is found in very small amounts in normal adult tissues. In patients with cancers of the colon, bladder, breast, and pancreas, the levels are higher. CEA is thought to be released into the bloodstream by tumors. Finding CEA, however, is not thought to be proof of cancer.

carcinogen /kärsin′əjin/, a substance that can cause the growth of cancer.

carcinogenesis /kär′sinəjen′əsis/, the process of causing cancer. Compare **oncogenesis sarcomagenesis, tumorigenesis.**

carcinogenic /kär′sinəjen′ik/, referring to the ability to cause cancer. Also called **cancerigenic, cancerogenic.**

carcinoid /kär′sinoid/, a small yellow, cancerous tumor that may grow in the stomach lining. It secretes substances that affect the nerves. The secretions often cause flushing, diarrhea, cramps, skin trouble, problems breathing, uneven heart beat, and heart disease. Also called **argentaffinoma, Kulchitsky-cell carcinoma.** See also **argentaffin cell, carcinoid syndrome.**

carcinolysis /kär′sinol′isis/, the killing of cancer cells, as by chemotherapy.

carcinoma /kär′sinō′mə/, pl. **carcinomas, carcinomata,** any cancerous tumor that starts with the cells that cover inner and outer body surfaces. Carcinomas invade surrounding tissue and spread to far regions of the body. It crops up most often in the skin, large intestine, lungs, stomach, prostate gland, cervix, and breast. The tumor is usually firm, uneven and has nodes, with a well-defined edge in some places.

carcinoma en cuirasse /äN′kēräs′/, a rare cancer that occurs along with advanced breast cancer. It is known by progressive growth of fibers in the tissues. It causes the skin of the chest, neck, back, and sometimes the stomach to become rigid. Another type of carcinoma en cuirasse develops with cancer of the rectum. In this type the belly becomes encased in a rigid, fibrous shell.

carcinoma fibrosum. See **scirrhous carcinoma.**

carcinoma gigantocellulare. See **giant cell carcinoma.**

carcinoma in situ, a precancerous tumor that has not invaded the surrounding tissues, but looks like it is invasive cancer. Such tumors are often seen on the cervix. They also occur in the anus, lung tissue, mucous membranes in the mouth, throat, eye, lip, penis, the wall of the uterus, vagina, and in skin growths in the aged (senile keratosis). Cervical carcinoma in situ is treated with success in various ways. These can include cryosurgery, electrocautery, and hysterectomy. Also called **cancer in situ, intraepithelial carcinoma, preinvasive carcinoma.**

carcinomatosis, an abnormal state known by the vast spread of cancer throughout the body.

carcinosarcoma /kär′sinōsärkō′mə/, pl. **carcinosarcomas, carsinosarcomata,** a cancerous tumor made of two kinds of cancer cells that are called carcinoma and sarcoma. Tumors of this type may occur in the throat, thyroid gland, and uterus.

carcinosis /kärsinō′sis/, the growth of many cancers throughout the body.

carcinostatic /kär′sinōstat′ik/, referring to the slowing or halting of the growth of a cancer.

card-, cardio-, a combining form meaning 'heart.'

-cardia, a combining form referring to a type of heart action or place.

cardiac, 1. referring to the heart. 2. referring to a person with heart disease. 3. referring to the part of the stomach that is joined by the esophagus.

cardiac aneurysm. See **ventricular aneurysm.**

cardiac angiography, a way to make an x-ray record of heart function. A material that will show on an x-ray film is injected into arteries, veins, or heart chambers. The anatomy of the heart and direction of blood flow can be studied, and diagnosis can be made.

cardiac anomalies. See **congenital heart disease.**

cardiac apnea, abnormal, short-term absence of breathing, as in Cheyne-Stokes respiration. The apnea alternates with periods of deep, rapid breathing.

cardiac arrest, a sudden stopping of heart output. The blood stops flowing and delivery of oxygen does not get to vital tissues. Carbon dioxide builds up in the tissues, and tissue cell functions fail. Heart and lung revival is needed right away to prevent permanent heart, lung, kidney, and brain damage. Also called **cardiopulmonary arrest.** See also **cardiac standstill, cardiopulmonary resuscitation.**

cardiac arrhythmia, an abnormal rate or rhythm of contractions of the upper (atria) or lower (ventricles) chambers of the heart. The state may be caused by a number of things. These can include a defect in the pacemaker function; failure of electrical conduction; increased energy need, as in exercise or fever. Cardiac arrhythmias are controlled by a number of drugs, as beta-blockers and calcium blockers. Kinds of arrhythmia include **bradycardia, extrasystole, heart block, premature atrial contraction, premature ventricular contraction, tachycardia.**

cardiac atria. See **atrium of the heart.**

cardiac atrophy, a breaking down of the heart muscle.

cardiac auscultation, the exam of the heart by listening to the heart sounds with a stethoscope.

cardiac catheterization, a test in which a long fine tube (catheter) is passed into the heart through a large blood vessel in an arm or a leg. A catheter nearly 4 feet long is passed through a cut into the vein. It is then passed into either the right upper chamber (atrium), the left lower chamber (ventricle) of the heart, or other parts to be studied. The catheter is guided by the doctor who watches its course on a fluoroscope. X-ray films may also be taken. An electrocardiogram monitors the heart during the procedure. As the catheter tip passes through the chambers and vessels of the heart, the pressure of the flow of blood is watched. Samples of the blood are taken for testing. Cardiac catheterization is not supposed to be painful, but it is normal for the patient to worry. The patient should expect to ask questions and get support. The test requires up to 3 hours, and the patient has to lie still during the entire time. A young child may need a sedative in order to lie still. An antibiotic may be given the day before to reduce the risk of infection. After the test, the patient may run a fever for a few hours, and there may be pain at the site of the incision.

★OUTCOME: Many conditions may be identified and assessed by using cardiac catheterization. These include hereditary heart disease, narrowing of the heart valves, and valve failure. Among the risks of the test are infection, uneven heart beat, (cardiac arrhythmia), and swelling of a vein (thrombophlebitis).

cardiac compression. See **cardiac tamponade.**

cardiac conduction defect, any impairment in the electric signals that control the pumping of the heart. Defects may occur in special fibers of the heart (the sinus node, the atrioventricular node, the bundle of His, the left or the right fiber bundles, or the Purkinje fibers). See also **heart block.**

cardiac cycle, the cycle of the heart from the start of one beat until the start of the next. The cycle begins with the electrical signal from special heart fibers (the sinoatrial node). The signal travels the pathways that run through the heart muscle. This causes the heart chambers, first the atria and then the ventricles, to contract. The cycle ends when the heart fibers become charged for the next contraction. The whole cycle lasts about 0.8 seconds.

cardiac decompensation, a condition of heart failure in which the heart is unable to provide enough blood to all the cells of the body. Causes may include heart attack, high blood pressure, infection, poisons, or faulty heart valves.

cardiac dyspnea, a loss of breath linked with the first stages of heart failure. It happens when the heart is unable to keep up with the increased oxygen needs during exercise.

cardiac failure, a state in which the heart cannot pump enough blood to meet the needs of the body. See also **congestive heart failure.**

cardiac hypertrophy, an enlargement of the heart.

cardiac impulse, the movement of the chest caused by the beating of the heart. It is easy to feel and easy to record.

cardiac massage, a repeated, rhythmic compression of the heart by outside force. Cardiac massage may be applied directly to the heart during surgery, or through the chest during resuscitation by pressing the chest with force. Cardiac massage is done when the heart stops beating or when an abnormally fast rhythm occurs (ventricular fibrillation). Also called **heart massage.** See also **cardiopulmonary resuscitation.**

cardiac monitoring, an electronic instrument that provides continuous reading of the heart on an oscilloscope. Each contraction of the ventricle is indicated by either a flashing light or a sound. The equipment also has an alarm system that is triggered by heart beats above or below normal rates. See also **electrocardiography.**

cardiac murmur, an abnormal heart sound usually caused when one or more valves fail to function normally. In general, many murmurs heard when the heart contracts are not abnormal. Most murmurs that occur when the heart rests are dangerous. Also called **heart murmur.**

cardiac muscle, the heart muscle that has qualities of both skeletal muscle and smooth muscle fibers. Its fibers look like those of skeletal muscle but are only one third as large when measured through the middle. However, cardiac muscle works on its own without the person being aware of it, which is how smooth muscle fibers work.

cardiac output, a measure of the amount of blood put out by the heart in a given space of time. A normal heart in a resting adult puts out from about 2.5 to 4 quarts (2.5 to 4.0 liters) of blood per minute. An output at rest of less than 2.5 liters usually indicates that something is wrong with the heart. Cardiac output is measured in many ways. One way is to measure the amount of oxygen in blood samples taken from a patient whose breathing has been measured for oxygen.

cardiac pacemaker. See **pacemaker.**

cardiac palpation, a way to examine the heart by feeling the vibrations through the chest at certain spots between the ribs near the breastbone.

cardiac plexus, a set of nerves near the arch of the main trunk where the system of arteries begins (aorta). It has nerve fibers that both speed up the heart rate (sympathetic fibers) and slow the heart rate (parasympathetic fibers). Both types of nerves follow along with the arteries of the heart (accompany the coronary arteries). They go into the heart, and end in the fibers that control electrical signals of the heart.

cardiac pressures, the blood pressures in the heart chambers (atria and ventricles) and nearby blood vessels as measured during catheterization. See also **cardiac catheterization.**

cardiac reflex, a change in the heart in response to a stimulus.

cardiac reserve, the potential of the heart to increase output and blood pressure above its normal level in response to bodily needs.

cardiac resuscitation. See **cardiopulmonary resuscitation.**

cardiac sphincter, a ring of muscle fibers where the gullet (esophagus) joins the stomach. Its function is to keep the stomach contents from backing up into the gullet.

cardiac standstill, the complete stopping of contractions and output of blood by the heart. See also **cardiac arrest.**

cardiac stimulant, any drug that increases heart action. Drugs such as digitalis, lanatoside, and ouabain increase the force of contractions and slow the heart rate. This allows more time for the heart to relax and fill with blood between beats.

cardiac tamponade, compression of the heart produced by the collection of blood or fluid in the sac around the heart. This can result when a blood vessel in the heart breaks or by a wound to the heart. Signs of cardiac tamponade may include neck veins that stand out, low blood pressure, decreased heart sounds, fast breathing, and weak or absent pulses. The patient can be anxious and restless, tending to sit upright or lean forward. The skin may be pale, gray, or blue. Also called **cardiac compression.**

cardiac ultrasound, a method used to test heart and blood vessel (cardiovascular) problems. The device is placed over the chest. Its high-pitched sound wave is bounced off the heart. This makes a picture of the heart chambers and valves.

cardiac valve. See **heart valve.**

cardialgia, any pain in the region of the heart. The term is used even if the heart is not directly involved. Also called **cardiodynia.**

cardiectasis, stretching of the heart.

cardiectomy, removing the area of the stomach where it joins the gullet (esophagus).

Cardilate, a trademark for a drug used to treat smothering chest pain, which is called angina pectoris (erythrityl tetranitrate).

cardinal, referring to the main feature of an organ or its function.

cardinal movements of labor, the sequence of movements by the infant as it comes down through the pelvis during labor and birth.

cardinal position of gaze, one of the positions to which the normal eye may be turned. Each position depends on certain eye muscles and nerve fibers. The positions include to the left, to the right, up, up and to the right, up and to the left, down, down and to the right, and down and to the left.

cardinal symptom. See **symptom.**

cardio-, cardia-, a combining form referring to the heart.

cardioaccelerator, any drug that speeds up the heart.

cardioangiology, a specialty in which the heart and blood system are the main course of study.

cardiocairograph, a test in which x-ray films of the heart are made at any point in its cycle.

cardiocele, an event in which the heart pushes through the muscle that holds it in place above the stomach (diaphragm), or through a nearby wound.

cardiochalasia, a state in which the muscle of the gullet (esophagus) is relaxed. This allows the stomach contents to back up into the gullet.

cardioclasis, a rupture of the heart.

cardiodiosis, the dilation of the heart end of the stomach.

cardiodynia. See **cardialgia.**

cardiogenic shock /kär′dē-ōjen′ik/, a form of shock caused when the heart fails to supply enough blood to the body. The state is linked with heart attack (myocardial infarction) and heart failure. Cardiogenic shock is an emergency that needs quick treatment. It is deadly about 80% of the time. Treatment may include giving fluids in the vein, or drugs. Devices, as pacing catheters, are also used. Compare **hypovolemic shock.** See also **electric shock, shock.**

cardiogram. See **electrocardiogram.**

cardiography /kär′dē·og′rəfē/, the technique of making cardiograms.

cardiologist, a doctor who finds and treats heart problems.

cardiolysis /kär′dē·ol′isis/, a procedure to separate scar tissue (adhesions) that constrict the heart. The ribs and breastbone are cut into, and the sac around the heart is cut from the membrane on the inside of the breastbone.

cardiomegaly /kär′dē·ōmeg′əlē/, enlargement of the heart caused most often by high blood pressure within the heart. It can also occur in arteriovenous fistula, congenital aortic stenosis, ventricular septal defect, patent ductus arteriosus, and Paget's disease. An enlarged heart is normal in athletes.

cardiomyopathy /kär′dē·ōmī·op′əthē/, any disease that affects the heart muscle. Examples include alcoholic cardiomyopathy and infiltrative cardiomyopathy, which is caused by deposits of substances in the heart muscle. *Secondary cardiomyopathy* refers to a problem that is linked to another form of heart disease or illness, as high blood pressure.

cardiomyopexy /kär′dē omī′əpeksē/, a surgical procedure in which the blood supply to the chest muscles is connected directly to the arteries supplying the heart.

cardionephric, referring to the heart and kidneys.

cardioneurosis, a state of mental upset that occurs with heart symptoms. They may have mental or unknown causes. The state may be set off by a heart condition or the fear of heart disease. The symptoms are chest pains or fluttering heart beat.

cardiopath, a person with heart disease.

cardiopericarditis, a hot, red swelling of the heart and the sac around the heart (pericardium).

cardiophobia, an abnormal fear of heart disease. See also **cardioneurosis.**

cardiophony, the use of a device, as a stethoscope, to listen to the heart sounds.

cardioplasty /kär′dē·ōplas′tē/, a surgical procedure to stretch the muscle (cardac sphincter) that closes the opening between the esophagus and the stomach. It is done when spasms of this muscle prevent food from reaching the stomach.

cardioplegia, paralysis of the heart, which may be caused by drugs, low body heat, or electrical excitement used in order to operate on the heart. See also **cardiac standstill.**

cardiopulmonary, referring to the heart and the lungs.

cardiopulmonary arrest. See **cardiac arrest.**

cardiopulmonary bypass, a technique used in heart surgery in which blood is sent through plastic tubes from the heart and lungs. A pump adds oxygen to the blood and returns it to the patient's blood system.

cardiopulmonary resuscitation (CPR), a basic emergency method of lifesaving. Artificial respiration and heart massage is used to re-start the heart and lungs. CPR is performed for cardiac arrest, electric shock, and drowning. Because permanent damage to the brain can occur if oxygen flow is not restored within about 4 minutes, it is vital that blood flow and breathing be kept up until trained help arrives. Chest compression presses the heart between the lower breastbone and the spine. During pressure, blood is forced into moving through the blood vessels. Blood refills the heart when the pressure is released. Mouth-to-mouth breathing is used at the same time to put oxygen in the blood, which is pumped through the body by heart massage. The American Heart Association, the American Red Cross, and other places offer CPR courses all over the United States. CPR can be done without equipment by one or two persons. Other persons not doing the CPR should call a doctor and ambulance. It is best if the rescue is handled by persons trained in CPR. CPR involves three actions: opening the airway, restoring breathing, and restoring blood flow. For an adult, CPR is done in the following way:
1) The patient is quickly placed on a hard flat surface, as a board or the floor.
2) Look at the patient closely. If unresponsive, the patient is tapped on the shoulder. The rescuer asks loudly, "Can you hear me? Are you all right?" If there is no response, assume the patient is not conscious.
3) Open the airway to the lungs. If the patient is lying face up, the tongue will drop back in the throat, blocking the airway. This can be fixed by tilting the head. To do this, place one hand beneath the patient's neck and the other on the patient's forehead and tilt up. This extends the neck and lifts the tongue from the back of the throat. However, if there is any sign of a neck injury, lift the lower jaw by placing the fingers behind the angles of the patient's jaw in front of the earlobes and move the lower jaw upward. If an airway device is handy, put it in with care. Otherwise, the head is held, either tilted back or with jaw lifted,

Emergency cardiopulmonary resuscitation (CPR)

Findings	CPR basic sequence	ABCs of action
1. No response	1. Call for help Stimulate or arouse	
2. Absence of respirations Cyanosis Dilated pupils Limp extremities	2. Open airway a. Head tilt, chin lift b. Back blows (if airway obstructed) c. Chest thrusts (if airway obstructed)	A—Open airway
3. Respirations still absent	3. Initiate artificial respiration a. Pinch nostrils & make a seal with rescuer's mouth; two quick breaths (1-1½ sec per breath)	B—Restore breathing
4. Pulse—not palpable	4. a. Palpate brachial artery in infants, carotid artery in children & adults b. Initiate external cardiac compressions & continue rescue breathing	C—Restore circulation
5. ECG ventricular fibrillation; ventricular tachycardia; asystole; electromechanical dissociation (EMD)	5. Drug therapy; defibrillation	D—Provide definitive treatment

Victim *must* be supported on hard surface; gastric emptying (decompression) is recommended only if the abdomen is so tense that ventilation is ineffective. Effective CPR is accompanied by improvement in skin color, pupillary constriction, spontaneous movement, and some gasping respirations. Effectiveness should be evaluated after 1 minute and periodically thereafter (every 1 to 3 minutes).

Adapted from the Supplement to Journal of the American Medical Association, August 1, 1980. Copyright 1980, the American Medical Association. Reprinted with permission from the American Heart Association.

Emergency cardiopulmonary resuscitation (CPR)

	Procedures		
Age	*Consideration*		
Infants (less than 1 year)	Breathing point	Mouth *and* nose	
	Pressure point	Midsternum—on line with nipples	
	Hands	Tips of 2 or 3 fingers	
	Compression distance	½ to 1 inch (1.3 to 2.5 cm)	
	Compression/ventilation C/V ratio	5/1 100C/20V/minute; use only slight hyperextension of neck; mouth or mask covers nose and mouth; use only small breaths from cheeks	
Children (1 through 8 years)	Breathing point	Mouth	
	Pressure point	Slightly below midsternum	
	Hands	Heel of one hand	
	Compression distance	1 to 1½ inches (2.5 to 3.8 cm)	
	Compression/ventilation C/V ratio	5/1 80-100C/15-20V/minute	
Older children and adults	Breathing point	Mouth	
	Pressure point	Lower half of sternum	
	Hands	Both	
	Compression distance	1½ to 2 inches (4 to 5 cm)	
	C/V ratio	Alone 15/2 2 Rescuer—5/1 80-100C/15-20V/minute	

throughout the procedure.

4) The rescuer should assess the need for artificial respiration by looking, listening, and feeling for signs of breathing. If the patient does not breathe on his or her own, regular mouth-to-mouth artificial respiration should start quickly.

5) To begin artificial respiration, pinch the patient's nostrils closed. The rescuer should put his or her mouth tightly around the mouth of the patient. Two quick breaths are forced into the patient's lungs. The rescuer's mouth is removed between each breath and the patient is allowed to exhale without help. The cycle is repeated every 5 seconds as long as the patient does not start breathing. If the chest does not expand, move the head and try again. If this does not work, the airway is blocked. If it looks like the airway is blocked, or the chest does not rise during resuscitation efforts, use the Heimlich maneuver or look in the patient's mouth for a foreign object. See also **Heimlich maneuver.**

6) Take the patient's pulse at the neck artery for 5 seconds and check for signs of heart stoppage right after the first four breaths are given. Absent or weak pulse at that time means that chest compression is needed.

7) To start compression, take a position facing the side of the patient. To find the right place to put the hands, uncover the patient's chest and find the lower end of the breastbone. Place the heel of one hand just above the tip of the breastbone. The other hand is placed on top of the first and the fingers are interlocked. With arms straight, the rescuer rocks back and forth from the hips, using enough downward pressure with the forward swing of the body to push down the adult patient's breast bone from 1½ to 2 inches. The fingers should be held so that they do not touch the ribs. (It is important to avoid hurting the victim.) After each compression, a rest is allowed for a time equal to the time of compression, but the hands must not be moved from their place on the chest. The cycle is repeated using a rate of 15 chest compressions to 2 breaths. A rate of about 60 compressions a minute should be maintained. The right rhythm may be found by counting "one and two and three," up to 15. If there are two persons, CPR is done with one person giving compressions and the other giving breaths, at a 5-to-1 ratio at a rate of 60 compressions a minute. Check results by feeling for the pulse in the neck and by watching for "pinking" of the skin, constriction of the pupils, and a return of breathing. If the person doing compressions gets tired, a switch may be made by changing the counting rhythm to "switch-one thousand, two-one thousand," up to "five-one thousand." At the end of that cycle, the person giving compressions moves the

patient's head and checks the pulse. The person at the head, after giving a breath, moves to the patient's side, and checks the pulse for 5 seconds. If the pulse is absent or weak, the person says, "No pulse. Continue CPR."

For children 8 years of age and older, the technique is like that for adults. In infants, the neck is not tilted back because soft cartilage and neck tissues can block the airway if the head is tilted too far. Put a hand beneath the shoulders of an infant to provide enough tilt. For mouth-to-mouth resuscitation, the rescuer's mouth should cover the infant's mouth and nose. The breath should be gentle and given about every 3 seconds. The infant's pulse is checked at the inside of the elbow. Chest compression for small infants is done with both thumbs on the middle of the breastbone while joining the fingers behind the infant's back. For an older infant and children up to 5 years of age, pressure is applied with two fingers on the middle of the breastbone with a sharp downward thrust. For children older than 5 years of age, the heel of one hand is used. Because the heart in infants and small children is higher in the chest than in adults, pressure should be applied to the middle of the breastbone and only to a depth of ½ to ¾ inch for infants, ¾ to 1 inch for young children, and 1½ to 2 inches for older children. The rate of chest compression for infants is 100 times per minute, with breaths given as quickly as possible after each 5 compressions – about one every 3 seconds. The rate of compression for children is 80 times per minute, with breaths given once every 4 seconds. Less air is needed for a child than for an adult. CPR is an emergency treatment used until medical help is available. Once started, it is kept up until one of the following occurs: breathing and blood flow are restored; someone else takes over; a doctor takes charge of the patient; the patient is handed over to the care of a hospital; or the rescuer is not able to continue. Even if CPR is begun as soon as possible and all steps are done correctly, there are some cases, as with severe emphysema or crushing chest injuries, in which it will not work. Even when done correctly, CPR may cause rib fractures in some patients. Other problems include fracture of the breastbone, liver injury, bruised lung, and other lung injuries. There is less danger of problems when the technique is correct.

cardiorrhaphy /kär′dē·ôr′əfē/, an operation in which the heart muscle is sewn up.

cardiospasm /kär′dē·ōspaz′əm/, a failure of the muscle at the end of the gullet (esophagus) to relax. This makes it hard to swallow and vomit. Surgery may be required to correct the defect.

cardiotachometer /kär′dē·ōtəkom′itər/, a device that watches and records the heartbeat over a long time.

cardiotomy /kär′dē·ot′əmē/, **1.** an operation in which the heart is cut into. **2.** an operation in which the heart or gullet end of the stomach is cut.

cardiotonic /kär′dē·ōton′ik/, a substance that makes the heart work better. Examples include drugs such as digitalis, digitoxin, and digoxin. They increase the force of contractions and slow the heart beat.

cardiotoxic, referring to a substance that has a poisonous or harmful effect on the heart.

cardiovascular /kär′dē·ōvas′kyələr/, referring to the heart and blood vessels.

cardiovascular assessment, a way to assess the state, function, and defects of the heart and blood flow. The patient's history of heart and blood flow problems is noted, including the onset, quality, length of time, and place of any pain. Also noted are weakness, fatigue, shortness of breath, fever, coughing, wheezing, and uneven heart beat. Questions are asked about fainting, stomach upset, swelling of the feet and hands, bluish skin, changes in sight, and whether the hands and feet ever feel numb or cold. The patient's appearance, color, posture, the rate and rhythm of the pulses, and the neck veins are observed. The blood pressure, temperature, and rate and type of breaths are checked. The sounds the heart makes are listened to closely. The sounds of the breath are checked. The color, temperature, and dryness or sweating of the skin are noted. The patient's level of awareness, reflexes, and responses to pain are noted. High blood pressure, weight, diabetes, and any lung and kidney problems are noted. Past heart surgery and illness are discussed. A number of tests are done on the blood itself as it relates to heart disease. A graph of the electrical signals of the heart may also be done (electrocardiogram). A thorough test of the heart and blood flow is an important part of a complete physical. It is vital to the care of a patient who has cardiovascular disease.

cardiovascular disease, any one of many defects that may cause problems with the heart and blood vessels. Some kinds of cardiovascular disease are **atherosclerosis, cor pulmonale, rheumatic heart disease, syphilitic heart disease,** and **systemic hypertension.** In the United States cardiovascular disease is the main cause of death. It accounts for more than 50% of all deaths from disease every year. More than a quarter of a million persons under 65 years of age in the United States die each year from this disorder.

cardiovascular system, the network of structures, which include the heart and the blood vessels, that pumps and carries the blood through the body. The system includes thousands of miles of blood vessels (arteries, capillaries, and venules). There are many controls in the system to ensure that the blood is sent to the places where it is most needed and at the proper rate. The arteries deliver nutrients to the fluids that surround the cells, and the veins take away waste products from the cells. The cardiovascular system works closely with the lungs and related structures, (respiratory system), to transport oxygen from the lungs to the tissues and carry carbon dioxide to the lungs to be exhaled. Special nerves control the heart rate and blood pressure so that constant changes are made to deal with the needs of the body. Many things, as diet, exercise, and stress, affect the cardiovascular system.

cardioversion, restoring of the heart's normal rhythm by giving an electric shock through two metal paddles placed on the patient's chest. Cardioversion is used to treat atrial fibrillation and for severe arrhythmias. The electric voltage is given by placing one of the metal paddles, covered with a thick layer of special paste, below the heart on the left side of the chest. The other paddle is placed over the upper right chest. The device is first set at a low level of voltage. If the normal rhythm of the heart does not resume, shocks of up to 400 watts per second can be given. The patient must sign an informed consent before treatment can start. Diuretics and digitalis are withheld for 24 to 72 hours. Nothing is given by mouth for 6 to 8 hours before the treatment. A sedative is given an hour before cardioversion. Afterwards, the patient must stay in bed. A constant graph of the heart's electric impulses is watched (electrocardiographic monitoring). Oxygen is given if needed. Cardioversion will usually work to restore the heart's normal rhythm.

carditis /kärdī′tis/, an inflammation of the muscles of the heart. It usually results from infection. Chest pain, uneven heartbeats, failure of the blood system, and damage to the heart may occur.

caries /ker′ēz/, decay, breaking down, and destruction of a bone or tooth. Kinds of caries include **dental caries, radiation caries, spinal caries.**

carina /kərē′nə/, *pl.* **carinae,** any structure shaped like a ridge or boat keel, as the carina of the windpipe (trachea), which sticks out from the lowest portion.

cariocas /kär′ē ō′kəs/, a form of sideways movement in which one leg is still, and the other is brought repeatedly in front of, then behind the still leg.

cariogenic /ker′ē·ōjen′ik/, tending to make caries.

carisoprodol, a drug used to relieve muscle spasm.

★CAUTION: Porphyria or known allergy to this drug or to drugs like it prohibits its use.

★ADVERSE EFFECTS: Among the more serious side effects are loss of sense of balance, fatigue, weakness, problems with eyesight, confusion, and allergic reactions.

carminative /kärmin'ətiv/, a substance that relieves bloating due to gas and painful spasms, especially after meals. Oils of anise, bitter almond, cinnamon, fennel, peppermint, spearmint, and wintergreen were once used as carminatives but are rarely used in modern medicine except as flavorings.

carmustine /kärmus'tin/, an anticancer drug used alone or with other chemotherapeutical drugs. Carmustine is used to treat brain tumors, multiple myeloma, Hodgkin's disease, and non-Hodgkin's lymphomas. Also called **BCNU.**

carnivore, an animal that belongs to the order *Carnivora,* classified as a flesh eater, with teeth, simple stomach, and short intestine for a meat diet. **–carnivorous,** *adj.*

carotene /kar'ətin/, a red or orange compound found in carrots, sweet potatoes, milk fat, egg yolk, and leafy vegetables. Carotene is changed to vitamin A in the body. A body that cannot digest carotene may become lacking in vitamin A. See also **vitamin A.**

carotenemia /kar'ətinē'mē·ə/, the presence of too much carotene in the blood. This results in yellow appearance of the blood and skin.

carotenoid /kərot'ənoid/, any of a group of red, yellow, or orange pigments that are found in some animal tissue. They can also be found in foods, as carrots, sweet potatoes, and leafy green vegetables. Many of these substances, as carotene, are needed to make vitamin A in the body. Others, as lycopene and xanthophyll, do not form vitamin A.

carotid /kərot'id/, referring to the carotid artery. The carotid artery is a blood vessel that begins at the large artery of the heart (aorta) and runs straight up through the neck. About an inch above the collar bone it branches into the outer carotid and the inner carotid arteries. The carotid artery pulse can be felt just below the jaw bone.

carotid body, a small structure that contains nerve tissue at the branch of the carotid arteries. The carotid body controls the oxygen content of the blood.

carotid body reflex, a normal chemical reflex that begins when there is decreased oxygen in the blood or increased carbon dioxide. The carotid body (respiratory center) sends nerve signals to the brain's breathing center. The center sends back nerve signals that increase the breathing rate. See also **aortic body reflex.**

carotid body tumor, a benign round, firm growth that occurs at the branch of the common carotid artery. The tumor usually has no symptoms, but it sometimes causes dizziness, nausea, and vomiting, especially if it blocks the flow of blood. It may be removed in some cases.

carotid pulse, the pulse of the carotid artery, which can be felt by gently pressing a finger in the groove between the voice box (larynx) and the muscle in the neck.

carotid sinus, an enlargement of the artery wall at the branch of the common carotid artery. It holds nerve ends that respond to changes in blood pressure.

carotid sinus reflex, the decrease in the heart rate as a normal response to pressure on the carotid artery where it branches.

carotid sinus syndrome, a short-term fainting spell that is sometimes seen with convulsions. It is caused by the strength of the carotid sinus reflex.

carotodynia /kərot'ōdin'ē·ə/, a soreness along the length of the common carotid artery.

carpal /kär'pəl/, referring to the wrist (carpus).

carpal tunnel, a channel in the wrist for the middle nerve (median nerve), and the tendons of the hand.

carpal tunnel syndrome, a common, painful defect of the wrist and hand. It is caused by pressure on the middle nerve in the carpal tunnel. The syndrome is seen more often in women, especially in pregnant and in menopausal women. Symptoms may result from a blow, swelling, a tumor, rheumatoid arthritis, or a small carpal tunnel that squeezes the nerve. The middle nerve (median nerve) serves the palm and the thumb side of the hand. Pressure on the nerve causes weakness, pain when the thumb is bent toward the palm, and burning, tingling, or aching that may spread to the forearm and the shoulder. Weakness and wasting of muscles may occur from lack of use, getting in the way of full use of the thumb and fingers. Pain may be infrequent or constant and is often most intense at night. Drugs given by injection often bring quick relief from bad pain. An operation to relieve nerve pressure usually corrects the syndrome for good.

carpometracarpal (CMC) joint, any of the joints of the wrist formed between the bones of the wrist and the bones of the middle part of the hand.

carpopedal spasm, a spasm of the hand, thumbs, foot, or toes that is sometimes seen with muscle cramps, twitching, and convulsions (tetany).

carpus /kär'pə/, the wrist, made up of eight bones arranged in two rows.

carrier, 1. a person or animal who carries and spreads disease, as typhoid fever, to others but who does not become ill. **2.** one who carries a gene that has no effect unless it is combined with the gene of another person (recessive gene).

Carrión's disease. See **bartonellosis.**

Carroll Quantitative Test of Upper Extremity Function, a test that measures the ability to grasp and lift objects of different sizes and shapes. It also shows how well a person can perform general arm and hand movements required for the activities of daily living.

carrying angle, the angle between the upper arm and the forearm when the arm is fully extended.

car sickness. See **motion sickness.**

cartilage, a tissue that connects and supports. It is made of cells and fibers, found mostly in the joints, the chest, and stiff tubes of all sorts, as the voicebox (larynx), windpipe (trachea), nose, and ear. Kinds of cartilage are **hyaline cartilage, white fibrocartilage, yellow cartilage. –cartilaginous,** *adj.*

cartilage graft, the transplantation of cartilage. It is used to correct ear and nose defects in children and to treat severe injuries in adults.

cartilage-hair hypoplasia, a genetic defect that is marked by dwarfism, which is caused by too little growth of the cartilage. Other qualities are defects of the skeleton, and very sparse, short, fine, brittle hair that is often light in color. The state is found mostly among Amish people in North America.

cartilaginous joint, a joint that can move slightly. In it, the cartilage joins the bone. An example of a cartilaginous joint is the line at which the pubic bones meet.

caruncle /kär′ungkəl/, a small piece of flesh that protrudes, as one of the caruncles that are left when the membrane that covers the vagina is broken (hymen).

carunculae hymenales, remains of a broken hymen that stick out from the skin around the mouth of the vagina. Also called **hymenal tags.**

cascade, any process that happens in stages. Each stage depends on the stage that came before, and together they often have a greater effect.

cascara sagrada /kasker′ə səgrä′də/, a drug made from the bark of the *Rhamnus purshianus* tree. It is used to treat constipation. ★CAUTION: Symptoms of appendicitis, blocked or torn bowels, tightly-packed feces (fecal impaction), or known allergy to this drug prohibits its use. It is not given to nursing mothers. ★ADVERSE EFFECTS: Among the more serious side effects are bleeding, muscle cramps, dizziness, and dependence on the drug.

caseation /kā′sē·ā′shən/, a form of tissue death in which the area looks like crumbly cheese. It is common in tuberculosis.

case-control study, a type of scientific investigation that studies the lives of patients with a certain medical problem, as heart disease, and compares them to a group of persons who have not developed that problem. The two groups are similar in age, sex, and other personal data. They are examined to determine what factors (cigarette smoking, coffee drinking, etc.) might account for the disease in the first group.

case fatality rate, the number of deaths known to be caused by any certain disease. It is given as a percentage of the total number of known cases of the disease.

case management, the assignment of a health-care provider to assist a patient in obtaining all necessary health and social services.

cast, 1. a stiff, solid dressing of plaster of Paris or other material. It is formed around a limb or other body part to keep it from moving while it heals. **2.** a mold of a part or all of a patient's teeth and inner jaw for fitting false teeth, caps, bridges or dentures. **3.** a small structure made when mineral or other substances collect on the walls of kidneys, bronchia, or other organs. Casts often show up in urine or blood collected for laboratory tests. **4.** also called **strabismus.** the switch of an eye from the normal lines of vision.

cast brace, a combination of a brace with a cast at a joint.

cast core, a metal casting that uses a post in the root canal of a tooth for holding a false tooth crown in place.

Castellani's paint. See **carbol-fuchsin solution.**

casting, 1. the act of encasing a body part in a cast. **2.** (in dentistry) the process by which crowns, inlays, and other metallic devices are produced.

casting tape, an adhesive tape used for shaping lightweight casts.

castor oil, an oil from the castor bean seed that is used as a laxative. It is given for constipation and for cleansing the bowel before examination. ★CAUTION: Symptoms of appendicitis, blocked or torn bowels, and tightly-packed feces (fecal impaction), prohibit its use. It is not to be used during menstruation or pregnancy. ★ADVERSE EFFECTS: Among the most serious side effects are rectal bleeding and laxative dependence. Nausea, cramps, and dizziness also may occur.

castration, the removal of one or both testicles or ovaries. It is usually done to reduce the production of hormones that may cause the growth of cancer cells in women with breast cancer and in men with cancer of the prostate. The removal of both ovaries or testicles (gonads) causes the patient to become sterile. See also **oophorectomy, orchiectomy.**

castration anxiety, the fear of harm or loss of the genitals. It is often caused by guilt over forbidden sexual desires. It may also be caused by some difficult or frightening event, as a bad embarrassment, loss of a job, or loss of power over other people. Also called **anxiety complex.** See also **anxiety neurosis.**

cast saw, a saw used to cut through a plaster cast.

cast shoe, a shoe worn over a foot that is encased in a plaster cast.

cast stabilization, the use off rods, pins, broom handles, or other devices to lend strength to a cast.

cast syndrome, a group of patient signs that indicates a fear of having a part of the body encased in a plaster cast.

CAT /kat/, a short term for **computerized axial tomography.**

catabasis /kətab'əsis/, *pl.* **catabases,** the phase in which a disease declines and health begins to return.

catabiosis, the normal aging of cells.

catabolism /kətab'əliz'əm/, a complex, chemical process of the body in which energy is released for use in work, energy storage, or heat production. The energy is released in the cells by breaking down complex substances into simple compounds. Compare **anabolism.** –**catabolic,** *adj.*

catagen. See **hair.**

catalase, an enzyme, found in most living cells. It speeds up (catalyzes) the break down of hydrogen peroxide to water and oxygen.

catalepsy /kat'əlep'sē/, an abnormal state in which a trancelike level of awareness and rigid muscles occur. It occurs in hypnosis and in some physical and mental defects, as schizophrenia, epilepsy, and hysteria.

catalysis /kətal'əsis/, an increase in the rate of any chemical reaction that is caused when a certain chemical that is not part of the reaction is added to the process to speed it up (catalyst). The catalyst does not change in the process even though it affects it. Compare **negative catalysis.** See also **catalyst.** –**catalytic,** *adj.*

catalyst /kat'əlist/, a substance that speeds up the rate of a chemical reaction without being changed by the process. See also **enzyme.**

catamnesis /kat'amnē'sis/, the medical history of a patient from the beginning of an illness. Compare **anamnesis.**

cataplexy /kat'əplek'sē/, a state in which sudden muscle weakness and loss of muscle tone occur. It is caused by emotions, as anger, fear, or surprise. It is linked with narcolepsy, a desire to sleep that cannot be controlled. –**cataplectic,** *adj.*

Catapres, a trademark for a drug used to treat high blood pressure (clonidine hydrochloride).

cataract, a disease of the eye that gets worse and worse, in which the lens loses its clearness. A gray-white film can be seen in the lens, behind the pupil. Most cataracts are caused by the functions of the body breaking down. This occurs most often after 50 years of age. Trauma, as a puncture wound, may result in cataracts. Sometimes, contact with poisons, as dinitro-phenol or naphthalene causes cataracts. **Congenital cataracts** may be inherited or caused by a virus infection during the first three months of pregnancy. If cataracts are not treated, sight is slowly lost. At first vision is blurred; then, bright lights glare, and images may appear double or distorted. Cataracts common to old age (**senile cataracts**) can be treated by removing the lens and wearing special contact lenses or glasses. The soft cataracts of children and young adults may be either cut and drained or broken up by the use of high pitched sound waves (ultrasound). The eye is then flushed and the fragments are removed through a small cut.

catarrh, *obsolete.* inflammation and draining of the mucous membranes.

catastrophic care, a type of medical care that involves intensive, very technical life-support systems for a severely ill or hurt patient.

catastrophic health insurance, health insurance that pays for the cost of severe or long-term injury or illness.

catastrophic reaction, the confused response to a bad shock or a sudden threatening state. This reaction often occurs in the victims of car crashes and disasters.

catatonia /kat'ətō'nē·ə/, a state of not being able to move due to a problem in the nerves of the muscles, which become very stiff. Catatonia is less often marked by improper, erratic actions. See also **catatonic schizophrenia.** –**catatonic,** *adj.*

catatonic excitement, a state of extreme agitation that may occur when a patient can no longer remain completely still.

catatonic schizophrenia, a form of schizophrenia in which times of extreme withdrawal are followed by times of extreme excitement. While in the withdrawal stage, the person does not speak, and stupor, rigid muscles, blocking, and catalepsy (cerea flexibilitas) may be seen. While in the stage of excitement, the person's aimless, constant actions may range from mild agitation to violence. See also **catatonia.**

catatonic stupor, a state marked by a lack of response; it may be related to a patient's fear of losing the ability to control his or her impulses.

cat-bite fever. See **cat-scratch fever.**

catch-up growth, a child's faster growth rate after a time of slowed growth that is caused by a lack of something, as severe malnutrition or illness. Catch-up growth, which is common in infants born before they are due, involves a fast increase in weight, length, and size of head. This growth keeps up until the normal growth pattern is resumed. The degree of illness and its length of time may result in some problem with growth or in a defect, as in brain tissue.

cat-cry syndrome, a rare, inherited defect known at birth by a kittenlike cry caused by a problem of the voicebox (larynx). The state is linked with other qualities that include low birth weight, small head, "moon face," wide-set eyes that do not work together (strabismus), and low-set misshaped ears. Also called **cri-du-chat syndrome** /crēdoōshä′/, **chromosome 5p-syndrome.**

catecholamine /kat′əkəlam′in/, any one of a group of chemicals made by the body that work as important nerve transmitters. Catecholamines are also made by chemists as drugs. The main catecholamines made by the body are dopamine, epinephrine (also called adrenaline), and norepinephrine. Norepinephrine and epinephrine are made by the adrenal medulla glands. Epinephrine opens up blood vessels that serve muscles. Norepinephrine slightly closes down these blood vessels. Both compounds excite the heart. Dopamine is found mainly in certain types of nerve tissue in the brain (basal ganglia). The main job of catecholamines is to prepare the body to act—the "flight or fight" syndrome—which includes increased blood pressure, faster heart beat, faster breathing. At the same time other processes shut down, as digestion. Synthetic catecholamines are used to raise blood pressure and excite the heart in emergencies.

cat-eye syndrome, a rare, inherited defect in which the pupils of the eye look like the slitlike pupils of a cat. A closed anus, heart defects, and severe mental retardation may also be present.

catgut, a thread that does not dissolve, made from the intestines of sheep. Catgut is used to stitch up wounds in surgery.

catharsis /kəthär′sis/, **1.** a cleaning out. **2.** the process of bringing memories of things or events that were not pleasant to the surface of thought. This can be done with the technique of free association, often used with hypnosis and hypnotic drugs. Also called **psychocatharsis.** See also **abreaction.**

cathartic /kəthär′tik/, referring to a substance that aids bowel movement by exciting intestinal waves (peristalsis), increasing the bulk of feces, making the feces soft, or adding slick fluid to the wall of the intestines. The term *cathartic* implies a fluid bowel movement; this is in contrast to *laxative,* which implies a soft, formed stool. Cathartics that increase intestinal waves, usually by lightly scraping membranes of the intestine, include certain plant substances, as aloe. Saline cathartics, as sodium sulfate, magnesium sulfate, and magnesium hydroxide, dilute the contents of the intestines by holding water. Suppositories that are made of sodium biphosphate, sodium acid pyrophosphate, and sodium bicarbonate cause a bowel movement when the salts form carbon dioxide and the expanding gas excites the bowels to move. Also called **coprogogue.** See also **laxative.** **–catharsis,** *n.*

catheter /kath′ətər/, a hollow, flexible tube that can be put into a vessel or space in the body to take out or to add fluids. Most catheters are made of soft plastic or rubber and may be used for treatment or tests. Kinds of catheters include **acorn-tipped catheter, Foley catheter, intrauterine catheter.**

catheter hub, a threaded plastic connection at the end of intravenous (IV) tubing.

catheterization, putting a catheter into a body cavity or organ to add or take out fluid. The most common practice is putting a catheter into the bladder through the urethra to empty it before surgery. It is also used when a sterile urine sample is needed. Kinds of catheterization are **cardiac catheterization, hepatic vein catheterization, laryngeal catheterization.** See also **female catheterization, Foley catheter, male catheterization.** **–catheterize,** *v.*

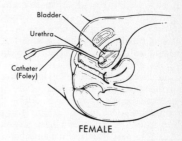

FEMALE

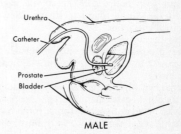

MALE

Catheterization (urethral)

cathexis /kəthek′sis/, to attach importance and feeling to a set idea, person, or object.

cathode, the negative pole of an electric circuit.

cathode ray, a stream of electrons given off by the negative electrode when the cathode is hit by positive ions. Examples include a cathode ray tube, an oscilloscope, and a television picture tube.

cathode-ray oscilloscope, a device that makes a picture of electric pulses by means of the screen of a cathode-ray tube. Oscilloscopes have many uses in medicine. For example, brain waves and heartbeats can be displayed in order to watch and test their functions.

cathode-ray tube (CRT), a tube that shines a beam onto a spot on a screen coated with a special substance that glows (phosphor). This makes a picture on the face of the tube.

catling, a long, sharp, double-edged knife used in amputation.

CAT scan. See **computerized axial tomography.**

cat-scratch fever, a disease that may be caused by a virus. It results from the scratch or bite of a cat that looks healthy. The first signs are swelling and bumps filled with pus near the scratch. Lymph nodes in the neck, head, groin, or armpits swell 2 weeks later. The symptoms can last for months. Also called **cat-bite disease.**

cat's eye amaurosis, blindness in one eye in which a bright reflection from the pupil is seen. The pupil is normally dark. The reflection is caused by a white mass in the eye. It is caused by a swelling or a cancerous tumor.

caudad /kô′dad/, toward the tail or end of the body, away from the head. Compare **cephalad.**

cauda equina, the nerve roots that come out from the end of the spinal cord and go down the spinal canal through the lower part of the spine and tailbone (coccyx). The cauda equina looks like a horse's tail.

caudal anesthesia, the use of a local drug to numb the senses in the lower part of the spinal canal (caudal portion). It is used during labor and childbirth. This type of drug is also used for surgery on the rectum and in surgery on the genitals or urinary tract. Caudal anesthesia has largely been replaced by anesthesia injected under the skin (epidural anesthesia). See also **regional anesthesia.**

caudate, having a tail.

caudate process, a small, raised tissue that comes out of the lower part of the tail end of the liver.

caul, the intact bag of waters (amniotic sac) that surrounds a baby at birth. The sac usually breaks open during the course of labor or birth. When it remains whole it must be torn or cut to allow the baby to breathe. In the past, pieces of the caul were sold to sailors as a good luck charm that would protect from death by drowning.

cauliflower ear, a thick, deformed ear caused by being hit over and over, as suffered by boxers.

caumesthesia /kô′məsthē′zhə/, a problem in which a patient has low body heat but feels a sense of intense heat.

causal connecting statements, a process in which a client is encouraged to identify the cause and effect between events that have affected the client's specific feelings, behavior, or responses.

causalgia /kôzal′jə/, a feeling of severe burning pain, sometimes with local redness of the skin.

It is caused by damage to a sensory nerve.

causality, referring to one event causing another. This process can be known in advance and can be watched. Causality is hard to prove; some experts think it is not possible to prove causality.

cause, anything that has an effect.

caustic, any substance that destroys living tissue, or causes burning or scarring, as silver nitrate, nitric acid, or sulfuric acid.

caustic poisoning, the accidental swallowing of strong chemicals resulting in burns and tissue damage to the mouth, esophagus, and stomach. The patient experiences immediate pain and swelling. The pulse may be weak and rapid. Breathing becomes shallow and the airway may swell shut. Complications of shock, perforation of the esophagus, and swelling of the throat leading to suffocation may be fatal. The patient should be hospitalized immediately. Recommended first aid is to drink large amounts of water and to remove any clothing that may have come in contact with the chemical. Giving "neutralizing" substance is not recommended as it may cause a heat-producing chemical reaction in the stomach. See also **acid burn, alkali burn.**

cautery /kô′tərē/, a device or substance that scars and burns the skin or other tissues.

cautery knife, an electric knife that cuts tissue and seals it with heat so it will not bleed.

cavalry bone. See **rider's bone.**

cavernous, having holes or hollow spaces. See also **cavernous hemangioma.**

cavernous body of the clitoris. See **corpus cavernosum.**

cavernous body of the penis. See **corpus cavernosum.**

cavernous hemangioma, a benign tumor that is present at birth. It is a red-blue spongy mass with blood vessels. The scalp, face, and neck are the most common sites, but these tumors have been found in the liver and other organs. Cavernous hemangiomas on the surface of the skin are brittle and can get infected easily if the skin is broken. Treatment includes x-ray therapy, sclerosing solutions, and surgery. Also called **angioma cavernosum, cavernoma.** Compare **capillary hemangioma, nevus flammeus.**

cavernous lymphangioma. See **lymphangioma cavernosum.**

cavernous rale, an abnormal hollow, metal-like sound heard when listening to the chest with a stethoscope. It is caused by in and out movement of a lobe of a lung while breathing. It means there is a disease.

cavernous sinus, one of a pair of unevenly shaped channels for blood vessels between the bone of the skull and the membrane covering the skull (dura mater). It is one of the five sinuses in the lower front portion of the skull that drain the blood from the skull membrane into the large vein in the neck (jugular vein).

cavernous sinus syndrome, a defect marked by swelling of the membrane that lines the eye (conjunctiva), the upper eyelid, and the root of the nose, and by deadening of the nerves that serve the eye. It is caused by a thrombosis of the cavernous sinus.

cavernous sinus thrombosis, a blood clot in the cavernous sinus. It is usually the result of infections near the eye or nose. Symptoms are swelling of the eye, blood vessel problems in the eye, and eye muscles that twitch. The infection may spread to the fluid of the brain and spinal cord (cerebrospinal fluid), and to the membranes that cover the brain and spinal cord (meninges). Treatment is with antibiotics and, sometimes, with drugs that slow the clotting action of the blood. Prevention includes leaving alone pimples or other sores around the nose and central face.

cavitary, denoting the presence of one or more hollow spaces.

cavitation, the making of hollow spaces in the body, as those made in the lung by tuberculosis.

cavity, 1. a hollow space in a larger structure, as the space that holds the lower organs of the body (peritoneal cavity), or the mouth (oral cavity). 2. *nontechnical.* a space in a tooth formed by decay of the tooth (caries).

cavity classification, the listing of cavities that refers to the tooth surfaces on which they occur, as labial, buccal, or occlusal; type of surface, as pitted or smooth; listing of cavity type by number as proposed by G.V. Black. See also **artificial classification cavity.**

cavosurface angle, in dentistry, the angle made where the wall of a drilled cavity meets the outer surface of the tooth.

cavum /kā'vəm/, *pl.* **cava** /kā'və/, 1. any hollow or cavity. 2. the major vein that runs through the trunk and returns to the heart (vena cava).

Cb, symbol for **columbium.**

CBC, short for **complete blood count.**

CBF, short for *cerebral blood flow.*

CBS, short for **chronic brain syndrome.**

CCU, short for **coronary care unit.**

Cd, symbol for **cadmium.**

CDC, short for **Centers for Disease Control.**

Ce, symbol for **cerium.**

CEA, short for **carcinoembryonic antigen.**

ceasmic teratism, a birth defect in which parts of the body that should be fused are not, as in cleft palate.

cecal /sē'kəl/, 1. referring to the top part of the large intestine (cecum). 2. referring to a blind spot in the field of vision.

cecal appendix. See **vermiform appendix.**

Ceclor, a trademark for an antibiotic drug (cefaclor).

cecocolostomy /sē'kōkəlos'təmē/, an operation that connects the upper and lower part of the large intestine (the cecum and the colon).

cecoileostomy /sē'kō·il'ē·os'təmē/, an operation that connects the lower part of the small intestine with the upper part of the large intestine, the ileum to the cecum. Also called **ileocecostomy** /il'ē-ōsēkos'təmē/.

cecostomy /sēkos'təmē/, an operation that makes an opening from the abdomen into the cecum. It is done as a short-term measure to relieve blocked intestines in a patient who cannot have major surgery.

cecum /sē'kəm/, the first part of the large intestine.

Cedilanid-D, a trademark for a drug that makes the heart pump harder. (deslanoside).

CeeNU, a trademark for an anticancer drug (lomustine).

cef-, a combining form for a cephalosporin.

cefaclor, a drug made from the fungus *Cephalosporium* (cephalosporin antibiotic). It is used to treat infections.
★CAUTION: Known allergy to drugs made from this fungus prohibits its use. It is used with caution in patients who are allergic to penicillins.
★ADVERSE EFFECTS: Among the most serious side effects are allergies, and diarrhea, nausea, and vomiting.

cefadroxil monohydrate, a drug made from the fungus *Cephalosporium* (cephalosporin antibiotic). It is used to treat bacterial infections.
★CAUTION: Known allergies to drugs made from this fungus prohibit its use. It is used with caution in patients who are allergic to penicillins.
★ADVERSE EFFECTS: Among the most serious side effects are allergies, and diarrhea, nausea, and vomiting.

Cefadyl, a trademark for an antibiotic (cephapirin).

cefamandole nafate, a drug made from the fungus *Cephalosporium* (cephalosporin antibiotic). It is used to treat bacterial infections.
★CAUTION: Known allergy to drugs made from this fungus prohibits its use. It is used with caution in patients who are allergic to penicillin.
★ADVERSE EFFECTS: Among the most serious side effects are allergies, blood clots in the legs (phlebitis), and pain when given in the muscle.

cefazolin sodium, an antibacterial drug made from the fungus *Cephalosporium.* It is used to treat a number of infections.
★CAUTION: Known allergy to drugs made from this fungus prohibits its use. It is used with caution in patients who are allergic to penicillin.

★ADVERSE EFFECTS: Among the more serious side effects are pain at the site where it is given, and allergies.

Cefizox, a trademark for a cephalosporin antibiotic (ceftizoxime).

Cefobid, a trademark for a cephalosporin antibiotic (cefoperazone).

cefonicid sodium, a cephalosporin-type antibiotic given by injection. It is given for infections of the lower respiratory or urinary tract, skin, bones and joints, blood, and before surgery to prevent infection.
★CAUTION: A history of allergy to cephalosporins or penicillin prohibits its use.
★ADVERSE EFFECTS: Pain and irritation may occur at the injection site. Occasionally, allergic reactions and stomach distress occur.

cefoperazone sodium, a cephalosporin antibiotic used to treat lung infections, bowel, skin, and female reproductive tract infections and blood poisoning caused by bacteria.
★CAUTION: Allergies to drugs made from the fungus *Cephalosporium* prohibit its use.
★ADVERSE EFFECTS: Among the most serious side effects are itching, rash, blood defects, and skin reactions to the shot.

ceforanide, a cephalosporin-type antibiotic given by injection. It is given for infections of the lower respiratory or urinary tract, skin, bones and joints, blood, and before surgery to prevent injection.
★CAUTION: A history of allergy to cephalosporins or penicillin prohibits its use.
★ADVERSE EFFECTS: Allergic reations and stomach distress may occur.

cefotaxime sodium, a cephalosporin antibiotic used to treat infections of the lungs, genitals, urinary tract, bowels, skin, bones and joints, and central nervous system and blood poisoning caused by bacteria.
★CAUTION: Allergy to drugs made from the fungus *Cephalosporium* prohibits its use.
★ADVERSE EFFECTS: The most common side effects are itching, bowel trouble, fungal infections, and skin reactions to the shot.

cefoxitin sodium, a cephalosporin antibiotic used to treat bacterial infections.
★CAUTION: Known allergy to drugs made from the fungus *Cephalosporium* prohibits its use. It is used with caution in patients who are allergic to penicillins.
★ADVERSE EFFECTS: Among the most serious side effects are allergies, blood clots in the legs, (phlebitis), and muscle pain where the shot is given.

ceftizoxime sodium, a cephalosporin antibiotic used to treat bacterial infections.
★CAUTION: Known allergy to this drug prohibits its use. It is used with caution in patients who are allergic to penicillin.
★ADVERSE EFFECTS: Among the most serious side effects are allergies, blood disorders, and pain at the place where the shot is given.

cefuroxime sodium, a cephalosporin antibiotic used to treat lung, urinary tract, and skin infections, blood poisoning caused by bacteria, meningitis, gonorrhea, and to prevent infections after surgery.
★CAUTION: Allergy to drugs made from the fungus *Cephalosporium* prohibits its use.
★ADVERSE EFFECTS: Among the most common side effects are itching, rash, blood defects, and skin reactions to the shot.

cel-, coel-, 1. a combining form that means 'a cavity of the body.' **2.** a combining form that means 'a swelling or tumor, hernia.'

Celestone, a trademark for a drug used to treat severe disorders, as lung disease, leukemia, allergies, rheumatic disease, and eye disease (betamethasone).

celiac artery, a thick branch of the blood vessel that serves the belly (abdominal aorta). It starts below the muscle that holds the lungs above the stomach (diaphragm). The celiac artery divides into three arteries that serve the stomach, the liver, and the spleen.

celiac disease, a defect in the chemistry of food breakdown that is present from birth. A patient with this defect cannot digest the gluten of some grain foods. The disease affects adults and young children, who may suffer from a swollen belly, vomiting, diarrhea, muscle wasting, and extreme fatigue. A symptom is a pale, foul-smelling stool that floats on water due to its high fat content. The patient may also be unable to digest lactose. Leaving all milk products out of the diet will help this problem. Most patients do well with a high-protein, high-calorie, gluten-free diet. Rice and corn are good in place of wheat. Any vitamin or mineral shortage can be helped with vitamin pills. Also called **celiac sprue, gluten-induced enteropathy, nontropical sprue.** Compare **malabsorption syndrome.**

celiac plexus. See **solar plexus.**

celiac rickets, growth and bone defects that result when the patient cannot absorb fat and calcium. See also **celiac disease, rickets.**

celio-, a combining form referring to the belly region.

celiocolpotomy /sē′lē·ōkəlpot′əmē/, a cut into the belly region through the vagina.

celioma /sēlē·ō′mə/, a tumor in the belly.

celioscope. See **laparoscope.**

cell, the basic unit of all living tissue. Cells are made of a nucleus, cytoplasm, and organelles held together by a cell membrane. Within the nucleus are the nucleolus (containing RNA) and chromatin granules (containing protein and DNA) that grow into chromosomes, which determine hereditary traits. Organelles in the cytoplasm include the endoplasmic reticulum, ribosomes, the Golgi complex, mitochondria, lysosomes, and the centrosome. Some cells lack a nucleus when they are mature, as red blood cells.

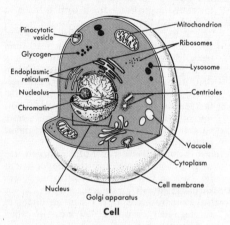

Pinocytotic vesicle
Mitochondrion
Ribosomes
Glycogen
Endoplasmic reticulum
Lysosome
Nucleolus
Centrioles
Chromatin
Vacuole
Cytoplasm
Cell membrane
Nucleus
Golgi apparatus

Cell

cell biology, the science that deals with the structures, processes, and functions of cells, especially human cells.

cell body, the part of a cell that contains the nucleus and cytoplasm around it. The cell body does the work that keeps the cell alive.

cell cycle, the series of events that occur during the growth and division of cells.

cell death, 1. the death of a cell. **2.** the point in the process of dying at which the cells of the body no longer perform their work.

cell division, the constant process by which a cell divides into two cells. Also called **mitosis.** Compare **meiosis.**

cell-mediated immune response, an allergy that does not show up right away. It is the response of special white blood cells (sensitized T lymphocytes) rather than by antibodies. Cell-mediated immune reactions deal with fighting off certain bacteria, fungi, and viruses, cancer cells, and other foreign protein or tissue. A common type of this response is skin rash from poison ivy. Also called **cellular hypersensitivity reaction, type IV hypersensitivity.**

cell membrane, the outer wall of a cell. It often has threads that stick out and also contains the cell's cytoplasm. The cell membrane is so thin and fragile it is very hard to see with a light microscope and can be studied in detail only with an electron microscope. The membrane takes care of the exchange of materials between the cell's cytoplasm and the area around it. Also called **plasma membrane.**

cellular hypersensitivity reaction. See **cell-mediated immune response.**

cellular immunity, the growth of special white blood cells (T lymphocytes) after exposure to a foreign substance (antigen). These T cells go to work each time they meet the same substance. Cellular immunity helps the body to resist infection caused by viruses and some bacteria. For example, a person who has had chickenpox will not get the disease a second time. Cellular immunity also plays a role in delayed allergic responses. It is involved in resistance to cancer, some diseases of the immune system, graft rejection, and some allergies. Also called **cell-mediated immunity.** Compare **humoral immunity.**

cellulitis, an infection of the skin that usually stays in one place, as the lower leg. The symptoms are heat over the area, redness, pain, and swelling, and occasionally fever, chills, and headache. Abscess and tissue destruction usually follow if antibiotics are not taken.

cellulose /sel'yoolōs/, a colorless, transparent solid carbohydrate that is the main part of the cell walls of plants. It is nondigestible by humans. However, it provides the bulk needed for proper functioning of the stomach and intestines. See also **dietary fiber.**

cell wall, the structure that covers and protects the cell membrane of some kinds of cells, as certain bacteria and all plant cells.

Celontin, a trademark for a drug used to prevent convulsions (methsuximide).

celothelioma. See **mesothelioma.**

Celsius (C) /sel'sē·əs/, a temperature scale in which 0° is the freezing point of water and 100° is the boiling point of water at sea level. Also called **centigrade.** Compare **Fahrenheit.**

cement, 1. a sticky, mucilagelike substance that helps neighboring tissue cells stick together. **2.** any of a variety of dental materials used to fill cavities or to hold bridgework or other dental prostheses in place. **3.** a material used to position an artificial joint in adjacent bone.

cemental fiber, any one of the many fibers that extend from the teeth to the bone.

cement base, a layer of insulated dental cement. It is sometimes medicated. It is pressed into the bottom of a prepared cavity to protect the pulp and reduce the bulk of fillings or crowns.

cementoblastoma /simen'tōblastō'mə/, a cell that is involved in the growth of cementum.

cementoma /sē'mentō'mə/, a pooling of cementum at the tip of a tooth. It is probably caused by injury.

cementopathia, an abnormal condition of the teeth caused by dead cementum. Cementopathia contributes to the swelling (periodontitis) and breakdown (periodontosis) of the tissues that support the teeth.

cementum, the bonelike connective tissue that covers the roots of the the teeth and helps to support them.

cen-, a combining form meaning 'common.'

cenesthesia /sē′nesthē′zhə/, the general sense of existing, based on all the various stimuli and reactions throughout the body at any specific moment.

cenogenesis, the development of traits that are absent in earlier forms of a species, usually as an adaptation to the environment.

censor, 1. a person who evaluates books, newspapers, plays, works of art, speech, or other means of expression in order to cut out certain kinds of information. 2. a form of psychological suppression that allows unconscious thoughts to rise to consciousness only if they are heavily masked.

cente-, a combining form meaning 'puncture,' as in amniocentesis.

center, 1. the middle point of the body. 2. a group of nerve cells with a common function, as the center in the brain that controls the heartbeat.

center of gravity, the midpoint or center of the weight of a body or object. In the standing adult, the center of gravity lies in the middle of the body at a level between the belly button and the pubic bone.

Centers for Disease Control (CDC), a federal agency of the United States government that offers facilities and services for the investigation, identification, prevention, and control of disease. It is concerned with all aspects of the study of the causes of disease (epidemiology) and the laboratory diagnosis of disease. Originally concerned only with communicable diseases, the CDC's interests today include environmental health, smoking, hunger, poisoning, and problems of health in the workplace.

centi-, a combining form meaning 'a hundred or a hundredth,' as in centiliter.

centigrade (C). See **Celsius.**

centimeter (cm) /sen′timē′tər/, a metric unit of measurement. It is equal to one hundredth of a meter, or 0.3937 inches.

centimeter-gram-second system (CGS, cgs), an internationally accepted scientific system of expressing length, mass, and time in basic units of centimeters, grams, and seconds. The CGS system is slowly being replaced by the International System of Units based on the meter, kilogram, and second.

centipede bite, a wound produced by the poison claws and the jaws of a centipede, a wormlike insect with many pairs of legs. The bite of a few species, particularly in the southern United States, may cause painful swelling, fever, headache, vomiting, and dizziness.

centipoise, a measure of the thickness (viscosity) of a liquid, equal to one-hundredth of a poise.

For example, the thickness of glycerine is 1490 centipoise, compared with 1.005 centipoise for water.

central, referring to or situated at a center.

central amaurosis, a form of blindness. It is caused by a disease of the central nervous system.

central canal of spinal cord, a tunnel that runs the entire length of the spinal cord. It has most of the body's fluid of the brain and spinal cord. This fluid flows into the canal from a space in the brain. Bleeding in the brain may form blood clots that block drainage of the fluid from the space. Lumbar puncture is often done to get samples of fluid for diagnostic purposes. However, the spinal cord ends at the first lumbar vertebra (about level with the bottom of the rib cage). The fluid is drawn from an area lower on the spine. See also **lumbar puncture.**

central chemoreceptor, any of the sensory nerve cells or chemical receptors that are located at the base of the brain. Also called **medullary chemoreceptors.**

central chondrosarcoma, a cancerous tumor of cartilage that forms inside a bone. Also called **enchondrosarcoma.**

central control hypothesis, a concept that the nervous system below the level of the cerebral cortex is controlled by mechanisms that are very similar to those of animal ancestors.

central electrode, a key part of a radiation detection instrument. It consists of a positively-charged rigid wire in the center of a gas-filled cylinder. The electrode attracts electrons given off due to radiation and converts them into an electric current.

central nervous system (CNS), one of the two main divisions of the nervous system of the body. It is made up of the brain and the spinal cord. The central nervous system deals with information to and from the peripheral nervous system. It is the main network of coordination and control for the entire body. The brain controls many functions and sensations, such as sleep, sexual activity, muscle movement, hunger, thirst, memory, and the emotions. The spinal cord contains various types of nerve fibers from the brain and acts as a switching and relay terminal for the peripheral nervous system. The 12 pairs of cranial nerves emerge directly from the brain. The nerves of the peripheral system leave the spinal cord separately between the vertebrae of the backbone. However, they unite to form 31 pairs of spinal nerves containing sensory fibers and motor fibers. Sensory nerves carry impulses to the spinal cord and brain. Motor nerves carry impulses (or "commands") from the central nervous system to the muscles and glands. The brain contains more than 10 billion nerve cells. Billions of other cells help form the soft, jellylike substance of the brain. Flowing through many cavities of the central nervous system is the fluid of the brain and spine. This fluid helps to protect the central nervous system from injury. It affects the rate of breathing through cells that measure its content of carbon dioxide. The brain and the spinal cord are made up of gray matter and white matter. The gray matter has mainly nerve cells and linked filaments. The white matter is made up of bundles of mainly insulated (myelinated) nerve fibers. The central nervous system grows from the neural tube of the embryo, which first appears in the third week of pregnancy. The cavity of the neural tube is kept after birth in the spaces (ventricles) of the brain and in the central canal of the spinal cord. Compare **peripheral nervous system.** See also **brain, spinal cord.**

central nervous system depressant, any drug that lessons the activity of the central nervous system (CNS), such as alcohol, barbiturates, and sleeping pills. Depressants, especially the tranquilizers, are the most widely given drugs throughout the world. These drugs work by depressing nerve activity throughout the CNS by decreasing the amount of chemicals that carry nerve impulses. Alcohol affects the CNS more than any other part of the body. All depressants can be abused, particularly through the use of unlawfully gotten depressants. Constant use of these drugs can make a condition in which the person's body needs the drugs to feel normal. This dependence leads to compulsive drug use. The compulsive use of barbiturates, tranquilizers, and related drugs is believed to be bigger than that of morphine or heroin. The most abused depressants are the barbiturates, especially pentobarbital, secobarbital, glutethimide, methyprylon, and methaqualone. These substances have popular street names on the illicit market, as "reds" (secobarbital) and "yellows" (pentobarbital). Sudden withdrawal of CNS depressants that have been used in high doses for prolonged periods can be fatal. Withdrawal treatment commonly involves substituting pentobarbital, then gradually reducing the dosage over a 10-day to 3-week period.

central nervous system stimulant, a substance that speeds up the activity of the central nervous system (CNS). CNS stimulants work by increasing the rate of nerve impulses or by blocking substances that would calm the nervous system. Many natural and artificial chemicals stimulate the CNS. Only a few are used in therapy. Caffeine, a potent CNS stimulant, is used to help restore mental alertness and overcome depressed breathing. It may cause nausea, nervousness, ringing in the ears, tremor, abnormal heart beats, increased urination, and visual disturbances. Amphetamines have been

used to treat long-term drowsiness and overweight. However, amphetamines have a high potential for abuse. They may cause dizziness, restlessness, rapid heart beat, high blood pressure, headache, mouth dryness, an unpleasant taste, digestive disorders, and hives. Amphetamines are given for the overactivity (hyperkinetic child syndrome) because some stimulants have a calming effect on children. Some are used to stimulate the breathing center and to restore consciousness after anesthesia or for overdose of depressants. Also called **analeptic.**

central nervous system syndrome (CNS syndrome), a group of nerve and emotional symptoms. They are caused by a massive whole-body dosage of radiation. The symptoms include hysteria and disorientation that increases during the last 24 to 48 hours before death.

central nervous system tumor, a growth of the brain or spinal cord that usually does not spread beyond the central nervous system. It may invade other tissues and have widespread effects on body functions. Brain tumors are about 4 times more common than those arising in the spinal cord. From 20% to 40% of brain tumors have spread from a main cancer in the breast, lung, stomach and intestines, kidney, or skin. See also **brain tumor, spinal cord tumor.**

central neurogenic hyperventilation (CNHV), a pattern of rapid and regular breathing at a rate of about 25 per minute. This occurs in patients who are in coma. Increasing regularity, rather than rate, shows a greater depth of coma.

central placenta previa, a problem of childbirth in which the placenta is implanted in the lower part of the uterus so that it completely covers the narrow lower end of the uterus (cervix). As the cervix opens during labor, the placenta is slowly separated from the blood vessels in the lining of the uterus. This results in bleeding that usually begins slowly, is painless, and continues to heavy bleeding that is life-threatening to the mother and the baby. An emergency cesarean section is usually done to save both lives. The condition may be discovered before bleeding begins by ultrasound or by vaginal examination in the normal course of prenatal care. See also **placenta previa.**

central ray (CR), the portion of the x-ray beam that is directed toward the center of the film or of the object being radiographed.

central scotoma, an area of blindness or lowered vision involving the central area of the retina.

central sleep apnea, a condition in which a person stops breathing during sleep because of reduced output from the central nervous system. It may be related to a tumor, polio, or other causes.

central tendon, a broad sheet of connective tissue (muscles, tendons, and ligaments) that runs across the middle of the body below the lungs. It is connected to the spine, ribs, and breastbone, and it forms the diaphragm.

central venous catheter, a tube that is used to measure **central venous pressure.** It is threaded through the veins of the body until its tip rests in the superior vena cava or right atrium of the heart.

central venous pressure (CVP), the blood pressure in the large veins of the body. It is measured with a pressure gauge and a **central venous catheter.**

central venous pressure (CVP) monitor, a device for measuring and recording the blood pressure inside a large vein by means of a catheter and a pressure gauge.

central venous return, the blood from the body's veins that flows into the right upper chamber (atrium) of the heart through the major vein in the trunk (vena cava).

central vision, vision that results from images falling on the center of the retina.

Centrax, a trademark for a drug that relieves anxiety (prazepam).

centrifugal /sentrif′ōōgəl/, referring to a force that is directed outward, away from a central point or axis, as the force that keeps the moon in its orbit around the earth.

centrifuge /sen′trifyōōj′/, a device for separating components in a liquid by spinning the mixture at high speeds. Centrifugal force causes the heavier substances to move to one part of the container, leaving the lighter substances in another. Blood is centrifuged, for example, for giving transfusions of just plasma.

centrilobular /sen′trəlob′yələr/, referring to something situated at the center of a lobe.

centriole /sen′trē·ōl′/, an organ within a cell, usually as a part of the center of a cell (centrosome). Often occurring in pairs, centrioles are linked to cell division. Under a light microscope, the centrioles appear as tiny dots. An electron microscope shows they are tiny cylinders positioned at right angles to each other. Their walls are made up of nine bundles of fine tubules, three tubules to a bundle. The precise function of centrioles is still unclear.

centripetal /sentrip′ətəl/, **1.** referring to a direction, as a sensory nerve impulse traveling toward the brain. **2.** the direction of a force pulling an object toward the center or an axis of rotation, as opposed to a centrifugal force.

centro-, centri-, a combining form meaning 'center.'

centromere /sen′trəmir/, a specialized, constricted region of the chromosome. It joins two chromosome halves (chromatids) to each other and attaches to the spindle fiber in cell reproduction. During cell division the centromeres split longitudinally, half going to each of the new daughter chromosomes.

centrosome, a region present in animal cells and in some plants. It is located near the nucleus and is involved in cell division.

centrosphere, a condensed area of cytoplasm surrounding the centrioles in the centrosome of a cell.

cephalad /sef′əlad/, a direction that is toward the head, away from the end or tail. Compare **caudad.**

cephalalgia /sef′əlal′jē·ə/, headache, often combined with another word to describe the type of headache, as histamine cephalalgia. See also **histamine headache.**

cephalexin /sef′əlek′sin/, a cephalosporin antibiotic used to treat certain infections.
★CAUTION: Known allergy to any cephalosporins prohibits its use. It is used cautiously in patients who are allergic to penicillin.
★ADVERSE EFFECTS: Nausea, diarrhea, and allergic reactions may occur.

cephalgia. See **cephalalgia, headache.**

cephalhematoma /sef′əlhē′mətō′mə, -hem′ətō′- mə/, swelling caused by the pooling of blood under the scalp. It may begin to form in the scalp of a baby during labor. It may slowly become larger in the first few days after birth. It is usually a result of trauma, often from forceps. Compare **caput succedaneum, molding.**

cephalic /sifal′ik/, referring to the head.

cephalic presentation, a classification of a baby's position during labor in which the head is at the narrow lower end of the uterus (cervix). Cephalic presentation is usually further qualified by the part of the head presenting, as the back (occiput) or front (bregma).

cephalic vein, one of the four superficial veins of the arm. It begins in the network of veins in the hand and winds upward to end at a vein near the shoulder.

cephalocaudal, referring to the length of the body, or the relationship between the head and the lower end of the spine.

cephalomelus /sef′əlom′ələs/, a deformed fetus. It has a structure resembling an arm or a leg pushing outward from the head.

cephalometry /sef′əlom′ətrē/, the scientific measurement of the head. It may be done in dentistry to determine orthodontic procedures for straightening the teeth.

cephalopelvic, referring to the relationship between a fetus's head and the mother's pelvis.

cephalopelvic disproportion (CPD), a condition in which a baby's head is too large or a mother's birth canal too small to allow normal labor or birth. In **relative CPD,** the size of the baby's head may be within normal limits but larger than average. Alternatively, the size of the mother's birth canal is within normal limits but smaller than average, or both. Relative CPD is often overcome by shaping of the head, the forces of labor, or by the use of forceps to effect childbirth. In **absolute CPD,** the baby's head is definitely large, or the mother's birth canal is very small. This makes vaginal birth impossible. See also **clinical pelvimetry, x-ray pelvimetry.**

cephalosporin /sef'əlōspôr'in/, an antibiotic originally derived from the fungus *Cephalosporium acremonium.* Cephalosporins are similar in chemical structure to penicillins.

cephalothin sodium /sef'əlōthin/, a cephalosporin antibacterial used to treat many infections.
★CAUTION: Known allergy to any cephalosporins prohibits its use. It is used with caution in patients who are allergic to penicillin.
★ADVERSE EFFECTS: Among the more serious side effects are pain at the site of injection and allergic reactions.

cephalothoracopagus /sef'əlōthôr'əkop'əgəs/, a twin fetal monster united at the head, neck, and chest.

cephapirin, an antibiotic used to treat various infections, including blood poisoning (septicemia), heart infection (endocarditis), bone infection (osteomyelitis), and infections of the breathing tract, urinary tract, and skin.
★CAUTION: Known sensitivity to cephalosporin antibiotics prohibits its use.
★ADVERSE EFFECTS: Among the most serious side effects are anemia and other blood disorders and allergic reactions.

cephradine, a cephalosporin antibacterial used to treat certain bacterial infections.
★CAUTION: Known allergy to any cephalosporins prohibits its use. It is used carefully in patients who are allergic to penicillin.
★ADVERSE EFFECTS: Nausea, diarrhea, and allergic reactions may occur.

cer-, a combining form meaning 'wax,' as in cerumen.

ceramics, the technology of making dental restorations from fused porcelain and other glasslike materials.

cercaria /sərker'ē-ə/, *pl.* **cercariae,** a tiny, wormlike form of the class Trematoda. It develops in a freshwater snail. It is released into the water and swims toward the sun, rising to the surface of the water in the warmest part of the day. Cercariae enter the body of a human, usually by direct invasion through the skin, or through a cut or other break in the skin. They form lumps (cysts). They end their growth in many organs of the body. Each species tends to go to a particular organ, as *Fasciola hepatica,* which becomes a liver trematode (fluke). See also **fluke, schistosomiasis.**

cerclage /sərkläzh'/, **1.** a procedure in which the ends of a fractured bone or the chips of a broken kneecap are bound together with a wire loop or a metal band. This holds the bone parts in position until the break is healed. **2.** a procedure in which a silicone band is applied around the white of the eye (sclera) to restore

contact between the retina and the blood vessel layer (choroid) when the retina is detached. **3.** an obstetric procedure in which stitches (suture) are used to hold the narrow lower end of the uterus (cervix) closed to prevent spontaneous abortion. The band is usually released when the pregnancy is at full term. This allows labor to begin. See also **incompetent cervix.**

cerea flexibilitas /sirē'ə flek'sibil'itas/, a psychiatric condition, often found in catatonic schizophrenia. The arms and legs stay for an indefinite period of time in the positions in which they are placed. Also called **flexibilitas cerea, waxy flexibility.** See also **catalepsy.**

cerebellar /ser'əbel'ər/, referring to a part of the brain (cerebellum).

cerebellar angioblastoma, a tumor in a part of the brain (cerebellum). It is made up of a mass of blood vessels. It sometimes appears as a lump (cyst).

cerebellar artery occlusion, blockage of one of the arteries leading to part of the brain that controls movement. (cerebellum). It may result in loss of awareness of pain and temperature, numbness of the face, and paralysis or lack of coordination on one side of the body.

cerebellar atrophy, a wasting of a part of the brain that controls movement (cerebellum).

cerebellar cortex, the outer layer of gray matter of a part of the brain (cerebellum). It covers the white substance in the core.

cerebellar cortical degeneration. See **alcoholic nutritional cerebellar degeneration.**

cerebeller speech, abnormal speech caused by diseases of a part of the brain (cerebellum). It is marked by slow, jerky, and slurred pronunciation of words. The tone may be intermittent and explosive or monotonous and unvaried in pitch.

cerebellum /ser'əbel'əm/, *pl.* **cerebellums, cerebella,** a part of the brain located at the base of the skull behind the brain stem. It consists of two cerebellar lobes, one on each side, and a middle section called the vermis. Three pairs of stalks link it with the brain stem. The cerebellum is concerned with coordinating voluntary muscular activity, as walking, and maintaining equilibrium.

cerebral, referring to the brain (cerebrum).

cerebral aneurysm, a ballooning of an artery in the brain (cerebrum). It is commonly the result of inborn weakness of the artery wall. Cerebral aneurysms may also be caused by infection, as bacterial endocarditis or syphilis, by tumors, hardening of the arteries, and injury. Cerebral aneurysms may occur in infancy or old age. They may be as small as a pinhead or as large as an orange. Most are the size of a pea. Depending on its size and location, a cerebral aneurysm may cause headache, drowsiness, confusion, dizziness, and weakness and pain of the face. Ringing in the ears, vision problems, stiff neck, and partial paralysis also occur. Since about half of all cerebral aneurysms break, the patient is closely watched for signs of brain bleeding. Very small aneurysms seldom break. The patient is treated by being placed in a bed, with the head raised at a 45-degree angle. He or she is kept quiet in a dark room. Drugs may be given. The pulse, blood pressure, breathing and nervous system function, as unevenly widened eye pupils, are checked often. An icebag may be used to relieve headache. Cooling measures may be ordered to lessen blood flow to the brain and decrease the risk of a break of the aneurysm. The patient is turned gently every 2 to 4 hours and may need to be fed. Nonstrenuous exercises of the arms and legs are done to maintain function. A sample of cerebrospinal fluid is examined for blood, which indicates the aneurysm has ruptured. A x-ray test (angiogram) will show the exact location of the aneurysm. If surgery is needed, the usual procedure involves opening the skull (craniotomy) and clamping the aneurysm off from the flow of blood. If the aneurysm is too large to be clamped, a plastic coating may be applied to support the weakened artery. When the patient is too ill to survive a craniotomy, the neurosurgeon may clamp the common carotid artery to reduce blood flow to the area of the aneurysm, provided other blood vessels can supply enough blood to the brain.

cerebral angiography, an x-ray test for seeing the blood vessels of the brain. A dye (radiopaque contrast material) is injected into an artery, and a series of x-rays are taken at certain intervals.

cerebral anoxia, a condition in which too little oxygen reaches the brain. This state, which is caused by failure of circulation, can exist for no more than 4 to 6 minutes before permanent brain damage occurs.

cerebral cortex, a thin layer of gray matter on the surface of the brain (cerebrum). It has brain cells that integrate higher mental functions, general movement, stomach functions, and behavioral reactions. Research has described more than 200 different areas and 47 separate functions of the cerebral cortex. The motor area has been studied in detail, because its stimulation with electrodes causes muscles to contract. The left cerebral hemisphere is dominant in right-handed people, and those who are left-handed have dominant right hemispheres (see cerebral dominance). The motor speech area is better developed in the left hemisphere of right-handed persons, for example. Its destruction causes loss of speech (aphasia) or other speech defects. Stimulation of the frontal area affects circulation, breathing, widening of the pupils, and other activity. Also called **pallium.**

cerebral dominance, the role of each of the two halves of the cerebrum (cerebral hemispheres) in the integration and control of different functions. The left hemisphere houses the logical, reasoning activities and controls reading, writing, speech, and analytic activities. The right hemisphere concerns imagination, intuitions, creativity, spatial skills, art, and left-hand control. In 90% of the population, the left cerebral hemisphere dominates the ability to speak, write, and understand spoken and written words. In the other 10% of the population, either the right hemisphere or both hemispheres dominates. The right cerebral hemisphere also dominates the integration of certain sounds other than speaking, as the sounds of coughing, laughter, crying, and melodies. The right cerebral hemisphere perceives touch stimuli and visual relationships better than the left cerebral hemisphere. See also **Brodmann's areas.**

cerebral edema, a pooling of fluid in the brain tissues. It may be caused by an infection, tumor, injury, or poison. Early symptoms are involuntary contraction of muscles, widening of

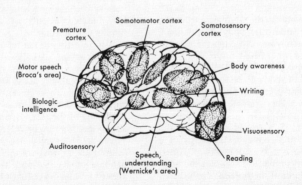

Cerebral cortex

pupils of the eye, and gradual loss of consciousness. It is a possibly fatal condition that requires emergency medical care.

cerebral embolism, a blood clot that stops the flow of blood through vessels of the brain. This results in lack of oxygen in cells beyond the clot. See also **cerebrovascular accident.**

cerebral evoked potential. See **evoked potential (EP).**

cerebral gigantism, an abnormal condition with excess weight and size at birth, too rapid growth until 4 or 5 years old, and then change to normal growth. Also called **Sotos' syndrome.**

cerebral hemiplegia, paralysis of one side of the body caused by a tumor in the brain.

cerebral hemisphere, one of the halves of the brain (cerebrum). The two cerebral hemispheres are divided by a deep groove at the top but are connected at the bottom by the corpus callosum. Prominent grooves further subdivide each hemisphere into four major lobes.

cerebral hemorrhage, bleeding from a blood vessel in the brain. Three criteria used to classify cerebral hemorrhages are: location, the kind of vessel involved, and the cause. Each kind of cerebral hemorrhage has its own symptoms, some of which include headache, partial paralysis, loss of consciousness, nausea, vomiting, and seizures. Most cerebral hemorrhages occur deep in a cerebral hemisphere. They are caused by the breaking of a hardened artery as a result of high blood pressure. Other causes of rupture include inborn ballooning of brain arteries (aneurysm) and head injury. Bleeding may lead to destruction of brain tissue. Extensive bleeding leads usually to death. Blood may be found in the spinal fluid. A CAT scan may be done to find the place of the tumor and to keep the bleeding apart from a blood clot or other disorder. Surgery is often necessary to stop the bleeding in order to prevent death. The person is kept without movement. The neck is held straight to allow adequate blood flow to and from the head. Recovery from the condition is often complete. Physical therapy and speech therapy may be needed during recovery. Depending on the extent and the location of the damaged tissue, residual effects may include loss of speech or understanding speech (aphasia), diminished mental function, or loss of the function of one of the special senses. See also **subarachnoid hemorrhage.**

cerebral nerve. See **cranial nerve.**

cerebral palsy, a motor nerve disorder. It is caused by a permanent brain defect or an injury at birth or shortly thereafter. The symptoms depend on the area of the brain involved and the extent of damage. Milder cases have spastic paralysis of the legs or both limbs on one side and normal intelligence. More severe cases have widespread loss of normal muscle control, seizures, numbness, mental retardation, blocked speech, vision, and hearing. The disorder is usually linked to too early or abnormal birth and lack of oxygen during birth, causing damage to the nervous system. Abnormalities in breathing, sucking, swallowing, and responsiveness are usually visible soon after birth. However, the stiff, awkward movements of the infant's limbs may be overlooked for several months. Walking is usually delayed, and when the child tries to walk, the walk has a scissorslike quality. The arms may be affected only slightly but the fingers are often spastic. Some reflexes are too strong. There may be slurred speech, and delay in acquiring bowel and bladder control. There also may be slow movements of the face and hands. Early identification of the disorder is important so that an exercise and training program can be started. Treatment may include braces, correction by surgery of deformities, speech therapy, and many drugs that relax the muscles and drugs that prevent convulsions. Many patients can lead near-normal, independent lives with the proper therapy. Even the severely affected can benefit from training and learn self-care activities, as washing, dressing, and feeding. Also called **congenital cerebral diplegia, Little's disease.**

cerebral perfusion pressure (CPP), a measure of the amount of blood flow to the brain. It is the difference between the pressure in the brain and the blood pressure in the arteries of the body.

cerebral tabes. See **general paresis.**

cerebral thrombosis, a clotting of blood in any brain blood vessel.

cerebral vascular. See **cerebrovascular.**

cerebrocerebellar atrophy, a breakdown of a part of the brain (cerebellum) caused by certain nutritional diseases.

cerebroid /ser'əbroid/, looking like the substance of the brain.

cerebroma /ser'əbrō'mə/, any unusual mass of brain tissue.

cerebromedullary tube. See **neural tube.**

cerebroretinal angiomatosis /ser'əbrōret'ənəl, sərē'brō-/, a hereditary disease of small tumorlike growths in the retina of the eye and part of the brain (cerebellum). Similar growths on the spinal cord, pancreas, kidneys, and other organs are also common. Seizures and mental retardation may be present.

cerebroside /ser'əbrōsīd/, any of a group of fatty carbohydrates found in the brain and other parts of the nervous system.

cerebrospinal /ser'əbrōspī'nəl, sərē'brō-/, referring to the brain and the spinal cord.

cerebrospinal fluid (CSF), the fluid that flows through and protects the brain and the spinal canal. The clear colorless fluid has small amounts of proteins, glucose, and electrolytes.

Changes in the carbon dioxide content of CSF affect the breathing center in the brain, helping to control breathing. A brain tumor may stop the flow of the fluid. This results in a form of water on the brain (hydrocephalus). Other blockages of the flow of cerebrospinal fluid, as those caused by blood clots, result in more serious complications. Examination of CSF is important in diagnosing diseases of the central nervous system. Samples of the fluid are taken by inserting a needle between the third and the fourth lumbar vertebrae (lumbar puncture) and drawing out a small amount.

cerebrospinal nerves, the nerves that begin in the brain (12 pairs) and spinal cord (31 pairs).

cerebrotendinous xanthamosis. See **van Bogaert's disease.**

cerebrovascular /ser'əbrōvas'kyələr, sərē'brō-/, referring to the blood vessels and blood supply of the brain.

cerebrovascular accident (CVA), an embolus (blood clot) or bleeding in the brain. This results in lack of oxygen to the brain tissues that are normally supplied by the vessels. The aftereffects of a cerebrovascular accident depend on the location and extent of damage. Paralysis, weakness, speech defect, inability to understand language, or death may occur. Symptoms usually diminish somewhat after the first few days as brain swelling subsides. Physical therapy and speech therapy may restore much lost function. Also called **stroke.**

cerebrum /ser'əbrəm, sərē'brəm/, *pl.* **cerebrums, cerebra,** the largest and uppermost section of the brain, divided by a deep groove into the left and the right halves of the brain (cerebral hemispheres). At the bottom of the groove the hemispheres are connected by the corpus callosum. The internal structures of the hemispheres join with the brain stem through the cerebral stalks. Each cerebral hemisphere is made up of the large outer cerebral cortex layer (the "gray matter" of the brain), the underlying white substance, the internal basal ganglia, and certain other structures. The surface of the cerebrum is convoluted and lobed. The cerebrum has sensory and motor functions, and functions linked to integration of many mental activities. It makes a variety of electrical waves that can be recorded (electroencephalogram). These brain waves can be used to diagnose brain problems or to identify changed states of consciousness. They can also show brain death. Some of the other processes that are controlled by the cerebrum are memory, speech, writing, and emotional response. See also **cerebral cortex, cerebral hemisphere.** –**cerebral,** *adj.*

cerium (Ce), a gray rare earth element. Its atomic number is 58. Its atomic weight is 140.13. A compound of cerium (cerium oxalate) is used as a sedative, to relieve nausea, and to control coughing.

cerium nitrate, a drug applied to the skin of burn patients to control infections.

ceroid /sir'oid/, a golden, waxy pigment appearing in the stomach and intestines, the nervous system, and the muscles. It is also sometimes found in the livers of people with cirrhosis of the liver.

certification, a process in which a person, an institution, or an educational program is evaluated and seen as meeting certain standards. Certification is usually made by a nongovernmental agency. The purpose of certification is to make sure that the standards met are those necessary for the safe and ethical practice of the profession or service.

certified milk, raw milk that is handled and marketed in accordance with state health laws. The milk must be made by disease-free cows, which are regularly inspected by a veterinarian. The cows are milked by sterilized equipment in hygienic surroundings. The milk must have less than a certain low bacterial count. The milk must not be older than 36 hours when delivered.

Certified Nurse-Midwife (CNM), a person who is educated in the disciplines of nursing and midwifery. He or she is certified by the American College of Nurse-Midwives. Nurse-Midwifery practice is the care of normal women before, during, and after labor. It includes care of the newborn. See also **midwife.**

certified registered nurse anesthetist (CRNA). See **nurse anesthetist.**

certify, 1. to guarantee that certain requirements have been met based on expert knowledge of significant facts. **2.** to claim, by a legal process, that someone is insane. **3.** to claim the fact of someone's death in writing, usually on a form as required by local authority.

Cerubidine, a trademark for an anticancer drug (daunorubicin hydrochloride).

ceruloplasmin /sirōō'lōplaz'min/, a substance in blood plasma that carries most of the body's copper.

cerumen /sirōō'mən/, a yellowish or brownish waxy substance. It is made by sweat glands in the ear canal. Also called **earwax.**

ceruminolytic /sirōō'mənolit'ik/, referring to a drug or other substance used to dissolve earwax.

ceruminosis /sirōō'minō'sis/, excess buildup of earwax in the outer ear canal. It can cause discomfort, hearing loss, and irritation leading to an ear infection. Removal of excess cerumen is done by inserting a wax softening agent. This is followed by carefully flushing the ear with an ear syringe.

ceruminous gland /sirōō'minəs/, one of a number of tiny structures in the outer ear canal. It is believed to be a type of sweat gland. They release a waxy cerumen instead of watery sweat.

cervical /sur'vikəl/, referring to the neck or a necklike structure, as the narrow lower end of the uterus (cervix).

cervical abortion, spontaneous expulsion of a fetus implanted on or near the narrow lower end of the uterus (cervix).

cervical adenitis, an abnormal condition with large, tender lymph nodes of the neck. It often occurs with infections of the throat.

cervical amputation, the surgical removal of the cervix.

cervical canal, the opening within the uterine cervix. It protrudes into the vagina. The canal is a passageway through which the menstrual flow escapes. It is completely widened during labor. The infant passes through this canal when childbirth is done vaginally. Many diagnostic and therapeutic procedures need widening of the canal, including obtaining samples of the uterine lining (endometrial biopsy), curettage (D&C), or radium implantation to treat cancer. Sperm must travel upward through the canal to reach the uterus and fallopian tubes. The mucus that is released by cervical glands changes in appearance and consistency through the menstrual cycle.

cervical cancer, a cancerous tumor of the uterine cervix. It can be detected in the early, curable stage by the Papanicolaou (Pap) test. Factors linked to the growth of cervical cancer are sexual activity at an early age, having many sexual partners, genital herpesvirus infections, and multiple pregnancies. Poor obstetrical and gynecological care are other factors. Early cervical tumor growth is usually without symptoms. However, there may be a watery vaginal release or some spotting of blood. Advanced tumors may cause a dark, foul-smelling vaginal release, leakage from bladder or rectal canals (fistulas), weight loss, and back and leg pains. Pap smears of cervical cells are very important in screening. Final diagnosis may require examination with an instrument with a magnifying lens (colposcope) and study of tissue obtained by biopsy. Carcinoma in situ (that is, not yet invading the tissue) is thought to be a forerunner of invasive cancer. Cervical cancer invades the tissues of nearby organs. It may spread cancer cells through lymph channels to distant sites, including the lungs, bone, liver, or brain. Treatment depends on the kind and the extent of the cancer. It also depends on the age of the woman, and her general health. Also considered are her wishes about keeping her reproductive function. Invasive tumors are treated with x-ray therapy or surgery (hysterectomy).

cervical cap, a birth-control device. It is made up of a small rubber cup fitted over the narrow lower end of the uterus (uterine cervix). It prevents sperm from entering the cervical canal. Some experts claim it is as effective as the diaphragm. It may be more comfortable than the diaphragm. It can be left safely on the cervix for days or weeks and remain effective. Accurate initial fitting by a trained person is needed. Practice by the user may be required to put the cap into proper position on the cervix. The cap has become a popular contraceptive in Europe.

cervical cauterization, the destruction, usually by heat or electric current, of the outer tissues of the cervix.

cervical conization, the removal of a cone-shaped section from the cervix. See also **cone biopsy.**

cervical disk syndrome, a spinal disorder. It is marked by compression or irritation of the cervical nerves around the neck and shoulders. Cervical disk syndrome may be caused by ruptured disks, degenerative disk disease, or by neck injuries. Most cervical disk syndromes are caused by injuries that overextend the vertebrae. Fluid usually pools around the injured area. Pain, the most common symptom, usually centers around the neck area. It also may radiate down the arm to the fingers. The pain may increase sharply with coughing, sneezing, or movement of the neck, head, or arms. Other symptoms linked to cervical disk syndrome include numbness, headache, blurred vision, decreased skeletal movement, weakened hand grip. Wasting, weakness, and slowed reflexes also occur. X-ray examination may show some minor misalignment of the vertebrae. Treatment may include keeping the neck in a neck brace to lessen irritation and to provide rest for the injured area. Other treatment may include special exercises, heat therapy, and being placed in traction. Mild pain relievers are usually successful in controlling the pain, especially when movement is prevented. Surgery is usually advised only when symptoms last despite nonsurgical treatment. The outcome for this condition is usually good. However, the return of symptoms is common. Also called **cervical root syndrome.** See also **ruptured intervertebral disk, whiplash injury.**

cervical endometritis, a swelling of the inner lining of the narrow lower end of the uterus (uterine cervix). See also **endometritis.**

cervical erosion, a condition in which the cell layer (epithelium) of the narrow lower end of the uterus (cervix) is eroded as a result of infection or trauma, as childbirth. Early treatment is desirable to avoid possible cancer later. It is made up of tissue destruction (cauterization) and douches.

cervical fistula, an abnormal passage from the narrow lower end of the uterus (uterine cervix) to the vagina or bladder. It may be caused by cancer, x-ray therapy, surgical injury, or injury during childbirth. A cervical fistula connecting with the bladder permits leakage of urine. This causes irritation, odor, and embarrassment. When surgical repair is not possible, the patient is advised to take sitz baths and use a deodorizing douche or powder. The patient is also advised to wear plastic pants or a protective apron. See also **branchial fistula.**

cervical mucus method of family planning. See **ovulation method of family planning.**

cervical os. See **external cervical os, internal cervical os.**

cervical plexus, the network of nerves formed by divisions of the first four cervical nerves in the neck.

cervical plexus anesthesia, nerve block between the second cervical nerve and the sixth cervical vertebra. This method is used for operations on the area between the jaw and collarbone. Complications may include vertebral artery bleeding, phrenic nerve block or paralysis (the phrenic nerve controls the diaphragm), or nerve block of the voice box manifested by sudden hoarseness.

cervical polyp, an outgrowth of tissue lining the cervical canal. It is usually attached to the wall of the canal by a slender skin flap. Often there are no symptoms. However, polyps may cause bleeding, especially from contact during intercourse. Polyps are most common in women over 40 years of age. The cause is not known. A polyp is removed during surgery by turning the polyp on its stalk while pulling gently until it tears off. Little bleeding and prompt healing usually follow.

cervical smear, a small amount of the secretions and cells scraped from the narrow lower end of the uterus (cervix) with a sterile device. For a Pap smear, it is taken from the tissues of the uterine cervix and from the vaginal walls. The specimen is spread on a glass slide. It is then sent to a laboratory for microscopic examination.

cervical spondylosis, a disease involving breakdown of the vertebrae and disks in the neck. It results in compression of the associated nerve roots. It causes pain, loss of feeling in the arm and shoulder and stiffness of the neck.

cervical stenosis, a narrowing of the passage that leads between the body of the uterus and the opening of the cervix.

cervical triangle, one of two triangular areas formed in the area of the neck by the midline of the throat, the muscle in the neck, and the lower jaw.

cervical vertebra, one of the first seven segments of the spinal (vertebral) column at the top of the spine. They are smaller than the thoracic and the lumbar vertebrae. The first cervical vertebra (called the atlas) supports the head. The seventh cervical vertebra is above the collarbones. It has a very long, bony extension that is nearly horizontal. It can be felt with the fingers. See also **vertebra.**

cervicitis /sur'visī'tis/, sudden or long-term inflammation of the narrow lower end of the uterus (uterine cervix). **Acute cervicitis** is an infection marked by redness, swelling, and bleeding of the cervix. Symptoms do not always occur. They may include any or all of the following: a large amount of foul-smelling release from the vagina, pelvic pressure or pain, slight bleeding with intercourse, and itching or burning of the outer genitals. The main causes are *Trichomonas vaginalis, Candida albicans,* and *Haemophilus vaginalis.* Specific antibiotics may be effective. Acute cervicitis tends to be a returning problem because of re-exposure to the germ, ineffective treatment, multiple sexual partners, or poor general health. **Chronic cervicitis** is a persistent inflammation of the cervix. It usually occurs among women in their reproductive years. Symptoms include a thick, irritating, foul-smelling discharge, that may, in severe cases, go together with pelvic pain. The cervix is congested and swollen. Lumps (cysts) are often present. There may be old cuts from childbirth. A Pap smear is taken before treatment is started. Antibiotics are seldom effective. The symptoms of mild chronic cervicitis may lessen with creams or suppositories. However, the underlying condition will not change. The most effective treatments are hot or cold cautery to remove the diseased tissue. See also *Candida albicans,* **cautery, cervical cancer, cervical polyp.**

cervicodynia /sur'vikōdin'ē·ə/, pain in the neck. Also called **trachelodynia.**

cervicofacial actinomycosis. See **actinomycosis.**

cervicouterine /sur'vikōyōō'tərin/, referring to the narrow lower end of the uterus (cervix).

cervicovaginitis, an inflammation of the cervix and vagina.

cervicovesical /sur'vikōves'ikəl/, referring to the cervix of the uterus and the bladder.

cervix /sur'viks/, the part of the uterus that protrudes into the cavity of the vagina. The cervix is divided into two parts: the supravaginal (above the vagina) portion and the vaginal portion. The outside of the supravaginal portion is next to the bladder. It is separated from it by a band of tissue. The vaginal portion of the cervix projects into the vagina. It has the cervical canal. The mucous membrane lining of the cervix is broken by numerous ridges, deep glandular cavities, little lumps (cysts), and tiny projections (papillae).

cesarean hysterectomy, a surgical operation in which the uterus is removed at the time of cesarean section. It is done most often for complications of cesarean section, usually severe bleeding. Less often it is done to treat a disease, as a cancer. It is rarely done for sterilization because the danger of bleeding is greater when both procedures are performed together.

cesarean section, a surgical procedure in which the abdomen and uterus are cut open for childbirth. It is done when abnormal conditions are judged likely to make vaginal birth dangerous for mother or child. About 15% of births in the United States are by cesarean section. The operation is performed less frequently in other countries. The maternal death rate is 0.1% to 0.2%. Reasons for the operation include severe bleeding from placenta abnormalities (placenta previa or abruptio placenta), severe toxemia (preeclampsia), fetal distress (such as from the umbilical cord around the neck), a baby too large to fit through the pelvis, a breech or transverse (sideways) presentation, and very difficult labor. A previous birth by cesarean section is no longer considered a good reason for doing it again in future births. Cesarean birth is less traumatic for babies than a difficult forceps delivery. The cut in the skin of the abdomen may be horizontal or vertical. Because she must begin mothering while she is recovering from major surgery, the mother needs special care that provides for both her medical needs and her need to nurture her new baby. See also **classical cesarean section, extraperitoneal cesarean section, low cervical cesarean section.**

cesium (Cs) /sē′zē-əm/, an alkali metal element. Its atomic number is 55; its atomic weight is 132.9. Like other alkali metals cesium gives off electrons when exposed to visible light. They are used in photoelectric cells and in television cameras.

cesium 137, a radioactive material with a half-life of 30.2 years. It is used in x-ray therapy as a source of gamma rays. Cesium 137 is used to treat various cancers.

cestode. See **tapeworm.**

cestode infection, cestodiasis. See **tapeworm infection.**

Cetacaine, a trademark for an anesthetic available as a spray, ointment, gel, or liquid. It is used to relieve pain of mucous membranes.

cetyl alcohol /sē′til/, a fatty alcohol. It is used as an emulsifier and stiffening agent in creams and ointments.

cetylpyridinium chloride, an antiinfection substance used as a skin cleanser. It is given to prevent infection of the skin or mucous membranes.

★CAUTION: Known allergy to this drug prohibits its use. It is inactivated by soap, serum, and tissue fluids. Therefore, the surface of the skin must be clean and well-rinsed.

Ce-Vi-Sol, a trademark for a vitamin C (ascorbic acid) supplement.

cevitamic acid. See **ascorbic acid.**

Cf, symbol for **californium.**

CGS, cgs, abbreviation for **centimeter-gram-second system.**

Ch¹, the symbol for **Christchurch chromosome.**

Chaddock reflex, an abnormal reflex. It is induced by firmly stroking the skin of the forearm on the side opposite the thumb. The stroking causes the wrist to flex and the fingers to spread like a fan. This reflex occurs on the affected side in partial paralysis. Compare **Gordon reflex, Oppenheim reflex.** See also **Babinski's reflex.**

Chaddock's sign, a variation of the Babinski reflex. It is induced by firmly stroking the side of the foot. This causes the great toe to extend and the other toes to fan. It is seen in disease of an area of the brain (pyramidal tract).

Chadwick's sign /chad′wiks/, the bluish color of the vulva and vagina that develops after the sixth week of pregnancy as a normal result of congestion of the blood vessels. It is an early sign of pregnancy.

chafe, an irritation of the skin by friction, as when rough material rubs against an unprotected area of the body.

Chagas' disease /chag′əs/, a parasitic disease. It is caused by protozoal organisms carried to humans by the bite of bloodsucking insects. It may occur in sudden or persistent form. The sudden form is common in children and rare in adults. It is marked by a sore from the bite, by fever, weakness, large spleen and lymph nodes, fluid pooling in the face and legs, and rapid heart beat. This form disappears within 4 months unless complications, as inflammation of the brain (encephalitis), develop. The long-term form may cause heart muscle disorders or expansion of the esophagus or colon. Also called **African sleeping sickness, African trypanosomiasis, Brazilian trypanosomiasis, Chagas-Cruz disease, Cruz trypanosomiasis, South American trypanosomiasis.** See also **trypanosomiasis.**

Chagres fever /chag′ris/, an arbovirus infection. It is carried to humans through the bite of a sandfly. The disease is rarely fatal. The symptoms are fever, headache, and muscle pains of the chest or stomach. There may be nausea and vomiting, giddiness, weakness, sensitivity to light, and pain on moving the eyes. The infection lessens within a week. Treatment includes pain relievers, bed rest, and plenty of fluids. The disease is most common in Central America. Also called **Panama fever.**

chain, 1. a length of several units linked together, as a polypeptide chain of amino acids. 2. a group of individual bacteria linked together, as streptococci formed by a chain of cocci. 3. the relationship of certain body structures, as the chain of small bones in the middle ear. Each of the small bones moves in order in response to vibration of the eardrum, thus carrying the sound to the inner ear.

chain reaction, 1. a chemical reaction that makes a compound needed for the reaction to continue. 2. an atomic reaction that continues itself by continuing the splitting of nuclei and the release of atomic particles, which cause more nuclear splitting.

chain reflex, a series of reflexes, each aroused by the preceding one.

chain-stitch suture, a continuous surgical stitch in which each loop of the series of stitches (suture) is secured by the next loop.

chalasia /kəlā′zhə/, the abnormal relaxation of a cardiac muscle (sphincter), which is the junction of the esophagus with the stomach. This results in the stomach contents backing up into the esophagus. Infants with this disorder vomit after every feeding. Most grow out of it by about 6 months of age. Treatment in infancy includes feeding several small meals a day to avoid bloating of the stomach and holding the baby upright while giving the feeding. Adults who develop chalasia have heartburn and, sometimes, vomiting. Complications include ulcer of the esophagus, pain, and bleeding. Treatment is made up of elevating the head of the bed 6 inches. Alcohol, coffee, fats, chocolate, and cigarettes must be avoided. Treatment includes antacids and antiulcer drugs, as cimetidine. Surgery may be needed if complications develop. See also **gastroesophageal reflux.**

chalazion /kəlā′zion/, a small swelling of the eyelid. It results from obstruction of the glands in the eyelid. It often requires surgery for correction. Compare **hordeolum, sty.**

chalice cell. See **goblet cell.**

chalicosis /kal′ikō′sis/, a lung disease caused by breathing in calcium dust. It is usually caused by breathing in pure calcium dust, not dusts from marble, limestone, or Portland cement. It results in breathing problems, such as breathlessness, cough, and rapid, shallow breathing.

chalkitis /kalkī′tis/, a swelling of the eyes. It is caused by rubbing the eyes with the hands after touching or handling brass. Also called **brassy eye.**

challenge, a way of testing a person's sensitivity to a substance. The person is injected with a sample of the substance to determine if the immune syustem reacts to it by producing antibodies.

chamaeprosopy /kam′əpros′əpē/, a facial appearance marked by a low brow and a broad face.

chamber, a hollow but not always empty space or cavity in an organ. An example is the upper and lower (atrial and ventricular) chambers of the heart.

Chamberlen forceps, one of the earliest kinds of obstetric forceps. It was introduced in the 17th century.

CHAMPUS, abbreviation for **Civilian Health and Medical Programs for Uniformed Services.**

chancre /shang′kər/, **1.** also called **venereal sore.**

A skin sore, usually from syphilis. It begins as a small lump and grows into a red, bloodless, painless ulcer with a scooped-out appearance. It heals without treatment. It leaves no scar. Two or more chancres may develop at the same time, usually in the genital area but sometimes on the hands, face, or other area. The chancre has *Treponema pallidum* (syphilis) and is highly contagious. **2.** an ulcerated area of the skin that marks the point of infection of a nonsyphilitic disease, as tuberculosis. Compare **chancroid.** See also **syphilis.**

chancroid /shang′kroid/, a highly contagious, sexually carried disease caused by infection with *Haemophilus ducreyi.* It usually begins as a pimple, usually on the skin of the external genitals. The chancroid grows and ulcerates. If untreated, the infection spreads, causing swollen lymph glands in the groin. A skin test is used to diagnose this condition. Sulfonamide drugs are given to treat chancroid. Because the ulcer looks like syphilis and other venereal infections (lymphogranuloma venereum), the diagnosis must be made before treatment begins in order to avoid obscuring other infections. Compare **chancre.**

change of life, *informal.* the end of the female reproductive period; menopause.

channel, a passageway or groove that passes fluid, as the central channels that connect the small arterial branches (arterioles) with the small veins (venules).

channel ulcer, a rare type of peptic ulcer found in the pyloric canal, which is between the stomach and the first segment of the intestine (duodenum). See also **peptic ulcer.**

chapped, referring to skin that is roughened, cracked, or reddened by exposure to cold or excess evaporation of sweat. Stinging or burning sensations are often felt with chapped skin. Prevention is by protection against exposure to cold and wind. Treatment includes avoiding frequent washing, replacing ordinary soaps and detergents with super-fatted soaps, and applying softening drugs (emollients). Compare **frostbite.** **–chap,** *v.*

character, the integrated group of traits and behavioral tendencies that enable a person to react in a relatively consistent way. Character, as contrasted with personality, implies choice and morality.

character analysis, a systematic investigation of the personality of an individual with special attention to psychological defenses and motivations. Character analysis is usually done to better behavior.

character disorder, a persistent, habitual, badly adaptive, and socially unacceptable pattern of behavior and emotional response. Also called **character neurosis.** See also **antisocial personality disorder.**

charcoal. See **activated charcoal.**

Charcot-Bouchard aneurysm /shärkō′boōshär′/, a small, round ballooning (aneurysm) of a small artery in the cerebral cortex or basal ganglia of the brain. These aneurysms can cause massive bleeding in the brain. Charcot-Bouchard aneurysms often occur in patients with very high blood pressure.

Charcot-Leyden crystal /shärkō′lī′dən/, a crystalline structure found in the sputum of patients suffering from bronchial asthma. They are also found in the feces of dysentery patients. Also called **asthma crystal, leukocytic crystal.**

Charcot-Marie-Tooth atrophy /shärkō′mərē′-tooth/, a progressive hereditary disorder with breakdown of the nerves and muscles of the lower legs. This results in clubfoot, foot drop, and muscular incoordination.

Charcot's fever /shärkōz′/, a returning liver disease (jaundice) and stomach pain on the right upper side linked to swelling of the bile ducts. It is caused by a gallstone becoming lodged in the bile ducts.

Charcot's joint. See **neuropathic joint disease.**

charlatan, a totally unqualified person posing as an expert, as a person pretending to be a physician. Also called **quack.**

Charles' law. See **Gay-Lussac's law.**

charley horse, a painful condition of the quadricep or hamstring muscles in the back of the thigh. It is marked by soreness and stiffness. It is the result of a strain, tear, or bruise of the muscle. It is often linked to great physical efforts. Compare **cramp.**

chart, *informal.* a patient record.

charta /kär′tə/, a piece of specially treated paper. A charta can be treated with medicine for outer use or with a chemical for a special purpose, as litmus paper.

chauffeur's fracture, any fracture of the wrist, caused by a twisting or a snapping type injury.

CHC, abbreviation for *community health center.*

check ligament. See **alar ligament.**

check-up, a thorough study of the health of an individual.

Chediak-Higashi syndrome /ched′ē·ak·higä′shē/, an inherited disorder. It is marked by partial absence of pigmentation (albinism), abnormal white blood cells, nervous system problems, returning infections, and early death.

cheek, a fleshy rise, especially the fleshy parts on both sides of the face between the eye and the jaw and the ear and the nose and mouth. Also called **bucca.**

cheesewasher's lung, a lung disease. It is caused by an allergic reaction to the mold of cheese. The condition is prevented by avoiding cheese mold. No treatment is needed.

cheilitis /kīlī′tis/, swelling and cracking of the lips. There are several forms including those caused by excessive exposure to sunlight, aller-gic sensitivity to cosmetics, and vitamin lack. Compare **cheilosis.**

cheilo-, cheil-, a combining form referring to the lip.

cheilocarcinoma /kī′lōkär′sinō′mə/, a cancerous tumor of the lip.

cheiloplasty /kī′ləplas′tē/, correction by surgery of a defect of the lip.

cheilorrhaphy /kīlôr′əfē/, a surgical procedure that stitches the lip, as in the repair of a cleft lip or a cut lip.

cheilosis /kīlō′sis/, a disorder of the lips and mouth. It is marked by scales and cracks. It results from a lack of riboflavin (vitamin B_2) in the diet.

cheiralgia /kəral′jə/, a pain in the hand, especially the pain linked to arthritis. **–cheiralgic,** *adj.*

cheiro-, cheir-, chir-, chiro-, a combining form referring to the hand.

cheiromegaly /kī′rōmeg′əlē/, extremely large hands. **–cheiromegalic,** *adj.*

cheiroplasty /kī′rōplas′tē/, an operation involving plastic surgery of the hand.

chelate /kī′lāt/, a chemical compound made up of a central metal ion and an organic molecule. It is ordered in ring formation. It is used in chemotherapy for metal poisoning.

chelation /kīlā′shən/, a chemical reaction in which a metal combines with another chemical to form a ring-shaped molecular complex. See also **chelate.**

cheloid. See **keloid.**

cheloidosis. See **keloidosis.**

chemabrasion /kem′əbrā′zhən/, a way of treating scars or other skin problems by applying chemicals that remove the top layer of skin cells. See also **chemical cauterization, chemosurgery.**

chemical, a substance made up of elements that can react with other substances. A substance produced by or used in chemical processes.

chemical action, any process in which natural elements and compounds react with each other to produce a chemical change or a different compound. For example, hydrogen and oxygen combine to produce water.

chemical antidote, any substance that reacts chemically with a poison to form a compound that is harmless or less harmful. There are few true antidotes. Treatment of poisoning depends largely on destroying the toxic agent before it can be absorbed by the body. Specific antidotes include naloxone for opiates and N-acetylcysteine for acetaminophen.

chemical burn, tissue damage caused by exposure to a strong acid or alkali, as phenol, creosol, mustard gas, or phosphorus. Emergency treatment includes washing the surface with large amounts of water to remove the chemical. If the damage is more than slight and superficial, the patient should be immediately transported to a medical facility. See also **acid burn, acid poisoning, alkali burn, alkali poisoning.**

chemical cauterization, the breakdown or burning of living tissue by a caustic chemical, as potassium hydroxide. Cauterization is done to remove severely infected or damaged tissue so that healthy tissue can grow. Also called **chemocautery.**

chemical energy. See **energy.**

chemical equivalent, a drug with similar amounts of the same ingredients as another drug.

chemical gastritis, an inflammation of the stomach. It is caused by swallowing a chemical compound. Treatment depends on the substance ingested. Gastric lavage (washing out the stomach) is often advisable. However, neither lavage nor drugs to cause vomiting are given in cases involving the most corrosive poisons. Compare **corrosive gastritis, erosive gastritis.**

chemical mediator, a substance, such as acetylcholine, that transfers messages from one nerve cell to another (a neurotransmitter).

chemical name, the name of a drug by its chemical structure.

chemical warfare, the waging of war with poisonous chemicals and gases.

cheminosis /kem′ənō′sis/, any disease caused by a chemical.

chemistry, the science dealing with the elements, their compounds, and the chemical structure and interactions of matter. Kinds of chemistry include **inorganic** and **organic chemistry.**

chemistry, normal values, the amounts of various substances in the normal human body. Normal values are determined by testing a large sample of people thought to be healthy.

chemo-, a combining form referring to a chemical or to chemistry.

chemonucleolysis, a method of dissolving the cartilage between the vertebrae of the spine (intervertebral disk) by injecting a substance, such as chymopapain. The procedure is used mainly to treat a protruded (herniated) disk.

chemoprophylaxis, the use of antibiotics to prevent infections from beginning or from spreading from one part of the body to another.

chemoreceptor, a sensory nerve cell that is activated by chemicals. One example is the chemoreceptor in the main artery in the neck (carotid artery) that is sensitive to carbon dioxide in the blood, signaling the breathing center in the brain to increase or decrease breathing.

chemoreflex, any reflex triggered by the stimulation of chemical receptors. For example, the carotid artery and aorta respond to changes in carbon dioxide, hydrogen, and oxygen levels in the blood. See also **chemoreceptor.**

chemosis /kimō′sis/, an abnormal swelling of the mucous membrane covering the eyeball and lining the eyelids. It is usually the result of trauma or infection. A blockage of normal lymph flow may be the cause of chemosis. Also called **conjunctival edema.**

chemosurgery, the destruction of cancerous, infected, or dead (gangrenous) tissue by applying chemicals. The technique is used to remove skin cancers.

chemotaxis, a response of an organism of moving toward or away from a chemical stimulus.

chemotherapeutic agent, a substance used to treat diseases. The term usually refers to drugs used to treat cancer by slowing or stopping the growth of tumors.

chemotherapy, the treatment of disease with chemicals or drugs. The term is most often used in treating cancer. The drugs interfere with DNA synthesis by the tumor. Thus they kill off new cells as the tumor grows. However, normal body cells are destroyed as well. So the drugs are given for short periods of time, followed by a rest to allow the body to recover. The typical side effects of chemotherapy are hair loss, nausea and vomiting, diarrhea, skin rash, mouth ulcers, severe anemia, and extreme weakness. There are four basic classes of anticancer drugs: alkylating agents (such as carmustine, bisulfan, cyclophosphamide, chlorambucil), antimetabolites (methotrexate, 6-mercaptopurine, 5-fluorouracil), antibiotics (actinomycin-D, bleomycin, mithramycin), and alkaloids (vincristine, vinblastine). The drugs are most often used in combination. Chemotherapy is often started after surgery or radiation treatments. Chemotherapy has been very successful in certain types of cancer, as chronic lymphoblastic leukemia, Hodgkin's disease, Burkitt's lymphoma, Wilms' tumor, and after mastectomy.

chenodeoxycholic acid, an acid found in bile. It is given to dissolve gallstones. See also **ursodeoxycholic acid.**

cherry angioma, a bright red skin tumor that is ½ to 2½ inches in size. It occurs most often on the trunk. However, it may be found anywhere on the body. These are very common. More than 85% of people over the age of 45 have cherry angiomas. Also called **capillary angioma, De Morgan's spots, senile angioma.**

cherry red spot, an abnormal red circular area of the retina of the eye. It is surrounded by white tissue. It is linked to cases of retinal artery disorders. It sometimes appears in people with Tay-Sachs disease. Also called **Tay's spot.**

cherubism /cher′əbiz′əm/, an abnormal hereditary condition. It is marked by continuous swelling at the angles of the lower jaws, especially in children. In some cases of cherubism, the entire jaw swells and the eyes turn up. This promotes the cherubic facial appearance. The condition tends to worsen during adult life.

chest. See **thorax.**

chest cavity. See **body cavity.**

chest lead, a conductor attached to an electrocardiograph with the electrode placed on the chest to pick up heart sounds.

chest pain, a physical complaint that may be symptomatic of heart disease or of disease of the lungs. The source of chest pain may also be musculoskeletal, gastrointestinal, or psychological. More than 90% of severe chest pain is caused by coronary heart disease, compression of a spinal nerve, or a psychological disturbance. Because of its link to serious, life-threatening heart disease, chest pain causes extreme anxiety. This tends to mask other symptoms that would aid in diagnosis and treatment. Evaluation of chest pain requires determining the quality of the pain (dull, sharp, or crushing). The site of the pain (in the center or side of the chest) must be located. It also must be determined how long the pain has persisted, how it has developed, and whether it has occurred in the past. It is important that the person with chest pain describe the spread of pain to other parts of the body and identify factors that worsen or relieve the pain, as physical efforts, emotional distress, or deep breathing. Musculoskeletal conditions that can cause chest pain include rib fractures, swelling of the rib cartilage, and muscle strain. Stomach and intestine conditions linked to chest pain include swelling of the esophagus (esophagitus), peptic ulcers, and swelling of the pancreas. (See Table on pp. 164-165.)

chest tube, a tube inserted into the chest cavity through the skin for removing air or fluid or pus. It is commonly used after chest surgery and lung collapse.

chewing gum diarrhea. See **osmotic diarrhea.**

chewing reflex, repeated chewing motions seen when the mouth is stimulated. It is a sign of injury in brain-damaged adults.

Cheyne-Stokes respiration (CSR) /chān'stōks'/, an abnormal pattern of breathing. It is marked by periods of breathlessness and deep, fast breathing. The breathing cycle begins with slow, shallow breaths that slowly increase to abnormal depth and speed. Breathing becomes slowly less and shallower, climaxing in a 10- to 20-second period without breathing before the cycle is repeated. Each cycle may last from 45 seconds to three minutes. The cause of Cheyne-Stokes respiration is a complex change in the functioning of the breathing center in the brain. Changes in blood gases, especially an increase in carbon dioxide, may be the cause. This pattern of breathing may occur in a patient who has taken a drug overdose. It occurs more often during sleep. Compare **Biot's respiration.**

CHF, abbreviation for **congestive heart failure.**

Chiari-Frommel syndrome /kē·är'ēfrom'əl/, a hormonal disorder. It occurs after a pregnancy in which weaning the baby does not spontaneously end milk production. The syndrome is usually the result of a decrease in pituitary gonadotropins and an excess of pituitary prolactin. It may go together with lack of menstruation. Treatment includes hormonal therapy and investigation to determine if a pituitary tumor exists.

Chiari's syndrome. See **Budd-Chiari syndrome.**

chiasm /kī'azəm/, the crossing of two lines or tracts, as the crossing of the optic nerves at the optic chiasm.

chickenpox, a serious, highly contagious viral disease. It is caused by a herpes virus, varicella zoster virus (VZV). It occurs mainly in young children. It is marked by crops of itching and blisterlike eruptions on the skin. The disease is carried by direct contact with the blisters or by droplets spread from the breathing tract of infected persons, usually in the early stages of the disease. The fluid and scabs from the blisters are infectious until entirely dry. Also called **varicella.** The diagnosis is usually made by physical examination and by the characteristic appearance of the disease. The incubation period averages 2 to 3 weeks. It is followed by slight fever, mild headache, malaise, and loss of appetite occurring about 24 to 36 hours before the rash begins. The early period is usually mild in children. It may be severe in adults. The rash begins as flat red spots and develops in a day or two to raised bumps. Finally, it leads to blisters surrounding a reddened base and containing clear fluid. Within 24 to 48 hours the blisters turn cloudy. They are easily broken, and become encrusted. They erupt in crops so that all three stages are present at the same time. They appear first on the back and chest; spread to the face, neck, and limbs; and occur only rarely on the soles and palms. In severe cases, blisters in the throat may cause breathing difficulty and pain with swallowing. Fever, swollen lymph glands, and extreme irritability from itching are other symptoms. The symptoms last from a few days to 2 weeks. Routine treatment is made up of bed rest, drugs to reduce fever, and applications of wet compresses. Calamine lotion, or a paste made from baking soda and water to control itching and antihistamines by mouth are given to relieve itching. Infected blisters may be treated with antibiotics if the secondary bacterial infection is extensive. People who are susceptible and at risk for severe disease when exposed to the infection may be protected with immune globulin. Babies born to women who develop chickenpox within 5 days of birth are especially likely to get a severe case of the disease. One attack of the disease gives permanent immunity. However, herpes zoster virus (HZV), like all herpes viruses, lies dormant in certain sensory nerve roots follow-

Differential diagnosis of chest pain

Cause	Onset of pain	Characteristic of pain	Location of pain
Acute myocardial infarction	Sudden onset; lasts more than 30 minutes to 1 hour	Pressure, burning, aching, tightness, choking	Across chest; may radiate to jaws and neck and down arms and back
Angina	Sudden onset; lasts only a few minutes	Aches, squeezing, choking, heaviness, burning	Substernal: may radiate to jaws and neck and down arms and back
Dissecting aortic aneurysm	Sudden onset	Excruciating, tearing	Center of chest; radiates into back; may radiate to abdomen
Pericarditis	Sudden onset or may be variable	Sharp, knifelike	Retrosternal: may radiate up neck and down left arm
Pneumothorax	Sudden onset	Tearing, pleuritic	Lateral side of chest
Pulmonary embolus	Sudden onset	Crushing (but not always)	Lateral side of onset
Hiatal hernia	Sudden onset	Sharp, severe	Lower chest: upper abdomen
Gastrointestinal disturbance or cholecystitis, reflux esophagitis	Sudden onset	Gripping, burning	Lower substernal and upper abdomen
Degenerative disk (cervical or thoracic spine) disease	Sudden onset	Sharp, severe	Substernal: may radiate to neck, jaw, arms, and shoulders
Degenerative or inflammatory lesions of shoulder, ribs, scalenus anterior	Sudden onset	Sharp, severe	Substernal: radiates to shoulder
Hyperventilation	Sudden onset	Vague	Vague
Pleurisy	Gradual onset	Sharp, knifelike	Unilateral side of chest, usually can isolate the area
Costochondritis	Variable	Sharp, tearing	Pain in area of cartilage between ribs

ing a main infection. The virus is sometimes reactivated later in life (usually after age 50), with the eruption following the path of a nerve on the trunk, face, or limbs. Chickenpox in childhood is usually benign. Few cases need hospitalization. It may be serious or fatal in people with less resistance, as those getting chemotherapy or radiotherapy for cancer. Common complications are secondary bacterial infections, as abscesses, pneumonia, and blood poisoning. Hemorrhagic varicella (tiny hemorrhages that may occur in the vesicles or surrounding skin) is another complication. Less common complications are swelling of the brain (encephalitis), Reye's syndrome, blood disorders, and liver disease (hepatitis).

chiclero's ulcer /chikler'ōz/, a kind of American leishmaniasis caused by a protozoal parasite, *Leishmania mexicana*. It is common among the workers in the Yucatan and Central America who harvest chicle (an ingredient in chewing gum) from the forest. The disease is marked by skin ulcers on the head that usually heal spontaneously by 6 months. Ulcers on the ear, however, may last for years. They may cause scarring and deformities. See also **American leishmaniasis, leishmaniasis.**

chief cell, 1. also called **zymogenic cell.** any of the cells lining the stomach glands that secrete pepsin and intrinsic factor, which is needed for the absorption of vitamin B_{12} and the normal growth of red blood cells. Severe anemia is caused by the absence of intrinsic factor. **2.** any of the cells with pale-staining cytoplasm and a large nucleus that form the main substance of the pineal gland. **3.** any of the cells, within the parathyroid glands, that have pale, clear cytoplasm and a large nucleus.

History	Pain worsened by	Pain relieved by	Other
40 to 70 years of age; may or may not have history of angina	Movement, anxiety	Nothing; no movement, stillness, position, or breath holding; only relieved by medication (morphine sulfate)	Shortness of breath, diaphoresis, weakness, anxiety
May have history of angina; circumstances precipitating; pain characteristic; response to nitroglycerin	Lying down, eating, effort, cold weather, smoking, stress, anger, worry, hunger	Rest, nitroglycerin	Unstable angina appears even at rest
Nothing specific except that pain is usually worse at onset			Blood pressure difference between right and left arms, murmur of aortic regurgitation
Short history of upper respiratory infection or fever	Deep breathing, trunk movement, maybe swallowing	Sitting-up, leaning forward	Friction rub, paradoxic pulse over 10 mm Hg
None	Breathing		Dyspnea, increased pulse, decreased breath sounds, deviated trachea
Sometimes, phlebitis	Breathing		Cyanosis, dsypnea, cough with hemoptysis
May have none	Heavy meal, bending, lying down	Bland diet, walking, antacids, semi-Fowler position	
May have none	Eating, lying down	Antacids	
May have none	Movement of neck or spine, lifting, straining	Rest, decreased movement	Pain usually on outer aspect of arm, thumb, or index finger
May have none	Movement of arm or sholder	Elevation and arm support to shoulder, postural exercises	
Hyperventilation, anxiety, stress, emotional upset	Increased respiratory rate	Slowing of respiratory rate	Be *sure* hyperventilation is from nonmedical cause!
May have history of viral infection, pneumonia, TB	Inspiratory effort, deep breathing, coughing	Analgesics, regional anesthesia	Dyspnea, may hear friction rub
Variable	Inspiratory effort, deep breathing, coughing	Analgesics, regional anesthesia	

chief complaint, a statement made by a patient describing his or her most important symptoms of illness or dysfunction; the reason for seeking medical attention.

chief resident, a senior resident physician who acts temporarily as the clinical and administrative director of the house staff in a department of the hospital.

chief surgeon, a surgeon appointed or elected head of the surgeons on the staff of a health-care facility.

chigger /chig'ər/, the larva of *Trombicula* mites found in tall grass and weeds. It sticks to the skin. It causes irritation and severe itching. Also called **harvest mite, red mite.**

chigoe /chig'ō/, a flea found in tropical and subtropical America and Africa. The pregnant female flea burrows into the skin of the feet. It causes a swelling that may lead to spontaneous amputation of a toe.

chikungunya encephalitis /chik'ən·gun'yə/, a virus infection. It is marked by a high fever that begins suddenly, muscle aches, a rash, and pain in the joints. It is carried by the bite of a mosquito. It occurs mainly in Africa, Asia, and on some of the Pacific islands, including Guam.

chilblain /chil'blān/, redness and swelling of the skin caused by excess exposure to cold. Burning, itching, blistering, and ulceration, similar to a burn, may occur. Treatment includes protection against cold and injury, gentle warming, and avoiding tobacco. Also called **pernio.** Compare **frostbite.**

child, 1. a person of either sex between the time of birth and adolescence. 2. an unborn (fetus) or recently born (neonate or infant) human being. 3. an offspring or descendant.

child abuse, the physical, sexual, or emotional mistreatment of a child. It often results in per-

Guidelines for identifying potential child abusers

One or both parents were often abused as children. Studies indicate more than 90% of abusive parents were abused children.

Parents tend to be lonely adults, attracted to each other as they search for loving parent figures.

Extreme personal and social isolation. These parents lack group and community integration and most often lack family support.

Unstable marital relationship. Parents lack positive feedback and support.

Low self-esteem.

Parent-child role reversal. The parents want the infant to meet their unfulfilled needs for mothering.

Unrealistic expectations of infants. Parents expect children to act older.

Parents unable to reach out and ask for help.

Special traits that make a child vulnerable to abuse

Usually young child, under 3 years of age.

Something different about child (i.e., pregnancy or delivery uncomfortable, child unwanted, preamture birth).

Child is extremely irritable or cries often.

Birth order. Most often the first or last child is abused.

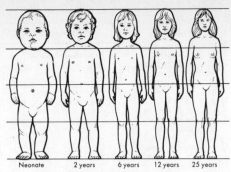

Neonate   2 years   6 years   12 years   25 years

Child development and proportion

manent physical or psychiatric injury, mental impairment, or, sometimes, death. Child abuse occurs mostly with children less than 3 years of age. Factors that contribute to child abuse include stressful environmental circumstances, as poor socioeconomic conditions, inadequate physical and emotional support within the family, and any major life change or crisis, especially those crises arising from marital strife. Parents that abuse their children often have unsatisfied needs and difficulty in forming healthy relationships. Unrealistic expectations of the child, and a lack of nurturing experience also often occur. Many of those parents are neglected or abused in their own childhoods. Obvious physical marks on a child's body, as burns, welts, or bruises, and signs of emotional distress, including symptoms of failure to thrive, are common signs of neglect or abuse. Compare **child neglect.** See also **battered child syndrome.**

child bearing period, the reproductive period in a woman's life, from puberty to menopause. It is the time during which she is physically able to bear children.

childbed fever. See **puerperal fever.**

childbirth. See **birth.**

childbirth center, a health facility where prenatal care and childbirth services are available to women who are healthy and have normal, uncomplicated pregnancies. The health-care team includes nurse-midwives, obstetricians, pediatricians, and other health professionals.

child development, the various stages of physical, social, and psychological growth that occur from birth to adulthood.

childhood, the period in human development that extends from birth until the beginning of puberty.

childhood aphasia, inability to speak or understand language because of a brain dysfunction in childhood.

childhood-onset pervasive developmental disorders, problems with thinking, mood, the ability to cooperate with other people, and behavior. They begin between the ages of 30 months and 12 years.

childhood polycystic disease (CPD). See **polycystic kidney disease.**

childhood schizophrenia, a form of schizophrenia. It begins before puberty. It may be caused by either organic brain damage or environmental conditions. It is marked by withdrawal into fantasy, obsessional attachments and failure to communicate verbally. Repetitive gestures, emotional unresponsiveness, and a severely blocked sense of identity also occur. Two kinds of childhood schizophrenia are **early infantile autism** and **symbiotic infantile psychotic syndrome.**

childhood triad, three types of behavior—fire setting, bedwetting, and cruelty to animals. When a child consistently performs all three, it may be a sign of future antisocial behavior.

child psychology, the study of the intellectual, emotional, and behavioral development of children.

child welfare, any service sponsored by the community or special organizations that provide for the physical, social, or psychological care of children in need.

chill, 1. the sensation of cold from exposure to a cold environment. 2. an attack of shivering with paleness and a feeling of coldness. Often it occurs at the beginning of an infection and goes together with a fast rise in body temperature.

Chilomastix /kī′lōmas′tiks/, a genus of flagellate protozoa, a common intestinal parasite of humans that does not cause disease.

chimera /kimir′ə, kīmir′ə/, an organism whose body has cells from different zygotes (fertilized eggs). This can occur naturally, as in twins. It can also happen artificially, as in a tissue graft. Compare **mosaic.**

chimerism /kimir′izəm/, in bone-marrow transplant, a state in which the donor's bone marrow and the host's cells are compatible. It is a state free of graft-versus-host disease.

chimney-sweeps' cancer. See **scrotal cancer.**

chin, the raised triangle-shaped part of the jawbone below the lower lip. It is formed by the lower teeth and jaw.

Chinese restaurant syndrome, a reaction that occurs immediately after eating food with the flavor additive monosodium glutamate. Symptoms are tingling and burning sensations of the skin, facial pressure, headache, and chest pain.

chip, a relatively small piece of a bone or tooth.

chip fracture, any small fracture that detaches from the bone. It usually involves a bone near a joint.

chiralgia /kəral′jə/, a pain in the hand, usually not from nerve injury or disease.

chirality. See **handedness.**

chiroplasty /kir′əplas′tē/, a surgical procedure that takes a hand that has been injured or deformed from birth and restores it to normal use.

chiropodist /kirop′ədist, shir-/, a health professional trained to diagnose and treat diseasesand disorders of the feet. A chiropodist may be awarded a degree of D.S.C. (Doctor of Surgical Chiropody) or Pod.D. (Doctor of Podiatry) after completing premedical studies and 4 years of study in an accredited college of podiatry. Internship is optional. However, a graduate must pass an examination and receive a state license before being allowed to practice. Also called **podiatrist.**

chiropody /kirop′ədē, shir-/, the study of disorders of the feet and the practice of treating these disorders.

chiropractic /kī′rōprak′tik/, a system of therapy. It is based on the theory that the state of a person's health is determined by the condition of the musculoskeletal and nervous systems. Treatment given by chiropractors involves manipulation of the spinal column. Some practitioners take x-rays for diagnosis. They use physiotherapy and diet. Chiropractic therapy does not use drugs or surgery. A chiropractor is awarded the degree of Doctor of Chiropractic (D.C.) after completing premedical studies followed by 4 years of training in an approved chiropractic school. Compare **allopathic.**

chirospasm. See **writer's cramp.**

-chirurgia. See **-surgery.**

chisel fracture, any fracture in which a bone fragment becomes detached from the head of the radius in the forearm.

Chlamydia /kləmid′ē·ə/, a genus of microorganisms that live as parasites within the cell. They have a number of properties in common with both viruses and some bacteria. They are clas-

sified as specialized bacteria. Two species of *Chlamydia* have been recognized. Both cause diseases in humans. *Chlamydia trachomatis* is an organism that lives in the membrane lining the eye (conjunctiva) and the lining of the urine passage (urethra) and lower end of the uterus (cervix). It is responsible for swelling of the conjunctiva (inclusion conjunctivitis) venereal disease (lymphogranuloma venereum), and eye disease (trachoma). It is one of the most common sexually transmitted diseases in North America. It is often a cause of sterility. *Chlamydia psittaci* is an organism that infects birds. It causes a type of pneumonia in humans. See also **psittacosis.** –**chlamydial,** *adj.*

chloasma /klō·az′mə/, tan or brown coloring, particularly of the forehead, cheeks, and nose. The condition is commonly linked to pregnancy and the use of birth-control pills. Also called **mask of pregnancy, melasma.**

chlor-, a combining form meaning 'green.'

chloracne /klôrak′nē/, a skin condition. It is marked by blackheads and pimples in people who are in contact with chlorinated chemical compounds, as cutting oils, paints, varnishes, and dioxin. The condition usually affects the face, arms, neck, and any other exposed areas.

chloral hydrate, a sedative and sleep inducer. It is used to relieve the inability to sleep (insomnia), anxiety, or tension.
★CAUTION: Liver or kidney disorders or known allergy to this drug prohibits its use.
★ADVERSE EFFECTS: Among the more common side effects are upsets of the stomach and intestines, skin rash, excitability, and low blood pressure.

chlorambucil, an alkylating agent. It is used to treat a variety of cancers, including chronic lymphocytic leukemia and Hodgkin's disease.
★CAUTION: Severe anemia or known allergy to this drug prohibits its use. It is not given during the first three months of pregnancy or within 28 days of other chemotherapy or radiation therapy.
★ADVERSE EFFECTS: Among the more serious side effects are severe anemia, disturbance of stomach and intestines, skin rash, and liver disease.

chloramphenicol, an antibacterial and antiricksettsial drug. It is used to treat a variety of serious infections.
★CAUTION: Mild or unidentified infections, pregnancy, breast feeding, or known allergy to this drug prohibits its use.
★ADVERSE EFFECTS: Among the more serious side effects are blood disorders and severe anemia.

chlorcyclizine hydrochloride /klôrsī′klizin/, an antihistamine. It has been used for nasal congestion, sinus infection, and hayfever. As a cream, it is also used for skin conditions.

chlordane poisoning. See **chlorinated organic insecticide poisoning.**

chlordiazepoxide /klôr′dī·az′əpok′sīd/, a minor tranquilizer. It is used to treat anxiety, nervous tension, and alcohol withdrawal symptoms.
★CAUTION: Psychosis, eye disease (glaucoma), or known allergy to this drug prohibits its use.
★ADVERSE EFFECTS: Among the more serious side effects are withdrawal symptoms occurring on discontinuation of treatment. Drowsiness and weakness commonly occur.

chlorhexidine, an antimicrobial agent. It is used as a surgical scrub, hand rinse, and antiseptic for the skin.

chlorhydria, a high level of hydrochloric acid in the stomach.

-chloric, a combining form referring to chlorine.

chloride /klôr′īd/, a chemical compound with chlorine.

chloriduria, a high level of chlorides in the urine.

chlorinated organic insecticide poisoning, poisoning resulting from inhaling, swallowing, or absorbing through the skin insecticides with chlorophenothane, as DDT, heptachlor, dieldrin, and chlordane. It is marked by vomiting, weakness, malaise, convulsions, tremors, rapid heart beats, breathing failure, and fluid in the lungs.

chlorine (Cl) /klôr′ēn/, a yellowish-green, gaseous element of the halogen group. Its atomic number is 17; its atomic weight is 35.453. It has a strong, distinctive odor. It is irritating to the breathing tract. It is poisonous if swallowed or inhaled. It occurs in nature chiefly as a component of sodium chloride in sea water and in salt deposits.

chloroform /klôr′əfôrm′/, a nonflammable liquid. It was the first gas anesthetic to be discovered. Because it is easy to give—often just a medicine dropper and a handkerchief face mask—it is still the principal general anesthetic in many underdeveloped countries. In these countries anesthesia equipment for the newer agents is not available. Chloroform is a dangerous anesthetic drug, however. Delayed poisoning, even weeks after apparently complete recovery, can occur. Serious eye damage is often reported.

chloroformism, the habit of inhaling chloroform for its narcotic effect.

chloroleukemia /klôr′ōlōōkē′mē·ə/, a kind of myelogenous leukemia in which body fluids and organs get a green color. See also **myelogenous leukemia.**

chlorolymphosarcoma /klôr′ōlim′fōsärkō′mə/, pl. **chlorolymphosarcomas, chlorolymphosarcomata,** a greenish tumor of bone marrow (myeloid) tissue. It occurs in patients with myelogenous leukemia.

chloroma /klôrō′mə/, pl. **chloromas, chloromata,** a cancerous, greenish tumor. It occurs anywhere in the body in patients with myelogenous leukemia. The green pigment has no definite function. Also called **granulocytic sarcoma, green cancer.**

Chloromycetin, a trademark for an antibacterial and antirickettsial drug (chloramphenicol).

chlorophyll /klôr′əfil/, a plant pigment that absorbs light and changes it to energy. Chlorophylls a and b are found in green plants. Chlorophyll c occurs in brown algae. Chlorophyll d occurs in red algae. See also **photosynthesis.**

chlorophyll test. See **Boas' test.**

chloroprocaine /klôr′ōprō′kān/, a local anesthetic with a chemical structure similar to procaine.

chloroquine /klôr′əkwīn′/, an antimalarial drug used to treat malaria, amebiasis outside the intestines, rheumatoid arthritis, some forms of skin disease (lupus erythematosus), and allergic reactions to light.
★CAUTION: Visual changes, porphyria, or known allergy to this drug prohibits its use.
★ADVERSE EFFECTS: Among the more serious side effects are disturbances of the stomach and intestines, headache, visual disturbances, and itching.

chlorothiazide, a diuretic and antihypertensive used to treat high blood pressure and water retention.
★CAUTION: Kidney dysfunction or known allergy to thiazide or sulfonamide drugs prohibits its use.
★ADVERSE EFFECTS: Among the more serious side effects are loss of potassium, high blood sugar, and excess uric acid in the blood. Allergic reactions may occur.

chlorotrianisene, an estrogen used to treat menopausal symptoms, prostatic cancer and to dry up breast milk after childbirth.
★CAUTION: Liver dysfunction, blood clots, unusual vaginal bleeding, known or suspected pregnancy, cancer that is stimulated by estrogen, or known allergy to this drug prohibits its use.
★ADVERSE EFFECTS: Among the more serious side effects are stomach and intestinal distress and breakthrough bleeding. In men, breast enlargement, decreased sexual interest, and impotence can occur.

chlorpheniramine maleate, an antihistamine used to treat a variety of allergic reactions, including nasal swelling, skin rash, and itching.
★CAUTION: Asthma or known allergy to this drug prohibits its use. It is not given to newborn infants or nursing mothers.
★ADVERSE EFFECTS: Among the more serious adverse reactions are skin rash, allergic reactions, and rapid heart beat. Drowsiness and dry mouth commonly occur.

chlorpromazine /klôrprō′məzēn/, a tranquilizer and antinausea drug used to treat psychotic disorders, severe nausea and vomiting, and intractable hiccups.

chlorpropamide, an oral antidiabetic drug used to treat mild, stable non-insulin-dependent diabetes mellitus.

chlorprothixene /klôr′prōthik′sēn/, a drug used to treat psychotic disorders.

★CAUTION: Parkinson's disease, taking depressant drugs, liver or kidney failure, low blood pressure, or known allergy to this drug prohibits its use.

★ADVERSE EFFECTS: Among the more serious side effects are low blood pressure, liver toxicity, a variety of nervous system reactions, blood disorders, and allergic reactions.

chlortetracycline hydrochloride, an antibiotic. It is used to treat many infections.

★CAUTION: Kidney or liver dysfunction, pregnancy, or known allergy to this drug or to other tetracycline drugs prohibits its use.

★ADVERSE EFFECTS: Among the more serious side effects are stomach and intestines disturbances, sensitivity to sunlight, additional infections, and allergic reactions. Discoloration of teeth may occur in children exposed to this drug before 8 years of age.

chlorthalidone, a diuretic and antihypertensive. It is used to treat high blood pressure and fluid pooling.

★CAUTION: Inability to urinate or known allergy to this drug, to other thiazide drugs, or to sulfonamide drugs prohibits its use.

★ADVERSE EFFECTS: Among the more serious side effects are low calcium levels, high blood sugar, excess urea in the blood, and allergic reactions.

Chlor-Trimeton, a trademark for an antihistamine (chlorpheniramine maleate).

chlorzoxazone /klôrzok′səzōn/, a skeletal muscle relaxant. It is used to relieve muscle spasms.

★CAUTION: Known allergy to this drug prohibits its use.

★ADVERSE EFFECTS: Among the more serious side effects are liver disease (jaundice) and bleeding in the stomach and intestines.

choanal atresia /kō′ənəl/, a birth defect in which a bone or membrane blocks the passageway between the nose and the throat. The defect is usually repaired by surgery. It is done soon after birth.

choke, to interrupt breathing by compression or obstruction of the throat or windpipe.

choke damp. See **damp.**

chokes, a breathing condition that occurs in decompression sickness. Decompression sickness occurs from reduction of the surrounding pressure by deep-sea diving or flying at high altitudes. The chokes are marked by shortness of breath, chest pain and a cough caused by bubbles of gas in the blood vessels of the lungs. If not treated promptly by chamber recompression, death can result.

choking, the condition in which a breathing passage is blocked by constriction of the neck, an obstruction in the windpipe, or swelling of the throat. It is marked by sudden coughing. A red face that rapidly becomes bluish from lack of oxygen is also noted. The person cannot breathe and clutches his or her throat. Emergency treatment requires removing the obstruction and resuscitation if necessary. See also **Heimlich maneuver.**

cholangeostomy /kōlan′jē·os′təmē/, a surgical operation to form an opening in a bile duct.

cholangiocarcinoma /kōlanm′jē·okär′sinō′mə/, a cancer of the liver occurring mainly in patients who have had an intestinal disease (ulcerative colitis) or an infestation of parasites (liver flukes). Diagnosis is made by examining a piece of liver tissue. The expectation of recovery is poor.

cholangiogram /kōlan′jē·əgram′/, an x-ray of the bile ducts. A cholangiogram is routinely performed as a part of biliary-tract surgery, before or after the procedure.

cholangiography /kōlan′jē·og′rəfē/, a special x-ray procedure for viewing the major bile ducts. A special dye is injected slowly into a vein. X-rays are taken of the region of the gallbladder. If the gallbladder has not been removed, a fatty meal may then be given and further x-rays taken to show contraction of the gallbladder. During and after surgery, the dye is injected into the common bile duct through a T-tube placed in the incision to drain the bile. The purpose is to discover any small gallstones still in the system. Cholangiography cannot be used if the patient has severe liver disease or jaundice, because the dye will not be concentrated and released into the bile. A sedative is often given before the x-ray. A local anesthetic is injected at the site of needle puncture. A burning sensation occurs as the dye is injected, but it lasts a short time. Bile peritonitis is occasionally a complication of T-tube cholangiography. See also **cholecystography.**

cholangiohepatoma /kōlan′jē·ōhep′ətō′mə/, a liver cancer that has a mixture of liver cells and bile duct cells.

cholangiolitis /kōlan′jē·əlī′tis/, inflammation of the fine tubules of the bile ducts.

cholangioma /kōlan′jē·ō′mə/, a cancer of the bile ducts.

cholangitis /kō′lanjī′tis/, inflammation of the bile ducts. It is caused either by bacterial invasion or by blocking of the ducts by stones or a tumor. The condition is marked by severe pain in the right upper stomach, liver disease (jaundice) if an obstruction is present, and intermittent fever. See also **biliary calculus.**

chole-, chol-, cholo-, a combining form referring to the bile.

cholecalciferol. See **vitamin D₃.**

cholecystectomy /kō'lisistek'təmē/, the removal by surgery of the gallbladder. Surgery may be delayed while the swelling is treated. A cholecystogram is done to confirm the diagnosis. Under general anesthesia, the gallbladder is removed. The bile duct is tied off. The common duct is searched and any stones found are removed. A T-tube is placed in the incision temporarily to drain bile to the outside of the body. Usually after about 10 days it is removed. The most common complication is a disruption of the liver or other ducts of the biliary system. This needs surgical correction. Wound infection, bleeding, bile leakage, and liver disease (jaundice) may also occur. See also **cholecystitis, cholelithiasis.**

cholecystitis /kō'lisistī'tis/, sudden or long-term inflammation of the gallbladder. **Acute cholecystitis** is usually caused by a gallstone that cannot pass through the bile duct. Pain is felt in the right upper part of the stomach. It goes together with nausea, vomiting, belching, and intestinal gas (flatulence). Diagnosis is usually made with x-rays. This is useful in ruling out appendicitis, intestinal obstruction, peptic ulcer, and other upper stomach disorders. Surgery is the usual treatment. **Chronic cholecystitis,** the more common type, has a slower beginning. Pain, often felt at night, may follow a fatty meal. Complications include gallstones, swelling of the pancreas, and cancerous growth (carcinoma) of the gallbladder. Again, correction is usually by surgery. See also **biliary calculus, cholecystectomy, cholelithiasis.**

cholecystogram /kō'lisis'təgram'/, an x-ray of the gallbladder. It is made after swallowing a dye, usually iodine.

cholecystography /kō'lisistog'rəfē/, an x-ray examination of the gallbladder. At least 12 hours before the study the patient has a fat-free meal and swallows a tablet containing iodine. The iodine material may also be injected into a vein. The iodine is released by the liver into the bile in the gallbladder. The patient then may consume a fatty meal. This stimulates the gallbladder to contract, expelling bile and the dye into the bile duct. Additional x-rays are taken about an hour later.

cholecystokinin /kol'isis'təkī'nin/, a hormone produced by cells of the small intestine. It stimulates contraction of the gallbladder and the release of enzymes from the pancreas.

choledocholithiasis. See **biliary calculus.**

choledocholithotomy /kōled'ōkō'lithot'əmē/, a surgical operation to make an incision in the common bile duct to remove a stone.

Choledyl, a trademark for a bronchi widener (bronchodilator) used to treat asthma (oxtriphylline).

cholelithiasis /kō'lilithī'əsis/, the presence of gallstones in the gallbladder. The condition affects about 20% of the population over age 40. It is more common in women. Many patients complain of general stomach discomfort, burping, and intolerance to certain foods. Other patients have no symptoms at all. See also **biliary calculus, cholecystitis.**

cholelithic dyspepsia /kō'lilith'ik/, an abnormal condition marked by sudden attacks of indigestion linked to the dysfunction of the gallbladder. See also **dyspepsia.**

cholelithotomy /kō'lilithot'əmē/, a surgical operation to remove gallstones through an incision in the gallbladder.

cholera /kol'ərə/, a serious bacterial infection of the small intestine. It is marked by severe diarrhea and vomiting, muscular cramps, and dehydration. The disease is spread by water and food that have been contaminated by feces of infected persons. The symptoms are caused by toxic substances made by the bacterium, *Vibrio cholerae.* The profuse, watery diarrhea (as much as a quart or a liter an hour) depletes the body of fluids and minerals. Complications include circulatory collapse, destruction of kidney tissue, and pooling of acid (acidosis). Mortality is as high as 50% if the infection is untreated. Treatment includes antibiotics and restoring fluids and electrolytes with intravenous solutions. A cholera vaccine is available for people traveling to areas where the infection is common. Other preventive measures include drinking only boiled or bottled water and eating only cooked foods. See also *Vibrio cholerae, Vibrio gastroenteritis.*

cholera vaccine, an agent used to immunize persons against cholera.

★CAUTION: Acute infection, use of corticosteroids, or known allergy to this drug prohibits its use.

★ADVERSE EFFECTS: The most serious side effect is an allergic reaction.

choleric /kol'ərik, kəler'ik/, having a hot temper or an irritable nature.

cholestasis /kō'listā'sis/, interruption in the flow of bile through any part of the biliary system, from liver to intestine. It is very important for the physician to discover whether the cause is within the liver (intrahepatic) or outside it (extrahepatic). Intrahepatic causes include liver disease (hepatitis), drug and alcohol use, and pregnancy. Extrahepatic causes may be an obstructing gallstone or tumor in the common bile duct or cancer of the pancreas. Symptoms of both types of cholestasis include swelling of the liver (jaundice), pale and fatty stools, dark urine, and intense itching of the skin. If liver disease is suspected, liver biopsy can confirm the suspicion, and attempts can be made to treat the underlying disorder. Extrahepatic cholestasis usually requires surgery. See also **cholestatic hepatitis, hyperbilirubinemia of the newborn. –cholestatic,** *adj.*

cholestatic hepatitis /kō'listat'ik/, inflammation of the liver from infection that causes interruption of the flow of bile in the bile ducts. Symptoms include jaundice and itching. These signs usually abate when the hepatitis becomes less. See also **cholestasis, hepatitis.**

cholesteatoma /kōles'tē·ətō'mə/, a lump (cyst) in the middle ear. It occurs as an inborn defect or as a complication of an ear infection (otitis media).

cholesterase, an enzyme in the blood and other areas of the body that forms cholesterol and fatty acids.

cholesterol, substance found in animal fats and oils, egg yolk, and the human body. It is most common in the blood, brain tissue, liver, kidneys, adrenal glands, and fatty covers around nerve fibers. It helps to absorb and move fatty acids. Cholesterol is necessary for the making of vitamin D on the surface of the skin. It is also needed for the making of various hormones, including the sex hormones. It sometimes hardens in the gallbladder to form gallstones. Cholesterol is found almost only in foods from animals and is constantly made in the body, mainly in the liver and the kidneys. High amounts of cholesterol in the blood may be linked to the development of cholesterol deposits in the blood vessels (atherosclerosis). Also called **cholesterin.** See also **high-density lipoprotein, low-density lipoprotein, vitamin D.**

cholesterolemia, the presence of too much cholesterol in the blood.

cholesterol metabolism, the making and breakdown of cholesterol in the body. Cholesterol is quickly absorbed from foods. It is also made in the liver and most other tissues in the body. As more cholesterol is eaten less is produced. Cholesterol is passed from the body by the liver fluids.

cholesterolosis /kəles'tərəlō'sis/, a rare condition, found in about 5% of patients with long-term swelling of the gallbladder (cholecystitis). It produces deposits of cholesterol in the lining of the gallbladder. Cholesterolosis is often linked to gallstones. See also **cholecystitis.**

cholestryl ester storage disease, a genetic disorder in which certain fats accumulate in body tissues. The disease may not show symptoms or may show an enlarged liver and spleen and fat in bowel movements. The cause is a lack of an enzyme that breaks down these fats. There is no specific treatment.

cholestyramine, a substance that increases cholesterol uptake by cells causing a lowering of blood cholesterol levels.

cholestyramine resin, a drug used to reduce too much cholesterol in the blood (hyperlipoproteinemia) and for itching resulting from partial blockage of the liver fluids.

★CAUTION: Complete blockage of the liver fluids or known allergy to this drug prevents its use.

★ADVERSE EFFECTS: Among the worst side effects are severe constipation, stomach problems, and loss of vitamins A, D, and K.

choline /kō'lēn/, one of the B complex vitamins, essential for the use of fats in the body. It is a large part of the nerve signal carrier (acetylcholine). It stops fats from being deposited in the liver and helps the movement of fats into the cells. The richest sources of choline are liver, kidneys, brains, wheat germ, brewer's yeast, and egg yolk. Lack of choline leads to cirrhosis of the liver, resulting in bleeding stomach ulcers, damage to the kidney, high blood pressure, high blood levels of cholesterol, cholesterol deposits in blood vessels (atherosclerosis), and hardening of the arteries (arteriosclerosis). See also **inositol, lecithin.**

choline esters, a group of drugs that act in places in the body where acetylcholine is responsible for transmitting nerve impulses.

cholinergic, 1. referring to nerve fibers that release a nerve signal carrier (acetylcholine) at the connections of muscles and nerves. 2. the tendency to pass on or to be stimulated by a nerve signal carrier (acetylcholine). Compare **adrenergic, anticholinergic.**

cholinergic blocking agent, any drug that blocks the action of the nerve signal carrier (acetylcholine) and similar substances.

cholinergic crisis, a severe weakness of the muscles and breathing difficulty caused by too many nerve signal carriers (acetylcholine). This condition is seen in patients suffering from diseases with severe muscle weakness.

cholinergic nerve, a nerve that releases the nerve signal carrier acetylcholine so that the signal is carried to another nerve.

cholinergic urticaria, an abnormal and usually temporary reaction of the skin. It is often associated with sweating in persons exposed to stress, strong exertion, or hot weather. The condition is marked by small, pale, itchy pimples surrounded by reddish areas.

cholinesterase /kō'lines'tərās/, an enzyme that causes the breakdown of one of the B complex vitamin forms (acetylcholine).

choliopancreatography, the x-ray study of the bile and pancreatic ducts.

Cholografin, a trademark for a dye (iodipamide) used to study the gallbladder.

Choloxin, a trademark for a drug used to reduce excess cholesterol in the blood (dextrothyroxine sodium).

chondral /kon'drəl/, referring to cartilage.

chondrectomy /kondrek'təmē/, the surgical removal of cartilage.

chondritis /kondrī'tis/, any swelling affecting the joints.

chondro-, chondr-, chondri-, a combining form referring to cartilage.

chondroangioma /kon′drō·an′jē·ō′mə/, a harmless tumor containing blood vessels and cartilage.

chondroblast /kon′drōblast/, any one of the cells that develops from the connective tissue of the embryo and forms cartilage. Also called **chondroplast.**

chondroblastoma /kon′drōblastō′mə/, a benign tumor formed from simple cartilage cells. It develops most often in growth areas of the thigh bone (femur) and upper arm bone (humerus) in young men. Also called **Codman's tumor.**

chondrocalcinosis /kon′drōkal′sinō′sis/, a type of arthritis in which calcium deposits are found in the joints of hands and feet. Chondrocalcinosis is similar to gout. It is often found in patients over 50 who have long-term joint disease (osteoarthritis) or diabetes. Also called **pseudogout.** Compare **gout, gouty arthritis.**

chondrocostal /kon′drōkos′təl/, referring to the ribs and the cartilages of the ribs.

chondrocyte /kon′drəsīt/, any one of the cartilage cells in the body.

chondrodysplasia /kon′drōdisplā′zhə/, a gentic disease marked by abnormal growth at the ends of bones, particularly the long bones of the arms and legs. Bones of the hands and feet may be similarly affected.

chondrodysplasia punctata, a genetic form of dwarfism marked by skin lesions, a pug nose, and an abnormal pattern of bone formation at the ends of bones when viewed by x-ray. One type of this condition is fatal and is marked by noticeable limb shortening. The other form is marked by bones of different lengths.

chondrodystrophia calcificans congenita, an inherited defect that affects the growth of long bones. This defect can be seen on x-ray films of newborn infants. Dwarfism, shortening of muscles, cataracts, mental retardation, and short stubby fingers develop as the infant grows into childhood. Also called **chondrodystrophia fetalis calcificans, Conradi's disease.**

chondrodystrophy /kon′drōdis′trəfē/, a group of illnesses in which cartilage changes to bone, especially in the long bones. Patients are dwarfed, with normal trunks and short arms and legs. See also **achondroplasia.**

chondroectodermal dysplasia /kon′drō·ek′ tədur′ məl/, a genetic form of dwarfism marked by a shortening of the bones of the arms and legs, heart abnormalities, and extra fingers and toes. Also called **Ellis-van Creveld syndrome.**

chondrofibroma /kon′drōfibrō′mə/, a fiberlike tumor containing cartilage elements.

chondrogenesis /kon′drōjen′əsis/, the growth of cartilage. **–chondrogenetic,** *adj.*

chondroid /kon′droid/, resembling cartilage.

chondrolipoma /kon′drōlipō′mə/, a harmless tumor found in the connective tissues of embryos. This tumor contains fat and cartilage elements.

chondroma /kondrō′mə/, *pl.* **chondromas, chondromata,** a fairly common, harmless tumor of cartilage cells. These cells grow slowly inside cartilage (enchondroma) or on the surface (ecchondroma).

-chondroma, a combining form referring to a harmless cartilage tumor.

chondromalacia /kon′drōmələ′shē·ə/, a softening of cartilage. **Chondromalacia fetalis** is a deadly inherited form of the condition that results in stillborn infants. The stillborn infant is born with soft, pliable limbs. **Chondromalacia patellae** occurs in young adults after knee injury and consists of swelling and pain that can be seen on x-ray films.

chondromatosis /kon′drōmətō′sis/, a condition defined by the presence of many tumors of the cartilage.

chondromyxofibroma /kon′drōmik′sōfibrō′mə/, a benign tumor that grows from connective tissues that form cartilage. The tumor is typically a firm, grayish-white, somewhat rubbery mass. These tumors tend to occur in the knee and small bones of the foot. Also called **chondromyxoid fibroma.**

chondrophyte /kon′drōfīt′/, an abnormal mass of cartilage. **–chondrophytic,** *adj.*

chondroplast. See **chondroblast.**

chondroplasty /kon′drōplas′tē/, the surgical repair of cartilage.

chondrosarcoma /kon′drōsärkō′mə/, a cancerous tumor of cartilage cells. This tumor occurs most often on long bones, the pelvis, and the shoulder. The usual tumor is a large, smooth, well-defined growth.

chondrosarcomatosis /kon′drōsär′kōmətō′sis/, a condition with numerous cancerous tumors of cartilage.

chondrotomy /kondrot′əmē/, a surgical process for dividing a cartilage.

CHOP, an anticancer drug combination of four separate drugs.

chord-, a combining form meaning string or cord.

chordae tendineae, *sing.* **chorda tendinea,** strong fibrous bands in the heart that attach the corners of the heart valves to the muscles of the lower heart chambers (ventricles). They prevent the valves from protruding into the upper heart chambers (atria) as the heart beats.

chordal canal. See **notochordal canal.**

chorda spinalis. See **spinal cord.**

chorda umbilicalis. See **umbilical cord.**

chordee /kôr′dē, kôr′dā/, a birth defect of the genital and urinary systems. The penis curves, caused by a fiberlike band of tissue instead of normal skin along the shaft of the penis. This is often linked to a defect in the placement of the urinary opening on the penis (hypospadias). It is surgically corrected in early childhood. The surgery improves the appearance of the genitals and constructs an organ that allows the boy to urinate in a standing position. It also produces a sexually functional organ.

chordencephalon /kôrd′ensef′əlon/, the part of the central nervous system that develops in the early weeks of pregnancy from the nerve tube. It later becomes the nerves of the spinal cord that control senses and movement.

chorditis /kôrdī′tis/, **1.** swelling of a spermatic cord. **2.** swelling of the vocal cords.

chordoma /kôrdō′mə/, a rare, inherited tumor of the brain. It is usually found in the center of the brain. Although it grows slowly it spreads very easily. Surgical removal is rarely possible.

chordotomy /kôrdot′əmē/, an operation in which parts of the spinal cord are surgically divided to relieve pain.

chorea /kôrē·ə/, a condition of uncontrolled, purposeless, rapid motions. Typical movements are bending and extending the fingers, raising and lowering the shoulders, or grimacing. In some forms the person is also irritable, emotionally unstable, weak, and restless. The causes vary and include bacterial infection and genetic disorders. See also **chorea gravidarum, Huntington's chorea, Sydenham's chorea.** –**choreic** /kôrā·ik/,*adj.*

chorea gravidarum, a form of uncontrolled, purposeless, rapid motions (chorea). It occurs during a first pregnancy to women who had a minor form of the disorder (Sydenham's chorea) as a child. Similar symptoms may develop in a woman taking birth-control pills. The disorder usually disappears after pregnancy, although it may reappear in future pregnancies.

chorea minor. See **Sydenham's chorea.**

choreiform /kərē′əfôrm′/, resembling the rapid jerky movements linked to chorea.

choreoathetoid cerebral palsy /kôr′ē·ō·ath′ətoid/, a form of cerebral palsy marked by both jerky twitching and slow, snakelike movements.

chorio-, a combining form referring to the membrane that protects the fetus (chorion).

chorioadenoma /kərē′ō·ad′inō′mə/, a tumor of the outer membrane protecting the fetus (chorion).

chorioamnionic /kôr′ē·ō·am′nē·ot′ik/, referring to membranes protecting the fetus.

chorioamnionitis, swelling in the fetal membranes caused by organisms in the fluid surrounding the fetus (amniotic fluid).

choriocarcinoma /kôr′ē·ōkär′sinō′mə/, a cancer that develops from the membranes protecting the fetus, usually from a cystic mole. Less often it grows following an abortion, during a normal or tubal (ectopic) pregnancy, or from a tumor of the genitals. The tumor most often first appears in the uterus as a soft, dark red, crumbling mass. It may attack and destroy the wall of the uterus and spread through lymph or blood vessels. It then forms more tumors in the wall of the vagina, vulva, lymph nodes, lungs, liver, and brain. The urine often contains much more of the hormone chorionic gonadotropin than is usual in pregnancy. The hormone level returns to normal when the tumor is completely removed. This form of cancer is more common in older than in younger women and responds to chemotherapy. Rarely, this type of cancer may develop in a tumor of the testicles or the pineal gland. Chemotherapy is usually not effective in treating these tumors. Also called **chorioblastoma, chorioepithelioma, chorionic carcinoma, chorionic epithelioma.**

choriocele /kôr′ē·əsēl′/, a hernia or bulging of tissue in the back (choroid layer) of the eyeball.

chorioepithelioma. See **choriocarcinoma.**

choriogenesis /kôr′ē·ōjen′əsis/, the growth of the outer membrane surrounding the fetus (chorion). This membrane at first contains fluid and loose pieces of tissue. As pregnancy proceeds, this membrane continues to expand around the fetus as it grows. In this way it protects the fetus and separates it from the wall of the uterus. –**choriogenetic,** *adj.*

chorion /kôr′ē·on/, one of the membranes surrounding the fetus. It is the outermost of two layers of membrane containing fluid and the fetus. The chorion forms the placenta connecting the mother and fetus (umbilical cord). Compare **amnion.** See also **amniotic sac.**

chorionic gonadotropin (CG), a hormone released by cells in the placenta, the tissue connecting the mother and fetus. This hormone causes the fertilized egg to release estrogen and progesterone, important hormones in preparing the uterus to accept the fetus. Chorionic gonadotropin is also used to treat some cases of undescended testicles. It also can help the ovary of an infertile woman to release an egg (ovum). Also called **human chorionic gonadotropin (HCG).** See also **gonadotropin.**

chorionic plate, the part of the connecting tissue between the mother and fetus (placenta) that produces projections (chorionic villi) that attach to the uterus while the placenta is still being formed.

chorionic villi, tiny projections on the surface of the membrane surrounding the fetus (chorion) that enter the blood supply of the lining of the uterus and help form the placenta.

chorioretinitis /kôr′ē·ōret′ini′tis/, swelling of the outer membrane and retina of the eye, usually as a result of infection. The symptoms are blurred vision, sensitivity to light, and distorted images. Also called **choroidoretinitis.**

chorioretinopathy /kôr′ē·ōret′ənop′əthē/, a disease of the eye that involves the outer membrane of the eye (choroid) and the retina. Swelling does not occur.

choroid /kôr′oid/, a thin membrane, richly supplied with blood, that covers the white of the eyeball. It begins near the iris and wraps around the back of eye. The choroid supplies blood to the retina. It conducts nerves and arteries to the front of the eye.

choroidal malignant melanoma, a tumor of the membrane surrounding the eyeball (choroid) that causes the retina to separate from the eye. The tumor is shaped like a mound or mushroom and requires complete removal of the eyeball. It also often causes increased pressure in the eye and loss of vision (glaucoma).

choroiditis /kôr'oidī'tis/, a swelling of the outer membrane of the eye (choroid). See also **chorioretinitis.**

choroidocyclitis /kôroi'dōsiklī'tis/, an unusual swelling of the eye that affects the outer membrane and the process that controls focusing of the lens.

choroid plexectomy /pleksek'təmē/, surgery to reduce the making of fluid in the area of the brain and spine. This is usually done to newborn infants whose bodies make too much of this fluid, causing it to collect in the skull (hydrocephalus).

choroid plexus, any one of the tangled masses of tiny blood vessels found in several parts of the brain.

Christchurch chromosome (Ch¹), an abnormally small chromosome that is linked to long-term leukemia centered in the lymph tissues. It has also been found in patients with various other inherited defects. See also **Philadelphia chromosome.**

Christmas disease. See **hemophilia B.**

Christmas factor. See **factor IX found in the blood.**

chromaffin /krō'məfin/, a structure that stains strongly with chromium salts. This refers to the cells of the adrenal glands. Also called **chromaphil** /krō'məfil/.

chromaffin body. See **paraganglion.**

chromaffin cell, any one of the special cells linked to sympathetic nerves, which produce the "flight or fight" response. The chromaffin cells of the central adrenal glands secrete the nerve stimulus carriers epinephrine and norepinephrine, which increase heart rate, raise blood pressure, increase breathing, and slow digestion. They are most highly responsive to stress.

chromaphil. See **chromaffin.**

chromatic, 1. referring to color. 2. able to be stained by a dye. 3. referring to chromatin. Also **chromatinic.**

chromatic dispersion, the splitting of light into its wavelengths or frequencies. A prism is often used to separate and study the different colors.

chromatid /krō'mətid/, one of the two identical threadlike fibers of a chromosome. It results when the chromosome reproduces itself. The two chromatid fibers making up each chromosome are joined in the center. During cell di-

vision, it divides lengthwise to form identical chromosomes.

chromatid deletion, the breakage of a chromatid.

chromatin /krō'mətin/, the material in the center of a cell (nucleus) that forms the chromosomes. It is made up of fine, threadlike strands of DNA attached to protein. It stains easily with basic dyes. During cell division, parts of the chromatin condense and coil to form the chromosomes. See also **chromatid, euchromatin, heterochromatin. −chromatinic,** *adj.*

chromatin-negative, referring to the centers of cells (nuclei) that lack sex chromatin. This is distinctive of the normal male.

chromatin nucleolus. See **karyosome.**

chromatin-positive, referring to the centers of cells (nuclei) that contain sex chromatin. This is distinctive of the normal female.

chromatism /krō'mətiz'əm/, 1. an abnormal condition in which the person suffers hallucinations and sees colored lights. 2. abnormal pigmentation.

chromatogram /krōmat'əgram'/, the results of a chromatography.

chromatography /krō'mətog'rəfē/, any one of several processes for dividing gases or dissolved chemicals. Once separated, they can be studied for their reactions to various stimuli. Some kinds of chromatography are **column chromatography, gas chromatography, paper chromatography. −chromatographic,** *adj.*

chromatopsia /krō'mətop'sē·ə/, 1. a visual defect that makes colorless objects appear touched with color. 2. a form of color blindness in which the patient may not see various colors correctly. It may be caused by a lack of one or more of the cells in the retina or from incorrect color messages being carried. The most common defect in color sense is the lack of ability to tell red from green, a defect in about 10% of men and 1% of women. Everyone is color blind in very dim light because the cells of the retina that are sensitive to color (cone cells) do not receive enough stimulation. In very dim light only the retinal cells that have the capacity to distinguish black from white (rod cells) are stimulated to act. Some color blind patients cannot see any color, seeing everything as gray. Very few persons are color blind to blue. Compare **chromesthesia.**

chromatosis, a condition of abnormal skin coloring in any part of the body. See also **chloasma, vitiligo.**

chromesthesia /krō'misthē'zhə/, 1. the color sense that depends on the mix of wavelengths in the light that enters the eye. It also depends on the response of the different cells in the retina linked with color vision (cone cells). One theory of color vision states that one type of cone cell responds to green light, a second to red light, a third to blue light. The human eye can distinguish hundreds of colors that combine the basic light wavelengths for red, green, and blue. Some of the retinal cones can react to all visible wavelengths. Different degrees of reaction of all the cones can produce all the colors known to humans. Defects in the cones cause various kinds of color blindness. **2.** an abnormal condition in which the patient confuses other senses, as taste and smell, to be sensations of color. Compare **chromatopsia.**

chromhidrosis /krō'midrō'sis/, a rare disorder in which the sweat glands secrete colored sweat. The sweat may be yellow, blue, green, or black and often also glows (fluoresces). A cause is regular exposure to copper, catechols, or ferrous oxide.

-chromia, a combining form referring to a state or condition of color.

-chromic, -chromatic, 1. a combining form meaning the number of colors seen by the eye. **2.** a combining form meaning a specific color of the blood indicating the hemoglobin content. **3.** a combining form meaning the ability of bacteria and tissues to be stained. **4.** a combining form meaning a specified skin color as a symptom of disease.

chromic myopia, a kind of color blindness in which colors can be distinguished only when the object is close to the eye.

chromium (Cr), a hard, brittle, metallic element. It does not occur naturally in pure form but exists with iron and oxygen in chromite. Traces of chromium occur in plants and animals. This element may be important in human nutrition, especially in digestion of carbohydrates. Workers in chromite mines are susceptible to a long-term lung disorder (pneumoconiosis) caused by breathing chromite dust.

chromium alum, a chemical commonly used to develop x-ray film when done by hand.

chromobacteriosis /krō'məbaktir'ē·ō'sis/, a very rare, usually fatal infection caused by a bacterium *(Chromobacterium violaceum)*. These bacteria are found in fresh water in tropic and subtropic regions. They enter the body through a cut in the skin. The symptoms are fever, liver abscesses, and severe exhaustion. Early diagnosis, surgical drainage of abscesses, and giving the drug chloramphenicol greatly improve the chance of survival.

chromoblastomycosis /krō'mōblas'tōmīkō'sis/, an infectious skin disease caused by a fungus. Symptoms include itching, warty bumps that develop in a cut or other break in the skin. These first appear as a small dull-red bump, slowly becoming a large ulcerlike growth. Over weeks or months, more warty growths may appear on the skin. Treatment includes surgical removal and, in some cases, applying antibiotics to the skin. Also called **chromomycosis, verrucous dermatitis.** See also **mycosis.**

chromogen, a substance that absorbs light, producing color.

chromomere /krō'əmir/, beadlike structures that are part of a chromosome during the early stages of cell division. Also called **idiomere.** See also **granulomere.**

chromomycosis. See **chromoblastomycosis.**

chromonema, /krō'mənē-'mə/, a twisted thread in a chromosome to which beadlike structures (chromomeres) attach. It forms the central part of the chromosome during cell division. Also called **chromoneme** /krō'mənēm/. See also **chromosome.** **–chromonemal,** *adj.*

chromophilic /krō'məfil'ik/, meaning a cell, tissue, or microorganism that is easily stained. Compare **chromophobic.**

chromophobic /krō'məfō'bik/, meaning a cell, tissue, or microorganism that is not easily stained, particularly certain cells of the pituitary gland. Compare **chromophilic.**

chromophobic adenoma, a tumor of the pituitary gland made up of cells that do not stain with dyes. Diabetes insipidus and other conditions caused by lack of one or more pituitary hormones are linked to this tumor. Also called **chromophobe adenoma.**

chromosomal aberration, any change in the normal structure or number of any of the chromosomes. This can result in birth defects ranging from mild to severe. In humans, a number of physical disabilities are linked to defects of both the non-sex chromosomes (autosomes) and the sex chromosomes. Some of these include Down's syndrome, Turner's syndrome, and Kleinfelter's syndrome. See also specific syndromes.

chromosomal nomenclature, a system used to identify the groupings of chromosomes in a person. The system features the number of chromosomes, sex, and the lack or addition of a specific chromosome or part of a chromosome. The grouping for a normal female is 46,XX, and for a normal male, 46,XY (X and Y are sex chromosomes). Any defect in the normal number or structure of the chromosomes can be indicated by this system.

chromosome /krō'məsōm/, any one of the threadlike structures in the center of a cell (nucleus) that carries genetic information. Each is made up of a double strand of twisted DNA (deoxyribonucleic acid). Along the length of each strand of DNA lie the genes, which contain the genetic material that controls the inheritance of traits. Chromosomes are studied after staining with dyes. In cell division, chromosomes reproduce themselves, forming two identical chromosomes called sister chromatids. These separate to become the chromosomes of the two new cells. In this way each new cell has a full set of chromosomes. Each species has a certain number of chromosomes. Humans have 46 chromosomes. These include

22 pairs of nonsex chromosomes (autosomes) one pair of sex chromosomes. Each parent contributes one sex chromosome. **–chromosomal,** *adj.*

chromosome banding. See **banding.**

chromosome complement, the normal number of chromosomes found in the cells of any given species. In humans it is 46. These consist of 22 pairs of nonsex chromosomes (autosomes) and one pair of sex chromosomes.

chromosome mapping. See **mapping.**

chromosome puff, a band of chromatin material that collects on a giant chromosome. It indicates that DNA or RNA is being made at that point. Such bands appear at certain points on chromosomes at distinct stages of growth in insects. They are important in the study of genetics.

chronaxie /krō'naksē/, the least amount of electric current needed to excite nerve or muscle tissue.

chronic /kron'ik/, referring to a disease or disorder that develops slowly and persists for a long period of time. It can sometimes remain for the person's lifetime. Chronic glaucoma is an example of this type of disease. Compare **acute.**

chronic airway obstruction, a type of breathing disorder in which there may be a long expiration and inspiration through pursed lips. At rest, the patient appears to breathe at a normal rate and shows no signs of distress. It is often seen in emphysema and chronic bronchitis.

chronic alcoholism, a condition that results from the regular use of alcohol in extreme amounts. This disease involves complex cultural, psychological, social, and physical factors. Alcoholism usually damages the person's health and ability to function normally in society. Symptoms of the disease include loss of appetite, diarrhea, weight loss, nerve and psychiatric problems (most often depression). Serious breakdown of the liver frequently leads to cirrhosis. Treatment depends on how severe the disease and its symptoms become. Withdrawal from alcohol should be done in a hospital because withdrawal symptoms can be severe. These may include trembling muscles, weakness, sweating, and delirium. Death can also result. Improved eating habits and tranquilizers are used to aid freedom from dependency. Drugs and psychotherapy often help further abstinence. The anesthesiologist should be told of the alcoholism in a patient undergoing surgery. Alcohol can reduce the effects of anesthetics. Support for the alcoholic and the family is offered by such organizations as Alcoholics Anonymous, Al-Anon, and Alateen. Rehabilitation facilities are also open to alcoholics. Compare **acute alcoholism.** See also **alcoholism.**

chronic appendicitis, a type of appendicitis in which previous swelling has caused thickening or scarring of the appendix.

chronic brain syndrome (CBS), an abnormal condition that is caused by damage to the brain tissue. The symptoms are loss of memory and disorientation. It may occur in several diseases (dementia paralytica, cerebral arteriosclerosis, brain trauma, and Huntington's chorea).

chronic bronchitis, a very common respiratory disease that causes severe weakness. The glands of the windpipe (trachea) and the large airways of the lungs (bronchi) produce too much mucus. This results in a cough that produces mucus (expectoration). The condition has a strong link to smoking and air pollutants. The disease was formerly seen almost only in men. It is becoming more common in women who smoke. A deep cough, often with wheezing, is always found. This is followed by breathing difficulty with exercise. The disease is noted for frequent pus-forming infections of the lungs. Difficult breathing results from narrow airways and often brings lung failure. Heart failure is a common result. Some patients develop too many red blood cells caused by lack of oxygen. Sharp attacks of breathing distress with rapid, labored breathing, long exhaling, large cough, and bluish skin can result. Patients who suffer from these symptoms are called "blue bloaters." It is usual to give antibiotics during the acute attack of symptoms. Drugs that open the airways (bronchodilators) are given to prevent the condition from getting worse. Heart failure is managed by restricting salt in the diet, diuretics, and sometimes digitalis. Patients with chronic bronchitis should be vaccinated against influenza and lung infections. Low-flow oxygen is often used in the home. Exercise, especially walking, and therapy are often given. See also **asthma, chronic obstructive pulmonary disease, cor pulmonale, emphysema, respiratory failure.**

chronic care, a type of medical care that concentrates on lasting care of people with long-term disorders. This care may be given either at home or in a medical facility. It includes medical treatment, as well as helping the patients to care for themselves and to eat properly. Physical therapy is also used to prevent loss of function.

chronic carrier, a person who acts as host to disease organisms for a long period of time. These persons do not display any signs of disease.

chronic chorea. See **Huntington's chorea.**

chronic cystic mastitis. See **fibrocystic disease.**

chronic disease, a disease that lasts a long period of time. This is different from the course of an acute disease, which attacks suddenly and ends quickly. The symptoms of chronic disease are usually less severe than those of the acute form of the same disease. Chronic disease may result in complete or partial disability.

chronic glomerulonephritis, a noninfectious disease that affects a part of the kidney (glomerulus). The disease causes protein and blood in the urine, gathering of fluid in the tissues, and less urine. The symptoms develop slowly, but the disease progresses to high blood pressure, fatigue, itching, nausea, and vomiting. This ends with kidney failure. Control of high blood pressure by salt restriction and drugs is helpful. However, transplanting a new kidney and dialysis are the only treatments in the later stages. The cause of the disease is unknown. See also **postinfectious glomerulonephritis, subacute glomerulonephritis, uremia.**

chronic hypoxia, a slow decrease in the amount of oxygen flow to cells resulting from lung diseases, heart disorders, or blood loss. Symptoms may include fatigue, sluggish mental responses, and the inability to perform physical tasks. If untreated, it may lead to cyanosis and disability.

chronic illness, any illness that persists over a long period of time and affects physical, emotional, intellectual, social, or spiritual functioning.

chronicity, a state of being chronic.

chronic lingual papillitis, a disorder of the tongue that causes it to swell. It sometimes also involves the cheeks and roof of the mouth (palate). The symptoms are scattered red patches, thinning of the nipplelike bumps (papillae), on the tongue, severe burning pain, and loss of tissue cells. The disorder affects middle-aged persons, especially women. It can come and go in attacks and remissions for weeks or months. Also called **Moeller's glossitis.**

chronic lymphocytic leukemia (CLL), a cancer of the tissues that form blood (the bone marrow and the lymph nodes). In this disease small, long-lived white blood cells grow in bone marrow, blood, liver, and lymph nodes. CLL is rare under the age of 35 and is more common in men than in women. The symptoms begin slowly. They are malaise, fatigue, loss of appetite, weight loss, night sweating, and enlarged spleen. Most patients can continue normal activities for years; 25% die of unrelated diseases. There is no cure for CLL. Slowing of the growth of the disease (remission) may be brought about by chemotherapy or by x-ray therapy.

chronic mucocutaneous candidiasis, an abnormal condition and rare form of infection caused by the yeast *Candida* (candidiasis). The infection causes sores on the skin, viral infections, and repeated infections in the lung. This disease usually occurs during the first year of life but can develop as late as the 20s. It affects both men and women and is linked to an inherited defect of the body's immune system. ★DIAGNOSIS: Chronic mucocutaneous candidiasis may cause large round sores on the skin, the mucous membranes, the nails, and the vagina. Viral infections linked to this disease may lead to abnormal hormone levels and hepatitis. Infections of the mouth, nose, and roof of the mouth (palate) may cause problems with speech and eating. Other problems linked to the disease include diabetes, Addison's disease, thyroid deficiency, and pernicious anemia. Some patients also develop psychiatric problems because of disfigurements and hormone imbalances that cause disorders. These hormone disorders can result in low blood levels of calcium, abnormal liver function, high blood sugar, iron deficiency, and abnormal vitamin B_{12} absorption.

★TREATMENT: Chronic mucocutaneous candidiasis does not react to agents that kill fungus being placed on the skin. Hormone disorders linked to the disease must be treated separately. Most success in treating severe cases has been with an antibiotic that kills fungus (amphotericin B) given in the vein. However, care must be used because amphotericin B is highly poisonous to kidneys. Some patients respond fairly well to the transplant of thymus from a fetus. Plastic surgery may also be part of the treatment to correct disfigurements caused by the disease. Treatment may also include extra iron to correct the anemia.

chronic myelocytic leukemia (CML), a malignant cancer of tissues that make blood (bone marrow and lymph nodes). It causes a rapid growth of grainlike white blood cells. The disease occurs most often in mature adults and begins slowly. The symptoms of CML are fatigue, heat intolerance, bleeding gums, skin sores, weight loss, and upset stomach. Also found are uric acid in the blood and growth in size of the spleen. Therapy with a cancer drug taken by mouth is usual, but advanced CML does not react well to chemotherapy. Also called **chronic granulocytic leukemia (CGL), chronic myelogenous leukemia (CML), chronic myeloid leukemia, splenomedullary leukemia, splenomyelogenous leukemia.**

chronic nephropathy, a disorder resulting in damage to the kidney. The condition frequently has more than a single cause, as diabetes and a bacterial infection. In some cases, the cause may be unknown. Symptoms include large volumes of urine, swelling, and protein and blood in the urine. Treatment varies, depending on the cause of the disease. See also **kidney disease.**

chronic obstructive pulmonary disease (COPD), an incurable condition in which lungs are able to take in less and less air over a period of time. The symptoms are problems in breathing while exercising, difficulty in breathing in or out deeply, and sometimes a long-term cough. The condition may result from chronic bronchitis, emphysema, asthma, or chronic bronchiolitis. It is made worse by cigarette smoking and air pollution. Also called **chronic obstructive lung disease.**

chronic (open-angle) glaucoma. See **glaucoma.**

chronic pain, pain that continues or returns over a long period. It can be caused by a number of diseases or abnormal conditions, as rheumatoid arthritis. Chronic pain is often less severe than acute pain. The patient with chronic pain usually does not have increased pulse and rapid breathing because these nervous system reactions to pain cannot be sustained for a long time. Many persons with chronic pain have an impulse to control their surroundings. They cannot control their disease so they try to control other people and their conditions. They may be called "uncooperative" or "manipulative." Others with chronic pain may withdraw from their surroundings and think only of their illness, ignoring their family, their friends, and the outside world. Scarring, continuing psychological stress, and the frequent need for drugs can slow treatment of patients with chronic pain. Compare **acute pain.** See also **pain intervention, pain mechanism.**

chronic tuberculous mastitis, a rare infection of the breast that results from the spread of tuberculosis from the ribs. With this disease tuberculosis is also found elsewhere in the body.

chronic undifferentiated schizophrenia, a condition marked by the symptoms of more than one of the classic types of schizophrenia—simple, paranoid, catatonic, or hebephrenic. See also **acute schizophrenia.**

chrono-, chron-, a combining form referring to time.

chronograph, a device that records small units of time, as a stopwatch.

chronologic, arranged in the order of occurrence. Also **chronological.**

chronologic age, the age of a person stated as the amount of time that has passed since birth. For example, the age of an infant is stated in hours, days, or months, and the age of children and adults is stated in years.

chronotropism /krənot′rəpiz′əm/, anything that affects the rhythm of a function of the body, as interfering with the rate of heartbeat.

chrysarobin /kris′ərō′bin/, a substance obtained from the wood of araboa trees and used to treat skin diseases, as psoriasis.

chrysotherapy /kris′ōther′əpē/, the treatment of any disease with gold salts. **—chrysotherapeutic,** *adj.*

Chua K'a, a counseling system to relieve muscle tension. It emphasizes the cleansing of mind and emotions.

Churg-Strauss /churg′strous′/, an allergy in which tumorlike masses appear, usually in the lungs. This often involves the circulatory system.

Chvostek's sign /khvôsh′teks/, an abnormal spasm of the face muscles when the facial nerve is lightly tapped. This spasm occurs in patients who have low blood calcium. It is a sign of a disorder of the nerves supplying the muscles (tetany.)

chyle /kīl/, the cloudy liquid that results from digestion in the small intestine. Consisting mainly of fats, chyle passes through fingerlike bulges in the small intestine (lacteals). It then goes into the lymph system for transport to the blood veins.

chyli-. See **chylo-.**

-chylia, a combining form referring to a condition of the digestive juices.

chyloid /kī′loid/, similar to the cloudy liquid (chyle) that fills the fingerlike bulges (lacteals) of the small intestine during the digestion of fatty foods.

chylomicron /kī′lōmī′kron/, very small drops of the fats that measure less than 0.5 microns (which is 0.001mm or 0.00004 inch) in diameter. They are made in the stomach and bowel and carry food particles through the wall of the intestine into the bloodstream. They then carry the nourishment through the body. The chylomicron drops are removed by the liver.

chylothorax /kī′lōthôr′aks/, a condition in which fluid caused by digestion in the intestine (chyle) makes its way through the thoracic duct in the chest to the space around the lungs. The cause is usually an injury to the neck or a tumor that attacks the thoracic duct. Treatment is surgical repair of the duct.

chylous ascites, an abnormal collection of digestive fluid (chyle) in the space between the stomach wall and the other organs (peritoneal cavity). Chylous ascites results from blockage in the thoracic lymph duct in the chest. This blockage may be caused by a tumor or by a break of a lymph vessel. Also called **ascites adiposus, chylosus ascites, chyliform ascites, fatty ascites, milky ascites.** See also **ascites.**

chyluria /kīloor′ē·ə/, milky appearing urine caused by the presence of digestive juices from the intestine (chyle).

chyme /kīm/, the thick and gummy contents of the stomach during digestion of food. Chyme then passes into the beginning of the small intestine (duodenum), where more digestion takes place.

chymopapain, an enzyme found in the tropical fruit papaya. It is used to treat ruptured or herniated vertebral disks.

chymotrypsin /kī′mōtrip′sin/, an enzyme, produced by the pancreas, that speeds the breakdown of milk protein (casein) and gelatin. It is used to treat digestive problems in which the enzyme is deficient or totally gone.

chymotrypsinogen /kī'mōtripsin'əjən/, a substance made in the pancreas. It is turned into the digestive enzyme chymotrypsin by trypsin.

C.I., abbreviation for **color index.**

cibophobia /sē'bə-/, an abnormal aversion to food or to eating.

cicatricial stenosis, the narrowing of a duct or tube caused by scar tissue.

cicatrix /sik'ətriks, sikā'triks/, scar tissue that is pale, tight, and firm. As the skin begins to heal it becomes red and soft.

ciclopirox, an antifungal drug used to treat ringworm (tinea) and yeast (candidiasis) infections.

★CAUTION: Known allergy to this drug prohibits its use.

★ADVERSE EFFECTS: Among the most serious side effects are allergy of the skin.

cicutism /sik'yōōtiz'əm/, poisoning caused by water hemlock. The symptoms are lack of oxygen, which results in blue skin, widened pupils, convulsions, and coma.

-cide, -cid, a combining element meaning 'killing.'

cigarette drain, a drain to allow fluids to escape from a wound or surgical cut. It is made from a piece of gauze drawn into a narrow tube.

cigarette smoking, the breathing in of the gases generated by slowly burning tobacco in cigarettes. The practice stems from the effect on the nervous system of the nicotine contained in the smoke. In addition to nicotine, nearly 1000 other chemicals have been identified in cigarette smoke, many of which have been shown to cause cancer. Cigarette smoke is considered more dangerous than pipe or cigar smoke because it is less irritating and more likely to be breathed in deeply. See also **lung cancer, nicotine.**

ciguatera poisoning /sē'gwəter'ə/, food poisoning that results from eating fish infected with the ciguatera poison. The poison comes from tiny creatures that the fish eat. Older, larger fish have greater poisons. Over 400 types of fish from the Caribbean and South Pacific are thought to carry this poison. The poison is believed to block nerve signals. Symptoms are vomiting, diarrhea, tingling or numbness of arms and legs and the skin around the mouth, itching, muscle weakness, and pain. Symptoms last 6 to 18 hours. Abnormal nerve sensations may last for months. Cold liquids feel hot to the mouth and throat. No treatment has been developed.

cilia /sil'ē-ə/, *sing.* **cilium, 1.** the eyelashes. **2.** small, hairlike projections on the outer layer of some cells, helping processing by making motion in a fluid. **–ciliary,** *adj.*

ciliary body, the part of the eye that joins the iris with the blood vessel layer (choroid).

ciliary gland, one of the many tiny sweat glands found in several rows on the eyelids. These glands lie near the eyelashes. Bacterial infection of one or more of the ciliary glands causes sties. Also called **gland of Zeiss.** Compare **tarsal gland.**

ciliary margin, the outer border of the iris of the eye.

ciliary movement, the waving motion of the hairlike projections on the lining of the passages in the lungs.

ciliary mucus transport, the movement of particles from the upper respiratory tract. These particles are breathed in and become trapped in mucus secreted by the cells of the upper airways of the lungs. These cells also have hairlike projections that sweep the mucus upward, out of the lungs.

ciliary muscle, a partly clear, round band of smooth muscle fibers of the eye. These help adjust the eye to view near objects.

ciliary process, any one of about 80 tiny projections on the back surface of the iris. They form a frill around the edge of the lens of the eye. See also **ciliary body.**

ciliary reflex. See **accommodation reflex.**

ciliary ring, a small, grooved band of tissue, about ⅕″ (4 mm) wide. This forms the back of the ciliary body of the eye.

ciliary zone, the outer round area on the front surface of the iris of the eye.

Ciliata /sil'ē-ā'tə/, a type of tiny primitive creature (protozoa) that has cilia through its whole life. The only important ciliate in humans is the intestinal parasite *Balantidium coli,* which causes dysentery.

ciliate /sil'ē-it/, having cilia, as certain cells of the body or Ciliata.

ciliated epithelium, any protective tissue that has cilia on its surface.

ciliospinal reflex /sil'ē-ōspī'nəl/, a normal reflex caused by scratching or pinching the skin of the back of the neck. This results in widening (dilation) of the pupils. Also called **pupillary-skin reflex.**

cimetidine, a drug used to treat duodenal ulcer, pancreatitis, and oversecretion of stomach acid.

Cimex lectularius. See **bedbug.**

cinchona /singkō'nə, sinchō'nə/, the trees and shrubs of the *Cinchona* species, which is found in South America. The bark contains quinine and quinidine. The bark is also called Peruvian bark.

cinchonism /sin'kōniz'əm/, a condition caused by eating too much cinchona bark or substances made from it. Symptoms are deafness, headache, dimmed eyesight, ringing in the ears, and giddiness. See also **quinine.**

cine-, kine-, kinesio-, a combining form referring to movement.

cineangiocardiogram /sin'ē·an'jē·ōkär'dēōgram'/, a picture of the cardiovascular system. It is made by combining x-ray, fluoroscopic, and motion picture techniques.

cine film /sin'ē/, a special type of film used to record x-ray procedures using dyes.

cineradiography /sin'irā'dē·og'rəfē/, injecting a dye into the body that is absorbed by parts of the body. The images made by these parts are then projected onto a screen. They are then filmed with a movie camera.

cingulate /sing'gyəlit/, having an area that usually has crossway markings.

cingulate sulcus. See **callosomarginal fissure.**

cingulectomy /sing'gyōōlek'təmē/, the surgical removal of part of the bundle of nerve fibers (cingulate gyrus) in the front part of the brain.

cingulotomy /sing'gyōōlot'əmē/, brain surgery to relieve constant pain. The operation stops the nerves in the bundle of nerve fibers (cingulum gyrus) by applying heat or cold to the tissues.

cinnamon, the strong-smelling inner bark of several species of *Cinnamomum,* a tree found in the East Indies and China. Saigon cinnamon is often used as a stimulant, a spice, or to help intestinal gas. **–cinnamanic,** *adj.*

CIPM, abbreviation for **Comité International des Poid et Mesures.**

circadian dysrhythmia, the stress effects of jet lag, or rapid travel through several time zones.

circadian rhythm /surkā'dē·ən, sur'kədē'ən/, the biologic clock in humans based on a 24-hour cycle. At regular intervals each day, the body becomes hungry or tired, active or peevish. Body temperature is highest in the afternoon or evening. It drops to its lowest point from 2 A.M. to 5 A.M.. Heart beat, blood pressure, breathing, urine flow, hormones, and enzymes rise and fall in a rhythmic pattern. Interference with this rhythm can cause impatience, less mental alertness, problems with sleep, stomach upsets, and rapid heartbeat. Jet lag is a common cause of circadian disturbance. So are some sleeping disorders (insomnia). It has been discovered that certain drugs affect the body more at certain times during the day than at others. As more is learned about this, it may be possible to determine more exact doses.

circinate /sur'sināt/, having a ring-shaped outline or form.

circle of Carus. See **curve of Carus.**

circle of Willis, blood vessel tracks at the base of the brain. It is formed by the joining of five arteries.

CircOlectric (COL) bed, a trademark for an electric bed that can be rotated up 210 degrees. This type of bed is used in orthopedics and for patients with severe burns. The bed is made up of a strong, aluminum, round frame and a back straight frame inside the circle. The patient is "sandwiched" and placed between the two straight frames during rotation. The bed can be rotated to move the patient from an upright position to a flat one. It can also turn the patient from his or her back to front. There are many advantages of the COL bed. It is easier to change the position of the patient in the bed. It also helps to slowly move the cardiovascular patient to an upright position before walking. The COL bed also permits more patient comfort during position changes after orthopedic and hip surgery. It also reduces the problems caused by too much bedrest in elderly patients. Compare **Foster bed, hyperextension bed, Stryker wedge frame.**

circuit, a course or path, most often one through which an electric current flows. Current flows through a closed circuit and stops if the circuit is open or broken.

circuit training, a method of physical exercise in which activities are arranged in sets so that the participant moves quickly from one activity to another with a minimum of rest between sets.

circular bandage, a bandage wrapped around an injured part, usually an arm or leg.

circular fiber, any one of the many fibers in the gums that circle the teeth. Compare **alveolar fiber, apical fiber.**

circular fold, one of the many ring-shaped, multi-sized folds in the small intestine. Circular folds are formed by mucous tissue. Most of the folds make less than a full turn around the inside of the intestine. Others curve along the wall, making as many as three turns. Also called **plica circularis, valve of Kerkring.**

circulation, movement of a substance in a round course so that it returns to its starting point. An example is the circulation of blood through the arteries and veins.

circulation time, the time it takes for blood to flow from one part of the body to another. This time is obtained by injecting a dye or radioactive atoms (radioisotope) into a vein and timing how long it takes to return to the same point in the body. Also a substance such as saccharin can be injected. Then the time it takes to travel to the tongue is noted.

circulatory failure, failure of the cardiovascular system to supply enough blood to meet the needs of the cells. One cause is the abnormal function of the heart, such as from a heart attack. Other causes are not enough blood in the body, as in severe bleeding, or from collapse of the blood vessels, such as in blood poisoning. See also **shock.**

circulatory fluid. See **blood, lymph.**

circulatory system, the network of vessels through which the blood circulates. See also the Color Atlas of Human Anatomy.

circulus arteriosus minor, the small artery circling the outer rim of the iris.

circum-, a combining form meaning 'around.'

circumanal /sur′kəmā′nəl/, referring to the area around the anus.

circumcision, a surgical removal of the foreskin of the penis or, rarely, the hood of the clitoris. Circumcision is often performed on newborn boys in spite of a lack of known medical benefit. There is also a small but real risk of complications. Circumcision can be performed on adult males to treat tightness of the foreskin (phimosis) and swelling of the penis (balanitis). Circumcision is required by the religions of about one-sixth of the people of the world.

circumcorneal, referring to the area of the eye surrounding the cornea.

circumduction /sur′kəmduk′shən/, 1. the round movement of a limb or the eye. 2. the motion of the head of a bone in a socket, as the hip joint. Circumduction is one of the four basic kinds of motion of the joints of the skeleton. Compare **angular movement, gliding, rotation.** See also **joint.**

circumferential fibrocartilage, fiberlike cartilage (fibrocartilage) rims that surround the edges of certain joint cavities, as the hip and the shoulder. The rims deepen such holes and protect their edges.

circumferential implantation. See **superficial implantation.**

circumlocution, the use of a different word or no word at all to avoid revealing that a word has been forgotten.

circumoral /sur′kəmôr′əl/, referring to the part of the face around the mouth.

circumscribed scleroderma. See **morphea.**

circum-speech, the behaviors that are linked to conversation. They include body language, keeping of personal space between persons, handsweeps, head nods, and activity, as walking or knitting, while carrying on a conversation.

circumstantiality, a disorder in which a person is unable to separate important from unimportant facts while describing an event. The person may include every detail and so lose his or her train of thought. Very often the person may need to have questions repeated. Circumstantiality may be a sign of chronic brain dysfunction. Compare **flight of ideas.**

circus movement, 1. an abnormal involuntary rolling or somersaulting. It is caused by injured parts of the brain that control body posture. 2. an abnormal circular walk caused by injury to the brain or other nerve centers.

cirrhosis /sirō′sis/, a long-term disease in which the liver becomes covered with fiberlike tissue. This causes the liver tissue to break down and become filled with fat. All functions of the liver then decrease, as making of glucose, processing drugs and alcohol, and vitamin absorption. Stomach and bowel function and making of hormones are also affected. Blood flow through the liver is blocked, causing back pres-

sure. It also leads to high blood pressure in the large vein of the liver and bleeding of the esophagus (esophageal varices). Fluid in the abdomen (ascites) and enlarged spleen may also occur. Unless the cause of the disease is removed, coma, bleeding in the stomach and bowels, and kidney failure occur. Cirrhosis is most often the result of long-term alcohol abuse. It can also be the result of malnutrition, hepatitis, or other infection. The symptoms of cirrhosis are nausea, appetite loss, weight loss, light-colored stools, weakness, stomach pain, varicose veins, and noticeable veins (often on the face). X-ray tests, physical examination, and blood tests of liver function are done to watch the growth of the disease. Treatment includes a balanced diet rich in protein, vitamins (especially folic acid), rest, and total avoidance of alcohol. The liver is able to restore itself, unless too much tissue is destroyed, but recovery may be very slow. Kinds of cirrhosis are **biliary cirrhosis, fatty cirrhosis, posthepatic cirrhosis.** See also **hepatic coma. –cirrhotic,** adj.

cirsoid aneurysm. See **racemose aneurysm.**

cisplatin, an anticancer drug used to treat many types of cancer, as cancerous tumors of the testicles, prostate, and ovaries.
★CAUTION: Kidney failure, hearing loss, or known allergy to this drug prohibits its use.
★ADVERSE EFFECTS: The most serious adverse effects are poisoning, severe nausea, appetite loss, vomiting, and allergic reactions.

cisterna /sistur′nə/, pl. **cisternae,** a cavity that holds lymph or other body fluids.

cisterna chyli, a widening at the beginning of the thoracic lymph duct, which is near a vertebra in about the middle of the back. It receives the two lymph ducts along the lower spine and the intestinal lymph duct.

cisternal puncture, insertion of a needle into a space containing fluids of the brain and spine (cerebellomedullary cistern) near the base of the skull. The purpose is to take out the fluid for examination.

cisterna subarachnoidea, any one of many spaces in the brain that hold fluid from the brain and spine (cerebrospinal fluid).

cistron /sis′tron/, a portion of DNA that is the smallest unit that can carry genetic information. The cistron is the same thing as a gene. –cistronic, adj.

cisvestitism /sisves′titiz′əm/, wearing clothing correct for the sex, but not the age, occupation, or status of the wearer. An example is a male bookkeeper wearing a male police uniform.

Citanest Hydrochloride, a trademark for a local anesthetic (prilocaine hydrochloride) one that affects only a small area of the body.

citrate /sit′rāt, sī′trāt/, any salt of citric acid.

citric acid /sit′rik/, a white, crystal-like organic

acid that dissolves in water and alcohol. It is taken from citrus fruits, especially lemons and limes, or from decaying sugars. Citric acid is used to flavor foods, carbonated drinks, and medicinal products, as laxatives. It is also used to prevent scurvy.

citrin /sit′rin/, a crystal-like substance that is used as a source of bioflavonoid, which maintains the walls of small blood vessels.

citrovorum factor. See **folinic acid.**

citrullinemia, a disorder caused by the lack of an enzyme used in the breakdown of certain amino acids. The clinical features include vomiting, convulsions, and coma. It is treated with a low-protein diet.

C/kg, a unit of radiation exposure representing coulombs per kilogram of air.

Cl, symbol for **chlorine.**

Claforan, a trademark for an antibiotic (cefotaxime sodium).

clairvoyance /klervoi′əns/, the alleged ability to be aware of objects or events without the use of the physical senses, as sight or hearing. Also called **clairsentience.** See also **extrasensory perception, parapsychology, telepathy.**

clamp, an instrument with notched tips and locking handles. It is used to grip, hold, join, support, or compress an organ or vessel. In surgery, clamps are most often used to control bleeding.

clamp forceps. See **pedicle clamp.**

clam poisoning. See **shellfish poisoning.**

clang association, the mental connection between unrelated ideas that is made because the two words sound similar. This happens often during manic-depression (bipolar disorder). Also spelled **klang association.**

clapping, a form of massage alternating the cupped palms in a series of rapid, sharp blows.

clarification, (in psychology) a technique to help the patient identify gaps or inconsistencies in his or her statements.

clarify, to clear a cloudy liquid. This is done by allowing the particles to settle, by adding something to make the particles settle, or by heating. **–clarification,** *n.*

Clark's rule, a rule for calculating the correct dose of a drug for a child. The formula is: weight in pounds/150 × adult dose. See also **pediatric dosage.**

clasp, **1.** a fitting that is fastened over a tooth to hold a partial denture in place. **2.** any surgical device for holding tissues together, especially bones.

clasp-knife reflex, an abnormal reflex in which a spastic arm or leg can not be moved and then suddenly jerks, like the the blade of a jackknife. It indicates damage to the brain's involuntary control system.

Class II biological safety cabinet, a container that recirculates air through a filter. It is usu-

ally located in a hospital pharmacy where drugs are mixed in order to protect personnel from exposure to harmful chemicals.

classic cesarean section, surgically delivering a baby through a vertical incision, running from below the navel to above the pubic bone. For many doctors this is the fastest method of cesarean delivery and is often used in emergencies. However, it results in a weaker scar. There is also more bleeding during surgery than from the low cervical cesarean section (the "bikini cesarean"). Compare **extraperitoneal cesarean section.** See also **cesarean section.**

classical conditioning, a form of learning in which an object or event that used to hold no special meaning now causes a predictable response. Also called **respondent conditioning.** See also **conditioned reflex.**

classic apraxia. See **ideomotor apraxia.**

classic tomography, a method that moves the x-ray source and the x-ray film during exposure. This produces an image with only one clear layer, the other layers being blurred. See also **computerized axial tomography.**

classic typhus. See **epidemic typhus.**

claudication, a pain of the legs with cramps in the calves caused by poor circulation of blood in the legs. The condition is often linked to hardening of the arteries (atherosclerosis) and may include lameness or limping. Intermittent claudication is a form of the disorder that occurs only at certain times, often after a period of walking. It is relieved by rest.

claustrophobia /klôs′trə-/, a great fear of being trapped in closed or narrow places. This fear is seen more often in women than in men. Sometimes it can be traced to some very frightening event involving closed spaces, usually occurring in childhood. However, in many cases the cause is unknown. It is often possible to treat this disorder by slowly changing the patient's behavior toward the feared situation. This is called behavioral conditioning.

claustrum /klôs′trəm/, *pl.* **claustra, 1.** a barrier, as a membrane that partly closes an opening. **2.** a thin sheet of gray matter in the brain.

clavicle /klav′ikəl/, the collarbone. It is a long, curved, horizontal bone just above the first rib, forming the front portion of the shoulder. It starts to form before any other bone in the body but does not totally unite with the breastbone (sternum) until about the twenty-fifth year. It is shorter, thinner, less curved, and smoother in women than in men. In persons who perform regular heavy manual labor, it becomes thicker, more curved, and more ridged for muscle attachment.

clavicular notch /kləvik′yələr/, one of a pair of oval dips found on either side of the top end of the breastbone (sternum). Each clavicular notch joins with the collarbone (clavicle) from the same side.

clavus. See **corn.**

clawfoot. See **pes cavus.**

clawhand, a hand seriously bent into a fixed position. Also called **main en griffe** /menäNgrif'/

claw-type traction frame, an orthopedic device that holds various pieces of traction equipment, such as pulleys, ropes, and weights, to various parts of the body. It consists of metal uprights, one at the head of the bed and the other at the foot, supporting an overhead metal bar. Compare **Balkan frame, IV-type traction frame.**

clean-catch specimen, a urine sample that is as free of bacteria as possible on routine urination.

cleansing enema, an enema, usually composed of soap suds, given to remove all formed fecal matter from the large intestine.

clearance, the removal of a substance from the blood by the kidneys. Kidney function can be tested by measuring how much of a specific substance appears in the urine in a given length of time.

clear cell, 1. a type of cell found in the parathyroid gland but not colored by the normal tissue stains used for microscopic examination. 2. the main cell of most cancerous tumors of the kidney and sometimes of tumors of the ovaries and parathyroid glands.

clear cell carcinoma, 1. a cancerous tumor of the kidney. The cancerous cells contain a large amount of clear cytoplasm. See also **renal cell carcinoma.** 2. an uncommon cancer of the ovary with cells having clear cytoplasm.

clearing test, a test of a joint's range of motion in order to reproduce symptoms. If the range of motion is normal and no symptoms are reproduced, the joint is cleared of causing any problem.

clear-liquid diet, a diet that supplies fluids and results in little waste. It consists mostly of dissolved sugar and flavored liquids, as ginger ale, sweetened tea or coffee, fat-free broth, plain gelatin, and strained fruit juices. The diet is usually given for a limited amount of time, as for one day after surgery.

cleavage, the series of repeated cell divisions of the egg (ovum) immediately after fertilization. A mass of cells is formed into an embryo capable of growth.

cleavage cavity. See **blastocoele.**

cleavage fracture, any broken bone that splits cartilage when a small piece of bone separates from a part of the upper arm bone (humerus).

cleavage line, any one of a number of lines in the skin that mark the basic structural pattern and tension of the skin tissue. They are present in all areas of the body but are visible only in certain sites, as the palms of the hands and soles of the feet. In general, the lines run in the direction in which the skin is most loose. Also called **Langer's line.**

cleavage nucleus. See **segmentation nucleus.**

cleavage plane, 1. the area in a fertilized egg (ovum) where cell division takes place; 2. any point in the body where organs or structures can be separated with the least amount of damage to surrounding tissue.

cleft, 1. divided. 2. a crack, most often one that begins in the embryo.

cleft foot, an abnormal condition in which the division between the third and fourth toes extends into the foot.

cleft lip, a birth defect consisting of one or more clefts in the upper lip. This results from the failure of the upper jaw and nasal area to close in the embryo. Also called **harelip.** See also **cleft palate.**

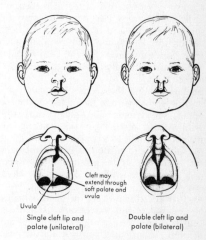

Cleft may extend through soft palate and uvula

Uvula

Single cleft lip and palate (unilateral)

Double cleft lip and palate (bilateral)

Cleft lip and palate

cleft-lip repair, the surgical correction of any birth defects in the upper lip known as cleft lips.

★METHOD: A cleft lip may sometimes be fixed during the infant's first 48 hours of life. Some surgeons follow a "rule of 10" and perform the operation when the child is 10 weeks old, weighs 10 or more pounds, and has an accepted level of hemoglobin in the blood. After surgery the infant is given breathing support until breathing is normal. A wire bow is laid along the infant's upper lip and taped to the cheeks to prevent pulling on the stitches. The infant is given clear liquids and juices through a syringe or special feeding unit. Milk products, solids, and a nipple or pacifier are not allowed. The diet and manner of feeding may vary, but the infant is normally fed with the head up and burped after every ounce of food.

Elbow restraints are worn at all times to prevent the infant from touching the lip.

★OUTCOME: This technique works very well in repairing cleft lips. In some cases a second operation is required to get rid of the scar.

cleft palate, a birth defect in which there is a hole in the middle of the roof of the mouth (palate). This results from the failure of the two sides to join during the development of the embryo. The crack may be complete, going through both the hard and soft palates into the nasal area, or it may go only partly through. The condition occurs about once in every 2,500 live births and affects females more than males. It is often linked to a cleft in the upper lip. These two problems are the most common disorders of the skull and face, making up half of the total number of defects. Feeding is done best with special feeding devices. Surgical repair of the defect is normally not begun until the first or second year of life. It is then normally done in steps. Long-term problems after surgery may include problems with speech, hearing loss, improper tooth growth and alignment, long-term breathing and ear infections, and some emotional and social problems. See also **cleft lip.**

cleft-palate repair, the surgical correction of a hole present at birth in the middle of the roof of the mouth (palate). Cleft palates range from a simple split in the tag of skin hanging from the palate (uvula) to a large hole through both the soft and hard palate and through the upper jaw. A cleft lip is often present as well. Repair of a cleft palate is usually done in the child's second year.

★METHOD: After surgery the child is kept in an atmosphere with lots of moisture and oxygen. This involves use of an oxygen tent until breathing is normal. Elbow restraints are used to prevent the child from touching the mouth. Clear liquids and juices are given by cup only; straws, nipples, pacifiers, utensils, or toys may not be put in the mouth. Milk products or solids are normally not given. The child is fed in a high chair, when possible, and a bib is used to catch drooling. Little mouth care is given; the teeth are not brushed.

★OUTCOME: Depending on the extent of a cleft palate, it may be repaired in one or several operations. Some experts believe that early repair of a defect in the bony palate can lead to structural problems. In these cases they may advise delaying the operation until the child is between 5 and 7 years of age and has more bone growth. Successful repair often greatly improves the child's breathing, eating, speech, and appearance.

cleft uvula, birth defect in which the flap of skin hanging from the palate (uvula) is split into two halves.

cleidocranial dysostosis /klē′dōkrā′nē·əl/, a rare,

abnormal hereditary condition characterized by defective hardening (ossification) of the skull bones and by the complete or partial absence of the collarbones (clavicles). The latter allows the shoulders to be brought together. Also called **cleidocranial dysplasia.** See also **dysostosis.**

clemastine, an antihistamine used to treat symptoms of allergy, as sneezing, runny nose and eyes, and itching.

Cleocin, a trademark for a substance that kills bacteria (clindamycin).

cleptomania. See **kleptomania.**

click, an extra heart sound that occurs during heart contraction (systole). See also **ejection click, systolic click.**

client-centered therapy, a method of group or individual psychotherapy. In this method the role of the therapist is to listen to the words of the client and then restate them without judging or interpreting them.

client interview. See **patient interview.**

climacteric melancholia. See **involutional melancholia.**

climate, the average conditions of the weather in any place. Climate may be considered in the diagnosis and treatment of some illnesses, especially those affecting breathing. –**climatic,** *adj.*

climax, a peak of intensity, such as a sexual orgasm or the high point of a fever.

climbing fiber, a type of nerve fiber that carries impulses to the balance center of the brain (cerebellum).

clindamycin hydrochloride, a drug that kills bacteria used to treat certain serious infections.

clinic, **1.** a department in a hospital where persons not needing to stay in the hospital receive medical care. Formerly it was called a dispensary. **2.** a group practice of doctors, as the Mayo Clinic. **3.** a meeting place for doctors and medical students, where lessons can be given at the bedside of a patient or in a similar place.

clinical, referring to direct, bedside medical care.

clinical crown, the part of a tooth that is covered by enamel and can be seen in the mouth.

clinical cytogenetics, the branch of gene study (genetics) that looks at the connection between abnormal chromosomes and disease.

clinical diagnosis, a diagnosis based on the facts learned from the medical history and physical examination alone, without use of laboratory tests or x-ray films.

clinical disease, a stage in the history of an illness. It begins with physical changes that produce familiar symptoms of a disease.

clinical genetics, a branch of the study of genes (genetics) that looks at inherited disorders. It studies the possible genetic factors that may cause the onset of a disease. Also called **medical genetics.**

clinical horizon, a point in a disease at which detectable symptoms first begin to appear. Compare **subclinical.**

clinical humidity therapy, respiratory therapy in which water is added to gases to make them more comfortable to breathe.

clinical laboratory, a laboratory in which tests are done to help diagnose a patient's illness. Such laboratories use material, as blood or skin samples, obtained from patients for testing. This differs from research laboratories where animal and other sources of test material are also used.

clinical nurse specialist (CNS), a registered nurse who holds a master of science degree in nursing (M.S.N.). A CNS has advanced knowledge and clinical skills in a specific area of nursing and health care.

clinical pathology, the laboratory study of disease by a pathologist. Among the many branches of clinical pathology are study of blood (hematology), microorganisms (bacteriology), chemistry, and immune systems (serology).

clinical pelvimetry, determining the size of the birth canal by feeling specific bony landmarks in the pelvis and estimating the distances between them. This is usually done by a midwife or obstetrician during the first vaginal examination of a pregnant woman.

clinical psychology, the branch of psychology that deals with diagnosis, treatment, and prevention of personality and behavior problems.

clinical research center, an organization that studies and describes medical cases. Such centers are often linked to a medical school or teaching hospital. They normally have extensive laboratory equipment. Staffs of physicians and medical technicians specialize in many areas. Clinical research centers often offer free or low-cost care for patients taking part in research programs. These centers often produce important new medical information.

clinical specialist, a doctor or nurse who has advanced training in a certain field of medicine. These include nurse-midwife, pediatrician, or radiologist.

clinical thermometry, a way of determining temperature in heated tissue.

clinical trials, organized studies to provide clinical data for assessment of a treatment.

Clinitest, a trademark for tablets used to test the urine for sugar.

clino-, a combining form meaning 'to bend or make lie down.'

clinocephaly /klī′nōsef′əlē/, a birth defect in which the upper surface of the skull dips in the middle, making it saddle-shaped.

clinodactyly /klī′nōdak′təlē/, a birth defect characterized by one or more fingers that are bent to either side.

clinometer /klīnom′ətər/, an instrument used to measure the movement of the eyes toward the nose as an object is brought closer to the face. Also called **clinoscope.**

Clinoril, a trademark for a drug to decrease swelling (sulindac).

clip, a surgical device used to line up the edges of a wound and to stop bleeding, especially of the small blood vessels.

Clistin, a trademark for an antihistamine (carbinoxamine maleate).

clitoris /klit′əris/, the female structure that corresponds to the penis. It is a pea-shaped projection made up of nerves, blood vessels, and erect tissue. It is partially hidden by the vaginal lips (labia minora). The clitoris is very sensitive to touch and is important in the sexual excitement of the female.

CLL. See **chronic lymphocytic leukemia.**

cloaca /klō·ā′kə/, *pl.* **cloacae,** an opening at the end of a structure (hindgut) in an embryo that develops into the rectum, the bladder, and the genitals.

cloacal septum. See **urorectal septum.**

clocortolone pivalate, a corticosteroid used on the skin to treat swelling.

★CAUTION: Viral and fungal diseases of the skin or circulation disorders prohibits its use.

★ADVERSE EFFECTS: Among the more serious side effects are those that may occur from too much use. Irritation of the skin may occur.

clofibrate /klō′fəbrāt/, a drug used to treat high levels of cholesterol, triglycerides, or both in the blood.

Clomid, a trademark for a fertility drug (clomiphene citrate).

clomiphene citrate /klō′məfēn/, a drug that causes ovulation. It is used mainly to treat infertility in women.

★CAUTION: Abnormal bleeding from the vagina, liver disturbance, or known allergy to this drug prohibits its use.

★ADVERSE EFFECTS: Among the more common side effects are blurred vision, upset stomach, rashes, and stomach pain. Ovaries may become larger.

clomiphene stimulation test, a test to study gonad function in males who show signs of abnormal sexual development. It helps to discover if there is disease of the hypothalamic or pituitary areas. It can also help discover a tumor of the pituitary. See also **clomiphene citrate, gonadotropins.**

clonal selection theory. See **antibody specific theory.**

clonazepam /klōnaz′əpam/, an anticonvulsant used to prevent seizures in petit mal epilepsy and other disorders involving seizures.

clone, a group of cells or organisms that have identical genes. They are a result of cell division.

clonidine hydrochloride /klō'nədēn/, a drug given to help relieve high levels of anxiety (antihypertensive). It is used to reduce high blood pressure.

clonorchiasis /klō'nôrkī'əsis/, an infestation of parasites (liver flukes). See also **Clonorchis sinensis, schistosomiasis.**

Clonorchis sinensis /klōnôr'kis sinen'sis/, a type of tapeworm called the Chinese or Oriental liver fluke. It is obtained by humans from eating raw or undercooked freshwater fish. The fluke is inactive in the skin of fish. Only after it enters the body of a warmblooded animal can it mature and produce eggs. These parasites infect the body and cause swelling. They can involve the liver, which can lead to cirrhosis. Infection from these flukes is called clonorchiasis.

clonus /klō'nəs/, abnormal activity of the nerves sending signals to the muscles. In this disorder the person cannot control rapid tensing and relaxing of muscles. Compare **tonus.** **–clonic,** *adj.*

C-loop, a loop of bowel formed by surgery with a C-shape.

closed amputation, removal of a limb (amputation) in which flaps of muscle and skin are used to make a cover over the end of the bone. It is done only when no infection is present. A hard dressing may be applied. The patient is often fitted for an artificial limb (prosthesis) right after surgery. Compare **open amputation.**

closed-angle glaucoma. See **glaucoma.**

closed bite, an abnormal overbite of the teeth. Compare **open bite.**

closed-chain, referring to a compound in which the carbon atoms are bound together to form a closed ring.

closed-circuit helium dilution, a technique for measuring lung volumes by having the patient breathe in a known amount of helium and measuring its final concentration.

closed drainage. See **drainage.**

closed group, a group in which all members are admitted at the same time so that all members are at the same stage of therapy. If a member should drop out, that place will remain unfilled.

closed system, a system that does not interact with its surroundings.

closed-system helium dilution method, a technique for measuring lung volumes by inhaling a known amount of helium and measuring its final concentration.

closed-wound suction, draining fluids, as blood and pus from surgical wounds. Such fluids slow the healing of wounds and often cause infection. Removing these fluids helps draw healing tissues together. Closed-wound suction devices most often are made of containers attached to suction tubes and suction pumps. After flushing out the wound to remove blood clots and debris, the surgeon places a tube in the wound. It is then brought out through healthy tissue, about 2 inches from the wound. When the suction tube is in place, the wound is closed and a dressing is put on. Closed-wound suction usually continues for 2 or 3 days after surgery or until the wound stops oozing fluid. Closed-wound suction is often used after chest surgery.

clostridial /klostrid'ē·əl/, referring to bacteria that form spores and need no oxygen to live. They are of the genus *Clostridium.*

Clostridium, a genus of bacteria of the Bacillaceae family. These bacteria form spores and need no oxygen to live. *Clostridium novyi, C. septicum,* and *C. bifermentans* are involved in gangrene. *C. botulinum* causes botulism. *C. perfringens* causes food poisoning, swelling, and wound infections. *C. tetani* is the cause of tetanus.

closure /klō'zhər/, the surgical closing of a wound by stitching it together. These stitches are called sutures. See also **flask closure, velopharyngeal closure.**

clot. See **blood clot.**

clotrimazole, a drug used to treat a number of simple fungus infections. It is also used for yeast infections of the vagina.

★CAUTION: Known allergy to this drug prohibits its use. Avoid contact with eyes.

★ADVERSE EFFECTS: The most serious side effects are severe allergic reactions of the skin.

clotting time, the time required for blood to form a clot. It is tested by putting a small amount of blood in a glass tube. The first clot is noted and timed. This simple test has been used to diagnose hemophilia, a serious clotting disease. It will not detect mild clotting disorders. Its chief use is in watching over treatment with anticlotting drugs. Also called **coagulation time.**

cloud baby, a newborn who looks well and healthy but carries bacteria or viruses. The infant may spread these into the air when breathing. This may cause disease among other infants in the hospital nursery.

clove, the dried flower bud of *Eugenia caryophyllata.* It contains an oil used as a dental pain reliever, a germ killer, and a salve. Clove is also used to treat nausea, vomiting, and intestinal gas. It is best known as a spice.

cloverleaf nail, a surgical nail shaped like a cloverleaf. It is used especially to repair breaks of the thigh bone (femur).

cloverleaf skull deformity, a birth defect characterized by a skull with three lobes. The defect is caused by premature closing of the soft spots of the skull (sutures) during development. The condition is associated with water on the brain (hydrocephalus), facial abnormalities, and skeletal deformities. Also called **kleeblattschädel deformity syndrome** /klä′blochä′dəl/.

cloxacillin sodium, a drug that kills bacteria used to treat certain serious infections. It is most helpful in treating bacteria resistant to penicillin.

clubbing, an abnormal enlargement of the tips of the fingers and toes. Clubbing is common in patients with cyanotic heart disease and long-term lung disease. It also may occur with cirrhosis, colitis, long-term dysentery, and thyroid disorders. Clubbing is most easily seen in the fingers. Advanced clubbing is obvious, but early clubbing is difficult to see. The fingers and toes are full, fleshy, and the skin may break away easily.

clubfoot, a birth deformity of the foot, sometimes resulting from crowding in the uterus. In a clubfoot the bones in the front part of the foot are misaligned. In 95 percent of clubfoot deformities the front half of the foot turns in and down (**equinovarus**). In the rest of the defects the front part of the foot turns out and up (**calcaneovalgus** or **calcaneovarus**). Treatment depends on the extent of the defect. Splints and casts in infancy may completely correct the clubfoot. In other cases, surgery in several steps may be done. See also **talipes.**

club hair, a hair in the final stage of the growth cycle. See also **hair.**

clubhand, a disorder present from birth in which the hand develops as a widened stump with stunted fingers.

cluster breathing, a breathing pattern in which fast breathing is followed by a period of not breathing. This is linked to a tumor or disease in the brain stem.

cluster headache. See **histamine headache.**

cluttering, a speech defect in which words are rapid, confused, nervous, and uneven. Letters or syllables may be reversed or left out. The condition is often linked to other language disorders, as problems in learning to speak, read, and spell. It is also seen in some personality and behavior problems.

Cm, symbol for **curium.**

CMAJ, abbreviation for *Canadian Medical Association Journal.*

CMF, an anticancer drug combination of cyclophosphamide, methotrexate, and fluorouracil.

CMV, abbreviation for **cytomegalovirus.**

CNA, abbreviation for **Canadian Nurses' Association.**

CNM, abbreviation for **Certified Nurse-Midwife.**

CNP, abbreviation for **community nurse practitioner.**

CNS, abbreviation for **central nervous system.**

CNS sympathomimetic, a drug, as cocaine, whose action imitates the action of the sympathetic nervous system.

Co, symbol for **cobalt.**

CO, 1. the symbol for carbon monoxide. **2.** abbreviation for cardiac output.

co-, col-, com-, con-, cor-, a combining form meaning 'together, with.'

CO₂, symbol for **carbon dioxide.**

Coactin, a brand name for the antibiotic amdinocillin.

coagulase /kō·ag′yəlās/, an enzyme produced by bacteria, particularly *Staphylococcus aureus.* It helps to form blood clots.

coagulation /kō·ag′yəlā′shən/, **1.** clotting; the process of turning a liquid into a solid, especially the blood. **2.** the hardening of tissue, as with electricity (electrocoagulation) or light (photocoagulation).

coagulation current, an electric current given by a needle ball or other point that hardens tissue. See also **electrocautery, electrocoagulation.**

coagulation factor, one of 13 elements in the blood that help to form blood clot. See also **blood clotting, coagulation, fibrinogen, hemophilia A, hemophilia B, hemophilia C, prothrombin, thromboplastin,** and see **factor IV** through **factor XIII.**

coagulation time. See **clotting time.**

coagulopathy /kō·ag′yəlop′əthē/, any disorder of the blood making it difficult for blood to coagulate.

coal tar, a substance put on the skin. It is used to treat long-term skin diseases, as eczema and psoriasis.

★CAUTION: Known allergy to this drug prohibits its use.

★ADVERSE EFFECTS: Among the most severe effects are skin irritation and skin allergic reactions.

coal worker's pneumoconiosis. See **anthracosis.**

coaptation splint /kō·ap′shən/, a small splint fitted to a broken limb to keep the fragments of bone in place. A longer splint usually covers the small one to provide for more support.

coarct /kō·ärkt′/, the act of narrowing or constricting, especially a blood vessel.

coarctation /kō·ärktä′shən/, a narrowing or contraction of the walls of a blood vessel, as the aorta.

coarctation of the aorta, a birth defect of the heart in which the major artery (aorta) is narrowed. This results in higher blood pressure on one side of the defect and lower pressure on the other side. In its most common form it causes high blood pressure in the arms and head and low blood pressure in the legs. Symptoms include dizziness, headaches, fainting, nose bleeds, and muscle cramps in the legs during exercise. Diagnosis is based on the blood pressure changes in the upper and lower body, and x-ray tests. Surgical repair is done even for minor defects because of possible complications. These include breaking of the aorta, high blood pressure, infections of the lining of the heart (endocarditis), bleeding in the brain, and heart failure.

coarse, a wide range of movements, as those linked to tremors and uncontrolled movements of the muscle.

coarse fremitus, a rough, loud vibration of the chest wall as a person breathes in and out.

coat, 1. a membrane that covers the outside of an organ or part. **2.** one of the layers of a wall of an organ or part, especially a canal or a vessel.

cobalamin /kōbôl'əmin/, a common term for part of the vitamin B_{12} complex. See also **cyanocobalamin.**

cobalt (Co), a metallic element found in certain minerals. Cobalt is a part of vitamin B_{12}, and is found in most foods. It is easily absorbed by the stomach and intestines. Research has shown that this element is common in the human diet. The amount the body needs is not known. Lack of enough cobalt in humans does not seem to happen. Giving a form of cobalt seems to help some patients with anemia. This is because cobalt helps to make red blood cells. A radioactive form is also used to treat cancer.

cobalt 60 (^{60}Co), (in radiotherapy) a radioactive atom (isotope) of cobalt. Its mass number is 60. ^{60}Co gives off high-energy gamma rays. It is the radioactive source most often used in x-ray treatment for cancer.

Coban, a brand name for an elastic pressure wrap applied to reduce swelling in an injured finger.

coca, a species of South American shrubs native to Bolivia and Peru. It is also grown in Indonesia. Some people of those areas dry and chew the leaves as a stimulant. It is a natural source of cocaine. See also **ecgonine.**

cocaine hydrochloride, a white crystal-like powder used as a local anesthetic. It was taken from coca leaves but now can also be made. It is commonly used to examine and treat the eye, ear, nose, and throat. The drug slows bleeding. Long or frequent use may damage the mucous membranes.

★CAUTION: Too much stimulation of the central nervous system may result from use with some drugs. Cocaine is not given to patients with severe heart disease, thyroid disease, or low blood pressure.

★ADVERSE EFFECTS: Among the most severe side effects are excitement, mental depression, and restlessness. Also found are tremors, dizziness, nausea, vomiting, high blood pressure, stomach cramps, chills, fever, coma, or death from lung failure.

★NOTE: Cocaine is a narcotic (Schedule II) drug under the Controlled Substances Act.

cocarcinogen, a substance that becomes cancerous only when combined with another substance.

cocci-, cocco-, a combining form meaning 'seed or berry'. It refers to a round bacterial cell.

coccidioidomycosis /koksid'ē·oi'dōmīkō'sis/, an infectious disease caused by breathing in spores of the fungus *Coccidioides immitis*. These spores are carried on dust particles in the wind. The disease occurs in hot, dry regions of the southwest United States. It is also found in Central and South America. The early symptoms of infection resemble the common cold or influenza. These symptoms then disappear for a period of time. Later new problems develop that last for weeks to years. These include low fever, appetite and weight loss, bluish skin, and breathing difficulty. Also found are blood in the spit, skin sores, and arthritic pain in the bones and joints. Also called **desert fever, desert rheumatism, San Joaquin fever, valley fever.**

coccidiosis /kok'sidē·ō'sis/, a parasitic disease found in tropical and subtropical regions. It is caused by swallowing eggs of a tiny organism (*Isospora belli* or *I. hominis*). Symptoms include fever, malaise, stomach pain, and watery diarrhea. The infection usually lasts 1 to 2 weeks and health returns. No specific treatment has been found. Compare **coccidioidomycosis.**

coccus /kok'əs/, *pl.* **cocci,** a bacterium that is round, spheric, or oval. –**coccal,** *adj.*

coccyg-, coccygo-, a combining form meaning 'coccyx.'

coccygeal vertebra, one of the four parts of the spinal column that join to form the adult coccyx. Compare **cervical vertebra, lumbar vertebra, sacral vertebra, thoracic vertebra.** See also **coccyx, vertebra.**

coccygeus /koksij'ē·əs/, one of the muscles in the floor of the pelvis. It is a band of muscle and fibers. This band stretches across the pelvic cavity like a hammock. Compare **levator ani.**

coccygodynia /kok'sigōdin'ē·ə/, a pain in the tailbone area of the body.

coccyx /kok'siks/, *pl.* **coccyges** /koksī'jēz/, kok'sijēz/,the small bone (tailbone) at the very end of the spine. It is joined to the end of the spine (sacrum) by a disk of cartilage. Between three and five vertebrae join to form the coccyx in early life. The coccyx fuses with the sacrum by adulthood.

cochineal /koch'inēl'/, a red dye made from the dried female insects of the species *Coccus cacti*. The dye has been used in coloring medicines.

cochlea /kok'lē·ə/, a small bone of the inner ear and the organ of hearing. It is coiled 2½ times into the shape of a snail shell. This bone has many small holes through which pass the nerve-carrying signals from the ear to the brain (acoustic nerve). The cochlea connects with the organs of the acoustic nerve. –**cochlear** /kok'lē·ər/,*adj.*

cochlear canal, a spiral tunnel in the organ of hearing (cochlea) of the inner ear.

cochlear toxicity, harmful effects of drugs that may result in hearing disorders, as ringing in the ears (tinnitus) and loss of hearing.

cockroach, a common name for certain insects that infest homes, workplaces, and other areas inhabited by humans. Cockroaches carry bacteria and the eggs of parasitic worms.

cockscomb papilloma, a harmless, small red tag that may grow from the uterine cervix during pregnancy. It disappears after delivery.

cocktail, *informal.* a mixture of drugs, usually in a liquid, to relieve pain. Cocktails are sometimes given to cancer patients. See also **Brompton's cocktail.**

cockup splint, a splint used to prevent movement at the wrist while keeping the fingers free to move.

cocontraction, the shortening, at the same time, of muscles that control opposite movements at a joint in an effort to strengthen a position. Also called **coinnervation.**

code, 1. a system of signals for passing on information, as a genetic code. 2. *informal,* a signal used to call a special team to revive a patient. This is done without alarming patients or visitors. Compare **decode, encode.**

code of ethics, a set of rules to which members of a profession are expected to conform. See also **Hippocratic Oath.**

codeine, a narcotic used to relieve mild pain, to treat diarrhea, and to stop coughing.
★CAUTION: Known allergy to this drug prohibits its use.
★ADVERSE EFFECTS: Among the most common side effects are constipation, nausea, drowsiness, and allergic reactions. High doses can affect breathing and circulation. The drug can be addictive.

code team, a team of specially trained and equipped people. This team is called to revive patients suffering from sudden heart and lung failure. The procedure is called cardiopulmonary resuscitation. A code team normally includes a physician, registered nurse, respiratory therapist, and pharmacist.

cod-liver oil, a pale-yellow, fatty oil from the fresh livers of codfish. It may also come from other related species. It is a rich source of vitamins A and D and is useful for treating a lack of those vitamins. It is also used to treat abnormal absorption of calcium and phosphorus. See also **osteomalacia, rickets, tetany.**

Codman's tumor. See **chondroblastoma.**

coel-, a combining form referring to the colon.

coelenteron, *pl.* **coelentera,** the digestive cavity of certain simple animals, as the hydra and jellyfish. See also **archenteron.**

coelom, the body cavity of the developing embryo.

coelosomy, a birth defect in which the stomach and bowels protrude from the body cavity.

coenzyme /kō·en′zīm/, a substance that combines with other substances to form a complete enzyme. Coenzymes include some of the vitamins, as B_1 and B_2.

coffee, the seeds of *Coffea arabica, C. liberica,* and *C. robusta* trees. These trees grow in almost all tropical areas. Coffee beans contain caffeine and are used to make a stimulating drink. Coffee has been used to treat headache, long-term asthma, and drug poisoning.

coffee-and- . . . , a method of treatment for long-term psychiatric patients living at home. Patients meet regularly with professional staff. The setting is social and informal. Patients gain mutual support and encouragement. Coffee and something to eat may be served.

coffee-ground vomitus, vomit that looks dark brown, like coffee grounds. It is made up of gastric juices and old blood. This is a symptom of slow bleeding in the stomach and upper bowels. Compare **hematemesis.**

coffee worker's lung, a lung condition caused by an allergic reaction to the dust of the coffee bean. See also **organic dust.**

Cogentin, a trademark for a drug used to treat Parkinson's disease (benztropine mesylate).

cognition, the mental process of knowing, thinking, learning, and judging.

cognitive development, the process by which an infant becomes an intelligent person. As it grows the infant gains knowledge. It also develops the ability to think, learn, reason, and abstract. See also **psychosexual development, psychosocial development.**

cognitive dissonance, a state of mental stress. This comes from learning new information that conflicts with old ideas or knowledge.

cognitive function, a mental process by which one becomes aware of ideas. It involves perception, thinking, reasoning, and remembering. Compare **conation.**

cognitive learning, learning to acquire problem-solving skills. This also refers to intelligence and conscious thought.

cognitive psychology, study of the development of thought, language, and intelligence.

cognitive therapy, various ways of treating mental and emotional disorders. These include behavior therapy, existential therapy, Gestalt therapy, and transactional analysis.

cogwheel rigidity, an abnormal stiffness in muscle tissue. It is marked by jerky movements when the muscle is made to stretch.

coherence, 1. the property of sticking together, as the molecules of a substance. 2. the logical pattern of speech and thought of a normal, stable person.

cohesiveness, 1. (in psychiatry) a force that attracts members to a group and causes them to remain in the group. **2.** (in dentistry) a property of pure gold that allows it to be used as a filling material.

cohort,   a group of people who share a characteristic, as age or sex.

cohort study,   a study comparing facts about specific groups of people. An example would be a study of children born in 1975 and the children born in 1955. See also **prospective study.**

coil.   See **intrauterine device.**

coiled tubular gland,   a gland that has a coiled, tube-shaped part that releases fluid. An example would be the sweat glands.

coil-spring contraceptive diaphragm,   a type of diaphragm for birth control. The flexible metal spring of the rim is coiled and round. This kind of diaphragm is given to women whose vaginal muscles offer good support, and whose uterus is not tipped back or forward. It is also given to women with a normal-size vagina with an abnormally deep arch behind the pubic bone. Compare **arcing-spring contraceptive diaphragm, flat-spring contraceptive diaphragm.** See also **contraceptive diaphragm fitting.**

coinnervation.   See **cocontraction.**

coitus /kō′itəs/,   the sexual union of two people of opposite sex. The penis is inserted into the vagina, usually resulting in orgasm. Also called **coition, copulation, sexual intercourse.** –**coital,** *adj.*

coitus interruptus.   See **withdrawal method.**

Colace,   a trademark for a stool softener (docusate sodium sulfosuccinate).

colation,   filtering or straining, as urine being strained for medical examination.

COL bed.   See **CircOlectric (COL) bed.**

colchicine /kol′chəsēn/,   a drug used to treat gout. It is also given to prevent gouty arthritis attacks.

★CAUTION: Ulcer, ulcerative colitis, or known allergy to this drug prohibits its use. The drug is very strong. It is not given to elderly, weakened patients nor to people with long-term kidney, liver, heart, or stomach and intestine disease.

★ADVERSE EFFECTS: Among the most serious side effects are severe stomach and bowel pain, diarrhea with blood, severe anemia, nerve disorders, liver failure, and hair loss.

cold,   **1.** the absence of heat. **2.** also called **common cold.** a contagious viral infection of the upper respiratory tract. The symptoms are stuffy nose, watery eyes, low fever, and aching. It is treated with rest, aspirin, decongestants, and drinking a lot of fluids.

cold abscess,   an infection that does not show the usual signs of heat, redness, and swelling.

cold agglutinin,   a substance that fights disease in the body (antibody) found on the surface of red blood cells in certain diseases. It may cause the cells to clump at temperatures below 39°F

(4° C). It may also break down the red blood cells. It does not occur when the body is at its normal temperature.

cold bath,   a bath in which the water temperature is about 50° F (10° C) to 65° F (18° C). Cold baths are used mainly to reduce body temperature.

cold-blooded,   referring to animals not able to control body heat, as fishes, reptiles, and amphibians. They have body temperatures that are near the temperatures of the areas in which they live. Also called **poikilothermic.** Compare **warm-blooded.**

cold cautery.   See **cryocautery.**

cold caloric irrigation,   a procedure for testing brainstem function. It is done by pouring a cold salt solution into the ear canal with the head at a 30° angle. This causes jerky but regular eye movements in a normal patient. Absence of the reaction may be a sign of a disease of the brainstem. See also **Barany test.**

cold environment,   surroundings in which the temperature is below 50° F (10° C). Nearly two-thirds of the world's population, including most of North America, Europe, and Asia north of India, lives in a naturally cold environment for at least a part of each year. The human body must be kept warm or it will not function well at temperatures below 59° F (15° C). The hands and fingers lose their sense of touch, and more errors and accidents occur. The body reacts by narrowing the blood vessels near the skin to retain body heat. As a result, the skin, arms, and legs feel cooler. If body temperature continues to drop, the person shivers and muscles become tense in an effort to conserve heat.

cold hemoglobinuria.   See **hemoglobinuria.**

cold injury,   any of several abnormal conditions caused by exposure to cold temperatures. These conditions are often serious. See also **chilblain, frostbite, hypothermia, immersion foot.**

cold-pressor test,   a test for the tendency to develop high blood pressure (essential hypertension). One hand of the person is placed in ice water for about 60 seconds. A large rise in the blood pressure or a delay in the return of normal pressure when the hand is taken from the water is watched for. If either takes place, it is believed that the person may develop hypertension.

cold sore.   See **herpes simplex.**

cold-wet-sheet pack,   a form of therapy for agitated patients. The patient is wrapped in cold, wet sheets, which are then warmed by body heat. This has been shown to be soothing for very agitated patients.

colectomy /kəlek′təmē/,   surgical removal of part or all of the large intestine (colon). This is done to treat cancer of the colon or severe long-term ulcerative colitis. See also **abdominal surgery.**

Colestid, a trademark for a drug used to lower cholesterol in the blood (colestipol hydrochloride).

colestipol hydrochloride, a drug that reduces high blood levels of cholesterol. It is used to treat high cholesterol and xanthoma.
★CAUTION: Blockage of the gallbladder or known allergy to this drug prohibits its use.
★ADVERSE EFFECTS: Among the more serious side effects are skin rash, constipation, and lack of vitamins A, D, and K.

colic /kol'ik/, sharp pain resulting from twisting, blockage, or muscle spasm of a hollow or tubelike organ. These can include a ureter or the intestines. Kinds of colic include **biliary colic, infantile colic, renal colic.**

colicinogen /kol'isin'əjən/, a gene in some strains of the bacteria *Escherichia coli.* It causes release of colicin, an antibiotic deadly to other strains of the bacterium. Also called **colicinogenic factor.**

coliform /kol'ifôrm/, referring to the bacteria that live in the intestines of humans and other animals.

colistimethate sodium, a drug that fights bacteria. It is used to treat some stomach and bowel infections and skin infections.

colistin sulfate, a drug that fights bacteria used to treat infections of the outer ear. It is taken by mouth for serious infections and to treat swelling of the stomach and bowels caused by *Escherichia coli* infections.
★CAUTION: Known allergy to this drug prohibits its use.
★ADVERSE EFFECTS: Among the more serious side effects are breathing arrest, kidney poisoning, and nerve and muscle disorders.

colitis, a general term for inflammation of the large intestine. This can refer to either one of the irritable bowel syndromes. It can also mean one of the more serious long-term bowel diseases. Irritable bowel syndrome is marked by colicky pain and diarrhea or constipation. These may often be caused by emotional stress. Treatment includes reducing stress and sticking to a diet that may include bland foods and less roughage than is usual. Because persons with colitis may be irritated by different foods, a diet is created for each patient. Inflammatory bowel disease is characterized by abscesses in the bowel, severe diarrhea, bleeding, and ulcers of the mucous membrane of the intestine. Weight loss and pain are great. Kinds of inflammatory bowel disease include **Crohn's disease, ulcerative colitis.** –colitic, *adj.*

collagen /kol'əjən/, a protein consisting of bundles of tiny fibers. Collagen forms connective tissue. These include the white inelastic fibers of the tendons, the ligaments, the bones, and the cartilage. –**collagenous** /kəlaj'ənəs/,*adj.*

collagenase ointment, a drug used to treat bed sores, burns, and other skin disorders.

collagen disease, any one of many disorders marked by swelling and breakdown of fiber in connective tissue. Some collagen diseases are polyarteritis nodosa, disseminated lupus erythematosus, rheumatic fever, arteritis, and ankylosing spondylitis.

collagenoblast /kəlaj'ənōblast'/, a cell that forms collagen. It can also change into cartilage and bone tissue.

collagenous fiber, the tough, white fibers that make up much of the connective tissue of the body. These fibers contain collagen. They are often arranged in bundles that strengthen the tissues in which they are found.

collagen vascular disease, any of a group of disorders in which swelling occurs in small blood vessels and connective tissue. The cause of most of these diseases is unknown. Hereditary factors and deficiencies, environmental factors, infections, and allergies may be involved. Common features of most of these diseases include arthritis, skin sores, and swelling of the eyes. Further features are infection of the membrane around the lungs (pleuritis), skin nodules, infection of the heart (myocarditis) and of the kidneys (nephritis). Diseases included in this category are mixed connective tissue disease, polyarteritis nodosa, polymyositis, rheumatic fever, rheumatoid arthritis, scleroderma, and systemic lupus erythematosus. Also called **connective tissue disease.**

collapse, 1. *nontechnical.* a state of extreme depression or of total exhaustion caused by physical or emotional problems. 2. an abnormal condition marked by shock. 3. the abnormal sagging of an organ.

collar, any structure that circles another, usually around its neck. The periosteal bone collars that form around the ends of young bones are an example.

collarbone. See **clavicle.**

collateral, 1. secondary or accessory. 2. a small branch, as any one of the arterioles in the body.

collateral pulp canal, a branch of the pulp canal that comes out of the root of a tooth at a place other than the tip.

collecting tubule, any one of the many straight small tubes of the kidney that take urine into the renal pelvis, which is at the center of the kidney. The collecting tubules drain the urine from the twisted tubules in the walls of the kidney. They then join one another at intervals along the path to the renal pelvis. The collecting tubules are important in keeping the fluid balance of the body by letting water seep through their membranes. Antidiuretic hormone in the blood allows water to pass through the membranes. If no antidiuretic hormone is present in the blood, the membranes do not allow the water to pass. This creates high water content in the urine. See also **Bowman's capsule, kidney.**

collective bargaining, the use of action by a group of employees to discuss working conditions and wages with an employer.

collective unconscious, that portion of the unconscious common to all people. Also called **racial unconscious.** See also **analytic psychology.**

collector, a device for collecting fluids from the bronchi of the lungs and the esophagus for laboratory examination.

college, 1. an organization of persons with common training and interests. Examples are the American College of Nurse-Midwives, the American College of Cardiology, or the American College of Surgeons. **2.** an institution of higher learning.

Colles' fascia /kol'ēz/, a strong, smooth sheet of tissue with stretchy fibers that fills a groove between the scrotum and the thigh in a man or between the labia and the thigh in a woman.

Colles' fracture, a break of one of the bones in the forearm (radius). It occurs 1 inch above the wrist and is easy to recognize by the hand position that it causes.

colliquation /koll'ikwā'shən/, the breakdown of a tissue of the body into liquid. It is normally linked to dead tissue.

colliquative /kol'ikwā'tiv/, marked by the release of a great amount of fluid. This is common when wounds become infected.

collision tumor, a tumor formed by two separate growths close to each other. See also **carcinoma.**

collodion /kəlō'dē·ən/, a clear or slightly cloudy, clear liquid that dries to a strong film. It is highly resistant to fire. Collodion is used to cover surgical wounds.

collodion baby, a newborn baby whose skin is covered with a scaly, dry membrane. See also **harlequin fetus, lamellar exfoliation of the newborn.**

colloid /kol'oid/, **1.** referring to a state of matter in which large molecules remain suspended in a liquid or other material. They neither mix in or settle to the bottom. **2.** a gelatinlike substance in the body that resembles glue. Compare **solution, suspension.**

colloidal sulfur, finely ground sulfur that is used to treat acne and other skin disorders.

colloid bath, a bath in water that contains substances as bran, gelatin, or starch. Colloid baths are often used to relieve irritation and swelling of the skin. See also **emollient bath.**

colloid goiter, a thyroid gland that has become very large and soft. The gland's pouchlike cavities (follicles) are swollen with colloid.

colloid osmotic pressure, an abnormal condition of the kidney. It is caused by the pressure of large particles that will not pass through a membrane. Also called **oncotic pressure.**

colo-, colon-, a combining form referring to the colon.

coloboma /kol'əbō'mə/, a birth defect in which a cleft extends along the edge of the eyeball. This affects the iris, ciliary body, or the blood vessel layer (choroid).

colon /kō'lən/, the part of the large intestine that extends to the rectum. The colon takes the contents of the small intestine, moving them to the rectum by contracting. Much water is added to the foodstuff by the stomach and small intestine during digestion. The colon absorbs most of this water through the walls. This firms the feces as they move into the rectum. **–colonic** /kəlon'ik/, *adj.*

colonic fistula, an abnormal passage from the colon to the surface of the body or to another organ or structure. Long-term swelling of the intestines may cause a passage (fistula) between two loops of bowel. An opening from the colon to the surface of the skin may be made surgically after a part of the bowel is removed. This surgery is common when a cancerous section or badly infected sore in the bowel is removed. See also **colostomy.**

colonic irrigation, a procedure for washing the inner wall of the large intestine by filling it with water, then draining it. It is not considered an enema.

colonization, the presence and growth of bacteria on the surface of the skin without any tissue damage.

colonoscopy /kō'lənos'kəpē/, the visual examination of the lining of the large intestine using a long, lighted instrument (colonoscope).

colon stasis. See **atonia constipation.**

colony, 1. a mass of microorganisms that grows from a single cell. This mass is grown in a special substance called a culture. **2.** a mass of cells in a culture.

colony counter, a device used for counting colonies of bacteria growing in a culture. It usually consists of a transparent plate divided into grid sections. Petri dishes containing colonies of bacteria are placed over the plate, and the numbers of colonies in each grid are counted.

coloproctitis, an inflammation of both the large intestine and the rectum. Also called **colorectitis.**

coloptosis, the dropping down of the large intestine.

Colorado tick fever, a relatively mild virus infection that is carried to humans by the bite of a tick. It is most common in the spring and summer throughout the Rocky Mountains, especially in Colorado. Symptoms occur in two phases between which there are no symptoms. They include chills, fever, headache, pain in the eyes, legs, and back, and sensitivity to light. Painkillers can be given for headache and other pains. Also called **American mountain fever, mountain fever, mountain tick fever.** Compare **Rocky Mountain spotted fever.**

color blindness, the inability to clearly tell one color from another. In most cases it is not a blindness but a weakness in seeing colors distinctly. There are two forms of color blindness. **Daltonism** is the most common form. It is marked by an inability to tell reds from greens. It is an inherited disorder that affects males. **Total color blindness,** or **achromatic vision,** is marked by an inability to perceive any color at all. Only white, gray, and black are seen. It may be the result of a defect in the cells that see colors (cones) in the retina. See also **deutan color blindness.**

color dysnomia /disnō′mē·ə/, an inability to name colors, even though the person can match and tell them apart. It may be caused by damaged speech centers in the brain (expressive dysphasia).

colorectal cancer /kō′lərek′təl/, a cancerous tumor of the large intestine. It is marked by dark, sticky stools containing blood and a change in bowel habits. Cancerous tumors of the large bowel usually occur after the age of 50. They are slightly more frequent in women than in men and are almost as common as lung cancer in the United States. Japan and rural Africa have low rates of colorectal cancer, whereas the United States and other developed Western countries have very high rates. This suggests that a diet high in carbohydrates and beef and low in roughage may be a factor. People who have long-term ulcerative colitis, diverticulosis, and polyps of the colon have a greater risk of developing this type of cancer. People who have inhaled asbestos fibers or who have been exposed to high levels of radiation are more likely than others to develop colorectal cancer. Rectal tumors may cause pain, bleeding, and a feeling of fullness, even after a bowel movement. They may spread slowly

through lymph channels and veins, and may sag through the anus. Some tumors constrict the intestine, causing partial blockage resulting in flat or pencil-shaped stools. Tumors in the ascending colon are usually large growths that can be felt on physical examination. They generally cause severe anemia, nausea, and constipation and diarrhea. Surgical treatment of colorectal cancer may involve removing the tumor, the surrounding colon, and the attached tissues. The remaining intestinal segments are sewed together whenever possible. Otherwise, a colostomy is performed. Tumors of the lower two-thirds of the rectum usually require removing the entire rectum. Radiation treatments may be given both before and after surgery and for tumors that cannot be removed.

colorimetry /kol′ərim′ətrē/, **1.** measurement of the intensity of color in a fluid or substance. **2.** measurement of color in the blood to determine the content of hemoglobin. **–colorimetric,** *adj.*

color index (C.I.), the ratio between the amount of hemoglobin and the number of red blood cells in a sample of blood.

color vision, the perception of color. Color is seen as the cones in the retina react to changing intensities of red, green, and blue light. This process is not completely understood. Some experts believe there are three specialized types of cones that each reacts to red, green, or blue light. Some retinal cones respond to the entire color spectrum. See also **color blindness.**

colosigmoidoscopy /kō′ləsig′moidos′kəpē/, the visual examination of the large intestine using an instrument consisting of a tube and a light (sigmoidoscope).

colostomate /kəlos′təmāt/, a person who has a colostomy.

colostomy /kəlos′təmē/, surgical creation of an opening for feces to pass through the abdomi-

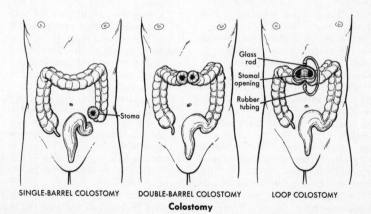

SINGLE-BARREL COLOSTOMY   DOUBLE-BARREL COLOSTOMY   LOOP COLOSTOMY

Stoma

Glass rod
Stomal opening
Rubber tubing

Colostomy

nal wall. An opening is made in the colon, and it is brought to the surface of the skin. Colostomies are performed for cancer of the colon and noncancerous tumors that block the bowel. They may also be done in the case of severe wounds to the stomach and bowels. A colostomy may be "single-barreled" with one opening or "double-barreled" with two loops opening onto the skin. The latter is done when the lower bowel is completely blocked or in paralyzed people to help with daily care. A temporary colostomy may be done to divert feces from a swollen area after surgery to allow it to heal. A type of colostomy is **loop colostomy**. Compare **enterostomy**.

colostomy irrigation, a procedure used by people with a colostomy (colostomates) to clear the bowel of feces and to help set up a regular schedule of bowel evacuation.

★METHOD: Daily irrigation usually begins 7 to 10 days after the operation. This is done as the patient sits on a toilet. A thin tube, or catheter, coated with petroleum jelly is gently placed in the opening (stoma) about 3 inches. A bag containing between a pint and a quart of warm solution is held 12 to 18 inches above the stoma. The fluid then flows slowly into the colon. The fluid is kept in the colon for several minutes and then drained out through a bag that is directed into the toilet. From 30 to 45 minutes is allowed for draining.

★PATIENT CARE: Colostomy irrigation should be learned while the person is a patient in the hospital. The patient is urged to report any symptoms of obstruction or problems with the stoma. A public health nurse may be found in many areas for home visits if help is needed. Most larger communities have organizations of persons who have colostomies. These offer educational and emotional support for new patients.

colostrum /kəlos'trəm/, the fluid released by the breast during pregnancy before milk production (lactation) begins. Colostrum is a thin, yellow fluid that contains white blood cells, water, protein, fat, and carbohydrate.

colotomy /kōlot'əmē/, a surgical cut into the large intestine, usually through the belly.

colpalgia /kolpal'jə/, a pain in the vagina.

colpitis, a vaginal inflammation.

colpectomy, the surgical removal of the vagina.

colpo-, colp-, kolpo-, kysth-, kystho-, a combining form referring to the vagina.

colpocystitis, an inflammation of the vagina and urinary bladder.

colpocystocele /kol'pəsis'təsēl/, the dropping down of the urinary bladder, causing it to push on the wall of the vagina.

colpohysterectomy, surgical removal of the uterus (hysterectomy) by way of the vagina. See also **hysterectomy**.

colporrhaphy, stitching of the vagina, usually to narrow the vagina.

colposcope /kol'pəskōp/, a lighted instrument for direct visual examination of the vagina and cervix.

colposcopy /kolpos'kəpē/, an examination of the vagina and cervix using a colposcope.

colpotomy, any surgical cut into the wall of the vagina.

columbium, former name for **niobium**.

Coly-Mycin M, a trademark for a drug that fights bacteria (colistimethate sodium).

coma, a state of deep unconsciousness. It is marked by the absence of eye movements, response to pain, and sounds. The person cannot be awakened. Coma may result from injury, brain tumor, serious infectious disease with brain inflammation, or blood vessel disease. It may also result from poisoning, diabetic acidosis, or intoxication. See also **Glasgow Coma Scale, unconscious**.

comatose, in a coma, or abnormally deep sleep, caused by illness or injury.

combat fatigue, a psychological disorder resulting from the physical and mental stress of warfare. It is usually temporary but sometimes leads to permanent neurosis. Combat fatigue is marked by anxiety, depression, irritability, memory and sleep disorders, and other similar symptoms. Also called **combat neurosis, war neurosis**. See also **posttraumatic stress disorder, shell shock**.

combination chemotherapy, the use of two or more anticancer drugs at the same time.

combined anesthesia. See **balanced anesthesia**.

combined cycling ventilator, a respirator that has more than one mechanism to control the breathing rate.

combined modality treatment, the use of anticancer drugs combined with surgery and/or radiation.

combined oxygen, the oxygen that is attached to hemoglobin in the blood.

combined patterns, a method of testing the function of a patient's nerves and muscles by observing how coordinated the patient is when performing certain movements of his or her body, arms, and legs.

combined system disease, a disorder of the nervous system caused by a lack of vitamin B_{12}. The disorder causes anemia and breakdown of the spinal cord and the nerves. There is also difficulty in walking, feeling of vibration in the legs, and a loss of sense of body position. Also known as **subacute combined degeneration of the spinal cord**. See also **pernicious anemia, vitamin B_{12}**.

combining form, a part of a word, often taken from Latin or Greek. It may be a root, a prefix, or a suffix, or all three.

combustion, the process of burning, which may give off light and heat. Oxygen is needed for burning but does not burn itself. The amount and pressure of oxygen control the rate of burning.

COMDU, abbreviation for **cardiac monitor and diagnostic unit.**

comedo /kom′idō/, *pl.* **comedones** /komidō′nēz/, blackhead, the basic sore of acne. Comedones are caused by a buildup of skin cells and oil in the pouch or follicle (from which a hair grows). It is dark because of the effect of oxygen on the skin oil, not because of dirt. Compare **milium.**

comedocarcinoma /kom′idōkär′sinō′mə/, a cancerous tumor of the milk ducts of the breast. Since the growth is confined in the milk ducts, the complete cure after surgery is better than for most other types of breast cancer.

comedogenicity /kom′idōjənis′itē/, the ability of certain drugs, such as steroids, to produce acne.

comfort, alteration in: pain, pain resulting from biological, chemical, physical, or psychological injury. The only way of detecting pain in another person is by the verbal or nonverbal communication of that person.

comfort measure, any action taken to increase comfort of the patient. Examples might be a back rub, a change in position, or warming a stethoscope or a bedpan before use.

Comité International des Poids et Mesures (CIPM) /kômitä′ aNternäsyōnäl′ dä pô·ä′ ā mesYr′/, a group of scientists that meet regularly to define the international (SI) units of physical amounts. Examples of these units are the volume of a liter, the length of a meter, or the precise amount of time in a minute. See also **SI units.**

command automatism, a condition in which a patient responds mechanically and without judgment to commands. This condition is seen in hypnosis and certain psychotic states.

command hallucination, a psychotic condition in which the patient hears and obeys voices that command him or her to perform certain acts. The hallucinations may cause the patient to behave in dangerous ways.

commensal /kəmen′səl/, an organism living on or in another. This organism does not harm the host. Both organisms may benefit from the relationship. Some bacteria in the digestive tract of humans help to process food. They also produce B vitamins needed for normal health while not hurting the host. Compare **parasite, synergist.**

comminuted, crushed or broken into pieces.

comminuted fracture, a fracture in which there are several breaks in the bone. This creates many bone fragments.

commissure /kom′isoŏr, -syoŏr/, **1.** a band of nerves or other tissue that cross from one side of the body to the other, usually connecting two structures. **2.** a site where two parts of the

body are joined, as the corner of the eye or lips.

commissurotomy /kom′ishoŏrot′əmē/, surgically dividing a fiberlike band or ring connecting parts of a body structure. This is often done to separate the thickened flaps of a narrowed mitral valve in the heart.

commitment, 1. the placement of a patient in a hospital or other facility designed to deal with the patient's special needs. See also **institutionalize. 2.** the legal act of admitting a mentally ill patient to an institution for psychiatric treatment. The process usually involves court action. This act is based on medical evidence that the person is mentally ill. See also **certification. 3.** a pledge or promise to do something in the future. It often refers to fulfilling an agreement. It is widely used in some forms of psychotherapy or marriage counseling.

common bile duct, the duct formed by the joining of the gallbladder (cystic) duct and liver (hepatic) duct.

common carotid artery, one of the major arteries bringing blood to the head and neck. The external carotid supplies the face, scalp, and most of the neck and throat tissues. The internal common carotids supply the brain, ears, and eyes.

common carotid plexus, a network of nerves on the common carotid artery. Branches accompany the blood vessels of the skull.

common cold. See **cold.**

common hepatic artery, an artery that branches off the aorta as it goes through the area of the stomach. Its five branches supply blood to the stomach, small intestines, and liver.

common iliac artery, a division of the abdominal aorta that divides into external and internal iliac arteries. These supply blood to the pelvis and legs.

common iliac node, a node in one of the seven groups of lymph nodes. These serve the stomach, bowels, pelvis.

common iliac vein, one of the two veins that pass through the pelvic area. It joins the inferior vena cava, which carries blood from the lower part of the trunk to the heart.

communicability period, the usual time in which an infected person is most likely to spread the infection to others. For measles, this period is from 4 days before the rash appears until 5 days after symptoms begin.

communicable, contagious; spread by direct or indirect contact, as a communicable disease.

communicable disease, any disease carried from one person or animal to another by direct or indirect contact. Direct contact includes touching any discharge from the body, as saliva. Indirect might include contact through something else, as drinking glasses, toys, water, or insects. To control a communicable disease, it is important to identify the organism causing the disease and prevent its spread. The infected person must be treated and others must be protected from contact with the organism. Many communicable diseases, by law, must be reported to the local health department. Also called **contagious disease.** See also **infectious disease.**

Communicable Disease Center, former name of the **Centers for Disease Control.**

communicating hydrocephalus. See **hydrocephalus.**

communication, transferring a message, especially from one person to another. Communication may be verbal or nonverbal. It may occur directly, as in a conversation, or by a gesture. It also may occur indirectly, spanning space and time, as in writing and reading. See also **kinesics.**

communication channels, any gesture, action, sound, written word, or visual image used to carry messages.

communication, impaired verbal, a condition that in some way affects the ability to speak. It may be caused by lack of blood to the brain, brain tumor, tube in the throat, or removal of the voice box. It may also be caused by a physical defect, as a cleft palate, or a psychosis. It may even apply to language barriers. The symptoms include slurring, stuttering, and problems in forming words or in expressing thoughts. Disorientation may also occur.

communication theme, a concept or idea that ties together elements of communication. Kinds of communication themes include **content theme, mood theme, interaction theme.**

community, a group of people who live in an area and who share common interests.

community-acquired infection, an infection acquired from one's typical surroundings or from use of medications. It is different from an infection acquired in the hospital (nosocomial infection).

community health nursing, a field of nursing that blends patient health care and public-health nursing. A community health nurse seeks to prevent, as well as cure, disease. This field is also concerned with rehabilitation.

community medicine, a branch of medicine concerned with the health of the members of a community or region.

community mental health, a treatment program based on the idea that a wide range of mental health services should be available to all members of the community.

community mental health center (CMHC), a community-based center that provides complete mental health care. This includes outpatient and inpatient care.

community nurse practitioner (CNP), a nurse who has completed advanced study in community nursing.

community psychiatry, the development of a program of mental health care for residents within a community. See also **community mental health center.**

compact bone, hard, dense bone that is usually found on the surface of bones.

companionship, placing a staff member or another patient with a disturbed patient. This is to provide support and to protect patients from hurting themselves or others.

comparative anatomy, the study of the structure and function of all living animals. It compares the various stages of growth in different animals. For example, the adult stage in some animals may resemble the youth stage in others. See also **applied anatomy, ontogeny, phylogeny.**

comparative embryology, the study comparing the embryos of various species during growth.

comparative physiology, the study comparing the physical processes in various species. The purpose is to find basic physical relationships between members of the animal and plant kingdoms.

comparative psychology, 1. the study comparing human behavior and animal behavior. **2.** the study of the differences in behavior among various peoples.

compartment syndrome, a condition caused by inward pressure of an artery reducing blood supply. It can result in a permanent contraction of the hand or foot. This may also cause a break in the hand or foot with or without a fracture. See also **Volkmann's contracture.**

compatibility, 1. the ability to live together in harmony. **2.** the orderly, efficient mixing of elements from one system with those of another. **3.** the ability of several drugs to work together without harming the patient. **4.** the degree to which the body's defense system will accept foreign matter, as blood or organs. Usually, perfect compatibility exists only between identical twins.

Compazine, a trademark for a drug used to treat nausea and psychosis (prochlorperazine).

compensated flow meter, a respiratory therapy device that accurately records the amount of air delivered to a patient.

compensated gluteal gait, a common abnormal walk linked to a weak muscle deep inside the buttock (gluteus medius). It results from an attempt to shift body weight off the affected hip. Also called **gluteal gait.**

compensated heart failure, an abnormal heart condition in which the body tries to compensate for heart failure. This may include increased nerve stimulation of the heart, increasing blood flow to the heart, and enlargement of the heart. This process may be helped by return of blood to the heart, giving digitalis or diuretics. See also **heart failure.**

compensating current, an electric current that counteracts a muscle current.

compensating curve, the curve of alignment of the biting surfaces of the teeth. It is used to ensure that the molar teeth meet properly. It also provides balancing contacts on dentures.

compensation, 1. correction of a defect or loss of the body by the increased output of another part. **2.** the process of keeping enough blood flow in spite of heart or circulatory problems. Failure of the heart to pump enough blood indicates a diseased heart muscle. **3.** a complex defense mechanism to avoid a feeling of inferiority. This can be achieved by putting forth great effort to overcome a handicap. Another way is to scorn the lack of quality. A kind of compensation is **dosage compensation.** See also **overcompensation.**

compensation neurosis, an unconscious process by which one keeps the symptoms of an injury or disease. This is done in order to receive other gains, especially money. Compare **malingering.**

compensatory hypertrophy, an increase in the size or function of part of the body. This is done to counterbalance a defect. See also **compensated heart failure.**

compensatory pause, a longer than normal pause between two heartbeats, usually after a premature beat.

competence, the ability of any part of the body to do what is required of it.

competent community, a population that is aware of its resources and options, able to make reasonable decisions on topics affecting the entire group, and to cope with problems facing the group. The group is an example of positive mental health.

competitive displacement, an interaction between two drugs in which one drug prevents the action of the other. When two drugs act in this manner, it is important to take them at different times so that both drugs may have their desired effects.

competitive identification, the unconscious modeling of one's personality on that of another. This is done in order to outdo the other person. See also **identification.**

competitive inhibitor, a substance that stops an enzyme reaction.

complaint, *informal.* any illness, problem, or symptom identified by the patient. The chief complaint is often the reason that the person seeks health care.

complement, complex proteins in the blood that bind with substances that defend the body (antibodies) against foreign invaders (antigens). Complement is involved in reactions, as severe allergic reaction (anaphylaxis). See also **antibody, antigen, antigen-antibody reaction, immune gamma globulin.**

complement abnormality, deficiency or defect of any of the parts of a **complement.** Patients with complement abnormalities are more likely to get infections and collagen vascular diseases. It is difficult and often expensive to diagnose complement abnormalities.

complementary feeding, an extra feeding given to an infant who is still hungry after breast feeding.

complementary transactions, (in psychiatry) interactions that may continue indefinitely as the parties involved keep acting from the same level of understanding.

complement cascade, a process in which one **complement** interacts with another in a certain pattern. The cascade effect causes fluid to build up in a cell. This buildup of fluid then breaks the cell.

complement fixation, a reaction in which a foreign invader (antigen) combines with an antibody and its complement. This causes the complement to become active. Complement-fixation tests are used to diagnose infectious diseases, as syphilis and viral illnesses. See also **complement, immune system, immunity, Wassermann test.**

complement-fixation test (C-F test), any blood test in which complement-fixation is found. This confirms the presence of a certain foreign invader in the body (antigen). The Wasserman test is a C-F test for syphilis.

complete abortion, the ending of pregnancy in which the fetus or embryo is completely removed. Because nothing remains in the uterus, a D and C (dilation and curettage) is not necessary. Compare **incomplete abortion.**

complete bed bath, a bath in which the entire body of a patient is washed while the person is still in bed. See also **blanket bath.**

complete blood count (CBC), the number of red and white blood cells per cubic millimeter of blood. A complete blood count is performed on all patients admitted to the hospital. It is one of the most valuable diagnostic tests. The count can be done by staining a smear of blood on a slide and counting the types of cells under a microscope. Most laboratories use an electronic counter. See also **differential white blood cell count, erythrocyte, hematocrit, hemoglobin, leukocyte.**

complete breech, a position of the fetus in the womb in which the buttocks and feet are toward the birth canal. The position of the fetus is the same as in a normal head-first position, but upside down. Compare **frank breech.** See also **breech birth.**

complete fistula, an abnormal passage from an inner organ or structure to the surface of the body. It may also go to another organ or structure.

complete fracture, a bone break that completely severs the bone across its width.

complete health history, a history of a patient's health patterns. It includes a history of the present illness and of any previous illness. Also listed are social and occupational history, sexual history, and a family health history. See also **health history.**

complete rachischisis, a rare birth defect in which there is a fissure of the entire spinal column and spinal cord. See also **spina bifida.**

complete response (CR), the total disappearance of a tumor.

complex, 1. a group of chemical molecules that are related in structure or function. **2.** a combination of symptoms of disease that forms a syndrome. **3.** a group of linked ideas, with strong emotional overtones. These ideas affect a patient's attitudes.

complex carbohydrate, a sugar or starch made up of a large number of glucose molecules.

complex cavity, a cavity that involves more than one side of a tooth.

complex fracture, a fracture in which the soft tissue around the bone is severely damaged.

complex spatial relations, an idea of how one part of an object is positioned in relation to another part of the object.

compliance, fulfillment by the patient of the treatment prescribed.

complication, a disease or injury that occurs during the treatment of an earlier disorder. A complication frequently will extend the time needed to recover from the original disorder.

component, a part of a larger unit.

component drip set, a device used for running fluids into a vein. It includes plastic tubing, drip chamber, and filter.

component syringe set, a device used for delivering fluids into a vein. It includes plastic tubing, two slide clamps, a Y-connector, and a needle syringe.

component therapy, transfusion in which only certain blood components are given. In this way it is possible to transfer more of the blood component than would be found in whole blood. Compare **plasmaphoresis.** See also **packed cells, pooled plasma.**

composite core, a buildup of resin to hold an artificial tooth crown.

compos mentis, the quality of having a healthy mind. Compare **non compos mentis.**

compound, 1. a substance made up of two or more elements that cannot be separated. **2.** any substance made up of two or more ingredients. **3.** to make a substance by combining ingredients, as a drug. **4.** referring to an injury marked by several factors.

compound aneurysm, a widening of a part of the wall of an artery. Some of the layers are bloated, and others are broken. Also called **mixed aneurysm.**

compound fracture, a break in which the broken end or ends of the bone tear through the skin. Also called **open fracture.**

compound melanocytoma. See **benign juvenile melanoma.**

compound tubuloalveolar gland, a gland with more than one duct for fluids, as a salivary gland.

comprehensive care. See **holistic health care.**

compress, a soft pad, usually made of cloth. It is used to apply heat, cold, or drugs to the surface of a body. A compress also may be placed over a wound to help stop bleeding. Compare **dressing.**

compressed air hazards. See **decompression sickness.**

compressibility factor, a measurement, relating to respirators, of the amount of inhaled and exhaled air that does not reach the patient because it is trapped inside the respirator.

compressible volume, a measurement, relating to respirators, of the amount of inhaled and exhaled air that does not reach the patient due to expansion of flexible tubing in the equipment.

compression, the act of applying pressure to an area of the body. A tumor or bleeding may cause compression of brain tissue, for example.

compression fracture, a bone break, most often found in a short bone. It breaks apart bone tissue and collapses the bone. The bones of the spine (vertebrae) are often sites of compression fractures.

compression neuropathy, any of several disorders in which nerves are damaged by severe pressure or injury. The symptoms are numbness, weakness, or paralysis.

compressive atelectasis, the inability of a section of lung to move air in and out because high pressures have caused that area of the lung to collapse. This condition may result from a blood clot in the lung.

compressor naris, the part of the nasal muscle that draws the nostril walls inward. Compare **dilatator naris.**

compromise, an action involving a change in a person's behavior, as in taking a different course of action to reduce stress or conflict that might have resulted if the first course were followed.

compromise body image, a new body image that a patient acquires as an adjustment to a new physical problem. A compromise body image changes the unacceptable features of the condition to make them more acceptable to the patient.

compromised host, a patient who is not able to resist infection. This may be due to defective immune system or severe anemia. A severe disease or condition, as cancer or general poor health, may also be involved.

compulsion, an irresistible impulse to perform an irrational act. The impulse is usually the result of an obsession. A kind of compulsion is **repetition compulsion.** Compare **phobia.** See also **obsession.** –**compulsive,** *adj.*

compulsive idea, a returning, irrational idea that persists in the mind. It often results in a compelling need to perform some improper act. Also called **imperative idea.**

compulsive personality, a type of personality in which a person is obsessed with clinging to rigid standards. The person is usually very reliable, inhibited, and inflexible. He or she may work extremely hard and be unable to relax or relate to people.

compulsive personality disorder, a condition in which a compulsive personality interferes with everyday work and normal behavior. The patient is preoccupied with order, rules, and detail. The disorder is marked by excessive devotion to work and clinging to a system of behavior. The patient cannot make decisions when faced with unexpected situations. See also **compulsive personality, obsessive-compulsive neurosis.**

compulsive polydipsia, a neurotic, compelling urge to drink large amounts of liquid. The condition is emotional. It is not caused by any physical disorder or lack. Extreme cases can result in death. See also **polydipsia.**

compulsive ritual, a series of acts a patient feels must be carried out. This is done even though he or she knows the behavior is useless and inappropriate. Failure to complete the acts results in extreme anxiety. See also **obsessive-compulsive neurosis.**

compuphobia, a fear of working with computers.

computerized axial tomography (CAT). See **computerized tomography (CT).**

computerized tomography (CT), a technique for examining internal structures of the body. The examination is painless and requires no special preparation. Computerized tomography produces a highly accurate picture that shows relationships of structures to each other. Tumors, blood clots, bone displacement, and gathering of fluid can be detected. This technique can be used on the brain, chest, stomach, and pelvis. Also called **computerized axial tomography (CAT), computerized transverse axial tomography.**

conation, the mental process marked by desire, impulse, voluntary action, and striving. Compare **cognition.** –**conative,** *adj.*

-conazole, a combining form indicating a miconazole-type drug that acts against fungi.

concatenates, long molecules that result from repeating the same molecular subunit.

concave-convex joint relationship, the shape of the two bone surfaces forming a joint as they meet. One surface is usually rounded inward like a bowl (concave), and the other is rounded outward like a sphere (convex). The convex surface rests in the concave surface.

concavity, the rounded, inward curving of an organ or body part.

concealed accessory pathway, an abnormal muscular tract between the upper and lower heart chambers. It allows blood to pass in only one direction. It is present in the Wolff-Parkinson-White syndrome.

conceive, to become pregnant.

concentrate, 1. to decrease the amount of a liquid and increase its strength. This is done by removing the inactive ingredients (usually water) through evaporation. 2. a substance, especially a liquid, that has been strengthened and reduced in volume.

concentric contraction, a form of muscle contraction that occurs in rhythmic activities. See also **isotonic exercise.**

concentric fibroma, a fiberlike tumor surrounding the uterus.

concept, an abstract idea or thought that begins and is held in the mind. –**conceptual,** *adj.*

conception, 1. the beginning of pregnancy. This is usually taken to be the instant that a sperm enters an egg (ovum). 2. the act or process of fertilization. 3. the process of creating an idea. 4. the idea created.

conception control. See **contraception.**

conceptional age, the number of weeks since conception of an embryo. Because the exact time of conception is difficult to know, conceptional age is said to be two weeks less than the pregnancy (gestational) age.

conceptual disorder, an inability to think productively or form ideas.

conceptus, the result of conception. It includes the fertilized egg and its enclosing membranes. See also **embryo, fetus.**

concha, a body structure that is shell shaped, like the area around the opening of the ear canal.

concoction, a remedy that has been prepared from heating a mixture of two or more drugs or substances.

concomitant symptom, any symptom that accompanies a patient's main symptom.

concordance, the appearance of one or more traits in both members of a pair of twins. Compare **discordance.** –**concordant,** *adj.*

concreteness, the content of a communicaton that is not vague. It expresses specific feelings, behaviors, experiences, and situations.

concrete operation, an idea based on real things rather than abstract thoughts.

concrete thinking, a stage in the development of the thinking process in the child. During this phase, thought becomes more logical. The child is able to classify, sort, order, and organize facts but is not able to deal with abstractions. Problem solving is based on what is seen.

The literal meaning of words is still present. This stage occurs between 7 and 11 years of age. It is preceded by the ability to combine different beliefs (syncretic thinking), and followed by abstract thinking.

concurrent disinfection, the daily disposal of infected material or equipment.

concurrent sterilization, fixing an infant feeding formula. All ingredients and equipment are sterilized before mixing the formula.

concussion, 1. a violent jar or shock, as caused by a blow or explosion. 2. *informal.* **brain concussion.**

condensation, 1. the change that occurs when steam cools to water. 2. (in psychology) a process often present in dreams in which two or more ideas are represented by a single symbol.

condensation nuclei, particles, as dust, in the air. These particles provide a site for water vapor to condense, and at high humidities, they produce fogs and hazes.

condenser, a dental tool for pressing filling material into a tooth cavity.

condition, 1. a state of being. It refers to physical and mental health or well-being. 2. to train the body or mind. This is done through certain exercises and repeated exposure to a state or thing. See also **classical conditioning.**

conditional discharge, a leave of absence or release from a psychiatric hospital in which certain behaviors are expected from the patient. The original commitment order remains in effect, and the patient will be required to return to the hospital if the behaviors are not followed.

conditioned avoidance response, a reaction that is learned in order to avoid an unpleasant stimulus. This response may be either conscious or unconscious.

conditioned escape response, a reaction that is learned in order to stop or to escape from an unpleasant stimulus. This response may be either conscious or unconscious.

conditioned orientation response (COR), a response used in hearing tests for children under the age of 2 years. A toy moves or lights up when a testing sound is made. The child learns to look at the toy when he or she hears a sound and is rewarded by the toy moving.

conditioned reflex, a response developed slowly by linking a behavior with a specific, repeated stimulus. An example is Pavlov's experiment in which a dog drools at the ringing of a bell. This is achieved if the bell is rung before every feeding.

conditioned response, an automatic reaction to a stimulus that has been learned through training. Such responses can be physical or psychological. They are caused by exposure to the stimulus or event. This is done over and over

until the response is automatic. Compare **unconditioned response.** See also **classical conditioning.**

conditioning, a form of learning in which a response to a stimulus is developed. Kinds of conditioning are **classical conditioning, instrumental conditioning, operant conditioning.**

condom, a soft, flexible sheath used to prevent conception during sexual intercourse. It is placed over the penis and stops semen from entering the vagina. Condoms are also used to avoid transmitting infection. They are made of plastic, rubber, or skin. Also called **prophylactic,** *(informal)* **rubber.**

conduct disorder, (in psychiatry) unacceptable behavior in a teen-ager that would be considered criminal in an adult.

conduction, 1. a process in which heat is carried from one substance to another. 2. the process by which a nerve signal is carried.

conduction anesthesia, a loss of feeling, especially pain, in a part of the body. It is caused by injecting a local anesthetic into a nerve. This stops the nerve signals from moving up and down the nerve. Also called **block anesthesia, nerve block anesthesia.**

conduction aphasia, a speech disorder in which the patient has problems in self-expression. Words can be understood but the patient may mix words similar in sound or meaning. He or she cannot repeat things, spell, or read aloud. The patient is alert and aware of the problem. A common cause is a blood clot in part of the middle brain artery. See also **aphasia.**

conduction system, a special type of tissue in the heart that is able to rapidly carry electrical impulses.

conduction velocity, the speed that an electrical impulse can be carried through certain tissue.

conductive hearing loss, hearing loss in which sound does not travel well to the sound organs of the inner ear. The volume of sound is less, but the sound remains clear. If volume is raised, hearing is normal. Compare **sensorineural hearing loss.**

conductive tissue. See **nerve.**

conductor, 1. any substance that can easily carry an electrical current. 2. (in psychiatry) a family therapist who uses his or her own personality to give direction to the family in therapy.

conduit, 1. a passage that has been made to connect two organs or different parts of the same organ. 2. a tube for carrying water from one region to another.

condylar fracture /kon'dilər/, any break of the round end of a hinge joint. This type of break most often occurs at the elbow or knee. A small bone fragment that includes the condyle often breaks off.

condyle /kon'dīl/, a rounded, knucklelike bump at the end of a bone. Muscles attach to this bump and join the bone to nearby bones.

condyloid joint, a joint in which a condyle fits into an oval cavity, as the wrist joint. Also called **articulatio ellipsoidea.** Compare **ball-and-socket joint, pivot joint, saddle joint.**

condyloma /kon′dilō′mə/, a wartlike growth on the anus, vulva, or penis.

condyloma acuminatum, *pl.* **condylomata acuminata,** a soft, wartlike growth common on the genitals. It is caused by a virus and is carried by sexual contact. Also called **acuminate wart, venereal wart.**

condyloma latum, a flat, moist, wartlike growth that appears in secondary syphilis. It is found in the groove between the thighs or on the penis.

cone, 1. a cell that receives light in the retina of the eye and causes a person to see colors. There are three kinds of retinal cones, one for each of the colors blue, green, and red. Other colors are seen by combining these three colors. **2.** a cone-shaped device used to focus x-rays on a small bit of tissue. See also **cone biopsy.** –**conic, conical,** *adj.*

cone biopsy, surgical removal of a cone-shaped piece from the cervix. The cone of tissue is examined to help make a diagnosis. This is most often used to test for cancer. See also **biopsy, cone.**

cone of light, 1. a reflection seen during an ear examination when light is shined through the eardrum. **2.** the light entering the pupil of the eye and forming an image on the retina.

confabulation, the invention of events, often told in a detailed and convincing way. This is done in order to fill in and cover up gaps in the memory. It occurs mainly as a way of defense. It is quite common in alcoholics and persons with head injuries or lead poisoning. Also called **fabrication.**

confession, the act of telling another about a real or imagined misdeed to relieve feelings of guilt.

confidentiality, the act of not telling certain information to anyone but another authorized person.

configurationism. See **Gestalt psychology.**

confinement, 1. a state of being held in a specific place. This is done in order to obstruct or reduce activity. **2.** the final phase of pregnancy during which labor and childbirth occur. See also **puerperium.**

confinement deprivation, an emotional problem that may result when a person is separated from his or her usual surroundings or denied contact with familiar persons or objects. It may occur when a person is confined to a single hospital room.

conflict, 1. mental tension resulting from conflicting thoughts, ideas, goals, or desires. **2.** a painful mental state caused by such conflicting forces. This state is made worse by not being able to resolve the conflicts. This kind of stress is found to some degree in every person. Kinds of conflict include **approach-approach conflict, approach-avoidance conflict, avoidance-avoidance conflict, extrapsychic conflict, intrapsychic conflict.**

confluence of the sinuses, a wide junction of veins in the skull.

confrontation test, a test of a person's vision in which the patient looks straight ahead and responds when objects are moved into his or her line of sight.

confusion, a mental state in which a patient is unsure of time, place, or person. This causes bewilderment and lack of orderly thought. The patient is also not able to make decisions. It often indicates an organic mental disorder. It may, however, appear with severe emotional stress and some psychological problems. –**confusional,** *adj.*

confusional insanity. See **amentia.**

confusional state, a mild form of fear and anxiety that may result in an elderly person or person with brain disease when placed in unfamiliar surroundings. The confusion may be marked by the inability to perform normal daily activities, memory loss, and unacceptable speech and behavior.

congener /kon′jənər/, several things that are similar in structure, function, or origin. Examples are muscles that function the same way, or drugs that are similar in effect.

congenital, present at birth, as a congenital defect.

congenital absence of sacrum and lumbar vertebrae, a rare, abnormal condition present at birth. It may be mild, involving the lack of the lower part of the tailbone (coccyx). In the severe form, it may involve the lack of the triangular bone that attaches to the pelvis (sacrum) and all the last five vertebrae. These cases display large deformities and nerve disorders. Symptoms may include short heights, flattened buttocks, or muscle paralysis. There may also be muscle wasting in the legs, foot deformities, and loss of feeling, especially below the knees.

congenital adrenal hyperplasia, a group of disorders resulting in the overgrowth of the adrenal gland and an increase in production of the adrenal gland hormones. Treatment involves cortisone and surgery. See also **adrenal virilism, macrogenitosomia, pseudohermaphroditism.**

congenital amputation, the absence of a limb or part at birth. It is due to a defect in development. See also **amputee.**

congenital anomaly, any defect present at birth, particularly a structural one. These may be inherited, obtained during pregnancy, or inflicted during childbirth. Also called **birth defect.**

congenital cardiac anomaly, any defect of the heart or great vessels existing from birth. Congenital heart disease is a major cause of new-born problems. Other than problems resulting from a premature birth, it is the most common cause of death in the newborn. The defect is found in eight to 10 out of every 1,000 live births. Approximately 90% of all deaths from the disease occur during the first year of life. Congenital heart defects may result from genetic causes. They may also result from the mother being exposed to certain chemicals or drugs. The basic symptoms are slow growth, frequent lung infections, rapid breathing and heart beat, bluish skin, and heart murmurs. Kinds of congenital cardiac anomalies include **atrial septal defect, coarctation of the aorta, tetrology of Fallot, transposition of the great vessels, tricuspid atresia, ventricular septal defect.** See also **aortic stenosis, patent ductus arteriosus, pulmonic stenosis, valvular stenosis.**

congenital cytomegalovirus disease. See **cytomegalic inclusion disease.**

congenital dermal sinus, a channel present at birth. It extends from the surface of the body- and passes between two vertebrae of the lower spinal column to the spinal canal.

congenital dislocation of the hip, a birth defect in which the top of the thigh bone (femur) does not fit into the hip socket. This is due to a very shallow hip socket. Treatment consists of keeping the thigh angled to the side. This causes the top of the femur to press into the center of the socket, deepening it. Also called **congenital dysplasia of the hip, congenital subluxation of the hip.** See also **Frejka splint.**

congenital glaucoma, a rare form of glaucoma in infants and young children. It is caused by a birth defect that blocks the flow of fluid that bathes the eyeball. This increases the pressure inside the eye. The condition gets worse with age, usually affects both eyes, and may damage the optic nerve. It is corrected surgically. Also called **buphthalmos, hydrophthalmos.**

congenital goiter, a swelling of the thyroid gland at birth. It may be caused by a lack of enzymes needed to make the hormone thyroxine.

congenital heart disease. See **congenital cardiac anomaly.**

congenital nonspherocytic hemolytic anemia, a large group of blood disorders caused by similar inherited diseases. Most are linked to a condition called hemolysis. This is when hemoglobin, which carries oxygen, is separated from the red blood cell. Compare **hemolytic anemia, spherocytic anemia.** See also **elliptocystosis, heme, sickle cell anemia.**

congenital pulmonary arteriovenous fistula, a direct passage (fistula) between the arteries and veins of the lung. This condition is present at birth. It permits blood that contains no oxygen

to enter the circulation. There may be several fistulas in any part of the lung. Surgery can correct the defect if it can be reached.

congenital scoliosis, an abnormal curve of the spine that is present at birth. It is not always noticeable until later in childhood. The defect increases with growth and age. The degree of deformity varies greatly. It is usually diagnosed with the use of x-ray tests. Treatment of the defect may be surgical or nonsurgical. Some nonsurgical treatments are exercise programs and the use of braces to support the body. See also **scoliosis.**

congenital short neck syndrome, a rare birth defect of the neck portion of the spine. The neck vertebrae are joined usually in pairs, into one piece of bone. This results in decreased neck motion and length. Nervous system complications are caused by deformities of the vertebrae. The extreme shortness of the neck is the most common sign of this defect. This allows little motion, bending, and rotation. Pain, paralysis, or numbness may occur when the defect squeezes the nerve roots. Congenital short neck syndrome may require no treatment. Mild symptoms can be helped with traction, casts, or neck collars. Surgery may be needed to relieve nervous system problems. Also called **Klippel-Feil syndrome** /klipel′fel′, klip′əlfīl′/.

congenital subluxation of the hip. See **congenital dislocation of the hip.**

congestion, abnormal collection of fluid in an organ or body area. The fluid is often blood, but it may be bile or mucus.

congestive atelectasis, severe congestion of the lung. It results in bleeding, stiffness of the lungs, difficult breathing, and lung failure. A sudden, severe, widespread infection is the main cause. Congestive atelectasis may result from injury, near drowning, or breathing stomach acids. Breathing certain chemicals, as chlorine or ammonia, or use of certain drugs, may also be causes. Also called **adult respiratory distress syndrome, hemorrhagic lung, pump lung, stiff lung, wet lung.**

congestive heart failure (CHF), circulatory congestion caused by heart disorders. It develops over a length of time and is linked with salt and water balance and kidney function. Sudden congestive heart failure may occur after a heart attack. Lung congestion may result. The condition may cause chest pains similar to those of a heart attack. Common symptoms of congestive heart failure include difficulty breathing, high blood pressure, and swelling of the legs and hands. Treatment of this condition includes rest, oxygen, digitalis, and diuretics. See also **heart failure.**

conglomerate silicosis, a severe disorder marked by masses of mineral dust in the lungs, causing severe shortness of breath and coughing. It usually causes a heart problem (cor pulmonale).

Congress for Nursing Practice, a unit of the American Nurses' Association concerned with the activities and the legal concerns of nursing practice, the importance of nursing practice to the community, and how new health-care trends affect nursing practice.

congruent communication, a pattern of expression in which a person delivers the same message by his or her words and body language.

conic papilla. See **papilla.**

conization, the removal of a cone-shaped piece of tissue.

conjoined tendon. See **inguinal falx.**

conjoined twins, two fetuses that grow from the same egg and are physically joined at birth. The defect may be mild. A serious form is when the fetuses share a large part of their body. Another serious form is when a small, partly formed fetus is joined to a more fully formed one. Conjoined twins result when cell division is incomplete during early development. Whether one or both can live depends on the extent of the fusion and the degree of growth of the fetuses. See also **Siamese twins.**

conjoint family therapy, a form of group therapy in which an entire family is seen by a therapist at once and the issues and problems raised are then discussed.

conjugate, a measurement of the female hip bones to determine if the fetus will have enough room to enter the birth canal.

conjugated estrogen, a form of estrogen given to relieve symptoms of menopause, as hot flashes or vaginal swelling. It is also used to treat failure of the ovaries. Conjugated estrogen provides relief in cancer of the prostate and some kinds of breast cancer. Used with other drugs it may slow the growth of bone fragility (osteoporosis) in women after menopause. Long-term use of estrogen can be dangerous. It increases the risk of cancer of the uterus, gallbladder disease, and blood clots. Female sex hormones should not be taken during pregnancy. This can damage the fetus. Adverse effects of conjugated estrogens are bleeding from the vagina, tender breasts, and nausea. Headaches, water retention, and acne may also result.

conjugated protein, a protein molecule joined to a nonprotein substance.

conjugation, a form of sexual reproduction in one-celled organisms. Two cells join and transfer genetic information.

conjunctiva /kon′jungktī′və/, two membranes in the eye. The **palpebral conjunctiva** lines the inner surface of the eyelids. It is thick, dull, and supplied with blood vessels. The **bulbar conjunctiva** covers the front part of the white of the eye (sclera). It is thin and transparent.

conjunctival burns, chemical burns of the surface of the eye and the inside of the eyelids. Emergency treatment involves bathing the eyes with large amounts of water until the chemical is washed away. The eye should be seen and treated by a physician.

conjunctival edema. See **chemosis.**

conjunctival reflex, a way of protecting the eye. The eyelids close whenever the front of the white of the eye is touched. Compare **corneal reflex.**

conjunctival test, a test to identify substances that cause allergic reactions (allergens). A small amount of an allergen is placed in the eye. If the patient is allergic to the allergen, the eye waters and turns red in 5 to 15 minutes. See also **allergy testing.**

conjunctivitis /kəjungk′tivī′tis/, swelling in the front of the white of the eye (conjunctiva). This is caused by infection, allergy, or outside factors. Red eyes, a thick discharge, sticky eyelids in the morning, and swelling without pain are the symptoms. Treatment depends on the cause. It may include antibiotics (drugs to fight bacteria), or corticosteroids. Also called **pinkeye.** See also **choroiditis, uveitis.**

connecting fibrocartilage, a disk of fiberlike cartilage between many joints. It is common between joints with little movement, as the spinal vertebrae. Each disk is made of rings of fiberlike tissue separated by cartilage. The disk swells outward if it is pressed by the vertebrae on either side. Compare **circumferential fibrocartilage, interarticular fibrocartilage, stratiform fibrocartilage.**

connective tissue, tissue that supports and joins other body tissue and parts. It also carries materials for processing, nutrition, and waste release. Various kinds of cells are found in this tissue, as plasma cells and white blood cells. Kinds of connective tissue are **bone, cartilage, fibrous connective tissue.**

Conor's disease. See **Marseilles fever.**

Conradi's disease. See **chondrodystrophia calcificans congenita.**

consanguinity, a hereditary or "blood" relationship between persons. These persons share a common parent or ancestor.

conscience, 1. the moral sense of what is right and wrong. This includes the ability to judge one's own actions. 2. the superego.

conscious, 1. able to respond to outside stimuli. This includes being awake, alert, or aware of one's surroundings. 2. that part of mental functioning that is aware of thoughts, ideas, and emotions. Compare **preconscious, unconscious.**

consciousness, an awareness of one's self and one's surroundings.

conscious proprioception, an awareness of the location and movement of body parts.

conscious sedation. See **awake anesthesia.**

consecutive angiitis, swelling of blood or lymph vessels. This results from swelling in surrounding tissues.

consensual, related to a reflex action in which stimulation of one part of the body results in a response in another part.

consensual reaction to light, the narrowing of the pupil of one eye when the other eye is exposed to light. Compare **direct reaction to light.** See also **light reflex.**

consensually validated symbols, symbols that are accepted by enough people that they have an agreed-upon meaning.

consenting adult, an adult who willingly agrees to participate in an activity with one or more other adults. The term is usually applied to sexual activity.

consequences, responses to particular behaviors that either strengthen or weaken them. Praise would strengthen a behavior, while punishment would weaken a behavior.

conservation of energy, a law of physics. It states that the total amount of energy in a closed system stays constant.

conservation of matter, a law of physics. It states that the amount of matter in the universe is constant. It can not be created or destroyed. Also called **conservation of mass.** See also **conservation of energy.**

consolidation, **1.** combining of separate parts into a single whole. **2.** the process of becoming solid. This is seen in pneumonia when the lungs become firm and will not stretch.

consolidation of individuality and emotional constancy, (in psychiatry) one of Mahler's phases of development beginning at the end of the second year.

constancy, the fact that some features of an object (such as shape) do not change even if other features (such as color or size) do.

constant positive airway pressure. See **continuous positive airway pressure (CPAP).**

constant pressure generator, a machine that maintains a constant air pressure at all times while a patient breathes in.

constant touch, a way to test the sense of touch by pressing an object to various areas of an injured body part.

constipation, problems in passing stools. Among the physical causes are intestinal blockage, a disease of the colon (diverticulitis), and tumors. Constipation may occur in elderly or bedridden patients who do not move much. For constipation not caused by disease, a diet of fruits, vegetables, and lots of water is advised. The patient should exercise lightly, if possible. This helps to develop regular bowel habits. See also **atonia constipation.** **–constipated,** *adj.*

constitutional delay, a time in the development of a child during which growth may be stopped. In some cases this delay may be caused by illness or a stressful event, and growth will continue later. The child may or may not make up for the lost growth. A form of constitutional delay is linked to some types of dwarfism.

constitutional psychology, the study of the link between psychological makeup and body form and function.

constitutive resistance, the resistance of bacteria to certain antibiotics that is carried in the bacteria's genes. As the bacteria divide, this resistance is passed on to the offspring. However, this resistance cannot be transferred to other species of bacteria.

constriction, an abnormal closing or reduction in the size of an opening or passage of the body. An example is the narrowing of a blood vessel (vasoconstriction). See also **stenosis.**

constriction ring, a band of muscle in the uterus that contracts around part of the fetus during labor. This often follows early breakage of the membranes around the fetus. This can interfere with labor. Compare **pathologic retraction ring.**

constrictive pericarditis, a thickening of the membrane surrounding the heart (pericardium) and caused by scarring of the membrane or the membrane becoming more fiber-like. The membrane becomes rigid and resists the normal expansion of the heart when it fills with blood.

constrictor, a muscle that causes the narrowing of an opening, as the muscles that control the size of the pupil of the eye.

constructional apraxia, inability to copy patterns or designs by drawing or moving objects.

constructive aggression, asserting oneself in response to a threatening action. This is done in order to protect and keep oneself safe. See also **aggression.**

consultation, a process in which the advice of a specialist is requested to identify ways to handle problems in patient management or in the planning and carrying out of health-care problems.

consultee-centered communication, expert advice given to a health-care worker (the consultee) to improve their ability to function more effectively in dealing with patients.

consumption, a term for tuberculosis now out of date.

consumption coagulopathy. See **disseminated intravascular coagulation (DIC).**

contact, **1.** the touching or bringing together of two surfaces, as those of upper and lower teeth. **2.** bringing together two patients so that an infectious organism can transfer from one to the other. This can be done by direct or indirect contact, as touching food or clothes.

contact dermatitis, skin rash resulting from exposure to either an irritating or allergic substance. In the first type, an irritant, as detergent or acid, causes a sore much like a burn. Treatment is to flush the area immediately with water. In the allergic type, the reaction is delayed. Symptoms are swelling, blisters, and large amounts of fluid in the body tissues. Poison ivy is a common example of this type. Treatment includes steroid creams and soothing or drying lotions. The irritating or allergic substance should be avoided. Also called **dermatitis venenata.** Compare **atopic dermatitis.** See also **delayed hypersensitivity.**

contact factor. See **factor XII.**

contact lens, a small, curved plastic lens shaped to fit the patient's eye. It is used to correct poor vision. Contact lenses float on the film of tears over the cornea. They must be handled with great care to avoid damage to the eyes. Various types of contact lenses include hard lenses, soft lenses, extended-wear lenses, and tinted lenses.

contact shield, a protective device placed over the eyes or sexual organs of a patient undergoing an x-ray procedure. The shield is made of metal or other material.

contagious, communicable, as a disease that is carried by direct or indirect contact. **–contagion,** *n.*

contamination, a condition of being soiled, stained, touched, or exposed to harmful agents, as the entry of bacteria into a previously clean or sterile area.

continence, 1. the ability to control the function of the bowel and urinary bladder. 2. the use of self-restraint, particularly in regard to sexual intercourse.

continent ileostomy, an opening in the small intestine. This opening drains into a pouch surgically made in the abdominal area. Body waste gathers in this pouch and is then drained from the body when it is full. The patient is able to do this without help. The tip of a thin tube (catheter) is placed into the pouch. The other end of the catheter is in the toilet, at least 12 inches below the pouch. Drainage may take up to 15 minutes to complete. A continent ileostomy has several advantages. These include the lack of unpleasant odors and the convenience of not having a drainage bag outside the body.

contingency contracting, a formal pact between a psychotherapist and a patient receiving behavior therapy. This pact specifies the results of certain actions by both parties.

contingency management, techniques used in behavior therapy. They attempt to alter a responsive behavior by controlling the results.

continuity theory, a concept that a person's personality does not change as the individual ages, with the result that his or her behavior becomes more predictable.

continuous anesthesia, a way of blocking nerve signals to an area below the naval. It is used for operations or labor. A small tube is inserted into the back near the base of the spine. Through this tube a small amount of an anesthetic solution is given at intervals. Also called **fractional anesthesia.**

continuous bath. See **continuous tub bath.**

continuous fever, a fever that remains constant for a long period of time. Compare **intermittent fever.**

continuous negative chest wall pressure, a pressure lower than the pressure of the surrounding air applied to the chest wall during the entire breathing cycle. This eases breathing.

continuous positive airway pressure (CPAP), breathing assisted by an outside flow of air. The air flows steadily throughout the breathing cycle. This is done for patients who are not able to keep enough oxygen in the blood without help. CPAP may be given through a tube inserted into the throat (endotracheal tube) or tube in the nose. It may also be given by way of a hood over the patient's head. Respiratory distress syndrome in the newborn is often treated with CPAP. Also called **continuous positive pressure breathing.** Compare **positive end expiratory pressure.**

continuous reinforcement, a schedule of reinforcement where reinforcement is offered each time the desired response is obtained.

continuous tremor, small, regular, purposeless movements that continue during rest. They may disappear briefly during voluntary movements. The trembling seen in Parkinson's disease is a typical continuous tremor. Compare **intention tremor.** See also **tremor.**

continuous tub bath, a bath, usually given to treat some skin conditions. The patient remains in a bath of lukewarm water in which drugs have been mixed. The bath is tedious and may be unpleasant for the patient. The solution is changed completely every 4 hours.

contra-, a combining form meaning 'against.'

contraception, a technique for preventing pregnancy. This may be done with a drug, device, or by blocking a process of reproduction. Contraception permits sexual union without resulting in pregnancy. Kinds of contraception are **cervical cap, condom, contraceptive diaphragm, intrauterine device, natural family planning method, oral contraceptive, spermatocide, sterilization.** Also called **birth control, conception control, family planning.** See also **planned parenthood.**

contraceptive, any device or technique that prevents pregnancy. See also **contraception.**

contraceptive diaphragm, a birth-control device made up of a thin rubber disk fastened to a flexible ring. It is inserted in the vagina together with jelly or cream that kills sperm. The diaphragm covers the cervix so that sperm cannot enter the uterus. This prevents pregnancy. About five to 10 unplanned pregnancies occur in 100 women using the method properly. The main advantages are that it has no side effects and that it needs to be used only during intercourse. There are reported disadvantages. These include claims that it is messy, it is uncomfortable for some people, and insertion may interfere with making love. The diaphragm must be left in place for at least 6 to 8 hours after intercourse. It must also be used for every act of intercourse. Diaphragms are manufactured in seven standard sizes. Kinds of diaphragms are **arcing spring, coil spring, flat spring.** Also called **diaphragm.**

contraceptive diaphragm fitting, a procedure in which a contraceptive diaphragm is selected to fit a certain woman. This is done in a doctor's office or clinic. Proper fitting takes into account the size and shape of the vagina, the position of the uterus, and the muscle support in the vagina. When the correct size has been found, the woman is taught to insert it herself. A new fitting is necessary if the woman gains

Contraceptives in common use, their modes of action, and female/male involvement

Contraceptive	Woman	Man	Mode of action	Involvement time Periodic	Daily
Natural family planning Rhythm/calendar	X		Couple cooperation: abstinence during fertile periods	Mathematic formula calculated once every month	
BBT	X		Couple cooperation: abstinence during fertile periods	Ovulation determined from daily record of BBT	X
Cervical mucus	X		Couple cooperation: abstinence during fertile periods	Ovulation determined from daily record of cervical mucus characteristics	X
Symptothermal	X	Assists	Couple cooperation: abstinence during fertile periods	Combination of BBT, cervical mucus observation, and record of secondary symptoms by couple	X
Oral contraceptives	X		Suppress ovulation by inhibiting hypothalamus and pituitary	Ingestion of OC at same time each day; physical examination by physician every 6 mo	X
Norplant	X		Suppresses ovulation and alters cervical mucus and endometrium maturation	Capsules inserted surgically (under local anesthetic) into arm just below the skin. It is effective for 5 years.	
IUDs (unmedicated)	X		Prevent implantation within uterus	Inserted into uterus by trained person; placement checked often; IUD changed every 2-3 yr, prn	
Mechanical barriers Diaphragms	X		Prevent sperm migration into uterus	Inserted into vagina over cervix before intercourse	
Cervical cap	X		Prevents sperm migration into the uterus	Inserted into vagina over cervix before intercourse	
Condoms		X	Prevent sperm migration into uterus	Applied to penis before intercourse	
Chemical barriers: foams, gels, suppositories*	X	X	Destroy sperm or make them immobile within vaginal vault	Inserted into vagina before each intercourse; applied with diaphragm or condom	
Fertility awareness	X	X	Family planning method combined with a barrier method of contraception		
Vaginal sponge	X		Releases spermicide Blocks cervical opening Absorbs semen	Inserted into upper vagina before intercourse; can be left in place to provide protection for 24 hr	

*Chemicals may be combined with other forms of contraception to enhance their effectiveness (e.g., Cu-7 IUD; spermicide with diaphragm or condom).

or loses more than 20 pounds or if she has an abortion or a vaginal delivery.

contraceptive effectiveness, the success of a method of contraception in preventing pregnancy. It is best expressed as the number of pregnancies per 100 women per year. A contraceptive method that results in a pregnancy rate of less than 10 pregnancies per 100 women per year is considered effective. See also **pregnancy rate, woman-year.**

contraceptive method, any act, device, or drug for preventing pregnancy. See also **cervical cap, condom, diaphragm, intrauterine device, natural family planning method, oral contraceptive, spermatocide, sterilization.**

contractile ring dysphagia, an abnormal condition marked by difficulty in swallowing. It is caused by an overreactive muscle band in the throat. This produces painful sticking feelings under the breastbone. Compare **dysphagia lusoria, vallecular dysphagia.**

contractility, the ability of the heart to contract when properly stimulated.

contraction, 1. a reduction in size, especially of muscle fibers. 2. an abnormal shrinkage. 3. a rhythmic tightening of the muscles in the upper part of the uterus during labor. Contractions are mild in early labor. They become quite strong late in labor, occurring as often as every 2 minutes and lasting more than a minute. Contractions make the uterus smaller and squeeze the fetus through the birth canal. 4. abnormal smallness of the birth canal. This can cause difficult labor (dystocia). See also **clinical pelvimetry, dystocia, x-ray.**

contracture, an abnormal condition of a joint. The joint is bent and will not move. This is usually a permanent condition. Contractures are caused by shortening and wasting away of muscle fibers or by loss of the normal stretchiness of the skin. Extensive scar tissue over a joint can cause contracture. See also **Volkmann's contracture.**

contraindication, a factor that prohibits a certain treatment for a specific patient due to some condition of the patient. For example, pregnancy is a contraindication for giving the antibiotic drug tetracycline.

contralateral, affecting the opposite side of the body.

contrast, differences between two areas next to each other in an image. Contrast is important in helping a radiologist to see image detail.

contrast bath, a bath in which the patient places a part of the body, as, the hands or feet, in hot and then cold water. This is used to increase the blood flow to a certain area.

contrast enema. See **barium enema.**

contrast examination, an x-ray study that uses dyes to make internal organs visible on x-ray film. Barium and iodine dyes are often used.

contrast medium, a dye injected into the body that illuminates inner structures that are hard to see on x-ray films.

control, to use restraint or maintain influence over a situation. This is seen in the conscious suppression of impulses used in self-control.

control cable, a stainless steel wire used to move an artificial limb.

control gene, a gene that controls the duplication of structural gene.

control group. See **group.**

controlled area, a part of a hospital or other health facility where radioactive materials are used. It is designed with barrier shielding that decreases the radiation exposure of the rest of the facility.

controlled association, 1. a direct connection of ideas as the result of a specific stimulus. 2. a process of releasing repressed ideas. This is done in response to words spoken by a psychoanalyst. Also called **word association.**

controlled oxygen therapy, the administration of oxygen to a patient on a timed schedule as if oxygen were a drug. The smallest amount of the gas to produce the desired effect is given.

controlled ventilation, the use of a breathing machine to replace natural breathing by the patient.

control of hemorrhage, stopping the flow of blood from a break in a blood vessel.
★METHOD: There are many ways to control hemorrhaging. These include direct pressure over the wound, use of a tourniquet, or putting pressure on the blood vessel above the wound. Direct pressure can be applied so that the edges of the wound are brought together. A tourniquet is applied above the bleeding only in the most drastic emergency. This is because lack of oxygen to the tissues may cause cell-death, requiring amputation. See also **tourniquet.**

contusion, an injury that does not break the skin, it is caused by a blow and marked by swelling, discoloration, and pain. Applying cold immediately may reduce the swelling and pain. Also called **bruise.** Compare **ecchymosis.**

convalescence, the period of recovery after an illness, injury, or surgery.

convalescent home. See **extended care facility.**

convection, the spread of heat through a gas or liquid. This is done by the circulation of heated particles.

convergence, the movement of two objects toward a point between them, as the turning of the eyes inward to see the tip of the nose.

convergent evolution, the growth of similar structures or functions within widely different species. This occurs in response to similar environments.

convergent strabismus. See **esotropia.**

conversion, 1. changing from one form to another. **2.** correcting the position of a fetus during labor. This is most often done when the infant's face or brow is against the cervix. The doctor moves the baby so that the head is against the cervix. **3.** an unconscious defense mechanism in which emotional conflicts are repressed. These are then changed into physical symptoms having no physical cause.

conversion disorder, a kind of hysterical neurosis. Emotional conflicts are repressed and change into symptoms of illness. However, the symptoms have no physical cause. Common symptoms are blindness, loss of feeling, increased sensitivity, or involuntary muscle movements (as tics or tremors). More severe symptoms are paralysis, loss of voice, hallucinations, trance and rigidness (catalepsy), choking, and breathing difficulties. The person who has conversion disorder firmly believes the physical condition exists. Also called **conversion hysteria, conversion reaction.**

convulsion, a sudden, violent, uncontrollable contraction of a group of muscles. Convulsions may occur in episodes, as in epilepsy. They also may occur once, such as after a brain concussion.

Cooley's anemia. See **thalassemia.**

cooling, reducing body temperature. This is done by applying a cooling blanket, cold moist dressings, ice packs, or an alcohol bath. Below-normal body temperature may be produced in a patient before some kinds of surgery. This reduces the rate of the body functions. Very high fevers of any cause may be treated with cooling techniques. See also **alcohol bath, hypothermia, hypothermia blanket.**

Coomb's positive hemolytic anemia, a form of anemia resulting from the destruction of red blood cells before the end of their normal life span. See also **antiglobulin test.**

Coombs' test. See **antiglobulin test.**

cooperative play, any organized play among a group of children. Activities are planned to achieve some goal. This usually takes place among older children. Compare **associative play, parallel play, solitary play.**

coordinated reflex, a series of muscular actions with a purposeful, set progression. An example is the act of swallowing.

COPD, abbreviation for **chronic obstructive pulmonary disease.**

coping, a process by which a person deals with stress, solves problems, and makes decisions.

coping ability, the degree to which a person is able to deal with the stress of daily life. The stress can be either physical or psychological. Coping is done through the use of both conscious and unconscious tools.

coping, ineffective family: compromised, a lack of emotional support for the patient from a family member or friend. This deficiency makes it hard for the patient to cope with the current health problem. The nonsupportive person may feel fear, grief, or anxiety that blocks the support to the patient.

coping, ineffective family: disabling, negative attitudes and behavior of the family or person who is important to the patient. The cause of the problem is often feelings of grief, anxiety, guilt, hostility, or despair by the significant person. Symptoms of this problem include neglect of the patient, intolerance, rejection, and adoption of the symptoms of the patient. There may also be a marked distortion of reality in regard to the patient's health problem.

coping, ineffective individual, a problem in coping with crisis situations or personal weakness. This is marked by a failure to fill a role or meet one's basic needs. There may also be a change in ability to take part in society. Other symptoms may be destructive behavior, excessive use of defense tools, a change in ways of communicating, and too many accidents and illnesses.

coping mechanism, any effort used to reduce stress; the factors that allow an individual to recover emotionally following a stressful experience.

coping resources, the characteristics of a person, group, or environment that are helpful in assisting individuals to deal with stress.

coping style, the way in which a person responds to stressful events.

COPP, an anticancer drug combination consisting of three different drugs (cyclophosphamide, procarbazine, and prednisone).

copper (Cu), a soft, metallic element essential to good health. Copper deficiency in the body is rare. Little is needed daily, and it is easily obtained from a number of foods. Too much copper in the body can result from some diseases. See also **ceruloplasmin, hepatolenticular degeneration.**

copperhead, a poisonous snake found mainly in the southeastern United States. The snake is reddish-brown with dark bands. It is responsible for nearly 40% of the snake bites in the United States. Few of its bites result in death. Pain, swelling, fang marks, and a bruise are usually produced. Immediate treatment is to place a tight band above the bite. The band should not be tight enough to stop the flow of blood to the limb. The fang marks are cut and the venom is sucked out. The wound is then allowed to bleed freely. The victim should be given antivenin if necessary. The drug is usually needed only for children and older people. See also **coral snake, cottonmouth, rattlesnake.**

Copper T, the brand name for an intrauterine device (IUD)—a device that is inserted into the uterus to prevent pregnancy. It is recommended only for women over 25 who have been pregnant, have one sexual partner, and who have not had pelvic inflammatory disease.

copro-, copr-, kopr-, kopra-, a combining form referring to feces.

coprolalia /kop'rōlā'lē·ə/, the excessive use of obscene words.

coproporphyria /kop'rōpôrfir'ē·ə/, a rare hereditary disorder in which large amounts of nitrogen substances (porphyrins) are released in the feces. Attacks may be caused by certain drugs, as barbiturates and steroids. These attacks are marked by stomach and nervous system disorders. Patients are often helped by a high-carbohydrate diet.

coproporphyrin /kop'rōpôr'firin/, the nitrogen substances normally released in the feces.

copulation. See **coitus.**

cor, 1. the heart. 2. relating to the heart.

coracobrachialis /kôr'əkōbrā'kē·al'is/, a shoulder muscle that functions by pulling the shoulder back.

coracoid process, the thick, curved part of the upper edge of the shoulder blade (scapula). The pectoralis minor muscle stretches between this process and the ribs. Compare **acromion.**

coral snake, a poisonous snake with red, black, and yellow bands. It is native to the southern United States. Bites are rare and do not always cause pain. However, nerve, muscle, and breathing problems may be severe. Coralsnake antivenin and oxygen are the normal emergency treatments.

Coramine, a trademark for a stimulant (nikethamide). This drug is used to treat breathing and nervous system problems and circulatory failure.

cord, any long, rounded, flexible structure. The body contains many cords, as the vocal, spinal, nerve, and umbilical cords. Cords serve many purposes, depending on location and need. **–cordal,** *adj.*

Cordarone, a brand name for an oral drug that controls the rhythm of the heart (amiodarone hydrochloride).

corditis /kôrdī'tis/, an abnormal swelling of the sperm cord with pain in the testicles. It is often caused by an infection in the urethra or by a tumor. Other causes are a collection of fluid in the testicles (hydrocele) and varicose veins in the scrotum (varicocele). Injury to the groin often causes a blood clot in the cord.

Cordran, a trademark for a drug to treat itching and skin inflammation (flurandrenolide).

core gender identity. See **gender identity.**

Corgard, a trademark for a drug used to treat high blood pressure and angina. (nadolol).

Cori's disease /kôr'ēz/, a rare disease that causes large deposits of glycogen in the liver, muscles, and heart. Glycogen is a type of sugar molecule needed for energy. Signs are a swollen liver, low blood sugar, and acidosis. It may also sometimes result in stunted growth. Symptoms can be controlled with frequent, small meals rich in carbohydrate and protein. See also **glycogen storage disease.**

corium /kôr'ē·əm/, the layer of skin, just below the outer layer (epidermis). It contains blood and lymph vessels, nerves and nerve endings, glands, and hair follicles.

corkscrew esophagus, a disorder of the throat (esophagus). Normal contractions are replaced by spastic movements. They may occur when swallowing or for no reason. They may also be caused by swallowing stomach acid backing up into the esophagus. Difficulty in swallowing, weight loss, and severe pain over the upper chest all mark the disorder. There is also a corkscrew image on x-ray pictures. Treatment may include drugs to fight the contractions, avoidance of cold fluids, or surgical correction. Compare **achalasia.** See also **dysphagia.**

cork worker's lung, a lung disease caused by an allergic reaction to cork dust. Also called **suberosis.** See also **organic dust.**

corn, a cone-shaped horny mass of thickened skin on the toes. Corns result from long-term friction and pressure. The conical shape of the corn presses down on the skin beneath, making it thin and tender. There are two types of corns. The hard corn is most often found on the outside of the little toe or the upper surfaces of the other toes. The soft corn is found between the toes and kept soft by moisture. Treatment includes relief from the pressure and surgical or chemical removal. Also called **clavus.** Compare **callus.**

cornea /kôr'nē·ə/, the transparent front part of the eye. It is a fiberlike structure with five layers. The cornea is dense and even in thickness. It projects like a dome beyond the white of the eye (sclera). The amount of curve varies in different persons and it can also change since the cornea tends to flatten with age.

corneal abrasion, the rubbing off of the outer layers of the cornea.

corneal grafting, transplanting corneal tissue from one human eye to another. This procedure can improve vision in persons with scars or warps of the cornea. It is also performed when an ulcer going through the cornea is removed. Also called **keratoplasty.**

corneal loupe, a magnifying device designed for examining the cornea.

corneal reflex, a way of protecting the eye in which the eyelids close when the cornea is touched. People who wear contact lenses may have a less or no corneal reflex. Compare **conjunctival reflex.**

cornification, thickening of the skin by a buildup of dead cells.

corn pad, a device that helps relieve the pressure and pain of a corn. It transfers the pressure to surrounding areas. Corn pads are made of flexible fabric and shaped in a number of ways.

cornual pregnancy, a type of pregnancy outside the uterus (ectopic pregnancy). The fertilized egg stays in the portion of the fallopian tube that is within the top of the uterus. Also called **interstitial pregnancy.** See also **ectopic pregnancy.**

corona /kərō′nə/, **1.** a crown. **2.** a crownlike projection as a projection of a bone. **–coronal, coronoid,** *adj.*

coronal plane. See **frontal plane.**

coronal suture, the joining line (suture) between the bones of the skull that crosses the top of the skull from temple to temple.

corona radiata, *pl.* **coronae radiatae, 1.** a network of fibers that passes through the outer layer of the brain (cerebral cortex) and mingles with the fibers of the white matter (corpus callosum). **2.** a group of cells that surrounds one of the layers (the zona pellucida) of the egg (ovum).

coronary /kôr′ənerē/, **1.** referring to circling structures, as the coronary arteries; referring to the heart. **2.** a nontechnical term for a heart attack.

coronary arteriovenous fistula, an unusual birth defect that affects the heart. It is marked by a direct joining (fistula) between a coronary artery and the right upper or lower chamber, or the major vein returning to the heart (vena cava). In simple cases there may be no ill effects. A severe case may result in growth failure, lack of tolerance for exercise, difficulty breathing, and anginal pain. A loud continuous heart murmur is also a symptom. Surgical closure is safe and effective.

coronary artery, one of a pair of arteries that branch from the major artery of the heart (aorta). These are the left and the right coronary arteries. These arteries and their branches supply blood to the heart. Because of this, any disorder affecting them can be serious or sometimes fatal.

coronary artery disease, any abnormal condition that may affect the arteries of the heart. This refers especially to those that reduce the flow of oxygen and nutrients to the heart muscle. The most common kind of coronary artery disease is coronary atherosclerosis. This is a form of hardening of the arteries (arteriosclerosis) in which fat (cholesterol) is deposited in the artery walls. This can lead to blood clots and heart attack. This disease has increased greatly in the last 50 years and is now a leading cause of death in the Western world. The disease is not always linked to the aging process and affects more men than women. It also occurs more often in whites, the middle-aged or elderly, and rich countries. Coronary atherosclerosis affects more younger women today than in the past. This is possibly due to the effects of increased cigarette smoking, stressful office jobs, and the use of birth control pills. The disease occurs most often in populations with regular diets high in calories, fat (especially saturated fat), cholesterol, and refined carbohydrates. Cigarette smokers are two to six times more likely to develop this disease or to die from it than nonsmokers. This risk also seems to be related to the number of cigarettes smoked per day. People who smoke pipes and cigars do not seem to develop the disease as often as cigarette smokers. High blood pressure is also a common related cause in atherosclerosis. Other risk factors include heavy alcohol use, obesity, lack of exercise, shortage of vitamins C and E, living in large urban areas, heredity, climate, and viruses. ★DIAGNOSIS: Angina pectoris is the classic symptom of coronary artery disease. It results from blockage of an artery, causing lack of oxygen to part of the heart. Angina is a crushing pain under the breastbone that travels to the left arm, neck, jaw, and shoulder blade. It often follows physical exercise, emotional excitement, or exposure to cold. The amount of pain and length of an attack varies. Long, intense angina is often a sign of a heart attack. Diagnosis of coronary artery disease is usually based on patient history, an electrocardiogram (ECG) during angina, exercise tests, and x-ray test (angiography) of the heart. ★TREATMENT: Treatment of coronary artery disease commonly includes giving of nitrate drugs (as nitroglycerin or isosorbide dinitrate) or propranolol. Bypass surgery may use vein grafts to bypass the diseased arteries. Another type of surgery is angioplasty, which opens the blocked arteries. Prevention of this disease is very important. Keeping a normal weight, reducing salt, fats, and cholesterol intake, regular exercise, stopping smoking, and reducing stress are steps everyone should take. Others include controlling high blood pressure and reducing blood clots. High blood pressure may be controlled with diuretics or other drugs. Studies on aspirin as a drug to prevent clotting are promising. However, regular doses of aspirin can cause side effects, some of them serious. Any drug should be taken only with a doctor's approval.

coronary artery fistula, a birth defect involving an abnormal passage (fistula) between an artery of the heart and the right side of the heart.

coronary autoregulation, the widening of an artery of the heart. This happens in response to lack of oxygen to the heart muscle.

coronary bypass, open-heart surgery to relieve a blocked heart artery. An artificial tube or part of a blood vessel is attached to the diseased coronary artery, then connected to the aorta, bypassing the damaged artery. The operation is often done on patients with coronary artery disease. It improves the blood supply to the heart muscle, eases the work of the heart, and helps anginal pain. Two or three grafts are most often done when several areas are blocked.

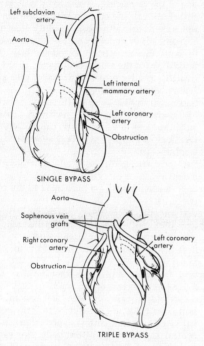

SINGLE BYPASS

TRIPLE BYPASS

Coronary bypass

coronary care unit (CCU), a specially equipped hospital area designed to treat patients with sudden, dangerous heart conditions. Such units contain equipment to revive and watch patients. The staff is trained in heart emergencies. See also **intensive care unit.**

coronary collateralization, the development of new blood vessels in areas of the heart where the blood flow is decreased.

coronary occlusion, a blockage of any one of the heart arteries. The most common cause is buildup of fat deposits in the arteries (atherosclerosis), sometimes with blood clots (thrombosis). These deposits narrow the channel, reduce the blood flow, and lead to heart attacks. In certain heart diseases spasms of an artery can narrow the opening and block blood flow. This causes symptoms of a heart attack, as crushing pain under the breastbone that spreads to the arms, jaw, and neck. Occlusions that lead to heart attack are common. Delayed treatment often results in death. Almost half of the deaths caused by heart attacks occur before the person gets to the hospital, often within 1 hour of the beginning of symptoms.

Occlusions often lead to irregular heart beats. Some types also cause fainting. Treatment includes drugs to correct irregular heart beat, nitroglycerin to relieve pain, oxygen, and bed rest. A temporary pacemaker may also be implanted. See also **coronary artery disease.**

coronary sinus, the wide channel, in the left upper heart chamber (atrium). It is about 1 inch long.

coronary thrombosis, a blood clot (thrombus) that blocks a coronary artery, often causing heart attack and death. They most often form in parts of arteries with fat deposits. This has led many to believe that persons with (atherosclerosis) are more likely to get thrombis.

coronary vein, one of the veins of the heart. It takes blood from the capillaries of the heart to the right upper heart chamber (atrium).

coronavirus /kôr′ənəvī′rəs/, a member of a group of viruses. Several types can cause severe breathing illnesses.

coroner /kôr′ənər/, a public official who looks into the causes and events of a death, especially one resulting from unnatural causes. Also called **medical examiner.**

corpse, the body of a dead human.

cor pulmonale /kôr pŏŏl′mənal′ē/, an abnormal condition of the heart. It is marked by swelling of the right lower chamber (ventricle) of the heart. This results from high blood pressure (hypertension) of the lung circulation. Long-term cor pulmonale increases the size of the right ventricle because it cannot adjust to a rise in pressure as easily as the left ventricle. In some patients, however, the disease also increases the size of the left ventricle. Some of the diseases linked to cor pulmonale are cystic fibrosis, myasthenia gravis, heart disease, and swelling of the lung arteries (pulmonary arteritis). Chronic obstructive pulmonary disease and emphysema are others. Cor pulmonale accounts for about 25% of all types of heart failure. The disease affects middle-aged and elderly men more than women. It may occur in children linked with cystic fibrosis, hemosiderosis, scleroderma, nervous system diseases affecting lung muscles, or disorders of the breathing control center in the brain.

★DIAGNOSIS: Some of the early signs of cor pulmonale include constant cough, difficulty breathing, fatigue, and weakness. As the disease grows worse, breathing difficulty may become more severe. Signs of this condition include water retention, swollen neck veins, and rapid heart beat. A weak pulse and low blood pressure may result from decreased heart function. The patient may in turn be awake or drowsy.

★TREATMENT: Treatment tries to increase oxygen, increase exercise tolerance, and correct the defect if possible. The outcome is usually poor, however. This is because cor pulmonale is most often the result of an incurable disease, chronic obstructive pulmonary disease. Treatment includes bed rest, digitalis, drugs to fight lung infection, oxygen, low-salt diet, a small amount of fluids, diuretics, and anticlotting drugs.

★PATIENT CARE: Treatment of cor pulmonale requires a careful diet of many small meals. The amount of fluids drunk daily must be limited. Digitalis poisoning is often a danger. The patient must be alert to the symptoms. These include appetite loss, nausea, vomiting, and seeing yellow halos around images. The cor pulmonale patient must avoid mixing with crowds and taking drugs that can harm breathing, as sedatives.

corpus cavernosum /kôr'pəs/, a type of spongy tissue in the penis or clitoris. The tissue becomes filled with blood during sexual excitement.

corpuscle, /kôr'pəsəl/, **1.** any cell of the body. **2.** a red or white blood cell. Also called **corpuscule. –corpuscular,** *adj.*

corpus luteum, *pl.* **corpora lutea,** a mound of yellow tissue that forms in the ovary. It occurs in the wall of the ovary where an egg (ovum) has just been released. Its purpose is to release hormones to help prepare the body for pregnancy. If the egg is impregnated, it grows larger and lasts for several months. If the egg is not impregnated, it shrinks and is shed during menstruation.

corpus spongiosum, one of the cylinders of spongy tissue that form the penis. The corpus spongiosum is on the bottom side of the penis and contains the urethra.

corpus vitreum. See **vitreous humor.**

corrected pressure, a measurement of pressure that takes into consideration any changes in humidity that may occur when the pressure is changing.

corrective emotional experience, a process by which a patient gives up old patterns of behavior and learns or relearns new patterns by dealing with early feelings and needs that had not been resolved.

corrective exercise, a program of physical therapy. Its purpose is to restore normal function to diseased, defective, or injured parts of the body. Also called **therapeutic exercise.** See also **exercise, osteopathy.**

Corrigan's pulse, a throbbing pulse. A great surge is felt followed by a complete lack of force or fullness in the artery. This kind of pulse occurs when a person is greatly excited. It is also found in various heart disorders, and as a result of hardening of the arteries (arteriosclerosis).

corrosive, 1. eating away a substance or tissue, especially by chemical action. **2.** a substance that eats away a substance or tissue. **–corrode,** *v.,* **corrosion,** *n.*

corrosive gastritis, a severe inflammatory condition of the stomach. It is caused by swallowing an acid, alkali, or other corrosive substance, which then eats away the lining of the stomach. The amount of damage and correct treatment depends on what was swallowed and how long it remained in the stomach. Compare **chemical gastritis, erosive gastritis.** See also **acid poisoning, alkali poisoning.**

corrugator supercilii, one of the three muscles of the eyelid. It draws the eyebrow downward and inward, as in a frown. Also called **corrugator.** Compare **levator palpebrae superioris, orbicularis oculi.**

cortex, *pl.* **cortices** /kôr'tisēz/, the outer layer of a body organ or other structure.

cortic-, a combining form pertaining to the cortex or bark.

cortical apraxia. See **motor apraxia.**

cortical blindness, blindness that results from injury to the visual center brain cortex.

cortical bone, bone that contains 70% to 90% minerals.

cortical fracture, any break that involves the outer layer (cortex) of the bone.

corticosteroid /kôr'tikōstir'oid/, any one of the hormones made in the outer layer of the adrenal gland (adrenal cortex). They influence or control key functions of the body, as making carbohydrates and proteins, working of the heart and lung systems, and functions of the muscles, kidneys, and other organs. The release of these hormones increases during stress, especially in anxiety and severe injury. Too much of these hormones in the body is linked with various disorders, as Cushing's syndrome. The skeletal muscles need the correct amount the corticosteroids to work normally. Corticosteroids can also be given to patients to help certain disorders, as swelling or failure of the glands to make enough for the body. These drugs are commonly referred to as **steroids.** Steroids can cause very severe side effects, as extreme changes in behavior.

corticotropin. See **adrenocorticotropic hormone.**

corticotropin-releasing factor (CRF), a hormone secreted by the hypothalamus of the brain into the bloodstream. CRF triggers the release of another hormone, ACTH, from the pituitary gland.

cortisol, a steroid hormone found naturally in the body, that reduces swelling. Also called **hydrocortisone.**

cortisone, a steroid hormone made in the liver. It can also be made artificially and is used to treat swelling.

Corti's organ. See **organ of Corti.**

Cortisporin, a trademark for a drug used in the eyes for infection and inflammation.

Corynebacterium /kôr'inēbaktir'ē·əm/, a common group of rod-shaped, curved organisms. The most common disease-causing types are *Corynebacterium acnes,* found in acne sores, and *C. diphtheriae,* the cause of diphtheria. See also *Propionibacterium.*

coryza. See **rhinitis.**

Cosmegen, a trademark for an anticancer drug (dactinomycin).

cosmetic surgery, repair of skin or tissues, usually around the face and neck. It is generally done to correct a defect, remove a scar or birthmark, or correct the effects of aging on the skin. The surgery is usually done with a local anesthetic. Kinds of cosmetic surgery include **rhinoplasty, rhytidoplasty.** Compare **plastic surgery.**

costal, 1. referring to a rib. 2. located near a rib or on a side close to a rib.

costal cartilage. See **cartilage.**

Costen's syndrome. See **temporomandibular joint pain dysfunction syndrome.**

costi-, cost-, costo-, a combining form referring to a rib.

costochondral /kos'təkon'drəl/, referring to a rib and its cartilage.

costophrenic (CP) angle, the angle at the bottom of the lung between the diaphragm and the chest wall.

costotransverse articulation, any one of the gliding joints between the ribs and vertebrae linked to them. This excludes the eleventh and twelfth ribs.

costovertebral, relating to a rib and the spinal column.

cosyntropin, a man-made form of the hormone ACTH, used to diagnose and treat diseases in which there is a decrease in the function of the adrenal glands, such as Addison's disease.

Cotazym, a trademark for a drug that replaces enzymes in the pancreas (pancrelipase).

cot death. See **sudden infant death syndrome.**

cottonmouth, a poisonous snake often found near waters and swamps of the southeastern United States. The symptoms of the bite are rapid swelling, severe pain, coloring of the skin at bite marks, and weakness. Antivenin and oxygen are the usual treatments. Also called **water moccasin.**

cotyledon, one of the segments on the surface of the placenta that attaches to the uterus. A normal placenta may have 15 to 20 cotyledons.

cough, a sudden, forceful release of air from the lungs. Coughing clears the lungs and throat of irritants and fluid. It also prevents breathing foreign matter into the lungs. It is a common symptom of diseases of the chest and throat. Tuberculosis, lung cancer, and bronchitis can cause long-term coughing. Ear infection, congestive heart failure, and heart-valve disease may be linked with severe coughing. Long-term coughing can be helped by reducing irritants in the air. Added moisture in the air (humidity) can also help. Cough-control drugs may be given.

cough fracture, any break of a rib, caused by violent coughing. This most often happens to the fifth or seventh rib.

Coulter counter /kōl'tər/, a trademark for an electric device that identifies, sorts, and counts the kinds of cells in a small sample of blood. These devices are used in laboratories to diagnose blood disorders.

Coumadin, a trademark for an anticlotting drug (warfarin sodium, also called coumarin).

coumarin /kōō'mərin/, an anticlotting drug used to prevent and treat various kinds of blood clots (thrombosis and embolism). A serious side effect can be bleeding in the body (hemorrhage). It should not be used where this is a risk. Also called warfarin sodium.

counseling, the act of providing advice or guidance to a patient or a patient's family. It helps the patient recognize and cope with stress and eases relationships between the patient and the family, significant others, or the health-care team. See also **genetic counseling.**

counterconditioning, a process used in behavioral therapy in which a learned, disruptive response is replaced by one that is more acceptable.

countercurrent, a change in the direction of flow of a fluid.

counterinjunction, (in transactional analysis) an instruction from a parent that may be difficult to follow because it conflicts with previous parental instructions. For example, the person may obey an earlier injunction to avoid close relationships, then be instructed later to "grow up and get married."

counterphobic behavior, a reaction to a phobia by a patient who seeks exposure to the types of situations that bring on his or her phobic symptoms.

countersociety, a group that opposes the established society in which it exists. An example is a street gang that may have its own role models, goals, system of values, and language that is not shared by the established society.

countertraction, a force that pulls against traction, as the force of body weight. Countertraction is begun slowly by changing the position of a patient and by adding or by removing weights from weight hangers.

countertransference, the conscious or unconscious emotional response of a psychotherapist or analyst to a patient. See also **transference.**

countertransport, the transport of two different substances across the same membrane at the same time. Each moves across the membrane in opposite directions.

coup /kōō/, any blow to the body. It is most

often used with a French word indicating a type of blow or wound. A **coup de sabre** /kōodəsäb′r(ə)/ means a wound similar to a sword cut. A **coup de soleil** is a sunstroke. A **coup sur coup** /kōosΥrkōo′/ refers to giving a drug in small amounts over a short period of time rather than in one large dose. A **contre coup** /kôNtrəkōo′/ means an injury most often linked to a blow to the skull. The force of the blow carries through the skull to the other side of the head where the bruise or break appears.

couples therapy, Counseling in which couples, who may be married or unmarried but living together, undergo therapy together.

coupling, the act of coming together, joining, or pairing.

coupling interval, the interval between the main heart beat and a premature heart beat.

Courvoisier's law /kōorvô·äzē·āz′/, the rule that the gallbladder is smaller than usual if a gallstone blocks the common bile duct. However, the gallbladder is enlarged if the common bile duct is blocked by something else, as cancer of the pancreas.

couvade /kōoväd′/, a custom in some cultures whereby the husband imitates labor while the wife is giving birth.

Couvelaire uterus /kōo′vəler′/, a bleeding condition of the uterus that may occur after sudden tearing loose of the placenta (abruptio placenta). The uterus turns purple and does not contract well. Also called **uteroplacental apoplexy.** See also **abruptio placenta.**

Cowling's rule, a way of finding the dose of a drug for a child. It uses this formula: (age at next birthday/24) × adult dose. See also **pediatric dosage.**

Cowper's gland /kou′pərz/, either of two pea-sized glands found at the end of the urine canal (urethral sphincter) of the male. They consist of several lobes with ducts that join and form a single duct. Also called **bulbourethral gland.** Compare **Bartholin's gland.**

cowpox, a mild infectious disease marked by a rash with pus-filled blisters. It is caused by the vaccine virus transferred to humans from infected cattle. Cowpox infection usually makes a person immune to smallpox. See also **smallpox, vaccinia, variola.**

coxa adducta, coxa flexa. See **coxa vara.**

coxal articulation, the ball-and-socket joint of the hip, it consists of the head of the thigh bone (femur) in the cup-shaped hole in the pelvis (acetabulum). These are attached by seven ligaments, which permit very extensive movements. Also called **hip joint.** Compare **shoulder joint.**

coxa magna, an abnormal widening of the head and neck of the thigh bone (femur).

coxa plana. See **Perthes' disease.**

coxa valga, a hip defect in which the thigh bone (femur) angles out to the side of the body.

coxa vara, a hip defect in which the thigh bone (femur) angles toward the center of the body. Also called **coxa adducta, coxa flexa.**

coxsackievirus /koksak′ē-/, any of 30 different viruses that infect the intestines (enterovirus). These cause a number of symptoms and affect mostly children during warm weather. These infections are linked to many diseases. These include hand, foot, and mouth disease, infection of the heart, infection of the membrane around the brain, and several diseases linked to skin eruptions. Treatment is relief of symptoms. See also **viral infection.**

CPAP, abbreviation for **continuous positive airway pressure.**

CPD, 1. abbreviation for **cephalopelvic disproportion. 2.** abbreviation for **childhood polycystic disease.** See **polycystic kidney disease. 3.** abbreviation for **congenital polycystic disease.**

CPK isoenzyme fraction, One of several chemicals released into the blood following a heart attack. The increase of a form of CPK (Creatinine phosphokinase) in the blood is a diagnostic clue to heart damage. See also **lactate dehydrogenase (LDH), serum glutamic oxaloacetic transaminase (SGOT).**

CPPB, abbreviation for **continuous positive pressure breathing.**

CPR, abbreviation for **cardiopulmonary resuscitation.**

Cr, symbol for **chromium.**

crab louse, a type of body louse infesting the hairs of the genital area and is often carried between persons by sexual contact. Also called *Pediculus pubis (informal),* **crab.** See also **pediculosis.**

crackle, a fine, bubbling sound heard when listening to breath sounds through a stethoscope. It is heard when watery secretions are present in the lungs.

cradle cap, a common swelling condition of the head and face (seborrheic dermatitis). It affects infants and consists of thick, yellow, greasy scales on the scalp. Treatment is to rub oil or ointment into the scalp at night. A shampoo is used in the morning.

cramp, 1. a spastic and often painful contraction of one or more muscles. **2.** a pain similar to a muscle cramp. Kinds of cramps include **cane-cutter's cramp, fireman's cramp, miner's cramp, stoker's cramp, writer's cramp.** See also **charley horse, dysmenorrhea, heat cramp, wryneck.**

cranial arteritis. See **temporal arteritis.**

cranial nerves, the 12 pairs of nerves emerging from the cranial cavity through openings in the skull. They are referred to by Roman numerals and named as follows: (I) olfactory, sense of smell; (II) optic, sight; (III) oculomotor, eye muscles; (IV) trochlear, eye muscles; (V) trigeminal, jaws, chewing; (VI) abducens, eye muscles; (VII) facial, taste; (VIII) acoustic,

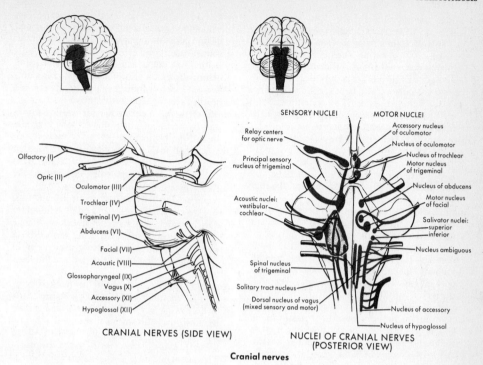

CRANIAL NERVES (SIDE VIEW)   NUCLEI OF CRANIAL NERVES
                                         (POSTERIOR VIEW)

Cranial nerves

hearing; (IX) glossopharyngeal, throat, swallowing; (X) vagal, heart, lungs, digestion; (XI) accessory, upper spine; (XII) hypoglossal, tongue, speaking.

cranio-, a combining form referring to the skull or cranium.

craniocervical, referring to the area at the back of the head where the skull meets the neck. The number of nerves and blood vessels and the flexibility of the neck lead to many disorders of this area.

craniodidymus /krānē·ōdid′iməs/, a two-headed fetal twin monster in which the bodies are fused.

craniofacial dysostosis, an abnormal hereditary condition. It is marked by bone defects, eye defects, parrot-beaked nose, and jaw defects. See also **dysostosis.**

craniohypophyseal xanthoma /krā′nē·ōhī′pōfiz′-ē·əl/, a condition in which cholesterol is deposited in the bones, as in Hand-Schüller-Christian disease.

craniometaphyseal dysplasia, an inherited bone disorder marked by thickened bones in the nasal area, skull and jaw, and pinching of the cranial nerves as they pass through the bones of the head. The long bones have clublike ends. The patient may have frequent sinus infections and colds, and jaws that do not fit together properly.

craniopagus /krā′nē·op′əgəs/, twins that are joined at the heads. Fusion can occur at the forehead, top, or back of the skull. Also called **cephalopagus.**

craniopharyngeal /krā′nē·ōfərin′jē·əl/, referring to the skull and the throat.

craniopharyngioma /krā′nē·ōfərin′jē·ō′mə/, an inherited tumor of the pituitary gland, it appears most often in children and adolescents. The tumor is solid and ranges in size from less than half an inch to more than 3 inches. It may expand into the brain, where it often becomes calcified. The tumor may alter pituitary function, damage the eye nerves, and result in water on the brain (hydrocephalus). It may also disrupt control of the nervous system. Increased pressure in the brain, severe headaches, vomiting, stunted growth, defective vision, impatience, sleeping a lot, and genitals that do not develop are often linked to the tumor in children. Appearance of the tumor after puberty often results in absence of menstruation in women and loss of sexual interest in men.

craniostenosis /krā′nē·ōstənō′sis/, a birth defect of the skull. It results from premature closing of the junctures (sutures) between the skull bones. The extent of the defect depends on which sutures close and when the closure occurred. Impaired brain growth may or may not be involved. Surgery is necessary to relieve pressure on the brain when several sutures are fused. Surgery may also be done to improve appearance. See also **brachycephaly, oxycephaly, plagiocephaly, scaphocephaly. –craniostenotic,** *adj.*

craniotabes /krā′nē·ōtā′bēz/, thinness of the top and back of the skull of a newborn. The condition is common. The bones feel brittle when pressed with the fingers. The condition disappears with normal eating and growth but may persist in infants who develop rickets.

craniotomy /kran′ē·ot′əmē/, any surgical opening into the skull. It may be done to relieve pressure in the brain, to control bleeding, or to remove a tumor. A curved cut is made in the skin, holes are drilled in a circle, and the flap of bone is removed.

craniotubular, referring to an overgrowth of bone that results in an abnormal contour and increased bone hardness.

cranium /krā′nē·əm/, the bony skull that holds the brain. It is made up of eight bones: frontal, occipital, sphenoid, and ethmoid bones, and paired temporal and parietal bones. **–cranial,** *adj.*

crankcase spool catheter, a special, elastic hollow tube (catheter) stored in a plastic spool. This makes insertion of the tube easier. It is used for prolonged feeding through a vein. The crankcase-spool catheter is less irritating than a regular catheter. It allows greater body movement and lessens the risk of blood clots. It may, however, cause complications, as blockage, swollen vein (phlebitis), infection, and catheter sensitivity.

crash cart, a cart carrying emergency equipment, as suction devices, sutures, surgical instruments, sponges, and others.

cravat bandage /krəvat′/, a triangular bandage, folded lengthwise. It may be used to control bleeding or to tie splints in place.

crawling reflex. See **symmetric tonic neck reflex.**

C-reactive protein (CRP), a protein not normally found in the blood. It is present in many severe swelling conditions. CRP appears within 24 to 48 hours after swelling begins and disappears when swelling is suppressed by salicylates and steroids. Also called **serum C-reactive protein.**

cream, **1.** the part of milk rich in butterfat. **2.** any fluid mix that is very thick. Creams are often used to apply medicine to the surface of the body. Compare **ointment.**

crease, a wrinkle formed by a folding back of tissue, as on the palm of the hand.

creatine /krē′ətēn, -tin/, an important nitrogen compound made in the body. It combines with phosphorus to form high-energy phosphate.

creatinine /krē·at′inēn, -nin/, a substance formed from the making of creatine. It is common in blood, urine, and muscle tissue. See also **creatine.**

creatinine height index (CHI), a measurement of the creatinine level in urine collected over a 24-hour period. This is an indication of the amount of muscle present and can indicate malnutrition if the value is low, especially in young males.

credentials, a set of standards, as certification, identifying that a person or institution has professional recognition in a specific field of health care.

credé's method, a technique for causing urination by pressing on the lower belly over the area of the bladder.

Crede's prophylaxis, a 1% silver nitrate solution dropped into the eyes of newborn infants. This is done to prevent gonorrhea infection of the eyes, which can result in blindness. State laws requiring this have greatly reduced blindness.

creep, an effect on metals and other solid materials in which they become longer or change shape as a result of a load being applied for a long time. For example, creep can occur in dental fillings that have been in place for some time.

creeping eruption, a skin disorder marked by irregular, wandering red lines. These are made by burrowing larvae of hookworms and certain roundworms. The worms make their way into the body when people walk barefoot where these parasites are known to be common. Treatment includes giving antiparasite drugs. In some cases the worms are surgically removed from the skin. Also called **larva migrans.**

cremaster /krimas′tər/, a thin muscle layer covering the spermatic cord through which sperm travels. The function of the cremaster is to pull the testicles up toward the body in response to cold or stimulation of nerves.

cremasteric reflex /krē′məster′ik/, a nerve reflex triggered by stroking the skin of the upper inner thigh in a male. This normally causes the testicle to draw up toward the body. The reflex is lost in certain nervous system diseases. See also **superficial reflex.**

crenation /krinā′shən/, notches or scalloped edges on an object. Red blood cells exposed to a salt solution become notched and shriveled. They are then called crenated red blood cells. **–crenate, crenated,** *adj.*

creosol, an oily liquid that is one of the active compounds in creosote. It should not be confused with cresol.

creosote, a flammable, oily liquid with a smoky odor that is used as a wood preservative. It can cause a variety of health problems, ranging from cancer and damage to the eye to convulsions, skin problems, and dizziness. Persons who work with treated wood are at the greatest risk of exposure. See also **phenol poisoning.**

crepitus /krep′itəs/, **1.** the noisy release of smelly gas from the intestine through the anus. **2.** a sound heard in gas gangrene or the rubbing together of bone fragments in damaged joints. Also called **crepitation**.

cresol /krē′sol/, a liquid obtained from coal tar. It is used as an antiseptic and disinfectant and is poisonous.

CREST syndrome /krest/, abbreviation for **calcinosis, Raynaud's phenomenon, esophageal dysfunction, sclerodactyly,** and **telangiectasis.** This syndrome may occur in patients with disease of the connecting tissues (scleroderma).

cretin dwarf /krē′tən/, a person in whom short height is caused by a severe lack of thyroid hormone during infancy. Also called **hypothyroid dwarf.** See also **cretinism.**

cretinism /krē′təniz′əm/, a condition marked by severe lack of thyroid function during infancy, it is often linked to other hormone defects. Signs of cretinism include dwarfism, mental deficiency, puffy facial features, a large tongue, navel hernia, and lack of muscle coordination. Early treatment with thyroid hormone can restore normal body growth, but it may not prevent mental retardation. The use of iodized salt dramatically reduces the incidence of cretinism in a population.

Creutzfeldt-Jakob disease /kroits′feltyä′kôp/, a rare degeneration of the brain caused by an unknown slow virus. The disease occurs in middle age and is fatal. Symptoms are dementia, muscle wasting, and various uncontrolled movements. Deterioration is obvious week to week. Death usually occurs within a year. Transmission between humans is rare.

CRF, abbreviation for **corticotropin-releasing factor.**

crib death. See **sudden infant death syndrome.**

cribriform carcinoma. See **adenocystic carcinoma.**

cricoid /krī′koid/, **1.** having a ring shape. **2.** a ring-shaped cartilage in the voicebox (larynx), it moves as the pitch of the voice raises or lowers.

cricopharyngeal /krī′kōfərin′jē·əl/, referring to the cricoid cartilage and the upper part of the esophagus (pharynx).

cricopharyngeal incoordination, a defect in the normal swallowing reflex. The cricopharyngeus muscle keeps the top of the esophagus closed except when the person swallows, vomits, or belches. Disease or injury can cause this complex series of nerve and muscle actions to malfunction. This may make the patient choke, swallow air, vomit fluid into the nose, or have difficulty swallowing food. See also **dysphagia.**

cricothyrotomy /krī′kōthīrot′əmē/, an emergency surgical cut into the larynx to open the throat in a choking person. A small vertical cut is made just below the Adam's apple and above the cricoid cartilage. The wound is then spread open with an object as a retractor. A tube is usually inserted through the opening. Compare **tracheostomy.**

cri du chat syndrome. See **cat-cry syndrome.**

Crigler-Najjar syndrome /krig′lərnaj′är/, a hereditary defect in which an enzyme (glucuronyl transferase) is deficient or absent. The condition is marked by jaundice and severe disorders of the central nervous system. See also **hyperbilirubinemia of the newborn.**

crime, any act that breaks a law and may include criminal intent.

Crimean-Congo hemorrhagic fever /krīmē′ən/, a virus (arbovirus) infection carried to humans through the bite of a tick. The symptoms include fever, dizziness, muscle ache, vomiting, headache, and other nervous system disorders. In severe cases, bleeding from the skin and mucous membranes, as the mouth and nose, bloody sputum or vomit, and blood-tinged feces may be seen. Blood may have to be given to replace lost blood; otherwise, treatment is supportive. See also **hemorrhagic fever, Omsk hemorrhagic fever.**

criminal abortion, the intentional ending of pregnancy under any condition not allowed by law. See also **induced abortion.**

criminal psychology, the study of the mental processes, reasons for acting, and behavior of criminals.

crisis, 1. a turning point for better or worse during a life. A crisis is most often noted by a marked change in the strength of symptoms. **2.** events that strongly affect the emotional state of a person, as death or divorce. See also **crisis intervention.**

crisis intervention, help given to solve a mental problem. The goal is to restore the patient to the level of coping that existed before the crisis.

crisis intervention unit, a group trained in emergency treatment and in methods for giving mental help to a patient during a period of crisis, as suicide attempts or drug abuse. Such groups are found in community hospitals, health-care centers, or as special units, as suicide-prevention centers, and are open 24 hours a day.

crisis resolution, (in psychiatry) the development of effective coping devices to handle a stressful situation.

crisis theory, a way of defining and explaining the events that occur when a person faces a problem that appears to have no solution.

crisscross inheritance, inheriting traits from the parent of the opposite sex.

crista supraventricularis /kris′tə soo′prəven′-trik′yəooler′is/, the muscle ridge on the inside wall of the right lower chamber (ventricle) of the heart. Compare **moderator band.**

criterion, pl. **criteria,** a standard or rule by which something is measured or by which a diagnosis is made. Criteria (the plural form is commonly used) are sets of rules against which something may be measured, as health-care practices.

critical care. See intensive care.

critical organs, tissues that are the most reactive to radiation, as the sex glands, lymph organs, and intestine. The skin, cornea, and lens of the eye, mouth, esophagus, vagina, and cervix are the next most reactive organs to radiation.

critical period of development, a specific time during which a person's surroundings have their greatest impact on that person's development.

critical temperature, the highest temperature at which a substance can exist as a liquid.

CRNA, abbreviation for certified registered nurse anesthetist. See also nurse anesthetist.

Crohn's disease, a long-term swelling bowel disease of unknown cause that most often affects the lower part of the small intestine (ileum), the main part of the large intestine (colon), or both structures. Diseased parts may be separated by normal bowel parts. Also called regional enteritis. Compare ulcerative colitis. See also colitis, ileitis.
★DIAGNOSIS: Crohn's disease is marked by many attacks of diarrhea, severe stomach pain, nausea, fever, chills, weakness, and appetite and weight loss. Children with the disease often have slowed growth. The diagnosis of Crohn's disease is based on symptoms, x-ray studies, and a special test (endoscopy). The disease is easily confused with ulcerative colitis.
★TREATMENT: Steroid drugs and antibiotics are used to control symptoms. In patients who are underfed because of the disease, feeding through the vein is often done to give nutrition for the body and to rest the bowel. Removal of the diseased part of the bowel gives some relief, but the disease is likely to return.
★PATIENT CARE: Patients with Crohn's disease are often depressed because the disease is long-lasting. Continued support is needed in helping the patient cope.

cromolyn sodium, a drug used to prevent bronchial asthma. The drug has no effect after an attack has started.
★CAUTION: Known allergy to this drug prohibits its use.
★ADVERSE EFFECTS: Lung spasms, wheezing, a stuffy nose, throat irritation, and other allergic reactions may occur.

Cronkhite-Canada syndrome, an abnormal inherited condition of growths (polyps) in the intestines with skin defects, as nail wasting, hair loss and excess amounts of skin color. In some patients it also has faulty intestine activity and a lack of blood calcium, potassium, and magnesium.

cross, any method of crossbreeding or any animal or organism made from crossbreeding. Kinds of crosses include dihybrid cross, monohybrid cross, polyhybrid cross, trihybrid cross.

cross-bite tooth, any of the back teeth that allow the cusps of the upper teeth to fit in the central grooves of the lower teeth.

crossbreeding, the making of offspring by the mating of individuals from different varieties, strains, or species. See also inbreeding. –crossbred, adj.

crossed extension reflex, a reflex normally present in the first 2 months of life, it is demonstrated by the straightening of one leg when the foot of the other leg is stimulated.

crossed reflex, any nerve reflex in which stimulating one side of the body causes a response on the other side.

cross-eye. See esophoria.

cross fertilization, the joining of male and female cells from different species or varieties to form hybrids.

crossmatching of blood, a means used by blood banks to find out whether donated blood can be used by a patient. This is done after the samples have been matched for major blood type, as A, B, AB, and O. Serum from the donor's blood is mixed with red cells from the patient's blood, and cells from the donor are mixed with serum from the patient. If clumping (agglutination) occurs, a foreign (antigenic) substance is present and the bloods are not usable. If no agglutination occurs, the donor's blood may safely be given to the patient. Compare blood typing. See also ABO blood groups, Rh factor, transfusion, transfusion reaction.

cross resistance, the resistance of a bacteria to an antibiotic to which it has never been exposed, caused by the development of resistance to another antibiotic. For example, bacteria that develop a resistance to polymixin B may also be resistant to colistin even though they have never been exposed to it.

cross-sectional anatomy, the study of the relation of the structures of the body to each other. This involves examining cross sections of the tissue or organ. Compare surface anatomy.

cross sensitivity, a sensitivity to one substance that makes a person sensitive to another substance that has a related chemical structure. For example, a person who develops an allergic reaction to a certain antibiotic may also develop an allergic reaction to antibiotics with a similar chemical structure.

cross tolerance, the decreased effects of usual doses of drugs that develops after exposure to another drug. An example is the cross tolerance that develops between alcohol and barbiturates.

croup /kroop/, a virus infection of the upper and lower breathing tract that occurs mostly in infants and young children aged 3 months to 3 years of age. Croup occurs after another upper breathing tract infection. The symptoms are hoarseness, fever, a distinct "barking" cough, and many degrees of breathing distress from blockage of the windpipe. Parainfluenza viruses, respiratory syncytial viruses (RSV), and influenza A and B viruses are the usual causes. Also called **acute laryngotracheobronchitis, angina trachealis, exudative angina, laryngostasis.** Compare **acute epiglottitis.** **–croupous, croupy,** *adj.*

★DIAGNOSIS: Infection is carried by airborne particles or by contact with infected fluids. The acute stage starts rapidly, most often occurs at night, and may be triggered by exposure to cold air. The child becomes irritable, gets a barking cough, and, in severe cases, a pale or blue skin. The child's condition often gets better in the morning, but it may get worse at night.

★TREATMENT: Treatment is bed rest, drinking a lot of fluids, and relieving airway blockage. Children with mild infections are treated at home with vaporizers, humidifiers, or steam from hot running water in a closed bathroom to relieve the spasm of the windpipe and to loosen up fluids. It may be necessary to put children in the hospital who have high fevers, breathing distress, and bluish or pale skin. A tube in the throat to open the airway may be necessary. Humidity and oxygen are often given. Fluids are often given in the vein to avoid tiring the child and the possibility of vomiting, because this would risk the child breathing the vomit. Drugs are not given. To prevent chilling, many changes of clothing and bed linen are needed because of the humid air. In most children the condition is mild and runs its course in 3 to 7 days. The infection may spread to other areas of the breathing tract, causing problems, as bronchiolitis, pneumonia, and ear infections.

Croupette, a trademark for a device that gives cool humidity with oxygen or compressed air. It is used for children from 1 month to 10 years of age. The Croupette is made up of a machine that lets out a fine spray with attached tubing that connects to a canopy. The patient is placed under the canopy, and ice can be added to the ice compartment. The Croupette helps relieve lack of oxygen, make sputum more fluid, and cool the child's environment. It is often used to treat croup, bronchiolitis, cystic fibrosis, asthma, laryngitis, dehydration after surgery, and extremely high fever.

crown, **1.** the upper part of an organ or structure, as the top of the head. **2.** the part of a human tooth that is covered by enamel.

crowning, the phase at the end of labor in which the baby's head is seen at the opening of the vagina. The labia are stretched around the head during crowning just before birth.

crown/root ratio, the ratio of the crown to the root of a tooth.

CRP, abbreviation for **C-reactive protein.**

crucial bandage. See **T bandage.**

cruciate ligament of the atlas, a crosslike ligament that attaches the top spinal bone (atlas) to the base of the skull above and connecting to the second spinal bone (axis) below.

crude birth rate, the number of births per 1,000 people in a population during 1 year. Compare **birth rate, refined birth rate, true birth rate.**

crural, referring to the leg, particularly the upper leg or thigh.

crureus. See **vastus intermedius.**

crus cerebri /ser′əbrī, -brē/, a part of the brain made of nerve fibers that pass from the center of the brain (cerebral cortex) to form the nerve bundles of the pons. Also called **basis pedunculi cerebri.**

crush syndrome, 1. a severe, near-fatal condition caused by a major crushing injury, it occurs when there is destruction of muscle and bone tissue, severe bleeding, and fluid loss. These injuries cause shock, bloody urine, kidney failure, and coma. Treatment includes giving fluids and electrolytes in the vein, antibiotics, pain relievers, and oxygen. Intensive care with close watching of all vital functions is often needed. **2.** a severe problem caused by heroin overdose. It is marked by coma, water buildup, blockage of the blood system, and lymph channel blockage.

crust, a solid, hard outer layer formed by the drying of body fluids. Crusts are common in skin conditions, as eczema, impetigo, seborrhea, and during the healing of burns and sores; a scab.

crutch, a wooden or metal staff. The most common kind reaches almost to the armpit to aid a patient in walking. A padded, curved surface at the top fits under the arm, and a crossbar is gripped by the hand to hold up the body.

Crutchfield tongs, a device put into the skull to hold the head and neck straight. The device is used in patients with broken necks (cervical vertebrae).

★METHOD: The tongs are placed into small bur holes drilled in each side of the skull. The surrounding skin is stretched and covered with a dressing. A rope attached to the tongs is set up with a pulley, and 10- to 20-pound weights are hung at the other end. The places where the tongs are placed are checked and cleaned every 1 to 2 hours. The patient is turned and helped in deep breathing every other hour and is given scalp and skin care every 2 to 4 hours. The bed linen is kept dry and smooth, an air mattress or sheepskin is used, and back rubs are given to prevent bed sores. Passive exercises of the limbs are done. Sandbags may be used to prevent the patient from sliding to the head of the bed.

★OUTCOME: A patient may have his or her body kept straight by Crutchfield tongs for weeks before surgery is done. During an oper-

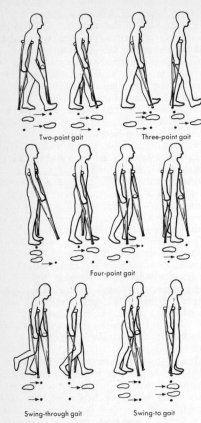

Two-point gait   Three-point gait

Four-point gait

Swing-through gait   Swing-to gait

Crutch gaits

ation on the spinal cord, the tongs may be left in place for proper alignment.

crutch gait, a type of walk used by a person on crutches by bearing weight on one or both legs and on the crutches. In a three-point gait, weight is placed on the good leg, then on both crutches, then on the good leg. Touchdown and movement to full-weight bearing on the leg are usual. Four-point gait is stable but means bearing weight on both legs. Each leg is used after each crutch. Two-point gait uses each crutch with the opposite leg. The swing-to and swing-through gaits are often used by patients who are partly paralyzed with weight-supporting braces on the legs. Weight is placed on the supported legs; the crutches are placed one stride in front of the patient, who then swings to that point or through the crutches to a spot in front of them.

crutch palsy, a loss of sensation or control of the muscles that straighten the elbows and wrist. It is a result of a crutch pressing into the armpit and may be temporary or permanent.

Cruz trypanosomiasis. See **Chagas' disease.**

cry, 1. a sudden, loud, willful or automatic sound in response to pain, fear, or a startle reflex. **2.** weeping, because of pain or as a response to depression or grief.

crying vital capacity (CVC), a measurement of the amount of air breathed in and out while an infant is crying. The CVC may be important in caring for infants with lung diseases.

cryo-, cry-, crymo-, a combining form referring to cold.

cryoanesthesia /krī′ō·an′isthē′zhə/, freezing a part to deaden nerve feelings to pain during brief minor surgery.

cryocautery /krī′ōkô′tərē/, applying any substance, as solid carbon dioxide, that destroys tissue by freezing. Also called **cold cautery.**

cryogen /krī′əjən/, a chemical that causes freezing. It is used to destroy diseased tissue without injury to nearby structures. Kinds of cryogens include **carbon dioxide, freon, liquid nitrogen,** and **nitrous oxide. –cryogenic,** *adj.*

cryoglobulin /krī′ōglob′yo͞olin/, a plasma protein that settles out and clumps together at low temperatures and dissolves at body temperature.

cryoglobulinemia /krī′ōglob′yo͞olinē′mē·ə/, an abnormal condition in which cryoglobulins are in the blood. The disorder occurs in a cancer (multiple myeloma) and fluid buildup (angioneurotic edema).

cryonics /krī·on′iks/, the ways in which cold is applied for many treatments, as brief local anesthesia.

cryostat, Used in testing tissues, a device made up of a special knife used for freezing and slicing samples of tissue for study.

cryosurgery, use of subfreezing temperature to destroy tissue. Cryosurgery is used to destroy nerve cells in the thalamus to treat Parkinson's disease, to destroy the pituitary gland to halt the progress of some kinds of spreading cancer, and to treat many cancers and skin disorders. The process is also used to heal the edges of a detached retina in the eye and to remove cataracts.

cryotherapy /krī·ōther′əpē/, a treatment using cold to destroy cells. Skin tags, warts, actinic keratosis, and dermatofibromas are some of the common skin disorders treated by cryotherapy.

crypt, a blind pit or tube on a surface. Some kinds of crypts are **anal crypt, dental crypt, synovial crypt.**

cryptitis /kriptī′tis/, swelling of a space (crypt), most often an anal crypt, often seen with pain, itching, and spasm of the sphincter.

crypto-, crypt-, krypto-, a combining form meaning 'hidden.'

cryptocephalus /krip′tōsef′ələs/, a malformed fetus that has a small, undeveloped head.

cryptococcosis /krip′tōkokō′sis/, an infection

caused by a fungus, *Cryptococcus neoformans,* it spreads through the lungs to the brain, skin, bones, and urinary tract. In North America it is most likely to affect middle-aged men in the southeastern states. Tumors filled with a jelly-like material grow in organs and under the skin. First symptoms may be coughing or breathing problems. After the fungus spreads to the brain lining, nervous system symptoms may develop, as headache, blurred sight, and difficulty speaking. Also called **Buschke's disease, European blastomycosis, torulosis.**

Cryptococcus, a genus of yeastlike fungi that reproduces by budding rather than by making spores. Many nonharmful species of *Cryptococcus* are found in the soil and on the skin and mucous membranes of people who are well. Certain disease-causing species exist; *C. neoformans* is the most important. See also **fungus, yeast.**

cryptodidymus /krip'tōdid'əməs/, joined twins in which one fetus is small, undeveloped, and hidden in the body of the other more fully formed fetus.

crypt of iris, any of the small pits in the iris of the eye along its outside margin. Also called **crypt of Fuchs.**

cryptomenorrhea /krip'tōmenôrē'ə/, an abnormal condition in which the products of menstruation stay in the vagina because of a closed hymen. The disorder can also be caused by a blockage in the cervical canal that holds the products in the uterus. The symptoms are signs of menstruation with very little or no flow and sometimes severe pain. If the flow is completely blocked, menstrual flow may back up into the pelvic space causing infected bowels (peritonitis), pain, scar tissue, and tissue shedding (endometriosis). **–cryptomenorrheal,** *adj.*

cryptophthalmos /krip'təfthal'məs/, a defect of a fetus with complete joining of the eyelids, most often found with defects in form or lacking eyes.

cryptorchidism /kriptôr'kidiz'əm/, failure of one or both of the testicles to move down into the scrotum. If descent does not occur by 1 year of age, hormones may be given. If not successful, surgery (orchipexy) will likely be done before the boy is 5 years of age. Also called **undescended testis.**

cry reflex, a normal response of a baby to pain, hunger, or the need for attention. The response may be absent in a premature baby or one in poor health.

crystal, a solid inorganic substance with the atoms or molecules in a regular, repeating three-dimension pattern. The exact pattern marks the shape of the crystal. **–crystalline,** *adj.*

crystalline lens /kris'təlin, -līn/, a clear structure of the eye that is in a capsule. It is located between the iris and the fluid in the eyeball (vitreous humor). The lens is a biconvex structure with the back surface more convex than the front. It is attached to the ciliary body and retina by ligaments that adjust the shape of the lens. This allows the lens to keep an object focused on the retina. For distant sight the lens thins, and for near sight it thickens. See also **eye.**

crystalloid, a substance in a solution that can be pushed through a sievelike membrane. Compare **colloid.**

crystalluria, the presence of crystals in the urine, this condition may cause urinary-tract infections.

Crystodigin, a trademark for a drug used to strengthen a weak heart muscle and correct irregular heart beats (digitoxin).

Cs, symbol for **cesium.**

CSF, abbreviation for **cerebrospinal fluid.**

CT, abbreviation for **computerized tomography.**

Cu, symbol for **copper.**

Cuban itch. See **alastrim.**

cubital, referring to the elbow or forearm.

cuboid bone, the foot (tarsal) bone on the outside of the foot next to the heel bone. Also called **os cuboideum.**

cue, a stimulus that makes a person respond or determines how a person responds.

cuff, a device placed around the upper arm and expanded with air during a blood-pressure examination. See also **cuffed endotracheal tube, Dacron cuff.**

cuffed endotracheal tube, a tube placed during surgery to keep the airway open so that the anesthetic and oxygen can be given. This type of endotracheal tube has a balloon at one end that is filled to tighten the fit of the tube in the airway. The balloon forms a cuff that prevents stomach contents from passing into the lungs. It also prevents the anesthetic gas from leaking back from the lungs. The pressure of a cuffed tube often causes sore throat after general anesthesia.

cul-de-sac /kul'dəsak, kYdesok'/, a blind pouch.

cul-de-sac of Douglas, a pouch formed by the part of the membrane lining the abdomen and organs (peritoneum) that are in the pelvis. Also called **pouch of Douglas, rectouterine pouch.**

culdocentesis /kul'dōsentē'sis/, the use of a needle puncture or a cut through the vagina to remove fluid or pus from the abdominal cavity.

culdotomy /kuldot'əmē/, a cut or needle puncture through the vagina into a small pouch in the lower abdominal cavity (cul-de-sac of Douglas).

Culex /koo'leks/, a type of mosquito that may spread viral encephalitis and filariasis.

Cullen's sign, the appearance of faint, irregularly formed patches when bleeding under the skin occurs around the navel. The discolored skin is blue-black and becomes greenish-brown or yellow. Cullen's sign may appear 1 to 2 days after loss of appetite and the severe stomach pains begin that are the signs of pancreatitis. Compare **Grey Turner's sign.** See also **pancreatitis.**

cult, a specific group of beliefs, rites, and ceremonies practiced by a social group in relation to some particular person or object. A cult is often considered to have a magical or religious significance.

cultural assimilation, a process by which members of an ethnic minority group lose cultural characteristics that separate them from the main cultural group.

cultural event, a communication that takes place every time one member of a society interacts with another member.

cultural healer, a member or an ethnic or cultural group who uses traditional methods of healing rather than modern scientific methods to provide health care for other members of the group or members of another ethnic minority group.

cultural relativism, a concept that what appears normal or healthy changes from one cultural group to the next. The differences are caused by the different situations and customs of the cultural groups.

culturally relativistic perspective, an ability to understand the behavior of other cultures. See also **transcultural nursing.**

culture, 1. (in microbiology) a laboratory test involving the growth of bacteria or other cells in a special growth broth. See also **medium.** 2. (in psychology) a set of learned values, beliefs, customs, and behavior shared by a group of interacting individuals.

culture-bound, referring to a health belief that is specific to a culture, as belief in certain kinds of prayer or the "evil eye."

culture procedure, any of several ways for growing colonies of microorganisms in a laboratory. Cultures are grown to note an organism and to find out which antibiotics are effective in fighting infections.

culture shock, the mental effect of a drastic culture change in the life of a person. The patient may have feelings of helplessness, discomfort, and confusion when trying to adapt to a different culture with unfamiliar practices, values, and beliefs.

cumulative, increasing by steps with an eventual total that may go past the expected result.

cumulative action, 1. the increased action of a treatment or drug when given repeatedly, as the cumulative action of a regular exercise program. 2. the increased effect of a drug when repeated doses build up in the body.

cumulative dose, the total dose that builds up from repeated exposure to radiation or a radioactive drug.

cumulative gene. See **polygene.**

cune-, a combining form referring to a wedge.

cuneate /kyōō′nē-āt/, wedge-shaped. The term is used in describing cells of the nervous system.

cuneiform /kyōōnē′əfôrm′/, (of bone and cartilage) wedge-shaped.

cuneiform bone. See **triangular bone.**

cunnilingus /kun′əling′gəs/, the stimulation of a woman's sex organs by her partner's mouth.

cup arthroplasty of the hip joint, surgery to replace the head of the thigh bone (femur) with a metal or plastic mold to relieve pain and increase motion in arthritis or to correct a deformity. The patient is given general anesthesia, and the damaged bone is removed. The cup-shaped space of the pelvis where the femur fits (acetabulum) and the head of the femur are reshaped. A metal cup is placed between the two and becomes the surface where the femur fits. After surgery the patient's leg is held in traction to hold it at an angle away from the body (abduction) and rotated inward to keep the disk in place in the acetabulum. Continued abduction is needed for 6 weeks. The patient gets strong physical therapy. Crutches are needed to avoid bearing the full weight for 6 months, and an exercise program must be followed for several years. Compare **hip replacement.** See also **arthroplasty, knee replacement, osteoarthritis, plastic surgery.**

cupping, a technique of applying a suction device to the skin to draw blood to the surface of the body.

cupping and vibrating, a way to help remove mucus and fluid from the lungs. It is used to prevent pneumonia, often after surgery. ★METHOD: The patient is placed on the side with the head lower than the chest. Cupping is done by rhythmic tapping on the back over the lungs with cupped hands. Cupping is begun gently and is increased in force as the patient is able to stand it. Vibration is done by placing the hands over the ribs, tensing and contracting the muscles to cause vibrations as if having a shaking chill. Cupping is never done over breast tissue, over the spine, or below the ribs because it causes discomfort and can damage soft tissue. After it is done, the patient is helped to a sitting position and asked to breathe deeply at least three times and to cough at least twice. See also **postural drainage.** ★OUTCOME: The patient can breathe more deeply and with less effort, and the danger of pneumonia is reduced.

Cuprimine, a trademark for a drug used to treat rheumatoid arthritis, kidney stones, and poisoning by heavy metals (D-penicillamine).

cupulolithiasis /kyōō′pyōōlōlithī′əsis/, a severe, long-lasting dizziness brought on by moving the head to certain positions. There are many causes, among them ear infection, ear surgery, or injury to the inner ear. In addition to extreme dizziness, symptoms are nausea, vomiting, and muscle imbalance. Also called **postural vertigo**.

curare /kyŏŏrä′rē/, a substance taken from tropical plants of the genus *Stryknos*. It is a very strong muscle relaxer that acts by preventing nerve signals from moving across the junctions. Large doses can cause complete paralysis, but this is most often short-term with drugs. The substance is used with general anesthesia. See also **tubocurarine chloride**.

curariform /kyŏŏrä′rifôrm′/, **1.** chemically like curare. **2.** having the effect of curare.

cure, 1. restoring the health of a patient with a disease or other disorder. **2.** the favorable result of treating a disease or other disorder. **3.** a course of treatment, a drug, or another method used to treat a medical problem.

curet /kyŏŏret′/, a surgery device shaped like a spoon or scoop for scraping and removing material from an organ, space, or surface.

curettage /kyŏŏr′ətäzh′/, scraping material from the wall of a space or other surface, this procedure is done to remove tumors, abnormal tissue, or to get tissue for microscopic tests. It may be done with a blunt or a sharp knife (curet) or by suction.

curie (Ci, c) /kyŏŏr′ē/, a unit of radioactivity used before using the becquerel (Bq) as the SI unit. It is equal to 3.70×10^{10} Bq.

-curium, a combining form for a substance that blocks the functioning of the junction between nurves and muscles.

curium (Cm), a radioactive metal element. Its atomic number is 96; its atomic weight is 247.

Curling's ulcer, an ulcer of the upper small intestine (duodenum) that grows in patients who have severe burns on the surface of the body. Also called **Curling's stress ulcer.** See also **milk therapy.**

current, 1. a flowing or streaming movement. **2.** a flow of electrons along a conductor in a closed circuit; an electric current. **3.** a certain electric activity of the heart that allows blood to flow. Other currents in the body include abnerval current, action current, axial current, centrifugal current, centripetal current, compensating current, demarcation current, and electrotonic current. See also **alternating current, direct current, volt, watt.**

current of injury. See **demarcation current.**

Current Procedural Terminology (CPT), a system developed by the American Medical Association for making standard the terms and codes used to describe medical services and methods.

Curschmann spiral /kŏŏrsh′mon/, one of the coiled fibers of mucus sometimes found in the sputum of patients with asthma.

curtain effect, (in radiology) a stain on an x-ray film caused by chemicals that were not properly squeezed from the film during development.

curvature myopia, a type of nearsightedness caused by an excess curve of the cornea in the eye.

curve of Carus, the normal axis of the opening at the base of the pelvis. Also called **circle of Carus.**

curve of occlusion, the curve of the biting surfaces of the teeth. See also **alignment, reverse curve.**

curve of Spee, the lining up of the biting surface of the teeth. The curve begins at the tip of the lower canine, follows the cusps of the premolars and molars on the cheek side of the teeth, and continues to the front border of the jaw.

cushingoid /kŏŏsh′ingoid/, having the traits of Cushing's disease.

Cushing's disease /kŏŏsh′ingz/, a disorder marked by the very high release of adrenocorticotropic hormone (ACTH) by the pituitary gland. The symptoms are fat pads on the chest, upper back, and face; water buildup; high blood sugar; round "moon" face; muscle weakness; purplish streaks on the skin; infection; fragile bones; acne; and heavy growth of hair on the face. The high blood sugar most often does not respond to treatment, and diabetes mellitus may become a long-term condition. The cause is often a tumor on the pituitary gland. Treatment is to surgically remove the tumor or shrink the tumor by x-ray treatments. Also called **hyperadrenalism.** Compare **Cushing's syndrome.**

Cushing's syndrome, a disorder resulting from making excess ACTH by the pituitary gland caused by large doses of steroid drugs over a period of several weeks or longer. The patient has high blood sugar levels, is overweight, and has a round "moon" face, fat pads, a pad of fat on the chest and stomach, lowered sex hormone levels, muscle wasting, water buildup, low potassium levels, and some emotional change. The skin may be highly colored and fragile; minor infections may become severe and long-lasting. Children with the disorder may stop growing. Lowering or changing the drug may relieve the symptoms. Also called **hyperadrenocorticism.** See also **Addison's disease, Cushing's disease, Nelson's syndrome.**

cusp, 1. a sharp or rounded projection that rises from the chewing surface of a tooth. **2.** any one of the small flaps on the valves of the heart.

cuspid tooth. See **canine tooth.**

cuspid valve. See **atrioventricular valve.**

cuspless tooth, a tooth without cusps on its surface.

custodial care, nonmedical, long-term care given most often for invalids and patients with chronic diseases. Kinds of custodial care include **board, room, personal assistance.**

cutaneous /kyōōtā′nē·əs/, referring to the skin.

cutaneous absorption, the taking up of substances through the skin.

cutaneous anaphylaxis, a strong skin reaction of allergy. It occurs as a raised, red area (wheal and flare) that is caused by a foreign material (antigen) injected into the skin of an allergic patient.

cutaneous horn, a hard, skin-colored projection of the skin, most often on the head or face. It may be a forerunner of cancer and is usually removed.

cutaneous larva migrans, a skin condition caused by a hookworm, *Ancylostoma braziliense,* a parasite of cats and dogs. Its eggs are placed in the ground with the feces of infected animals, grow into larvae, and invade the skin of people. They are usually picked up by going barefooted, although they can enter through skin anywhere on the body. The larvae rarely grow into adult hookworms in the human body. As the larvae move through the skin, a trail of swelling follows the burrow, causing severe itching. Infections often occur if the skin has been broken by scratching. Also called **creeping eruption.**

cutaneous leishmaniasis. See **oriental sore.**

cutaneous lupus erythematosus. See **discoid lupus erythematosus.**

cutaneous membrane. See **skin.**

cutaneous papilloma, a small brown or flesh-colored tag of skin, occurring most often on the neck of an older person. Also called **cutaneous tag, skin tag.**

cutdown, cutting into a vein to insert a polyethylene tube (catheter), this procedure is done when a vein cannot be entered with a needle. It is also given for nutrition (hyperalimentation) therapy when highly packed solutions are given. The skin is cleaned before it is done. After the catheter is removed, the cut is stitched shut, and a sterile dressing is applied. See also **hyperalimentation, venipuncture.**

cuticle /kyōō′təkəl/, **1.** skin. **2.** the sheath of a hair sac (follicle). **3.** the thin edge of thick skin at the base of a nail.

cutis laxa /kyōō′təs/, abnormally loose, relaxed skin resulting from a lack of stretchy fibers in the body. This is most often inherited.

cutis marmorata. See **livedo.**

cutting oil dermatitis, a skin disorder that affects machinists and others who use cutting oils as coolants and lubricants. Exposure to the oil blocks the pores of the skin, leading to irritation; sometimes infections may result from small metal particles in the oil.

CVA, 1. abbreviation for **cerebrovascular accident. 2.** abbreviation for **costovertebral angle.**

CVP, 1. abbreviation of **central venous pressure. 2.** an anticancer drug combination of three different drugs (cyclophosphamide, vincristine, and prednisone).

cyanide poisoning, poisoning resulting from swallowing or breathing in cyanide from substances as bitter almond oil, wild cherry syrup, prussic acid, hydrocyanic acid, or potassium or sodium cyanide. The symptoms are rapid heart beat, tiredness, seizures, and headache. Cyanide poisoning may result in death within 1 to 15 minutes. Treatment includes flushing the stomach out, giving amyl-nitrite, oxygen, and sodium thiosulfate.

cyano-, cyan-, a combining form meaning 'blue.'

cyanocobalamin /sī′ənōkōbal′əmin/, a red, crystal-like substance that can be dissolved in water, important as a vitamin. It is used in processing protein, fats, and carbohydrates, normal blood making, and nerve function. The first substance with cobalt found to be vital to life, cyanocobalamin cannot be made in a laboratory but can be taken from cultures of *Streptomyces griseus.* Rich dietary sources are liver, kidney, meats, fish, and dairy products. A lack is most often caused by the lack of a substance made in the small intestine (intrinsic factor). Intrinsic factor is needed for the taking up of cyanocobalamin from the digestive tract. A lack of cyanocobalamin results in pernicious anemia and brain damage. Also called **antipernicious anemia factor, extrinsic factor, LLD factor, vitamin B_{12}.** See also **intrinsic factor, pernicious anemia.**

cyanomethemoglobin /sī′ənōmethē′məglō′bin/, a form of hemoglobin formed during nitrite therapy for cyanide poisoning.

cyanosis /sī′ənō′sis/, bluish discoloration of the skin and mucous membranes from lack of oxygen. The cause can be hemoglobin without oxygen in the blood or a defect in the hemoglobin molecule, as in methemoglobin. **–cyanotic,** *adj.*

cyanotic congenital defect, a heart defect present from birth that allows the mixing of oxygen-rich and oxygen-poor blood resulting in a bluish color to the skin and lips (cyanosis).

cyclacillin, a penicillin antibiotic used to treat bacteria infections.

★CAUTION: Known allergy to the penicillin drugs prohibits its use.

★ADVERSE EFFECTS: Among the most serious side effects are allergic reactions and severe diarrhea and nausea. Skin rash may also occur.

cyclamate /sī′kləmāt/, an artificial sweetener with no food value, it was taken from the market in the United States because it caused cancer in laboratory animals.

cyclandelate /sīklan′dəlāt/, a drug that widens the blood vessels, it is used to treat blockage of blood flow or blood vessel spasm.

★CAUTION: Pregnancy or known allergy to this drug prohibits its use.

★ADVERSE EFFECTS: Rapid heart beat, stomach upset, and flushing may occur.

Cyclapen-W, a trademark for a penicillin antibiotic (cyclacillin).

cycle. See **menstrual cycle.**

cyclencephaly /sĭk'lənsef'əlē/, a birth defect marked by the fusion of the two parts of the brain (cerebral hemispheres).

cyclic adenosine monophosphate, a cyclic nucleotide, a compound that is important in hormone transport. It is involved in the action of many hormones. Also called **cyclic AMP, adenosine 3':5'-cyclic phosphate.**

-cycline, a combining form for an antibiotic made from tetracycline.

cyclitis /siklī'tis/, swelling of the focusing part of the eye (ciliary body). Cyclitis causes redness of the white (sclera) next to the cornea of the eye.

cyclizine hydrochloride, an antihistamine used to treat or prevent motion sickness.

★CAUTION: Asthma or known allergy to this drug prohibits its use. It is not given to newborn infants or nursing mothers.

★ADVERSE EFFECTS: Among the more serious side effects are skin rash, allergic reactions, and rapid heart beat. Drowsiness and dry mouth commonly occur.

cyclo-, cycl-, a combining form meaning 'round, recurring'; often in referring to the eye.

cyclobenzaprine hydrochloride, a muscle relaxing drug used to treat muscle spasm.

cyclocephalic, cyclocephalous, cyclocephaly. See **cyclopia.**

Cyclocort, a trademark for a steroid drug used to treat itching and swelling of the skin (amcinonide).

cyclomethycaine sulfate, a local anesthetic used on intact mucous membranes before tests are done on the area using instruments.

Cyclopar, a trademark for an antibiotic (tetracycline).

cyclophosphamide, a drug used to treat many cancers and to prevent rejection in organ transplants.

cyclopia /sīklō'pē-ə/, a defect in a fetus marked by a joining of the eye sockets into a single space with one eye. The condition is often seen with other head and face defects. Also called **cyclocephaly, synophthalmia.** –**cyclops,** n.

cycloplegic /sī'klōplē'jik/, **1.** referring to a drug or treatment that causes paralysis of the muscles of the eye that focus the lens (ciliary muscles). **2.** one of a group of drugs used to paralyze the ciliary muscles of the eye for tests or surgery.

cyclopropane /sī'klōprō'pān/, a highly flammable and explosive anesthetic gas. Cyclopropane is a good pain killer and relaxes skeletal muscles. It is not very harmful, has few side effects, and acts rapidly. The gas is now used for anesthesia only when traits of other anesthetic drugs prohibit their use in a specific patient.

cycloserine /sī'klōser'ēn/, an antibiotic used to treat active tuberculosis of the lungs and other parts of the body.

★CAUTION: Seizures, depression, severe anxiety, psychosis, severe kidney disease, excess use of alcohol, or known allergy to this drug prohibits its use.

★ADVERSE EFFECTS: Among the most serious side effects are tremor, drowsiness, seizures and mental changes.

Cyclospasmol, a trademark for a drug that widens blood vessels, it is used to treat hardening of the arteries, thrombophlebitis, night leg cramps, and Raynaud's phenomenon (cyclandelate).

cyclosporin, any of a group of drugs made from certain fungi. These drugs tend to fight fungal infections, reduce fever, and suppress the immune system by primarily affecting the T lymphocytes. Also spelled **ciclosporin.**

cyclosporine, a drug that slows down the immune system. It is used in transplant surgery to prevent rejection. Also spelled **ciclosporin.**

cyclothymic disorder, a mild form of manic depressive (bipolar) disorder.

cyclothymic personality, **1.** a personality marked by extreme swings in mood from joy to depression. **2.** a patient who has this disorder. Also called **bipolar disorder.**

cyclotomy /sīklot'əmē/, a surgical procedure to correct a defect in the ciliary muscle of the eye, which controls the size of the pupil.

Cylert, a trademark for a drug used to treat overactive children (pemoline).

cylindrical grasp, the normal position of the hand and fingers when holding cylindrical objects, as a glass tumbler, railing, or pot handle. The fingers close around the object, which rests against the palm of the hand. While children learn to control this grasp, it occurs as a reflex in infants.

cylindroma. See **adenocystic carcinoma.**

cyproheptadine hydrochloride, an antihistamine used to treat many allergic reactions, including stuffy nose, skin rash, and itching.

Cyprus fever. See **brucellosis.**

Cys, abbreviation for **cysteine.**

cyst, a closed sac in or under the skin lined with skin tissue and containing fluid or semisolid material, as a **sebaceous cyst.**

cystadenocarcinoma /sis'tədē'nəkär'sinō'mə/, a type of tumor of the pancreas. Clinical features include pain in the stomach and a mass in the stomach that can be felt by pressing on the stomach wall or seen with an ultrasound procedure or CT scan. This tumor is treated by removal of the tumor or the complete pancreas.

cystadenoma /sis'tadinō'mə/, pl. **cystadenomas, cystadenomata, 1.** a benign skin tumor (adenoma) linked to a tumor with cysts (cystoma). **2.** an adenoma with many cysts. The cysts may contain blood, clear fluid, or thick, sticky fluid.

cystathioninemia /sis'təthī'ənine'mē·ə/, an inherited disorder caused by the lack of an enzyme that breaks down the amino acid methionine. Some patients may show no symptoms while others may show signs of mental retardation. This disorder is treated with large doses of vitamin B_6 (pyridoxine).

cystectomy /sistek'təmē/, a kind of surgery in which all or a part of the bladder is removed. This is most often done for cancer of the bladder.

cysteine (Cys) /sis'tēn/, an amino acid found in many proteins in the body, including keratin. It is an important source of sulfur for many body actions.

cystic acne. See **acne conglobata.**

cystic carcinoma, a cancer tumor with sacs (cysts) or cystlike spaces. Tumors of this kind occur in the breast and ovary.

cystic duct, the duct through which bile from the gallbladder passes into the common bile duct.

cysticercosis /sis'tisərkō'sis/, an infection by the larval stage of the pork tapeworm *(Taenia solium)* or the beef tapeworm *(T. saginata).* The eggs are swallowed and hatch in the intestine. The larvae invade the tissue under the skin, brain, eye, muscle, heart, liver, lung, and lining of the abdomen (peritoneum). The early phase of the infection is marked by fever, tiredness, and muscle pain. Years later, seizures and personality change may appear if the brain is affected, and hardening and destruction of local structures are seen in other infested parts of the body.

cysticercus /sis'tiser'kəs/, a form of a tapeworm in the larval stage of its development.

cystic fibroma, a fiberlike tumor in which saclike (cystic) breakdown has occurred.

cystic fibrosis, an inherited disorder of the glands that secrete through ducts (exocrine glands), it causes the glands to make very thick releases of mucus. The result is excess sweat with electrolytes, more substances in saliva, and overactivity of the part of the nervous system that controls automatic actions. The glands most affected are those in the pancreas, the breathing system, and the sweat glands. Cystic fibrosis is often diagnosed in infancy or early childhood. It occurs mainly in whites. The earliest symptom is often a blockage of the small bowel by thick stool that appears in newborns (meconium ileus). Other early signs are a long-term cough, many foul-smelling stools, and constant upper lung infections. The best diagnosis is made by the sweat test, which shows high levels of both sodium and chloride. Because there is no known cure, treatment is directed at preventing lung infections, which are the most common cause of death. Drugs that thin the mucus, lung drugs, and mist tents are used to help turn the thick mucus more liquid. Chest physical therapy, as draining and breathing exercises, can also dislodge fluids. Antibiotics may be used to prevent infections. When the pancreas does not release enough enzymes, pancreatic enzyme supplements must be taken at each meal. Other important dietary needs are enough calories, a high amount of protein, less fat, and multivitamins plus extra vitamins A and E. Life expectancy in cystic fibrosis has improved greatly over the past few decades. With early diagnosis and treatment, most patients can expect to reach adulthood. Also called **fibrocystic disease of the pancreas, mucoviscidosis.**

cystic goiter, a swelling of the thyroid gland.

cystic lymphangioma, a saclike (cystic) growth made by lymph vessels. Usually inborn, it most often occurs in the neck, armpit, or groin of children. Also called **cystic hygroma, lymphangioma cysticum.**

cystic myxoma, a tumor of the connective tissue that has had a saclike breakdown (cystic degeneration).

cystic neuroma, a tumor of nerve tissue that has broken down and become saclike (cystic). Also called **false neuroma.**

cystic tumor, a tumor with spaces or sacs with a semisolid or a liquid material.

cystine /sis'tin/, an amino acid found in many proteins in the body, including keratin and insulin.

cystinosis /sis'tinō'sis/, an inborn disease marked by amino acid (cystine) deposits in the liver, spleen, bone marrow, and cornea in the eye. Other symptoms include sugar and proteins in the urine, rickets, kidney defects, and slowed growth. Also called **cystine storage disease, Fanconi's syndrome.** See also **cystine.**

cystinuria /sis'tinōōr'ē·ə/, **1.** high amounts of an amino acid (cystine) in the urine. **2.** an inherited defect of the kidney filtering tubes, marked by excess urinary release of cystine and many other amino acids. In high amounts, cystine forms kidney or bladder stones.

cystitis /sistī'tis/, an inflammation of the urinary bladder and ureters. The symptoms are bloody urine and pain, and the need and desire to urinate often. It may be caused by a bacterial infection, stone, or tumor. Depending on the diagnosis, treatment may be antibiotics, drinking more liquids, bed rest, drugs to control bladder spasms, and, when needed, surgery.

cysto-, cyst-, cysti-, cystido-, a combining form referring to the bladder, or to a sac (cyst).

cystocele /sis'təsēl/, sagging of the urinary bladder through the wall of the vagina. Compare **rectocele.**

cystogram /sis'təgram'/, a series of x-ray films of the bladder and ureters.

cystoma /sistō'mə/, *pl.* **cystomas, cystomata,** any

tumor or growth with sacs (cysts), as one in or near the ovary.

cystometry /sistom'ətrē/, the study of bladder workings by use of a **cystometer** /sistom'ətər/, an instrument that measures ability in relation to changing pressure. The method, **cystometography** /sis'tōmətog'rəfē/, measures the amount of pressure placed on the bladder at many capacities. The results of the measurements are traced on a **cystometogram** /sis'tōmet'əgram'/.

cystosarcoma phyllodes, a breast tumor that is not cancerous but tends to grow rapidly and recur if not completely removed.

cystoscope /sis'təskōp'/, an instrument for testing and treating disorders of the urinary bladder, ureters, and kidneys. It consists of an outer covering with a lighting system, a viewing scope, and a passage for tubes (catheters) and surgery devices. **–cystoscopic,** adj.

cystoscopy /sistos'kəpē/, the direct examination of the urinary tract with a special device (cystoscope) placed in the urethra. Before the test, the patient either is given a tranquilizer or is put to sleep. For the test, the bladder is filled with air or water and the cystoscope is put into place. In addition to testing, cystoscopy is used for taking samples of tumors or other growths and for removing growths (polyps). After the test, the patient is watched for the common problems of injury and signs of urinary infection.

Cystospaz, a trademark for an antispasm drug used to treat urinary-tract disorders (hyoscyamine).

cystourethrogram /sis'təyo͞orē'thrəgram'/, an x-ray procedure in which an iodine dye is used to help see the urinary bladder and urethra.

cyt-, cyto-, a combining form referring to a cell or a cytoplasm.

Cytadren, a trademark for a drug used to slow down adrenal-gland action in some patients with Cushing's syndrome (aminoglutethimide).

cytarabine, an anticancer drug used to treat short-term and long-term myelocytic leukemia, lymphocytic leukemia, and erythroleukemia. Also called **arabinosylcitosine, cytosine arabinoside.**

★CAUTION: Known allergy to this drug prohibits its use.

★ADVERSE EFFECTS: The most serious side effects are severe anemia, swelling of the mouth and blood vessels, liver damage, and fever. Stomach problems may occur.

-cythemia, -cythaemia, a combining form referring to a condition involving cells in the blood.

cytoarchitecture, the normal pattern of cells in a tissue or organ, as in the cerebral cortex. **–cytoarchitectural,** adj.

cytobiotaxis. See **cytoclesis.**

cytocentrum. See **centrosome.**

cytochemism /sī'tōkem'izəm/, the chemical action in a living cell, as the many reactions to chemicals.

cytochemistry /sī'tō-/, the study of the many chemicals in a living cell and their actions.

cytocide, any substance that destroys cells. **–cytocidal,** adj.

cytoclesis /sī'tōklē'sis/, the impact of one cell on the action of other cells. Also called **cytobiotaxis. –cytocletic, cytobiotactic,** adj.

cytoctony /sītok'tənē/, destroying cells, as killing cells in culture by viruses.

cytode /sī'tōd/, the most simple type of cell, made up of a protoplasm without a nucleus, as a bacterium.

cytodieresis /sī'tōdī·er'isis/, pl. **cytodiereses,** cell division, as by mitosis. **–cytodieretic,** adj.

cytogene /sī'təjēn/, a particle in the cytoplasm of a cell that reproduces itself. Taken from genes, this particle can carry inherited data. **–cytogenic,** adj.

cytogenesis /sī'tōjen'əsis/, the beginning, growth, and dividing of cells. **–cytogenetic, cytogenic,** adj.

cytogenetics /sī'tōjənet'iks/, the branch of genetics that studies the cell parts that concern heredity, mainly the chromosomes.

cytogenic gland, a gland that releases living cells, as the testicles and ovaries.

cytogenics. See **cytogenetics.**

cytohistogenesis /sī'tōhis'tōjen'əsis/, the growth and making of cells. **–cytohistogenetic,** adj.

cytoid /sī'toid/, like or looking like a cell.

cytoid body, a small white spot on the retina of each eye in patients with systemic lupus erythematosus. It is seen by using a special device (ophthalmoscope) to examine the eyes.

cytokerastic /sī'tōkəras'tik/, referring to cell growth from a lower to a higher form, or from a simple to a more complex form.

cytokinesis /sī'tōkinē'sis, -kīnē'sis/, the changes that occur in the cytoplasm during cell division and fertilization. **–cytokinetic,** adj.

cytologic map /sī'tō-/, a picture of the placement of genes on a chromosome.

cytologic sputum examination, a microscopic examination of secretions coughed up from the lungs; a search for cells that may be cancerous or otherwise abnormal.

cytology /sītol'əjē/, the study of cells, their growth, beginnings, structure, action, and diseases.

cytolymph. See **hyaloplasm.**

cytolysin /sītol'isin/, a substance that dissolves foreign (antigenic) cells. Kinds of cytolysin are **bacteriolysin, hemolysin.**

cytolysis /sītol'isis/, pl. **cytolyses,** the destruction of a living cell, mainly by breaking down the outer lining (membrane). A kind of cytolysis is **immune cytolysis. –cytolytic,** adj.

cytomegalic inclusion disease (CID) /sī'tōme-gal'ik/, an infection caused by a virus (cytomegalovirus), a "salivary gland" virus related to the herpes viruses. Mainly an inherited disease of newborn infants, CID is marked by a very small head, slowed growth, liver and spleen defects, hemolytic anemia, and broken long bones. See also **cytomegalovirus (CMV) disease, TORCH syndrome.**

cytomegalovirus (CMV) /sī'tōmeg'əlōvī'rəs/, a member of a group of large herpes-type viruses that can cause many diseases. It causes serious illness in newborns and in patients being treated with drugs that slow down the immune system, as after an organ transplant. See also **cytomegalic inclusion disease, TORCH syndrome.**

cytomegalovirus (CMV) disease, a virus infection caused by a virus (cytomegalovirus). The symptoms are fatigue, fever, swollen lymph glands, pneumonia, and liver and spleen defects. Another infection with many bacteria and fungi often occurs as a result of slowing down the immune response, a common effect of herpesviruses. See also **cytomegalic inclusion disease (CID).**

Cytomel, a trademark for a thyroid hormone drug used to treat an underactive thyroid gland (liothyronine sodium).

cytometry /sītom'ətrē/, counting and measuring cells, as blood cells. **–cytometric,** *adj.*

cytomitome /sī'təmī'tōm/, the network of fibers in the cytoplasm of a cell, as opposed with that in the nucleoplasm. See also **karyomitome.**

cytomorphology /sī'tō-/, the study of the many forms of cells and the structures they contain.

cytomorphosis /sī'tōmôr'fəsis/, *pl.* **cytomorphoses,** the many changes that occur in a cell during the course of its life cycle, from the first stage until death.

cyton, /sī'tən/, the cell body of a nerve, or the part of a nerve with the nucleus and its surrounding cytoplasm. Also called **cytone** /sī'tōn/.

cytophoresis /sī'tōfôr'əsis/, a process of removing red or white blood cells or platelets from patients with certain blood disorders.

cytophotometer /sī'tōfətom'ətər/, a device for measuring light density through stained parts of cytoplasm. It is used for locating and labeling chemicals in cells.

cytophysiology /sī'tō-/, the study of the workings of a cell, as opposed to the workings of organs or tissues.

cytoplasm /sī'təplaz'əm/, all of the substance of a cell other than the nucleus. See also **cell, nucleus.**

Cytosar-U, a trademark for an anticancer drug (cytarabine).

cytosine /sī'təsin/, a substance that is an important part of DNA and RNA, it occurs in small amounts in most cells. See also **thymine, uracil.**

cytosine arabinoside. See **cytarabine.**

cytoskeleton /sī'tō-/, the parts in the cytoplasm, as the tonofibrils, keratin, and other microfibrils, that act as a support system in a cell, as a skin cell.

cytotoxic, referring to a chemical compound or drug that kills or damages tissue cells.

cytotoxic drug, any drug that blocks the growth of cells in the body. These drugs, compounds, as the alkylating drugs and the antimetabolites, are able to destroy abnormal cells while saving as many normal cells as possible. They are commonly used in chemical treatments. Cytotoxic drugs can themselves cause cancer, so they are used only for a short time.

cytotoxin /sī'tōtok'sin/, a substance that has a harmful effect on some cells. A substance that defends the body against foreign bodies (antibody) may act as a cytotoxin. **–cytotoxic,** *adj.*

cytotrophoblast /sī'tōtrof'əblast'/, the inner layer of cells of the early fetus (embryo). Also called **Langhans' layer.** Compare **syncytiotrophoblast. –cytotrophoblastic,** *adj.*

Cytoxan, a trademark for an anticancer drug (cyclophosphamide).

CY-VA-DIC, an anticancer drug combination of four different drugs. (cyclophosphamide, vincristine, doxorubicin, and decarbazine.

D

d, symbol for one tenth

da, symbol for the multiple 10.

DA, abbreviation for **developmental age.**

D & C, abbreviation for **dilatation and curettage.**

dacarbazine, a drug used to treat cancerous melanoma, sarcoma, and Hodgkin's disease.
★CAUTION: Known allergy to this drug prohibits its use.
★ADVERSE EFFECTS: Among the more serious side effects are severe anemia, intestinal symptoms, kidney and liver failure, hair loss, and fever.

dacryo-, dacry-, a combining form referring to tears.

dacryoadenitis /dak′rēōad′ən′tis/, an inflammation of the gland of the eye that produces tears (lacrimal gland).

dacryocyst /dak′rəsist/, a tear sac at the inner corner of the eye. It is a normal feature.

dacryocystectomy /dak′rē·ōsistek′təmē/, removal of part or all of the tear sac.

dacryocystitis /dak′rē·ōsistī′tis/, an infection of the tear sac caused by blockage of the duct that drains into the nose (nasolacrimal duct). The symptoms are tearing and discharge from the eye.

dacryocystorhinostomy /dak′rē·ōsis′tôrīnos′təmē/, a surgical procedure for restoring drainage into the nose from the tear sac. This is done when the duct draining into the nose (nasolacrimal duct) is blocked.

dacryostenosis /dak′rē·ōstinō′sis/, an abnormal narrowing of the duct that drains into the nose (nasolacrimal duct). This occurs either as a birth defect or as a result of infection or trauma. See also **dacryocystitis.**

dactinomycin, an antibiotic used as an anticancer drug to treat a variety of forms of cancer, including Wilms' tumor and rhabdomyosarcoma in children.
★CAUTION: Herpes zoster infection or known allergy to this drug prohibits its use.
★ADVERSE EFFECTS: Among the more serious side effects are severe anemia, severe intestinal problems, swelling of the rectum, hair loss, and ulcers of the mouth.

dactyl /dak′til/, a digit (finger or toe).

-dactyl, a combining form meaning digit (finger or toe).

dactylitis, a painful inflammation of the fingers or toes, usually in patients with sickle cell anemia or certain infectious diseases, as syphilis or tuberculosis.

daily adjusted progressive resistance exercise (DAPRE), a program of exercises that allows for individual differences in the rate at which patients regain strength in an injured or diseased body part.

Dakin's solution, a solution for killing bacteria (antiseptic).

Dalmane, a trademark for a drug that produces sleep or has a calming effect (flurazepam hydrochloride).

daltonism /dôl′təniz′əm/, *informal.* a form of red-green color blindness, is inherited as a sex-linked trait. Also called **protanopia.**

damp, a harmful gas found in caves and mines. **Black damp** or **choke damp** is caused by coal seams soaking up the oxygen in the tunnels. **Fire damp** is made up of explosive gases. **White damp** is another name for carbon monoxide.

danazol, a manufactured drug that stops pituitary hormones, used to treat endometriosis.
★CAUTION: Genital bleeding, heart, liver, or kidney malfunction, or known allergy to this drug prohibits its use. Danazol is not used in pregnancy or during nursing.
★ADVERSE EFFECTS: Among the most serious side effects are muscle spasms, nausea, weight gain, acne, water retention, oily skin, voice changes, and other masculinizing effects.

dance reflex, a normal response in the newborn infant to make walking motions when held upright with the feet touching a surface. The reflex, which disappears by about 3 to 4 weeks of age, is replaced by controlled, deliberate movement. Also called **step reflex, stepping reflex.**

dance therapy, (in psychology) the use of body movements or dance to express feelings.

dander, dry scales shed from the skin or hair of animals or the feathers of birds. Dander may cause an allergic reaction in some persons.

dandruff, scaly material (dead skin) shed from the scalp. Treatment with a dandruff (keratolytic) shampoo is often given to soften and remove the scales.

dandy fever. See **dengue fever.**

Dandy-Walker cyst, a brain lump (cyst) that occurs with water on the brain (hydrocephalus). Diagnosis of the defect is made with CAT scan, x-ray, or tests, ventriculogram. See also **hydrocephalus, shunt.**

Danocrine, a trademark for a drug that suppresses the action of the pituitary gland (danazol).

danthron, a laxative used to treat constipation and empty the bowels before x-ray tests or surgery.
★CAUTION: Abdominal pain, nausea, or vomiting prohibits its use. Danthron is not recommended for nursing mothers.
★ADVERSE EFFECTS: Among the most serious

side effects are dizziness, irregular heart rate, stomach cramps, and increased bowel activity.

Dantrium, a trademark for a drug that relaxes muscles and is used in anesthesia (dantrolene sodium).

dantrolene sodium, a drug that relaxes muscles, used to treat muscle spasms resulting from injury to the spinal cord or brain. This drug is not used for spasm from rheumatic disorders. ★CAUTION: Liver malfunction or allergy to this drug prohibits its use. ★ADVERSE EFFECTS: The most serious side effect is possible liver poisoning. Common reactions include confusion, drowsiness, diarrhea, dizziness, fatigue, and muscle weakness. Side effects may continue for several days.

DAPRE abbreviation for **daily adjusted progressive resistance exercise.**

dapsone (DADPS), a drug used to treat leprosy. ★CAUTION: Pregnancy or known allergy to this drug prohibits its use. ★ADVERSE EFFECTS: Among the more serious side effects are red blood cell disorders, episodes of active disease, nervous system disorders, nausea, loss of appetite, and skin rash.

-dapsone, a combining form for drugs used to treat mycobacterial infections.

Daraprim, a trademark for a drug used to treat malaria (pyrimethamine).

Darbid, a trademark for a drug used to treat peptic ulcers (isopropamide iodide).

Darier's disease. See **keratosis follicularis.**

dark adaptation, an increase in the ability of the sensory cells of the eye to detect light when a person is in a dark environment. The process is accompanied by an increase in size of the pupil to let more light in.

dark-adapted eye, an eye in which the pupil has widened, making it more sensitive to dim light.

darkroom, a room in a hospital or other facility for the storage and processing of materials that cannot be exposed to light, as x-ray film.

Darvon, a trademark for a drug that relieves pain (propoxyphene hydrochloride).

Darvon Compound, a trademark for a combination drug containing a pain reliever (propoxyphene hydrochloride) and APC (aspirin, phenacetin, and caffeine).

Darwinian reflex. See **grasp reflex.**

Darwinian theory, the theory proposed by Charles Darwin. It states that evolution results from the process of natural selection of the plants and animals best able to survive in their environment. Also called **Darwinism.** Compare **Lamarckism.**

data acquisition system (DAS), a radiation detection device that measures the amount of radiation passing through a patient.

data clustering, the grouping of information from the patient's health history, physical examination, and laboratory results in order to make a diagnosis.

data retrieval, the recovery of information from an organized filing system, as a computer, index card file, or color-coded record folders.

data source, the source of information regarding a patient's level of wellness and health patterns.

data validation, the process of determining whether information gathered during a patient health evaluation is complete and accurate.

date/acquaintance rape, a sexual assault or rape by a person the victim knows. This may include a date, employer, friend, or acquaintance. See also **rape.**

daughter chromosome, either of the two spiral threads that make up a chromosome (chromatids). They separate, then go to opposite ends of the cell before cell division. Each contains the complete genetic information of the original chromosome.

daunorubicin hydrochloride, an antibiotic used to treat cancer, particularly leukemia and tumors of the nervous system. ★CAUTION: Severe anemia caused by drugs or known allergy to this drug prohibits its use. ★ADVERSE EFFECTS: Among the most serious side effects are severe anemia and heart poisoning. Intestinal disorders, swelling of the mouth, and hair loss are common.

Davidson regimen, a method of treating longterm constipation in children, it involves developing regular bowel habits and identifying bowel disease or blockage.

day blindness. See **hemeralopia.**

daydream, a fantasy that a person has while awake. Normal daydreams usually center on the direct fulfillment of a person's wishes.

day health care services, centers that provide health services to adult patients who are mobile but do not require constant hospital care.

day hospital, a psychiatric center that offers a program during the day for patients released from hospitals.

day patient. See **inpatient.**

day sight. See **nyctalopia.**

Daytop Village, a treatment community for patients dependent on heroin. Treatment includes education, training, and rehabilitation rather than use of methadone or other drugs.

db, abbreviation for **decibel.**

D.D.S., abbreviation for *Doctor of Dental Surgery.*

DDT (dichlorodiphenyltrichloroethane), a substance once used worldwide as a major insecticide, most often in agriculture. DDT does not break down naturally in the environment. In recent years, its use has been restricted because DDT is a danger to the environment.

DDT poisoning. See **chlorinated organic insecticide poisoning.**

DE, abbreviation for **dose equivalent.**

D.E.A., 1. abbreviation for **Drug Enforcement Administration.** 2. abbreviation for **Drug Enforcement Agency.**

dead-end host, any animal from which a parasite cannot escape to continue its life cycle.

dead fetus syndrome, a condition in which a fetus has died but remains in the mother's uterus for more than 6 weeks. The condition leads to a blood-clotting disorder. Delivery of the fetus usually causes massive bleeding. See also **disseminated intravascular coagulation.**

dead space, a hole that can remain after the incomplete closure of a wound. Blood can collect in the cavity and delay healing. See also **anatomic dead space, physiologic dead space.**

deaf-mute, a person who is unable to hear or speak.

deafness, a condition of partial or complete loss of hearing. In assessing deafness, the patient's ears are examined to determine the cause of the hearing loss. Deafness may be caused by sound waves that are blocked (conductive) or because nerves are damaged (sensory), which can be temporary or permanent. It is also determined whether the deafness is inborn or a condition acquired in childhood, adolescence, or adulthood. The effect of aging is considered in older adults. Patients are also judged on their adjustment to the deafness. Some accept the handicap, while some react with fear, frustration, depression, anger, or hostility. See also **conductive hearing loss, sensorineural hearing loss.**
★DIAGNOSIS: Many conditions and diseases may cause deafness. More than 50% of people over 65 years of age have hearing loss in both ears. The person with a slight hearing loss may be unaware of the problem at first. As the loss increases, the person may then try to hide or deny it. An older person with hearing loss usually has both sensory and conductive hearing loss. High sounds are hard to hear, and some letter sounds, as /s/ and /f/, become difficult to tell apart. A severe or sudden hearing loss usually causes the person to seek help. If the loss is sudden, confusion, fear, and even panic are common. The person's speech becomes loud and slurred. Most children born deaf also have a disturbance of visual perception. They are more dependent and less mature emotionally and socially. Reading and writing are learned with more difficulty.
★TREATMENT: The treatment of deafness depends on the cause. Simply removing hardened wax from the ear canal may greatly improve hearing. Hearing aids, amplifying the sound, or lip reading may be useful. Speech therapy is helpful in teaching a person to speak and can also help a person retain the ability to speak.
★PATIENT CARE: To communicate with a deaf patient who lip-reads, one must speak slowly and clearly and use simple phrases. The speaker should avoid shouting, chewing gum, or covering the mouth while speaking. When speaking with a person who uses a hearing aid, the speaker should stand or sit where the lips are visible to the deaf person. If the person uses sign language, an interpreter may be needed. The newly deaf person should know about lip reading and sign language classes, and of organizations for the deaf.

death, the absence of life. **Apparent death** is the end of life as indicated by the absence of heart beat or breathing. **Legal death** is the total absence of activity in the brain, heart, and lungs, as observed and declared by a physician.

death instinct, inborn behavior that tends to be self-destructive.

death rate, the number of deaths that occur in a specific group of people within a specific time period. Death rate is usually expressed as the number of deaths per 1,000 persons per year.

death rattle, a sound produced by air that moves through mucus in the throat of a dying person. It occurs after the cough reflex is lost.

death trance, a state in which a person appears to be dead but is not.

debilitating, referring to a disease or injury that weakens or disables a person.

debility, feebleness, weakness, or loss of strength. See also **asthenia.**

debride /dibrēd'/, to remove dirt, and damaged tissue from a wound or a burn. This prevents infection and aids healing. In treating a wound, this is the first step in cleaning it. –**debridement** /debrēdmäN'/,*n.*

debris /dəbrē'/, the dead, diseased, or damaged tissue, plus other material, that is removed when a wound is treated.

Debrox, a trademark for drops that soften ear wax and aid its removal (carbamide peroxide).

dec-, **1.** a combining form meaning 'ten.' **2.** a combining form meaning 'tenth.'

Decadron, a trademark for a steroid drug used to treat swelling (dexamethasone).

Deca-Durabolin, a trademark for a male hormone used to build tissue after severe injuries, to control the spread of breast cancer, and bone weakness (nandrolone decanoate).

decalcification, a loss of calcium salts from the teeth and bones, caused by malnutrition, failure of the body to absorb nutrients (malabsorption), or other factors. This condition may result, especially in older people, from a diet that lacks enough calcium. Malabsorption is caused by a lack of vitamin D, necessary for the body to absorb calcium, by a lack of stomach acids, and other disorders. See also **calcium, mineral.**

decanoic acid. See **capric acid.**

decerebrate posture /dēser'əbrāt/, the position of a patient in which the arms are extended and turned toward the body and the legs are extended with the feet flexed downward. The posture is usually seen in patients who are in a coma.

deci-, a prefix meaning $\frac{1}{10}$, as in deciliter.

decibel (db), a unit of measure of the intensity of sound. A decibel is ¹/₁₀ of a bel; an increase of 1 bel is approximately double the loudness of a sound.

decidua /disij'oo·ə/, the skinlike tissue of the inner lining of the uterus, it surrounds the fetus during pregnancy and is shed after childbirth. Decidua is also shed during menstruation.

decidua basalis, the skin like tissue of the inner lining of the uterus (decidua) that is beneath the implanted egg (ovum). Also called **decidua serotina.**

decidua capsularis, the tissue of the inner lining of the uterus (decidua) covering the implanted egg (ovum). Also called **decidua reflexa.**

decidual endometritis /disij'oo·əl/, an inflammation or infection of any part of the inner lining of the uterus (decidua) during pregnancy. See also **endometritis.**

decidua menstrualis, the inner lining of the uterus (decidua) shed during menstruation.

decidua reflexa. See **decidua capsularis.**

decidua serotina. See **decidua basalis.**

decidua vera, the tissue of the inner lining of the uterus (decidua) except for those areas beneath (decidua basalis) and above (decidua capsularis) the implanted egg (ovum).

deciduoma /disij'oo·ō'mə/, a tumor of the lining of the uterus that tends to develop after a pregnancy. It may be benign or cancerous.

deciduous tooth /disij'oo·əs/, any one of the 20 teeth that appear normally during infancy, often called baby teeth. In most children the first deciduous tooth appears through the gum about 6 months after birth. Then one or more erupt about every month until all 20 have appeared. The deciduous teeth are usually lost between the ages of 6 and 13. Also called **milk tooth, primary dentition.** Compare **permanent tooth.** See also **predeciduous dentition, teething, tooth.**

Declomycin, a trademark for a drug that kills bacteria (demeclocycline hydrochloride).

decoction, a liquid medicine made by boiling substances, as plants and herbs, in water. Herbal remedies are usually decoctions. See also **concoction.**

decompensation, the failure of a system, as cardiac decompensation in heart failure.

decomposition, the breakdown of a substance into simpler chemical forms.

decompression, 1. a technique used to readjust a person to normal atmospheric pressures after exposure to higher pressures. For example, it is used for deep-sea divers. 2. the removal of pressure caused by gas or fluid in a body cavity, as the stomach or intestine.

decompression sickness, a painful, sometimes deadly condition caused by nitrogen bubbles forming in the body tissue. This sickness, most often found in deep-sea divers, caisson workers, and aviators, is caused by moving too

quickly from areas of higher atmospheric pressures to lower pressures, as divers coming up from the bottom of the ocean too fast. Disorientation, severe pain, and fainting result. Treatment is to return the patient quickly to an environment of higher pressure and gradually reduce the pressure to allow the body time to adjust (decompression). Also called **bends, caisson disease.** Compare **barotrauma.**

decongestant, 1. referring to a substance or procedure that reduces congestion or swelling. 2. a drug used to reduce congestion or swelling, especially of the nasal passages.

decontamination, the process of making a person, thing, or place free of viruses, molds, and bacteria; radiation; or dangerous substances.

decorticate posture /dēkôr'tikāt/, the position of a patient in which the arms are bent at the elbows and at the wrists. The legs also may be bent. This position is seen in patients in comas and indicates an injury in the midbrain.

decorticate rigidity. See **decorticate posture.**

decortication /dēkôr'tikā'shən/, the removal of the center (cortical) tissue of an organ or structure.

decrement, a decrease or stage of decline. For example, the term may be applied to the final part of a labor contraction, when the uterus relaxes and the pain is eased.

decubitus /dikyoo'bitəs/, a reclining or flat position, as lying on one side. See also **decubitus care, decubitus ulcer.**

decubitus care, preventing and treating sores that form over bony parts of the body (decubitus ulcers). They occur in patients not able to move around, especially the elderly, the obese, and the seriously ill. These ulcers occur on pressure areas, most often on the bottom of the spine, elbows, heels, outer ankles, inner knees, hips, shoulder blades, and ear rims.
★METHOD: Decubiti may be prevented by turning the patient every 2 hours, keeping the skin dry, and watching pressure areas for signs of redness. Care for decubitus ulcers, which can take a long time to heal, involves cleaning the area and applying special drugs to the ulcers. Large areas of ulcers can be life-threatening. Prompt and continued care of early ulcers can prevent infection and promote healing.

decubitus posture, the position a bedridden patient takes to relieve pressure on the lower spine, heels, or other body area subject to bedsores (decubitus ulcers). The patient usually lies on his or her side.

decubitus projection, (in radiology) a position for taking an x-ray picture of the chest or belly of a patient who is lying down. The x-ray tube is held horizontal.

decubitus ulcer, a swollen sore or ulcer of the skin over a bony part of the body, results from prolonged pressure on the part. Decubitus ulcers are most often seen in patients not able to move around easily, as the elderly, infirm, or severely ill. The sores are graded by stages of severity: Stage I: The skin is red and does not return to normal with relief of pressure. Stage II: The skin is blistered, peeling, or cracked, though damage is still minor. Stage III: The skin is broken and tissue under the skin may also be damaged, and drainage may be seen. Stage IV: A deep, craterlike ulcer has formed. The full thickness of skin and the underlying tissues are destroyed. Prevention of decubitus ulcers is an essential aspect of care. See **decubitus care for prevention and treatment.**

decussate /dəcus'āt/, to cross in the form of an X, as certain nerve fibers from the retina that cross at the optic chiasm. **–decussation,** *n.*

deep brachial artery, a branch of each of the brachial arteries, which pass from the heart deep into the arm. These supply blood to the bones and muscles of the upper arm.

deep-breathing and coughing exercises, the exercises taught to a person to improve or keep breathing functions. This is especially important after long periods of no activity or after general anesthesia. Pain from the incision after surgery in the chest or stomach often restricts normal breathing. See also **cupping and vibrating, postural drainage.**
★METHOD: The person is helped to a comfortable position, either lying down or sitting up. Breathing in through the nose and out through the mouth are encouraged. After taking a deep breath, the patient is asked to cough. If pain prevents the person from coughing deeply, a series of short barklike coughs may be encouraged.

deep coma. See **coma.**

deep fascia, an intricate series of feltlike membranes that split and join in a complex network around the skeleton. Compare **subcutaneous fascia, subserous fascia.**

deep heat, the application of heat to treat deep body tissues, as muscles and tendons. Shortwave therapy or ultrasound may be used.

deep palmar arch, the end of the radial artery in the lower arm. It joins the end of the ulnar artery, which also travels down the lower arm, in the palm of the hand.

deep sensation, the awareness of pain, pressure, or tension in the deep layers of the skin, muscles, or joints. These sensations are carried to the brain by way of the spinal cord. Compare **superficial sensation.**

deep structure, (in neurolinguistics) the deeper experience and meaning to which words may refer.

deep temporal artery, an artery on the front of each side of the head.

deep tendon reflex (DTR), a quick contraction of a muscle when its tendon is sharply tapped by a finger or rubber hammer. Absence of the reflex may be caused by damage to the muscle, the nerve, nerve roots, or the spinal cord. A violent reflex may be caused by disease of the nervous system or by overactive thyroid gland. Kinds of DTRs include **Achilles tendon reflex, biceps reflex, brachioradialis reflex, patellar reflex, triceps reflex.**

deep vein, one of the many veins that accompany the arteries. The vein and artery are usually wrapped together in a sheath. Compare **superficial vein.**

deep vein thrombosis, a condition involving a blood clot (thrombus) in a deep vein. The areas most often affected are the lower back and the thigh. Symptoms include tenderness, pain, swelling, warmth, and change in skin color. The condition may be life-threatening. The goal of treatment, which includes bed rest and anti-clotting drugs, is to prevent the blood clot from moving toward the lungs.

deep x-ray therapy, the use of x-rays to treat internal cancers, as Wilms' tumor of the kidney and Hodgkin's disease.

deerfly fever. See **tularemia.**

defecation /def'ikā'shən/, the ridding of feces from the digestive tract through the rectum. See also **constipation, diarrhea, feces.**

defecography /def'əkog'rəfē/, an x-ray procedure for viewing the rectum and lower intestines of children who are unable to control their bowel movements. The child sits on a toilet or potty that x-rays can pass through. Barium is injected through an enema tube, and the tube is left in place until the child indicates that he or she feels the urge to move the bowels. The bowel movement may be recorded on videotape for review and study.

defense mechanism, an unconscious, intrapsychic reaction that offers protection from a stressful situation. Kinds of defense mechanisms include **compensation, conversion, dissociation, displacement, sublimation.** Also called **ego-defense mechanism.**

defensin, a substance with natural antibiotic effects found in human blood cells. There are three types of defensins. Other animal species have similar substances. Defensins, which work against viruses, fungi, and bacteria, are believed to weaken their target cells by making their cell membranes porous.

defensive radical therapy, (in psychology) a treatment method that uses encouragement to help the patient avoid self-defeating behavior.

deferent duct. See **vas deferens.**

deferoxamine mesylate, a drug used to treat iron overdose.
★CAUTION: Kidney disease or inability to urinate prohibits its use.
★ADVERSE EFFECTS: Among the most serious side effects are low blood pressure, rapid heart beat, painful or difficult urination, visual difficulties, and allergic reactions.

defervescence /di'fərves'əns/, the dropping or disappearance of a fever. **–defervescent,** *adj.*

defibrillate /difī'brilāt, difib'-/, to stop very rapid contractions (fibrillation) of the heart. This is usually done by giving an electric shock to the heart through the chest wall. See also **defibrillation.**

defibrillation /difī'brilā'shən/, the process of stopping very rapid contractions of the heart (fibrillation) by delivering a direct electric shock to the patient's heart with a defibrillator. Defibrillation by electric shock is a common emergency procedure.

defibrillator /difī'brilā'tər, difib'-/, a device that delivers an electrical shock to the heart through the chest wall.

deficiency disease, a condition resulting from the lack of one or more essential nutrients in the diet. It can be caused by failure of the body to absorb the nutrients from food or digestive problems. Compare **malnutrition.** See also **avitaminosis.**

deficit, a deficiency, or difference, from what is normal. For example, a patient may have an oxygen deficit.

definitive host, any animal in which the reproductive stages of a parasite develop. The female *Anopheles* mosquito is the definitive host for malaria. Humans are definitive hosts for pinworms and tapeworms. Also called **primary host.** Compare **dead-end host, intermediate host, reservoir host.** See also **host.**

definitive treatment, any treatment generally accepted as the specific cure of a disease. Compare **expectant treatment, palliative treatment, supportive treatment.**

defloration, the rupture of the hymen, a membrane inside the vagina. It may occur during sexual intercourse, a physical examination, or by surgery.

deformity, a condition of being distorted or flawed. A deformity may affect the body in general or just part of it and may be the result of disease, injury, or birth defect.

degenerative chorea. See **Huntington's chorea.**

degenerative disease /dijen'ərətiv/, any disease in which there is decay of structure or function of tissue. Some kinds of degenerative disease are **arteriosclerosis, osteoarthritis.**

degenerative joint disease. See **osteoarthritis.**

degeneration, the gradual decay of normal cells and body functions.

degloving, the exposure of the lower jawbone in oral surgery.

deglutition /di'glo͞otish'ən/, swallowing.

deglutition apnea, the normal absence of breathing during swallowing.

dehiscence /dihis'əns/, the separation of a surgical cut (incision). It may also refer to the splitting open of a closed wound.

dehydrate /dihī'drāt/, **1.** to remove or lose water

from a substance. **2.** to lose excessive water from the body. **–dehydration,** *n.*

dehydrated alcohol, a clear, colorless liquid containing at least 99.5% ethyl alcohol. Also called **absolute alcohol.**

dehydration, 1. the large loss of water from the body tissues. Dehydration may occur after prolonged fever, diarrhea, vomiting, and any condition where there is rapid loss of body fluids. It is of particular concern in infants, young children, and the elderly. **2.** completely removing water from a substance.

dehydration fever, a fever that often occurs in newborns. It is thought to be caused by dehydration. Also called **inanition fever.** Compare **inanition, starvation.**

dehydration of gingivae, the drying of gum (gingival) tissue, often the result of breathing through the mouth. This condition lowers the resistance of the gum tissue to infection.

deinstitutionalization, releasing certain long-term mentally ill patients into the local community.

Deiter's nucleus, a part of the brainstem (base of the brain).

déjà vu /dāzhävY', -vē', -vo͞o'/, French. the feeling that one is encountering an event or place that has been experienced before. The phenomenon, normal in everyone, occurs more often in certain emotional and physical disorders. Déjà vu results from some unconscious emotional connection with the present experience. Compare **jamais vu, paramnesia.**

Dejerine-Sottas disease /dezh'ərinsot'əz/, a rare inherited disorder in which the sensory and muscle nerves disintegrate in the first few years of life. Weakness, numbness, loss of feeling pain, and touch occur. There is no specific treatment. Also called **progressive interstitial hypertrophic neuropathy.**

deka (da), a prefix meaning the number 10, as in dekagram.

de Lange's syndrome. See **Amsterdam dwarf.**

delayed dentition. See **retarded dentition.**

delayed echolalia, a speech pattern often seen in schizophrenia. Words and phrases are repeated meaninglessly. It occurs hours, days, or even weeks after the original words are heard.

delayed hypersensitivity reaction. See **cell-mediated immune response.**

delayed language, a child's failure to begin to use language at the expected age. It is usually caused by a hearing deficit, brain injury, or emotional disturbance.

delayed postpartum hemorrhage, bleeding that occurs more than 24 hours after childbirth. It is most often caused by fragments of the placenta still in the uterus, a tear of the cervix or vagina, or the uterus remaining expanded. See also **postpartum hemorrhage.**

delayed sensation, a feeling that is not experienced until sometime after stimulation. See also **sensation,** def.1.

delayed treatment seeker, (in psychology) a person who delays seeking treatment until months or years after a troubling event, as a rape. The person usually seeks treatment after a related event, as the anniversary of the attack.

Delecato-Doman theory, a theory about the treatment of disabled or mentally retarded children. The theory states that the child must pass through a series of developmental levels. In the first five steps, the child moves from infantile reflexes to walking. The sixth step is development of dominance of one side of the brain.

deletion, the loss of genetic material due to a piece of chromosome breaking off.

deletion syndrome, any of a group of birth defects that result from the loss of genetic material.

Delhi boil. See **oriental sore.**

deliberate biologic programing, the Hayflick theory of aging. The theory is based on studies that show that human cells die after dividing a certain number of times.

deliberate hypotension, a process in which a drug is given to reduce blood pressure briefly during surgery. This reduces bleeding, making vessels and tissues more visible to the surgeon.

délire de toucher /dälir'dətŏŏshä'/, French. a powerful urge to touch or handle objects.

delirium /dilir'ē·əm/, **1.** a state of great excitement or enthusiasm. **2.** a serious mental disorder marked by confusion, speech disorders, anxiety, excitement, and often hallucinations. The condition is caused by an upset in brain functions that can result from many physical disorders. These include nutritional or hormone disorders, exposure to various poisons (as gas, drugs, or alcohol), stress, or high fever.

delirium tremens (DTs), a serious and sometimes fatal psychotic reaction to sudden withdrawal of alcohol in the alcoholic. The reaction may follow an alcoholic binge during which no food was eaten. It can also be triggered by a head injury, infection, or withdrawal of alcohol after extended drinking. Symptoms include loss of appetite and difficulty in sleeping. This is followed by excitement, mental confusion, hallucinations, fear, and anxiety. There may also be body tremors, fever, increased heart rate, perspiration, stomach pain, and chest pain. The episode generally lasts from 3 to 6 days and is a medical emergency. A deep sleep often follows. Sedatives and tranquilizers are useful for calming the patient.

delirious mania, an extreme form of the excited (manic) state. The patient's activity is so frenzied and confused that it is difficult to detect a link between his or her behavior and underlying emotions.

delivery, the birth of a child.

delivery room, a unit of a hospital for childbirth.

DeLorme technique, a method of physical exercise with weights. The person repeats a set of exercises with rest periods in between. The technique involves the use of heavier weights and fewer repetitions in later exercise sets.

delta-9-tetrahydrocannabinol (THC), the active ingredient of marijuana (cannibas), it has been used to treat some cases of nausea and vomiting caused by cancer chemotherapy. See also **cannabis.**

delta optic density analysis, a method for diagnosing anemia in a fetus. If the fetus is severely anemic, delivery is often advised if the fetus is old enough to survive. Otherwise, fetal blood transfusions may be needed.

delta wave, 1. the slowest of the four types of brain waves. Delta waves are "deep-sleep waves" linked with a dreamless sleep from which the person is not easy to awaken. Also called **delta rhythm.** Compare **alpha wave, beta wave, theta wave. 2.** in study of the heart (cardiology), a part of the tracing of a heart beat on an electrocardiogram.

deltoid, 1. in the shape of a triangle. **2.** referring to the deltoid muscle that covers the shoulder.

deltoid muscle, a large, thick muscle that covers the shoulder joint. It bends, extends, rotates, and moves the arm away from the body. The deltoid attaches to the collarbone, several points of the shoulder blade, and the upper arm bone (humerus). Also called **deltoideus.**

delusion, a belief or perception held to be true by a person even though it is illogical and wrong. Kinds of delusion include **delusion of being controlled, delusion of grandeur, delusion of persecution, nihilistic delusion, somatic delusion.** Compare **illusion.**

delusion of being controlled, the false belief that one's feelings, thoughts, and acts are controlled by something else. This is seen in various forms of schizophrenia. See also **delusion.**

delusion of grandeur, the wild exaggeration of one's importance, wealth, power, or talents. This is seen in some disorders, as megalomania, general paresis, and paranoid schizophrenia. See also **delusion.**

delusion of persecution, a morbid belief that one is being mistreated and harassed by unknown enemies. This is seen in paranoia and paranoid schizophrenia. See also **delusion.**

delusion of poverty, (in psychology) a person's false belief that he or she is poor.

delusion of reference. See **idea of reference.**

delusion stupor, a state in which a patient is unresponsive and lethargic; seen in catatonic schizophrenia.

demarcation current, an electric current that flows from an uninjured to an injured end of a muscle. Also called **current of injury.**

Demazin, a trademark for a respiratory, combination drug containing a stimulant (phenylephrine hydrochloride) and an antihistamine (chlorpheniramine maleate).

deme /dēm/, a small, closely related group of organisms or people, it occupies a small area and is marked by interbreeding. Also called **genetic population.**

demecarium bromide, a drug used to treat a type of disorder in the eye (open-angle glaucoma).
★CAUTION: Swelling of the eye, some types of glaucoma, asthma, peptic ulcer, epilepsy, recent heart attack, or known allergy to this drug prohibits its use.
★ADVERSE EFFECTS: Very slow heart beat, diarrhea, eye irritation, low blood pressure, or headaches can occur.

demeclocycline hydrochloride, an antibiotic used to treat a number of infections, it is often given when penicillin cannot be used.
★CAUTION: Kidney or liver disorders, pregnancy, or known allergy to this drug prohibits its use. It is also not given to young children.
★ADVERSE EFFECTS: blood disorders, intestinal problems, excessive sensitivity to light, and allergy may occur.

dementia /dimen'shə/, a disorder in which mental functions deteriorate and break down, grows worse with time and is marked by personality change, confusion, and lethargy. Thinking, reason, memory, and judgment are also affected. The cause is usually brain disease. Kinds of dementia include **Alzheimer's disease, dementia paralytica, Pick's disease, secondary dementia, senile dementia, toxic dementia.**

dementia paralytica. See **general paresis.**

dementia praecox /prē'koks/, a term for schizophrenia, no longer used. See **schizophrenia.**

Demerol, a trademark for a narcotic drug that relieves pain (meperidine).

Demerol Hydrochloride, a trademark for a narcotic drug that relives pain (meperidine hydrochloride).

demigauntlet bandage /dem'igônt'lit/, a glovelike bandage, it covers only the hand and leaves the fingers free. See also **gauntlet bandage.**

demineralization, a decrease in the amount of minerals or salts in tissues. This occurs in certain diseases.

democratic style, a leadership style in which group members participate in making decisions to reach group goals.

demography /dəmog'rəfē/, the study of human populations, particularly the size, distribution, and characteristics of members of population groups. Demography is applied in studies of health problems involving ethnic groups, populations of a specific geographic region, or religious groups with special dietary restrictions.

demonstrative, a type of behavior that accompanies and illustrates speech. See **circum-speech.**

De Morgan's spots. See **cherry angioma.**

Demser, a trademark for a drug that reduces high blood pressure (metyrosine).

demulcent /dimul'sənt/, an oily substance used to sooth and reduce irritation of the skin.

Demulen, a trademark for a birth-control pill. It contains an estrogen (ethinyl estradiol) and a progestin (ethynodiol diacetate).

demyelination /dimī'əlinā'shən/, the destruction of the covering (myelin sheath) of a nerve.

denaturation, 1. a change in the basic nature or structure of a substance. 2. the process of making a food or drink unfit for human consumption. The denatured substance may still be used for other purposes, as a solvent.

denatured alcohol, ethyl alcohol made unfit for drinking. This is done by adding several poisonous chemicals.

dendrite /den'drīt/, a structure that extends from the cell body of a nerve (neuron). These receive signals that are sent on to the cell body. The number of dendrites varies with the functions of a neuron. Compare **axon.**

dendritic keratitis, a serious herpes virus infection of the eye. It causes an open sore of the surface of the eye that looks like a tree with knobs at the ends of the branches. Light sensitivity, pain, and swelling of the eyelid are usual. Treatment includes applying certain drugs to the sore or removing the sore by surgery.

dengue fever /deng'gē, den'gā/, a serious virus infection given to humans by the *Aedes* mosquito, it occurs in tropical and subtropical regions. The disease, which usually causes fever, rash, and severe head, back, and muscle pain, most often occurs in two phases. In the first attack, the patient has a fever, weakness, headache, sore throat, muscle pains, and swelling of the hands and feet. The second attack follows a day after these symptoms stop. It is marked by a return of fever and by a bright-red rash. The infection clears up without treatment, though it may take patients several weeks to recover. Also called **Aden fever, bouquet fever, breakbone fever, dandy fever, solar fever.** See also *Aedes,* **arbovirus.**

dengue hemorrhagic fever shock syndrome (DHFS), an often fatal form of dengue fever. It is marked by shock with collapse, clammy arms and legs, a weak pulse, breathing problems, and the symptoms of dengue fever. Severe bleeding, bruises, small reddish spots on the skin, and bloody vomit, urine, and feces may occur. This is followed by failure of the circulatory system.

denial, 1. refusal of something requested or needed, often resulting in physical or emotional deficiency. 2. an unconscious defense mechanism. Certain thoughts and feelings that cause emotional conflict are avoided. Denial often involves failure to admit what is true or real.

Denis Browne splint, a splint to correct clubfeet (talipes equinovarus). The splint is a curved bar attached to the soles of a pair of high-top shoes. It is most often put on nightly in late infancy.

denitrogenation, the removal of nitrogen from the lungs and body tissues while a person is breathing pure oxygen.

Denman's spontaneous evolution, a natural, unaided turning of the fetus in the womb just before birth. As the fetus drops in the pelvis, it turns from a crossway position to a bottom-down position (breech).

dens, *pl.* **dentes** /den'tēz/, a tooth or toothlike structure. See also **dentition, tooth.**

dense fibrous tissue, a connective tissue made up of strong, nonstretchy bundles of fibers that are a shiny white color. These combine to make up tendons, membranes covering organs and bones, and parts of the skin.

dens in dente /den'tə/, a defect of the teeth, found chiefly in the incisors of the upper jaw. The defect is marked by channels or grooves in the enamel.

dens serotinus. See **wisdom tooth.**

dental, referring to a tooth or teeth.

dental abscess, a pocket of infectious material that forms in bone or soft tissue of the jaw, resulting from infection caused by tooth decay or injury. Symptoms include pain that is made worse by eating hot or cold food, or pressure caused by closing the jaw firmly. If left untreated, the infection may spread to other structures of the mouth and jaw. Treatment may include painkillers, antibiotics, root-canal therapy, or removal of the tooth.

dental alveolus /alvē'ələs/, a tooth socket in the lower (mandible) or upper (maxilla) jaw.

dental amalgam, a combination of several metals used for filling tooth cavities.

dental anesthesia, any of several anesthetic procedures used in dental surgery. Local anesthetics injected into the jaw are the most common.

dental anomaly, a defect in which one or more teeth are not normal in form or position.

dental arch, the curve formed by the grouping of a normal set of teeth.

dental assistant, a person who assists a dentist and may help with dental care or other general duties in the office.

dental calculus, a deposit of calcium and food on the teeth.

dental caries, destruction of the tooth enamel, caused by the interaction of food, as starches and sugars, with bacteria to form deposits (dental plaque). This material clings to the teeth. Plaque eventually causes breaks in the enamel of the tooth. This process, if untreated, leads to deep cavities and infection of the inside of the tooth and the nerves. Removal of plaque by a dentist eliminates the source of decay. Treatment of dental caries includes removing the decayed material with a drill, then filling the cavity with silver or other material. Dental caries are often called "cavities" or "tooth decay." Kinds of dental caries include **active caries, arrested caries, primary caries, secondary caries.**

dental crypt, the space taken up by a developing tooth.

dental engine, a hand instrument to which various rotating tools or drills can be fitted. It is driven by an electric motor.

dental erosion, the destruction of a tooth that causes variously shaped channels or holes. The surfaces of these depressions, unlike those of cavities, are hard and smooth.

dental extracting forceps, a type of pliers used for pulling teeth.

dental filling, *informal.* material placed into a prepared tooth cavity.

dental film, x-ray film made for dental use.

dental fistula, an abnormal passage that goes from the end of the root of the tooth through the gum to the surface. This allows infected fluid to drain out. Also called **alveolar fistula.**

dental floss, a waxed or unwaxed thread used to clean tooth surfaces and spaces between the teeth.

dental granuloma, a disorder in which a mass of grainy tissue is surrounded by a fiberlike cover. This mass is attached to the bottom of a tooth. The condition is seen when the inner tissue of the tooth (pulp) is diseased.

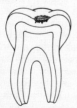 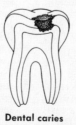 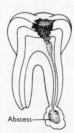

Dental caries   Abscess

dental hygienist, a person trained to provide minor dental services, including cleaning the teeth, taking x-ray films, and applying drugs when needed.

dental implant, a plastic or metal device that is placed inside the jaw to provide permanent support for fixed bridges or dentures. An implant is used when the patient does not have a large enough bony ridge to support a denture.

dental plaque. See **bacterial plaque.**

dental pulp, a small amount of connective tissue, blood vessels, and nerves located in a chamber within a tooth. See also **pulp canal, pulp cavity.**

dental restoration. See **restoration.**

dental root cyst. See **periodontal cyst.**

dental sealants, plastic films that are applied to the chewing surfaces of teeth; used to cover the pits and to seal grooves where food becomes trapped.

dental technician, a person who makes dentures, false teeth, and tooth retainers as ordered by a dentist.

dentate fracture /den'tāt/, any break that causes jagged bone ends that fit together like the teeth of gears.

dentate nucleus, a structure within the balance center (cerebellum) of the brain. It appears to be responsible for voluntary movement and, in part, for ongoing movement.

denticle, a hardened deposit in the inside (pulp chamber) of a tooth. Also called **endolith, pulp stone.**

dentifrice /den'tifris/, commonly called "toothpaste," a substance used with a toothbrush for cleaning and polishing the teeth. It may also contain drugs to prevent tooth decay.

dentigerous cyst /dentij'ərəs/, one of three kinds of cysts; a sac filled with thick fluid. This cyst covers the top (crown) of a tooth that has not yet emerged from the gum.

dentin /den'tin/, the chief material of teeth. It surrounds the inner part of the tooth (pulp) and is covered by the enamel. Dentin is harder and denser than bone. Also spelled **dentine.**

dentinogenesis /den'tinōjen'əsis/, the formation of the chief material of the teeth (dentin). –**dentinogenic,** *adj.*

dentinogenesis imperfecta, a hereditary disorder of the teeth. Brown teeth material (dentin) overgrows and fills in the center of the tooth. The teeth have short roots and wear rapidly. The disorder affects both baby (deciduous) and permanent teeth. Early corrective dentistry should be done. The condition is often linked to growth of brittle bones (osteogenesis imperfecta) and other disorders affecting bone, connective tissue, and teeth.

dentist, a person who is educated and licensed to practice dentistry. Training consists of 2 to 4 years in an undergraduate college and a passing score on a Dental Aptitude Test (DAT).

This is followed by 3 to 4 years at a dental college. Written and practical examinations must be passed to obtain a state license.

dentistry, practice of preventing and treating diseases and disorders of the teeth and gums. This includes repairing teeth and replacing missing teeth. It also includes detecting signs of diseases, as tumors, that would require treatment by a doctor. There are eight dental specialties, each needing extra training after graduation from a dental college. These are **endodontics, oral pathology, oral surgery, orthodontics, pedodontics, periodontics, prosthodontics,** and **public health dentistry.**

dentition, 1. the development and appearance of the teeth. 2. the arrangement, number, and kind of teeth as they appear in the mouth.

PRIMARY TEETH	Eruption (mo)	Shedding (yr)
Central incisor	9.6	7.5
Lateral incisor	12.4	8
Cuspid (canine)	18.3	11.5
Bicuspid	15.7	10.5
Molar	26.2	10.5
Molar	26.0	11
Bicuspid	15.1	10
Cuspid (canine)	18.2	9.5
Lateral incisor	11.5	7
Central incisor	7.8	6

SECONDARY TEETH	Eruption (yr)
Central incisor	7.35
Lateral incisor	8.45
Cuspid (canine)	11.35
First bicuspid	10.2
Second bicuspid	11.05
First molar	6.3
Second molar	12.25
Third molar	(17-21) Variable
Third molar	11.9
Second molar	6.05
First molar	11.2
Second bicuspid	10.5
First biscuspid	10.35
Cuspid (canine)	7.5
Lateral incisor	6.4
Central incisor	(17-21) Variable

Dentition

dentoalveolar abscess /den'tō·alvē'ələr/, the gathering of pus in the jawbone around a tooth.

dentofacial anomaly, a defect of the mouth structure in form, function, or position.

dentogenesis imperfecta /den'tōjen'əsis/, 1. a genetic disturbance of the main material of the teeth (dentin), marked by rapid wear and a milky look to the teeth. 2. a bone and connective tissue disorder (mesodermal dysplasia) that affects the main material of the teeth (dentin) and may be hereditary. It is linked to growth of brittle bones (osteogenesis imperfecta). 3. a genetic condition that produces defective dentin but normal tooth enamel.

dentogingival fiber /den'tōjinji'vəl/, any one of the many fibers that spread like a fan, fastening the root of a tooth to the gum. These fibers hold the tooth in place.

dentogingival junction, the junction between the surface of the teeth and the gum (gingiva).

dentulous dental arch, a dental arch that contains natural teeth.

denture /den'chər/, an artificial tooth or a set of teeth that are not permanently fastened in the mouth. Compare **fixed bridgework.**

denture base, the part of a denture that fits over the gum and holds the artificial teeth.

denturist, a person who performs the same type of work as a dental technician, as making dentures, false teeth, and tooth retainers. This work is not ordered by a dentist, but is provided directly to clients. In the United States, practice is only allowed in a few states. See also **dental technician.**

Denver Articulation Screening Examination (DASE), a test to judge the ability to speak clearly. It is given to children between 2½ and 6 years of age.

Denver Developmental Screening Test (DDST), a test for assessing development in children from 1 month to 6 years of age. The level of motor, social, and language skills is judged by comparing the child's performance with the average performance of other children.

deodorant, 1. destroying or covering up odors. **2.** a substance that destroys or masks odors. Common deodorants fight underarm, breath, vaginal, or room odors.

deossification /dē·os'ifikā'shən/, the loss of mineral matter from bones.

deoxyribonucleic acid (DNA) /dē·ok'sirī'bōnōō-klē'ik/, a large molecule, mainly the chromosome of a cell. It is the carrier of genetic information. Also called **desoxyribonucleic acid.** See also **nucleic acid, ribonucleic acid.**

Depakene, a trademark for a drug used to treat convulsions (valproic acid).

Department of Health and Human Services (DHHS), a cabinet-level department of the U.S. government, it includes the Food and Drug Administration (FDA), the Office of Consumer Affairs, Office of Civil Rights, Administration on Aging, Public Health Service, Indian Health Service, Social Security Administration, and the National Institutes of Health.

Department of Transportation (DOT), a cabinet-level department of U.S. government, it is responsible for national transportation policy, including maritime, railroad, aviation, and highway safety. It also regulates the transport of dangerous materials, as medical gases.

dependence, the state of being addicted to drugs or alcohol. As time passes, more and more of the substance is needed to prevent withdrawal.

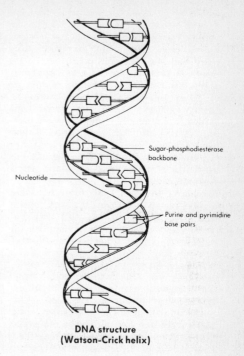

Nucleotide

Sugar-phosphodiesterase backbone

Purine and pyrimidine base pairs

DNA structure (Watson-Crick helix)

dependent, relying on someone or something for help, support, and other need. For example, a child is dependent on a parent, a drug addict is dependent on a drug. **–depend,** v., **dependence,** n.

dependent differentiation. See **correlative differentiation.**

dependent intervention, a therapeutic action by a health professional based on the written or verbal orders of another health professional. For example, a physical therapist may prescribe treatment based on a physician's diagnosis of the patient's condition.

dependent personality, behavior in which there is an excessive need for attention, acceptance, and approval from other people.

dependent personality disorder, a mental state in which a person lacks self-confidence and is unable to function independently.

depersonalization, the loss of a sense of personal identity, often involving a feeling of strangeness about oneself. This often results from anxiety. See also **alienation, depersonalization disorder.**

depersonalization disorder, an emotional disorder in which there is a loss of the feeling of personal identity (depersonalization). Everything becomes dreamlike. The body may not feel like one's own, and important events may be watched with detachment. It is common in some forms of schizophrenia and in severe depression.

depilation/dep'ilā'shən/, the removal of hiar from the body. It may be temporary, as in shaving. It may also be permanent, as by electrolysis, which destroys the hair root. Also called **epilation. -depilate,** *v.*

depilatory, /dipil'ətôrē/, referring to a substance or procedure that removes hair.

depot, 1. any area of the body in which drugs or other substances, as fat, are stored until needed. **2.** a drug that is injected in the body and is slowly absorbed over a period of time into the blood.

depot injection, an injection of a drug into the muscle that is released gradually over a period of several days.

depressant, a drug that tends to decrease the activity of a part of the body, as a heart depressant.

depressed fracture, any break of the skull in which pieces of bone are below the surface of the skull.

depression, 1. a depressed area or hollow; downward movement. **2.** a decrease of body activity. **3.** an emotional state in which there are extreme feelings of sadness, dejection, lack of worth, and emptiness. The obvious signs range from a slight lack of motivation and failure to concentrate to severe changes of body functions. The causes of depression can be hereditary or drug-related. Lack of balance of hormones or diet can also be causes. Depression can result from diseases, as nervous system disorders, infection, or cancer. See also **bipolar disorder. -depressive,** *adj.*

depressor, any drug that reduces activity when applied to nerves and muscles. See also **depressant.**

depressor septi, one of the three muscles of the nose. It narrows the nostril.

deprivation, to keep something away from someone. In experimental psychology, animal or human subjects may be deprived of something in order to study their reactions.

depth perception, the ability to judge depth or the distance between objects. Vision from both eyes is essential to this ability.

de Quervain's fracture, /də kərvānz'/, break of the navicular bone in the top of the foot with dislocation of the lunate bone.

de Quervain's thyroiditis, a swelling condition of the thyroid. It is marked by tenderness of the gland, fever, difficulty swallowing, fatigue, and severe pain in the neck, ears, and jaw. The disorder, which often occurs after a viral infection of the lungs, tends to come and go. Treatment may include drugs to fight swelling, as aspirin. Steroids are given for prolonged or severe cases. Also called **giant cell thyroiditis, granulomatous thyroiditis, subacute thyroiditis.**

derailment, a pattern of speech seen in schizophrenic patients. Disconnected, unrelated ideas replace logical and orderly thought patterns.

derby hat fracture See **dishpan fracture.**

dereflection, a technique of psychology. A person's mind is taken off one goal by diverting it to another. This often results in the person accomplishing the original goal.

dereistic thought /dē'rē·is'tik/, a thought pattern in which fantasy is not influenced by logic, experience, or reality.

derivative, 1. anything that is obtained from another substance. For example, penicillin is derived from a fungus. **2.** a molecule that is chemically altered from its original form.

derived lipid, a fat (lipid) derived from the breakdown of other fats, including fatty acids.

dermabrasion, /dur'məbrā'zhən/, a treatment for removing scars on the skin. Wire brushes or sandpaper are used. This is done to reduce facial scars of severe acne and to remove tattoos.

Dermacentor, a group of ticks. It includes ticks that transmit Rocky Mountain spotted fever and other infectious diseases. See also **Lyme disease.**

dermatitis, /dur'mətī'tis/, an inflammation of the skin marked by redness, pain, or itching. The condition may be long-term or sudden. Treatment depends on the cause. Some kinds of dermatitis are **actinic dermatitis, contact dermatitis, rhus dermatitis, seborrheic dermatitis.**

dermatitis exfoliativa neonatorum. See **Ritter's disease.**

dermatitis herpetiformis, a long-term skin disease with groups of itchy red bumps or blisters that leave deeply colored spots. It is sometimes linked to cancer in an inner organ or stomach disease.

dermatitis medicamentosa See **drug eruption.**

dermatitis venenata. See **contact dermatitis.**

dermato-, derma-, dermat-, dermo-, a combining form referring to the skin.

dermatocyst /dur'mətōsist'/, a fluid-filled tumor (cyst) of the skin.

dermatofibroma, /dur'mətōfibrō'mə/, *pl.* **dermatofibromas, dermatofibromata,** a painless, round, firm, and gray or red bump on the skin. It is most commonly found on the arms and legs and needs no treatment. Also called **fibrous histiocytoma.**

dermatoglyphics /dur'mətōglif'iks/, the study of the skin ridge patterns on fingers, toes, palms of hands, and soles of feet. These patterns are often called prints, as fingerprints. The patterns are used for identification. They can also help diagnose certain chromosome defects.

dermatographia, dur'mətōgraf'ē·ə/, an abnormal skin condition marked by large raised areas that result from drawing blunt objects across the skin. This condition makes the skin especially sensitive. It may be caused by certain foods or drugs. Also called **autographism, dermatographism, Ebbecke's reaction.**

dermatologist, a doctor specializing in disorders of the skin.

dermatology, the study of the skin, including the diagnosis and treatment of skin disorders.

dermatomycosis /dur'mətōmīkō'sis/, a mild fungus infection of the skin found on areas that are moist and covered by clothing, as the groin or feet. See also **dermatophytosis.**

dermatomyositis /dur'mətōmī-ōsī'tis/, a disease of the connective tissues marked by itching, swelling of the skin, and tenderness and weakness of the muscles. Muscle tissue is destroyed, often to the point where the patient may not be able to walk or perform simple tasks. Swelling of the eyelids and face and loss of weight are common symptoms.

Dermatophagoides farinae, a common household dust mite. It causes allergic reactions in sensitive persons. Bug killers and vacuum cleaning can help to control them. The mites thrive on skin, hair, pet foods, carpets, and bedding, as well as house dust.

dermatophyte /dur'ətōfit', dəmat'əfit/, any of several fungi that cause skin disease in humans. See also **dermatophytid,** specific fungal infections.

dermatophytid /dur'mətof'itid, dur'mətōfi'tid/, an allergic skin reaction marked by small blisters and linked to dermatomycosis.

dermatophytosis dur'mətō'fitō'sis, a mild fungus infection of the skin. On the trunk and arms it is commonly called "ringworm." The infection causes round scaly patches with slightly raised edges and clear centers. On the feet, small blisters, cracking and itching, occur; the condition is called "athlete's foot." Treatment includes drugs to fight fungus placed on the skin. See also **tinea.**

dermatoplasty /dur'mətōplas'tē/, a surgical procedure in which skin is transplanted to a part of the body that has been damaged by disease or injury.

dermatosclerosis, a skin disease in which patches of thick, leathery skin form. See **scleroderma.**

dermatosis /dur'mətō'sis/, any disorder of the skin that does not cause swelling. Compare **dermatitis.**

dermatosis papulosa nigra, a common abnormal skin condition in blacks marked by many noncancerous, tiny, dark bumps on the cheeks.

dermis. See **corium.**

dermoid /dur'moid/, **1.** referring to the skin. **2.** sometimes used to refer to a certain tumor (dermoid cyst).

dermoid cyst/, a tumor filled with fatty material and cartilage; has a fiberlike wall. More than 10% of all tumors on the ovary are dermoid cysts, which are most often noncancerous. Also called **organoid tumor, teratoid tumor.**

derotation brace, a device used to support and strengthen the knee. It has two parts: a single-joint hinged bar and a rotating pad. The pad is placed on the unstable side of the knee. The brace is custom-made for the person who wears it.

DES/, abbreviation for **diethylstibestrol.**

descending aorta, the main part of the large artery of the heart (aorta), it leads to the trunk of the body and supplies blood to many areas, including the throat, ribs, and stomach.

descending colon, the middle part of the large intestine (colon) that runs up and down.

descending urography. See **intravenous pyelography.**

descriptive anatomy, the study of the form and structure of various systems of the body, as the digestive system and the nervous system.

descriptive embryology, the study of the changes that occur in the fetus during pregnancy.

Desenex, a trademark for a drug used on the skin for the treatment of athlete's foot (undecylenic acid and zinc undecylenate).

desensitize, **1.** to make a person insensitive to any of the various foreign substances (antigens) that might cause an allergic reaction. **2.** to help to relieve an emotionally disturbed person become free of phobias and neuroses. This is done by talking about the fears and events that cause the problems. **3.** in dentistry, to reduce the pain in the teeth caused by irritating substances and temperature changes.

deserpidine /disur'pədēn/, a drug used to treat mild high blood pressure and anxiety.
★CAUTION: Depression, stomach ulcer, colon ulcers, or known allergy to this drug prohibits its use. It can react with other drugs to increase high blood pressure.
★ADVERSE EFFECTS: Among the more serious side effects are possible severe mental depression. This drug may cause dizziness, blurred vision, and fainting when a person stands up or stands still for a long time.

desert fever. See **coccidioidomycosis.**

desert rheumatism, a form of coccidioidomycosis that causes pain in the bones and joints.

Deseral Mesylate, a trademark for a drug used to treat too much iron in the body (deferoxamine mesylate).

desiccant /des'ikənt/, any drug or procedure that causes a substance to dry up. Also called **exsiccant.**

desiccate /des'ikāt/, to dry thoroughly.

desipramine hydrochloride, drug used to treat mental depression.

deslanoside /dislan'əsīd/, a drug used to treat heart failure and certain forms of irregular heart beats.
★CAUTION: Irregular heart contractions, rapid heart beat, or known allergy to this drug prohibits its use.
★ADVERSE EFFECTS: The most serious side effect is irregular heart beat.

desmocyte. See **fibroblast.**

desmoid tumor, a cancerous tumor of the muscle that may occur in the head, neck, upper arm, stomach, or legs.

desmopressin acetate, a drug that slows urine production in the kidneys; it is used to treat diabetes.
★CAUTION: Known allergy to this drug prohibits its use.
★ADVERSE EFFECTS: Among the most serious side effects are salt deficiency and too much water in the body. Mild effects, as headache, cramps, and stuffy nose, may also occur.

desmosis, any disease of the connective tissue.

desonide, a drug put on the skin to reduce swelling.
★CAUTION: Diseases of the skin, poor circulation, or known allergy to this drug prohibits its use.
★ADVERSE EFFECTS: The more serious side effects most often occur after using this drug for a long time. These include streaks in the skin, loss of skin color, and skin irritation.

desoximetasone, a drug put on the skin to reduce swelling.
★CAUTION: Diseases of the skin, poor circulation, or known allergy to this drug prohibits its use. The wound should not be sealed from the air with a bandage.
★ADVERSE EFFECTS: The more serious side effects most often occur after prolonged use. These include streaks in the skin, loss of skin color, and skin irritation.

Desoxyn, a trademark for a drug that stimulates the central nervous system on the body as a whole (methampehtamine hydrochloride).

desoxyribonucleic acid. See **deoxyribonucleic acid.**

desquamation /des′kwəmā′shən/, a normal process in which the top layer of the skin comes off in tiny pieces. Certain conditions, injuries, and drugs speed up desquamation. Also called **exfoliation.**

desquamative interstitial pneumonia, a disease of the breathing system in which dead cells accumulate in the lungs and tubes leading to them. Its symptoms are coughing, chest pain, weight loss, and difficult breathing. The disease is treated with steroid drugs and oxygen.

destructive aggression, an act of hostility not needed for self-protection; directed toward an object or person. See also **aggression.**

Desyrel, a trademark for a drug used to treat depression (trazodone).

detached retina. See **retinal detachment.**

detection bias, a potential error that can occur in studies of the spread of disease (epidemiology), caused by the use of a particular diagnostic technique or piece of equipment in the study. For example, the reported cancer rates may vary between regions or time periods. The difference may be caused by the use of tests to detect cancer, while the underlying rate of disease is actually the same.

detergent, a cleaning agent. See also **surfactant.**

deterioration, a gradual worsening, as of a patient's condition.

determinants of occlusion, the factors that influence proper closure of the teeth.

determinate cleavage, cell division of the fertilized egg (ovum) into sections that will each become a specific part of the embryo. Damage to any of the cells results in a malformed fetus. Also called **mosaic cleavage.** Compare **indeterminate cleavage.** See also **mosaic development.**

detoxification, removal of the poison from a substance or speeding up its removal from the body.

detoxification service, a hospital service that treats the effect of chemical poisons, as alcohol or drugs. Detoxification is the first step in helping people overcome their dependence (addiction) on these substances.

detriangle, (in psychology) a process by which one avoids becoming involved in a three-sided situation, either with two other people, or with another person and an object.

detrusor urinae muscle /ditoo′zər/, a complex of fibers that form the outer layer of the muscle coat of the bladder.

deutoplasm /doo′təplaz′əm/, the parts of the yolk that store nutrition. Also called **deuteroplasm.**

DEV, abbreviation for **duck embryo vaccine.** See also **rabies vaccine.**

development, 1. the gradual process of change from a simple to a more complex level. In humans the ability to adapt to our surroundings and to function in society is gained through growth and learning. 2. the series of events that occur in an organism from the time the egg is fertilized to the adult stage. -developmental, adj.

developmental age (DA), an expression of a child's development, stated in age and determined by accepted measurements. The child is judged by body size, social and psychological abilities, and motor skills. Mental and aptitude tests are also given. Compare **achievement age, developmental quotient, mental age.**

developmental agraphia, problem in a child's ability to learn to form letters and to write. Other learning is normal, and the child usually has no physical problems.

developmental anatomy, the study of the growth of an organism from a single cell to birth. Also called **embryology.**

developmental anomaly, any birth defect that results when the normal growth of the fetus is disturbed. Such defects can occur at any stage of development. They vary greatly in type and severity and may be caused by a number of things. These include chromosome abnormalities, drugs, diseases of the mother (such as measles), and environmental factors.

developmental crisis, a severe, usually temporary stress that prevents a person from moving to the next stage of psychosocial development. See also **psychosocial development.**

developmental disability (DD), a disorder that starts developing before 18 years of age. Most disorders of this type last the person's lifetime, but many can be treated. See also **congenital condition.**

developmental disorder, a form of mental retardation that develops in a child who has progressed normally for the first 3 or 4 years of life. The condition usually begins with a mild viral infection or other similar disease.

developmental dysfunction, an abnormal or slowed process of development, or its result.

developmental dyspraxia, a disorder in which a person's ability to plan nonroutine skilled movements is decreased.

developmental fog, (in radiology) an x-ray film that is dull, washed-out, and lacking in contrast. The fog may be caused by incorrect temperature, time, or concentration of chemicals during development.

developmental handling, the moving of a child through part or all of the sequence in which movement skills develop; done to enhance the child's ability to perform normal movements such as balance.

developmental model, a concept that outlines four stages of a patient's therapy for mental problems. In the first stage (orientation) the patient starts to recognize the problem with the help of the therapist. In the second stage (identification) a sense of closeness to the therapist develops. This allows them to work well together. In the third stage (exploitation) the patient assumes some control of the meetings and grows more independent. During the last stage (resolution) the patient is independent and no longer needs the therapist.

developmental physiology, the study of the physical processes as they relate to development in the early embryo.

developmental quotient (DQ), a child's developmental level as stated by a number. This is done by dividing the developmental age by the child's actual age. This figure is then multiplied by 100. Compare **intelligence quotient.** See also **developmental age.**

developmental task, a physical or mental skill that a person must learn during a certain age period in order to continue developing. For example, a baby must first learn to walk in order to develop a sense of independence.

developmental theory of aging, the idea that characteristics developed early in life tend to last into the later years.

deviance /dē'vē·əns/, behavior that is against the accepted standards of a group of people.

deviant behavior, actions that exceed the usual limits of accepted behavior. Such actions involve failure to comply with social norms.

deviate /dē'vē·it/, a person or an event that varies from the normal standard.

deviated septum, a condition affecting many adults in which the center section (septum) of the nose shifts to one side. The septum often shifts to the left during normal growth. This shift may be increased by a blow to the nose or by other problems. A severe shift of the septum may block the nasal passages and cause infection, sinusitis, shortness of breath, headache, or frequent nosebleeds.

device, an item other than a drug used to aid healing. Devices include splints, crutches, artificial heart valves, pacemakers, wheelchairs, hearing aids, and eye glasses.

devitalized, referring to tissues with reduced oxygen supply and blood flow.

devital tooth. See **pulpless tooth.**

dewar, (in nuclear magnetic resonance imaging) a double chamber used to maintain the equipment at very low temperatures. The outer chamber is filled with liquid nitrogen at a temperature of $-196°$ C ($-321°$ F). The inner chamber is filled with liquid helium at a temperature of $-270°$ C ($-454°$ F).

dew point, the temperature at which the air becomes saturated with moisture, which then condenses to liquid. In aerosol therapy, water may collect on containers, tubing, and other surfaces when the dew point is reached.

dexamethasone, a drug used to treat numerous swelling disorders.

dexchlorpheniramine maleate, a drug used to treat a number of allergic reactions. These include swelling of the nose, skin rash, and severe itching.

Dexedrine, a trademark for a drug that stimulates the central nervous system (dextroamphetamine sulfate).

dextrality. See **right-handedness.**

dextran, a form of liquid sugar (glucose) given in the vein.

dextro-, dextr-, a combining form meaning 'right.'

dextrocardia, the location of the heart on the right side of the chest, rather than the left. This may occur as a result of disease, or a person may be born with the defect.

dextromethorphan hydrobromide, a drug used to help stop coughing.
★CAUTION: Known allergy to this drug prohibits its use.
★ADVERSE EFFECT: The most serious side effect is breathing difficulty caused by large doses.

dextrose /dek'strōs/, a liquid sugar solution (glucose) given in the vein.

D.H.E.-45, a trademark for a drug used to treat migraine and certain other forms of headache (dihydroergotamine mesylate).

dhobie itch /dō′bē/, a skin infection caused by laundry marking fluids. See also **jock itch, jockstrap itch.**

di-, **1.** a combining form meaning 'two, twice.' **2.** a combining form meaning 'apart, away from.'

DiaBeta, a trademark for an oral drug taken by diabetics. Its generic name is glyburide.

diabetes /dī′əbē′tēz/, **1.** a disease affecting sugar use by the body. **2.** diabetes mellitus. See also **diabetic.**

diabetes insipidus /insip′idəs/, an uncommon type of diabetes disorder marked by extreme thirst and heavy urination. It is caused by a lack of enough of the hormone that limits the amount of urine made (ADH) and may also be caused by a failure of the kidneys to respond to ADH. The condition may be inborn, result from a kidney disorder, or just appear for no obvious reason. ★DIAGNOSIS: The disorder may begin quite suddenly, and the urine output may be as much as 2½ gallons in 24 hours. The patient seldom suffers from any other problems except the constant need to drink. A person with diabetes insipidus who is unconscious because of injury or surgery will still produce great amounts of urine. If enough fluids are not given, the patient becomes severely dehydrated and salt-depleted. ★TREATMENT: In mild cases, no treatment is necessary. Drugs may be given to help the kidneys respond to ADH. Drugs will also reduce the amount of urine.

diabetes mellitus (DM) /məli′təs/, a complex disorder caused by the failure of the pancreas to release enough insulin into the body. It may also be caused by a defect in the parts of cells that accept the insulin. The disease tends to run in families. There are four main types of diabetes mellitus. Type I diabetes is also called insulin-dependent diabetes, juvenile-onset diabetes, brittle diabetes, or ketosis-prone diabetes. This is the more serious form of the disease. Type I diabetes most often develops during childhood, although young adults also can develop this form. Type II diabetes is also called non-insulin-dependent diabetes, adult-onset diabetes, ketosis-resistant diabetes, or stable diabetes. Type II often develops in overweight adults. Type III, or gestational diabetes, occurs in some women during pregnancy. It disappears after childbirth, but many women later develop Type II diabetes. Type IV includes other types of diabetes linked to disease of the pancreas, hormonal changes, side effects of drugs, or genetic defects. ★DIAGNOSIS: The beginning of diabetes mellitus is sudden in children and usually slow in Type II diabetes. The symptoms include the need to urinate often, increased thirst, weight loss, and increased appetite. The levels of sugar in the blood and urine will be high. The eyes, kidneys, nervous system, and skin may be affected. Infections are common, and hardening of the arteries often develops. In childhood and in Type I diabetes, coma from not enough insulin (ketoacidosis) is a constant danger. ★TREATMENT: The goal of treatment is to maintain a sugar and insulin balance. Mild, early, or late onset of the disease can often be controlled by diet alone. Insulin tablets are sometimes used for Type II diabetes. In more severe diabetes, insulin is given in injections.

Classification of diabetes mellitus and descriptive characteristics for each type

Class	Clinical and associated factors and former terminology
Type I: insulin-dependent diabetes mellitus (IDDM)	Patients dependent on insulin to prevent ketosis; onset usually in youth but may occur in adults; associated with certain HLA types, islet cell antibodies are frequently present; formerly called juvenile-onset diabetes, ketosis-prone diabetes, brittle diabetes
Type II: noninsulin-dependent diabetes mellitus (NIDDM)	Patients not dependent on insulin to preserve life, although they may be treated with insulin (even if treated with insulin, they are still classified as NIDDM); ketosis resistant except in very special circumstances such as presence of infection; not HLA related; onset usually after 40 years of age but may occur in youth; serum insulin levels may be depressed, normal, or elevated; 60% to 90% of diabetics in this class are obese; formerly called maturity-onset diabetes, adult-onset diabetes, ketosis-resistant diabetes, and stable diabetes; class may be subdivided into two classes: (1) obese Type II, and (2) nonobese Type II
Type III: gestational diabetes mellitus (GDM)	Glucose intolerance occurs during pregnancy; group does not include known diabetics who become pregnant; after delivery, glucose intolerance may remain but not be serious enough to be treated or the patient may have characteristics of Type I or Type II diabetes, or glucose intolerance may disappear; patient is reclassified after delivery, formerly called gestational diabetes
Type IV: other types, includes diabetes mellitus associated with pancreatic disease, other hormonal abnormalities, drugs	Patients in this class must have diabetes mellitus and one of the other diseases, syndromes, or causal factors; formerly called secondary diabetes

The kind and amount of insulin given varies with the person's condition. Stress of any kind may require a change in the dose. See also **diabetic foot and leg care.**

★PATIENT CARE: The person with diabetes must understand that the effects are severe but can be prevented. Daily care must include staying on the proper diet, testing the urine for sugar, and taking the insulin at the correct times. Recognizing the symptoms of diabetic coma (ketoacidosis) is essential. These are restlessness, thirst, hot dry skin, rapid pulse, and nausea. The patient also learns to recognize the signs of too much insulin (insulin shock) and too little blood sugar. These are headache, nervousness, sweating, and slurred speech. The patient should avoid infection, carry a supply of sugar at all times, and wear a medical-alert tag. Regular exercise, not smoking, following the proper diet, and prompt treatment of infections will allow most people with diabetes to live healthy, normal lives.

diabetes, other types. See **other types of diabetes.**

diabetic /dī'əbet'ik/, **1.** referring to diabetes. **2.** a person who has diabetes mellitus.

diabetic amaurosis, blindness linked to diabetes, caused by bleeding into the retina (retinopathy). Cataracts are also common in Type I and Type II diabetes.

diabetic coma. See **diabetic ketoacidosis.**

diabetic diet, a diet for patients with diabetes mellitus. The diet usually limits sugar or simple carbohydrates. It increases proteins, complex carbohydrates, and unsaturated fats. Many persons with Type II diabetes can control their disease by diet alone and need not take insulin. The diet helps to keep the level of sugar in the blood stable. See also **diabetes mellitus, insulin.**

diabetic foot-and-leg care, the special care given to prevent the problems with blood circulation and infections that often occur in the feet and legs of diabetic patients.

★METHOD: The patient's legs and feet are examined daily for signs of dry, red, or cracked skin. Blisters, calluses, infection, blueness and swelling around varicose veins, and thick discolored toenails are also watched for. The feet are bathed daily in lukewarm water with mild soap, then dried gently with a soft towel. A lanolin-based lotion is applied. Vigorous rubbing and the use of alcohol are avoided. The toenails are cut straight across after the feet have been soaked in water. The feet should be kept dry at all times. Careful care of the feet and legs can prevent infection, skin ulcers, and gangrene.

diabetic ketoacidosis, a life-threatening condition that can occur in patients with diabetes mellitus. It is caused by failure to take insulin or anything that increases the body's need for insulin, as infection, surgery, injury, or stress.

Warning signs include a dull headache, fatigue, extreme thirst, pain below the breastbone, nausea, dry lips, sunken eyes, and a fruity breath odor. The temperature usually rises and then falls. The ketoacidosis is a medical emergency. The person should be taken to a hospital as soon as symptoms develop. Immediate treatment is to give insulin and replace fluids to help dehydration. Also called **diabetic coma.**

diabetic retinopathy, a disorder of the blood vessels in the retina of the eye, resulting in broken blood vessels in the eye. The disorder occurs most often in patients with long-term, poorly controlled diabetes. Repeated bleeding may result in partial or complete blindness. Treatment is to stop the bleeding of damaged blood vessels by laser beam (photocoagulation).

diabetic treatment, treatment of diabetes mellitus by means of insulin injections or drugs to lower levels of sugar in the blood.

diabetic xanthoma, the appearance of yellow bumps on the skin in uncontrolled diabetes mellitus. The skin disorder disappears when the disease is brought under control.

Diabinese, a trademark for a drug used to treat diabetes (chlorpropamide).

diacet, abbreviation for **carboxylate diacetate anion.**

diacetic acid. See **acetoacetic acid.**

diacondylar fracture /dī'əkon'dilər/, any break that runs across the top of a rounded bone projection (condyle).

diagnose, to determine the type and cause of a health condition. This is based on the patient's signs and symptoms, laboratory tests, and information about family and occupational background as recent injuries or exposure to dangerous substances.

diagnosis, pl. **diagnoses,** identification of a disease or condition. Physical signs, symptoms, history, laboratory tests, and procedures are used.

diagnostic, referring to a diagnosis.

diagnostic anesthesia, a procedure in which just enough anesthetic is given to permit mildly painful procedures to be performed. See also **awake anesthesia.**

diagnostician, a person skilled and trained in making diagnoses.

diagnostic position of gaze. See **cardinal position of gaze.**

diagnostic process, the act of determining a patient's health status and evaluating the factors that influence that health status.

diagnostic radiology, x-ray tests used to help make a diagnosis.

diagnostic radiopharmaceutical, a radioactive drug that allows images of body organs or structures to be obtained. In this way it is possible to tell if structures or functions are normal. The drug, given to the patient, emits radiation, which can be detected by a special machine. This process is used for diagnosis.

diagnostic related groups (DRG), groups of patients classified by their medical diagnosis. The classification is done to measure a hospital's delivery of care. DRGs are used by the federal government to determine Medicare payments for hospital care. They are based on diagnosis, procedures performed, age, and length of time in the hospital.

diagnostic services, acts related to the diagnosis made by a physician. These may be performed by nurses or other health professionals.

diagonal conjugate, the x-ray measurement of the distance between the lower part of the pubic bone and the most prominent part of the tailbone (sacrum). The measurement, which averages 12.5 to 13.0 cm, may also be taken by vaginal exam. See also **conjugate, true conjugate.**

dialect, a form of language different from other forms of the same language. Dialects differ from each other in pronunciation, grammar, and word meanings. Members of an ethnic group or people living in the same geographic area usually share a dialect.

Dialose, a trademark for a drug containing a stool softener (docusate potassium) and a laxative (casanthranol).

dialysate /dī·al′isãt/, a solution used in dialysis.

dialysis /dī·al′isis/, a procedure for removing certain elements from the blood, done by passing it through a dense membrane that filters out the unwanted elements by diffusion. Dialysis is used to remove poisons and drugs. It is also used in cases of kidney failure to remove the elements normally taken from the blood by the kidneys. See also **hemodialysis, peritoneal dialysis.**

dialysis dementia, a disorder that occurs in some patients undergoing dialysis; believed to be related to chemicals in the dialyzing fluid, drugs given to patients, or both.

dialysis disequilibrium syndrome, a disorder affecting cells that is sometimes caused by dialysis. The syndrome may be marked by brain or nervous-system disorders, irregular heart beat, and fluid in the lungs.

dialysis fluid, the solution that attracts the unwanted elements during dialysis, it flows on the other side of the membrane from the blood.

dialyzer /dī′əlī′zər/, **1.** a machine used in dialysis. **2.** a dense membrane in a dialysis machine. See also **hemodialysis, peritoneal dialysis.**

Diameter-Index Safety System (DISS), a system of connection between containers of medical gases and flow meters or regulators. To prevent accidental hookup of the wrong gas, each type of gas has connections of a specific size. Each type of gas and connector has a DISS number, as 1040 for nitrous oxide. See also **Pin-Index Safety System (PISS).**

Diamond-Blackfan syndrome, a rare inborn disorder evident in the first 3 months of life. This disorder is marked by severe anemia.

Diamox, a trademark for a drug (acetazolamide), used with other drugs in treating certain seizure disorders and to reduce eye pressure in glaucoma.

diapedesis /dī′əpidē′sis/, the passage of red or white blood cells through the walls of blood vessels. This occurs without damage to the vessels.

diaper rash, a skin irritation in the diaper area of infants, caused by contact with feces, urine, moisture, and heat. Treatment includes frequent diaper changes to keep the area dry, clean, cool, and exposed to air. Also called **diaper dermatitis.**

diaper restraint, a device used to provide traction of the legs when other methods do not work. Diaper restraints are often used to treat children with orthopedic disorders. They fit over the pelvic area like a diaper, with rings attached at the four corners. A strap is threaded through the rings and attached to the top of the bed.

diaphanoscopy /dī·af′ənos′kəpē/, examination of an inner structure with an instrument that makes body tissues visible. It is sometimes used in the diagnosis of breast tumors.

diaphonography /dī·af′ənog′rəfē/, a diagnostic technique using selected wavelengths of light and special equipment to examine the breast. The resulting pictures are still-frame images, like x-ray films. See also **diaphonoscopy.**

diaphoresis /dī′əfərē′sis/, profuse sweating that occurs with a fever, physical exertion, exposure to heat, or stress. Sweating is controlled by the nervous system and is mainly a way to control body temperature. However, the sweat glands on the palms and soles respond to emotional conditions. Also called **sweating.** See also **sudorific.**

diaphragm /dī′əfram/, **1.** a dome-shaped muscle that separates the chest cavity from the abdominal cavity. This muscle has holes through which pass the large artery (aorta), esophagus, and large vein (vena cava). The diaphragm aids breathing by moving up and down. When breathing in it moves down and increases the space in the chest. When breathing out it moves up, decreasing the volume. **2.** a contraceptive diaphragm. **3.** an opening that controls the amount of light passing through an optical device.

diaphragmatic hernia, the bulging of part of the stomach through an opening in the diaphragm. This occurs most often at the point where the throat passes through the diaphragm. In some cases the intestines may also bulge into the chest. A kind of diaphragmatic hernia is **hiatus hernia.** This is one of the most common disorders of the stomach and intestines. It occurs most often in middle-aged and elderly people. ★DIAGNOSIS: Symptoms usually include heartburn after meals, when lying down, and on exertion, especially when bending forward. There may be vomiting, difficulty swallowing, bloating of the stomach after eating, belching, rumbling in the intestines, rapid breathing, and a dull pain below the breastbone that extends to the shoulder. The continued backup of stomach fluids into the throat may lead to ulcers with bleeding. ★TREATMENT: The person with diaphragmatic hernia should eat bland food, in portions. The food should be chewed slowly and thoroughly, and one to two glasses of water should be drunk with a meal. Smoking should be avoided. The head should be raised with pillows when lying down or sleeping. Drugs may be ordered. If symptoms are severe and persist, the hernia may be repaired surgically.

diaphragmatic node, a lymph node located on the chest side of the diaphragm.

diaphragm pessary. See **pessary.**

diaphragm stethoscope, an instrument for listening to bodily sounds. It consists of a vibrating disk (diaphragm), which carries sounds through tubing to the ear. Also called **binaural stethoscope.** See also **stethoscope.**

diaphyseal aclasis /dī'əfiz'ē·əl ak'ləsis/, a rare and inborn defect that affects the skeletal system, marked by many bony protrusions (exostoses). The long bones are usually affected more severely and more often than the short bones. Various deformities may result. Diaphyseal aclasis is more common in boys than in girls. Although this disease is inborn, it is not usually evident until the child is 2 years of age or older. One form of the disorder, dyschondroplasia, causes dwarfism. Also called **hereditary deforming chondroplasia, multiple cartilaginous exostoses.**

diaphysis /dī·af'isis/, the shaft of a long bone. It consists of a tube of bone enclosing the bone marrow.

Diapid, a trademark for a pituitary hormone (lypressin), it is available as a nasal spray and used to treat excessive urination and other problems in diabetes insipidus.

diapositive. See **reversal film.**

diarrhea, the frequent passage of loose, watery stools, usually the result of increased activity of the large intestine (colon). The stool may also contain mucus, pus, blood, or large amounts of fat. Diarrhea is usually a symptom of some other disorder. It is a common symptom in some types of flu, food poisoning, and may occur after eating spicy foods. It is also a symptom of more severe diseases. These include various disorders, as tumors of the intestines, malabsorption syndrome, or milk intolerance. In addition, patients may complain of stomach

cramps and weakness. Untreated, diarrhea may lead to dehydration. Diarrhea may be accompanied by vomiting and various other symptoms. See also **dehydration. –diarrheal, diarrheic,** *adj.*

Diasone Sodium Enterab, a drug used to treat leprosy (sulfoxone sodium).

diastasis /dī·as'təsis/, the separation of two body parts that normally are joined together, as the separation of parts of a bone.

diastasis recti abdominis, the abnormal separation of the two rectus muscles along the center of the abdomen. In a newborn infant, the condition is the result of incomplete development. In an adult woman, it is often caused by many pregnancies or a multiple birth, as with triplets.

diastole /dī·as'təlē/, **1.** the period of time between contractions of the heart. During this state, blood enters the relaxed chambers of the heart to be pumped throughout the body. Compare **systole.** See also **diastolic blood pressure. –diastolic** /dī'əstol'ik/, *adj.*

diastolic /dī'əstol'ik/, referring to the blood pressure at the moment when the heart is most relaxed (diastole).

diastolic blood pressure, the lowest level of blood pressure measured between contractions of the heart. Diastolic pressures for a person will vary with age, sex, weight, and emotional state. Other factors that may have an affect are the time of day and whether the person has just finished a meal. In general, normal diastolic pressure for a young, healthy, resting adult is 70 to 80. This is expressed as the second number of the total blood pressure.

diastrophic /dī'əstrof'ik/, referring to a bent or curved condition of the bones or to distortion of other structures.

diastrophic dwarf /dī'əstrof'ik/, a person in whom short height is caused by any disorder of bone and cartilage. Linked to various deformities of the bones and joints, the condition may be inherited.

diathermy /dī'əthur'mē/, the production of heat in body tissues to treat certain disorders. This heat results from high-frequency electric currents. The currents are not intense enough to destroy tissues or to damage function. Diathermy is used to treat arthritis, bursitis, fractures, gynecological diseases, and swelling of the sinuses (sinusitis).

diathesis /dī·athē'sis/, *pl.* **diatheses,** an inherited condition of the body that makes it more susceptible to certain diseases or disorders than is normal. This condition seems to affect males more than females. For example, a varicose diathesis is a tendency to develop varicose veins.

diazepam, a sedative and tranquilizer used to treat anxiety, nervous tension, muscle spasm, and convulsions.

diazoxide /dī'əzok'sīd/, a drug used to reduce very high blood pressure in emergencies, it may also be used in some cases to treat low blood sugar.

Dibenzyline, a trademark for a drug used to improve circulation of the arms and legs in certain conditions (phenoxybenzamine hydrochloride).

dicalcium phosphate and calcium gluconate with vitamin D, a source of calcium and phosphorus used to treat low levels of calcium, especially in pregnancy and nursing.
★CAUTION: Poor thyroid function or known allergy to any of the ingredients of this drug prohibits its use.
★ADVERSE EFFECTS: There are no known side effects.

dicephaly /dīsef'əlē/, a birth defect in which the fetus has two heads.

dichlorodiphenyltrichloroethane. See **DDT.**

dichroic stain /dīkrō'ik/, an effect on an x-ray film caused by a colored chemical stain. The color on the film may range from yellow to purple, usually resulting from mistakes in film processing. See also **curtain effect.**

Dick-Read method. See **Read method.**

Dick test, a skin test for determining the lack of ability to resist scarlet fever. A small dose of the scarlet fever bacteria is injected under the skin. A small area of swelling and redness indicates that the person is not immune. Larger doses may then be given to create immunity.

dicloxacillin sodium /dī'kloksəsil'in/, a drug used to treat staph infections.

Dicor, a trademark for a ceramic dental material.

dicrotic notch, the time interval between the two peaks of a dicrotic pulse.

dicrotic pulse, a pulse with two separate peaks. The second is usually weaker than the first. Compare **bisferious pulse.**

dicumarol, a drug that prevents blood from clotting, used to prevent and treat blood clots.

dicyclomine hydrochloride, a drug used to treat ulcers.

Didrex, a trademark for a drug that decreases the appetite (benzphetamine hydrochloride).

Didronel, a trademark for a drug that regulates calcium in the body (etidronate disodium).

didym-, a combining form referring to a testicle.

didymitis /did'əmī'tis/, an inflammation in a testicle.

didymus /did'iməs/, a testis (male sex organ).

dieldrin /dī·el'drin/, a strong pesticide that is poisonous to humans and animals if eaten, inhaled, or absorbed through the skin. It causes dysfunction of the central nervous system and may cause cancer.

diencephalon /dī'encef'əlon/, the middle part of the brain

dienestrol /dī'ines'trôl/, an estrogen used to treat a lack of estrogen and wasting away of the vulva.
★CAUTION: Pregnancy, cancer of the breast, swelling of a vein, vaginal bleeding, or known allergy to this drug prohibits its use.
★ADVERSE EFFECTS: Among the more serious side effects are risk of cancer, swelling of a vein, tumor of the liver, blood clots, and gallbladder disease.

diet, 1. food and drink judged by nutritional value, composition, and effects on health. 2. food and drink restricted in type and amount for treatment or other purposes. 3. the usual amount of food and drink consumed. Compare **nutrition.** See also specific diets. **–dietetic,** *adj.*

dietary fiber, a term for substances found in plants the body does not digest. Fiber promotes healthy intestinal action and prevents constipation. It may also help protect against cancer of the large intestine (colon). Major sources of dietary fiber are vegetables, fruits, and whole grains. Also called **bulk, roughage.**

dietetic food, 1. a specially made low-calorie food, often containing artificial sweeteners. 2. a food prepared for any special need or restriction, of the diet, as food without salt or meals with no meat. See also **dietetics.**

dietetic food diarrhea. See **osmotic diarrhea.**

dietetics /dī'itet'iks/, the study of foods and their nutrients and how they relate to both health and disease.

diethyl ether. See **ether.**

diethylpropion hydrochloride, a drug that curbs the appetite, used to treat obesity.

diethylstilbestrol (DES), a hormone, made to be similar to estrogen. Also called **stilbestrol.**

diethylstilbestrol diphosphate, an anticancer drug used to treat cancer of the prostate, which cannot be treated by surgery.
★CAUTION: Inflammation of a vein, blood clot disorders, liver disorders, or stroke prohibits its use.
★ADVERSE EFFECTS: The most serious side effects are swelling of a vein, blood clots in the lungs or brain, jaundice, mental depression, severe skin rashes, changes in sexual interest, and dizziness.

dietitian, a person who has completed a special training in nutritional care of groups and persons.

Dietl's crisis /dē'təlz/, a sudden, very severe pain in the kidney, caused by rapidly drinking very large amounts of liquid, or by blockage in the tube that carries urine from the kidneys to the bladder. See also **hydronephrosis.**

differential absorption, (in radiology) the difference between x-rays that are absorbed by body tissue and those that are not. Differential absorption results in the image on the x-ray film.

For example, an image of an arm shows the bone clearly because bone tissue absorbs more x-rays than the surrounding tissue.

differential diagnosis, the process of telling the difference between two or more similar diseases. This is done by comparing their signs and symptoms. See also **diagnosis.**

differential growth, a comparison of the different growth rates of organisms, tissues, or structures.

differential white blood cell count, the number of different types of white blood cells (leukocytes) in a small blood sample. The different kinds of white cells are reported as percentages of the total examined. Compare **complete blood count.**

leukocyte, red cell indexes.

differentiation, 1. a process in development in which simple cells or tissues change to take on specific physical forms, functions, and chemical properties. **2.** taking on functions and forms different from those of the original. **3.** the distinguishing of one thing or disease from another, as in differential diagnosis.

diffuse, widely spread, as through a fluid.

diffuse goiter, an enlargement of all parts of the thyroid gland.

diffuse hypersensitivity pneumonia, swelling in the lungs caused by exposure to a foreign substance (allergen). The allergen may be from a fungus, bird droppings, animal fur, or wood dust. It may also result from a side reaction to a drug. The disorder is marked by cough, fever, difficulty in breathing, fatigue, and fluid in the lungs. Also called **allergic alveolitis, extrinsic allergic pneumonia.**

diffuse idiopathic skeletal hyperostosis, a joint disease in which the ligaments along the spinal column become hard and lose their ability to bend.

diffuse myocardial fibrosis, a type of heart disease in which fibrous tissue replaces normal heart muscle cells.

diffusing capacity, the ability of gas to pass through a permeable membrane, as the ability of oxygen to enter blood cells. Measured in terms of unit area and the pressure difference on the two sides of the membrane, diffusing capacity is affected by chemical reactions that may occur in the blood. Also called **diffusion factor, transfer factor of lungs.**

diffusing capacity of the lungs (D_L), the amount of gas that diffuses from the lung to the bloodstream each minute; measured in terms of the pressure difference on either side of the cell membrane. The average D_L value for oxygen is 20 ml/min/mm Hg (mercury).

diffusion, the process in which solid particles in a fluid move from an area with more particles to an area of fewer particles. This results in an even distribution of the particles in the fluid.

diffusion defect, an impairment of the diffusion of gases between the lungs and the bloodstream. It results in less oxygen entering the bloodstream. Causes include fibrosis, granuloma, edema, and growth of connective tissue.

diffusion deposition, the landing of a particle on a membrane or other part of the airway. It causes the particle to settle out of a vapor or gas.

diflorasone diacetate, a drug placed on the skin to reduce swelling.

★CAUTION: Virus and fungus diseases of the skin, poor circulation, or known allergy to this drug or to other steroids prohibits its use.

★ADVERSE EFFECTS: Among the more serious side effects are streaks, loss of color, or irritation of the skin.

diflunisal, a drug that relieves mild pain and swelling in the skeletal muscles.

★CAUTION: Allergy to aspirin and similar drugs that fight swelling or known allergy to this drug prohibits its use.

★ADVERSE EFFECTS: The most serious side effects are intestinal pain, diarrhea, ulcer, loss of appetite, and water retention.

digastricus /dīgas′trikəs/, one of the lower jaw muscles. It acts to open the jaw and to move the bone under the tongue (hyoid). Also called **digastric muscle.**

DiGeorge's syndrome /dijôrj′əz/, an inherited disorder marked by severe losses in the immune system and structural defects. The defects include notched low-set ears, small mouth, downward slanting eyes set far apart, and heart defects. There may also be a lack of the thymus and parathyroid glands. Death, often from infection, usually occurs before 2 years of age. Also called **thymic parathyroid aplasia.**

digest, 1. to soften by heat and moisture. **2.** to convert food into a form that can be absorbed by the body. This is done by chewing the food, adding water, and the action of stomach and intestinal fluids.

digestant, a substance, as pepsin, that is added to the diet to help a patient digest food.

digestion, the changing of food into substances able to be absorbed by the body. This takes place in the stomach and intestines. See also **digest. –digestive,** *adj.*

digestive fever, a slight rise in body temperature that normally occurs during digestion.

digestive gland, any one of the many structures that releases substances that break down food so that it can be absorbed by the body. Some kinds of digestive glands are the salivary glands, gastric glands, intestinal glands, liver, and pancreas.

digestive system, the organs, structures, and glands of the digestive tube of the body through which food passes. The digestive system includes the mouth, throat, stomach, and small and large intestines. See also the **Color Atlas of Human Anatomy.**

digestive tract, a muscular tube, about 30 feet (9 meters) long, which extends from the mouth to the anus. It includes the mouth, throat, stomach, small intestine, and large intestine. The tube, which is part of the digestive system of the body, includes several organs that release substances for digesting food. Also called **alimentary canal, digestive tube.** See also **digestive system.**

digital, referring to a digit, that is, a finger or toe.

digital angiography, a technique using computerized equipment to produce enhanced x-ray pictures of the heart. A material visible on x-rays is injected into a vein, and an image is made and stored in computer memory. Later images are made to show changes from the first image. The images are enlarged and displayed on a TV screen, recorded on videotape, and can be stored on a computer disk.

digital fluoroscopy, a technique for enhancing fluoroscopic images with a television system and high-speed processor.

digitalis, a drug that stimulates the heart, it is used to treat heart failure and certain forms of irregular heart beats.

digitalis glycoside. See **glycoside.**

digitalis therapy, giving the drug digitalis to a person with a heart disorder. Digitalis increases the force of heart contractions and produces a slower and more regular heart rate. Digitalis is given with extreme care, in the exact dosage, and at the exact times prescribed. The pulse is checked for a full minute before the drug is taken. Digitalis therapy can also reduce blood pressure, improve circulation, reduce water retention, and stop extremely rapid heart beat.

digitalization, giving the drug digitalis in doses large enough to produce the best effects without also producing poisoning symptoms.

digitalized, referring to a patient who has a therapeutic dose of a cardiac glycoside, as digitalis.

digitalizing dose, the amount of a cardiac glycoside, as digitalis, needed to digitalize a patient.

digital radiography (DR), a method of taking x-ray pictures that uses a computer to enhance and store the images. See also **digital angiography, digital fluoroscopy, digital tomosynthesis.**

digital tomosynthesis, a system of tomography (x-ray scanning) using a computer and digital fluoroscopy unit. The technique can view any plane of the body with only one scan. This reduces the amount of radiation the patient receives, as well as the time needed to perform the exam. See also **digital fluoroscopy.**

digitate /dij′itãt/, having fingers or fingerlike projections. See also **digital.**

digitate wart, a fingerlike, horny bump that grows from a pea-shaped base on the scalp or near the hairline.

digitoxin, a drug that stimulates the heart, it is used to treat heart failure and certain forms of irregular heart beats.

digoxin /dijok′sin/, a drug that stimulates the heart; used to treat heart failure and certain forms of irregular heart beats.

diGuglielmo's disease, diGuglielmo's syndrome. See **erythroleukemia.**

dihydroergotamine mesylate, a drug used to treat migraine headaches and certain other forms of headache.

★CAUTION: Heart disease, high blood pressure, liver or kidney disorders, blood poisoning, pregnancy, or known allergy to this drug prohibits its use.

★ADVERSE EFFECTS: Among the more serious side effects are gangrene, nausea, vomiting, diarrhea, headache, weakness, visual disturbances, and irregular heart beats.

dihydrotachysterol /dīhī′drōtəkis′tərol/, a form of vitamin D, it is used to treat calcium deficiency resulting from an underactive parathyroid gland.

★CAUTION: Low calcium levels linked to kidney malfunction, kidney insufficiency, or known allergy to this drug or to vitamin D prohibits its use. Caution is advised for nursing mothers.

★ADVERSE EFFECTS: The most serious side effect is an excess increase of calcium. An overdose may cause hardening of soft tissues, including those of the heart. Kidney or heart failure may also result.

dil-, -dil, a combining form for the names of a drug that causes widening of blood vessels.

Dilantin, a trademark for a drug used to prevent convulsions (phenytoin).

dilatation /dil′ətā′shən/, normal increase in the size of a body opening, blood vessel, or tube. An example is the widening of the pupil of the eye in dim light. See also **effacement, station.** **–dilatate, dilate** /dī′lãt/, v.

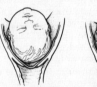

Partial dilatation   Complete dilatation (10 cm)

Cervical dilatation

dilatation and curettage (D & C), widening of the opening to the uterus (cervix) and scraping the lining (endometrium) of the uterus. A D & C is done to diagnose diseases of the uterus, to correct heavy vaginal bleeding, or to empty the uterus of substances from conception (as after a miscarriage or in an abortion). See also **abortion.**

dilatator naris, the portion of the muscle covering the nose (nasalis) that widens the nostril.

dilatator pupillae, a muscle that contracts the iris of the eye and widens the pupil.

dilator, a device used to widen a body opening or cavity. For example, a tent dilator is a sponge or bundle of seaweed used to dilate the opening to the uterus (cervix), and Barnes' dilator is a water-filled rubber bag that puts pressure on cavity walls.

Dilaudid Hydrochloride, a trademark for a drug that relieves pain (hydromorphone hydrochloride).

Dilor, a trademark for a drug that widens the openings of the air passages to the lungs (dyphylline).

diltiazem, a drug used to treat pain in the chest caused by physical exertion.
★CAUTION: Irregular heart beats, heart block, or low blood pressure prohibits its use.
★ADVERSE EFFECTS: Among the more serious side effects are water retention, irregular heart beats, very slow heart beats, low blood pressure, fainting, rash, headache, and dizziness.

diluent /dil'oo-ənt, dil'yoo-ənt/, a substance, usually a fluid, that makes a solution of mixture thinner, easier to pour or more watery.

dilute, referring to a solution in which there is a relatively small amount of substance dissolved (solute).

diluting agent, (in respiratory therapy) a substance that can thin mucus in the breathing tubes so it can be removed easily. Water and saline solution are both used as diluting agents.

dilution, making a less concentrated solution from a solution of greater concentration.

dimenhydrinate /dim'ənhī'drināt/, a drug used to treat nausea and motion sickness.
★CAUTION: Asthma or known allergy to this drug prohibits its use. It is not given to newborn infants or nursing mothers.
★ADVERSE EFFECTS: Among the more serious side effects are skin rash, allergic reactions, and very rapid heart beats. Drowsiness and dry mouth are common.

dimensional stability, (in radiology) the stiffness of the base used for x-ray films, and the film's resistance to warping or changing size or shape during processing.

dimercaprol /dī'mərkap'rol/, a drug used to treat Wilson's disease and severe arsenic, mercury, or gold poisoning. Previously called **British antilewisite (BAL).**
★CAUTION: Liver or kidney disorders, poisoning with certain metals, or known allergy to this drug prohibits its use.
★ADVERSE EFFECTS: Among the most serious

side effects are kidney damage, high levels of acid in the blood, convulsions, and abnormal heart functions. Mild reactions include pain at the injection site, nausea, excess salivation, and skin tingling.

Dimetane, a trademark for an antihistamine drug (brompheniramine maleate).

dimethindene maleate /dīmeth'indēn/, a drug used to treat a number of allergic reactions, including swelling of the nose, skin reactions, and itching.
★CAUTION: The drug is not given to newborn infants or to nursing mothers. Asthma or known allergy to this drug prohibits its use.
★ADVERSE EFFECTS: Drowsiness, skin rash, allergic reactions, dry mouth, and rapid heart beats commonly occur.

dimethoxymethylamphetamine (DOM), a psychedelic drug.

dimethyl carbinol. See **isopropyl alcohol.**

dimethyl sulfoxide (DMSO), a drug that reduces swelling, especially for the bladder. It also has been used on the skin to relieve sports injuries.
★CAUTION: Known allergy to this drug prohibits its use.
★ADVERSE EFFECTS: Among the most serious side effects are intestinal disturbances, intolerance of the eyes to sunlight, disturbance of color vision, and headache. A garliclike body odor and taste in the mouth may occur. When applied to the skin, it can cause skin irritations.

dinitrochlorobenzene (DNCB), a substance applied to the skin to test for a delayed allergic reaction; also used to treat skin cancers.

dioctyl calcium sulfosuccinate, dioctyl sodium sulfosuccinate. See **docusate.**

diode /dī'ōd/, (in radiology) an x-ray tube with two electrodes.

Dionysian, the attitude of one who is sensual, emotional, irrational, and not inhibited or influenced by normal social standards.

diopter /dī·op'tər/, a measure of the strength of a lens. It is equal to the reciprocal of the focal length of the lens, expressed in meters. For example, a lens with a focal length of 0.5 m has a diopter measure of 2.0 (1/0.5). When prescribed as a corrective lens for the eye, such a lens should make printed matter most clearly focused when held 0.5 m from the eye.

dioptric power, the strength of a lens, as measured in diopters.

diovular. See **binovular.**

diovulatory, routinely releasing two eggs (ova) during each ovarian cycle. Compare **monovulatory.**

dioxin /dī·ok'sin/, an ingredient in a certain herbicide used widely throughout the world to help control plant growth. Because of its high level of poison, it is no longer made in the United States. Exposure to dioxin is linked to a type of acne (chloracne) and porphyria cutanea tarda. Dioxin was an ingredient of Agent

Orange, sprayed by the U. S. military aircraft over areas of southeast Asia from 1965 to 1970 to kill concealing trees and shrubs. No safe exposure levels have been found. It has been strongly linked to many cancers and is very harmful to all living things. Also called **TCDD (2,3,7,8-tetrachlorodibenzopara-dioxin).**

DIP, abbreviation for **desquamative interstitial pneumonia.**

diphenhydramine hydrochloride, a drug used to treat motion sickness and a number of allergic reactions, including swelling of the nose, skin rash, and itching.

diphenidol, a drug used to treat vertigo and to control nausea and vomiting.
★CAUTION: Absence of urination or known allergy to this drug prohibits its use.
★ADVERSE EFFECTS: Among the most serious side effects are low blood pressure, hallucinations, and mental confusion.

diphenoxylate hydrochloride, a drug used to treat diarrhea and cramps of the intestines.
★CAUTION: Liver disease, diarrhea from antibiotics, or known allergy to this drug prohibits its use. It is not given to children under 2 years of age.
★ADVERSE EFFECTS: Among the more common side effects are stomach pain, intestinal blockage, skin rash, and nausea.

diphenylhydantoin. See **phenytoin.**

diphenylpyraline hydrochloride /dī'fenəlpī'rəlen/, a drug used to treat a number of allergic reactions, including swelling of the nose, skin rash, and itching.
★CAUTION: Asthma or known allergy to this drug prohibits its use. It is not given to newborn infants or nursing mothers.
★ADVERSE EFFECTS: Among the more serious side effects are skin rash, allergic reactions, and very rapid heart beats. Drowsiness and dry mouth are common.

2,3-diphosphoglyceric acid (DPG), a substance in red blood cells, it is a product of breakdown of sugar that regulates the flow of oxygen to the tissues.

diphtheria /difthir'ē·ə, dipthir'ē·ə/, a serious, contagious disease, it produces a poison throughout the body and a false membrane lining of the throat. The poison is very harmful to the tissues of the heart and central nervous system. The thick membrane lining the throat may interfere with eating, drinking, and breathing. The membrane may also occur in other body tissues. Lymph glands in the neck swell. If not treated, the disease is often fatal, causing heart and kidney failure. Patients are usually put in the hospital in isolated rooms. Immunization against diphtheria is available to all children in the United States. It is usually given early in infancy. See also **Schick test.**

diphtheria and tetanus toxoids (DT), a drug used for immunizing persons against diphtheria and tetanus.

diphtheria, tetanus toxoids, and pertussis vaccine (DTP), a drug used for immunizing children under 6 years of age against the diseases diphtheria, tetanus, and pertussis.

diphtheroid /dif'thəroid'/, referring to diphtheria.

diphyllobothriasis. See **fish tapeworm infection.**

Diphyllobothrium /dəfil'ōboth'rē·əm/, a type of large, parasitic, intestinal flatworms. The species that most often infects humans is *Diphyllobothrium latum,* a giant tapeworm found in freshwater fish of North America and Europe. See also **tapeworm infection.**

-dipine, a combining form for the name of a phenylpyridine vasodilator (drug that dilates blood vessels).

diplegia /dīplē'jə/, paralysis affecting the same parts on both sides of the body. One kind of diplegia is **facial diplegia,** which affects both sides of the face. Compare **hemiplegia. –diplegic,** adj.

diplo-, a combining form meaning double.

diploë /dip'lō·ē/, the spongy tissue between the skull bones.

diploid /dip'loid/, referring to anything that has two complete sets of chromosomes. In humans the normal diploid number is 46 (23 pairs). Compare **haploid. –diploidic,** adj.

diploma program in nursing, an educational program that trains nurses in a hospital, usually in 2 or 3 years.

diplopagus /diplop'əgəs/, joined twins that are more or less equally developed. One or several inner organs may be shared.

diplopia /diplō'pē·ə/, double vision, which may be caused by defective eye muscles or it may result from a disorder of the nerves that signal the muscles. A temporary diplopia is usually not serious and is common after a mild brain concussion. Also called **ambiopia, double vision.** Compare **binocular vision.**

diplornavirus, a double-stranded RNA virus that causes Colorado tick fever; related to the viruses that cause some colds.

diplosomatia /dip'lōsōmā'shə/, a birth defect in which fully formed twins are joined at one or more areas of their bodies. Also called **diplosomia.**

dipodia /dīpō'dē·ə/, a birth defect in which one or both feet are duplicated.

dipole /dī'pol/, a molecule with areas of opposite electric charges. For example, hydrogen chloride (salt), has areas of negative charge around the chloride part and positive charge around the hydrogen part.

diprop, abbreviation for **carboxylate diproprionate anion.**

diprosopus /dīpros'əpəs, dī'prəsō'pəs/, a malformed fetus with a normal body but with a double face showing varying degrees of development.

dipsomania, an uncontrollable craving for alcoholic beverages.

dipstick, a strip of paper treated with chemicals and dipped in urine or other fluids. It is used to analyze the contents of the fluid.

dipus /dī′pəs/, joined twins that have only two feet.

dipyridamole, a drug that increases blood flow to the heart, it is used for the long-term treatment of chest pain.

★CAUTION: The drug should be used with caution in patients with low blood pressure and those taking drugs that decrease blood clotting.

★ADVERSE EFFECTS: The side effects are mild and temporary. They include headache, dizziness, rash, nausea, and flushing.

direct-access memory, direct access to computer memory, as opposed to access through previously obtained data. The computer transfers information directly between its memory and peripheral devices, as printers. See also **random-access memory (RAM).**

direct antagonist, one of a pair of muscles that pull in opposite directions. Their combined action keeps the part from moving.

direct calorimetry, the measurement of the amount of heat made by the body's processes. This is a method of measuring energy released by the cells. Compare **indirect calorimetry.**

direct causal association, a cause-and-effect relationship between a disease and the cause of the disease.

direct contact, mutual touching of two persons or organisms. Many communicable diseases may be spread by the direct contact between an infected and a healthy person.

direct-exposure film, a type of x-ray film used to take pictures of thin body parts, such as the hands and feet, where structures are easily visible. The film is exposed directly rather than indirectly.

direct fracture, any bone break that occurs exactly at a point of injury.

direct gold, any form of pure gold that is placed directly into a prepared tooth cavity to form a filling.

directive therapy, an approach in psychoanalysis in which the therapist asks questions and offers interpretations. Compare **nondirective therapy.** See also **psychoanalysis.**

direct care nursing functions, nursing activities that are focused on a patient, patient's family, or group for whom the nurse is directly responsible.

direct-question interview, an interview in which the questions require only simple one- or two-word answers.

direct retainer, a clasp that fastens to a tooth to keep removable false teeth in place.

direct self-destructive behavior (DSDB), any type of suicidal behavior, it includes threats, attempts, or gestures, or the act of suicide itself. The intent of the action is death, and the person is aware of this.

dirofiliariasis /dī′rōfil′ərī′əsis/, an infection of a human by the dog heartworm, *Dirofilaria immitis.* The infection is transmitted by the bite of a mosquito. The organisms travel through the bloodstream to the lung, causing chest pain, coughing, and spitting of blood. The disease is rare among humans.

dis-, a combining form meaning 'reversal or separation.'

disability, the loss or damage of physical or mental fitness. Compare **handicap.**

disaccharidase deficiency. See **lactase deficiency.**

disaccharide, a sugar made up of two simple sugars, as lactose and sucrose.

disadvantaged, any person or group of people who lacks money, education, literacy, or other advantages.

disaster preparedness plan, a formal plan of action for the hospital staff in case of a disaster in the hospital or the surrounding community.

disc. See **disk.**

discharge, 1. also **evacuate, excrete, secrete.** to release a substance or object. **2.** to release a patient from a hospital. **3.** to release an electric charge. **4.** to release a burst of energy from or through a nerve. **5.** a release of emotions.

discharge summary, a report prepared by a physician at the end of a patient's hospital stay or series of treatments. The summary outlines the patient's problem and the diagnosis. It then lists the treatment given, the patient's response to it, and ends with suggestions for the patient after discharge.

disciform keratitis, an inflammatory condition of the eye, often following an attack of sores or ulcers of the cornea (dendritic keratitis). It is thought to be a response of the immune system to the herpes simplex virus that causes the ulcers. The condition is marked by a round film in the cornea, usually with swelling of the iris. The condition can lead to blindness if untreated. See also **herpes virus simplex.**

disclosing solution, a dye used to stain the teeth so that plaque and other deposits are visible. The dye is helpful in cleaning the teeth.

disco-, a combining form pertaining to a disk, disk-shaped.

discoid lupus erythematosus (DLE), a long-term disease that mainly affects the skin, marked by a red rash covered with scales and extending into the hair follicles. The rash is most often spread in a butterfly pattern covering the cheeks and bridge of the nose, but it may also occur on other parts of the body. On healing, the rash leaves scars that are either dark colored or very pale. If hairy areas are involved, hair loss may result. Sunlight triggers the skin rash and is often the first sign a person has DLE. Eye involvement is common. The cause of the disease is not certain. Some cases seem to be caused by certain drugs. DLE is at least five times more common in women than in men and occurs most often between 20 and 40 years of age. Treatment of the rash is steroid ointments or creams. When the rash is severe, drugs for malaria and oral steroids are given. The skin should be protected with a sunscreen at all times. Also called **cutaneous lupus erythematosus.** See also **systemic lupus erythematosus.**

discoid meniscus, an abnormal condition in which the cartilage (meniscus) of the knee is shaped like a disk rather than the normal half-moon. The outside of the cartilage is most often affected, although the inner part may also be involved. The condition occurs more often in children between 6 and 8 years of age. Common complaints are that a "clicking" occurs in the knee joint or that the knee joint gives way.

disconfirmation, an abnormal form of communication that negates, discounts or ignores information received from another person.

discordance, the appearance of one or more specific traits in only one member of a pair of twins.

discrete x-rays. See **x-ray.**

discus articularis, a small oval plate between the lower jaw bone (mandible) and the shallow depression in the jaw (mandibular fossa). Disalignment or injury to the plate can lead to pain in the lower jaw area, known as temporomandibular joint (TMJ) pain.

disease, 1. a condition of abnormal function involving any structure, part, or system of an organism. 2. a specific illness or disorder marked by a specific set of signs and symptoms, it may be due to heredity, infection, diet, or environment. Compare **condition, diathesis.**

disease prevention, procedures to protect people from health threats and their harmful results.

disengagement, 1. moving the part of the baby lowest in the pelvis in order to aid childbirth. See also **Kielland rotation, version and extraction.** 2. the detachment of oneself from other persons or responsibilities.

disengagement theory, the concept that person's tend to withdraw from society as they grow older.

dishpan fracture, a break that causes a hollow or depression in the skull. Also called **derby hat fracture.**

disinfectant, a chemical that can destroy bacteria.

disinfection, the process of killing disease-causing organisms or making them ineffective.

disintegrative psychosis, a mental disorder in children that usually occurs at 3 years of age and older, following normal development of speech, social behavior and other traits. After a vague illness, the child suddenly becomes irritable and suffers a loss of mental functions, eventually becoming severely retarded. The condition may be caused by a virus. There is no specific treatment.

disjunction, the separation of the paired chromosomes during cell division. Compare **nondisjunction.**

disk, 1. also spelled **disc.** A flat, round, platelike structure, as a joint (articular) disk or an optic disc. 2. a term for the cartilage between the backbones. Also called **discus.**

diskography, X-rays of the individual disks between the vertebrae of the spinal column. During this procedure, two needles are used to inject a small amount of iodine solution into the center of the disk while the patient is under a local anesthetic.

dislocation, the displacement of any part of the body from its normal position. This applies most often to a bone moved from its normal position with a joint. See also **subluxation.** –**dislocate,** v.

disodium edetate. See **edetate disodium.**

disopyramide phosphate /dī'sōpir'əmīd/, a drug used to treat irregular or very rapid heart beats.

disorganized schizophrenia, a form of schizophrenia that begins at a young age, usually at puberty. It is marked by a more severe decay of the personality than occurs in other forms of the disease. Symptoms include inappropriate laughter and silliness, odd mannerisms, talking and gesturing to oneself; bizarre and often obscene behavior and extreme social withdrawal. There are often fantastic hallucinations and delusions, which are most often of a sexual, religious, or paranoid nature. Also called **hebephrenia, hebephrenic schizophrenia.** See also **schizophrenia.**

disorientation, a state of mental confusion as to place, time, or personal identity.

disparate twins, twins who are different from each other in weight and other features.

dispersing agent, a chemical used to distribute the ingredients throughout the product, as in lotions with both oil and water.

dispersion, the breakup of finely divided material, as when particles of a substance are scattered throughout a fluid. Examples include gluelike substances, as proteins or starches (colloids), and gels, as egg white, soap, and gelatin, which consist of large molecules or clumps of molecules. These molecules are able to join with and hold large numbers of water molecules.

displaced fracture, a bone break in which two ends of the bone are separated from each other. The ends of broken bones often pierce through the skin.

displacement, 1. the state of being moved from the normal position. 2. an unconscious defense mechanism to avoid emotional conflict. Emotions or ideas are transferred from one object or person to another that is less threatening. Compare **sublimation.**

DISS, abbreviation for the **Diameter-Index Safety System.**

dissect, to cut apart tissues for study. Compare **bisect.** —**dissection,** *n.*

dissecting aneurysm, a widening of a part of an artery, most often the large artery of the heart (aorta). There is also a tear in one of the layers of the artery wall. Aortic dissecting aneurysms occur most often in men between 40 and 60 years of age, and 90% of these cases have high blood pressure. Symptoms include severe pain that may mimic a heart attack, lack of pulse in the neck or arm, and sometimes heart failure. Treatment is to remove the damaged part of the artery. See also **aortic aneurysm.**

disseminated intravascular coagulation (DIC), a severe disorder that results from too much of the body's clotting substance being made in response to disease or injury. DIC can be caused by blood poisoning (septicemia), severe low blood pressure, poisonous snake bites, cancer, childbirth emergencies, severe injury, or extensive surgery and bleeding. The disease or injury triggers clotting in the vessels. This then causes the body to make too much anticlotting substance. As a result, the clotting is followed by a lack of clotting factors, resulting in a failure of the blood to clot and bleeding. ★DIAGNOSIS: Widespread purple spots on the chest and stomach are a common first sign of DIC often followed by blood blisters, blue tinged hands and feet, and gangrene in the skin. There may be bleeding from cuts in the skin, blood in the feces and urine, fluid and clots in the lungs, low blood pressure, rapid heart beat, pulses, restlessness, convulsions, or coma. Blood is usually given to replace the clotting factors.

disseminated lupus erythematosus. See **systemic lupus erythematosus.**

disseminated multiple sclerosis. See **multiple sclerosis.**

dissemination, a phase of cancer in which cells spread (metastasize) to other parts of the body.

dissimilar twins. See **dizygotic twins.**

dissociation, **1.** the act of separating into parts or sections. **2.** an unconscious defense mechanism by which an idea or emotion is separated from the consciousness. In this way it loses emotional significance. See also **dissociative disorder, dissociative reaction.**

dissociative anesthesia, an anesthetic procedure in which a pain killer (analgesic) and a drug that produces amnesia are used. There is no loss of breathing function or throat reflexes. This form of anesthesia is used for short and simple surgery or diagnostic processes.

dissociative disorder, a type of hysterical neurosis. Emotional conflicts are denied to the point that a split in the personality occurs. This causes a confusion in identity. Symptoms include amnesia, sleep walking, flight from reality, dream state, or multiple personality. The disorder is caused by failure to cope with severe stress or conflict. It most often occurs suddenly, after a traumatic situation. Compare **conversion disorder.** See also **dissociation.**

dissolved gas, gas in a simple solution that has not reacted chemically with another solvent or combined with that solvent.

distal /dis'təl/, **1.** away from or being the farthest from a point of origin. **2.** away from or being the farthest from a central point of the body. For example, the distal phalanx is the bone at the tip of the finger. Compare **proximal.**

distal latency, (in electroneuromyography) the time between the stimulation of a muscle group (compound muscle) and the observed response. Normally, the time needed for the nerve impulse to travel is about 40 m/second in the legs and above 50 m/second in the arms. However, age, muscle disease, temperature and other factors can affect the time of the response.

distal muscular dystrophy, a rare form of muscular dystrophy that most often affects adults. It causes weakness and muscle wasting that begins in the arms and legs and then moves to the trunk and face. Also called **Gowers' muscular dystrophy.**

distal phalanx, any one of the small bones in the tips of the fingers and toes. Also called **ungual phalanx.**

distal radioulnar articulation, the pivotlike joint connecting the two bones of the lower arm (ulna and radius) at the wrist. The joint allows the wrist to rotate the lower arm. Also called **inferior radioulnar joint.** Compare **proximal radioulnar articulation.**

distal renal tubular acidosis (distal RTA), an abnormal condition marked by a severe acid buildup in the urine. This condition may result in excess calcium in the urine and kidney stones. Compare **proximal renal tubular acidosis.**

distal sparing, a condition in which the spinal cord remains intact below an injury or wound (lesion). The nerve pathway that reacts to stimulation (reflex arc) remains, but it is not controlled by the normal actions from the brain. This may result in jerky movements below the injury.

distance regulation, behavior that is related to the control of personal space. Most humans need a certain space between themselves and others. This space offers security but does not create a sense of isolation. The amount of social distance varies with different persons and in different cultures.

distance vision, the ability to see objects clearly from a distance, usually from more than 20 feet or 6 meters away.

distension, the state of being expanded or swollen.

distortion, **1.** (in psychology) the process of shifting or altering the perception of an experience. Distortions serve as personal beliefs of truth, validity, and right and wrong. Patient's distortions tend to influence their views of the world and themselves by changing negative perceptions into more favorable. **2.** (in radiology) an inaccuracy or false reading in an x-ray image that may be caused by variations in the size, shape or position of the object being viewed. Thick or curved objects result in greater distortion than thin, flat objects due to unequal magnification.

distraction techniques, procedures that prevent or lessen the feeling of pain by focusing attention on other unrelated feelings.

distributive analysis and synthesis, the process of psychotherapy that involves extensive analysis of a person's total past experiences.

district nurse. See **public health nurse.**

disulfiram, a drug used to discourage the drinking of alcohol, it is used to treat long-term alcoholism. The drug causes severe stomach cramping, severe perspiration, and nausea if alcohol is drunk.

disuse phenomena, the physical and psychological changes that result from not using part of the body; linked to immobility, especially in orthopedics. Patients who are treated for broken bones and other orthopedic disorders must often be confined to beds and immobilized in traction for long periods. Such patients often lack communication with others and lose motivation, and abilities because of lack of practice. Some studies have shown that young, healthy patients confined to bed rest for even 3 hours experience disturbances of time sense and memory. Some patients have even experienced hallucinations in feeling, hearing, and seeing. Pain and narcotic drugs commonly given in many illnesses may worsen the condition. Continued bed rest may lead to many physical problems as skin, muscle, stomach, cardiovascular, and breathing problems. The skin of the patient on long bed rest is commonly subjected to abnormal conditions, as pressure from the bed, moisture, friction, and inadequate nutrition. This can produce problems in blood circulation and lack of oxygen to the skin tissues (ischemia). Symptoms of ischemia are redness, pain, swelling and breaks in the skin. Elderly patients are often more susceptible to skin breakdown because of poor nutrition, lack of mobility, and generally poor skin condition. Tissue ischemia can occur in any patient in 1 or 2 hours. One of the biggest problems linked to extended bed rest or limited activity of a part of the body is wasting (atrophy), which may affect the bones and muscles. Unused muscles lose size and strength, often wasting away until they are unable to perform their vital functions of support and contraction. Another disuse phenomenon is contracture, which is a joint "freezing" in one position. Contractures occur when a limb is constantly flexed. A patient on bed rest will flex the knees and hips to relax muscles, especially when cold or in pain. The amputee often flexes the remaining portion of the limb for comfort or to reduce swelling. Continued flexion, however, will produce stiffness in the joint which, if not exercised, may become permanently contracted. Prevention of contractures includes daily manipulation and range-of-motion exercises, if possible. Constipation is also a disuse phenomenon that develops from the weakening of abdominal muscles required for normal bowel movements. This problem is often compounded by the horizontal position of the bed patient, diet changes, and narcotics and anesthetic agents, which slow the normal intestinal contractions. The immobilized patient may develop brittle bones (osteoporosis) because of a restricted diet and reduced mobility. Muscle action is required to maintain the blood flow to the bones. Without adequate blood flow, nutrients are not delivered to the bones. Immobile patients are particularly susceptible to diseases of the lungs, as pneumonia. Normal fluids of the breathing tract pool in the lungs of the patient on bed rest, creating a ripe medium for bacterial growth. Long bed rest also encourages certain cardiovascular problems, as the blood not flowing enough (venous stasis) in the pelvis and legs, loss of water, and clot formation. Some common measures to deal with disuse phenomena are better diet and nutrition, proper positioning and regular movement of the bed-rest patient. Good hygiene, careful skin care, and positive social interaction with the patient are some other measures that must be taken. See also **hypostatic pneumonia.**

Ditropan, a trademark for a drug that relieves spasms (oxybutynin chloride).

Diucardin, a trademark for a drug that lowers blood pressure and stimulates urine release (hydroflumethiazide).

Diupres, a trademark for a drug that stimulates urine release (chlorothiazide) and lowers blood pressure (reserpine).

diuresis /dī'yŏŏrē'sis/, increased formation and release of urine. Diuresis occurs in conditions as diabetes mellitus and diabetes insipidus. It is normal in the first 48 hours after childbirth. Coffee, tea, certain foods, diuretic drugs, and some steroids cause diuresis.

diuretic /dī'yŏŏret'ik/, a drug or other substance that promotes the formation and release of urine. Diuretics are given to lessen the volume of fluid in the treatment of many disorders, as high blood pressure, congestive heart failure, and water retention. Allergy to sulfur drugs prohibits use of this class of drug. Several side effects are common to all diuretics, including a decrease of fluid volume and electrolyte imbalance.

Diuril, a trademark for a drug that stimulates urine release (chlorothiazide).

diurnal, **1.** occurring during the day. Compare **nocturnal. 2.** a daily occurrence, as in the act of sleeping or eating.

diurnal mood variation, a change in a person's mood that is related to the time of day. These mood variations are often cited for the differences between "morning people" and "night people."

diurnal variation, the range of the release rate of a substance, as urine, being collected for laboratory analysis over a 24-hour period.

divergence, a separation or movement of objects away from each other, as when the eyes turn outward at the same time because of a defect in the outer eye muscles.

diverticular disease. See **diverticulitis, diverticulosis.**

diverticulitis /dī'vurtik'yŏolī'tis/, inflammation of one or more pouches (diverticula) in the wall of the large intestine (colon). It is caused by fecal matter seeping through the thin-walled diverticula. Swelling and abcesses form in the tissues surrounding the colon. With repeated swelling, the opening of the colon narrows and may become blocked. During an attack of diverticulitis, the patient will experience crampy pain, particularly in the lower abdomen, and fever. Mild and moderate attacks are treated with bedrest and antibiotics. Severe attacks require surgery. An opening between colon and body surface is created (colostomy) to rest the bowel for about 6 months. After this time, the colostomy is reversed. Compare **diverticulosis.**

diverticulosis /dī'vurtik'yŏolō'sis/, a pouchlike bulging through the muscular layer of the large intestine (colon) without inflammation, particularly in the sigmoid colon, which is above the rectum. Diverticulosis affects mainly people over age 50. It may be the result of the modern, highly refined, low-fiber diet. Most patients with this condition have few symptoms except for occasional bleeding from the rectum, gas, and vague stomach distress. Other reasons for bleeding, as cancer and bowel disease, must be ruled out. Barium enemas and proctoscopic examination are used to make the diagnosis. Diverticulosis may lead to diverticulitis. Treatment is to add roughage to the diet, rest, a heating pad to relieve discomfort, and sometimes medication to relieve the pain. See also **diverticulitis.**

diverticulum /dī'vurtik'yŏoləm/, *pl.* **diverticula,** a pouchlike bulging through the muscular wall of a tubular organ. A diverticulum may occur in the stomach, in the small intestine, or, most commonly, in the colon. See also **diverticulitis, diverticulosis, Meckel's diverticulum. –diverticular,** *adj.*

diving, the act of plunging under water for work or recreational purposes. The main health effects of this activity are the result of the increased pressure the body is subjected to as the surrounding pressure usually increases significantly below the water surface. Diving should be avoided by patients who suffer from obesity, diabetes, alcoholism, epilepsy, drug abuse, and breathing disorders, as nasal allergies. See also **decompression sickness, diving reflex.**

diving goiter, a large movable thyroid gland, located at times above the collarbone and at other times below it. Also called **plunging goiter, wandering goiter.**

diving reflex, an automatic change in the heart and blood vessels that occurs when the face and nose are immersed in water. This reflex causes the heart rate to decrease and the blood pressure to remain stable or increase slightly, while reducing blood flow to all areas of the body except the brain. This focus on maintaining blood flow to only the brain helps the body to conserve oxygen. The reflex occurs in humans and other animals.

division, **1.** an administrative unit in a hospital, as a division of medical nursing. **2.** the separation of something into two or more parts. A kind of division is **cell division.**

divorce therapy, a type of counseling designed to help divorced couples free themselves from their former relationship and curb harmful behavior toward each other or their children.

dizygotic /dī'zīgot'ik/, referring to twins from two fertilized eggs. Compare **monozygotic.** See also **twinning.**

dizygotic twins, two offspring born of the same pregnancy and developed from two eggs that were released from the ovary and fertilized at the same time. They may be of the same or opposite sex, differ both physically and in genetic traits, and have two separate placentas and membranes. The frequency of dizygotic twinning varies according to ethnic origin and age of the mother. They are most common in the black race and the least common in Orientals. Dizygotic twins are most common when the mother is 35 to 39 years old. The overall ratio is two-thirds dizygotic twinning to one-third twins born from one egg (monozygotic). Also called **binovular twins, dissimilar twins, false twins, fraternal twins, heterologous twins.** Compare **monozygotic twins.**

dizziness, a feeling of faintness or an inability to keep normal balance in a standing or seated position, sometimes linked to giddiness, mental confusion, nausea, and weakness. A patient who feels dizziness should be carefully lowered to a safe position on a bed, chair, or floor to avoid injury from falling. Compare **syncope.** See also **vertigo.**

DLE, abbreviation for **discoid lupus erythematosus.**

DM, abbreviation for **diabetes mellitus.**

D.M.D., abbreviation for *Doctor of Dental Medicine.*

DMSO, abbreviation for **dimethyl sulfoxide.**

DNA, abbreviation for **deoxyribonucleic acid.**

DNR, abbreviation for *do not resuscitate.* See **nocode.**

D.O., abbreviation for *Doctor of Osteopathy.* See **physician.**

dobutamine hydrochloride, a drug used to increase heart output in severe long-term congestive heart failure. It is also used in heart surgery.
★CAUTION: Narrowing of the large artery of the heart (aorta) or known allergy to this drug prohibits its use. It is not recommended for use in pregnancy.
★ADVERSE EFFECTS: Among the most serious side effects are effects on the heart, including too rapid heart beats (tachycardia), high blood pressure, irregular heart beats (arrythmias), and chest pain. Nausea, vomiting, and headache may also occur.

Dobutrex, a trademark for a drug used to increase heart output (dobutamine hydrochloride).

Doctor of Medicine, Doctor of Osteopathy. See **physician.**

doctrine of double effect, a belief that an evil or questionable act is morally acceptable if done to achieve a greater good and if certain conditions are in place.

docusate /dok′yoōsāt/, a stool softener used to relieve constipation.
★CAUTION: Symptoms of appendicitis, simultaneous administration of mineral oil, or known allergy to the drug prohibits its use.
★ADVERSE EFFECTS: No serious side effects are known.

Doederlein's bacillus, a bacterium present in normal vaginal discharge.

Dolene, a trademark for a painkiller (propoxyphene hydrochloride).

doll's-eye reflex, a normal response in newborns to keep the eyes stationary as the head is moved to the right or left. The reflex disappears as ability to focus the eyes develops.

Dolobid, a trademark for a drug that reduces swelling (diflunisal).

Dolophine Hydrochloride, a trademark for a narcotic painkiller (methadone hydrochloride).

dolor, physical pain, mental anguish or suffering from heat. It is one of the four signs of inflammation. The others are heat (calor), redness (rubor), and swelling (tumor).

DOM, abbreviation for **dimethoxymethylamphetamine.**

dome fracture, any bone break of the hip socket, which the thigh bone fits into (acetabulum).

dominance, a basic genetic principle stating that not all genes operate with equal strength. If two genes produce a different trait, as eye color, the gene that is expressed is dominant. See also **autosomal-dominant inheritance, independent assortment, recessive, segregation.** –**dominant,** *adj.*

dominant gene, one that produces a trait. Compare **recessive gene.**

dominant group, a social group that controls the system of values and rewards in a particular society.

dominant trait, an inherited characteristic, as eye color, likely to appear in children even if only one parent possesses it. Brown eye color will usually dominate if one parent has brown eyes, even though the other parent does not.

Donath-Landsteiner syndrome, a rare blood disorder marked by separation of hemoglobin from the red cells (hemolysis) minutes or hours after exposure to cold. Symptoms include dark urine, severe pain in the back and legs, headache, vomiting, and diarrhea. When the condition occurs with syphilis, treatment with pencillin may cure the disorder. Also called **paroxysmal cold hemoglobinuria.**

Donnatal, a trademark for a drug (phenobarbital) with a calming effect and three nerve blockers (hyoscyamine sulfate, atropine sulfate, and hyoscine hydrobromide). It is used to decrease the activity of the intestinal tract and relieve diarrhea.

donor, 1. a human or other organism that gives living tissue to another body, for example, blood for transfusion or a kidney for transplantation. 2. a substance that gives part of itself to another substance, as an electron donor. Compare **acceptor.** See also **universal donor.**

Donovan bodies, encapsulated rods of the species *Calymmatobacterium granulomatis.* They are present in the cells obtained from granuloma inguinale tissue. See also **granuloma inguinale.**

donut pad, a pad designed to protect an injured joint, it is cut to fit over the injury site and transfers the force placed on that body part to surrounding areas. Donut pads are most effective for protecting small areas, as the heel or the elbow.

dopa, a chemical substance produced by animals and plants. In humans, dopa leads to the production of epinephrine and norepinephrine. See also **dopamine hydrochloride, levodopa.**

dopamine hydrochloride /dō′pəmin/, a drug used

to treat shock, low blood pressure, and low heart output.

dopaminergic /dō'pəminur'jik/, having the effect of dopamine.

dope, *slang.* morphine, heroin, marijuana, or another illegal substance. It is taken for the calming, sleep-inducing, euphoric, or other mood-changing effects.

Doppler effect /dop'lər/, the apparent change in frequency of sound or electromagnetic waves as the source moves away from or toward an observer. The frequency increases as the source moves toward the observer and decreases as it moves away. An example is the rising pitch of the whistle of an approaching train and the falling pitch of a departing train.

Doppler scanning, a technique used in ultrasound to monitor the behavior of a moving structure, as flowing blood or a beating heart. The frequency of ultrasonic waves reflected from a moving surface is slightly different from that of the incident waves. The frequency shift gives information about the moving structure. Fetal heart detectors work on this principle.

Doriden, a trademark for a drug that induces sleep (glutethimide).

dornase, a natural protein substance that affects the makeup of DNA molecules, which are the chemical basis of heredity. Because as much as 70% of material coughed up from the lungs (sputum) consists of DNA, dornase is used in respiratory therapy to help break up this material in the airway passages. One of the main sources of dornase is beef pancreas.

dorsal /dôr'səl/, referring to the back or posterior. Compare **ventral.** See also **dorsiflect.** **–dorsum,** *n.*

dorsal cutaneous nerve, a nerve that is close to the surface of the foot and ankle, where it can be both seen and felt. Because of its location, this nerve is prone to injury and is the usual cause of pain in a sprained ankle.

dorsal decubitus position. See **supine.**

dorsal digital vein, one of the veins along the sides of the fingers. The veins from both sides of the fingers unite to form three dorsal metacarpal veins, which end in a dorsal vein network on the back of the hand.

dorsal inertia posture, a tendency of a sick or weak person to slip downward in bed when the head of the bed is raised. Because of mental indifference or loss of muscular strength, the person is often unable to adjust to a new position in the bed.

dorsal interventricular artery, the branch of the right coronary artery. It branches to supply both lower heart chambers (ventricles). Also called **right interventricular artery.**

dorsalis pedis artery, the continuation of the anterior tibial artery of the lower leg. It starts at the ankle joint, divides into five branches, and supplies various muscles of the foot and toes.

dorsalis pedis pulse, the pulse of the dorsalis pedis artery, felt between the first and second metatarsal bones on the top of the foot. It can be felt in approximately 90% of people.

dorsal rigid posture, a position in which a patient lying in bed holds one or both legs up to his chest. Often, only the right leg is involved. The position is used to relieve pain caused by appendicitis, peritonitis, kidney stones, or pelvic inflammation.

dorsal scapular nerve, one of a pair of nerve branches above the collarbone. It supplies the muscles of the shoulder blade (rhomboideus major and the rhomboideus minor) and sends a branch of nerves to the levator muscle in the neck.

dorsiflect /dôr'siflekt/, to bend or flex backward, as in the upward bending of the fingers, wrist, foot, or toes.

dorsiflexor /dôr'siflek'sər/, a muscle causing backward flexion of a part of the body, as the hand or foot.

dorsiflexor gait, an abnormal walk caused by weakness of the dorsiflexor muscles of the ankle. It is marked by footdrop and excess knee and hip flexion to allow the involved foot to clear during the swing phase. The sole of the foot also slaps forcibly against the ground. Compare **Trendelenburg gait.**

dorso-, dorsi-, a combining form referring to a dorsum or the back.

dorsodynia, back pain, particularly in the muscles of the upper back area.

dorsosacral position. See **lithotomy position.**

dorsum sellae, the back boundary of the large bone at the base of the skull (sphenoid), it is often used during physical examination to help locate the pituitary gland.

dosage, the size, frequency, and number of doses of a drug to be given to a patient.

dosage compensation, a genetic mechanism that counterbalances the number of X-linked gene doses in the sex chromosomes so that they are equal in both the male, which has one X chromosome, and the female, which has two. In mammals this occurs by genetic activation of only one of the X chromosomes in the cells of females. See also **Lyon hypothesis.**

dose, the amount of a drug or other substance to be given at one time. See also **absorbed dose.**

dose-limiting recommendations, the largest amount, or maximum permissible dose (MPD), of radiation exposure recommended for an individual. This amount may vary for different parts of the body. For example, the MPD for the arms of a person who is exposed to radiation daily will usually be much higher than the MPD for the rest of the body.

dose rate, the amount of radiation absorbed in a certain amount of time.

dose response, the range of the effects of a particular drug. On one end of the range is the minimum dose needed to produce an observable effect; at the other end of the range is the toxic dose level that results in adverse side effects.

dose-response relationship, (in radiology) a mathematical relationship between a dose of radiation and the body's reaction to it. In a linear dose-response relationship, the response is proportional to the dose, meaning that if the dose is double, the response is also doubled. In a linear non-threshold relationship, any dose, regardless of size, can cause a response.

dose threshold, the minimum amount of absorbed radiation that produces an effect.

dose to skin, the amount of absorbed radiation at the center of the irradiation field on the skin.

dosimeter /dōsim′ətər/, an instrument to detect and measure total radiation exposure.

double bind, a "no-win" situation that results when a person receives conflicting messages from someone who is crucial to his or her survival. This can occur when a verbal message differs from a nonverbal message. For example, a mother may insist that she is not angry about her child's behavior, yet indicate otherwise to the child by her actions.

double-blind study, an experiment made to test the effect of a treatment or drug. Groups of experimental and control subjects are used in which neither the subjects nor the investigators know which treatment is being given to which group. In a double-blind test of a new drug, the drug may be identified to the investigators only by a code.

double-contrast arthography, a method used to take x-rays of a joint in which two agents that are visible on x-rays are injected into the space surrounding the joint. A form of gas is usually combined with an iodine solution during this technique, most commonly used to x-ray the knee joint.

double-emulsion film, x-ray film coated with a gel on both sides.

double fracture, a fracture that has breaks or cracks in two places in a bone, resulting in more than two bone segments.

double innervation, being supplied by nerves that are part of the nervous system not under conscious control (autonomic nervous system) that lead to and away from organs. The purpose of these nerves are to operate at cross-purposes to keep the organs in a state of balance. The digestive system, the reproductive system, the urinary system, bronchioles, heart, and eyes are all doubly innervated.

double monster, a fetus that has developed from a single egg but has two heads, trunks, and multiple limbs. Also called **twin monster.**

double quartan fever, a form of malaria in which fever occurs in a repeating pattern of 2 days followed by one day of no symptoms. The pat-

tern is usually the result of infections by two species of the genus *Plasmodium.* One causes attacks of fever every 72 hours. The other causes attacks of fever every 48 hours. Compare **biduotertian fever.**

double tachycardia, the simultaneous but independent firing of two rapid heart contraction impulses. One impulse controls the upper chambers (atria) and one the lower chambers (ventricles).

double vision. See **diplopia.**

double-void, a procedure to test urine samples in which the first specimen is discarded and a second specimen, taken 30 to 45 minutes later, is used. This method provides accurate measurement of the amount of blood sugar (glucose) in the urine at that particular time.

douche /dōōsh/, a procedure in which a quart (liter) or more of a medicated solution or cleansing agent in warm water is flushed into the vagina under low pressure. Douching may be recommended for treating various pelvic and vaginal infections.

doughnut pessary. See **pessary.**

Douglas' cul-de-sac, a pouch formed by a fold of membrane lining the stomach (peritoneum) between the rectum and the uterus. Also called **excavatio rectouterina.**

Down's syndrome, a birth defect marked by mental retardation and many physical defects. Down's syndrome occurs in about 1 in 600 to 650 live births. It is more frequent in infants born to women over 35 years of age. The incidence is as high as 1 in 80 for offspring of women older than 40 years. Also called **mongolism, mongoloid idiocy, trisomy G syndrome, trisomy 21.** Infants with the syndrome are small with weak muscles. They have a small head with a flat back skull, a mongoloid slant to the eyes, depressed nose bridge, low-set ears, and a large, protruding tongue that is furrowed and lacks the central groove. The hands are short and broad with a single crease across the palm (called a simian crease). The fingers are stubby and slant to the side, especially the fifth finger. The feet are broad and stubby with a wide space between the first and second toes and a prominent crease on the sole. Other common defects in Down's syndrome are bowel defects, inborn heart disease, long-term breathing infections, and vision problems. Abnormalities in tooth development, and susceptibility to acute leukemia are other defects. The most significant feature of the syndrome is mental retardation, which varies considerably, although the average IQ is in the range of 50 to 60. The child is generally trainable and in many instances can be reared at home. They can live to middle or old age, although adults with Down's syndrome are prone to breathing infections, inflammation of the lungs (pneumonia), and lung disease. Care for the child with

Down's syndrome depends on the severity of physical defects and the degree of mental impairment. Prevention of the physical problems linked to the disorder is important. Food intake can present a problem because of difficulties caused by the large protruding tongue. The characteristic dry, cracked skin can result in skin breakdown. Long-term-care centers offer carefully planned programs to promote development of motor and mental skills. Since the potential of a child with Down's syndrome is greatest during infancy, a stimulation program of exercise based on the child's ability is necessary for teaching gross motor skills.

Downey cells, white blood cells (lymphocytes) identified in patients with infectious mononucleosis.

doxapram hydrochloride, a breathing stimulant, given to improve breathing after anesthesia, in drug overdose, and for long-term disease linked to an acute condition of excess carbon dioxide in the blood (hypercapnia).
★CAUTION: Seizure disorder, lung disease, coronary artery disease, high blood pressure, or known allergy to this drug prohibits its use.
★ADVERSE EFFECTS: Among the more serious side effects are convulsions, spasms of the bronchial tubes, heart symptoms, and swelling of veins (phlebitis).

doxepin hydrochloride /dok'səpin/, an antidepressant drug used to treat depression.

doxorubicin hydrochloride, an antibiotic drug used to treat several forms of cancer.

doxycycline, an antibacterial used to treat some infections.
★CAUTION: Kidney or liver dysfunction or known allergy to this drug or to other tetracyclines prohibits its use. It is not given during pregnancy or to children under 8 years of age.
★ADVERSE EFFECTS: Among the more serious adverse reactions are intestinal disturbances, excess reaction to sunlight (phototoxicity), potentially serious new infections, and allergic reactions. Discoloration of teeth may occur in children exposed to the drug before birth or under 8 years of age.

doxylamine succinate /dok'siləm'ēn/, an antihistamine used to treat acute allergic symptoms.
★CAUTION: Known allergy to this drug prohibits its use. It is not recommended for use during pregnancy or nursing nor given to children under 6 years of age.
★ADVERSE EFFECTS: Among the more serious side effects are sleepiness, poor muscle coordination (ataxia), excess rapid heart beat (tachycardia), anemia, and decrease in blood platelets.

DPG, abbreviation for **2,3-diphosphoglyceric acid.**

DPT vaccine, abbreviation for **diphtheria, tetanus toxoids, and pertussis vaccine.**

DQ, abbreviation for **developmental quotient.**

dracunculiasis /drakun'kyōōlī'əsis/, a parasitic infection caused by the worm (nematode) *Dracunculus medinensis.* It is marked by skin ulcers on the legs and feet that are produced by pregnant female worms. Intense itching and burning results from the ulcers. Patients are infected by drinking contaminated water or eating contaminated shellfish. Treatment is with antiparasite drugs. Also called **dracontiasis, guinea worm infection.**

drain, a tube or other opening used to remove air or a fluid from a body cavity or wound. The drain may be a closed system, designed to provide complete protection against contamination, or an open system.

drainage, the removal of fluids from a body cavity, wound, or other source of discharge by one or more methods. **Closed drainage** involves attaching a tube to the area to remove fluid to an airtight container, preventing contaminants from entering the wound or cavity. **Open drainage** is drainage in which discharge passes through an open-ended tube into a container. **Suction drainage** uses a pump to assist in removing fluid. **Tidal drainage** is drainage in which a body area is washed out by alternately flooding and then emptying it with the aid of gravity, a technique that may be used in treating a urinary bladder disorder. See also **postural drainage.**

drainage tube, a heavy-gauge tube (catheter) used to remove air or a fluid from a cavity or wound in the body. The tube may be attached to a suction device or it may simply allow flow by gravity into a container.

Draize test, a controversial method of testing the toxicity of drugs and other products to be used by humans. A small amount of the substance is placed in the eyes of rabbits. A substance that irritates the rabbit's eyes is considered a measure of the possible effect the product could have on similar human tissues.

-dralazine, a combining form for the name of a drug used to lower blood pressure (hypertension).

dram, a unit of mass equivalent to an apothecaries' measure of 60 grains or ⅛ ounce and to 1/16 ounce or 27.34 grains avoirdupois.

Dramamine, a trademark for an antihistamine used to prevent nausea and motion sickness (dimenhydrinate).

dramatic play, an activity in which a child fantasizes and acts out various adult social roles and situations, as rocking a doll, pretending to be a doctor or nurse, or teaching school. It is the main form of play among preschool children.

drape, a sheet of fabric or paper for covering all or a part of a person's body during a physical examination or treatment; usually the size of a small bed. **–drape,** *v.*

drawer sign, a sign that indicates a ruptured or torn knee ligament, tested by having the patient flex the knee at a right angle while the examiner grasps the lower leg just below the knee and moves the leg first forward, then away from the examiner. If the head of the large, inner bone between the knee and ankle (tibia) can be moved more than one-half inch from the joint, the ligament is considered to be ruptured or torn.

drawing, *informal.* a vague sensation of muscle tension.

drawsheet, a sheet that is smaller than a bottom or top sheet of a bed and is usually placed over the middle of the bottom sheet to keep the mattress and bottom linens dry. The drawsheet can be used to help turn or move a patient while in bed.

dream, 1. an order of ideas, thoughts, emotions, or images that pass through the mind during the rapid-eye movement stage of sleep. **2.** describing the sleeping state in which this process occurs. **3.** a creation of the imagination during wakefulness. **4.** the expression of thoughts, emotions, memories, or impulses repressed from the consciousness.

dream analysis, a process of gaining access to the unconscious mind by examining the content of dreams. It is usually done through the method of free association.

dream state, a condition of altered consciousness in which a person does not recognize the environment and reacts in a manner not like his or her usual behavior, as by flight or an act of violence. The state is seen in epilepsy and certain neuroses. See also **automatism, fugue.**

drepanocytic anemia. See **sickle cell anemia.**

dressing, a clean or sterile covering applied directly to wounded or diseased tissue. The purpose is to absorb secretions, protect from trauma, cover with a drug, keep the wound clean, or stop bleeding. Kinds of dressings include **absorbent dressing, antiseptic dressing, occlusive dressing, pressure dressing, wet dressing.**

Dressler's syndrome /dres'lərz/, an autoimmune disorder that may occur several days after severe heart attack. It is marked by fever, fluid in the lungs, joint pain, and swelling of the sac around the heart and the membrane around the lungs. The syndrome results from the body's immune system's response to a damaged heart.

DRG, abbreviation for **diagnosis-related group.**

drift, a change that occurs in a strain of virus so that variations appear periodically with alterations in the virus' qualities. Also called **antigenic drift.**

drifting tooth, any one of the teeth that migrate from normal position.

Drinker respirator, an airtight breathing machine consisting of a metal tank that encloses the entire body, except for the head. It is used for long-term therapy and provides artificial breathing by contracting and expanding the walls of the chest. Also called **artificial lung, iron lung.**

drip, 1. the process of a liquid or moisture forming and falling in drops. Kinds of drip are **nasal drip, postnasal drip. 2.** the slow but continuous flow of a liquid into the body, as into the stomach or a vein. **3.** to put a liquid continuously into the body.

drip gavage, a method used to feed patients a liquid-formula diet using a tube inserted through the nostrils into the stomach. The formula may be heated to approximately 100° F or given at room temperature. It is placed in a bottle suspended from a stand.

drip system, a device for putting specific volumes of solutions into a vein. It is set at a specific flow rate for a certain amount of time. See also **macrodrip, microdrip.**

drop, a small, ball-shaped amount of liquid. A drop may vary in size, depending on differences in temperature and thickness of the liquid and other factors. For treatment purposes, a drop is considered as having a volume of .06 to 0.1 ml, or 1 to 1.5 minims.

drop arm test, a test used to diagnose a tear in the upper tendon in the spine. If the patient is unable to slowly and smoothly lower the affected arm 90 degrees outward from the middle of the body, the tendon is considered to be torn.

drop attack, a brief interruption of blood flow to the brain that results in a person falling to the floor without losing consciousness. The episode may affect the person's sense of balance or muscle tone in the legs, leading to the fall. Weakness of the leg muscles or impairment of the hip or knee joint can contribute to the collapse. The condition is a form of transient ischemic attack (TIA).

droperidol /drəper'ədol/, a drug with a calming, sleep-inducing effect, used to decrease anxiety and pain before anesthesia (fentanyl).

drop foot, a condition in which the foot is flexed down and cannot voluntarily be flexed up. It is usually caused by nerve damage.

droplet infection, an infection gotten by inhaling disease-causing microorganisms that are in particles of liquid sneezed or coughed by another infected person or animal.

dropped foot. See **footdrop.**

dropper, a glass or plastic tube that is narrow at one end so that only one drop of medication is given at a time.

dropsy. See **hydrops.**

Drosophila /drōsof'ilə/, a genus of fly, including the Mediterranean fruit fly, *(Drosophila melanogaster,).* They are useful in genetic experiments because of their large chromosomes and their sensitivity to such environmental effects as exposure to radiation.

drowning, suffocation from being submerged in a liquid. See also **near drowning.**

drox, an abbreviation for **noncarboxylate hydroxide anion.**

drug, 1. any substance taken by mouth, injected into a muscle, the skin, a blood vessel, or a cavity of the body, or applied to the skin to treat or prevent a disease. Also called **medicine.** 2. *informal.* a narcotic substance.

drug absorption, the process by which a drug moves from the muscle, digestive tract or other site of entry through the body and into the bloodstream to the organ or tissue being treated.

drug abuse, the use of a drug for a nontherapeutic effect. Some of the most commonly abused drugs are alcohol, amphetamines, barbiturates, cocaine, methaqualone, and opium alkaloids. Drug abuse may lead to organ damage, addiction, and disturbed patterns of behavior. Some illegal drugs have no known therapeutic effect in humans. See also **drug addiction.**

drug action, the means by which a drug has a desired effect. Drugs are usually classified by their actions. For example, a vasodilator, which is prescribed to decrease the blood pressure, acts by widening the blood vessels.

drug addiction, a condition marked by an overwhelming desire to continue taking a drug because it produces a particular effect, usually an alteration of mental activity, attitude, or outlook. Addiction usually goes along with a tendency to increase the dose, a psychological or physical dependence, and harmful effects for the person and society. See also **alcoholism, drug abuse.**

drug allergy, allergy to a drug manifested by reactions ranging from a mild rash to severe allergic reaction and shock. The seriousness of the reaction depends on the person, the drug, and the dose. Allergic responses may be caused by any drug.

drug agonist, one of two similar drugs that may affect the same organ or tissue being treated, producing the same or a similar effect. If the drugs act on the same site within the body, the two products may affect or negate the potency of each other, requiring larger-than-usual doses to achieve the desired effect.

drug clearance, the elimination of a drug from the body, commonly as waste matter through the kidneys. The rate of clearance helps to determine the size and frequency of a dosage of a particular medication.

drug compliance, the reliability of a patient to use a prescribed drug exactly as ordered by a physician. Noncompliance occurs when the patient forgets or neglects to take the prescribed dosages at the recommended times or decides to stop taking the drug without consulting the physician.

drug dependence, a psychological craving for or a physical dependence on a drug resulting from habituation, abuse, or addiction. See also **drug abuse, drug addiction.**

drug dispensing, the preparation, packaging, labeling, record keeping, and transfer of a prescription drug to a patient or to one who is responsible for giving the drug.

drug distribution, the way the body absorbs a particular drug's molecules through various tissues after the chemical enters the bloodstream. Because of differences in the makeup of the drug, cell membrane functions and other tissue factors, most drugs are not equally distributed throughout all parts of the body. For example, the acid content of aspirin can affect the way it is distributed throughout the body, which will differ from the way a product with a high alkaline content will be absorbed.

drug-drug interaction, a change of the effect of a drug when given with another drug. The effect may be an increase or a decrease in the action of either drug. The effect may also be a side effect that is not normally linked to either drug.

Drug Enforcement Agency (D.E.A.), an agency of the Drug Enforcement Administration of the federal government. The D.E.A. enforces regulations regarding the import or export of narcotic drugs and certain other substances or the traffic of these substances across state lines.

drug eruption, any skin reaction or rash caused by a drug. Also called **dermatitis medicamentosa.** See also **fixed drug eruption.**

drug fever, a fever caused by the action of a drug, a complication of injecting a drug, or, an immune system reaction of antibodies to the drug. The fever usually begins between 7 and 10 days after the drug is begun. Temperature returns to normal within 2 days of stopping the drug. See also **Jarisch-Herxheimer reaction.**

drug-food interaction, the effect produced when a particular drug is taken at the same time as certain foods or beverages. Some drugs can react dangerously with certain food groups.

drug-induced parkinsonism, a syndrome that resembles the signs and symptoms of Parkinson's disease but is caused by the actions of drugs used to treat psychosis (antipsychotics). The condition is reversible. See also **parkinsonism.**

drug metabolism, the method by which the body chemically transforms a particular drug through the tissues to convert it into an agent that can treat a condition. For example, the body converts or metabolizes codeine into morphine.

drug potency, a measure of the effects of one drug compared to those of a similar drug of the same dosage. The drug that produces the greatest effect using the smallest dose is considered to have the greater potency.

drug rash, a skin rash usually caused by an allergic reaction to a particular drug. Nearly any drug can produce a skin reaction, either because the drug gradually accumulates in the body or because the body develops defenses to the medication. In allergies the rash does not occur the first time the drug is taken; instead, the effect is seen after repeated use of the same drug. Also called **dermatitis medicamentosa.** See also **fixed drug eruption.**

drug receptor, any part of a cell, usually an enzyme or large protein molecule, with which a drug molecule interacts to achieve a desired response or effect.

drug rehabilitation center, an agency that provides long-term care for a person with a chemical or drug dependancy so that he or she can gradually return to the community. See also **Daytop Village.**

drug sequestration, the process by which certain drugs are stored in the body tissues. For example, tetracycline, an antibiotic, is stored in bone tissue. Certain vitamins and other substances are stored in fat deposits within the body.

drug tolerance, a condition by which the cells adapt to a drug so that the body requires increasingly larger doses to produce the same effect originally achieved with smaller doses.

drug trial, the process of determining what dose of a specific drug is adequate and effective for the treatment of a particular patient. The trial ends with (1) an acceptable response after treatment; (2) negative results that cannot be tolerated; (3) a poor response after an appropriate blood level is reached; or (4) having given the drug for a specific time. The usual time required for the trial of a drug to treat depression (antidepressant) is 3 weeks, whereas the trial for a drug used to treat severe mental illness is 3 to 6 weeks.

dry catarrh, a dry cough with almost no sputum that occurs in severe coughing spells, it is linked to asthma and emphysema in older people.

dry dressing, a plain dressing with no medication applied directly to an incision or a wound to prevent contamination or injury or to absorb releases.

dry gangrene. See **gangrene.**

dry gas (D), (in respiratory therapy) a gas that contains no water vapor.

dry ice, a solid form of carbon dioxide, with a temperature of approximately $-140°$ F, it is used in treating various skin disorders to freeze an area, as in the removal of warts.

dry labor, *informal.* labor in which the water (amniotic fluid) has already escaped.

dry rale, an abnormal chest sound made by air passing through a narrowed bronchial tube in the lungs. Compare **amphoric breath sound, atelectatic rale, bubbling rale.**

Drysdale's corpuscle /drīz'dālz/, one of a number of transparent cells in the fluid of some lumps (cysts) of the ovary. Also called **Bennet's small corpuscle.**

dry skin, skin lacking moisture or oil often marked by a pattern of fine lines, scaling, and itching. Causes include too frequent bathing, low humidity, and low oil production in aging skin. Treatment includes bathing less often, increased humidity, bath oils, drugs that soften the skin such as lanolin and glycerine, and water-absorbing ointments. Also called **xerosis** /zērō'sis/.

dry tooth socket, a swelling condition of a tooth socket (alveolus) after the tooth has been pulled. Normally, a blood clot forms over the alveolar bone at the base of the tooth socket after a tooth is pulled. If the clot fails to form properly or becomes loose, the bone tissue is exposed and can become infected. This is usually a painful condition requiring pain relievers and sedatives. A dry socket is treated by packing the socket with gauze soaked with an antibiotic.

DSDB, abbreviation for **direct self-destructive behavior.**

DSM, abbreviation for *Diagnostic and Statistical Manual of Mental Disorders.*

DT, abbreviation for **diphtheria and tetanus toxoids.**

DTIC-Dome, a trademark for a drug used to treat cancer (dacarbazine).

DTR, abbreviation for **deep tendon reflex.**

DTs, abbreviation for **delirium tremens.**

duality of central nervous system control, a theory that the normal central nervous system (CNS) is regulated by a check-and-balance program that provides feedback to the body. The theory is based on studies of patient actions and reactions compared to the laws of basic physics. Proponents of the theory suggest that CNS disorders are caused by imbalances in the feedback system.

DUB, **1.** abbreviation for **dysfunctional uterine bleeding. 2.** a genetically determined human blood factor associated with immunity to certain diseases.

Dubin-Johnson syndrome /doo'binjon'sən/, a rare, long-term, hereditary disorder in which high levels of bilirubin appear in the blood. It produces liver disease (jaundice), abnormal liver pigmentation, and abnormal function of the gall bladder. It is caused by an inability of the liver to release several substances. See also **hyperbilirubinemia of the newborn, Rotor syndrome.**

Dubowitz assessment, a system of estimating the age from conception (gestational age) of a newborn child according to such factors as posture, ankle flexion upwards, and arm and leg recoil.

Duchenne-Erb paralysis. See **Erb's palsy.**

Duchenne's disease /dooshenz'/, a series of three different nervous system disorders: **spinal muscular atrophy, bulbar paralysis,** and **tabes dorsalis.** See also **muscular dystrophy.**

Duchenne's muscular dystrophy, a birth defect marked by progressive wasting of the muscles in the legs and pelvis, this disease affects mostly males. It accounts for 50% of all muscular dystrophy diseases. It is a sex- (X)-linked inborn disease that appears gradually between the ages of 3 and 5 years and spreads from the leg and pelvic muscles to the involuntary muscles. Linked muscle weakness produces a waddling walk and sway back. Muscles rapidly break down, and calf muscles become firm and large from fatty deposits. Affected children develop frozen flexed joints (contractures), have difficulty climbing stairs, often stumble and fall, and display winglike shoulder blades when they raise their arms. Such persons are usually confined to wheelchairs by the age of 12. Progressive weakening of heart muscle causes toorapid heart beats (tachycardia) and lung problems. Also called **pseudohypertrophic muscular dystrophy.**

Typical medical and family history may also suggest the disease. Confirming diagnosis is usually aided by a muscle biopsy showing fat and connective tissue deposits. There is no successful treatment of the disease. Orthopedic appliances, exercise, physical therapy, and surgery to correct contractures can help preserve mobility. Family members who are carriers should be cautioned about the risk of transmitting this disease. No form of muscular dystrophy can be detected by examination of the amniotic fluid during pregnancy (amniocentesis). However, this procedure can determine the sex of the fetus. It is often recommended for carriers who are pregnant.

★PATIENT CARE: The patient should avoid long periods of bed rest and inactivity to assure maximum physical activity. Splints, braces, grab bars, and overhead slings help the patient to exercise. A wheelchair helps to preserve mobility. Other devices that can increase comfort and help prevent footdrop include footboards, high-topped sneakers, and foot cradles. The patient should keep peer relationships. The parents should keep the child in school as long as possible. The Muscular Dystrophy Association offers support and assistance.

duct ectasia, an abnormal widening of a duct by fatty substances and cellular waste products. In the ducts of the breast that produce milk the condition may cause the area to become inflamed; this condition tends to affect women after menopause.

duck embryo vaccine. See **rabies vaccine.**

duck walk. See **metatarsus valgus.**

duct, a narrow tube structure, especially one through which material is released.

duct carcinoma, a cancer developed from the skinlike layer of ducts, especially in the breast or pancreas.

duction, the movement of one eyeball from one position to another position.

ductless gland, a gland lacking a duct. Endocrine glands, which release hormones directly into blood or lymph, are ductless glands.

duct of Rivinus /rivē′nəs/, one of the minor salivary gland ducts under the tongue. Compare **Bartholin's duct.**

duct of Wirsung. See **pancreatic duct.**

ductus /duk′təs/, *pl.* **ductus** /duk′toos/, a duct.

ductus arteriosus, a vessel in the fetus that joins the pulmonary artery directly to the descending aorta. It shuts down soon after the lungs inflate after birth. See also **ductus arteriosus.**

ductus deferens. See **vas deferens.**

ductus venosus, the vessel in the fetus passing through the liver and joining the umbilical vein with the large vein in the abdomen (inferior vena cava). Before birth, it carries highly oxygenated blood from the placenta to the fetal circulation. It closes shortly after birth as lung circulation is established and as the vessels in the umbilical cord collapse. See also **ductus arteriosus, foramen ovale.**

Duke's classification, a system of identifying tumors in the colon and rectum according to the degree of tissues involved and the spread of the diseases (metastasis). The system uses four classifications from A to D: A Duke's A tumor is one that is confined to the mucous membrane (mucosa) and the layer under the membrane (submucosa); a B tumor is one that has entered the surrounding muscles but has not affected the lymph glands; C tumors have invaded the surrounding muscles and spread to the surrounding lymph nodes; and D tumors are those that have spread to tissues in distant organs.

Dulcolax, a trademark for a laxative (bisacodyl).

dumdum fever. See **kala-azar.**

dumping syndrome, the combination of profuse sweating, nausea, dizziness, and weakness, it is experienced by patients who have had part of their stomachs removed (gastrectomy). Symptoms are felt soon after eating, when the contents of the stomach empty too rapidly into the first part of the small intestine (duodenum). A high-protein, high-calorie diet with small, frequent meals should prevent discomfort and ensure good nutrition. See also **gastrectomy.**

Duncan's mechanism, a technique for delivering the placenta with the maternal rather than the fetal surface first.

Dunlop skeletal traction, an orthopedic mechanism that helps immobilize the arm to treat abnormal shortening of the muscle or fracture of the elbow. The mechanism employs a system of traction weights, pulleys, and ropes. The system is attached to the bone with a pin or wire. It may be further secured by adhesive or nonadhesive skin-traction components. Compare **Dunlop skin traction.**

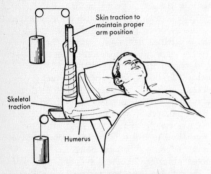

Dunlop skeletal traction

Dunlop skin traction, an orthopedic mechanism that helps immobilize the arm to treat abnormal shortening of the muscle or fracture of the elbow. The mechanism employs a system of traction weights, pulleys, and ropes. It is usually applied to one side of the arm but sometimes both sides. Dunlop skin traction may be applied as adhesive skin traction or nonadhesive skin traction. Compare **Dunlop skeletal traction.**

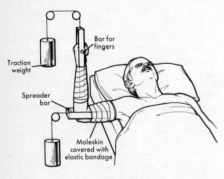

Dunlop skin traction

duodenal /dōō'ədē'nəl/, referring to the first part of the small intestine (duodenum).

duodenal bulb, the first part of the top portion of the duodenum, which looks like a bulb on x-ray views of the small intestine.

duodenal ulcer, an ulcer in the first part of the small intestine (duodenum), the most common type of peptic ulcer. See also **peptic ulcer.**

duodenography /dōō'ədənog'rəfē/, the process of taking an x-ray of the duodenum and pancreas, it usually requires that the patient be given a drug that paralyzes the duodenum to prevent muscular contractions. The procedure involves the use of two solutions that contrast on the x-ray film so that the organ presses against and outlines the head of the pancreas.

duodenojejunal flexure. See **angle of Treitz.**

duodenoscope /dōō'ədē'nəskōp'/, an instrument, usually fiberoptic, for the visual examination of the duodenum.

duodenum /dōō'ədē'nəm, dōō·od'inəm/, _pl._ **duodena, duodenums,** the shortest, widest, portion of the small intestine that joins the stomach at the pyloric valve. It is about 10 inches (25 cm) long. It is divided into superior, descending, horizontal, and ascending portions. Compare **jejunum, ileum.**

duplex transmission, the passage of a nerve impulse in both directions along a nerve fiber.

duplicating film, a film used in x-rays to copy an existing image by exposing it to ultraviolet light.

Dupuytren's contracture /dYpY·itraNz', dēpē· itranz'/, a progressive, painless thickening and tightening of tissue under the skin of the palm. It causes the fourth and fifth fingers to bend into the palm and resist extension. Tendons and nerves are not involved. Although the condition begins in one hand, both hands become affected. Of unknown cause, it is most frequent in middle-aged males.

Dupuytren's fracture. See **Galeazzi's fracture.**

Durabolin, a trademark for a steroid used to build up tissues damaged from severe disease or injury (nandrolone phenpropionate).

dural sac, the hidden pouch formed by the end of the dura mater at the lower end of the spinal cord.

dura mater /dōō'rə mā'tər, dyōō'rə/, the fiberlike, outermost of the three membranes surrounding the brain and spinal cord. The **dura mater encephali** covers the brain. The **dura mater spinalis** covers the cord. See also **meninges.**

Duranest, a trademark for a drug used to produce local anesthesia (etidocaine hydrochloride).

Durozier murmur, a heart murmur heard when a stethoscope is placed over a large artery and the artery is compressed. The murmur indicates that the patient suffers from high blood pressure or lack of sufficient blood to the aorta.

dust, any fine, particulate, dry matter. Kinds of dust are **inorganic dust, organic dust.**

Dutton's relapsing fever, an infection caused by a spirochete, _Borrelia duttonii,_ which is carried by a soft tick, *Ornithodoros moubata.* It is found in human dwellings in tropical Africa. The spirochete enters the skin through the tick bite. The symptoms are a high fever, chills, rapid heart beat, headache, joint and muscle pain, vomiting, and nervous system disorders. Also called **African relapsing fever, Dutton's disease.** See also **relapsing fever.**

Duverney's fracture /dōō´vurnăz´/, fracture of the pelvic bone (ilium) just below the spine.

dwarf, **1.** an abnormally short person, especially one whose bodily parts are not proportional. Kinds of dwarfs include **achondroplastic dwarf, Amsterdam dwarf, asexual dwarf, ateliotic dwarf, bird-headed dwarf, Brissaud's dwarf, cretin dwarf, diastrophic dwarf, phocomelic dwarf, pituitary dwarf, primordial dwarf, rachitic dwarf, renal dwarf, Russell dwarf, sexual dwarf, Silver dwarf, thanatophoric dwarf.** Also called **nanus. 2.** to prevent or slow normal growth.

dwarfism, the abnormal underdevelopment of the body, marked by extreme shortness. The condition is linked to numerous other defects and sometimes includes varying degrees of mental retardation. Dwarfism has numerous causes, including genetic defects, lack of hormones of either the pituitary or thyroid glands, chronic diseases (as rickets, kidney failure, and intestinal malabsorption defects), and psychosocial stress (as the maternal deprivation syndrome). See also **dwarf.**

dwarf tapeworm infection, a type of infection caused by the intestinal parasite *Hymenolepsia nana,* it occurs mainly in the southern United States and usually affects children who ingest the parasite's eggs by placing contaminated material in their mouths. The disease may not produce any symptoms, or it may cause stomach disorders or diarrhea. It is treated with the drugs niclosamide or paromomycin.

Dwyer cable instrumentation, one of the two most common surgical methods for correcting spinal curve (scoliosis). A device is inserted at the spine to help in keeping the corrected curvature, and the curved part of the spine is fused. The device is not usually removed unless there is displacement after the operation.

dyadic interpersonal communication, a process in which two people interact face to face as senders and receivers, as in a conversation.

Dyazide, a trademark for a drug containing two drugs that stimulate urine release (triamterene and hydrochlorothiazide).

Dyclone, a trademark for a drug used to produce local anesthesia (dyclonine hydrochloride).

dyclonine hydrochloride, a local anesthetic drug that also destroys bacteria and fungus. It is used for mouth pain, severe itching, insect bites, and minor skin burns and injuries.

dye, **1.** to apply coloring matter to a substance. **2.** a chemical compound that colors a substance to which it is applied. Various dyes are used as stains for tissues, as test reagents, as therapeutic agents, and to color drugs.

Dymelor, a trademark for a drug used to treat diabetes (acetohexamide).

dynamic cardiac work, the energy transfer that occurs during the process of ejecting blood from the lower heart chamber (ventricle).

dynamic equilibrium, the ability of a patient to adjust to movement of the body's center of gravity by changing the body's base of support.

dynamic ileus, a blockage of the intestines, which causes repeated and continuous muscle spasm activity. Also called **spastic ileus.**

dynamic imaging, (in ultrasonography) the imaging of a moving object that does not cause significant blurring of any one image yet still adequately represents a true movement pattern. Also called **real-time imaging.**

dynamic psychiatry, the study of how motivation, emotion, and biology determine human behavior.

dynamic range, **1.** (in radiology) the range of input signals or voltage used in x-ray imaging that results in a digital output. **2.** (in audiology) the range of loudness from the faintest sound a person can hear to the level of sound that causes pain.

dynamic response, the accuracy with which a monitoring system, as an electrocardiograph, will record the actual event being recorded.

dynamometer /dī´nəmom´ətər/, a device for measuring the amount of energy used in the contraction of a muscle or a group of muscles. For example, a squeeze dynamometer measures the force of the hand when squeezing the device.

Dynapen, a trademark for an antibacterial drug used to treat infections (dicloxacillin sodium).

dyne /dīn/, a unit of force that would accelerate a 1-gram mass to a velocity of 1 cm per second in 1 second. One dyne equals one-one-hundred-thousanth (10^{-5}) newton.

dynode /dī´nōd/, one of a series of plate-shaped parts in a device that detects radiation. Dynodes amplify electron pulses.

dyphylline, a drug that relaxes the bronchial muscle of the airway, it is used to treat acute bronchial asthma, bronchitis, and emphysema. ★CAUTION: It is used carefully in patients with ulcer or heart disease. Known allergy to this or to other xanthines prohibits its use. ★ADVERSE EFFECTS: Among the more serious side effects are distress of stomach and intestines, dizziness, too-rapid heart beat (tachycardia), headache, and palpitations.

Dyrenium, a trademark for a drug that stimulates urine release (triamterene).

dys-, a combining form meaning bad, painful, or disordered.

dysadrenia, abnormal adrenal gland function, it is marked by decreased production of hormones or by increased release of the gland. Also called **dysadrenalism.**

dysarthria /disär′thrē·ə/, difficult, poorly articulated speech, it results from interference in the control over the muscles of speech, usually because of damage to a motor nerve.

dysautonomia, a dysfunction of the autonomic nervous system, it can occur in patients with diabetes, Parkinson's disease, and other conditions. A common effect of dysautonomia is a drop in blood pressure when the patient lies down (orthostatic hypotension). Other symptoms are poor muscle coordination, impotence, incontinence, drooling, abnormal perspiration and tearing of the eyes, and sudden emotional swings.

dysbarism, a reaction to sudden changes in air pressure. For example, in high altitudes, people are exposed to low atmospheric pressures. The symptoms are similar to those of decompression sickness.

dysbetalipoproteinemia. See **broad beta disease.**

dyscholia /diskō′lē·ə/, any abnormal condition of the bile, either regarding the amount released or the condition of the contents.

dyschondroplasia. See **enchondromatosis.**

dyscrasia /diskrā′zhə/, an abnormal blood or bone marrow condition, as leukemia, aplastic anemia, or Rh incompatibility.

dyscrasic fracture /diskraz′ik/, any broken bone caused by the weakening of a specific bone as a result of a debilitating disease.

dysdiadochokinesia /dis′dī·ədō′kōkinē′zhə/, a lack of ability to perform rapidly alternating movements. For example, a patient may be unable to tap the fingers rhythmically on the knee. This condition is caused by a brain tumor.

dysentery /dis′inter′ē/, an inflammation of the intestine, especially of the large intestine (colon). It may be caused by chemical irritants, bacteria, protozoa, or parasites. The symptoms are frequent and bloody stools, stomach pain, and straining. Dysentery is common when sanitary living conditions, clean food, and safe water are not available. See also **amebic dysentery, shigellosis.**

dysesthesia /dis′esthē′zhə/, a common result of spinal cord injury, it consists of numbness, tingling, burning, or pain felt below the injury.

dysfunctional, unable to function normally, as a body organ or system. **–dysfunction,** *n.*

dysfunctional communication, a communication that results from inaccurate perception, faulty interpretations of information, and social isolation. Such communications are typical of emotionally ill persons and may prevent such patients from forming and maintaining relationships.

dysfunctional stereotype, a preconceived opinion (stereotype) that emphasizes the negative elements of a culture. For example, an Anglo person may perceive all Hispanic men in terms of the machismo ethic.

dysfunctional thought record, in psychology, a treatment technique in which a patient records his or her thoughts when a strong emotion is felt. The therapist and patient then review the record to find the causes of the thoughts and consider whether they are accurate.

dysfunctional uterine bleeding (DUB), uterine bleeding as a result of hormone imbalance rather than a disease.

dysgammaglobulinemia /disgam′əglob′yəlinē′mē·ə/, an inherited immune-deficiency disease. Patients have blood disorders and tend to have repeated infections. The cause is failure to produce substances needed to fight infections.

dysgenesis /disjen′əsis/, **1.** defective formation of an organ or part, primarily during early fetal (embryonic) development. Also called **dysgenesia. 2.** loss of the ability to reproduce. A kind of dysgenesis is **gonadal dysgenesis.** Compare **agenesis. –dysgenic,** *adj.*

dysgenitalism /disjen′itəliz′əm/, any condition involving the abnormal growth of the genital organs.

dysgerminoma, *pl.* **dysgerminomas, dysgerminomata,** a rare cancerous tumor of the ovary found in young women. Also called **embryoma of the ovary, ovarian seminoma.**

dysgraphia /disgraf′ē·ə/, a blockage of the ability to write, caused by a disease process.

dyshidrosis /dis′hidrō′sis, dis′hī-/, a condition in which abnormal sweating occurs.

dyskeratosis /dis′kerətō′sis/, an abnormal or too-early change of skin cells to keratin that may cause the skin to waste and become heavily pigmented. It can also cause mucous membranes to thicken and the eyes to become light-sensitive.

dyskinesia /dis′kinē′zhə/, impaired ability to make voluntary movements. **–dyskinetic** /-et′ik/, *adj.*

dyskinetic syndrome, a type of cerebral palsy involving a brain disorder. Patients have unusual movements of the arms, legs, and sometimes the trunk of the body. The movements tend to increase with emotional tension and decrease during sleep.

dyslexia /dislek′sē·ə/, a blockage of the ability to read, as a result of a variety of disorders, some of which are linked to the central nervous system. Dyslexic persons often reverse letters and words. They cannot determine the order of letters in written words. They also have difficulty determining left from right. Some reading experts believe the condition is a combination of reading problems. Compare **alexia. –dyslexic,** *adj.*

dysmaturity, 1. the failure of an organism to develop, ripen, or otherwise mature in structure or function. **2.** a fetus or newborn who is abnormally small or large for the length of pregnancy (age of gestation).

dysmelia /dismē'lyə/, a birth defect marked by missing or shortened arms and legs. This is linked to abnormalities of the spine in some individuals. See also **phocomelia.**

dysmenorrhea /dis'menərē'ə/, pain linked to menstruation. Primary dysmenorrhea is menstrual pain that results from the shape of the uterus and the process of menstruation. It is extremely common, occurring at least occasionally in almost all women. If the painful episode is mild and brief, it is thought normal and requires no treatment. In about 10% of women, dysmenorrhea is severe enough to cause episodes of partial or total disability. The cause in most cases is poorly understood. Various physical, nervous system, hormone, and psychological abnormalities have been suggested. Pain occurs typically in the lower stomach or back and is crampy. It comes in successive waves — apparently with intense uterine contractions and slight widening of the lower narrow end of the uterus. Pain usually begins just before, or at the beginning of, menstrual flow. It lasts from a few hours to one day or more. The pain may continue through the entire period. Pain is often linked to nausea, vomiting, and frequent bowel movements with intestinal cramping. Dizziness, fainting, paleness, and obvious distress may also occur. Treatment with an antiprostaglandin drug gives relief for many women if begun 1 to 3 days premenstrually and continued through the first day of the period. Oral contraceptives are also effective for many women. They are taken through the full monthly cycle. Strong painkillers or narcotics may be required. Secondary dysmenorrhea is menstrual pain that is caused by specific pelvic abnormalities, as abnormal tissue growth in the uterus (endometriosis, adenomyosis), long-term pelvic infection, chronic pelvic congestion, or fibroid tumors. Typically, the pain begins earlier in the cycle and lasts longer than the pain of primary dysmenorrhea. Painful bowel or bladder function may accompany the condition, depending on the location of the problem.

dysmetria /dismet'rē·ə/, an abnormal condition that prevents the affected person from properly estimating distances linked to muscular movements, as reaching for an object. See also **hypermetria, hypometria.**

dysmnesia. See **dysmnesic syndrome.**

dysmnesic syndrome /disne'sik/, a memory disorder in which the patient cannot learn simple new skills. The patient can, however, perform complex skills learned before the condition began. The disorder is caused by a disease or injury that affects brain tissues responsible for memory. The patient may make up stories about the recent past for which he or she has no memory. Also called **dysmnesia.**

dysmorphogenesis /dis'môrfōjen'əsis/, the development of ill-shaped or otherwise poorly formed body structures.

dysmorphophobia /dis'môrfō-/, **1.** a basic delusion of body image. **2.** the morbid fear of deformity or of becoming deformed.

dysostosis /dis'ostō'sis/, an abnormal condition marked by defective bone formation (ossification), especially by defects in the normal ossification of fetal cartilages.

dyspareunia /dis'pəroo'nē·ə/, an abnormal condition of women in which sexual intercourse is painful. The pain may result from abnormal conditions of the genitals, a psychological reaction to sexual union, rape, or incomplete sexual arousal. See also **vaginismus.**

dyspepsia /dispep'sē·ə/, a vague feeling of discomfort under the breastbone after eating. There is an uncomfortable feeling of fullness, heartburn, bloating, and nausea. Dyspepsia is not a distinct condition, but it may be a symptom of underlying intestinal disorder, as peptic ulcer, gallbladder disease, or long-term swelling of the appendix (appendicitis). **–dyspeptic,** *adj.*

dysphagia /disfā'jē·ə/, difficulty in swallowing, commonly linked to blockage or motor disorders of the esophagus. Patients with blockages as esophageal tumor or lower esophageal ring are unable to swallow solids but can tolerate liquids. Patients with motor disorders, as muscle problems related to esophagus (achalasia), are unable to swallow solids or liquids. See also **achalasia, aphagia, corkscrew esophagus.**

dysphagia lusoria, an abnormal condition marked by difficulty in swallowing and caused by compression of the esophagus from an abnormally placed right subclavian artery.

dysphasia /disfā'zhə/, difficulty speaking, not as severe as aphasia. It is usually the result of an injury to the speech area of the brain. Dysphasia is marked by lack of coordination in speaking and getting words out of order. It may follow a stroke or brain tumor and may go along with other language disorders, such as inability to write (dysgraphia).

dysphonia, an abnormality in the speaking voice, as hoarseness. Dysphonia puberum refers to the voice change that takes place in teen-age boys.

dysphoria, a disorder of mood. Patients feel depression and anguish.

dysplasia /displā'zhə/, an abnormal development of the body's tissues or organs, such as dwarfism.

dyspnea /dispnē'ə/, a shortness of breath or a difficulty in breathing, it may be caused by certain heart conditions, strenuous exercise, or anxiety. Compare **hyperpnea.** **–dyspneal, dyspneic,** *adj.*

dyspraxia /disprak'sē·ə/, a partial loss of the ability to perform skilled, coordinated movements. See also **apraxia.**

dysprosium (Dy), a rare earth metallic element. Its atomic number is 66; its atomic weight is 162.50. Radioactive isotopes of dysprosium are used in studies of the bones and joints.

dysproteinemia /disprō'tēnē'mē·ə/, an abnormality of the protein content of the blood.

dysraphic syndrome, a developmental problem involving the spinal cord. The neural tube of the fetus fails to fuse properly. See also **Arnold-Chiari syndrome.**

dysreflexia /dis'riflek'sē·ə/, an abnormal nerve or muscle condition, marked by abnormal reflexes. **–dysreflexic,** *adj.*

dysrhythmia /disrith'mē·ə/, any abnormality in a normal rhythmic pattern. This especially refers to irregularity in the brain waves or pattern of speech. Compare **arrhythmia.**

dyssebacea /disibā'shē·ə/, a skin condition marked by red, scaly, greasy patches on the nose, eyelids, scrotum, and lips. It results from a lack of vitamin B$_2$ and is most commonly seen in persons with long-term alcoholism, liver disease, long-term diarrhea, and protein malnutrition. Also called *(informal)* **shark skin.**

dysthymia /disthim'ē·ə/, a form of long-lasting depression that occurs in elderly people. Patients usually have physical disorders, loss of many loved ones, and long-term marital problems. Several episodes of depression may merge into chronic depression. The condition is sometimes treated with drugs.

dystocia /distō'shē·ə/, a difficult labor, it may be caused by an blockage or narrowing of the birth passage or an abnormal size, shape, or position, of the fetus.

dystonia, an impairment of muscle tone, often affecting the head, neck, and tongue. It is often a side effect of medication.

dystonia musculorum deformans /distō'nē·ə/, a rare genetic disorder marked by intense, irregular muscle spasms that contort the body. The muscles of the trunk, shoulder, and pelvis are commonly involved. The cause of this disorder is not known, but a biochemical dysfunction is suspected. The non-sex related form appears most often in Ashkenazic Jews. It starts between the ages of 5 and 15. It commonly begins with intermittent, spasmodic inversion of the foot, so that the patient has difficulty placing the heel on the ground when walking and develops an odd, bowing walk.

dystonic, referring to an excessive increase in muscle tone, often resulting in abnormal posture.

dystrophic calcification, the pooling of calcium salts in dead or broken-down tissues. Compare **metastatic calcification.**

dystrophy /dis'trəfē/, any abnormal condition caused by defective nutrition. The term is often applied to a change in muscles that does not involve the nervous system, as fatty break down linked to increased muscle size but decreased strength. Also called **dystrophia.** **–dystrophic** /distrof'ik/, *adj.*

dysuria /disyŏor'ē·ə/, painful urination, usually the result of a bacterial infection or blockage in the urinary tract. Dysuria is a symptom of such conditions as inflammation of the urine bladder (cyctitis), swelling of the urethra (urethritis), swelling of the prostate (prostatitis), urinary tract tumors, and some gynecological disorders. Compare **hematuria, pyuria.**

E

E, symbol for **expired gas.**

ear, the organ of hearing. The ear has three parts: the inner, middle, and outer ear. The outer ear is both the skin-covered cartilage that sticks out on either side of the head and the tube that leads from the outside of the head to the eardrum. The two parts of the outer ear focus sound waves on the eardrum. The middle ear, the space between the eardrum and the inner ear, is filled with air and holds three small bones called the hammer (malleus), anvil (incus), and stirrup (stapes). These bones pick up the vibrations caused by sound waves hitting the eardrum. The bones pass the vibrations on to the inner ear, which is filled with fluid and holds two organs. One of the organs gives a sense of balance (vestibular apparatus), the other picks up the sound vibrations from the inner ear fluid and carries them to the nerve endings that sense sounds.

earache, a pain in the ear that may be sharp, dull, burning, on and off, or constant. The cause does not have to be a disease of the ear, because infections and other disorders of the nose, mouth, throat, and jaw joint can cause pain in the ear. Infection of the ear, **otitis media,** can cause earache. Also called **otalgia, otodynia.**

eardrops, a liquid drug for treating various conditions of the ear, including inflammation or infection or hardened wax.

eardrum. See **tympanic membrane.**

Early and Periodic Screening Diagnosis and Treatment (EPSDT), a section of the Medicaid program that requires all states to run a program to determine the physical and mental defects of persons under 21 who are covered by the program and to provide short- and long-range treatment. See also **Medicaid.**

earth bath, covering a part of the body with warm sand or earth.

earwax. See **cerumen.**

eastern equine encephalitis. See **equine encephalitis.**

Eaton-agent pneumonia. See **mycoplasma pneumonia.**

Ebbecke's reaction. See **dermatographia.**

EBV, abbreviation for **Epstein-Barr virus.**

ec-, a combining form meaning 'out of.'

eccentric implantation, rooting of the fertilized egg in a fold of the wall of the womb (uterus). The fold then closes off from the main cavity.

eccentricity, behavior that is seen as odd or peculiar for a given culture or community, although not unusual enough to be considered dangerous or insane.

ecchondroma /ek′əndrō′mə/, a harmless tumor that grows on the surface of a cartilage or under bone covering (periosteum).

ecchymosis /ek′imō′sis/, *pl.* **ecchymoses,** darkening of an area of the skin or mucous membrane caused by blood leaking into the tissues under the skin. It occurs as a result of damage to the blood vessels or by brittle vessel walls. Also called **bruise.** Compare **contusion, petechiae.**

eccrine /ek′rin/, meaning a sweat gland that releases fluid through a duct to the surface of the skin. See also **exocrine.**

eccrine gland, one of two kinds of sweat glands in the skin. These glands are unbranched, coiled, and tubelike, and they are found throughout the skin covering of the body. They cool the body by evaporation of the fluid they release (sweat), which is clear, has a faint odor, and contains water, sodium chloride, and traces of albumin, urea, and other compounds. Compare **apocrine gland.**

eccyesis. See **ectopic pregnancy.**

ECG, **1.** abbreviation for **electrocardiogram. 2.** abbreviation for **electrocardiograph.**

echino-, a combining form meaning spines, or spiny.

echinococcosis /ekī′nōkokō′sis/, an attack, usually of the liver, by the larval stage of a tapeworm of the genus *Echinococcus.* Dogs are the main hosts of the adult worm. Sheep, cattle, rodents, and deer are the natural hosts for the larvae. Humans, especially children, can be attacked by larvae by swallowing eggs, which are shed in the stool of infected dogs. The disease is most common in countries where animals are raised with the help of dogs. Removal of the cysts is the only treatment. Also called **hydatid disease, hydatidosis.** See also **cysticercosis, tapeworm infection.**

Echinococcus /ekī′nōkok′əs/, a genus of small tapeworms that infects mostly dogs. See also **echinococcosis, hydatid cyst.**

echo beat, a heart beat that is restarted when an electric impulse returns to one of the chambers of the heart.

echocardiography /ek′ōkär′dē·og′rəfē/, a method of diagnosis that studies the structure and motion of the heart. Ultrasonic waves directed through the heart are reflected backward, or echoed, when they pass from one type of tissue to another, as from heart muscle to blood. This test can find tumors in the upper chambers and fluid in the sac around the heart (pericardial effusion). It can measure the parts of the lower chambers (ventricles) and spot problems with the movement of the valve between the upper and lower chambers on the left side of the heart (mitral valve). Also called **ultrasonic**

cardiography. See also **phonocardiograph, ultrasonography.**

echoencephalography /ek′ō·ensef′əlog′rəfē/, the use of ultrasound to study the brain. The method is useful for showing widening of the hollows (ventricles) and a major shift of the tissues between the hollows as a result of a growing tumor. See also **ultrasonography.** – **echoencephalographic,** *adj.*

echolalia /ek′ōlā′lyə/, **1.** also called **echophrasia, echo speech.** the automatic and meaningless repeating of another's words or phrases, especially as seen in schizophrenia. **2.** a baby's imitation of words produced by others. It occurs normally in early childhood development. –**echolalic,** *adj.*

echopraxia /ek′ōprak′sē·ə/, imitation of the body movements of another person, a behavior shown by some schizophrenic patients.

echoradiography /ek′ōrā′dē·og′rəfē/, a method of diagnosis using ultrasonography and various devices for visualizing inner parts of the body.

echothiophate iodide, a drug for the eyes used for long-term, open-angle glaucoma and some forms of crossed eyes. Patients with eye swelling, most types of open-angle glaucoma, or known allergy to this drug should not take it. Reactions to this drug include retinal detachment, nonreversible cataract, lens thickening, eye swelling, and cysts of the eyes.

echovirus /ek′ōvī′rəs/, a picornavirus linked to other infections. There are many echoviruses, and most are harmless. Bacterial or viral disease may be found with echovirus infection, as seen in aseptic meningitis that comes with some severe bacterial and viral infections.

eclampsia /iklamp′sē·ə/, the gravest form of poisoning of pregnancy, marked by grand mal convulsion, coma, high blood pressure, water retention, and protein in the urine. The symptoms of coming convulsions often include anxiety, pain under the breastbone, headache, blurred vision, continual and extremely high blood pressure, and increasingly overactive reflexes. Convulsions may be prevented by bed rest in a quiet, dimly lit room and by injecting a calming drug into the muscles. Treatment of a convulsion must include keeping the mother's airway open, protecting her against injury, and giving drugs to stop the convulsion and lower the blood pressure. Once this is done, the child can be born. Convulsions rarely happen after the child has been born. Eclampsia occurs in 0.2% of pregnancies, and the cause is not known.

ecology, the study of the interaction between living organisms and the various influences of their environment.

econazole, a drug that destroys fungus and is used to treat ringworm, candidiasis, and other fungus infections. Patients who are allergic to

this drug should not use it. Among the most serious reactions to the drug are skin irritation and allergy.

ecstasy, an emotional state marked by exultation, extreme delight, or frenzy. Compare **euphoria, mania.** –**ecstatic,** *adj.*

ECT, abbreviation for **electroconvulsive therapy.**

ecthyma /ek′thimə/, a deep form of impetigo marked by large boils, crusts, and sores circled by red skin. Staphylococci and streptococci bacteria are the cause. The skin of the legs is most often affected. Treatment includes rigid cleaning, wet bandages soaked with cool Burow's solution to soften and remove crusts, and drugs given by mouth or by shot. Compare **folliculitis, impetigo.**

ecto-, a combining form meaning 'outside.'

ectoderm, the outer of the three main cell layers of a young fetus (embryo). The ectoderm makes the nervous system; the organs of special sense, as the eyes and ears; the epidermis, and epidermal tissue, as fingernails, hair, and skin glands; and the mucous membranes of the mouth and anus. See also **embryo, endoderm, mesoderm.** –**ectodermal, ectodermic,** *adj.*

ectodermal cloaca, a part of the gut (cloaca) in the growing embryo that gives rise to the anus and anal canal. Compare **endodermal cloaca.**

ectomorph /ek′təmôrf′/, a person whose body is slender and fragile and whose most distinct parts are grown from the ectoderm. Compare **endomorph, mesomorph.** See also **asthenic habitus.**

ectoparasite /ek′tōper′əsīt/, an organism that lives on the outside of the body of the host, as a louse.

ectopic /ektop′ik/, **1.** referring to an object or organ located in an unusual place, away from its normal area. For example, an ectopic pregnancy is one that occurs outside the uterus. **2.** referring to an event occurring at the wrong time, as a premature heart beat.

ectopic pregnancy, an abnormal pregnancy in which the fertilized egg settles outside the womb (uterus). Kinds of ectopic pregnancy are **abdominal pregnancy, ovarian pregnancy, tubal pregnancy.** Also called **eccyesis** /ek′sī·ē′sis/.

ectrodactyly /ek′trōdak′təlē/, a birth defect marked by the lack of part or all of one or more fingers or toes. Also called **ectrodactylia, ectrodactylism.**

ectromelia /ek′trōmē′lē·ə/, a birth defect marked by the lack or faulty growth of the long bones of one or more of the arms or legs. Kinds of ectromelia are **amelia, hemimelia, phocomelia.** –**ectromelic,** *adj.,* **ectromelus,** *n.*

ectropion /ektrō′pē·on/, turning outward of an edge (eversion). The term usually refers to the eyelid, in which the lining of the eyelid is exposed. The condition may involve only the lower eyelid or both eyelids. The cause may be paralysis of the facial nerve or, in an older

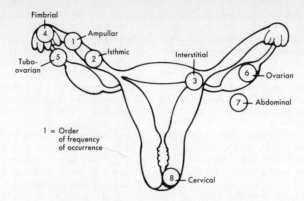

Fimbrial

Ampullar

Isthmic

Interstitial

Tubo-
ovarian

Ovarian

Abdominal

1 = Order
of frequency
of occurrence

Cervical

Ectopic pregnancy implantation sites

person, changes in the skin from aging. Compare **entropion.**

ECU, abbreviation for **extended care unit.**

eczema /ek'simə/, swelling of the outer skin of unknown cause. In the early stage it may be itchy, red, have small blisters, and be swollen, and weeping. Later it becomes crusted, scaly, and thickened. Eczema is not a distinct disease. See also **atopic dermatitis, nummular dermatitis.** **–eczematous,** *adj.*

eczema herpeticum, a skin disease with pus-filled blisters, it is caused by herpes simplex virus or vaccinia virus infection of a rash already present on the patient. Hospitalization is advised because this disease can be fatal. Also called **Kaposi's varicelliform eruption.**

eczematous conjunctivitis, swelling of eye tissue found along with many tiny open sores. The cause is thought to be a delayed allergic reaction to bacterial protein. If not treated, the disease may lead to ingrowth of small blood vessels in the cornea, eventually blocking sight.

ED, abbreviation for **effective dose.**

ED50, symbol for **median effective dose.**

EDB, abbreviation for **ethylene dibromide.**

EDC, abbreviation for **expected date of confinement.**

Edecrin, a trademark for a diuretic (ethacrynic acid).

edema /idē'mə/, the abnormal pooling of fluid in tissues. Edema may be caused by increased pressure in the capillaries, blocking of a vein (as in varicose veins, thrombophlebitis, or pressure from casts, tight bandages, or garters), congestive heart failure, kidney failure, liver cirrhosis, overactive adrenal glands (as in Cushing's syndrome), steroid therapy, and inflammatory reactions. Edema may also occur because of loss of serum protein in burns, draining wounds, excessive bleeding, nephrotic syndrome, or chronic diarrhea. Edema is seen in malnutrition, in allergic reactions, and in

blockage of lymph vessels caused by cancer or worms. Treatment of edema is directed at correcting the basic cause. Some drugs may be given to promote the removal of sodium and water. When a limb has edema because blood is pooling in a vein, raising the limb and wrapping it with an elastic stocking or sleeve helps the fluid move back into the vein and return to the heart. See also **anasarca, lymphedema.** **–edematous, edematose,** *adj.*

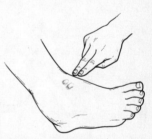

Pitting edema

edentulous /ēden'chələs/, toothless.

edetate disodium, a drug used to treat a serious condition resulting from excess calcium. It is also used for irregular heart beats and heart block resulting from reaction to the drug digitalis, and for lead poisoning.

★CAUTION: Patients who have low levels of calcium, kidney disease, or known allergy to this drug should not use it.

★ADVERSE EFFECTS: Among the more serious side effects to the drug are low levels of calcium, swelling of a vein linked to clotting, kidney damage, and excess bleeding linked to lowered ability of the blood to clot.

EDG, abbreviation for **electrodynogram.**

edge response function (ERF), the ability of a CT scan system to show a high-contrast edge, for example, the edge of the heart in contrast to nearby organs.

edgewise-fixed orthodontic appliance, an orthodontic appliance used to correct or improve a bad bite.

edrophonium chloride, a drug that acts to cancel the effect of the drug curare and is an aid in the diagnosis of myasthenia gravis. It is also used to treat severe reactions to curare and to slow rapid heart beats.

★CAUTION: Patients who have a blocked stomach or intestines, blocked kidneys or bladder, or who have low blood pressure, slow heart beats, or known allergy to this drug should not use it.

★ADVERSE EFFECTS: Among the most serious side effects are stopping of breathing, low blood pressure, slow heart beats, and spasms of the air passages.

Edsall's disease, a cramping condition that is the result of excess exposure to heat. Also called **heat cramp.**

Edwards' syndrome. See **trisomy 18.**

EEE. See **equine encephalitis.**

EEG, 1. abbreviation for **electroencephalogram.** **2.** abbreviation for **electroencephalography.**

effacement, the shortening of the cervix and thinning of its walls as it is stretched and widened by the fetus during labor. See also **birth, cervix, dilatation, station.**

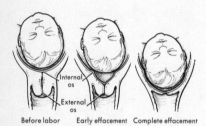

Internal os

External os

Before labor   Early effacement   Complete effacement

Cervical effacement

effective dose (ED), the dose of a drug that may be expected to have a specific effect.

effective half-life (ehl), the time needed for a radioactive element in an animal body to be diminished 50% as a result of the combined action of radioactive decay and biological elimination. See also **biologic half-life.**

efferent /ef'ərənt/, directed away from a center, as certain arteries, veins, nerves, and lymph channels. Compare **afferent.**

efferent duct, any duct through which a gland releases its fluids.

efficacy /ef'əkəsē/, the greatest ability of a drug or treatment to produce a result, regardless of dosage. Narcotics have a nearly identical effi-cacy but need various dosages to obtain the effect.

effleurage /ef'ləräzh'/, a method in massage in which long, light, or firm strokes are used, usually over the spine and back. Fingertip effleurage is a light technique done with the tips of the fingers in a circle pattern over one part of the body or in long strokes over the back or an arm, leg, hand or foot. Compare **pétrissage, rolling effleurage.**

effort syndrome, an abnormal condition marked by chest pain, dizziness, fatigue, and rapid, uneven heart beat. This condition is often found in soldiers in combat but occurs also in other persons. The symptoms of effort syndrome often mimic angina pectoris but are really anxiety states. Effort syndrome differs from angina pectoris because it includes cold, moist hands, sighing breaths, and chest pain after, rather than during, exercise. Also called **neurocirculatory asthenia.**

effusion, 1. the escape of fluid from blood vessels because of break or leaking, usually into a body hollow. The condition is usually a circulation or kidney disease and is often an early sign of heart disease. The term may be linked to an affected body area, as pleural effusion. See also **edema, transudate. 2.** the outward spread of a bacterial growth.

Efudex, a trademark for a drug used to treat cancer (fluorouracil).

egest /ijest'/, to release a substance from the body, especially to pass unabsorbed foods from the intestines. **–egesta,** *n. pl.,* **egestive,** *adj.*

ego /ē'gō, eg'ō/, **1.** the conscious sense of the self; those elements of a person, as thinking and feeling, that mark the person as an individual. **2.** the part of the self that experiences and maintains conscious contact with reality and which balances the primitive drives of the id and the demands of the superego with the social and physical needs of society. See also **id, superego.**

ego analysis, the intensive study of the ego.

ego boundary, a sense or awareness that there is a difference between the self and others. In some psychoses the person does not have an ego boundary and cannot tell the difference between his or her own personal feelings and other people's feelings.

egocentric, 1. seeing the self as the center of all experience and having little regard for the needs, interests, ideas, and attitudes of others. **2.** a person having these traits.

ego-defense mechanism. See **defense mechanism.**

ego-dystonic /ē'gōdiston'ik/, referring to the elements of a person's behavior, thoughts, and attitudes that are at odds with the standards of the ego and do not fit in with the total personality.

ego ideal, the image of the self which a person strives to be both consciously and unconsciously and against which he or she measures him or herself. It is usually based on a positive identification with the important and influential figures of early childhood years. See also **identification.**

egoism /ē'gō·iz'əm, eg'-/, **1.** an exaggeration of the importance of the self that takes the form of a willingness to gain an advantage at the expense of others. See also **egotism. 2.** the belief that individual self-interest is, or ought to be, the basic motive for all conscious behavior.

egoist /ē'gō·ist, eg'-/, **1.** a person who seeks to satisfy his or her own interests at the expense of others. **2.** a person who believes in the concept that all conscious action is justifiably motivated by self-interest. **–egoistic, egoistical,** *adj.*

ego libido, focusing of the sexual interest (libido) on the self; self-love, narcissism.

egomania, an extreme, long-term focus on the self and magnified sense of one's own importance.

ego strength, the ability to keep up the ego by a group of traits that together contribute to good mental health.

ego-syntonic /ē'gōsinton'ik/, referring to those elements of a person's behavior, thoughts, and attitudes that agree with the standards of the ego and are in line with the total personality. Compare **ego-dystonic.**

egotism /ē'gətiz'əm, eg'-/, a magnifying the importance of the self and the contempt of others. See also **egoism.**

egotist /ē'gətist, eg'-/, one who places too much importance on the self and is boastful, self-centered and arrogant.

egress /ē'gres/, the act of coming out or moving forward.

Egyptian ophthalmia. See **trachoma.**

Ehlers-Danlos syndrome /ā'lərzdan'ləs/, a hereditary tissue disease, marked by extremely stretchy skin, fragile tissue, and joints that allow bones to move too far in one or more directions. Minor injury may cause a large wound with little bleeding. Sprains, joint dislocations, and fluid pooling in the joints (synovial effusions) are common. Patients who have this condition usually live a normal length of time.

eicosansoic acid /ī'kōsənō'ik/, a type of fatty acid found in peanut oil, butter, and other fats.

eidetic /īdet'ik/, **1.** referring to the ability to visualize and reproduce accurately the image of objects or events previously seen. **2.** a person possessing such ability.

eidetic image, an unusually vivid, elaborate, and apparently exact mental image coming from a visual experience and happening as a fantasy, dream, or memory. See also **image.**

eighth cranial nerve. See **acoustic nerve.**

einsteinium (Es) /īnstī'nē·əm/, an artificial metallic element.

ejaculate /ijak'yəlit/, the semen released at one time. See also **ejaculation. –ejaculate** /ijak'yəlāt/, *v.*

ejaculation, the sudden release of semen from the male urethra, usually happening during intercourse, masturbation, and sleep (nocturnal emission). It is a reflex action in two phases: First, sperm fluid and releases from the prostate and bulbourethral gland are moved into the urethra; second, strong spasms (peristaltic) force ejaculation. The feeling of ejaculation is called orgasm. The fluid volume is usually less than 0.2 ounces (2 to 5 ml). Each milliliter usually contains 50 million to 150 million sperm. **–ejaculatory** /ijak'yələtôr'ē/, *adj.*

ejaculatory duct, the passage through which semen enters the urethra.

ejection clicks, sharp clicking sounds from the heart, which may be caused by the sudden swelling of a pulmonary artery, the abrupt widening of the large artery (aorta), or the forceful opening of the aortic valves (cusps). See also **ejection sounds.**

ejection fraction (EF), the proportion of blood that is released during each contraction of the lower heart chamber (ventricle) compared with the total volume of blood released by both ventricles.

ejection murmur. See **systolic murmur.**

ejection sounds, sharp clicking sounds heard early in contraction of the lower left ventricle (systole). They coincide with the beginning of either right or left ventricular systolic ejection and reflect either widening of the pulmonary artery or aorta, or the presence of valve problems. See also **ejection clicks.**

Ekbom syndrome. See **restless legs syndrome.**

EKG, abbreviation for **electrocardiogram.**

elaborate, a process by which a gland makes a complex substance from simpler substances. **–elaboration,** *n.*

Elase, a trademark for a combination drug containing enzymes (fibrinolysin and desoxyribonuclease). It is put on the skin to cure many infections and types of swelling.

elastance, 1. the quality of returning to an original form after pressure is removed. **2.** the degree to which an air-filled or fluid-filled organ, as a lung, bladder, or blood vessel, can return to its original size and shape when a force that widens or squeezes it is removed.

elastic bandage, a bandage of stretchy fabric that gives support and allows movement.

elastic band fixation, a method of treating breaks of the jaw using rubber bands to join metal splints or wires that are attached to the upper and lower jaws. The rubber bands pull the jaws together and align the teeth properly while the break heels. Rubber bands are thought to be safer than rigid wires.

elastic cartilage. See **yellow cartilage.**

elasticity, the ability of tissue to regain its original shape and size after being stretched or squeezed. Muscle tissue is generally thought of as elastic, because it is able to change size and shape and return to its original state.

elastin /ilas'tin/, a protein that forms the main part of yellow elastic tissue fibers.

elation, an emotion marked by extreme vigor, excitement, extreme joyfulness, optimism, and self satisfaction. It is considered to be abnormal when such an emotion does not realistically reflect a person's actual state.

Elavil, a trademark for an antidepressant drug.

elbow, the bend of the arm at the joint that connects the upper arm and forearm. It is a common site of swelling and injuries, especially injuries from playing sports. See also **elbow joint.**

elbow bone. See **ulna.**

elbow joint, the hinged joint of the arm. The bone of the upper arm (humerus) and the two bones of the forearm (ulna and radius) join at the elbow. The elbow joint allows the forearm to bend and extend and to roll from side to side. Also called **articulatio cubiti.**

elbow reflex. See **triceps reflex.**

Eldopaque, a trademark for a skin bleaching drug (hydroquinone).

elective, referring to a treatment done by choice but not required, as elective surgery.

elective abortion, ending a pregnancy, by choice, usually before the fetus has developed enough to live if born. It is chosen by the pregnant woman and performed at her request. Commonly (but incorrectly) called **therapeutic abortion.** See also **induced abortion, therapeutic abortion.**

elective induction of labor. See **induction of labor.**

electrically stimulated osteogenesis, a process of causing bone growth (osteogenesis) by implanting electrodes that send electric current to the bone. This is used for breaks that don't heal.

electric blood warmer, an electric device for heating blood before giving it in the vein. It is used for massive transfusions in which cold blood might put the patient into shock. The electric blood warmer has an electric heater and space for setting a disposable blood warming bag. The warmer also has a thermometer, which shows when the heating bag reaches the proper temperature of 99° F (37.6° C).

electric burns, the tissue damage that results from heat of up to 5,000° C given off by an electric current. The point of contact on the skin is burned, and the muscle and tissues under the skin may be hurt. If the burn is severe, circulatory and respiratory failure may occur and are treated before the burn. In this case, artificial respiration and cardiac resuscitation are performed as the person is taken rapidly to a medical facility.

electric cautery. See **electrocautery.**

electric shock, a damaged physical state caused by electric current passing through the body. It usually occurs from accidental contact with exposed parts of electric circuits in home appliances and power supplies. It may also result from lightning or contact with high-voltage wires. About 1,000 persons in the United States die from electric shock each year. The damage electricity does in passing through the body depends on the intensity of the electric current. Alternating current (AC), direct current (DC), and mixed current cause different kinds and degrees of damage in passing through body tissues. High-frequency current (measured in Hz, or Hertz) gives off more heat than low-frequency current and can cause burns, blood clotting, and tissue death. Low-frequency current can burn tissues if the area of contact is small and focused. Severe electric shock commonly causes unconsciousness, stopping of breathing, muscle spasms, bone breaks, and heart disorders. Even small electric currents passing through the heart can cause dangerously rapid heart beats. Treatment of severe electric shock commonly involves such measures as cardiopulmonary resuscitation, defibrillation, and giving electrolytes in the vein to help bring vital functions back to normal levels. See also **cardiogenic shock, hypovolemic shock.**

electric shock therapy. See **electroconvulsive therapy.**

electric spinal orthosis, an electric device that helps control curving of the spine (scoliosis) by stimulating the back muscles. The portable, battery-powered machine does not correct scoliosis, but it does stop the condition from getting worse.

electro-, a combining form meaning electricity.

electrocardiogram (ECG, EKG), a picture record made by an electrocardiograph.

electrocardiograph (ECG), a device used to record the electric activity of the heart to detect abnormal electric impulses through the muscle. Electrocardiography allows diagnosis of cardiac abnormalities. To make an ECG recording, the patient lies quietly on his or her back on a table. Leads are placed on certain spots on the patient's chest, usually with a gluey gel that helps send the electric impulse to the recording device. The ECG is also used for stress tests, which require that the patient be active (usually walking or running on a treadmill) while the machine is working. –**electrocardiographic,** *adj.*

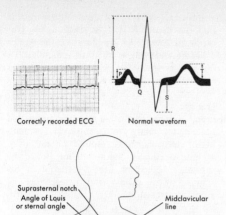

Correctly recorded ECG   Normal waveform

Suprasternal notch
Angle of Louis
or sternal angle

Midclavicular
line

Second rib
Second interspace

V_1
V_2
V_3
V_4
V_5
V_6

Landmarks for ECG 6-lead placement

Electrocardiogram (ECG)

electrocardiograph lead, 1. an electrode placed on part of the body and linked to an electrocardiograph. 2. a record, made by the electrocardiograph, that varies depending on the site of the electrode. Electrocardiography is generally performed with six leads placed over the heart and three leads placed at different points (one on each upper arm and one below a knee is common).

electrocautery /ilek′trōkô′tərē/, placing a needle that is heated by electric current on tissue. This destroys the tissue. The method is often used to remove warts or polyps. Also called **electric cautery, galvanic cautery, galvanocautery.** See also **diathermy.**

electrocoagulation /ilek′trōko·ag′yŏŏlā′shən/, a form of surgery in which tissue is hardened by high-frequency current from an electric cautery device through it. Also called **surgical diathermy.** Compare **electrodesiccation.**

electroconvulsive therapy (ECT), causing a brief convulsion by passing an electric current through the brain. It is used to treat some mental disorders, especially in patients who have not been helped by drug therapy. The patient has no memory of the shock. A side effect is both long-term and short-term memory loss. Also called **electric shock therapy, electroshock therapy.**

electrocution, death caused by an electric current passing through the body. See also **electric shock.**

electrode /ilek′trōd/, 1. a contact for bringing on or recording electric activity. 2. a substance that conducts an electric current from the body to measuring equipment.

electrodermal audiometry, a method of testing hearing in which a harmless electric shock is used to condition the subject to a pure tone. After that, the tone, coupled with the anticipation of a shock, causes a brief electric impulse in the skin. This is recorded, and the lowest intensity of the sound that produces the skin response is called the subject's hearing threshold.

electrodesiccation /ilek′trōdes′ikā′shən/, a technique in surgery in which tissue is burned away with an electric spark. It is used mainly for removing small surface growths and may also be used to remove abnormal tissue deep in the skin, in which case layers of skin are burned, then scraped away. The burning is done under local anesthesia.

electrodynograph (EDG) /ilek′trōdin′əgraf′/, an electronic device used to measure pressures made by the body as it moves. An EDG can measure pressures put forth by the human foot in walking, running, jogging, or climbing stairs.

electroencephalogram (EEG) /ilek′trō·en-sef′ələgram′/, a chart of the electric impulses made by the brain cells, as picked up by electrodes placed on the scalp. The brain waves recorded are called alpha, beta, delta, and theta rhythms, according to the frequencies they produce. Changes in brain-wave activity can show nervous system disorders, mental states, and level of consciousness. See also **encephalography.**

electroencephalograph /ilek′trō·ensef′ələgraf′/, an instrument that receives and records the electric impulses produced by the brain cells. It is a vacuum tube amplifier that magnifies the electric currents received by electrodes on the scalp. It then records the patterns on a chart. See also **electroencephalography.**

electroencephalography (EEG) /ilek′trō·ensef′əlog′rəfē/, the process of recording brain-wave activity. Electrodes are attached to areas of the patient's head. During the procedure the patient remains quiet, with eyes closed, and does not talk or move. In certain cases, however, some activities may be done, as breathing rapidly. The test is used to diagnose seizure disorders, brainstem disorders, tumors or clots, and impaired consciousness. During surgery on the nervous system, the electrodes can be set directly on the brain (intracranial electroencephalography) or placed within the brain tissue (depth electroencephalography) to detect injury or tumors. See also **electroencephalogram.** —**electroencephalographic,** *adj.*

electrogram /ilek'trōgram'/, record of electric activity of the heart as sensed by electrodes inside the heart chambers or on the surface of the heart.

electrohemodynamics (EHD) /ilek'trōhē'mō-dīnam'iks/,a method for measuring the workings of the blood-flow system of the body. This measures blood pressure in the arteries, the strength of nerve impulses, blood flow, and the ability of the system to hold and direct flowing blood.

electrohydraulic heart, a type of artificial heart in which the lower chambers (ventricles) are driven by the alternate pumping of a fluid rather than by compressed air. The heart is powered by a compact electric motor, which can be put in a patient's chest along with the hydraulic pump. See also **artificial heart, Jarvik-7 artificial heart.**

electrolysis, a process in which electric energy causes a chemical change in a solution or fluid. **–electrolytic,** *adj.*

electrolyte, an element or compound that, when melted or dissolved in water or other solvent, breaks up into ions and is able to carry an electric current. Electrolyte concentrations vary in blood plasma, in tissues, and in cell fluid. The body must have the correct amounts of the main electrolytes to use energy. For example, calcium (Ca^{++}) is needed to relax the heart muscles and contract the heart. Potassium (K^+) is needed to contract muscles and relax the heart. Sodium (Na^+) is needed to maintain fluid balance. Certain diseases, defects, and drugs may lead to a lack of one or more electrolytes. Watching the levels of electrolytes and replacement of fluids and electrolytes are part of care in many illnesses. **–electrolytic,** *adj.*

electrolyte balance, the balance among electrolytes in the body.

electrolyte solution, any solution with electrolytes that is made to give a patient. It may be given by mouth, rectally, or in the vein. The loss of potassium (K^+) from vomiting, diarrhea, or the action of certain drugs (as diuretics and steroids) is corrected by giving a solution high in potassium. Other electrolyte solutions with calcium, sodium, phosphate, chloride, or magnesium may be given to treat an imbalance due to disease, as long-term kidney disease or lack of insulin in diabetes (ketoacidosis).

electromagnetic radiation, every kind of electrical and magnetic radiation. It is thought of as a whole range of energy. It includes energy with the shortest wavelength, as gamma rays, to that with the longest wavelength, as long radio waves.

electromallet condenser, a device for packing down filling gold in prepared tooth cavities.

electromyogram (EMG), a record of the electric impulses in a muscle. It is made to look for problems. Electrodes are placed on the skin or a needle electrode is put into a muscle. The impulses are recorded. Some electromyograms show defects and help to pinpoint problems with motor nerves. See also **electroneuromyography.**

electron, 1. a particle with a negative charge that has a certain charge, mass, and spin. The number of electrons moving around the nucleus of an atom is equal to the atomic number of the substance. Electrons may be shared or exchanged by two atoms. After the exchange the atom becomes an ion. **2.** a negative beta particle given off from a radioactive substance. Compare **neutron, proton.** See also **atom, element, ion, proton, neutron.**

electronarcosis, general painkiller that does not use gases or drugs. The patient loses consciousness when an electric current is passed through the brain. The method is experimental.

electroneuromyography, a method to test and record nerve and muscle function using electric impulses to stimulate the nerves. Needle electrodes are put into the muscle, and electric current is passed through the electrodes. The results are recorded. The method helps with the study of nerve injury and reflex responses. See also **electromyogram.**

electronic fetal monitor (EFM), a device that allows the fetal heart beat and the contractions of the uterus to be observed. When used outside the body, two belts are put around the mother's belly, one to pick up heart beats and one to detect contractions. When done internally, the fetal heart is observed by clipping an electrode to the fetal scalp. The strength, number, and length of time of the uterine contractions are detected by a catheter inside the uterus. See illustration on p. 279.

electronic thermometer, a thermometer that gives temperature quickly by electronic means.

electron microscopy, using an electron microscope, a beam of electrons is focused by a special lens onto very thin tissue or other sample. A second lens takes the image and projects it onto a screen. The image is 1,000 times greater than with an optical microscope. It is two-dimensional because the specimen must be so thin. Also called **transmission electron microscopy.** Compare **scanning electron microscopy, transmission scanning electron microscopy.**

electronystagmography, a method of testing and recording eye movements by measuring the electric impulses of the eye muscles. See also **electroencephalogram, nystagmus.**

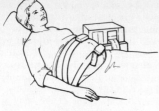

External fetal monitor

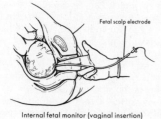

Fetal scalp electrode

Internal fetal monitor (vaginal insertion)

Electronic fetal monitors

electroporation, a process in which an electric current is used to make holes in cell membranes so alien DNA can enter the cells. See also **transfection.**

electroresection, a technique used to remove bladder tumors. An electric wire is put in through the urethra. A painkiller is given (anesthetic) before the technique is used.

electroshock therapy. See **electroconvulsive therapy.**

electrosleep therapy, a technique to bring about sleep, especially in mental patients. A low-level electric current is passed through the brain.

electrosurgery, surgery that is done with electric instruments. Kinds of electrosurgery include **electrocoagulation, electrodesiccation.**

electrotonic current, a current in a nerve sheath caused by an electric current within the nerve of a muscle.

eleidin, a clear protein substance that looks like keratin, found in the skin, mucous membrane, and other surface tissues.

element, one of more than 100 primary, simple substances that cannot be broken down by chemical means into any other substance. Each atom of any element contains a set number of electrons moving around the nucleus. The nucleus has a number of neutrons that may vary. A **stable element** has an equal number of neutrons and electrons and does not easily give up neutrons. A **radioactive element** does not contain a balanced number of electrons and neutrons, and gives off neutrons readily. See also **atom, compound, molecule.**

elephantiasis /el'əfəntī'əsis/, the last stage of a worm infestation (filariasis). It causes great swelling, usually of the genitals and the legs. The skin over the swelling becomes dark, thick, and coarse. See also **filariasis.**

eleventh cranial nerve. See **accessory nerve.**

elimination diet, a way to test for food to which a person is allergic. Certain foods are left out of the diet one at a time until the symptoms go away.

ELISA /əlīzə/, abbreviaton for **enzyme-linked immunosorbent assay.**

elixir, a clear liquid made of water, alcohol, sweeteners, or flavors mainly in drugs that are taken by mouth.

Elixophyllin, a trademark for a muscle relaxant used to make the airway passages open wider (theophylline).

elliptocyte, an oval-shaped red blood cell. See also **elliptocytosis.**

elliptocytosis, a mild defect of the blood in which there are increased numbers of elliptocytes. Less than 15% of the red cells appear in this form in normal blood. Small increases occur in certain anemias.

Ellis-van Creveld syndrome. See **chondroectodermal dysplasia.**

elope, *informal.* to leave a locked mental hospital without permission.

Elspar, a trademark for a drug used to treat cancer antineoplastic (asparaginase).

emaciation, extreme leanness caused by disease or lack of nutrition.

Embden-Meyerhoff defects /emb'denmī'ərhof/, a group of hereditary anemias caused by lack of certain enzymes. The condition causes abnormal red blood cells. The trait is recessive, and the anemia occurs only in persons who inherit a defective gene from each parent.

embedded tooth, a tooth that has not cut through the gums. It is usually completely covered with bone. Also called **imbedded tooth.** Compare **impacted tooth.**

embolectomy, a cut made in an artery to remove a clot (embolus). It is done as emergency treatment. The operation is done within 4 to 6 hours after pain has started, if possible. Clots may break away from the inflamed vein where they form. When this happens, they tend to lodge where major arteries join. More than half lodge in the large artery of the heart (aorta), in arteries of the legs, in the common arteries, or in the lung arteries.

embolism, a defect in which a clot (embolus) travels through the bloodstream and becomes lodged in a blood vessel, usually in the heart, lungs, or brain. The symptoms vary with the degree of blockage that the embolism causes, the type of embolus, and the size, nature, and location of the blocked vessel. Kinds of embolism include **air embolism, fat embolism.**

embolized atheroma, an embolized fat particle lodged in a blood vessel.

embolotherapy, a technique of blocking a blood vessel with a tube (catheter) that balloons at one end. It is used to treat bleeding sores within the body, and blood vessel defects. During surgery it is used to stop blood flow to a tumor.

embolus, *pl.* **emboli,** a foreign object, a large bubble of air or gas, a bit of tissue or tumor, or a piece of a blood clot that travels through the bloodstream until it becomes lodged in a vessel.

embryectomy, the removal of an embryo. It is done most often in pregnancy outside the uterus (ectopic pregnancy).

embryo /em′brē-ō/, **1.** any organism in the first stages of growth. **2.** in humans, the stage of growth between the time the fertilized egg is implanted in the uterus, which occurs about 2 weeks after conception, until the end of the seventh or eighth week of pregnancy. The period involves rapid growth, early growth of the major organ systems, and of the main external features. Compare **fetus, zygote. –embryonal, embryonoid, embryonic,** *adj.*

embryoctony, the intentional destruction of the embryo or fetus in the uterus. Also called **feticide.** See also **abortion.**

embryogenesis, the process in which an embryo forms from a fertilized egg. Also called **embryogeny.**

embryologic development, the stages in the growth and development of the embryo from the time of fertilization of the egg until about the eighth week of pregnancy. The stages are divided into two distinct periods. The first is embryogenesis, or the formation of the embryo. It occurs during the 10 days to 2 weeks after fertilization until the embryo is implanted in the wall of the uterus. The second period, organogenesis, involves emergence of the cells, tissues, organ systems, and the main outer features of the embryo. This second stage occurs from about the end of the second week to the eighth week of pregnancy. The fetal stage begins at about the ninth week of pregnancy. Embryogenesis starts shortly after fertilization when the sperm and egg fuse to form the zygote. It is mainly a process of cell division in which the cells begin to specialize and group into tissues and organs. At 8 weeks of development, the embryo looks human and is called a fetus. See also **prenatal development.**

embryology /em′brē-ol′əjē/, the study of the origin, growth, and function of an organism from the time it is fertilized to birth.

embryoma /em′brē-ō′mə/, *pl.* **embryomas, embryomata,** a tumor growing from embryonic cells or tissues.

embryoma of the ovary. See **dysgerminoma**

embryonal carcinoma, a very cancerous tumor that usually grows in gonads, especially the testicles. The tumor is a firm lump-filled mass with many bleeding areas. Bodies that look like

a 1- or 2-week-old embryo are sometimes seen in these tumors. See also **choriocarcinoma.**

embryonal leukemia. See **stem cell leukemia.**

embryonic abortion, ending a pregnancy before the twentieth week. Compare **fetal abortion.**

embryonic layer, one of the three layers of cells in the embryo: the endoderm, the mesoderm, and the ectoderm. From these layers, all of the structures and organs of the body grow. The endoderm is the first to appear, followed by the ectoderm. During the third week of pregnancy, the mesoderm forms between the ectoderm and the endoderm. The ectoderm grows into skin, nails, hair, and nervous system tissues. The mesoderm forms connective tissues, muscle, bones, and tissues of the vessels and lymph system. The endoderm grows into the lining of the stomach tract.

embryonic rest, a portion of embryonic tissue that stays in the adult. Such tissue may act as a sign for certain types of cancer. Also called **epithelial rest, fetal rest.**

embryopathy /em′brē-op′əthē/, any defect in the embryo or fetus as a result of problem with growth. A kind of embryopathy is **rubella embryopathy.**

embryotomy /em′brē-ot′əmē/, **1.** the tearing away of a fetus to remove it from the womb when normal delivery can not happen. **2.** the cutting up of an embryo for testing and checking.

embryotrophy /em′brē-ot′trəfē/, the feeding of the embryo. **–embryotrophic,** *adj.*

Emcyt, a trademark for a drug used to treat cancer of the prostate (estramustine phosphate sodium).

emergence, a stage in recovering from general anesthesia. It includes breathing and swallowing under one's own control and consciousness. See also **postoperative care.**

emergency, a serious situation that arises quickly and threatens the life or welfare of a person or a group of people, as a tornado or a health crisis.

emergency childbirth, a birth that occurs accidentally in or out of the hospital, without standard procedures. Symptoms of childbirth include increased bloody show, strong contractions, desire to bear down or to have a bowel movement, bulging of the bag of waters, or the baby's head showing at the vaginal opening. See childbirth.

emergency department, part of a health center that is set up to provide quick emergency care, especially for sudden acute illness or severe injury.

emergency doctrine, assumes a person agrees to treatment when in immediate danger and not able to approve of the care. It assumes that they would agree if they could.

Emergency Medical Service (EMS), a national network of services providing aid from the first response to the selected care. The staff is trained in emergency care. EMS is linked by a local and regional communications system. There is usually an emergency number.

Emergency Medical Technician (EMT), a person trained in and responsible for giving special emergency care and transporting victims of acute illness or injury to the proper place. In addition to basic life-support skills, the EMT is trained in removing trapped victims, driving emergency vehicles, basic anatomy, basic assessment of and care for injuries and illnesses, environmental emergencies, and childbirth. EMTs must have ongoing training in new procedures and be recertified every 2 years. See also **Emergency Medical Service.**

emergency medicine, a branch of medicine dealing with the diagnosis and care of conditions coming from injury or sudden illness. The patient is stabilized. Care is then given by the person's doctor or a specialist.

emergency room (E.R., ER), a hospital area set up to receive and treat patients suffering from sudden trauma or medical problems, as bleeding, poisoning, broken bones, heart attack, and breathing failure.

emergency theory, the theory that the body responds to an emergency by getting ready to run or fight. See also **flight-or-fight reaction.**

emesis. See **vomit,** def. 2.

Emete-con, a trademark for a drug used to prevent nausea and vomiting after anesthesia. (benzquinamide hydrochloride).

emetic /imet′ik/, **1.** referring to a substance that causes vomiting.

emetine hydrochloride /em′ətēn/, a powerful drug that kills amebas in the body. It is used to treat severe intestinal problems, open sores, and liver problems caused by amebas.
★CAUTION: Do not use this drug more than once in 6 to 8 weeks. Heart disease, nervous system problems, kidney disease, or known allergy to this drug prohibits its use.
★ADVERSE EFFECTS: Among the more serious side effects are heart irregularities, low blood pressure, nerve and muscle problems.

EMG, short for **electromyogram.**

EMG syndrome, an inherited problem marked by bulging eyes, enlarged tongue, and gigantism. It is often accompanied by larger organs, kidney problems, and larger cells in the adrenal gland. Also called **Beckwith-Wiedemann syndrome, exophthalmos-macroglossia gigantism syndrome.**

emissary veins /em′əserē/, the small vessels that connect the spaces in the membrane over the brain (dura) with the veins on the outside of the skull.

emission computed tomography (ECT), a form of tomography in which the positrons or gamma rays of a radioactive substance are recorded in detectors outside the body. A computer produces a cross-sectional image of the body from the information.

emmetropia /em′ətrō′pē·ə/, the state of normal (20/20) vision. Compare **amblyopia, hyperopia, myopia.** –**emmetropic,** *adj.*

emollient /imol′yənt/, a substance that softens tissue, especially the skin and mucous membranes.

emotion, the feeling part of awareness as compared with thinking. Physical changes, as illness, can come with changes in emotion, whether the feelings are conscious or not.

emotional abuse, the misuse of a person's feelings. As a result, one thinks less of oneself.

emotional care of the dying patient, the support of the dying patient and the family. The terminally ill person is helped to express feelings and worries about death. The patient needs gentle, realistic care. Not all questions need answers. The doctor and the patient's family must decide whether to tell the patient he or she is dying. The patient needs relief from pain, tender care, and attention through all the stages of dying. A period of denial, followed by anger, bargaining, depression, and, finally, acceptance are the stages the dying patient goes through. When the patient denies the truth and will not follow directions, one neither argues nor agrees with the person. During the stage of anger, the patient is encouraged to express the anger. In the period in which the patient tries to make bargains, as "If I could live until . . . ," it may help to discuss the importance of events and people in earlier life. When depression sets in, efforts to cheer the patient or stop the crying should not be made. The patient may want only the most beloved person to be present. In the final stage of acceptance, the patient may feel less pain and discomfort, become peaceful and accept care from people who are close. See also **stages of dying.**
★PATIENT CARE: The nurse has the major role in providing emotional care for the terminally ill patient in the hospital. He or she may help the family arrange for home care when the person wants or needs to die at home.
★OUTCOME: Sensitive care and support through all stages of dying may help the patient accept death more quickly and easily. The family often goes through like stages. Support and counseling may help the patient and the patient's family.

emotional illness. See **mental disorder.**

emotional need, a psychological need. It is often centered on such basic feelings as love, fear, anger, sorrow, anxiety, frustration, and depression. Emotional need requires the understanding and support of one person for another. Such needs occur in everyone. They often become greater during times of stress, physical and mental illness, and at various stages of life, as infancy, early childhood, and old age. Compare **dependency needs**. See also **emotion**.

emotional response, a response to a certain feeling. It occurs with physical changes that may or may not be obvious. However, they may cause some action or response. An example is crying as a response to death of a loved one. See also **emotion**.

emotional support, the sensitive, understanding approach that helps patients accept and deal with their illnesses, talk about their fears, take comfort from a caring person. It can help a patient to better care for him or herself. It is vital to respect the patient's needs, wants and independence. It helps to understand what the patient has gone through. Stock answers, as "Don't worry, everything will be ok," are not too useful. Avoid trying to change the patient or the patient's moods. Emotional support often helps the patient's mental and physical state. It often helps the patient to accept the illness, to adjust with less stress, and to cope with the changes that are needed.

empathy /em'pəthē/, the ability to know and to some extent share the emotions of another and to understand the meaning of that person's behavior. Compare **sympathy**. –**empathic,** *adj.,* **empathize,** *v.*

emphysema /em'fəsē'mə/, a defect of the lung system. It causes too much inflation of the lungs and destructive changes of the pouches where air exchange occurs (alveolar walls). This causes the lungs to become too rigid and handle less oxygen. When emphysema occurs early in life, it is often because of an inherited defect. Acute emphysema may be caused by the break in the air pouches due to hard efforts at breathing, as in bronchopneumonia, suffocation, whooping cough, and sometimes during labor. Long-term emphysema is often present with long-term bronchitis. A major cause of this is cigarette smoking. Emphysema is also seen after asthma or tuberculosis. In old age, the membranes waste and may collapse. This results in large air-filled spaces with less total surface area. The person may have shortness of breath, cough, blue-toned skin, trouble breathing while lying down, fast shallow breathing, unequal chest expansion, rapid heart beat, and a fever. Anxiety, high levels of carbon dioxide, lack of sleep, confusion, weakness, appetite loss, congestive heart failure, fluid in the lungs, and lung failure are common in advanced cases. The airway is kept open, and moist oxygen may be given. Drugs may be given. The patient is taught breathing exercises and is told to drink between 2 and 3 quarts (2,000 ml and 3,000 ml) of fluids daily. Movement should be limited to the patient's tolerance. Fatigue, constipation, and lung infection are to be avoided. A respirator and oxygen

equipment may be prescribed for the patient's use at home.

empiricism, a form of therapy based on personal experience, as trial and error, and the experience of others in the practice. –**empiric, empirical,** *adj.* –**empiricist,** *n.*

Empirin, a trademark for a combination drug that has two drugs to relieve pain and reduce fever (aspirin and phenacetin) and a drug that stimulates the nervous system (caffeine).

emprosthotonos /em'prosthot'ənəs/, a position of the body in which it is stiffly bent forward at the waist. It is the result of a long-term muscle spasm, most often seen with tetanus infection or strychnine poisoning.

empty sella syndrome, enlargement of the cavity inside the base of the skull. This cavity normally holds the pituitary gland. In this defect, the gland may be smaller than normal, or it may be absent. Symptoms of hormone imbalance may be present, but some patients show no symptoms. The defect is often seen in overweight, middle-aged women who have had many pregnancies. The cause is unknown.

empyema /em'pī·ē'mə, em'pē·ē'mə/, a collection of pus in a body cavity, especially the space between the lung and the membrane that surrounds it (pleural space). It is caused by an infection, as pleurisy or tuberculosis.

EMS, short for **Emergency Medical Service.**

EMT, short for **Emergency Medical Technician.**

emulsify, to mix a liquid into another liquid, making a suspension that has globules of fat. Bile is an emulsifier in the digestive tract. –**emulsification,** *n.*

emulsion, a mix of two liquids, made so that small droplets are formed, as oil and water.

E-Mycin, a trademark for an antibiotic (erythromycin).

enamel, a hard white substance that covers a tooth.

enamel hypocalcification, an inherited defect of the teeth in which the enamel is soft and lacks calcium. The teeth are chalky to the touch and the surfaces wear down quickly. A yellow or brown stain appears as the dentin under the enamel is showing. The defect affects both baby and permanent teeth.

enamel hypoplasia, a defect of the teeth in which the enamel is thin and lacking. There is lack of contact between teeth and rapid breakdown of biting surfaces. A yellowish brown stain appears where the dentin under the enamel is showing. The defect affects both baby and permanent teeth.

enanthema /en'anthē'mə/, a sore on the surface of a mucous membrane.

enarthrosis. See **ball-and-socket joint.**

encapsulated, referring to arteries, muscles, nerves, and other body parts that are enclosed in fiber or membrane sheaths. See also **fascia bulbi, synovial sheath.** –**encapsulate,** *v.*

encephalitis /ensef'əli'tis/, *pl.* **encephalitides** /-tidēz/, an inflammation of the brain. The cause is usually a virus infection that comes from the bite of an infected mosquito. It may also be caused by lead or other poisoning, or bleeding. **Postinfectious encephalitis** is the result of another infection, as chickenpox, influenza, or measles. It can also occur after smallpox vaccination. The symptoms are headache, neck pain, fever, nausea, and vomiting. Nervous system problems may occur, including seizures, personality change, short temper, laziness, paralysis, weakness, and coma. Treatment is with antibiotics for infections, steroids to reduce brain swelling, and fluids in the vein. Lead encephalitis is treated with drugs that bind (chelate) iron. When the disease involves the spinal cord and brain, the correct term is *encephalomyelitis.* Compare **meningitis.** See also **encephalomyelitis, equine encephalitis.**

encephalocele /ensef'ələsēl'/, bulging of the brain through an opening in the skull; hernia of the brain. This problem may be from a birth defect or trauma. See also **neural tube defect.**

encephalodysplasia, any birth defect of the brain.

encephalography /ensef'əlog'rəfē/, x-ray tests of the structures of the brain that contain fluid. The fluid of the brain and spine (cerebrospinal) is taken out and replaced by a gas, as air, helium, or oxygen. The method is used mainly for finding the site of cerebrospinal fluid blockage. Because the method is risky, it is used only when other methods do not provide a complete picture. Kinds of encephalography are **pneumoencephalography, ventriculography.** Also called **air encephalography.**

encephaloid carcinoma. See **medullary carcinoma.**

encephalomeningocele. See **meningoencephalocele.**

encephalomyelitis /ensef'əlōmī'əli'tis/, a disease of the brain and spinal cord in which there is fever, headache, stiff neck, back pain, and vomiting. Nervous system problems, seizures, paralysis, personality changes, a lowered level of awareness, coma, or death may occur. Permanent damage of the nervous system can result in seizure defects or lower mental function. Treatment is the same as for encephalitis. See also **encephalitis, equine encephalitis.**

encephalomyocarditis /ensef'əlōmī'ōkärdī'tis/, an infectious disease of the brain, spinal cord, and heart tissue. It is caused by a group of small RNA picornaviruses. Rodents are a major source of the infection. Human illness ranges from infection with no symptoms to severe encephalomyelitis. Symptoms are generally similar to those of poliomyelitis. Treatment is supportive. See also **picornavirus.**

encephalopathy /ensef'əlop'əthē/, any defect of the structure or function of brain tissues. It often refers to long-term defects in which there is a breakdown or death of tissue, as Wernicke's encephalopathy or Schilder's disease.

enchondroma /en'kəndrō'mə/, *pl.* **enchondromas, enchondromata,** a harmless, slow growing tumor of cartilage cells that grows near the ends of long bones. The growth of the tumor may cause the bone to bulge.

enchondromatosis /en'kəndrō'mətō'sis/, too much cartilage in the flared ends of many bones. This causes thinning of the bone. It also affects the length. See also **Maffucci's syndrome.**

enchondromatous myxoma, a tumor of the connective tissue, in which cartilage grows between the cells of connective tissue. See also **myxoma.**

enchondrosarcoma. See **central chondrosarcoma.**

enchondrosis. See **enchondroma.**

enchylema. See **hyaloplasm.**

encopresis /en'kōprē'sis/, a state of being unable to control bowel movements. —**encopretic,** *adj.*

encounter, the exchange between a patient and a psychotherapist, (as in existential therapy). It can also occur among members of a small group (as in encounter or sensitivity-training groups). Emotional change and growth occur when the members express their feelings.

encounter group, a small group of people who meet to increase self-awareness, promote growth, and improve communication. Members focus on being aware of their feelings and on learning how to express those feelings openly, honestly, and clearly. See also **group therapy, psychotherapy, sensitivity-training group.**

enculturation, the process of learning the concepts, values, and behavior of a certain culture.

encyst /ensist'/, to form a cyst or capsule. See also **cyst.** —**encysted,** *adj.*

endarterectomy /en'därtərek'təmē/, a method to remove the core (tunica intima) of an artery that has become thickened by fatty deposits (atherosclerosis).

endarteritis /en'därtərī'tis/, a disease of the inner layer of one or more arteries. The arteries may become partly blocked or completely blocked.

endarteritis obliterans, a defect in which the artery walls become inflamed. The lining grows, narrows the opening of the vessels, and blocks the smaller vessels.

end bud, a mass of cells that grows from the remains of the growing embryo. In humans it forms the tail end of the trunk. Also called **tail bud.**

end bulbs of Krause. See **Krause's corpuscles.**

endemic /endem'ik/, a disease or infection common to a geographic area or population. See also **epidemic, pandemic.**

endemic goiter, a swelling of the thyroid gland caused by lack of iodine in the diet. Lack of iodine leads to less output of thyroid hormone. The pituitary gland senses the lack and secretes larger amounts of thyroid-stimulating hormone. This causes the thyroid gland to get larger. The goiter may grow during the winter and shrink during the summer when more fresh vegetables that have iodine are eaten. Endemic goiter occurs sometimes in adolescents at puberty. It is more common in areas where there is little iodine in the soil, water, and food. The use of iodized salt can prevent this problem. Seafood is a very good source of iodine.

endemic typhus. See **murine typhus.**

endocardial cushion defect, any heart defect that results from the failure of the endocardial cushions in the fetal heart to fuse and form the wall that divides the upper chambers (atrial septum). See also **atrial septal defect, congenital cardiac anomaly.**

endocardial fibroelastosis /fī'brō·ē'lastō'sis/, a defect in which the wall of the lower left chamber of the heart (ventricle) grows too much. The tissue that lines the heart (endocardium) becomes thick and fibrous. This state often makes the capacity of the heart chamber larger, but it may also make it smaller.

endocarditis /en'dōkärdī'tis/, a defect in which the lining of the heart, (endocardium) and the heart valves become inflamed. The kinds of endocarditis are bacterial endocarditis, nonbacterial thrombotic endocarditis, and Libman-Sacks endocarditis. If not treated, all types of endocarditis are quickly fatal. They are often treated with success using drugs or surgery. See also **bacterial endocarditis, subacute bacterial endocarditis.**

endocardium /en'dōkär'dē·əm/, pl. **endocardia,** the lining of the heart chambers, it contains small blood vessels and a few bundles of smooth muscle. Compare **epicardium, myocardium.**

endocervical, referring to the inner part of the cervix and uterus.

endocervicitis /en'dōsur'visi'tis/, a defect in which the lining and glands of the uterine cervix become inflamed or swollen. See also **cervicitis.**

endocervix /en'dōsur'viks/, the membrane lining the canal of the uterine cervix.

endocrine fracture /en'dōkrīn, -krēn/, any break in a bone due to a weakness caused by an endocrine defect, as hyperparathyroidism.

endocrine system, the network of glands that do not have ducts and other structures that secrete hormones into the bloodstream. They affect the function of specific target organs. Glands of the endocrine system include the thyroid and the parathyroid, the pituitary, the pancreas, the adrenal glands, and the gonads. The pineal gland is also thought of as a endocrine gland because it lacks ducts, although its precise function is not known. The thymus gland, once thought of as an endocrine gland, is now classed with the lymph system. Secretions from the endocrine glands affect a number of functions in the body, as metabolism and growth. Endocrine glands also affect secretions of each other and of organs. Compare **exocrine.** See also **Color Atlas of Human Anatomy.**

endocrinology, the study of the form and function of the endocrine system and the treatment of its problems.

endoderm /en'dədurm/, the innermost of the cell layers that grow from the early embryo. From the endoderm comes the lining of the upper system, stomach tract, liver, pancreas, urinary bladder and canal, thyroid, ear cavity, tonsils, and parathyroid glands. The endoderm thus lines most of the internal organs and spaces. Compare **ectoderm, mesoderm.**

endodermal cloaca, a part of the hindgut (cloaca) in the growing embryo that forms the bladder and urogenital ducts. Compare **ectodermal cloaca.** See also **urogenital sinus.**

endogenous /endoj'ənəs/, coming from inside the body, as a disease caused by failure of an organ. Compare **exogenous.** —**endogenic,** adj.

endogenous carbon dioxide, carbon dioxide produced within the body by normal processes of respiration and digestion.

endogenous depression, a major mental defect characterized by a stubborn unhappy mood, worry, a short temper, fear, brooding, appetite and sleep trouble, weight loss, either too much or too little energy, feelings of no worth, guilt, trouble thinking clearly, delusions, and thoughts of death or suicide. Treatment includes the use of antidepressant drugs, followed by long-term psychotherapy. The patient may have to be protected from self-injury. Patients who do not respond to treatment with drugs are sometimes given electroconvulsive treatments. Also called **major depressive episode.** See also **bipolar disorder, depression.**

endogenous infection, an infection caused by an organism that has caused an illness before becoming active again. Coccidioidomycosis, histoplasmosis, and tuberculosis often occur again.

endogenous obesity, fatness due to malfunction of the endocrine or metabolic systems. Compare **exogenous obesity.** See also **obesity.**

endolith. See **denticle.**

endolymph /en'dəlimf/, the fluid in the ducts of the inner ear. The endolymph carries sound waves to the ear drum, and helps maintain balance. Compare **perilymph.**

endolymphatic duct, a passage in the inner ear filled with endolymph.

endometrial /en'dōmē'trē·əl/, **1.** referring to the lining of the uterus. **2.** referring to the uterine cavity.

endometrial cancer, a cancerous tumor of the lining (endometrium) of the uterus, it most often occurs in the fifth or sixth decade of life. Some reasons for the disease are a history of infertility, lack of ovulation, taking drugs with estrogen, and uterine growths. Women who have diabetes, high blood pressure, or are very overweight are also at greater risk. Vaginal bleeding that is not normal, especially after menopause, is the main symptom. There also may be lower belly and low back pain. A Pap test does not always show endometrial cancer because the tumor cells are rarely found outside the uterus in early stages of the disease. The disease is often tested for with a surgical exam of the uterus. Endometrial cancer may spread to the cervix, but rarely to the vagina. They often grow in the broad ligaments, fallopian tubes, and ovaries. Treatment is removal of the uterus (hysterectomy) and removal of both ovaries and fallopian tubes (salpingo-oophorectomy). X-ray therapy is usually given before and after surgery. High doses of a hormone may be given for advanced cases.

endometrial hyperplasia, an overgrowth of the lining of the uterus (endometrium), it is due to too much estrogen for too long and not enough progesterone. The estrogen may be made by the body or come from drugs. Estrogens act as growth hormone for endometrium. If the imbalance goes on for 3 to 6 months without stopping, the endometrium becomes thick. Over-long estrogen action occurs in women who do not ovulate, who are in menopause, and who receive drugs containing estrogen without added progestogen. Over-long action of estrogen in time will cause cystic growths or a precancerous state.

endometrial polyp, a bulb-like pouch on a stem that grows from the lining of the uterus (endometrium), and is usually harmless. Polyps are a common cause of vaginal bleeding in women during menopause. They are often liked with other uterine defects, as endometrial hyperplasia or fibroids.

endometriosis /en'dōmē'trē·ō'sis/, a growth of endometrial tissue outside the uterus, it is thought to occur in about 15% of women. Women who do not get pregnant until later in life are more likely to have the disease. The average age of women found to have endometriosis is 37. The disease is not common among black women. Pregnancy seems to prevent or correct this problem in some women. The causes of endometriosis are unknown. It is thought fragments of the lining of the uterus that come loose during menstruation back up into the belly cavity. There they attach, grow, and function. Fragments of this tissue may be found in the wall of the uterus or on its surface, in or on the tubes, ovaries, or pelvic area, or, sometimes in areas outside the pelvis. Tissue has been found in scars, the navel, the bowel, the lung, the eye, and the brain. When endometriosis occurs in a crucial place, it may cause dysfunction of the organ it is attached to. Intestinal blockage often occurs. Endometriosis functions in cycles. A menstrual breakdown occurs that results in bleeding within cysts, stretching of the cyst wall, and pain. The most typical symptom of endometriosis is pain, especially severe menstrual cramps and pain during sex, painful bowel movements, and soreness above the pubic bone. Pain is not always present, however. Other common symptoms include premenstrual vaginal bleeding, too much bleeding during menstruation, and infertility. Treatment of endometriosis in its milder forms may consist only of pain-relieving drugs, because many women will outgrow it or become pregnant. When the disease is worse, the treatment includes hormones or surgery to reduce the size and number of deposits, relieve symptoms, and correct infertility. Birth-control pills sometimes shrink the deposits.

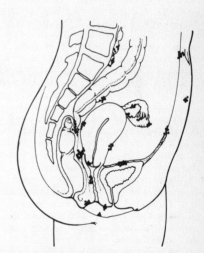

Common sites of endometriosis

endometritis /en'dōmitrī'tis/, a swelling of the endometrium. It is often caused by infection. Symptoms include fever, pain in the lower belly, discharge with a bad odor, and swelling of the uterus. It occurs most often after childbirth or abortion and in women fitted with an intrauterine contraceptive device (IUD). Endometritis may cause sterility because scars form, blocking the fallopian tubes. Septic abortion and childbirth (puerperal) fever are forms of endometritis, which caused many deaths before antibiotics and sterile techniques were used. A kind of endometritis is **decidua endometritis.** See also **pelvic inflammatory disease.**

endometrium /en'dōmē'trē·əm/, the mucous membrane lining of the uterus, consisting of three layers. The endometrium changes thickness during the menstrual cycle. Two of the layers are shed with each menstrual flow. The third layer provides the surface for the placenta to attach to during pregnancy. Compare **parametrium.**

endomorph /en'dəmôrf'/, a person whose body build is soft and round. The endomorph has a large trunk and thighs, tapering limbs, and fat throughout the body. Compare **ectomorph, mesomorph.** See also **pyknic.**

endoparasite /en'dōper'əsīt/, an organism that lives within the body of the host, as a tapeworm.

endophthalmitis /endof'thalmī'tis/, an inflammation of the inner eye. The eye becomes red, swollen, painful, and, sometimes, fills with pus. The vision is often blurred. This state may cause vomiting, fever, and headache. Endophthalmitis may be due to bacteria or fungus infection, trauma, allergy, drug or chemical poisoning, or vessel disease. Also called **endophthalmia.**

endophthalmitis phacoanaphylactica /fak'ō-an'əfilak'təkə/, a defect in which there is a short-term allergic response of the eye to itself, caused by an allergy of the eye to the protein in the lens. It often occurs after trauma to the lens or after a cataract operation. Other symptoms include swelling and soreness of the eye, severe pain, and blurred vision. The other eye may also be affected. Compare **uveitis.**

endophytic /en'dōfit'ik/, referring to the tendency to grow inward. An example is a tumor that grows on the inside of an organ.

endoplasmic reticulum, a vast network of membrane-enclosed tubes in the cytoplasm of cells. This tiny structure can be seen only with an electron microscope. The structure makes proteins and fats and aids in getting them to the rest of the cell.

endorphin /endôr'fin/, any one of the substances of the nervous system. Endorphins are composed of amino acids. They are made by the pituitary gland and act on the nervous system to reduce pain. They produce effects like that of morphine. Compare **enkephalin.**

endoscope, a device with a light, used to look at the inside of a body cavity or organ.

endoscopic retrograde cholangiography, an x-ray test for outlining the common bile duct. A flexible device with a light is placed in the common bile duct. A fluid that will show an x-ray is flushed into the duct, and a series of x-rays are taken. See also **cholangiography.**

endoscopy /endos'kəpē/, examination of the inside of organs and cavities of the body with an endoscope. See also **bronchoscopy, cystoscopy, gastroscopy, laparoscopy.** –**endoscopic,** *adj.*

endothelial myeloma /en'dōthē'lē·əl/, a cancerous bone marrow tumor (myeloma). Myelomas occur most often in the long bones, especially the legs. Young people between 10 and 20 years of age are most often affected. Pain, fever, and increased numbers of white blood cells usually occur. Amputation is necessary for large tumors. X-ray therapy and chemotherapy are standard treatments. Also called **Ewing's tumor.**

endothelium /en'dōthē'lē·əm/, the layer of cells that lines the heart, the blood and lymph vessels, and the fluid-filled cavities of the body. It is well supplied with blood and heals quickly.

endotoxin /en'dōtok'sin/, a poison contained in the cell walls of some bacteria. It is released when the bacterium dies. Fever, chills, shock, and a number of other symptoms result, depending on the condition of the infected person. Compare **exotoxin.**

endotracheal /en'dōtrā'kē·əl/, within or through the windpipe (trachea).

endotracheal anesthesia, gas anesthesia that is given through a tube into the windpipe and so into the lungs. General anesthesia is usually performed by endotracheal anesthesia. See also **endotracheal intubation, endotracheal tube.**

endotracheal intubation, inserting a large tube through the mouth or nose into the trachea (windpipe). An endotracheal tube may be used to keep an open airway or to prevent material from the stomach from getting into the lungs in the unconscious or paralyzed patient. It may also be used to suction fluid from the bronchial tree or when using a respirator. Endotracheal tubes may be made of rubber or plastic. See illustration on p. 287.

★METHOD: The endotracheal tube is inserted through the mouth or nose into the trachea. Once the tube is in place, it is taped in place and checked often to be sure it is in place.

endotracheal tube, a large tube (catheter) inserted through the mouth or nose and into the trachea, it is used for giving oxygen under pressure when breathing must be totally controlled. It is also used for general anesthesia.

endoxin /endok'sin/, a hormone made in the human body that is similar to the drug digoxin. Endoxin regulates the excretion of salt.

Enduron, a trademark for a drug that lowers blood pressure and increases urine output (methyclothiazide).

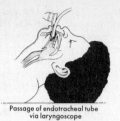

Passage of endotracheal tube
via laryngoscope

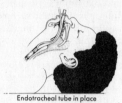

Endotracheal tube in place

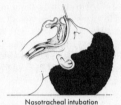

Nasotracheal intubation
Endotracheal intubation

Enduronyl, a trademark for a drug that increases urine output (methyclothiazide) and a
drug that lowers blood pressure (deserpidine).
It is used to treat heart conditions.

enema, a procedure in which a fluid is flushed
into the rectum for cleansing or treatment.
★METHOD: The solution is warmed to 99.0° F
(37.8° C) to 105° F (40.6° C) to avoid causing
cramps. The patient should lie on the left side
with knees drawn close to the chest. The tip of
the catheter is then lubricated gently inserted
3 to 4 inches (7.5 cm to 10 cm) into the rectum.
The enema is given slowly to avoid sudden
expansion that would cause spasm of the intestine. The tip of the catheter is taken out. The
fluid is held in by the patient as long as possible before expelling the fluid.

energy, the capacity to do work or to perform
vigorous activity. Compare **anergy.** **–ener-
getic,** *adj.*

enervation, **1.** lack of energy; weakness; lethargy.
2. removal of a complete nerve or of a section
of nerve.

en face /äNfäs´/, *French.* "face-to-face"; a position in which the mother's face and the infant's
face are about 8 inches apart. Examples are
when the mother holds the infant up in front
of her face and when she nurses the child.
Studies have shown that mothers seek eye-to-
eye contact, and that they will instinctively
move the baby to an en face position. In addi-

tion, infants prefer looking at a human face
over other objects. Babies are best able to focus at a distance of 8 to 10 inches.

enflurane /en´floŏrān/, a nonflammable anesthetic gas belonging to the ether family, it is
used for general anesthesia.

engagement, the point in childbirth when the
part of the fetus descending first comes down
into the mother's pelvis. This occurs roughly
half-way through labor.

English position. See **lateral recumbent position.**

engorgement, swelling or congestion of body tissues. An example is the swelling of breast tissue before the mother's milk comes in.

enkephalin /enkef´əlin/, one of two pain-
relieving substances made in the body. Researchers have found enkephalins in the pituitary gland, brain, and stomach and bowels. It
is believed that enkephalins can slow nerve
activity through the central nervous system.
They slow nerve signals to indicate pain, which
reduces the mental and physical sensation of
pain. Compare **endorphin.**

enomania. See **oinomania.**

enophthalmos /en´əfthal´məs/, retraction of the
eyeball into the socket. It is caused by an injury
or birth defect. **–enophthalmic,** *adj.*

Enovid, a trademark for a birth-control pill with
the female hormones estrogen (mestranol) and
progestin (norethynodrel).

Ensure, a trademark for a nutritional supplement that does not contain any milk product.
It does contain protein, carbohydrate, fat, vitamins, and minerals.

Entamoeba /en´təmē´bə/, a family (genus) of intestinal parasites. Several types are harmful to
humans. Also spelled *Entameba.*

Entamoeba histolytica, an organism that causes a
type of dysentery in humans. It can also infect
the liver. See also **amebiasis, amebic dysentery, hepatic amebiasis.**

enteric coating, a coating added to drugs taken
by mouth that need to reach the intestines.
The coating resists the effects of stomach
juices, which can destroy certain drugs.

enteric fever. See **typhoid fever.**

enteric infection, a disease of the intestine
caused by any infection. Similar symptoms may
be caused by bacteria, food poisoning, or allergic reactions to certain foods. Symptoms of
those infections are diarrhea, stomach pain,
nausea and vomiting, and loss of appetite.
There may be a great loss of fluid from severe
vomiting and diarrhea. Nothing should be
taken by mouth until vomiting has ceased. At
that time, a clear fluid diet may be given.

entericoid fever, a typhoidlike disease that
causes fever and swelling in the stomach and
bowels. See also **enteric infection, typhoid
fever.**

enteritis /en´tərī´tis/, swelling in the lining of the

small intestine. It can be caused by a number of things, including bacteria, viruses, and certain functional disorders. If the large intestine also becomes involved, it is called **enterocolitis.** Compare **gastroenteritis.**

entero-, enter-, a combining form referring to the intestines.

enterobacterial, referring to a type of bacterium found in the digestive tract.

Enterobacteriaceae /en′tirōbaktir′ē·ā′si·ē/, a family of bacteria that includes both harmless and harmful organisms. Among the most important disease-causing types are *Escherichia, Klebsiella, Proteus,* and *Salmonella.*

enterobiasis /en′tirōbī′əsis/, an infection by the common pinworm *(Enterobius vermicularis).* The worms infect the large intestine, and the females deposit eggs in the anal area, causing itching and insomnia. Because the eggs remain alive for 2 or 3 days, it is possible for an entire family to become infected by contact with bedclothes or hands of the patient. Treatment for the whole family may be necessary. Treatment with drugs usually completely rids the body of pinworms. Also called **oxyuriasis.**

Enterobius vermicularis, a common parasitic worm that resembles a white thread less than ½ inch long (between 0.5 and 1 cm). Also called **pinworm, seatworm, threadworm.**

enterochromaffin cell. See **argentaffin cell.**

enterococcus, *pl.* **enterocci,** any bacteria of the *Streptococcus* family that lives in the intestinal tract.

enterocolitis, a swelling of both the large and small intestines.

enterokinase /en′tirōkī′nās/, a substance in the intestines that helps the body absorb protein.

enterolith /en′tərōlith/, a stone found in the intestine. See also **calculus.**

enterolithiasis /en′tərōlithī′əsis/, the presence of stones (enteroliths) in the intestine.

enterostomy /en′təros′təmē/, surgery to produce an artificial opening in the small intestine. A hole is made in the intestine, and this is connected to a hole in the skin on the abdomen. The contents of the intestine empty through this opening (stoma). Compare **colostomy.**

enterovirus, a virus that flourishes mainly in the intestinal tract. Kinds of enteroviruses are **coxsackievirus, echovirus, poliovirus. –enteroviral,** *adj.*

Entozyme, a trademark for a combination drug containing bile salts and digestive enzymes (pancreatin and pepsin).

entrainment, a natural state in which a person will move with the rhythms of speech and movement from another person. Infants seem to move in time to the rhythms of adult speech. They do not move to random noises or words. Entrainment is thought to be important in the developing relationship of a mother and infant.

entrance block, an imaginary area around the heart's natural pacemaker. The entrance block protects the area from a stray electrical signal that might cause abnormal heart beats.

entropion, turning inward. The term is often used for a condition in which the edge of the eyelid turns inward toward the eye. **Cicatricial entropion** can occur in either the upper or lower eyelid as a result of scar tissue. **Spastic entropion** results from swelling or another factor that affects tissue strength. Swelling of the eyelid may be caused by an infection or by irritation from an inverted eyelash. Compare **ectropion.** See also **blepharitis.**

entropy /en′trəpē/, the tendency of a system to go from a state of order to a state of disorder. Living organisms tend to go from a state of disorder to a state of order in their development. This would appear to be a reverse of entropy. However, a living system uses energy, leaving less energy for work. The result is that entropy of the system increases.

ENT specialist, a doctor who specializes in treating the ear, nose, and throat. See also **otolaryngologist.**

enucleation, 1. removal of an organ or tumor in one piece. 2. removal of the eyeball. This is done in case of a cancerous tumor, severe infection, injury, or to control pain in glaucoma.

enuresis /en′yŏōrē′sis/, lack of ability to control the need to urinate, especially in bed at night.

environment, all of the many factors, including physical and psychological, that affect the life of a person. See also **biome, climate.**

environmental carcinogen, any of many natural or manufactured substances that can cause cancer. These substances may be chemical agents, physical agents, or certain hormones and viruses. They include arsenic, asbestos, uranium, vinyl chloride, radiation, ultraviolet rays, x-rays, and various things derived from coal tar.

environmental health, all of the aspects in and around a community that affect the health of the population.

Enzactin, a trademark for a drug applied to the skin to treat fungus (triacetin).

enzygotic twins. See **monozygotic twins.**

enzymatic detergent asthma, an allergic reaction that occurs in persons who are sensitive to alcalase, a substance found in some laundry detergents. In severe cases, the patient may suffer from inflammation of the small air sacs of the lung (alveoli). The most serious cases were originally found in workers in plants that produce detergents.

enzyme, a protein that speeds up or causes chemical reactions in living matter. Most enzymes are produced in tiny amounts and affect reactions that take place within the cells. Digestive enzymes, however, are made in large amounts and act outside the cells in the digestive tube.

enzyme-linked immunosorbent assay, a test commonly used to help in the diagnosis of AIDS infections. The test can detect the presence of antibodies of the HIV infection in blood or plasma. The test can only determine if the person was previously infected with HIV. The test is repeated if positive, since antibodies develop 6 to 12 weeks after infection. If positive, the Western Blot test is performed. See also HIV, Human immunodeficiency virus, Western Blot test.

eosinophil /ē′əsin′əfil/, a two-lobed white blood cell (leukocyte). Eosinophils make up 1% to 3% of the white blood cells of the body. They increase in number with allergy and some infections. Compare **basophil, neutrophil.** –eosinophilic, *adj.*

eosinophilia /ē′əsin′ōfil′ē-ə/, an increase in the number of eosinophils in the blood. This occurs in allergies and many swelling conditions.

eosinophilic /ē′əsin′əfil′ik/, referring to an eosinophilic leukocyte.

eosinophilic adenoma. See **acidophilic adenoma.**

eosinophilic enteropathy, a rare form of food allergy that causes nausea, stomach cramps and pain, diarrhea, hives, increased eosinophils in the blood, and eosinophils in the intestine.

eosinophilic granuloma, a growth marked by numerous eosinophils and white blood cells that destroy foreign material (histiocytes). The condition affects bone and lungs, usually in persons between 20 and 40 years of age.

eosinophilic leukemia, a cancerous tumor of white blood cells, mainly eosinophils. It resembles chronic myelocytic leukemia but is most often sudden and quick.

eosinophilic pneumonia, swelling of the lungs in which there is a buildup of white blood cells. It is marked by fluid in the lungs, fever, night sweats, cough, difficulty breathing, and weight loss. The disease may be caused by an allergy to fungus, plant fibers, wood dust, bird droppings, or other foreign substance. Compare **bronchopneumonia.** See also **asthmatic eosinophilia.**

ependyma, a layer that lines the central canal of the spinal cord and the chambers (ventricles) of the brain.

ependymal glioma, a large tumor composed of the tissue that supports nerve (glioma). It is well supplied with blood and located in the fourth chamber (ventricle) of the brain.

ependymoblastoma /ipen′dimōblastō′mə/, a cancerous tumor made up of simple cells from the lining (ependyma) of the chambers of the brain.

ependymocytoma. See **ependymoma.**

ependymoma /ipen′dimō′mə/, a tumor made up of specialized cells from the lining (ependyma)

of the chambers of the brain. Also called **ependymocytoma.**

ephapse /ef′aps/, a point of side-to-side contact between nerve fibers. Nerve signals may be passed through the walls of the nerves rather than through the space (synapse) between the ends of two nerves. Compare **synapse.**

ephaptic transmission /ifap′tik/, the passage of a nerve signal from one nerve to another through the membranes. This may be a factor in epileptic seizures. Compare **synaptic transmission.**

ephedrine, a stimulant drug that opens the airway passages. It is used to treat asthma and bronchitis and is also used as a nasal decongestant.

ephemeral fever, any fever that lasts only 24 to 48 hours and has an unknown cause.

epicanthus /ep′ikan′thəs/, a vertical fold of skin over the inner corner of the eye. It may be slight or marked. This is normal in Oriental people. Some infants with Down's syndrome also have the folds. Also called **epicanthal fold.**

epicardium /ep′ikär′dē-əm/, one of the three layers of tissue that form the wall of the heart. It is made up of a single sheet of cells that covers delicate connective tissue. Compare **myocardium.**

epicondylar fracture, any bone break that involves the knob on the end of a bone (epicondyle), as at the elbow.

epicondyle /ep′ikon′dəl/, a knuckle-like projection at the end of a bone.

epicondylitis /ep′ikon′dilī′tis/, a painful and sometimes disabling swelling of the muscle and tissues of the elbow. It is caused by repeated strain on the forearm. This is commonly known as a sports-related injury called "tennis elbow." See also **lateral humeral epicondylitis.**

epicranial aponeurosis, a fiberlike membrane that covers the skull between the muscles on top of the scalp. Also called **galea aponeurotica.**

epicranium, the complete scalp, including the skin, muscles, and tendon sheets. Compare **epicranius.**

epicranius, the muscle and tendon layer covering the top and sides of the skull from the back of the head to the eyebrows. It consists of broad, thin muscles connected by an extensive tendon sheet. Branches of the facial nerves can draw back the scalp, raise the eyebrows, and move the ears. Compare **epicranium.**

epidemic, 1. affecting a large number of people at the same time. 2. a disease that spreads rapidly through a part of the population. For example, an epidemic may affect everyone in a certain geographic area, (as a military base or a town), or everyone of a certain age or sex, (as the children or women of a region). Compare **endemic, epizootic, pandemic.**

epidemic encephalitis, any general swelling of the brain that occurs as an epidemic. Two kinds of epidemic encephalitis are **Japanese encephalitis, St. Louis encephalitis.** See also **encephalitis.**

epidemic hemoglobinuria. See **hemoglobinuria.**

epidemic hemorrhagic fever, a severe virus infection marked by fever and bleeding. The disorder develops rapidly and begins with fever and muscle ache. This is often followed by hemorrhage, blood vessel collapse, shock, and kidney failure. The virus is thought to be carried by mosquitoes, ticks, or mites. Among the various forms of epidemic hemorrhagic fevers are **Argentine hemorrhagic fever, Bolivian hemorrhagic fever, dengue hemorrhagic fever, Lassa fever, yellow fever.** See also specific viral infections.

epidemic myalgia, epidemic myositis. See **epidemic pleurodynia.**

epidemic parotitis. See **mumps.**

epidemic pleurodynia, an infection caused by a virus that mainly affects children. The symptoms include severe pain in the stomach or lower chest, fever, headache, sore throat, fatigue, and extreme muscle aches. The symptoms may continue for weeks or stop after a few days and recur weeks later. There is no specific treatment. Complete recovery is usual. Also called **Bornholm disease, devil's grip, epidemic myalgia, epidemic myositis.**

epidemic typhus, a severe infection caused by an organism of the *Rickettsia* family. The symptoms are prolonged high fever, headache, and a dark rash that covers most of the body. The organism infects the body as a result of the bite of the human body louse. The rickettsia is in the feces of the louse and enters the body when the bite is scratched. An intense headache and a fever reaching 104° F begin after a period of 10 days to 2 weeks. The rash follows. Further problems may include collapse of blood vessels, kidney failure, pneumonia, or gangrene. The death rate is high among older patients. Also called **classic typhus, European typhus, jail fever, louse-borne typhus.** Compare **murine typhus.** See also **Brill-Zinsser disease, rickettsia, typhus.**

epidemiologist, a physician or scientist who studies the spread, prevention, and control of disease in a community or a group of persons.

epiderm-, epidermo-, a combining form referring to the outer layer of the skin (epidermis).

epidermis /ep'idur'mis/, the outer layers of the skin, made up of an outer, dead portion and a deeper, living portion. Epidermal cells gradually move outward to the skin surface, changing as they go, until they become flakes. Altogether, these layers are less than one-hundredth of an inch (between 0.5 and 1.1 mm) thick. Also called **cuticle. –epidermal, epidermoid,** *adj.*

epidermoid carcinoma, a cancerous tumor in which the cells tend to behave much like the cells of the outer layer of the skin (epidermis). They then form horny cells called prickle cells.

epidermoid cyst, a common, noncancerous swelling under the skin. It is lined by packed outer skin cells. The cyst is filled with oil and dead cells. Also called **sebaceous cyst, wen.** Compare **pilar cyst.**

epidermolysis bullosa /ep'idurmol'isis/, a group of rare, hereditary skin diseases in which blisters develop, usually at sites of a wound. Severe forms may also involve mucous membranes and may leave scars and muscle weakness.

epidermophytosis, a fungus infection of the skin.

epididymis /ep'idid'imis/, *pl.* **epidiymides,** one of a pair of long, tightly coiled tubes that carry sperm from the testicles to the tip of the penis.

epididymitis /ep'idid'imi'tis/, swelling of the tubes that carry sperm from the testicles to the tip of the penis (epididymis). It may result from venereal disease, urinary-tract infection, or swelling or removal of the prostate.

epididymoorchitis /ep'idid'imō·ôrki'tis/, swelling of the tubes that carry sperm from the testicles to the tip of the penis (epididymis) and the testicles. See also **epididymitis, orchitis.**

epidural /ep'idoor'əl/, outside the outer membrane surrounding the brain and spinal cord (dura mater).

epidural anesthesia, the process of numbing the pelvic, stomach, genital, or other area. A local anesthetic is injected into the epidural space of the spinal column. Epidural anesthesia is commonly used during labor and childbirth.

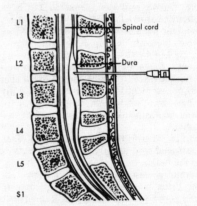

Epidural anesthesia

epidural blood patch, a patch to repair a tear in the outer membrane (dura mater) around the spinal cord. The tear is usually made by a needle during spinal anesthesia or other procedures. To form a patch, a small amount of the patient's blood is injected into the area of the hole. This blood forms a clot, covering the hole.

epidural space, the space immediately surrounding the membrane (dura mater) surrounding the brain or spinal cord.

Epifrin, a trademark for a stimulant drug (epinephrine hydrochloride).

epigastric node, a node in one of the groups of lymph nodes that serve the stomach, intestines, and pelvis. See also **lymph, lymphatic system, lymph node.**

epigastric region, the upper middle part of the abdomen, just below the breastbone. Also called **epigastrium.** See also **abdominal regions.**

epigastric sensation, a weak, sinking feeling of unclear cause. It is most often centered in the pit of the stomach but may occur elsewhere in the area of the stomach or intestines. See also **sensation,** def.1.

epigastrium. See **epigastric region.**

epigenesis /ep'ijen'əsis/, a theory of development in which the organism grows from a simple to more complex form. Compare **preformation.**

epiglottiditis. See **epiglottitis.**

epiglottis /ep'iglot'is/, the cartilagelike structure that overhangs the windpipe like a lid. It prevents food from entering the windpipe by closing while swallowing.

epiglottitis /ep'igloti'tis/, inflammation of the structure that prevents food from entering the windpipe while swallowing (epiglottis). Acute epiglottitis is a severe form of the condition, affecting mostly children. The symptoms are fever, sore throat, harsh breathing sounds, croupy cough, and a red swollen epiglottis. Also called **epiglottiditis.**

epilation. See **depilation.**

epilepsy, a group of nervous-system disorders. They are marked by repeated episodes of convulsive seizures, sensory disorders, abnormal behavior, blackouts, or all of these. All types of epilepsy have an uncontrolled electrical discharge from the nerve cells of the surface of the brain (cerebral cortex). Most epilepsy is of unknown cause. It may sometimes be linked to head injury, brain infection, brain tumor, blood vessel disturbances, intoxication, or chemical imbalance. See also **focal seizure, grand mal seizure, petit mal seizure, psychomotor seizure.**
★DIAGNOSIS: Seizures may occur several times a day to one every few years. They can occur during sleep or after stimulation, as a blinking light or sudden loud sound. Emotional disturbances also may cause seizures. Some people have odd visual effects (aura) before a seizure, but others have no warning symptoms. Most epileptic attacks are brief. They may affect the entire body or a small area. The muscles may contract and relax violently or only twitch slightly. Seizures are often followed by drowsiness or confusion. Diagnosis is made by observing the pattern of seizures. Partial (also called focal or jacksonian) seizures begin in a hand or foot and move up the limb. Mental confusion can last for several minutes or for hours or days. Petit mal attacks are marked by loss of consciousness for several seconds and eye or muscle fluttering. Grand mal seizures are the classic muscle contractions involving the entire body, loss of consciousness, and often loss of bowel control.
★TREATMENT: The kind of epilepsy determines the drug to prevent the seizures. If the cause is a tumor or metabolic imbalance, this is corrected. During an attack the patient should be protected from injury.
★PATIENT CARE: A person watching an epileptic attack should carefully note the nature of the seizure in order to tell the doctor. It is essential that the patient take the given drug as directed. Treatment must not be stopped without medical advice. The person should wear a medical identification tag. Most people who have epilepsy can control it with drugs and should expect to live a normal life. See also **anticonvulsant, aura, central nervous system stimulant, clonus, ictus, tonic.** –**epileptic,** *adj., n.*

International classification of epileptic seizures

Generalized seizures
- Tonic-clonic (grand mal)
- Absence (petit mal)
- Infantile spasms
- Other (myoclonic seizures, akinetic seizures, undetermined)

Partial seizures
- Simple partial seizures (e.g., disturbances in movement only)
- Complex partial seizures (psychomotor, other)
- Secondarily generalized seizures

From The Office of Scientific and Health Reports, National Institute of Neurological and Communicative Disorders and Stroke: Epilepsy: hope through research, NIH Publication No. 81-156, Bethesda, MD, July 1981, National Institutes of Health.

---

epileptic mania, *obsolete.* attacks of violence that occur right before, after, or in place of an epileptic seizure. See also **epilepsy, mania.**

epileptic stupor, the state of being unaware or unresponsive directly after an epileptic seizure.

epiloia. See **tuberous sclerosis.**

epimysium /ep'imiz'ē·əm/, a fiberlike cover around a muscle.

Epinal, a trademark for a stimulant drug (epinephryl borate).

epinephrine /ep'ənef'rin/, a drug that stimulates the adrenal glands and narrows the blood vessels. It is used to treat stuffy nose, to help extreme allergic reactions, and as a local anesthetic.

epinephryl borate, stimulant drug used to treat open-angle glaucoma.

★CAUTION: Narrow-angle glaucoma, absence of the lens of the eye, or known allergy to this drug bans its use.

★ADVERSE EFFECTS: Among the more severe side effects are very rapid heart beats, high blood pressure, headache, blurred vision, and allergic reaction.

epiphora. See **tearing.**

epiphyseal fracture, a break in the area at the end of a long bone where bone growth occurs. This results in separation of the head of the bone. Also called **Salter fracture.**

epiphysis /ipif'isis/, *pl.* **epiphyses,** the rounded head of a long bone, as in the arm or leg. During childhood it is separated from the shaft of the bone by the growth plate where bone growth occurs. When the bone stops growing, the growth plate becomes solid.Compare **diaphysis.** –**epiphyseal,** *adj.*

epipygus. See **pygomelus.**

episcleritis /ep'isklerī'tis/, swelling of the outer layers of the white of the eye (sclera).

episiotomy /epē'zē·ot'əmē/, a surgical procedure, performed during childbirth. The opening of the vagina is enlarged with a cut. This is done to aid delivery of the baby or to prevent stretching of the mother's muscles and connective tissues. Such stretching is thought to cause the bladder and uterus to relax and so decreases their ability to function. The incision is then closed after the baby is delivered.

episode, an incident that stands out from everyday life, as an episode of illness.

episodic care, a type of medical service in which care is given to a person for a certain problem. The patient does not remain for continued care. Emergency rooms provide episodic care.

epispadias /ep'ispā'dē·əs/, a birth defect in boys in which the urine canal (urethra) opens on the underside of the penis. Surgical correction is usually performed in the first few years of life. The defect in girls (fissure of the upper wall of the urethra) is quite rare. Compare **hypospadias.**

epistasis /epis'təsis/, suppression of the effects of a gene by another, more dominant gene. Compare **dominance.** –**epistatic,** *adj.*

epistaxis /ep'istak'sis/, bleeding from the nose. It is caused by irritation of the soft inner lining of the nose, violent sneezing, or fragile arteries in the nose. It may also be caused by long-term infection, injury, high blood pressure, leukemia, lack of enough vitamin K, or by picking of the nose. Epistaxis may result from tiny vessels breaking in the wall between the nostrils (nasal septum). This occurs most often in childhood. In adults, it is more common in men than in women and may be severe in elderly persons.

Nose bleeds may cause breathing distress, dizziness, and nausea, and may lead to fainting. Also called **nosebleed.**

★TREATMENT: The patient should breathe through the mouth and sit quietly with the head tilted a bit forward. The bleeding may be stopped by pinching the nose firmly with the fingers or by placing ice over the nose. Placing a cotton ball soaked in a drug that contracts blood vessels in the nose will also help. Epistaxis can often be prevented by using a vaporizer and gently covering the inner part of the nose with petroleum jelly.

epistropheus. See **axis.**

epithalamus /ep'ithal'əməs/, one of the parts of the thalamus, a part of the brain that passes on nerve signals for the senses and movement.

epithelioid leiomyoma /ep'ithē'lē·oid/, a rare tumor of smooth muscle which most often develops in the stomach.

epithelial rest. See **embryonic rest.**

epithelioma, a tumor derived from the epithelium.

epithelioma adenoides cysticum. See **trichoepithelioma.**

epithelium, the covering of the organs of the body, including the lining of vessels. –**epithelial,** *adj.*

epitheliofibril. See **tonofibril.**

epitympanic recess, one of two areas of the eardrum (tympanic) cavity. The other area is the tympanic cavity proper. Also called **the attic.**

epizootic /ep'izə·ot'ik/, a disease that infects the animals of a species in a certain area at the same time.

eponychium. See **cuticle,** def. 3.

epoophorectomy /ep'ō·of'ərek'təmē/, surgical removal of the epoophoron.

epoophoron /ep'ō·of'əron/, a structure that lies between the ovary and the uterine tube. It is made up of a few short tubules pointing toward the ovary and, on the other end, open into a duct. The epoophoron serves no apparent purpose. It is left over from embryonic development. Also called **parovarium.**

EPSDT, abbreviation for **Early and Periodic Screening Diagnosis and Treatment.**

Epsom salt. See **magnesium sulfate.**

Epstein-Barr virus (EBV) /ep'stīnbär'/, the herpes virus that causes mononucleosis ("kissing disease").

Epstein's pearls, small, white, pearl-like cysts that occur on both sides of the hard palate in newborn infants. They are normal and usually go away within a few weeks. Compare **Bednar's aphthae, thrush.**

e.p.t., a trademark for a home pregnancy test. It tests a substance found in the urine.

epulis /epyōō'lis/, any tumor or growth on the gum.

Equagesic, a trademark for a combination drug containing aspirin and a sedative (meprobamate). It is used to relieve pain accompanied by anxiety or tension.

equal cleavage, cell division of the fertilized egg into identical sizes, such as occurs in humans and most mammals. Compare **unequal cleavage.**

Equanil, a trademark for a sedative drug used to treat anxiety (meprobamate).

equilibration, the act of bringing new experiences into balance with the past in the mental development of a person.

equilibrium, 1. a state of balance caused by the equal action of opposing forces, as calcium and phosphorus in the body. **2.** a state of mental or emotional balance.

equine encephalitis /ē'kwin, ek'win/, an insect-carried virus infection. It causes inflammation of the nerve tissues of the brain and spinal cord. Symptoms are high fever, headache, nausea, vomiting, muscle aching, and nervous system signs as visual disturbances, tremor, lethargy, and disorientation. The virus is carried by the bite of an infected mosquito. Horses are the main host of the viruses that cause the infection. Humans are secondary hosts. **Eastern equine encephalitis (EEE)** is a severe form of the infection. It occurs along the eastern coast of the United States, lasts longer, and causes more deaths and disability. **Western equine encephalitis (WEE),** which occurs throughout the United States, is a mild, brief illness. **Venezuelan equine encephalitis (VEE),** which is also mild, is common in Central and South America, Florida, and Texas. See also **encephalitis, encephalomyelitis.**

Er, symbol for **erbium.**

ER, E.R., abbreviation for **emergency room.**

Erb-Duchenne paralysis. See **Erb's palsy.**

erbium (Er), a rare-earth, metallic element. Its atomic number is 68; its atomic weight is 167.26.

Erb's muscular dystrophy, a form of muscular dystrophy that first affects the shoulder muscles and, later, often involves the pelvic muscles. It is a gradually crippling disease that begins in childhood or adolescence. The disease is usually inherited and often affects both sexes.

Erb's palsy, a kind of paralysis caused by injury to the nerves branching off the spinal cord at the base of the neck (brachial plexus). It occurs most often in infants during delivery. The symptoms of Erb's palsy include numbness in the arm. Paralysis and wasting of the deltoid, biceps, and brachialis muscles occur. The arm on the affected side hangs loosely with the elbow pointed out and the palm toward the back. Physical therapy and splinting may be needed to improve function of the muscles and to prevent a frozen elbow (contracture). Also called **Erb-Duchenne paralysis.**

erectile /irek'til, -tīl/, capable of being raised to an erect position. The term usually describes the spongy tissue of the penis or clitoris. This tissue becomes erect when filled with blood. It also may be used when referring to the "goose bumps" on the skin (horripilation) in response to fear, anger, or cold.

erection, the condition of hardness, swelling, and raising of the penis. This may also describe the clitoris. Erection is usually caused by sexual arousal, but it also occurs during sleep or as a result of physical stimulation. Erection begins when extra blood enters the organ and blood pressure increases. This is also affected by mental and nerve reactions. See also **ejaculation, nocturnal emission, priapism.**

erector spinae. See **sacrospinalis.**

ergocalciferol. See **calciferol.**

ergoloid mesylates, a stimulant drug used to treat lessened mental ability of unknown cause, as in senility (senile dementia).
★CAUTION: Psychosis or known allergy to this drug prohibits its use.
★ADVERSE EFFECTS: Among the most serious side effects are irritation to the area under the tongue, passing nausea, and stomach disorder.

Ergomar, a trademark for a drug used to treat migraine headaches (ergotamine tartrate).

ergonovine maleate /ur'gōnō'vēn/, a drug used to contract the uterus to treat or prevent bleeding after birth or after an abortion. Also called **ergometrine maleate.**
★CAUTION: Pregnancy, blood vessel disease, high blood pressure, or known allergy to this drug forbids its use.
★ADVERSE EFFECTS: Among the more serious side effects are high blood pressure, nausea, headache, blurred vision, and allergic reactions. Death of the fetus may occur if the drug is given in pregnancy.

ergosome. See **polysome.**

ergosterol /urgos'tərôl/, a steroid of the vitamin D group. It is found in yeast, mushrooms, ergot, and other fungi. When treated with ultraviolet light it is changed into vitamin D_2. See also **calciferol, viosterol, vitamin D.**

ergot /ur'gət/, the food storage body of the fungus *Claviceps purpurea*. This fungus commonly infects rye and other cereal grasses. It contains ergot alkaloids.

ergot alkaloid, one of a large group of alkaloids found in the common fungus, *Claviceps purpurea*. This fungus grows on rye and other grains throughout the mild areas of the world. There are 3 types of these alkaloids, which include ergotamine, dihydroergotamine, and ergonovine. Ergotamine and dihydroergotamine are not as useful at causing uterine contractions as ergonovine. Therefore, ergonovine, given orally or in the vein, is used in obstetrics to treat or prevent bleeding after childbirth and to complete a partial miscarriage. Ergotamine, which is used to ease migraine headache, reduces the strength of pulses in the skull arteries.

ergotamine tartrate /urgot′əmēn/, a drug that narrows blood vessels and hastens labor. It is used to treat migraine headaches and after birth when the uterus lacks strength to contract on its own.
★CAUTION: Pregnancy, blood vessel disease, infection, or known allergy to this drug forbids its use.
★ADVERSE EFFECTS: Among the more serious side effects are vomiting, diarrhea, thirst, tingling of fingers and toes, and increased blood pressure. Death of the fetus may occur if the drug is given to a woman during pregnancy.

ergotherapy, the use of exercise to treat disease. The therapy also includes any treatment that increases the blood supply to a diseased or injured part, as massage or hot baths.

Eros, a term, used by Freud, for the instinct for survival. It includes self-preservation and survival of the species through reproduction.

erosion, the wearing away or slow and steady destroying of a tissue. Erosion may be caused by infection, injury, or other disease. It is usually marked by the appearance of an ulcer. See also **necrosis.**

erosive gastritis, a swelling condition marked by several erosions of the mucous membrane lining the stomach. Nausea, loss of appetite, pain, and stomach bleeding may occur. Treatment includes removing the irritating substance. See also **chemical gastritis, corrosive gastritis.**

erosive osteoarthritis. See **Kellgren's syndrome.**

eroticism, 1. sexual impulse or desire. **2.** the arousal or attempt to arouse sexual desire. Also called **erotism.** See also **anal eroticism, oral eroticism.**

erotomania, *obsolete.* a mental state of obsession with sexuality and sexual behavior.

erucic acid, a fatty acid that has been linked with heart disease. It is found in rapeseed oil and is used in some countries as a vegetable oil for salad dressings, margarines, and mayonnaise.

eructation, the act of bringing up air from the stomach with a typical sound. Also called **belching.**

eruption, the rapid growth of a skin rash, especially one caused by a virus or by a drug reaction.

eruptive fever, any disease marked by fever and a rash.

eruptive gingivitis, a gum swelling that may occur when the permanent teeth emerge.

eruptive xanthoma, a skin disorder linked with high fatty acid levels in the blood. A red or pale raised rash suddenly appears on the trunk, legs, arms, and buttocks.

erysipelas /er′isip′ələs/, a skin infection marked by redness, swelling, blisters, fever, pain, and swollen lymph nodes. It is caused by a species of streptococci. Treatment includes antibiotics, pain relievers, and dressings on the skin.

erysipeloid /er′isip′əloid/, an infection of the hands marked by blue-red bumps or patches and sometimes redness. It is caught by handling meat or fish infected with *Erysipelothrix rhusiopathiae.* Also called **fish-handler's disease.** Compare **erysipelas.**

erythema /er′ithē′mə/, redness or swelling of the skin or mucous membranes. It is the result of widening and clogging of capillaries near the skin surface. Examples of erythema are nervous blushes and mild sunburn. See also **erythroderma, rubor. −erythematous,** *adj.*

erythema chronicum migrans, a skin blemish that begins as a small bump. It spreads outward, extending by a raised, red edge that is clear in the center. It may be linked with **Lyme arthritis,** which is caused by the bite of a small tick.

erythema infectiosum, an acute infection, mainly of children. The symptoms are fever and a rash beginning on the cheeks and appearing later on the arms, thighs, buttocks, and trunk. As the rash spreads, earlier areas fade. Sunlight worsens the rash. It usually lasts about 10 days. Also called **fifth disease.**

erythema marginatum, a variety of **erythema multiforme** that occur in acute rheumatic fever. The symptoms are disk-shaped, non-itching, flat red areas on the skin. When they fade in the center, they leave raised edges.

erythema multiforme, an allergic condition marked by a rash on the skin and mucous membranes. A variety of sizes and shapes appear on the patient (multiforme) and include nodules, pimples, blisters, and bull's-eye-shaped areas. Erythema multiforme can occur with many infections, collagen diseases, drug reactions, allergies, and pregnancy. A severe form of this condition is known as **Stevens-Johnson syndrome.**

erythema nodosum, an allergy marked by blood vessel swelling. It causes reddened, tender bumps on both shins and, occasionally, on other parts of the body. The bumps last for several days or weeks and never become open sores. This disorder is often linked with mild fever, malaise, and pains in muscles and joints. This condition occurs with streptococcal infections, tuberculosis, sarcoidosis, drug allergy, and pregnancy.

erythema perstans, a continuous limited redness of the skin, often caused by a reaction to drugs.

erythema neonatorum, a common skin condition of newborns. A pink raised rash occurs that is often covered by blisters or pustules. The rash appears within 24 to 48 hours after birth, covers the chest, stomach, back, and diaper area, and disappears spontaneously after several days. Also called **toxic erythema of the newborn,** *(informal)* **flea bites.**

erythrasma /er'ithraz'mə/, a bacteria-caused skin infection of the armpit or groin regions. It causes irregular, reddish-brown raised patches. The disease does not cause any symptoms. It is more common in diabetics and responds quickly to the oral antibiotic erythromycin. Compare **intertrigo, tinea cruris.**

erythredema polyneuropathy. See **acrodynia.**

erythremia /er'ithrē'mēə/, an abnormal increase in the number of red blood cells.

erythrityl tetranitrate, a drug that dilates the blood vessels of the heart. It is used to treat chest pain resulting from heart disease.

★CAUTION: It is used with caution when glaucoma is present. Known allergy to this drug forbids its use.

★ADVERSE EFFECTS: Among the most serious side effects are low blood pressure, allergic reactions, headache, and flushing.

erythro-, a combining form meaning 'red.'

erythroblastosis fetalis, a type of anemia that occurs in newborns who have Rh positive blood, but whose mothers are Rh negative. The fetal blood as a foreign substance (antigen). Her blood forms antibodies against the fetal blood. As a result, red blood cells (erythrocytes) in the fetus's body are killed. This causes high levels of bilirubin in the fetus, the amniotic fluid, and the placenta. The antigen-antibody reaction rarely occurs with the first pregnancy, but there is greater risk with each succeeding pregnancy. However, if anti-Rh gamma globulin is given to the mother after delivery or abortion of an Rh positive fetus, the reaction is avoided in future pregnancies. Diagnosis of the disease during pregnancy is made by analyzing the bilirubin levels in the amniotic fluid. If erythroblastosis fetalis is found, the fetus can be given a transfusion inside the uterus or immediately after birth. Similar reactions involving the ABO blood groups can occur but are generally less severe. See also **hydrops fetalis, hyperbilirubinemia of the newborn, Rh factor.**

erythrocyte /erith'rəsīt'/, a red blood cell. It is a concave disk, microscopic in size (about 7 micrometers in diameter), and contains hemoglobin. As the main element of the circulating blood, its main function is to transport oxygen, which is carried by the hemoglobin. The number of cells per cu mm of blood is usually between 4.5 million and 5.5 million in men and between 4.2 million and 4.8 million in women. The number varies with age, activity, and environment. For example, an increase to a level of 8 million per cu mm can normally occur at over 10,000 feet above sea level. An erythrocyte usually lives for 110 to 120 days. It is then removed from the bloodstream and broken down in the body's cells. New erythrocytes are produced in the marrow of long bones at a steady rate so that a constant level is usually maintained. With acute blood loss, hemolytic anemia, or chronic lack of oxygen, erythrocyte production may increase greatly. Kinds of erythrocyte include **burr cell, discocyte, macrocyte, meniscocyte, spherocyte.** Also called **red blood cell, red cell, red corpuscle.**

erythrocyte sedimentation rate (ESR), a blood test that measures the rate at which red blood cells settle out in a tube of unclotted blood. It is stated in millimeters per hour. Blood is collected in a substance that prevents clotting. It is allowed to sit and form a sediment for 1 hour. The distance the erythrocytes have fallen in the tube is then measured. Elevated sedimentation rates indicate inflammation. Swelling alters the blood proteins, which makes the red blood cells clump together, becoming heavier than normal. The faster they fall to the bottom of the tube, the more severe the swelling. A series of ESR evaluations is useful in tracking the course of swelling in rheumatic diseases. When done with a white blood cell count, an ESR can indicate infection. Certain nonswelling conditions, as pregnancy, can also produce high sedimentation rates. Women normally have higher (faster) ESRs than men. Also called *(informal)* **sed. rate.** See also **inflammation.**

erythrocythemia /erith'rōsīthē'mē·ə/, a rise in the number of erythrocytes circulating in the blood.

erythrocytosis /erith'rōsītō'sis/, an abnormal rise in the number of circulating red cells. See also **polycythemia.**

erythroderma /erith'rōdur'mə/, any dermatitis linked with abnormal redness of the skin. Compare **erythema, rubor.**

erythroleukemia, a cancer-causing blood disorder marked by a excess production of red blood cells in bone marrow. Immature red blood cells in the bone marrow have bizarre, lobed nuclei. There are also abnormal immature erythrocytes in peripheral blood. Also called **diGuglielmo's disease, diGuglielmo's syndrome, erythromyeloblastic leukemia.**

erythromelalgia /erith'rōmilal'jə/, a rare disorder marked by attacks of blood vessel dilation. It is linked with burning, redness of the skin, and pain. **–erythromelalgic,** *adj.*

erythromycin /erith'rōmī'sin/, an antibiotic used to treat many bacterial infections, particularly infections that cannot be treated by penicillins.

★CAUTION: Liver disease or known allergy to this drug prohibits its use.

★ADVERSE EFFECTS: Among the more serious side effects are liver disease and allergic reactions.

erythromyeloblastic leukemia. See **erythroleukemia.**

erythrophobia, **1.** an anxiety disorder marked by an irrational fear of blushing or of displaying embarrassment. **2.** an unnatural fear of the color red.

erythroplasia of Queyrat /erith′rōplā′zhə/, a precancerous sore on or around the tip of the penis. It is a reddish patch on the skin and is usually surgically removed. See also **carcinoma in situ.**

erythropoiesis /erith′rōpō·ē′sis/, the process of erythrocyte production. The bone marrow produces cells with nuclei. These cells mature into erythrocytes without nuclei that contain hemoglobin. See also **erthrocyte, erythropoietin, hemoglobin, leukopoiesis. –erythropoietic,** *adj.*

erythropoietin (EPO) /erith′rōpō·ē′tin/, a hormone produced mainly in the kidneys. It is released into the bloodstream in response to low oxygen levels. The hormone controls the production of erythrocytes and is thus able to raise the oxygen-carrying capacity of the blood. See also **erythropoiesis.**

Es, symbol for **einsteinium.**

escape beat, an automatic beat of the heart that occurs when there is a pause in the dominant heart beat cycle. Escape beats act as safety mechanisms. Anything that causes a pause in the heart cycle may allow an escape to occur.

eschar /es′kär/, a scab or dry crust resulting from a burn, infection, or skin disease. **–escharotic,** *adj.*

escharonodulaire, escarronodulaire. See **Marseilles fever.**

Escherichia coli /eshirī′kē·ə kō′lī/, a species of bacteria of the family Enterobacteriaceae. *E. coli* normally lives in the intestines and is common in water, milk, and soil. It is the most frequent cause of urinary-tract infection and is a cause of serious infection in wounds.

escutcheon, the shieldlike pattern of the growth of pubic hair.

eserine, eserine sulfate. See **physostigmine.**

Esidrix, a trademark for a diuretic drug used to treat high blood pressure (hydrochlorothiazide).

Eskalith, a trademark for an antidepressant used to treat bipolar disorders (lithium carbonate).

Esmarch's bandage /es′märks/, a broad, flat, elastic bandage wrapped around an elevated arm or leg to force blood out of the limb. It is used before certain operations to create a blood-free area.

esophageal cancer /əsof′əjē′əl, es′ofä′jē·əl/, a cancer-causing tumor of the esophagus that occurs three times more often in men than in women and more often in Asia and Africa than in North America. Risk factors are heavy use of alcohol, smoking, betel-nut chewing, Plummer-Vinson syndrome, hiatus hernia, and inability to relax the muscle between the esophagus and the stomach (achalasia). A mold poison (aflatoxin) in grain and peanuts or a dietary deficiency of molybdenum may be involved. Esophageal cancer does not often cause any symptoms in the early stages. In later stages it causes painful swallowing, appetite and weight loss, vomiting, swollen lymph nodes in the neck, and often a nagging cough. Surgical treatment may require total or partial removal, with the diseased segment replaced by a Dacron graft or a section of the large intestine. If only the lower third of the esophagus is removed, the end may be attached to the stomach. X-ray therapy may heal early tumors and may effectively treat symptoms of advanced cancer. See also **esophagectomy.**

esophageal dysfunction, any disease or abnormality that interferes with normal functioning of the esophagus. Examples include difficulty swallowing, esophagitis, or sphincter incompetence. The condition is one of the main symptoms of scleroderma.

esophageal lead, an electrocardiographic conductor in which an electrode is placed within the esophagus. This helps to identify heart irregularities.

esophageal varices, a network of twisted veins at the lower end of the esophagus, which is enlarged and swollen as the result of high blood pressure within the portal vein in the abdomen. These vessels often form open sores and bleed. This is often a complication of cirrhosis of the liver.

esophagectomy /esof′əjek′təmē/, an operation in which all or part of the esophagus is removed. This may be required to treat severe, recurrent, bleeding esophageal varices.

esophagitis /esof′əjī′tis/, inflammation of the lining of the esophagus. It is caused by infection, irritation from a tube inserted through the nose to the stomach, or, most commonly, backflow of gastric juice from the stomach. See also **gastroesophageal reflux.**

esophagoscopy /esof′əgos′kəpē/, examination of the esophagus with an endoscope.

esophagus /esof′əgəs/, the muscular canal, 9½ inches long (about 24 cm), extending from below the tongue to the stomach. It is the narrowest part of the digestive tube. It is narrowest where it begins and at the point where it passes through the diaphragm. The esophagus is made up of a fibrous coat, a muscular coat and is lined with mucous membrane. Also called **gullet. –esophageal,** *adj.*

esophoria /es′əfôr′ē·ə/, deviation of one eye toward the other eye when the eyes are not focused on an object. Also called **cross-eye.** Compare **esotropia.**

esotropia /es′ətrō′pē·ə/, an inward deviation of one eye in relation to the other eye. Also called **convergent strabismus, cross-eye, inter-**

nal strabismus. Compare esophoria, exotropia. See also strabismus. −esotropic, adj.

ESP, abbreviation for extrasensory perception.

espundia /espun′dē·ə/, a form of American leishmaniasis that is most common in Mexico and Central and South America. It is caused by the protozoa Leishmania brasiliensis and is transmitted by the bite of sandflies. The first sign is a skin ulcer that often disappears on its own. This is followed by ulcers on the mucous membranes in the nose and mouth. Treatment includes antimony, infrared therapy, and x-ray treatment.

ESR, abbreviation for erythrocyte sedimentation rate.

essential amino acid, an organic compound that is not produced in the body but is essential for health in adults and growth in infants and children. Essential amino acids must be obtained from the diet. Adults require isoleucine, leucine, lysine, methionine, phenylalanine, threonine, tryptophan, and valine. Infants need these eight amino acids, plus arginine and histidine. Cysteine and tyrosine are considered semiessential. See also amino acid.

essential fatty acid, a polyunsaturated acid, as linoleic, linolenic, and arachidonic, that is essential in the diet for the proper growth and functioning of the body. It forms prostaglandins, which help organ muscles contract, regulate stomach acid, lower blood pressure, and regulate body temperature. Essential fatty acid also aids in fat transport and metabolism. It is necessary for the normal functioning of the reproductive system, hormone regulation, and for breaking up cholesterol deposits in the arteries. The best sources are natural vegetable oils (safflower, soy, and corn oils), margarines blended with vegetable oils, wheat germ, seeds (pumpkin, sesame, and sunflower), poultry fat, and fish oils, especially cod-liver oil. A deficiency of essential fatty acids causes changes in cell structure, resulting in slowed growth and other disorders. Symptoms include brittle and dull hair, nail problems, dandruff, allergies, and dermatitis, especially eczema in infants.

essential fever, any fever of unknown cause.

essential hypertension, high blood pressure for which no cause can be found and which is often the only disorder. High blood pressure is a health risk, especially for developing heart disease. Essential hypertension can be controlled by drugs. Also called primary hypertension. See also benign hypertension, malignant hypertension.

essential nutrient, the carbohydrates, proteins, fats, minerals, and vitamins necessary for growth and normal function. These substances are supplied by food, since some are not produced in the body in large enough amounts for normal health.

essential thrombocythemia. See thrombocytosis.

essential tremor, an uncontrollable fine shaking of the hand and head, especially during routine movements of the body. It is an inherited, family disorder that appears during adolescence or in middle age. It begins very slowly, then progresses until it is a more noticeable disorder. Also called familial tremor. Compare parkinsonism.

EST, abbreviation for electric shock therapy.

established name, the name given to a drug by the United States Adopted Names Council. The established name, which is usually shorter than the chemical name, is the name by which the drug is known to doctors, nurses and druggists. Also called generic name. See also chemical name, trademark.

Estar, a trademark for a coal tar substance used to treat eczema and psoriasis.

ester /es′tər/, a class of chemical compound formed by an alcohol bonding to one or more organic acids. Fats are esters, formed by the bonding of fatty acids with the alcohol glycerol.

esterase, any enzyme that splits esters.

esterified estrogen, a form of natural estrogen used to treat menstrual irregularities and symptoms of menopause. It is also used as a contraceptive.
★CAUTION: Pregnancy, known or suspected breast cancer, inflammation of a vein associated with clotting, vaginal bleeding of unknown origin, or known allergy to this drug prohibits its use.
★ADVERSE EFFECTS: Among the more serious side effects are gallbladder disease, blood clots, and a possible increase in risk of cancer.

Estinyl, a trademark for an estrogen used to treat postmenopausal breast cancer, menstrual cycle irregularities, cancer of the prostate, decreased function of sexual organs, for contraception, and to relieve menopausal symptoms (ethinyl estradiol).

estr-, the combining form for the name of an estrogen (female sex hormone).

Estrace, a trademark for an estrogen (estradiol).

estradiol /cs′trədī′ôl/, the most potent, naturally occurring human estrogen. It is also found in hog ovaries and in the urine of pregnant mares. Various esters of estradiol given in the muscle or orally are used as estrogens. See also estrogen.

Estradurin, a trademark for an estrogen used to treat cancer (polyestradiol phosphate).

estramustine phosphate sodium, a drug used to treat cancer of the prostate.
★CAUTION: Clotting disorders or known allergy to this drug prohibits its use.
★ADVERSE EFFECTS: The most serious side effects are stroke, heart attack, inflammation of a vein linked with clotting, clots in the lungs, and heart failure.

estrangement, emotional stress caused by the separation of a mother from her newborn child when the infant is ill, is premature, or has a birth defect. This prevents the mother from establishing a normal relationship with her child.

Estratab, a trademark for an estrogen (esterified estrogens).

Estraval, a trademark for an estrogen (estradiol valerate).

estriol /es'trē-ôl/, a relatively weak, naturally occurring human estrogen found in large amounts in urine. See also **estrogen**.

estrogen /es'trojən/, one of a group of hormonal steroid compounds that aid the development of female secondary sex traits (such as breast development). Human estrogen is produced in the ovaries, adrenal glands, testicles, and both the fetus and placenta. Estrogen prepares the wall of the uterus for fertilization, implantation, and nutrition of the early embryo after each menstrual period. Drugs containing estrogen are used in oral contraceptives, to treat postmenopausal breast cancer and prostatic cancer, and to inhibit production of breast milk. These drugs are also used to prevent miscarriage, treat brittle bones (osteoporosis), and ovarian disease. Estrogen is also given to relieve discomforts of menopause. Kinds of estrogen are **conjugated estrogen, esterified estrogen, estradiol, estriol, estrone. –estrogenic,** *adj.*

estrone /es'trōn/, a relatively strong estrogen. It is used to treat menstrual cycle irregularities, cancer of the prostate, blood vessel symptoms in menopause, and to prevent pregnancy.
★CAUTION: Swelling of a vein linked with clotting, abnormal genital bleeding, known or suspected pregnancy, or known allergy to this drug prohibits its use.
★ADVERSE EFFECTS: Among the more serious side effects are swelling of a vein linked with clotting, clot formation, and excess levels of calcium.

estropipate, an estrogen used to treat blood vessel symptoms of menopause, vaginitis linked with menopause, atrophy of the female genitalia, decreased function of the female sex organs and ovarian failure.
★CAUTION: Known or suspected cancer of the breast or estrogen-dependent cancer, pregnancy, inflammation of a vein linked with clotting, clotting disorders, undiagnosed abnormal genital bleeding, or complications from previous estrogen use prohibits its use.
★ADVERSE EFFECTS: Among the most serious side effects are a possible increased risk of cancer, gallbladder disease, and clotting disorders.

estrus, the cyclic period of sexual activity in mammals other than primates.

ethambutol hydrochloride, an antibiotic used to treat tuberculosis.
★CAUTION: Swelling of eye nerves or known allergy to this drug prohibits its use. It is not recommended for small children.
★ADVERSE EFFECTS: Among the most serious side effects are diminished vision and allergic reactions, as rashes.

ethanoic acid. See **acetic acid.**

ethanol, ethyl alcohol. See also **alcohol.**

ethaverine hydrochloride, a drug that relaxes smooth muscles to relieve spasm of the intestinal or urinary tract, spasms of the arteries, and decreased blood flow to the brain.
★CAUTION: Liver disease, heart beat irregularities, or known allergy to this drug prohibits its use. It is used with caution in patients who have glaucoma.
★ADVERSE EFFECTS: Among the more serious side effects are low blood pressure, abdominal distress, irregular heart beats, and headache.

ethchlorvynol /ethklôr'vənôl/, a drug with calming and sleep-inducing effects, it is used to treat insomnia.

ethene. See **ethylene.**

ether, a liquid used as a general anesthetic. Because it causes excellent relief of pain, and profound muscle relaxation, other supplementary drugs to relieve pain and block nerve and muscle are often unnecessary. It has an irritating, strong odor, is highly flammable and explosive, and often causes nausea and vomiting after surgery.

ethical drug, a drug available only by prescription and advertised only to physicians and other health professionals. Also called **prescription drug.** Compare **over the counter.**

ethinamate /ethin'əmāt/, a drug that produces sedation. It is used to treat insomnia.
★CAUTION: Known allergy to this drug prohibits its use. It is not recommended for pregnant women, for people under 15 years of age, or for persons with a history of drug abuse.
★ADVERSE EFFECTS: Among the more serious side effects are small hemorrhages into the skin, physical and psychological dependence, and skin rash.

ethinyl estradiol /eth'inil/, an estrogen used to treat postmenopausal breast cancer, menstrual cycle irregularities, cancer of the prostate, decreased function of sexual organs; for contraception; and to relieve blood vessel symptoms of menopause.
★CAUTION: Thrombophlebitis, abnormal genital bleeding, known or suspected pregnancy, or known allergy to this drug prohibits its use.
★ADVERSE EFFECTS: Among the more serious side effects are swelling of a vein associated with clotting, clot formation, and excess levels of calcium.

ethionamide /eth'ē-ənam'īd/, an antibacterial drug used to treat tuberculosis.

★CAUTION: Existing liver damage or known allergy to this drug prohibits its use. This drug should not be used in pregnancy.

★ADVERSE EFFECTS: Among the more serious side effects are skin rash, jaundice, and mental depression. Intestinal side effects are common.

ethmoidal air cell /ethmoi′dəl/, one of the many small, thin-walled cavities in the ethmoid bone of the skull.

ethmoid bone, the very light and spongy bone at the base of the skull that forms most of the walls of the upper part of the nasal cavity.

ethoheptazine citrate, a nonnarcotic drug used to relieve mild to moderate pain.

★CAUTION: Known allergy to this drug prohibits its use.

★ADVERSE EFFECTS: Among the most common side effects are stomach and intestine distress and dizziness.

ethology, the scientific study of the behavioral patterns of animals, especially in their native habitat.

ethopropazine hydrochloride, a drug used to treat parkinsonism and other nervous-system disorders.

★CAUTION: Narrow-angle glaucoma, asthma, blockage of the genitourinary or gastrointestinal tract, severe ulcerative colitis, or known allergy to this drug or to phenothiazines prohibits its use.

★ADVERSE EFFECTS: Among the more serious side effects are blurred vision, nervous-system effects, excessively rapid heart beats, dry mouth, decreased sweating, and allergic reactions.

ethosuximide, a drug that controls convulsions. It is used to treat petit mal epilepsy.

★CAUTION: Known allergy to this drug or to any succinimides prohibits its use.

★ADVERSE EFFECTS: Among the more serious side effects are abnormal blood conditions, disorders of the stomach and intestines, complications of blood cell formation, and systemic lupus erythematosus.

ethotoin /ethō′tō·in/, a drug that controls convulsions. It is used to treat grand mal and psychomotor seizures.

★CAUTION: Liver disease, blood disorders, or known allergy to this drug or to any hydantoin prohibits its use. It is not recommended for use during pregnancy or nursing.

★ADVERSE EFFECTS: Among the more serious side effects are blood disorders, nausea, fatigue, skin rash, and chest pain.

Ethril, a trademark for an antibacterial used to treat many bacterial infections, particularly infections that cannot be treated by penicillins (erythromycin stearate).

ethyl alcohol. See alcohol.

ethylene /eth′əlēn/, a colorless, flammable gas that is lighter than air and has a slightly sweet odor and taste. It was once used as a general anesthetic. It is slightly stronger than nitrous oxide.

ethylenediamine /eth′əlēndi·am′ēn/, a clear, thick liquid having the odor of ammonia. It is used as a solvent and an emulsifier. It is also mixed with a stabilizer with aminophylline, a drug for bronchial asthma, when the drug is injected.

ethylene dibromide (EDB), a liquid used as an insecticide and gasoline additive. Because it has been found to be a cause of cancer in animals, the Environmental Protection Agency has limited the use of EDB on grains and fruits intended for human use.

ethylene oxide, a gas used to sterilize surgical instruments and other supplies.

ethylestrenol, a steroid used to help rebuild body tissue in patients with severe diseases and injuries.

ethylnorepinephrine hydrochloride /eth′ilnôrep′inef′rin/, a drug that widens the airway passages. It is used to treat bronchial asthma.

★CAUTION: Known allergy to this drug or to similar drugs prohibits its use.

★ADVERSE EFFECTS: Among the more serious side effects are increased or decreased blood pressure, palpitations, and a rise in heart rate.

ethyl oxide, a colorless liquid solvent similar to diethyl ether, it is widely used in making drugs.

ethynodiol diacetate /eth′inōdī′ôl/, an oral contraceptive drug (progestin).

ethynodiol diacetate and ethinyl estradiol, an oral contraceptive drug.

★CAUTION: Swelling of a vein linked with clotting, heart disease, breast or reproductive organ cancer, or known allergy to either ingredient prohibits its use.

★ADVERSE EFFECTS: Among the more serious side effects are swelling of a vein, linked with clotting, tumors of the uterus, gall bladder disease, clot formation, and liver disorders.

ethynodiol diacetate and mestranol, an oral contraceptive drug.

★CAUTION: Swelling of a vein, linked with clotting, heart disease, breast or reproductive organ cancer, or known allergy to either ingredient prohibits its use.

★ADVERSE EFFECTS: Among the more serious side effects are swelling of a vein, linked with clotting, tumors of the uterus, gallbladder disease, clot formation, and liver disorders.

etidronate disodium /etid′rənāt/, a drug that regulates the metabolism of calcium. It is used to treat Paget's disease of bone, hardening of muscle into bone, and after total-hip replacement. Also called **sodium etidronate.**

★CAUTION: There are no known cautions.

★ADVERSE EFFECTS: Among the more serious side effects are bone pain at sites of Paget's disease, intestinal disturbances, and elevated levels of phosphate in the blood.

etiology /ē′tē·ol′əjē/, the study of all factors that

may be involved in the development of a disease. This includes the condition of the patient, the cause, and the way in which the patient's body is affected. Compare **pathogenesis.**

etomidate /etom'idāt/, a drug that produces sleep very quickly. It is used to start anesthesia.
★CAUTION: Allergy to the drug prohibits its use.
★ADVERSE EFFECTS: This drug may cause pain at the injection site and some movement during anesthesia.

Etrafon, a trademark for a combination drug containing a tranquilizer (perphenazine) and an antidepressant (amitriptyline hydrochloride).

Eu, symbol for **europium.**

eucaryon. See **eukaryon.**

eucaryosis. See **eukaryosis.**

eucholia /yōōkō'lē·ə/, the normal state of the bile. This includes the amount produced and the condition of the contents.

euchromatin /yōōkrō'mətin/, that part of chromosome material that is active in gene expression during cell division. See also **chromatin.** –**euchromatic,** adj.

euchromosome. See **autosome.**

eugenics /yōōjen'iks/, the study of methods for controlling the traits of future human populations through selective breeding.

euglobulin, a globulin that does not dissolve in distilled water. Compare **albumin, cryoglobulin.**

eugnathic anomaly /yōōnath'ik/, an abnormality of the teeth and their bone supports.

eukaryocyte /yōōker'ē·ōsit'/, a cell with a true nucleus. These cells are found in all higher organisms and in some microorganisms, including amebae, plasmodia, and trypanosomes. Also spelled **eucaryocyte.** Compare **prokaryocyte.** –**eukaryotic,** adj.

eukaryon /yōōker'ē·on/, **1.** a nucleus in a cell that is very complex, organized, and surrounded by a nuclear membrane. Eukaryons usually occur only in higher organisms. **2.** an organism containing a very complex, organized nucleus surrounded by a nuclear membrane and containing organelles. This is typical of all organisms except bacteria, viruses, and blue-green algae. Also spelled **eucaryon.** Compare **prokaryon.**

eunuch /yōō'nək/, a male whose testicles have been destroyed or removed.

eunuchoidism /yōō'nəkoidiz'əm/, deficiency of male hormone. The deficiency leads to sterility, abnormal tallness, small testicles, poor development of secondary sexual traits, lack of sexual desire, and impotence.

euphoretic /yōō'fəret'ik/, **1.** a substance or event tending to produce a condition of euphoria. **2.** a substance tending to produce euphoria, as LSD, mescaline, marijuana, and other hallucinogenic drugs.

euphoria /yōōfôr'ē·ə/, **1.** a feeling of well-being or elation. **2.** a greater-than-normal sense of physical and emotional well-being. It is not based on reality, is out of proportion to its cause, and is inappropriate to the situation. This is commonly seen in some forms of mental disorders, and in poisonous and drug-induced states. Compare **ecstasy.**

euploid /yōō'ploid/, **1.** referring to a person, organism, or cell with a chromosome number that is an exact multiple of the normal (haploid) number of the species. For example, diploid is two sets of chromosomes, triploid is three, tetraploid is four, and polyploid is having over two sets.

Eurax, a trademark for a drug used to treat scabies (crotamiton).

European blastomycosis. See **cryptococcosis.**

European typhus. See **epidemic typhus.**

europium (Eu), a rare earth, metallic element. Its atomic number is 63; its atomic weight is 151.96.

eustachian tube /yōōstā'shən/, a tube lined with mucous membrane that joins the nose-throat cavity (nasopharynx) and the inner ear (tympanic cavity). This tube allows air pressure in the inner ear to be equalized with the outside air pressure. When the air pressure change is sudden or extreme (such as in an airplane), causing the ears to stop up, swallowing will usually equalize the pressure. Also called **auditory tube.**

eustress /yōō'stres/, a good form of stress.

euthenics, the science that deals with improving the human species through the control of environmental factors, as pollution, malnutrition, disease, and drug abuse. Compare **eugenics.**

euthanasia /yōō'thənā'zhə/, deliberately bringing about the death of a person who is suffering from an incurable disease. Euthanasia can be performed actively, as by giving a lethal drug, or by allowing the person to die by not giving treatment. Euthanasia is both a legal and ethical issue that has received much attention in recent years. Legally, euthanasia is murder and therefore against the law. Also called **mercy killing.**

Euthroid, a trademark for a thyroid hormone used to treat underactive thyroid (liotrix).

euthymism /yōōthī'mizm/, the typical responses of normal moods.

Eutonyl, a trademark for an antidepressant drug used to treat high blood pressure (pargyline hydrochloride).

Eutron, a trademark for a combination drug containing a diuretic (methyclothiazide) and an antidepressant (pargyline hydrochloride). It is used to release high blood pressure.

evacuate, to discharge or remove a substance from a cavity, space, organ, or tract of the body. –**evacuation,** n.

evaporation, the change of a substance from a solid or liquid state to a gas. The process of evaporation is speeded by raising the temperature and lowering the atmospheric pressure. See also **boiling point.** **–evaporate,** *v.*

event-related potential (ERP), a type of brain wave that is a response to a specific stimulus. An example is a particular wave pattern that occurs whenever a patient hears a clicking sound. See also **evoked potential.**

evisceration, 1. the removal of the organs (viscera) from the abdominal cavity; disembowelment. **2.** the removal of the contents from an organ or an organ from its cavity. **3.** bulging of an internal organ through a wound or surgical incision, especially in the abdominal wall. **–eviscerate,** *v.*

evocation, a specific change in an early fetus (embryo) that occurs because of a single evocator. See also **induction.**

evocator, a specific chemical or hormone produced by embryonic tissue. The substance stimulates the embryo to grow and change.

evoked potential (EP), a tracing of a brain wave. It is measured by electrodes on the surface of the head at various places and recorded by an electroencephalograph (EEG). The EP, unlike the waves seen on the standard EEG tracing, shows response to specific stimulation. The parts of the brain that receive information about vision, hearing, or touch are electrically stimulated. This method is used during surgery to monitor the activity of the brain and nerves. The surgeon is thus able to avoid damage to the nerves. Evoked potentials are also used to detect multiple sclerosis and various disorders of hearing and sight. Kinds of evoked potentials include **brain stem auditory evoked potential, somatosensory evoked potential, visual evoked potential.** See also **brain electric activity map.**

evoked response. See **evoked potential.**

evoked response audiometry, a method of testing hearing. It is used to detect possible defects in the eighth cranial nerve and the brainstem.

evolution, 1. a slow, steady, orderly, continuous process of change from one condition to another. In humans, it includes all aspects of life, including physical, mental, social, cultural, and intellectual development. Evolution involves a steady movement from a simple to a more complex state. **2.** the theory of the origin and continuation of all plant and animal species, including humans. It includes their development from lower to more complex forms. This occurs by natural selection through genetic changes; and inbreeding. Kinds of evolution are **convergent evolution, determinant evolution, emergent evolution, organic evolution, orthogenic evolution, saltatory evolution.** **–evolutionist,** *n.*

evulsed tooth. See **avulsed tooth.**

Ewing's sarcoma, a cancerous tumor that develops in bone marrow, usually in long bones or the pelvis. It occurs most often in adolescent boys. The symptoms are pain, swelling, and fever. The tumor, a soft, crumbly grayish mass that may invade nearby soft tissues, is difficult to tell apart from other bone-marrow cancers. Also called **Ewing's tumor.** See also **neuroblastoma, reticulum cell sarcoma.**

Ewing's tumor. See **endothelial myeloma.**

exa-, a combining form that refers to the multiple 10^{18}.

exacerbation /igzas'ərbā'shən/, an increase in the seriousness of a disease or disorder. It is marked by greater intensity in the symptoms.

exanthema /ig'zanthē'mə/, a skin rash that often has the specific features of an infectious disease. Chicken pox, measles, roseola infantum, or rubella usually have particular types of exanthema. Also called **exanthem.** Compare **enanthema.** **–exanthematous,** *adj.*

exanthem subitum. See **roseola infantum.**

excess mortality, an early death, one that occurs before the average life expectancy for the person.

exchange transfusion in the newborn, giving whole blood in exchange for 75% to 85% of an infant's blood. The infant's blood is repeatedly drawn out in small amounts and replaced with equal amounts of donor blood. This is done to improve the oxygen-carrying ability of the blood in treating erythroblastosis fetalis. It removes Rh and ABO antibodies, sensitized red blood cells, and excess bilirubin. See also **erythroblastosis fetalis.**

★METHOD: Before exchange transfusion, nothing is given by mouth for 3 to 4 hours. The baby's limbs are held still and the blood is warmed. A needle is inserted into a vein, and the removing-replacing cycle of blood exchange is started. The procedure may be carried out under phototherapy lights. During the procedure the young patient is carefully watched for reaction symptoms: heartbeat less than 100 beats a minute, blue skin, low temperature, breathing abnormalities, vomiting, abdominal distention, or heart problems. The breathing and heart rates are checked every 5 minutes, the temperature every 15 to 30 minutes. After the procedure, the infant should be handled gently and as little as possible for 2 to 4 hours. Feeding can be started 4 to 6 hours after transfusion with a bottle having a soft nipple and a large enough hole to make nursing easy. The infant is fed slowly and his or her position is changed after each feeding.

★OUTCOME: An exchange transfusion is usually given only to a high-risk infant. The procedure often is very useful in treating the blood disorders in erythroblastosis in the newborn.

excise /iksīz'/, to remove completely, as surgically excising the tonsils. Compare **resect.**

excision, 1. the process of excising or removing. 2. the process by which a genetic element is removed from a strand of DNA.

excitability, the property of a cell that allows it to react to irritation or stimulation. An example is the reaction of a nerve to stimulation.

excitatory amino acids, amino acids that affect the central nervous system. In some cases, they may be poisonous to the nervous system. Examples are glutamate and aspartate, which are both substances that help transmit messages from one nerve cell to another (neurotransmitters) and cause the death of nerve cells. Amimo acids produced by plants and fungi can cause similar effects.

exciting eye, the eye that is mainly affected by an injury or infection, even though both eyes are disordered. Also called **inciting eye.**

excoriation /ekskôr'ē-ā'shən/, an injury to the surface of the skin or other part of the body caused by scratching or scraping.

excreta /ekskrē'tə/, any waste matter discharged from the body; feces or urine.

excrete, to remove a waste substance from the body, often through normal secretion, as a drug excreted in urine. **–excretion,** *n.*

excretion, the process of getting rid of substances by body organs or tissues. This is part of a natural metabolic activity. Excretion usually begins at the level of the cell where water, carbon dioxide, and other waste products of cells are emptied into the capillaries. The skin, for example, excretes dead skin cells by shedding them daily.

excretory, relating to the process of excretion.

excretory duct, a duct that conducts substances.

excretory urography. See **intravenous pyelography.**

exercise, 1. performing any physical activity for the purpose of conditioning the body, improving health, or maintaining fitness. Exercise can also be a type of therapy for correcting a deformity or restoring the body's functions to a state of health. 2. any action or skill that exerts the muscles and is performed repeatedly in order to develop or strengthen the body. 3. to use a muscle or part of the body in a repetitive way in order to maintain or develop its strength.

exercise electrocardiogram (exercise ECG), a stress test used to diagnose disease of the arteries of the heart. An exercise electrocardiogram is recorded while a person walks on a treadmill or pedals a stationary bicycle. Abnormal changes in heart function may appear during exercise. Some abnormalities will not show on ECG during rest.

exfoliation, peeling and flaking off of tissue cells. This is a normal process of the skin that occurs constantly. Exfoliation may be often seen in certain skin diseases or after a severe sunburn. See also **desquamation, exfoliative dermatitis.**

exfoliative cytology, the microscopic examination of dead cells for diagnosis. The cells are obtained from sores, sputum, secretions, urine, and other material. The cells may be removed with a syringe, scraping, a smear, or washings of the tissue. Compare **aspiration biopsy cytology.**

exfoliative dermatitis, any skin swelling in which there is too much peeling or shedding of skin. Causes include drug reactions, scarlet fever, leukemia, lymphoma, and certain swelling disorders of the skin.

exhalation. See **expiration.**

exhale, to breathe out or to let out with the breath. **–exhalation,** *n.*

exhaustion delirium, a madness that may result from long-term physical or emotional stress, fatigue, or shock. It is linked with severe metabolic or nutritional problems. See also **delirium.**

exhibitionism, 1. the flaunting of oneself or one's abilities in order to attract attention. 2. a disorder occurring in men in which the act of exposing the genitals to unsuspecting females in socially unacceptable situations is the preferred means of achieving sexual satisfaction. See also **paraphilia, scopophilia. –exhibitionist,** *n.*

eximer laser /ek'simir/, a small laser used to break up substances, as cholesterol deposits, without causing intense heat.

existential humanistic psychotherapy. See **humanistic existential therapy.**

existential psychiatry, a school of psychiatry based on the philosophy of existentialism. It emphasizes an analytical, total approach in which mental disorders are deviations within the total structure of a person's existence. Thus the mental disorders would not be caused by biological or cultural factors.

exit block, the failure of an electric impulse in the heart to travel from its point of origin and cause a heart beat.

exit dose, the amount of radiation on the opposite side of the body from where the x-ray beam is aimed.

Exna, a trademark for a diuretic drug used to treat high blood pressure (benzthiazide).

exocoelom. See **extraembryonic coelom.**

exocrine /ek'səkrin/, referring to the process of releasing outwardly through a duct to the surface of an organ or tissue or into a vessel. Compare **endocrine system.** See also **eccrine.**

exocrine gland, glands that open on the surface of the skin, organ, or into a vessel through ducts. These glands secrete specialized substances. Examples are the sweat glands and the oil (sebaceous) glands of the skin, and the salivary glands in the mouth. Exocrine glands are also found in the kidney, digestive tract, and mammary glands. See also **apocrine gland.**

exogenous /igzoj′ənəs/, beginning outside the body or an organ of the body or produced from external causes. For example, a disease caused by a bacterial or virus is exogenous. Compare **endogenous. −exogenic,** *adj.*

exogenous depression. See **reactive depression.**

exogenous hyperlipemia. See **Type I hyperlipidemia.**

exogenous obesity, overweight caused by greater calorie intake than the body needs. Compare **endogenous obesity.** See also **obesity.**

exon /ek′son/, the part of a DNA molecule that produces the code for the final messenger RNA.

exophoria /ek′səfôr′ē·ə/, deviation of one eye to the side. This occurs when the eyes are at rest. When focusing on an object, the deviation disappears. Compare **exotropia. −exophoric,** *adj.*

exophthalmia /ek′softhal′mē·ə/, an abnormal condition marked by a noticeable bulging of the eyeballs (exopthalmos). The condition is usually caused by a tumor pushing the eyeballs outward, bleeding or swelling of the brain or eye, paralysis or injury to the eye muscles, or clots in the sinuses (cavernous sinus thrombosis). It may also be caused by endocrine disorders (overactive thyroid gland) or by varicose veins within the eye. See also **exophthalmic goiter.**

exophthalmic goiter, exophthalmos occurring with goiter, a swelling of the thyroid gland around the Adam's apple. This disorder occurs in Graves' disease, a type of overactive thyroid gland disorder.

exophthalmometer /ek′səfthalmom′ətər/, an instrument for measuring the distance the eye bulges forward in exophthalmos.

exophthalmos-macroglossia-gigantism syndrome. See **EMG syndrome.**

exophytic /ek′sefit′ik/, referring to the tendency to grow outward. For example, an exophytic tumor grows on the surface of an organ or structure.

exophytic carcinoma, a cancerous skin tumor that looks like a wart.

exostosis /ek′səstō′sis/, an abnormal, harmless growth on the surface of a bone.

exotoxin /ek′sətok′sin/, a poison that is released or excreted by a living microorganism. Compare **endotoxin.**

exotropia /ek′sətrō′pē·ə/, the outward deviation of one eye in relation to the other. Compare **esotropia, exophoria.** See also **strabismus. −exotropic,** *adj.*

expectant treatment, therapy to relieve symptoms as they arise in the course of a disease, rather than treating the cause of the illness itself. An example of expectant treatment is amputating a leg with gangrene in a patient with diabetes. Compare **definitive treatment, palliative treatment, treatment.**

expectation of life, the probable number of years a person will live after a certain age. This is determined by the death rate in a specific geographic area. It may be adjusted by the person's health, race, sex, age, or other factors. Also called **life expectancy.**

expected date of confinement (EDC), the predicted date of a pregnant woman's delivery. Pregnancy lasts about 266 days (38 weeks) from the day of fertilization. Because the exact day of conception is usually unknown, the EDC is based on 280 days (40 weeks, 10 lunar months, or 9⅓ calendar months) from the first day of the last menstrual period (LMP). The EDC is arrived at by counting back 3 months from the first day of the LMP and then adding 7 days and 1 year. Thus, if the first day of a woman's LMP was July 18, 1985, one counts back 3 months to April 18, 1985, then adds 7 days and 1 year to arrive at an EDC of April 25, 1986. Because calendar months differ in length, this estimate may vary by a few days from the 280 days, but it is close enough. The expectant mother is advised that the EDC is only an estimate. The chances are that she will give birth within 2 weeks before or, more often, after the calculated date.

expectorant, 1. referring to a substance that aids coughing up mucus or other fluids from the lungs. Also called **mucolytic. −expectorate,** *v.*

expectoration, removing mucus, sputum, or fluids from the throat and lungs by coughing or spitting.

experimental medicine, a branch of medicine in which new drugs or treatments are tested for safety and effect by using animals or, in certain cases, human subjects.

experimental variable. See **independent variable.**

expiration, 1. breathing out. Expiration depends on the elastic qualities of lung tissue and the chest. Also called **exhalation.** Compare **inspiration. 2.** termination or death. **−expire,** *v.*

expiratory reserve volume (ERV), the largest amount of air that can be forced out of the lungs after a normal breath has been let out.

expired gas (E), air or any gas exhaled from the lungs.

explosive personality, behavior marked by episodes of uncontrolled rage and physical abusiveness in reaction to relatively minor stresses.

explosive speech, slow, jerky speech alternating with sudden loud words. This is often seen in brain disorders.

expression, 1. the indication of a physical or emotional state through facial appearance or tone of voice. **2.** the act of pressing or squeezing in order to expel something, as expressing milk from the breast.

expressive aphasia. See **motor aphasia.**

expulsive stage of labor, the second stage of labor, during which contractions of the uterus are accompanied by an urge to bear down. It begins after the cervix is completely widened. This stage ends with the complete delivery of the infant.

exsanguination, referring to a loss of blood.

exsiccant. See **desiccant.**

exsiccate. See **desiccate.**

extended care facility, an institution devoted to providing medical, nursing, or custodial care over a long period of time. Also called **convalescent home, nursing home.**

extended family, a family group consisting of the parents, their children, the grandparents, and other family members. The extended family is the basic family group in many societies.

extended insulin-zinc suspension, a long-acting insulin that is slowly absorbed and slow to act. It is used by some diabetics.

Extendryl, a trademark for a combination drug containing a stimulant (phenylephrine hydrochloride), an antihistamine, (chlorphenira mine maleate), and a nerve blocker (methscopolamine nitrate). It is used to treat nasal congestion.

extension, a movement allowed by certain joints of the skeleton that increases the angle between two adjoining bones. For example, extending the leg increases the angle between the thigh and the calf. Compare **flexion.**

extensor carpi radialis brevis, one of the muscles of the forearm, it acts to extend the hand.

extensor carpi radialis longus, one of the muscles of the forearm, it serves to extend and flex the hand toward the thumb.

extensor carpi ulnaris, one of the muscles on the side of the forearm, it acts to extend and flex the hand toward the little finger.

extensor digiti minimi, an extensor muscle of the forearm, it acts to extend the little finger.

extensor digitorum, the main muscle in the forearm that moves the fingers, it acts to extend the fingers and the wrist. Also called **extensor digitorum communis.**

extensor digitorum longus, a muscle located at the side of the calf. It extends the four small toes and flexes the foot up and out.

extensor retinaculum of the hand. See **retinaculum extensorum manus.**

extern, a medical or dental student who lives outside the institution but provides medical or dental care to patients. The services are provided as an extracurricular activity under the professional supervision of hospital staff members. Compare **intern.**

external, 1. being on the outside of the body or an organ. 2. acting from the outside. 3. referring to the outward or visible appearance. Compare **internal.**

external abdominal region. See **lateral region.**

external absorption, the taking up of substances through the mucous membranes or the skin.

external acoustic meatus, the canal of the outer ear. It is made of bone and cartilage, extending from the outside ear (auricle) to the eardrum (tympanic membrane). Also called **external auditory canal.**

external aperture of aqueduct of vestibule, an outer opening for the small canal leading from the vestibule of the inner ear.

external aperture of canaliculus of cochlea, an outer opening of the organ of hearing duct (cochlear channel). The aperture is in the temporal bone.

external aperture of tympanic canaliculus, the lower opening of the eardrum duct (tympanic channel) in the temporal bone.

external auditory canal. See **external acoustic meatus.**

external carotid artery, one of a pair of arteries with eight major branches supplying blood to the head and neck. It rises from the common carotid arteries.

external carotid plexus, a network of nerves around the external carotid artery. It is formed by the external carotid nerves from the upper spinal cord. Compare **common carotid plexus, internal carotid plexus.**

external cervical os, an external opening of the uterus that leads into the cervix. This opening is in the center of the rounded part of the cervix that projects into the vagina. Compare **internal cervical os.**

external conjugate, the distance measured with obstetric calipers from the dent below the lowest spine bone above the pelvis (lumbar vertebra) to the upper edge of the pubic bone. This is one of the measurements made early in pregnancy to determine the ease of childbirth. Also called **Baudelocque's diameter.**

external cuneiform bone. See **lateral cuneiform bone.**

external ear, the outer structure of the ear, consisting of the auricle and the external canal (acoustic meatus). Sound waves are funneled through the external ear to the middle ear. Compare **internal ear, middle ear.**

external fertilization, the union of male sperm and female egg outside of the bodies from which they originated. This occurs normally in fish and frogs.

external fistula, an abnormal passage between an internal organ or structure and the outside surface of the body.

external iliac artery, a division of the common iliac artery that descends into the thigh and becomes the femoral artery. The external iliac supplies the leg and is larger than the internal iliac. Compare **internal iliac artery.**

external iliac node, one of the lymp nodes that serves the abdomen and the pelvis. About 10 external iliac nodes, arranged in three groups, lie along the external iliac vessels. They drain lymph from several structures including the deep abdominal wall, part of the thigh, the prostate, and the vagina. Compare **common iliac node, iliac circumflex node, internal iliac node.** See also **lymph, lymphatic system, lymph node.**

external iliac vein, one of a pair of veins in the pelvis that join the internal iliac vein to form the two common iliac veins. Each external iliac vein begins at the groin, runs up along the brim of the pelvis, and ends near the tailbone where it joins the internal iliac vein. In many persons it contains at least one valve, and sometimes two. Compare **internal iliac vein.**

external jugular vein, one of a pair of large blood vessels in the neck that receive most of the blood from the surface of the skull and the deep tissues of the face. It runs down the neck and joins the subclavian vein. It contains two pairs of valves, one where it joins the subclavian vein and one about 1½ inches above the collarbone. Compare **internal jugular vein.**

external oblique muscle. See **obliquus externus abdominis.**

external perimysium. See **epimysium.**

external pin fixation, a method of holding together the fragments of a broken bone. Metal pins are inserted through the fragments. A compression device is attached to the pins outside the skin surface to keep them in place. Compare **internal fixation.**

external pterygoid muscle. See **pterygoideus lateralis.**

external radiation therapy (ERT), x-ray therapy with a beam outside the body. ERT is used most often to treat cancer. It is also used in the therapy of keloids and other skin conditions.

external rotation, turning outward or away from the midline of the body. For example, a leg is turned out when the toes point away from the body's midline.

external shunt, a device for passing a fluid from one chamber of the body to another. It consists of a tube or series of containers that removes fluid from one part and replaces it into another area. See also **hemodialysis, hydrocephalus.**

external version, a childbirth procedure in which a fetus is turned, usually from a breech to a head-first position. It is done by manipulating the fetus through the wall of the abdomen. Compare **version and extraction.**

exteroceptive, referring to stimulation that comes from outside the body. The term also refers to the nerves that are stimulated by outside events. Compare **interoceptive, proprioception.**

exteroceptor, any sensory nerve ending, as those found in the skin, mucous membranes, or sense organs, that responds to stimulation that comes from outside of the body. Examples of this type of stimulation are touch, pressure, and sound. Compare **interoceptor, proprioceptor.** See also **chemoreceptor.**

extrabuccal feeding, giving nutrients by means other than the mouth. Also called **extraoral feeding.** See also **gavage, intravenous feeding.**

extracapsular fracture, any bone break that occurs near a joint but does not directly involve the joint capsule. This type of break is very common in the hip.

extracellular, referring to outside a cell in spaces between cell layers. See also **cell, edema, interstitial.**

extracellular fluid (ECF), the part of the body fluid outside the tissue cells. This includes fluid in the spaces of tissues (the interstitial fluid) and blood plasma. The adult body contains nearly 3 gallons (11.2 liters) of interstitial fluid. This accounts for about 16% of body weight. In addition, there are about 3 quarts (2.8 liters) of plasma, which is about 4% of body weight. Plasma and interstitial fluid are very similar chemically. Together with fluid inside the cells (intracellular fluid), ECF helps control the movement of water and electrolytes throughout the body.

extracoronal retainer, 1. a kind of dental retainer that includes a cast restoration lying largely outside the crown (coronal) part of a tooth. It complements the contour of the tooth crown. **2.** a direct clasp type retainer that fastens on a tooth on its outer surface. It is used to retain and support a removable partial denture.

extracorporeal, something that is outside the body. An example is extracorporeal circulation in which venous blood is routed outside the body to a heart-lung machine and returned to the body through an artery.

extracorporeal technician. See **perfusion technologist.**

extract, to remove a tooth by means of elevators, forceps, or both. **–extraction,** *n.*

extradural /ek′trədŏŏr′əl/, outside the lining of the brain and spinal cord (dura mater).

extradural hemorrhage, bleeding in an area around but outside of the dura mater of the brain or spinal cord.

extraembryonic coelom, a space outside the developing embryo. It forms between the outer membrane (chorion) and the membrane over the amniotic cavity and yolk sac. Also called **exocoelom.**

extramedullary myeloma, a blood cell tumor that occurs outside of the bone marrow. It usually affects the abdominal organs or the nose, throat, and mouth. Also called **extramedullary plasmacytoma, peripheral plasma cell myeloma, plasma cell tumor.**

extramedullary myelopoiesis, the growth of bone marrow (myeloid) tissue outside of the bone marrow. Also called **ectopic myelopoiesis.**

extraocular /ek'strə-ok'yŏŏlər/, outside the eye.

extraocular muscle palsy, paralysis of the eye muscles. This may affect the following muscles: the superior, inferior, medial, and lateral rectus muscles, and the superior and the inferior oblique muscles. See also **strabismus.**

extraoral feeding. See **extrabuccal feeding.**

extraoral orthodontic appliance, a device secured to a part of the face, the neck, or the back of the head to place traction on the teeth or jaws. It is used for changing the relative positions of the teeth.

extraperitoneal, occurring or located outside the peritoneal cavity. The peritoneal cavity is formed by a membrane (peritoneum) lining the abdominal and pelvic walls and covering the organs.

extraperitoneal cesarean section, a method for surgically delivering a baby through an incision in the lower part of the uterus without entering the peritoneal cavity. This is done by pushing the fold of peritoneum out of the way and pushing the bladder downward. This procedure is performed to avoid spreading infection from the uterus into the peritoneal cavity. It is somewhat slower to perform than other cesarean operations. Compare **classical cesarean section, low cervical cesarean section.** See also **cesarean section.**

extrapyramidal /ek'strəpiram'ədəl/, referring to the nerves and fibers that coordinate and control movement. See **extrapyramidal system, extrapyramidal tracts.**

extrapyramidal disease, any of a large group of conditions marked by uncontrolled movement, changes in muscle tone, and abnormal posture. Disorders such as tardive dyskinesia, chorea, athetosis, and Parkinson's disease are extrapyramidal diseases.

extrapyramidal reaction, a response to a drug marked by symptoms of extrapyramidal disease. The reaction may persist or fade after stopping the drug.

extrapyramidal system, the part of the nervous system that controls movement. These nerves include the basal ganglia, substantia nigra, subthalamic nucleus, part of the midbrain, and the motor neurons of the spine. See also **extrapyramidal tracts.**

extrapyramidal tracts, the tracts of nerves from the brain to the spinal cord, that coordinate and control movement. Within the brain, the extrapyramidal tracts are nerve relays between the many motor areas of the brain. The extrapyramidal tracts are functional rather than anatomic units. They control and coordinate posture, position, support, and locomotor

mechanisms. The tracts cause contractions of muscle groups in sequence or at the same time. Compare **pyramidal tract.**

extrasystole /ek'strəsis'təlē/, heart beat that is abnormal in timing with respect to the normal rhythm of the heart.

extrauterine /ek'strəyŏŏtərin/, occurring or located outside the uterus, as an ectopic pregnancy.

extravasation /ikstrav'əsā'shən/, a passage into the tissues, usually of blood, serum, or lymph. Compare **bleeding.** See also **exudate, transudate.** –**extravasate,** v.

extraversion. See **extroversion.**

extrinsic allergic alveolitis, an swelling form of pneumonia that is caused by an immune reaction in an allergic patient. The reaction may be brought about by a variety of inhaled organic dusts, often those containing fungal spores. A wide variety of symptoms may occur, including difficulty breathing, fever, chills, malaise, and muscle aches. The symptoms usually develop 4 to 6 hours after exposure. Kinds of extrinsic allergic alveolitis include **bagassosis, farmer's lung, humidifier or air conditioner lung, mushroom worker's lung, suberosis.** Also called **hypersensitivity pneumonitis.** See also **Arthus reaction.**

extrinsic allergic pneumonia. See **diffuse hypersensitivity pneumonia.**

extrinsic asthma. See **allergic asthma.**

extrinsic factor. See **cyanocobalamin.**

extroversion, 1. the tendency to direct one's interests and energies toward things outside the self. **2.** the state of being mainly concerned with what is outside the self. Also spelled **extraversion.** Compare **introversion.**

extrovert, a person who is outgoing. Also spelled **extravert.** Compare **introvert.**

extrusion reflex, a normal response in infants to force the tongue outward when the tongue is touched. The reflex begins to go away by about 3 or 4 months of age. Before it fades, food must be placed well back in the mouth to be kept in and swallowed. Constant sticking out of a large tongue may be a sign of Down's syndrome.

exuberant callus. See **heterotopic ossification.**

exudate /eks'yŏŏdāt/, fluid, cells, or other substances that have been slowly discharged through small pores or breaks in cell membranes. Perspiration, pus, and serum are sometimes called exudates.

exudative /igzŏŏ'dətiv/, relating to the oozing of fluid and other materials from cells and tissues, usually as a result of swelling or injury.

exudative angina. See **croup.**

exudative enteropathy, diarrhea in diseases marked by swelling or destruction of intestinal lining. This occurs in Crohn's disease and ulcerative colitis, for example. See also **diarrhea.**

eye, one of a pair of organs of sight, located in bony hollows at the front of the skull. The eyes are embedded in fat and supplied by one of a pair of optic nerves from the forebrain. Certain structures that are associated with the eye are the muscles, the tough muscle covering (fascia), the eyebrow, the eyelids, the membrane lining the lids (conjunctiva), and the tear (lacrimal) gland. The eyeball has 3 layers that enclose 2 spaces separated by the crystalline lens. The smaller space in front of the lens is divided by the iris into two chambers, both filled with a liquid (aqueous humor). The back chamber is larger than the front chamber and contains the jellylike vitreous body. The outside layer of the eye consists of the transparent cornea in the front, which makes up one fifth of the layer. The lens, which is just behind the cornea, and the cornea focus images onto the retina. The white (sclera) makes up the other five-sixths of the outer layer. The middle layer is supplied with blood and consists of the choroid under the sclera, the ciliary body which focuses the lens, and the iris which controls the amount of light entering the eye. The inner layer of nervous tissue is the retina. Light waves passing through the lens strike a layer of rods and cones in the retina, creating impulses that are carried by the optic nerve to the brain. Also called **bulbus oculi, eyeball.**

eyebrow, 1. the arch of bone over the eye that separates the eye socket from the forehead. 2. the arch of hairs growing along the ridge formed by the bony arch over the eye socket.

eyeground, the back (fundus) of the eye. See also **funduscopy.**

eyelash, one of many small hairs (cilia) growing in double or triple rows along the border of the eyelids.

eyelid, a movable fold of thin skin over the eye. The eyelid contains eyelashes, ciliary glands that produce sweat, and meibomian glands that produce oil along its edge. It consists of loose connecting tissue containing a thin plate of fiber tissue lined with mucous membrane. The orbicularis oculi muscle and the oculomotor nerve control the opening and closing of the eyelid. Also called **palpebra.**

eye memory. See **visual memory.**

F

F_1, symbol for the offspring made by the mating of two unrelated individuals.

FA, 1. abbreviation for **fatty acid. 2.** abbreviation for **femoral artery. 3.** abbreviation for **folic acid.**

Fabere's test /fä′bāräz/, a test for pain of dysfunction in the hip and lower-back joints. The examiner applies pressure on the knee and on the opposite side of the lower spine while the patient moves the hip.

fabrication, (in psychology), a reaction in which a patient makes false statements to hide defects of memory. It is common in Korsakoff's psychosis and other disorders. See also **confabulation.**

Fabry's disease, Fabry's syndrome. See **angiokeratoma corporis diffusum.**

FAC, an anticancer durg. It is a combination of fluorouracil, doxorubicin, and cyclophosphamide.

face, 1. the front of the head from the chin to the brow. It includes the skin, muscles, and structures of the forehead, eyes, nose, mouth, cheeks, and jaw. **2.** to direct the face toward something. See also **en face.** –**facial,** *adj.*

face-bow, a device looking like a caliper, used to measure the jaws for making dentures.

facet, a flattened, highly polished wear pattern on a tooth.

facial artery, one of a pair of arteries that come from the external carotid arteries. They divide into four neck and five face branches, and supply the organs and tissues in the head.

facial diplegia, a nerve and muscle condition characterized by paralysis of many muscles of the face. See also **Möbius' syndrome.**

facial hemiplegia, paralysis of the muscles of one side of the face, with the rest of the body not being affected.

facial muscle, any of many muscles of the face. The five groups of facial muscles include the muscles of the scalp, the outside muscles of the ear, the muscles of the nose, the muscles of the eyelid, and the muscles of the mouth. Also called **muscle of expression.**

facial nerve, either of a pair of mixed sense and motor nerves that come from the brain stem. Also called **seventh cranial nerve.**

facial paralysis, the part or the total loss of use of the face muscles or the loss of feeling in the face. It may be caused by disease or by injury. The amount of paralysis depends on the nerves affected. See also **Bell's palsy.**

facial perception, the ability to judge the distance and direction of objects through the feeling felt in the skin of the face. It is commonly felt by those who are blind. Also called **facial vision.**

facial vein, one of a pair of veins that drain blood that has lost oxygen from the surface of the face back to the heart. Because the vein has no valves that prevent the backflow of blood, infections of the skin near the nose and mouth may cause a nerve disease (meningitis).

facial vision. See **facial perception.**

facies /fā′shē·ēs/, *pl.* **facies** /fā′shē·ēs/, **1.** the face. **2.** the surface of any body structure, part, or organ. **3.** the face's expression or appearance.

facilitation, increasing any action or function so that it is carried out with ease. Compare **inhibition.** See also **summation.**

facio-, a combining form for the face.

facitis /fasī′tis/, a noncancerous growth looking like a tumor that develops in the mouth tissues under the skin, usually in the cheek. It may be mistaken for a cancer tumor (fibrosarcoma).

factitial dermatitis, a self-caused skin rash usually done by the patient for some desired gain or as a sign of mental illness.

factitious disorders, conditions in which the patient produces symptoms on purpose to gain attention. The patient may continue to produce symptoms even when he or she knows the possible dangers.

factor I. See **fibrinogen.**

factor II. See **prothrombin.**

factor III. See **thromboplastin.**

factor IV, a symbol for calcium, as in the process of blood clotting.

factor V, a blood-clotting factor that occurs in normal plasma but is lacking in patients with a blood-clotting disease (parahemophilia). It is needed to change prothrombin rapidly to thrombin. Also called **proaccelerin.**

factor VI, a chemical agent that comes from factor V (proaccelerin), in blood clotting.

factor VII, a blood-clotting factor in the blood plasma and broken down in the liver if vitamin K is present. Also called **proconvertin.**

factor VIII, a blood-clotting factor in normal plasma but lacking in patients with a blood-clotting disease (hemophilia A). It is made up of two separate substances. The lack of one substance results in hemophilia A, and the other when lacking results in Von Willebrand's disease. See also **antihemophilic factor.**

factor IX, a blood-clotting factor in normal plasma but lacking in patients with a blood-clotting disease (hemophilia B). Also called **Christmas factor.**

factor IX complex, an antibleeding drug with factors II, VII, IX, and X given to treat a blood-clotting disease (hemophilia B). It is a protein that depends on vitamin K in the liver.

factor X, a blood-clotting factor that occurs in normal plasma but is lacking in some defects in blood-clotting. Factor X is made in the liver when vitamin K is present. Also called **Stuart-Power factor.**

factor XI, a blood-clotting factor in normal plasma. A lack of it results in a blood-clotting disease (hemophilia C).

factor XII, a blood-clotting factor in normal plasma. Also called **activation factor, contact factor, glass factor, Hageman factor.**

factor XIII, a blood-clotting factor in normal plasma. It acts with calcium to make a protein (fibrin) clot. Also called **fibrinase, fibrin stabilizing factor.**

facultative /fak′əltā′tiv/, being able to adapt to more than one condition.

facultative aerobe, an organism able to grow without oxygen but growing most rapidly in oxygen. Compare **obligate aerobe.** See also **aerobe.**

facultative anaerobe, an organism able to grow in oxygen but growing most rapidly without oxygen. Compare **obligate anaerobe.** See also **anaerobe, anaerobic infection.**

facultative parasite. See **parasite.**

faculty, any normal function or ability of a living organism, as being able to sense and recognize sense stimulations.

FAD, abbreviation for *fetal activity determination.*

Faget's sign /fazhāz′/, a falling pulse rate with a constant temperature, or a constant pulse with a rising temperature. It is a sign found in yellow fever. Also called **Faget's law.**

fagicladosporic acid /faj′iklad′ōspôr′ik/, a poison made by a fungus (Cladosporium epiphyllum). This fungus causes "black spots" on stored meat, a skin disease (tinea negra), and black decay of the brain.

Fahrenheit /fer′ənhīt/, a scale for measuring temperature in which the boiling point of water is 212° and the freezing point of water is 32° at sea level. Compare **Celsius.**

failure to thrive, slowed growth of an infant from conditions that affect normal body functions, appetite, and activity. Causes include birth defects, as in Turner's syndrome and other defects; major organ system defects; sudden illness; bad nutrition; and many psychological or social factors, as maternal deprivation syndrome.

faint, *nontechnical.* **1.** to lose consciousness, as in a fainting attack. **2.** a fainting attack. See also **syncope.**

faith healing, a belief that a person has the power to cause a cure or recovery from an illness or injury without using normal medical treatments. It assumes the healer has been given that power by a cosmic force.

falciform body. See **sporozoite.**

falciform ligament, a triangular of sickle-shaped ligament of the body, as a ligament of the liver (ligamentum falciform hepatis).

falciparum malaria /falsip′ərəm/, the most severe form of malaria, caused by a protozoa *(Plasmodium falciparum).* It is characterized by symptoms that include confusion, a large spleen, stomach upset, and anemia. Falciparum malaria does not last as long as other forms of malaria. If treatment is begun soon, the disease may be mild and the patient will recover. Later spells of the disease are uncommon, but death may result from dehydration and anemia.

fallopian tube /fəlō′pē·ən/, one of a pair of tubes opening at one end into the uterus and at the other end into the cavity over the ovary. Each tube is the passage through which an egg (ovum) is carried to the uterus and through which sperm move toward the ovary. The parts (fimbriae) at the open end of each tube drape in fingerlike bunches over the ovary. Also called **oviduct, uterine tube.**

Fallot's syndrome. See **tetralogy of Fallot.**

fallout, the spread of radioactive waste after a nuclear explosion.

false anorexia. See **pseudoanorexia.**

false labor. See **Braxton Hicks contractions.**

false negative, an incorrect result of a medical test or procedure that falsely shows the lack of a finding, condition, or disease. False negative results are more common than false positive results, because the person doing the test is more likely to fail to see a finding than to imagine seeing something that does not exist. Compare **false positive.**

false neuroma, **1.** a tumor that does not contain nerve elements. **2.** a lumpy tumor (cystic neuroma).

false nucleolus. See **karyosome.**

false pelvis, the upper part of the pelvis.

false personification, in psychiatry, the labeling and prejudgment of other persons without cause.

false positive, a test result that wrongly shows the presence of a disease or other condition. Compare **false negative.**

false rib. See **rib.**

false suture, a rigid, fiberlike joint in which rough edges form the connection between certain bones of the skull. Compare **true suture.**

false transactions, interaction between people in which communication is stopped or distorted because one person is using a different point of view (ego state) than expected.

false twins. See **dizygotic twins.**

false vertebrae, the lower parts of the spine (sacrum and coccyx). Also called **fixed vertebrae.**

false vocal cord, either of two thick folds of mucous membrane in the throat (larynx). Compare **vocal cord.**

FAM, a combination anticancer drug. It consists of fluorouracil, doxorubicin, and mitomycin.

familial, a disease in some families and not in others. It is usually but not always hereditary. Compare **acquired, congenital, hereditary.**

familial cretinism, a genetic disorder caused by an inborn error of body functions. It results from the lack of an enzyme that stops the making of thyroid hormone. Symptoms include lack of energy, slowed growth, and mental retardation. See also **cretinism.**

familial hypercholesterolemia, an inherited disorder marked by a high level of serum cholesterol, and early signs of hardening of the arteries (atherosclerosis). Patients with this disease at 50 years of age have three to 10 times greater risk of having heart disease than the general population. The disorder occurs in whites, blacks, and Orientals. Also called **hypercholesterolemic xanthomatosis, type II hyperlipoproteinemia.**

familial lipoprotein lipase deficiency. See **hyperchylomicronemia.**

familial polyposis, a condition marked by growths (polyps) in the colon and rectum. The disease, which has high cancer potential, is inherited. A kind of familial polyposis is **Gardner's syndrome.** See also **polyposis.**

familial spinal muscular atrophy. See **Werdnig-Hoffmann disease.**

familial tremor. See **essential tremor.**

family, 1. a group of people related by blood, as parents, children, and brothers and sisters. The term sometimes includes persons living in the same household or those related by marriage. 2. a group of persons having a common last name, as the Anderson family. 3. a category of animals or plants. Humans are members of the genus *Homo sapiens,* which is a part of the hominid family that, in turn, is a part of the primate order of mammals. See also **genetics, heredity.** –**familial,** *adj.*

family APGAR, a rating system used in family therapy. APGAR stands for Adaptability, Partnership, Growth, Affection, and Resolve, the categories on the questionnaire. Each family member indicates how satisfied her or she is in each category ranging from 0 to 2. The system is most often used in studies of families with elderly members.

family-centered care, health care that includes the health of an entire family and actions needed to keep or improve the health of the unit and its members.

family counseling, a program of information and guidance to members of a family. Counseling usually centers on a specific health problem, as care of a handicapped child or the risk of a genetic defect.

family disorganization, a breakdown of a family system. It may be caused by overburdened parents or by the loss of persons who served as role models or support systems. Family disorganization may lead to the loss of social controls that families usually impose on their members.

family dynamics, the forces at work within a family. They result in the family members' actions or systems.

family functions, activities in which the family acts as a whole. These include communication and problem-solving.

family ganging, an unethical medical practice in which the patient is urged or forced to involve the entire family in a program of health care even if the other family members do not need such care. The practice allows the health-care service to get insurance payments for all family members.

family history, a necessary part of a patient's medical history in which the patient is asked about the health of the other members of the family. Questions may include: "Has anyone in your family had tuberculosis? diabetes mellitus? breast cancer?" These questions are asked to find out about any diseases to which the patient may be at a high risk of getting.

family medicine, the branch of medicine that is concerned with the diagnosis and treatment of health problems in people of either sex and any age. Physicians who practice family medicine are often called family-practice physicians, family physicians, or, formerly, general practitioners.

family myths, myths that family members make up to help them deny the reality of family problems.

family nurse practitioner (FNP), a nurse who provides health care for families along with primary-care physicians.

family of origin, the family into which a person is born.

family of procreation, the family a person forms by marrying and having children.

family physician, 1. a physician who practices family medicine. 2. a general practitioner. See also **family medicine.**

family planning. See **contraception.**

family projection process, the means by which family members attribute their thoughts and impulses to other family members.

family structure, the composition and membership of a family. It also includes the pattern of relationships among family members. Knowledge of family structure may be helpful to health-care workers in planning care for a family member or for the entire family.

famine fever. See **relapsing fever.**

Fanconi's anemia, a usually inborn disorder marked by anemia in childhood or early adult life, bone problems, and birth defects. Also called **congenital pancytopenia, pancytopenia-dysmelia.**

Fanconi's syndrome, a group of disorders including kidney disease and sugar and phosphates in the urine. The condition is often marked by weak bones, excess acid in the urine, and low blood potassium. Two main types of the syndrome have been found. Idiopathic Fanconi's syndrome is inherited and usually appears in early middle age. Acquired Fanconi's syndrome is usually the result of poisoning from many sources, including the use of outdated tetracycline.

fan lateral projection, a technique for making an x-ray image of the hand so that the fingers do not touch. The patient places wedge-shaped sponges between the fingers. The image on the x-ray film has a fanlike pattern.

Fansidar, a trademark for an antimalaria drug (pyrimethamine and sulfadoxine).

fantasy, 1. the completely free play of the imagination; fancy. **2.** the mental process of changing undesirable experiences into imagined events to fulfill an unconscious wish, need, or desire or to express unconscious conflicts, as a daydream.

Faraday cage, a wire-mesh cage that surrounds a nuclear magnetic resonance scanner. It protects the scanner from stray radio waves, which can interfere with the results of the scan.

Farber test, an examination of newborn feces (meconium) for hair and skin cells. The fetus normally swallows amniotic fluid containing these proteins that then pass through the intestines to be released, usually after birth, in the first stools. The lack of hair or skin cells is a sign of blocked intestines.

Far Eastern hemorrhagic fever, a form of a bleeding fever (epidemic hemorrhagic fever) that is carried by a virus in a rodent. Symptoms are chills, fever, headache, stomach and bowel pain, nausea, vomiting, loss of appetite, and excess thirst. Shock may occur as the fever goes down. Thirst continues into the second week, there is a lack of urine, and the blood pressure returns to normal. Excess urination follows, resulting in an output of as much as 8 liters a day of urine. The death rate may be as high as 33%. There is no specific treatment.

far field. See **Fraunhofer zone.**

farmer's lung, a lung disorder caused by breathing dusts from moldy hay. It is a form of an allergic lung disease (pneumonitis) affecting individuals who have developed an allergy to the mold spores. Symptoms include coughing, nausea, chills, and fever.

farsightedness. See **hyperopia.**

FAS, abbreviation for **fetal alcohol syndrome.**

fascia /fash'ē·ə/, *pl.* **fasciae,** fiberlike connective tissue of the body that may be separated from other organized structures, as the tendons and the ligaments. It varies in thickness and weight and in the amounts of fat, fiber, and tissue fluid it contains. Kinds of fasciae are **deep fascia, subcutaneous fascia, subserous fascia.** –**fascial,** *adj.*

fascia bulbi, a thin membrane that surrounds the eyeball from the optic nerve to the pupil and allows the eyeball to move freely.

fascial compartment, a part of the body that is walled off by fiberlike (fascial) membranes. It usually contains a muscle or group of muscles or an organ, as the heart is contained by the mediastinum.

fascial membrane lamination, a pad of connective tissue that contains fat and sometimes a blood vessel or a lymph node.

fascicular neuroma, a tumor made up of covered (myelinated) nerve fibers. Also called **medullated neuroma.**

fasciculation /fasik'yŏŏlā'shən/, the uncontrollable twitching of a single muscle group served by a single motor nerve fiber or filament. The twitching may be felt and seen under the skin. It results from many drugs as a side effect with a normal dose or from an overdose. It also may be a symptom of a lack in the diet, cerebral palsy, fever, a nerve disease (neuralgia), polio, or rheumatic heart disease. Fasciculation of the heart muscle is known as fibrillation. –**fascicular,** *adj.,* **fasciculate,** *v.*

fasciculus /fəsik'yələs/, *pl.* **fasciculi,** a small bundle of muscle, tendon, or nerve fibers. The shape of fasciculi in a muscle is related to the power of the muscle and its range of motion. –**fascicular,** *adj.*

fasciitis /fas'ē·ī'tis/, **1.** an inflammation of the connective tissue. It may be caused by an infection, an injury, or an immune reaction. **2.** an abnormal, benign growth that resembles a tumor. It develops beneath the skin (usually in the cheek), normally grows rapidly, and then shrinks. It may be mistaken for a tumor (fibrosarcoma). Also called **fascitis.**

fascioliasis /fas'ē·ōlī'əsis/, an infection with a liver fluke (*Fasciola hepatica*), it is marked by stomach and bowel pain, fever, a liver disease (jaundice), hives, and diarrhea. One gets it by swallowing forms of the fluke found on water plants, as raw watercress. The disease is common in many parts of the world, including southern and western United States.

fasciolopsiasis /fas'ē·ōlopsī'əsis/, an infection of the intestines, common in the Far East, it is marked by stomach and bowel pain, diarrhea, constipation, and fluid pooling. It is caused by the fluke *Fasciolopsis buski*. One usually gets the disease by eating infected water plants, as raw water chestnuts.

fascioscapulohumeral dystrophy /fas'ē-ōskap'-yōōlōhyōō'mərəl/, one of the main types of muscular dystrophy. It is marked by wasting of the skeletal muscles, especially the muscles of the face, the shoulders, and the upper arms. This disease is not usually fatal but spreads to all the voluntary muscles and commonly causes a thick lower lip. It is an inherited disease that may be carried to males and females. Fascioscapulohumeral dystrophy usually occurs before 10 years of age but may also start during adolescence. Early symptoms include not being able to pucker the lips, abnormal face movements when laughing or crying, face flattening, not being able to raise the arms over the head, and, in infants, not being able to suck. No known treatment can halt the spread of this disease and the resulting muscle problems. Some measures that may help keep the muscles working are physical therapy, surgery, and the use of braces. The patient is helped to move by assisting with exercises. The patient with a dystrophy disorder often becomes constipated because activity is increasingly limited. High-protein, high-fiber diets and the use of stool softeners can help avoid constipation. Information about social services and financial help for patients and families can be gotten from the Muscular Dystrophy Association, Inc.

fasciotomy /fas'ē-ot'əmē/, a surgical cut into an area of fiberlike membranes (fascia).

fast-acting insulin, one of a group of insulin drugs in which the start of action is rapid, about 1 hour, and it lasts a short time, about 6 to 14 hours.

fastigium /fastij'ē-əm/, the highest point in the course of a fever, or the point in the course of an illness when the most symptoms are present.

Fastin, a trademark for a drug used to reduce appetite (phentermine hydrochloride).

fast-twitch (FT) fiber, a muscle fiber that can develop high tension rapidly. FT fibers are used for activities like sprinting, jumping, and weight lifting. See also **slow-twitch (ST) fibers.**

fat, 1. a substance made up of lipids or fatty acids and occurring in many forms ranging from oil to tallow. 2. a type of body tissue made up of cells containing stored fat (depot fat). Stored fat is usually called white fat, which is found in large cells, or brown fat, which consists of lipid droplets. Stored fat contains more than twice as many calories per gram as sugars and is a source of quick body energy. In addition, stored fat helps protect important organs. See also **adipose, obesity.**

fatal, referring to something, as an injury or disease, that inevitably leads to death.

fat cell lipoma. See **hibernoma.**

fat embolism, the blocking of an artery by a blob (embolus) of fat in the circulation. It may follow the breaking of a long bone, or less commonly, after injury to fat (adipose) tissue or to a fatty liver. Lipid functions are changed by the injury and cause the release of free fatty acids resulting in blood vessel swelling with blockage of many small lung and brain arteries. Fat embolism usually occurs 12 to 36 hours after the injury and is marked by severe chest pain, pale skin, breathing difficulty, rapid heartbeat, exhaustion, confusion, and, in some cases, coma. Classic signs of fat embolism are skin bleeding on the neck, shoulders, arm pits, and eye surfaces, appearing 2 or 3 days after the injury. There is no specific treatment for fat embolism; the patient is placed in a sitting position and given oxygen, drugs, blood transfusion, help in breathing, and other care.

FA test. See **fluorescent antibody test.**

father complex, a hidden desire to have sex with one's father. See also **Oedipus complex.**

father fixation, an abnormally close and often paralyzing emotional attachment to one's father. Compare **mother fixation.** See also **Freudian fixation.**

fatigability, a tendency to become tired quickly or easily. It may occur in types of cells that have periods of high activity.

fatigue, 1. a state of exhaustion or a loss of strength or endurance, as may follow excess physical activity. 2. an inability of tissues to respond to stimulations that normally cause muscles to contract or other activity. Muscle cells generally need a recovery period after activity. During this time cells restore their energy supplies and release waste products. 3. a sense of weariness or tiredness. 4. an emotional state linked to extreme or extended exposure to psychic pressure, as in battle or combat fatigue.

fatigue fever, a period of fever and muscle pain following overactivity. The symptoms are caused by a buildup of the waste products of muscle contractions and may last for several days.

fatigue fracture, any broken bone that results from excess physical activity and not from any specific injury. It commonly occurs in the foot (metatarsal) bones of runners.

fat metabolism, the biochemical process by which fats are broken down and used by the cells of the body. Fats provide more food energy than carbohydrates; 1 gram of fat provides 9 kilocalories of heat as compared with 4.1 kilocalories from 1 gram of carbohydrate. Before the final reactions in fat use can occur, fats must be changed into fatty acids and glycerol. The body also changes fats from fatty acids and glycerol or from compounds coming from glucose or amino acids. The body can build only saturated fatty acids. Essential unsaturated fatty acids can be gotten only from the diet. Certain hormones, as insulin and the glucocorticoids, control fat use.

fat pad, a mass of closely packed fat cells surrounded by fibrous tissue. A fat pad may have many small blood vessels and nerve endings.

fatty acid, any of several acids produced by the breakdown of neutral fats. Essential fatty acids are unsaturated molecules that cannot be produced by the body and must therefore be included in the diet. Kinds of essential fatty acids are **arachidonic, linoleic.** See also **saturated fatty acid, unsaturated fatty acid.**

fatty ascites. See **chylous ascites.**

fatty cirrhosis. See **cirrhosis.**

fatty infiltration, a normal phase of breast development. During this phase, fat accumulates in the breast tissue. Later in life, that fat buildup is normally reversed.

fatty liver, a buildup of fats in the liver. The causes include alcoholic cirrhosis, injecting drugs, and exposure to poisonous substances, as carbon tetrachloride and yellow phosphorus. Fatty liver is also seen in a nutrition disease (kwashiorkor) and is a rare problem of late pregnancy. The symptoms are loss of appetite, large liver, and stomach upset. The condition will usually disappear after the condition causing it is corrected or the drug causing it is no longer used. See also **cirrhosis.**

fauces /fô'ēz/, the opening of the mouth into the throat.

faucial isthmus /fô'shəl/, an opening between the throat and the mouth.

faulty restoration, any dental work that contains flaws, as overhanging or incomplete tooth fillings. Such faults may cause inflammatory diseases of the teeth and mouth.

favism /fā'vizəm/, an anemia caused by eating the beans or breathing in the pollen from the fava (*Vicia faba*) plant. Allergic persons show a lack of an enzyme glucose-6-phosphate dehydrogenase, usually the result of a hereditary blood disorder. Symptoms include dizziness, headache, vomiting, fever, a liver disease (jaundice), and often diarrhea. The condition is found mostly in persons whose familes are from southern Italy and is treated by blood transfusion and avoiding fava beans. See also **glucose-6-phosphate dehydrogenase deficiency.**

favus /fā'vəs/, a fungus infection of the scalp. More common in children than adults, the infection is caused by *Trichophyton* fungi. Favus is marked by thick, yellow crusts, a strong "mousy" odor, permanent scars, and loss of hair.

Fc fragment, the part of the molecule of an antibody that is left after the molecule is split by an enzyme. The Fc fragment is the stable part of the antibody, as opposed to the Fab portion. The Fc portion is also called the crystallizable fragment.

F.D.A., abbreviation for **Food and Drug Administration.**

fear, a feeling of dread that may result from natural or inborn causes, as a sudden noise, loss of physical support, pain, heights, or other stimulations.

febri-, a combining form referring to a fever.

febrifuge. See **antipyretic.**

febrile /fē'bril, feb'ril/, referring to high body temperature, as a febrile reaction to an infection.

febrile seizure, a seizure that occurs with high fever. Treatment depends on the patient's age and number of seizures. In children, recurring febrile seizures may be treated as epilepsy.

fecal fistula, an abnormal passage from the colon to the outside surface of the body. It results in a release of feces from an opening in the abdomen. Fistulas of this kind are usually created surgically in operations involving the removal of cancerous or severely injured or punctured bowel segments. See also **colostomy.**

fecal impaction, a buildup of hardened feces in the bowel that the individual cannot move naturally. Diarrhea may be a sign of fecal impaction because only liquid material is able to pass the blockage. Fecal impaction may cause urinary difficulty from pressure on the bladder. Treatment includes oil and cleansing enemas and breaking up and removing the stool by a gloved finger. Prevention includes enough bulk food, fluids, exercise, regular bowel habits, privacy for defecation, and occasional stool softeners or laxatives. See also **constipation, obstipation.**

fecalith /fē'kəlith/, a hard, impacted mass of feces in the colon. See also **atonia constipation, constipation.**

fecal softener, a drug that allows intestinal fluids to penetrate and soften the stool. Also called **stool softener.**

feces /fē'sēz/, mostly solid waste from the digestive tract. It is formed in the intestine and released through the rectum. Feces consist of water, food remains, bacteria, and fluids of the intestines and liver. Also called **stool.** See also **defecation.** –**fecal,** *adj.*

fecundation /fē'kəndā'shən, fek'-/, the act of fertilizing. –**fecundate,** *v.*

fecundity /fikun'ditē/, the ability to produce offspring, especially in large numbers and rapidly; fertility. –**fecund,** *adj.*

feeblemindedness. See **mental retardation.**

feeding, the act or process of taking or giving food. Kinds of feeding include **breastfeeding, forced feeding.** See also **alimentation, parenteral nutrition.**

fee-for-service, 1. a charge made for a professional activity, as for a physical examination or checking a patient's blood pressure. **2.** a system for paying for professional services in which the physician is paid for the particular service rather than getting a salary.

feel life, *nontechnical.* to experience movement.

feet. See **foot.**

Feldene, a trademark for an arthritis drug (piroxicam).

Feldenkrais therapy, (in psychiatry) therapy based on forming a good self-image through awareness and correction of body movements.

feldspar, a part of dental porcelain.

fellatio /fəlā'shēō/, oral stimulation of the genitals of a male.

felon, an open sore on the finger.

Felty's syndrome /fel'tēz/, a spleen disorder occurring with adult rheumatoid arthritis, with many infections. See **hypersplenism.**

female, referring to the sex that bears children; feminine.

female catheterization, removal of urine by means of a tube (catheter) put through the urethra into the bladder. It is done if voluntary urination is not possible. See also **catheterization, male catheterization.**

female reproductive system assessment, an examination of a woman's genital tract and breasts including past and present disorders. The woman is asked about lower stomach and bowel pain, cramps, vaginal bleeding, itching, swelling, redness, or a vaginal discharge. She is asked if she has pain during sexual intercourse and pain or burning on urination. Observations are recorded of her general appearance, temperature and blood pressure, weight, if the breasts are the same size, the feel of the breasts, lumps, and nipple color. The stomach area is examined for shape, stretch marks, scars, tumors, and bowel sounds. Swelling or redness of the external genitals, cervix, and lumps or tumors on the labia majora, the presence or lack of hymenal tags, and a bloody discharge are noted. The woman's age at the beginning of menstruation, the length, spacing, and regularity of cycles, and symptoms, as pain and excess bleeding, are recorded. The problems and outcome of each of the patient's pregnancies, the kind of childbirth, any abortion, and the date of menopause and linked symptoms are explored. The examination may include an examination by hand, Pap test, a base body temperature figure, doing tests on the vaginal discharge, tests on tissues, scraping and flushing out the uterus, and blowing material into the tubes. Laboratory studies may include levels of hormones, tests for sexually carried diseases, and thyroid function tests.

female sexual dysfunction, inability of a woman to have or enjoy satisfactory sexual intercourse and orgasm. Symptoms include pain, spasms, a complete inability to reach orgasm, and being unable to be aroused sexually. Causes include

anxiety, fear, and negative feelings about sexual arousal and intercourse. Compare **male sexual dysfunction.** See also **sexual dysfunction.**

feminist therapy, a form of therapy based on consciousness raising. It focuses on the presence of sexism and sex role stereotyping in society.

feminization, **1.** the normal growth or beginning of female sex characteristics. **2.** the beginning of female sex characteristics in a male. Feminization may be caused by tumor, advanced alcoholism, or by the use of estrogen therapy for cancer. Some testicle tumors may cause feminizing symptoms, and male breasts becoming larger may be caused by Klinefelter's syndrome and by certain drugs. Compare **virilization.** See also **pseudohermaphroditism.**

feminizing adrenal tumor, a tumor of the adrenal gland. Symptoms in males include breasts becoming larger and loss of ability to have sexual intercourse. The testicles often begin wasting, but the prostate and penis are usually normal in size. In women, these tumors are linked to early puberty.

femoral /fem'ərəl/, referring to the thigh (femur).

femoral condyle, one of a pair of large, flared projections at the lower end of the thigh bone (femur). They are covered with a thick layer of cartilage and join with the knee cap and large bone of the lower leg (tibia) at the knee joint.

femoral epiphysis, a secondary bone-forming center of the thigh bone (femur). Before the bones are mature, the epiphysis is separated from the main part of the femur by cartilage.

femoral hernia, a hernia in which a loop of intestine moves into the groin. Surgery (herniorrhaphy), is the usual treatment. See also **hernia.**

femoral nerve, the main nerve of the thigh.

femoral pulse, the pulse of the artery (femoral) felt in the groin.

femoral vein, a large vein in the thigh.

femur /fē'mər/, the thigh bone.

fenestra /fines'trə/, *pl.* **fenestrae,** an opening in a bandage or cast that is often cut out to reduce pressure or to give regular skin care.

fenestrated drape, a covering (drape) with a round or slitlike opening in the center.

fenestration, a surgery in which an opening is made to gain access to the space within an organ or a bone. Also called **window.** **–fenestrate,** *v.*

fenfluramine hydrochloride /fenfloor'əmēn/, a drug given to decrease the appetite in patients who are overweight.

★CAUTION: Glaucoma, alcoholism, high blood pressure, or known allergy to this drug prohibits its use.

★ADVERSE EFFECTS: Among the more serious

side effects are drug addiction, diarrhea, mental confusion, and depression.

fenoprofen calcium, a drug given to treat arthritis and other painful conditions.

★CAUTION: Kidney or stomach and intestine diseases, or known allergy to this drug, to aspirin, or to similar drugs prohibits its use.

★ADVERSE EFFECTS: Among the more serious side effects are stomach and intestine disturbances, peptic ulcers, dizziness, skin rash, and hearing problems. The drug interacts with many other drugs.

fenoterol, a drug used in respiratory therapy to reduce the patient's effort in breathing.

fentanyl citrate /fen'tənil/, a painkiller used with general anesthesia.

★CAUTION: Myasthenia gravis or known allergy to this drug prohibits its use.

★ADVERSE EFFECTS: Among the more serious side effects are drug addiction, itching, and throat spasm.

Feosol, a trademark for a blood builder (ferrous sulfate).

Fergon, a trademark for a blood builder (ferrous gluconate).

Ferguson's reflex, a contraction of the uterus after the cervix is stimulated. The reflex is important in labor.

fermentation, a chemical change caused by the action of an enzyme or microorganism.

fermentative dyspepsia /fərmen'tətiv/, impaired digestion linked to the fermenting of digested food. See also **dyspepsia.**

ferning test, a test for the presence of estrogen in the cervical mucus. High levels of estrogen cause the cervical mucus to dry on a slide in a fernlike pattern. In pregnancy testing, the fern pattern does not appear.

ferric, referring to a compound containing iron, as ferric chloride.

ferritin /fur'itin/, an iron compound found in the intestine, spleen, and liver. It contains over 20% iron and is essential for red blood cells.

ferro-, ferr-, ferri-, a combining form for iron.

ferromagnetic, referring to substances, as iron, nickel, and cobalt, that are strongly magnetic. Such substances may become magnetized by being exposed to a magnetic field.

ferrous sulfate, a blood building drug given to treat iron deficiency anemia.

★CAUTION: There are no cautions.

★ADVERSE EFFECTS: Among the most serious side effects are diarrhea and constipation.

fertile, **1.** able to reproduce or bear offspring. **2.** able to be fertilized. **3.** fruitful; not sterile. **–fertility,** *n.,* **fertilize,** *v.*

fertile eunuch syndrome, a hormone disorder of males in which the amount of sex hormone is not enough for spermatogenesis.

fertile period, the time in the menstrual cycle during which fertilization may occur. Sperm can live for 48 to 72 hours; the egg (ovum) lives

for 24 hours. Thus, the fertile period begins 2 to 3 days before ovulation and lasts for 2 to 3 days afterward.

fertility, the ability to have children.

fertility rate, the number of births per 1,000 women aged 15 through 44 in a particular population over a given period of time.

fertilization, the union of male and female gametes to form a zygote from which the embryo develops. The process takes place in the fallopian tube of the female when a sperm comes in contact with the egg (ovum).

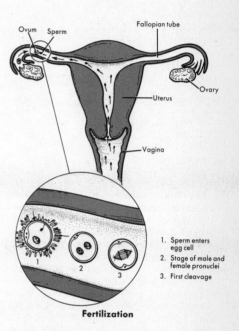

Fertilization

fertilization age. See **fetal age.**

fertilization membrane, a membrane surrounding the fertilized egg (ovum) that prevents entry by more sperm.

Festal, a trademark for a stomach and bowel drug containing digestive enzymes and bile parts.

festinating gait, a way of walking in which the person increases speed in an unconscious effort to "catch up" with a displaced center of gravity. It is common in persons with Parkinson's disease.

fetal abortion, end of pregnancy after the twentieth week but before the fetus is able to live outside of the uterus. Compare **embryonic abortion.**

fetal age, the age of the embryo from the time since fertilization. Also called **fertilization age.** Compare **gestational age.**

fetal alcohol syndrome, an infant disorder caused by the mother's intake of alcohol during preg-

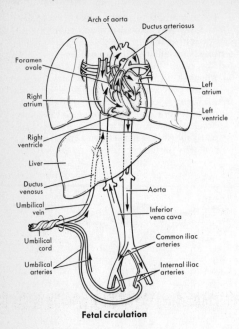

Fetal circulation

nancy. It often occurs when the mother drinks an amount equal to 3 ounces or more of pure alcohol each day. Affected children have defects of their heads and faces, arms and legs, and hearts. They also suffer from delayed growth and mental retardation.

fetal bradycardia, an abnormally slow fetal heart rate, usually below 100 beats per minute.

fetal circulation, the pathway of blood flow in the fetus. Blood-carrying oxygen from the placenta travels through the umbilical cord to the liver. The blood then flows to the heart. It goes through a hole between the right and left chambers (atria) of the heart. Blood-carrying oxygen is available for circulation through the left chamber (ventricle) to the head and upper body area. The blood returning from the head and arms enters the right chamber (ventricle)

and is pumped through the lung artery and into the large heart artery (aorta) for circulation to the lower parts of the body. The blood is returned to the placenta through the umbilical cord arteries.

fetal death, the death of a fetus in the uterus, or the death of a fetus that weighs at least 500 g or after 20 or more weeks of gestation.

fetal distress, a fetus with an abnormal heart rate or rhythm. If possible, the cause is found and corrected. Cesarean section may be necessary if the cause of the problem cannot be corrected.

fetal dose, the estimated amount of radiation a fetus receives during an x-ray examination of its mother. It is calculated in millirads (mrad) per 1,000 milliroentgens of skin exposure. It varies from less than 1 mrad when a leg or arm is examined to nearly 300 mrad when the x-ray beam is directed toward the pelvis.

fetal heart rate (FHR), the number of heart beats in the fetus per minute. The FHR is affected by many factors, including fever, contractions of the uterus, and drugs. The normal FHR is more than 100 beats per minute and less than 160 beats per minute.

fetal membranes, the structures that protect, support, and nourish the embryo and fetus (including the yolk sac, allantois, amnion, chorion, placenta, and umbilical cord).

fetal hemoglobin, hemoglobin F, the major hemoglobin present in the blood of a fetus and newborn. Hemoglobin F is present in small amounts in the blood of adults.

fetal hydantoin syndrome (FHS), a complex of birth defects caused by the mother's use of hydantoin drugs. Symptoms of FHS include lack of nails on the fingers or toes, mental retardation, slowed growth, and heart defects.

fetal lie, the relationship of the length of the fetus to the height of the mother. See also **fetal presentation.**

fetal lipoma. See **hibernoma.**

fetal position, the relationship of the body part of the fetus to the mother's pelvis. If a fetus comes out with the head directed to the back

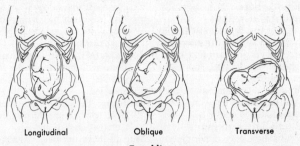

Longitudinal   Oblique   Transverse

Fetal lie

of the mother's right side, the fetal position is right occiput posterior (ROP). Compare **fetal attitude, fetal presentation.**

fetal presentation, the body part of the fetus that first appears in the pelvis.

fetal stage, the period from the end of the embryonic stage, after the seventh week of pregnancy, to birth, 38 to 42 weeks after the the last menstrual period.

fetal tachycardia, a fetal heart rate of 160 or more beats per minute for more than 10 minutes.

feticide. See **embryoctony.**

fetish, 1. any object or idea given unreasonable attention or worth. 2. any inanimate object or any part of the body not of a sexual nature that arouses erotic feelings.

fetishist, a person who believes in or receives erotic pleasure from fetishes.

fetofetal transfusion. see **parabiotic syndrome.**

fetography /fētog'rəfē/, x-ray films of the fetus in the uterus. See also **fetometry.**

fetology /fētol'əjē/, the branch of medicine that is concerned with the fetus. Also called **embryatrics.**

fetometry /fētom'ətrē/, the measurement of the size of the fetus, especially the size of the head and the body.

fetoplacental, referring to the fetus and the placenta.

fetoprotein, a substance that occurs naturally in fetuses and occasionally in adults as the result of certain diseases. Leukemia and other cancers are linked to **beta-fetoprotein** in the blood of adults. An increased amount of **alpha-fetoprotein** in the fetus shows nervous-system defects.

fetoscope /fē'təskōp'/, a stethoscope for hearing the fetal heart beat through the mother's stomach.

fetoscopy /fētos'kəpē/, observing a fetus in the uterus through a small incision in the abdomen.

fetotoxic, referring to anything that is poisonous to a fetus.

fetus /fē'təs/, the human child in the uterus following the embryonic period, usually from the eighth week after fertilization until birth. Compare **embryo.** See also **prenatal development.**

fetus acardiacus, fetus acardius. See **acardius.**

fetus anideus. See **anideus.**

fetus in fetu, a birth defect in which a small, imperfectly formed twin is contained within the body of the normal twin.

fetus papyraceus, a twin fetus that has died in the uterus and has been pressed flat against the uterine wall by the living fetus. Also called **paper-doll fetus, papyraceous fetus.**

fever, an abnormal temperature of the body above 98.6° F (37° C). Exercise, anxiety, and dehydration may increase the temperature of healthy people. Infection, nerve disease, can-

cer, anemia, and many drugs may cause fever. No single theory explains why the temperature is increased. Fever increases metabolism 7% per °C, meaning more food needs to be eaten. Convulsions may occur in children whose fevers tend to rise quickly. Confusion is seen with high fevers in adults and in children. It may begin quickly or gradually. The period of highest fever is called the stadium or fastigium. It may last for a few days or up to 3 weeks. See also **fever treatment, hyperpyrexia.**

fever blister, a cold sore caused by herpesvirus. Also called **herpes simplex.**

fever of unknown origin (FUO), a fever of at least 101° F (38.3° C) that lasts for at least 3 weeks without discovery of the cause in spite of at least 1 week of study.

fever therapy. See **artificial fever.**

fever treatment, the care of a patient with a high temperature. The patient is observed for rapid heart beat; a full, bounding pulse or a weak, thready pulse; rapid breathing; hot, dry skin; chills; headache; sweating; confusion; dehydration; tremors; convulsions; and coma. Treatment may include giving antibiotic, antifever, and sedative drugs. If the temperature is extremely high, an alcohol sponge bath, cooling tub bath, a cold wet sheet, or ice packs may be helpful. The patient's temperature is checked every 2 to 4 hours. The room temperature may be reduced, and air currents increased by a fan. Increased amounts of fluids are given, physical activity is reduced, and the skin is exposed to air.

FHR, abbreviation for **fetal heart rate.**

FHS, abbreviation for **fetal hydantoin syndrome.**

fiber diet, a diet that contains a great deal of fibrous material. Fiber, material that resists digestion, is found in vegetables, fruits, and cereals. It adds bulk to the diet and is thought to reduce the risk of bowel cancer.

fiberoptic bronchoscopy, examination of the bronchial tubes through a fiberoptic bronchoscope. Also called **bronchofibroscopy.** See also **bronchoscopy, fiberoptics.**

fiberoptic duodenoscope, an instrument for showing the inside of the stomach (duodenum).

fiberoptics, process by which an internal organ or space can be viewed, using glass or plastic fibers that reflect a magnified image. **–fiberoptic,** *adj.*

-fibrate, a combining form referring to compounds similar to a drug used to treat high cholesterol levels in the blood (clofibrate).

fibril /fī'bril/, a small threadlike structure that often is part of a cell.

fibrillation, involuntary contractions of a single muscle fiber or of an isolated group of nerve fibers.

fibrin /fī'brin/, a stringy protein that cannot be dissolved. It gives the semisolid character to a blood clot. Compare **fibrinogen.** See also **blood clotting, coagulation, fibrinolysis, thrombin.**

fibrinase. See **factor XIII.**

fibrinogen /fībrin'əjən/, a protein in the blood-clotting process that is converted into protein (fibrin) by thrombin when calcium is present. Also called **factor I.** Compare **fibrin.** See also **afibrinogenemia, blood clotting, fibrinolysis, thrombin.**

fibrinogenopenia, a lack of fibrinogen in the blood.

fibrinokinase /fī'brinōkī'nās/, an enzyme that starts up plasminogen. Also called **tissue activator, tissue kinase.**

fibrinolysin /fī'brinol'isin/, an enzyme that dissolves protein (fibrin). Also called **plasmin.** See also **fibrinolysis.**

fibrin-stabilizing factor. See **factor XIII.**

fibro-, a combining form referring to fiber.

fibroadenoma /fī'brō·ad'inō'mə/, pl. **fibroadenomas, fibroadenomata,** a tumor of the breast. It is round, movable, and firm. It occurs most frequently in women under 25 years of age and is caused by greater-than-usual amounts of estrogen.

fibroangioma. See **angiofibroma.**

fibroareolar tissue. See **areolar tissue.**

fibrocartilage, cartilage that is a dense mixture of white collagen fibers. Of the three kinds of cartilage in the body, fibrocartilage has the greatest strength. Fibrocartilaginous disks are found between the back bones. See also **elastic cartilage, hyaline cartilage.**

fibrocartilaginous joint. See **symphysis.**

fibrocystic breast disease, single or multiple lumps (cysts) in the breasts. The cysts are often harmless and fairly common, but they may be cancerous. Women with fibrocystic disease of the breast are at greater-than-usual risk of getting breast cancer later in life. Also called **chronic cystic mastitis.**

fibrocystic disease of the pancreas. See **cystic fibrosis.**

fibrocyte. See **fibroblast.**

fibroelastic tissue. See **fibrous tissue.**

fibroids /fī'broids/, a noncancerous tumor of the smooth muscle on the uterus. It appears firm, round, and gray-white. Multiple tumors of this kind develop most often in the wall of the uterus. They usually occur in women between 30 and 50 years of age. Also called fibromyoma uteri, leiomyoma uteri.

fibrolipoma, a tumor that contains both fibrouos and fatty material.

fibroma /fībrō'mə/, a noncancerous tumor largely made up of fiberlike or fully developed connective tissue. See also specific fibroma.

fibroma cutis, a fiberlike tumor of the skin.

fibroma durum. See **hard fibroma.**

fibroma molle. See **soft fibroma.**

fibroma thecocellulare xanthomatodes. See **theca cell tumor.**

fibromyoma uteri. See **fibroids.**

fibromyomectomy /fī'brōmī'omek'təmē/, surgical removal of a fibrous tumor (fibroma) from the uterus or other location.

fibromyositis /fī'brōmī'əsī'tis/, stiffness and joint or muscle pain, with swelling of the muscle tissues and the fiberlike connective tissues. The condition may develop after a weather change, infection, or injury. Kinds of fibromyositis include **lumbago, pleurodynia, torticollis.** See also **rheumatism.**

fibropapilloma. See **fibroepithelial papilloma.**

fibrosarcoma, a cancer that contains connective tissue, it develops suddenly from small bumps on the skin.

fibrosing alveolitis /fī'brōsing/, a lung disorder (alveolitis) with breathlessness and air hunger, occurring in rheumatoid arthritis and other diseases. See also **alveolitis.**

fibrosis /fibrō'sis/, **1.** a fiberlike connective tissue that occurs normally in the growth of scar tissue. It replaces normal tissue lost through injury or infection. **2.** the spread of fiberlike connective tissue over normal smooth muscle or other normal organ tissue. See also **cystic fibrosis, fibrositis.**

fibrositis /fī'brəsī'tis/, a swelling of fiberlike connective tissue. Symptoms include pain and stiffness of the neck, shoulder, and body. Fibrositis occurs in middle age. Compare **fibromyositis, myositis.**

-fibrous, a combining form meaning 'composed of fiberlike tissue.'

fibrous capsule, 1. the layer of tissue surrounding the joint between two bones. **2.** the tough membrane envelope surrounding some organs, as the liver. See also **synovial membrane.**

fibrous dysplasia, the fiberlike displacement of bone tissue. The kinds of fibrous dysplasia are monostotic fibrous dysplasia, and polyostotic fibrous dysplasia. Symptoms may include a limp, a pain, or a broken bone on the affected side. Girls affected may have an early start of menstruation and breast development. The involved leg may be shortened, and the classic 'shepherd's crook' deformity is common.

fibrous goiter, a large thyroid gland, marked by overgrowth of the capsule and connective tissue.

fibrous histiocytoma. See **dermatofibroma.**

fibrous joint, an immovable joint, as those of the skull segments, in which a fiberlike tissue may connect the bones.

fibrous thyroiditis, a replacement of normal thyroid tissue by dense fiberlike tissue. The gland becomes fixed to the muscles, nerves, blood vessels, and throat (trachea) by fiberlike tissue. The disease occurs more often in women than in men and usually shows up after 40 years of age. Symptoms include a sense of choking, breathlessness, and swallowing problems. Also called **ligneous thyroiditis, Riedel's struma, Riedel's thyroiditis.**

fibula /fib'yo͞olə/, a bone of the lower leg, next to and smaller than the shin bone (tibia). In relation to its length, it is the most slender of the long bones. Also called **calf bone.**

fictive kin, people who are regarded as members of a family even though they are not related by blood or marriage. Fictive kinship may bind people in ties of affection, concern, obligation, and responsibility.

FID, abbreviaton for **free induction display.**

field, a defined space, area, or distance. The field of vision is the total area a person can see with one eye without moving the eye. The binocular field is the area that can be seen with both eyes.

Fielder's myocarditis, a rare inflammation of the heart that may be caused by a virus infection. The infection is not related to a current or recent illness. It is usually fatal.

field fever, a form of infection (leptospirosis) caused by a germ *(Leptospira grippotyphosa)*. It affects mainly farm workers and is marked by fever, stomach and bowel pain, diarrhea, vomiting, listlessness, and eye inflammation. Also called **canefield fever.** See also **leptospirosis.**

fiery serpent, *informal. Dracunculus medinesis.* See also **dracunculiasis.**

fievre boutonneuses. See **African tick typhus.**

fifth disease. See **erythema infectiosum.**

fifth cranial nerve. See **trigeminal nerve.**

fight-or-flight. See **flight-or-fight reaction.**

figure 4 test. See **Fabere's test.**

figure-of-eight bandage, a bandage with successive laps crossing over and around each other like the figure eight. See also **bandage.**

fila-, a combining form referring to a thread, or threadlike.

filament, a fine, threadlike fiber. Filaments are found in most tissues and cells of the body and serve various functions.

filariasis /fil'ərī'əsis/, a disease caused by the presence of *Filaria* worms in the tissues of the body. Filarial worms are round, long, and threadlike and are common in most warm areas of the world. They tend to infest the lymph glands after entering the body through the bite of a mosquito or other insect. There is swelling and pain of the affected body area. After many years, an arm or leg may become greatly swollen and the skin coarse and tough. See also **elephantiasis.**

filariform /filer'ifôrm/, referring to a structure or organ that is threadlike.

-filcon, a combining form referring to a type of contact lens material.

file, a collection of related information kept together as a unit.

filling. See **dental filling.**

filling pressure, the pressure in the left lower chamber of the heart at the end of the time when the heart muscle is relaxed and the heart chambers are filled with blood (diastole).

film badge, a photographic film packet, worn by healthteam members when they work around radioactive materials. It is able to pick up radiation. It is used for estimating exposure to x-rays and other radioactive sources.

film development, the processing of photographic or x-ray film so the image shows. It involves wetting the film and bathing it in chemicals.

film on teeth, a collection of deposits attaching to the teeth. It contains microorganisms, tissue and blood cell elements, and other wastes. See also **plaque.**

film screen mammography, a breast x-ray technique that produces a fine image with low exposure to radiation.

filter, 1. a device or material through which a gas or liquid is passed to separate out unwanted material. 2. in radiology. a device added to an x-ray machine that removes low-energy x-rays that cannot reach the film. Examples include bow-tie, compensating, and conic filters.

filum /fī'ləm/, a threadlike structure. An example is the filum terminale at the lower end of the spinal cord.

fimbria, any structure that forms a border or edge that resembles a fringe.

fimbriae tubae, the branched, fingerlike border at the end of each of the fallopian tubes. The fimbriae have hairlike fibers (cilia) that move the egg (ovum) toward the uterus.

fimbrial tubal pregnancy, a kind of tubal pregnancy in which implantation occurs in the fringed (fimbriated) distal end of a fallopian tube. See also **tubal pregnancy.**

finger, any of the digits of the hand. The fingers are made up of a metacarpal bone and three bony hinges (phalanges). Some count the thumb as a finger, although it has one less bone. The digits of the hand are numbered 1 to 5, starting with the thumb.

finger agnosia, a nerve disorder in which a person cannot distinguish between stimuli applied to two different fingers without looking. It occurs in some types of dementia.

finger percussion. See **percussion.**

finger stick, the act of pricking the tip of the finger to obtain a small sample of blood from the small blood vessels (capillaries). Sometimes the hand is first soaked in warm water for 10 minutes to give the blood the properties of arterial blood.

Finnish bath. See **Russian bath.**

Fiorinal, a trademark for a group of drugs containing a sedative-hypnotic (butalbital), an analgesic, antifever, and anti-inflammatory (aspirin), an analgesic (phenacetin), and a stimulant (caffeine).

fire damp. See **damp.**

fireman's cramp. See **heat cramp.**

first aid, the care given to an injured or ill patient, usually where the victim was injured or became sick. It is the initial care given to the victim before medically trained people arrive or before the victim arrives to a health-care center. Attention is given first to the most critical problems: opening of an airway, the presence of bleeding, and heart function. The patient is kept warm and as comfortable as possible. The conscious patient is reassured and is asked for details of medical history, as diabetes, a known heart condition, or allergic reactions to drugs; if the patient is unconscious, a medical identification card, bracelet, or necklace is looked for. The patient is moved as little as possible, particularly if there is a possibility of broken bones. If there is vomiting, the patient's head is moved to a position for the vomit to exit easily to avoid having the patient breathe in the vomit. See also **cardiopulmonary resuscitation, control of hemorrhage, emergency medicine, emergency nursing.**

first generation scanner, an early type of CAT scan (computed tomography) device. It required up to 5 minutes for one scan.

first intention. See **intention.**

first cranial nerve. See **olfactory nerve.**

first rib, the highest rib in the chest. Its movement is responsible for raising and lowering the breast bone during breathing. During quiet breathing, first-rib movement is slight. During stress, it can increase the diameter of the chest.

fishmeal worker's lung, a lung inflammation that occurs in workers who are sensitive to fish meal. The symptoms are similar to those of other allergic conditions caused by dust.

fish poisoning, poisoning caused by eating fish that contains dangerous substances. Symptoms may range from nausea and vomiting to inability to breathe. Scromboid poisoning results from a poison produced by bacteria in mackerel, tuna, or bonito. The symptoms appear immediately. They include facial flushing, nausea and vomiting, stomach pain, and itching. Tetraodon poisoning is caused by a poison in puffer fish. It results in nerve and muscle problems. See also **ciguatera poisoning.**

fish skin disease. See **ichthyosis.**

fish tapeworm infection, an infection caused by a tapeworm (*Diphyllobothrium latum*). It is carried to humans when they eat infected raw or undercooked freshwater fish. Fish tapeworm infection is common in warm areas throughout the world and is found in the Great Lakes area of the United States. See also *diphyllobothrium,* **tapeworm infection.**

fiss-, a combining form referring to a split (cleft).

fission, the act of splitting into parts.

fissure /fish'ər/, **1.** a split or a groove on the surface of an organ. It often marks the division of the organ into parts, as the lobes of the lung. A fissure is usually deeper than a sulcus, but *fissure* and *sulcus* are often used as if they were the same thing. **2.** a cracklike break in the skin, as an anal fissure. Compare **sulcus.**

fissure fracture, any broken bone in which a crack extends into the outer layer of the bone but not through the entire bone.

fissure-in-ano, a painful cut at the margin of the anus.

fissure of Bichat. See **transverse fissure.**

fissure of Rolando. See **central sulcus.**

fissure of Sylvius. See **lateral cerebral sulcus.**

fistula /fis'chŏŏlə, -chələ/, an abnormal passage from an internal organ to the body surface or between two internal organs. Fistulas may occur in many sites from the mouth to the anus and may be made for treatment. An arteriovenous fistula is commonly made to get to the bloodstream for blood filtering (hemodialysis).

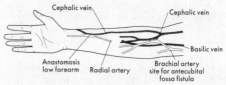

Fistula

fistula in ano. See **anal fistula.**

fit, 1. *nontechnical.* an attack or seizure. **2.** the sudden beginning of symptoms, as a fit of coughing. **3.** the manner in which one surface is placed next to another, as the fit of a denture to the gums.

Fitzgerald factor, a substance that may be needed for the interaction of two substances (factors XII and XI) in blood clotting.

fixating eye, the normal eye that can be focused in cases of eye wandering (strabismus). Compare **squinting eye.**

fixation, stopping at a certain stage of psychological and sexual growth, as anal fixation.

fixation muscle, a muscle that holds a part of the body in a position.

fixative, any substance used to bind, glue, or keep rigid.

fixed bridgework, a dental device using artificial teeth permanently attached in the upper or the lower jaw.

fixed combination drug, a group of mixtures with many ingredients giving specific amounts of two or more drugs at the same time.

fixed dressing, a dressing usually made of gauze with a hardening agent, as plaster of Paris or starch. It is applied to support or keep rigid a part of the body. The dressing is soaked in water, applied to the part to be held rigid, and allowed to harden. See also **cast.**

fixed idea, 1. a continuous, single-minded thought or notion. **2.** a confused idea that controls mental activity and continues despite evidence or logical proof that it is false. Also called **idée fixe** /idā′fiks′/.

fixed interval (FI) reinforcement, (in psychiatry), reinforcement repeated after a specific amount of time has elapsed.

fixed orthodontic appliance, a device cemented to the teeth or attached by an adhesive.

fixed phagocyte. See **phagocyte.**

fixed ratio (FR) reinforcement, in psychiatry, reinforcement given after a certain number of responses have occurred.

fixed vertebrae. See **false vertebrae.**

fixer, a chemical used to process photographic or x-ray film. It is applied after the film is developed to remove other chemicals and harden the emulsion.

flaccid /flak′sid/, weak, soft, and flabby; lacking normal muscle tone, as flaccid muscles.

flaccid bladder, a urinary bladder disorder. It is marked by continual filling and occasional overfilling of the bladder, lack of an urge to urinate, and unable to urinate at will. Compare **spastic bladder.**

flaccid paralysis, the weakening or the loss of muscle tone. Compare **spastic paralysis.**

flagell-, a combining form referring to a whiplike movement; tapping.

flagellant, a person who gets sexual pleasure from whipping or being whipped (flagellation).

flagellate /flaj′əlāt′, -lit/, a microorganism that moves itself by waving whiplike, thready fibers (filaments) as *Trypanosoma, Leishmania, Trichomonas,* and *Giardia.* See also **protozoa.**

flagellation, 1. the act of whipping, beating, or flogging. **2.** a type of massage given by tapping the body with the fingers. See also **massage.**

Flagyl, a trademark for an antiprotozoa drug (metronidazole).

flail chest, a chest in which many broken ribs cause the chest wall to be unstable. The lung under the injured area contracts on breathing in and bulges on breathing out. The condition, if uncorrected, leads to air hunger. Flail chest is marked by sharp pain; uneven chest expansion; shallow, rapid breathing; and reduced breath sounds. Problems are collapsed lung, shock, and the stopping of breathing. The treatment is to stabilize the inside of the chest wall with a mechanical lung. Chest tubes may be needed to remove air or fluid stopping the affected lung from expanding, and a tube may be used to provide food and fluids through the nose. Traction may be applied by attaching a steel wire to the ribs or breastbone and connecting the wire to a rope, pulley, and weight.

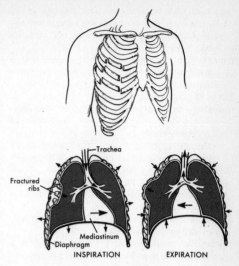

Flail chest

flank, the back part of the body between the ribs and the hip.

flapping tremor. See **asterixis.**

flare, 1. a red blush on the skin at the edge of a hives sore. **2.** the sudden worsening of a disease.

flaring of nostrils, a widening of the nostrils during breathing in, a sign of air hunger or breathing problems.

flashback, a phenomenon that happens to persons who have taken mind-altering drugs. The drug's effects are unexpectedly repeated later.

flat affect, the appearance or mood of a person who does not show emotion either verbally or nonverbally.

flat bone, any of the bones that provide the contours of the body. Examples are the ribs and bones of the skull.

flat electroencephalogram, a chart on which no tracings were recorded during a brain-wave test (electroencephalography). It indicates a lack of brain wave activity. Flat readings are a sign of brain death except in cases of central nervous system problems. Also called **isoelectric electroencephalogram.**

flatfoot. See **pes planus.**

flat-spring contraceptive diaphragm, a birth control device (diaphragm) with a metal spring that forms the rim. The diaphragm is given to a woman whose vaginal muscles give good support and whose uterus is in the normal position. Compare **arcing spring contraceptive diaphragm, coil spring contraceptive diaphragm.** See also **contraceptive diaphragm fitting.**

flatulence, an excess amount of air or gas in the stomach and intestines. It may cause the organs to bloat and in some cases mild to moderate pain.

flatus /flā′təs/, air or gas in the intestine that is passed through the rectum. See also **aerophagia.**

flat wart. See **verruca plana.**

flavoxate hydrochloride, a smooth, muscle-relaxing drug given for spastic conditions of the urinary tract.

★CAUTION: Stomach or bowel bleeding or blockage, urinary-tract blockage, or known allergy to this drug prohibits its use.

★ADVERSE EFFECTS: Among the more serious side effects are nervousness, nausea, stomach and bowel pain, and fever.

flea, a wingless, bloodsucking insect. Some species carry viruses to humans.

flea bite, a small puncture wound caused by a bloodsucking flea. Fleas may carry plague, murine typhus, and tularemia.

flea-borne typhus. See **murine typhus.**

Fleischner method /flīsh′nər/, a technique for producing x-ray views of the lungs. The patient leans backward from the waist.

Fletcher factor, a blood-clotting substance that interacts with two other blood-clotting substances (factor XII and Fitzgerald factor) and activates both of those substances.

Flexeril, a trademark for a muscle-relaxing drug (cyclobenzaprine hydrochloride).

flexibilitas cerea. See **cerea flexibilitas.**

flexion /flek′shən/, a movement allowed by certain joints of the skeleton. It decreases the angle between two connecting bones, as bending the elbow. Compare **extension.**

flexion jacket, a corset designed to prevent the spine from moving. It is made out of rigid material.

flexor carpi radialis, a muscle of the forearm. It flexes the hand.

flexor carpi ulnaris, a muscle of the forearm. It flexes the hand.

flexor digitorum superficialis, a large muscle of the forearm.

flexor retinaculum of the hand. See **retinaculum flexorum manus.**

flexure /flek′shər/, a normal bend or curve in a body part, as the curve of the spine.

flight into health, a reaction to an unpleasant physical sense or symptom. The person denies the reality of the symptom, insisting that nothing is wrong. See also **illness experience.**

flight of ideas, a continuous stream of talk in which the patient switches quickly from one topic to another, each subject being hard to understand and not related to the one before it. The condition is often a symptom of sudden manic states and schizophrenia. Compare **circumstantiality.**

flight-or-fight reaction, 1. the reaction of the body to stress. The nervous system and the adrenal gland increase the heart output, widen the pupils of the eyes, increase the rate of the heart beat, narrow the blood vessels of the skin, and cause an alert, aroused mental state. 2. a person's reaction to stress by either fleeing from a situation or staying and trying to deal with it.

flight to illness, in psychiatry, the patient's effort to convince the therapist taht he or she is too ill to end therapy. The patient tries to obtain continued support.

flip-flop, the digit system of computer memory. Data are recorded in one of two states, such as 0 or 1, yes or no, and + or −.

floater, one or more spots that appear to drift in front of the eye. It is caused by a shadow cast on the retina by material within the eyeball. Most floaters are leftovers of blood vessels that were in the eye before birth. The sudden beginning of several floaters may mean serious disease. Bleeding into the eye may cause a large number of big and little shadows and a red discoloration of vision. The cause is often injury, but sudden bleeding occurs in diabetes mellitus, high blood pressure, or brain disease. Cancer, loosening (detachment) of the retina, or other eye diseases may also cause bleeding. Retinal detachment also causes a sudden appearance of lightninglike floaters and reduced sight as a shower of red cells and color is released into the eyeball. *Technical name:* **muscae volitantes.**

floating kidney, a kidney that is not securely fixed in the usual location because of a birth defect or injury. Compare **ptotic kidney.**

floating rib. See **rib.**

flocculation test /flok′yo͞olā′shən/, a blood test for syphilis.

flocculent /flok′yo͞olənt/, clumped or tufted, as a cloud, or covered with a woolly, fuzzy surface.

flooding, a technique used to reduce anxiety linked to unreasonable fears (phobia). Exposure to the stimulation that causes anxiety makes a person able to resist that stimulation. Also called **implosive therapy.** Compare **systemic desensitization.**

floppy infant syndrome, a general term for childhood muscle diseases (juvenile spinal muscular atrophies), including Werdnig-Hoffmann and Wohlfart-Kugelberg-Welander diseases.

flora, microorganisms (viruses, bacteria, and fungi) that live on or in a body. They compete with disease-causing microorganisms and provide a natural immunity against some infections.

Florone, a trademark for an anti-inflammation drug (diflorasone diacetate).

Floropryl, a trademark for an eye ointment (isoflurophate).

flossing, the cleaning of tooth surfaces with stringlike waxed or unwaxed dental floss.

flotation device, a foam mattress with a gel-like pad in its center, designed to protect bony parts of the body and to even out pressure on the skin.

flotation therapy, a state of semiweightlessness caused by many types of hospital equipment. It is used in treating and preventing bed sores.

flow sheet, a report of changing factors in a patient's record, temperature, blood pressure, or weight and the treatments and drugs given.

flow-volume loop, a lung-function test system in which the patient breathes into a machine that measures the amount of air breathed in and out. It displays the information as a loop whose shape shows lung volume and other breathing functions.

floxuridine /floksyŏŏr′ədēn/, an anticancer drug given to treat cancers of the brain, breast, liver, and gallbladder.
★CAUTION: Infection, poor state of the diet, or known allergy to this drug prohibits its use.
★ADVERSE EFFECTS: Among the more serious side effects are bone-marrow disorders and sudden stomach and bowel problems, including nausea, vomiting, diarrhea, and mouth swelling.

flu, *informal.* **1.** influenza. **2.** any viral infection of the breathing or intestinal system.

fluctuant, pertaining to a wavelike motion felt when a body part containing a liquid is pressed.

flucytosine /floōsī′təsēn/, an antifungus drug given to treat certain fungus infections.
★CAUTION: Known allergy to this drug prohibits its use. Close watching is needed when giving this drug to patients with kidney disease.
★ADVERSE EFFECTS: Among the more serious side effects are stomach and bowel problems, including swelling of the intestines (enterocolitis) and liver disease.

fluid, 1. a liquid or gas that is able to flow and to adjust its shape to that of a container. **2.** a body fluid involved in moving electrolytes and other needed chemicals to, through, and from tissue cells. See also **blood, lymph, cerebrospinal fluid.**

fluid balance, a state of balance in which the amount of fluid taken in equals the amount lost in urine, feces, perspiration, and exhaled air.

fluid ounce, a measure of liquid volume in the apothecaries' system, equal to 8 fluidrams or 29.57 ml. See also **apothecaries' measure, metric system.**

fluid retention, a failure to eliminate extra fluid from the body. Causes may include kidney, heart, or metabolic problems. In simple cases, the condition can sometimes be corrected by water pills (diuretics) and a low-salt diet.

fluid therapy, the control of water balance in patients with poor kidney, heart, or metabolic function by carefully measuring fluid taken in against fluid lost each day.

fluke, a parasitic flatworm, as *Schistosoma.* See also **schistosomiasis.**

fluocinolone acetonide, a hormone cream given to reduce swelling.
★CAUTION: Bad circulation, viral and fungus diseases of the skin, or known allergy to this drug or to other steroid drugs prohibits its use.
★ADVERSE EFFECTS: Among the more serious side effects are various ones resulting from long-term or excess use of steroid drugs. Many allergic reactions may occur.

fluocinonide /floō′osin′ənīd/, an artificial steroid drug given to reduce swelling.
★CAUTION: Viral and fungus diseases of the skin, tuberculosis of the skin, or known allergy to this drug prohibits its use.
★ADVERSE EFFECTS: Among the more serious side effects are other infections, skin streaks, and skin swelling (contact dermatitis).

Fluonid, a trademark for a hormone cream (fluocinolone acetonide).

fluorescent antibody test (FA test), a test for syphilis and tuberculosis.

fluorescent microscopy, examination with a microscope using ultraviolet light rays to study specimens, as tissues or microorganisms. The specimens are stained with fluorescent dye. Also called **ultraviolet microscopy.** See also **fluorescent antibody test.**

Fluorescent Treponemal Antibody Absorption Test (FTA-ABS test), a blood test for syphilis. See also **fluorescent antibody test.**

fluoridation /flôr′idā′shən/, adding fluoride, especially to a public water supply, to reduce tooth decay. See also **fluoride.**

fluorine (F) /floō′ərēn/, an element added to the water supply of many areas to harden the tooth enamel and decrease cavities. Excess amounts of fluoride can spot the tooth enamel.

Fluoroplex, a trademark for an anticancer drug used on the skin (fluorouracil).

fluoroscope /floōr′əskōp′/, a device used for the immediate showing of an x-ray image. **–fluoroscopic,** *adj.*

fluoroscopic compression device, an object that can be placed on the patient's abdomen to compress the skin during the taking of an x-ray of the digestive tract.

fluorosis /floōrō′sis/, excess fluorine in the body. Unusually high amounts of fluorine in drinking water causes spotted discoloration and pitting of the enamel of the teeth in children. Severe long-term fluorine poisoning will lead to bone and joint changes in adults. See also **fluoridation, fluoride.**

fluorouracil /floō′ərōyoōr′əsil/, an anticancer drug given to treat cancerous diseases of the skin and internal organs.

Fluothane, a trademark for a general anesthetic (halothane).

fluoxymesterone /flōō·ok'simes'tərōn/, a steroid hormone used to treat breast cancer in females, and late puberty in males.
★CAUTION: Male breast or prostate cancer, liver disease, known or suspected pregnancy, or known allergy to this drug prohibits its use.
★ADVERSE EFFECTS: Among the more serious side effects are allergic shock, excess blood calcium, and liver disease (jaundice).

fluphenazine hydrochloride, a phenothiazine tranquilizer given to treat psychotic disorders.

flurandrenolide, an anti-inflammation drug.
★CAUTION: Bad circulation, viral and fungus diseases of the skin, or known allergy to this drug or to steroid drugs prohibits its use.
★ADVERSE EFFECTS: Many allergic reactions may occur.

flurazepam hydrochloride /flŏōraz'əpam/, a benzodiazepine minor tranquilizer given to treat an inability to sleep (insomnia).

flush, 1. a blush or sudden reddening of the face and neck. It may occur with a feeling of heat, as may be seen with fever, certain drugs, or an overactive thyroid gland (hyperthyroidism). **2.** a sudden, rapid flow of water or other liquid.

flutter, a rapid vibration that may interfere with normal function.

fly, a two-winged insect, some species of which carry viruses to humans.

fly bites, bites that may be caused by deer, horse, or sand flies. Such bites produce a small painful wound with swelling. Emergency treatment for fly bites includes cleaning the site and placing ice on it. The bite should be checked for infections, as biting flies often carry disease.

FMG, abbreviation for **foreign medical graduate.**

FML, a trademark for an eye medicine (fluorometholone).

FNP, abbreviation for **family nurse practitioner.**

foam bath, a bath in water containing a substance that covers the surface of the liquid. Air or oxygen is used to form the foam.

focal motor seizure. See **motor seizure.**

focal plane, the plane of tissue that is in focus for an x-ray film.

focal seizure, a motor nerve problem caused by abnormal electric activity in the brain. Focal seizures commonly begin as spasms in the face, hand, or foot and spread to other muscles. Symptoms may include chewing, lip-smacking, swallowing movements, and excess saliva. Seizures in the eye-turning area of the brain may begin with a forced turning of the head and eyes. Also called **Jacksonian seizure.** See also **epilepsy, motor seizure.**

focus, a specific location, as the site of an infection or the point at which a signal begins.

focused activity, a technique of actively focusing the patient toward coping abilities and away from negative ones.

fog nebulizer, (in respiratory care) a device that keeps the air moist by producing large amounts of particles.

foil pellet, a loosely rolled piece of gold foil, used for making dental devices, as a tooth cavity filling or tooth crown.

folacin. See **folic acid.**

folate deficiency. See **folic acid.**

Foley catheter /fō'lē/, a rubber tube (catheter) with a balloon tip placed in the bladder. This kind of catheter is used when continuous draining of the bladder is desired, as in surgery. See also **catheterization.**

folic acid /fō'lik, fol'ik/, a vitamin of the B complex group able to be dissolved in water. It is needed for cell growth and reproduction. It functions with vitamins B_{12} and C in the breakdown of proteins and in the making of hemoglobin. Folic acid also increases the appetite and causes the making of hydrochloric acid in the stomach. The vitamin is stored in the liver and may be made by bacteria in the stomach and intestines. Lack of folic acid results in poor growth, gray hair, mouth and tongue swelling, and diarrhea. Need for folic acid is increased in pregnancy, infancy, and by stress. Rich food sources include spinach and other green leafy vegetables, liver, kidneys, and whole-grain cereals. Also called **folacin, pteroylglutamic acid, vitamin B_9.**

folic acid deficiency anemia, a form of anemia caused by a lack of a vitamin (folic acid) in the diet.

folie /fōlē'/, a mental disorder.

folie à deux. See **shared paranoid disorder.**

folie circulaire. See **bipolar disorder.**

folie du doute /dYdŏōt'/, a psychological problem, marked by doubting, repeating a certain act or behavior, and not being able to make a decision.

folie du pourquoi /dYpŏōrkwô·ä'/, a psychological condition marked by continuously asking questions.

folie gemellaire /zhemeler'/, a psychotic condition that occurs at the same time in twins. The twins may not be living together or in close contact at the time.

folie raisonnante /rezônäNt'/, psychosis marked by seemingly logical thinking but lacking common sense.

folinic acid /fōlin'ik/, an active form of folic acid used to treat certain (megaloblastic) anemias. Also called **citrovorum factor, leucovorin.**

folk illnesses, health disorders that do not have scientific causes. The major groups are naturalistic illnesses caused by impersonal forces, as yin-yang, and personalistic illnesses caused by such forces as voodoo or evil eye.

follicle, a pouchlike recessed spot, as the dental follicles that surround the teeth before they emerge or the hair follicles within the skin. **–follicular,** *adj.*

follicle stimulating hormone (FSH), a pituitary gland hormone that stimulates the growth and aging of Graafian follicles in the ovary. It also causes the making of sperm (spermatogenesis) in the male. Also called **menotropins.**

follicular adenocarcinoma, a cancer that usually comes from the thyroid gland. It has a tendency to spread to the lungs and bones. See also **medullary carcinoma, papillary adenocarcinoma.**

follicular cyst, a lump (cyst) that comes from the tissue of a tooth bud.

follicular phase, the first of the menstrual cycle, when follicles in the ovary grow to prepare for the releasing of an egg.

folliculitis /fōlik′yōoli′tis/, swelling of hair follicles, as in sycosis barbae.

folliculoma. See **granulosa cell tumor.**

Follutein, a trademark for a placenta hormone (human chorionic gonadotropin).

fomentation, 1. a treatment for pain or swelling with a warm, moist application to the skin. 2. a substance that is used as a warm, moist application.

fomite, nonliving material, as bed linens, which may carry disease organisms.

Fone's method, a toothbrushing technique that uses big sweeping scrubbing circles over teeth, with the toothbrush held at right angles to the tooth surfaces.

fontanel /fon′tənel′/, a space between the bones of an infant's skull covered by tough membranes. The front fontanel, roughly diamond-shaped, remains soft until about 2 years of age. The back fontanel, triangular in shape, closes about 2 months after birth. Increased brain pressure may cause a fontanel to become tense or bulge. A fontanel may be soft and sunken if the infant is dehydrated. Also spelled **fontanelle.**

food, 1. any substance, usually of plant or animal origin, made up of carbohydrates, proteins, fats, and minerals and vitamins. It is swallowed or injected into the body and used to provide energy and to cause growth, repair, and good health. 2. nourishment in solid form, not liquid form.

food additives, substances that are added to foods to prevent spoiling, improve appearance, enhance the flavor, or increase the nutritional value. Most food additives must be approved by the FDA (Federal Drug Administration) after tests to determine if they could be a cause of cancer, birth defects, or other health problems. Examples include BHA (Butylated hydroxyanisole) and BHT (butylated hydroxytoluene), which are added to fats to slow spoiling.

food allergy, an allergic state resulting from a specific food substance. Symptoms of allergies to specific foods can include runny nose, bronchial asthma, hives, swelling, itching, head-ache, nausea, vomiting, diarrhea, stomach pains, constipation, and skin rashes. Allergic substances in foods are mostly proteins. The most common foods causing allergic reactions are wheat, milk, eggs, fish and other seafoods, chocolate, corn, nuts, and strawberries.

Food and Drug Administration (F.D.A.), a federal agency responsible for carrying out laws covering food, drugs, and cosmetics, as protection against the sale of unsafe or dangerous substances.

food contaminants, substances that make food unfit for humans to eat. Examples include bacteria, poisons, cancer-causing agents, substances causing birth defects, and radioactive materials. Also regarded as contaminants are basically harmless substances, as water, that may be added to food to increase its weight.

food-exchange list, a grouping of foods in which the carbohydrate, fat, and protein values are equal for the items listed. The list is used for meal planning in many diseases. The six groups of foods included on the list are milk, vegetables, fruits, bread, meat, and fats. Starchy vegetables are listed as bread exchanges; fish and cheese are meat exchanges.

food poisoning, a condition resulting from eating food infected by poisons or by bacteria containing toxins. Kinds of food poisoning include **bacterial food poisoning, ciguatera poisoning, Minamato disease, mushroom poisoning, shellfish poisoning.** See also **botulism, ergot alkaloid, phalloidine poisoning, toadstool poisoning.**

foot, the farthest part of the leg.

foot-and-mouth disease, a virus infection of animals, carried to humans by contact with infected animals or infected milk. Symptoms include headache, fever, and mouth and tongue blisters. The blisters go away in about 1 week, and total healing without scars is complete by 2 or 3 weeks. See also **picornavirus.**

footboard, a broad or open box placed at the foot of a patient's bed with its top above the mattress to prevent the weight of the top sheet and blankets from resting on the feet. The bottoms of the feet are positioned firmly against the board. This helps the bedfast patient retain normal posture and prevent footdrop. See illustration on p. 326.

footdrop, an inability to flex the foot backward. It is caused by damage to a leg (peroneal) nerve. Also called **dropped foot.**

footling breech, a position of the fetus in the uterus in which one or both feet are folded under the buttocks. One folded foot coming out is a single footling breech; both feet, a double footling breech. Compare **frank breech.** See also **breech birth.**

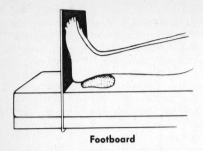

Footboard

foot-pound, a unit for measuring work or energy. One foot-pound is the amount of work needed to move 1 pound a distance of 1 foot.

foramen /fôrā'mən/, *pl.* **foramina,** an opening (aperture) in a membrane or bone.

foramen magnum, a passage in the skull (occipital) bone through which the spinal cord enters the spinal column.

foramen ovale, an opening in the wall between the right and the left chambers (atria) in the fetal heart. This opening provides a bypass for blood that would otherwise flow to the fetal lungs. The foramen ovale begins to close after the newborn takes the first breath and full circulation through the lungs begins. See also **ductus arteriosus.**

Forbes-Albright syndrome, a hormone disease marked by lack of menstruation (amenorrhea), and breast milk abnormalities. It is caused by a tumor of the front pituitary gland. See also **galactorrhea, pituitary gland.**

Forbes' disease. See **Cori's disease.**

force, energy applied so that it begins motion, changes the speed or direction of motion, or changes the size or shape of an object.

forced expiratory flow (FEF), the average flow of air measured while a person forces out as much air as possible after a deep breath.

forced expiratory volume (FEV), the volume of air that can be forced out in 1 second after taking a deep breath. Compare **vital capacity.**

forceed expired vital capacity (FEVC), the largest volume of air that can be forced out rapidly after taking a deep breath. Also called **time vital capacity.**

forced feeding, the giving of food by force, as nasal feeding, to persons who cannot or will not eat.

forced-inhalation abdominal breathing, a breathing therapy in which the patient is trained to breathe in through the nose forcefully enough to lift small weights placed on the stomach. It resembles the abdominal effort involved in normal breathing.

forceps, any of a large number of surgery instruments, all of which have two handles or sides, each attached to a blade. Forceps are used to grasp, handle, press, pull, or join tissue, equipment, or supplies. See specific forceps.

forceps delivery, a childbirth operation in which forceps are used to deliver a baby. It is done to help a difficult childbirth, to quickly deliver a baby with breathing problems, or, most often, to shorten normal labor. The blades of the forceps are put into the vagina one at a time and applied to opposite sides of the baby's head. The handles of the forceps are brought together so that the head is held firmly between the blades. The head is rotated, if necessary, and traction is carefully applied to draw the head from the birth passage. When the head has been delivered the forceps are removed and the delivery is completed by hand.

forceps rotation, a childbirth operation in which forceps are used to turn a baby's head in the birth canal. It may be done to help emergency birth or as the first step in a forceps delivery. Kinds of forceps rotation are **Kielland rotation, Scanzoni rotation.**

Fordyce's disease, the presence of enlarged oil glands in the linings of the lips, cheeks, gums, and genital areas. It is a common condition and may have no symptoms. Tiny, whitish-yellow raised spots (Fordyce spots) may appear on the inside of the cheek or gums.

fore-, a combining form meaning 'front or before.'

forearm, the part of the arm between the elbow and wrist. It contains two long bones, the radius and ulna.

forebrain. See **prosencephalon.**

forefinger, the first, or index, finger.

forefoot, the part of the foot that includes the bones in the middle of the foot (metatarsus) and the toes.

foreign body, any object or substance found in the body in an organ or tissue in which it does not belong.

foreign body obstruction, a disturbance caused by an object stuck in a body opening, passage, or organ. Most cases occur in children who breathe in or swallow a foreign object or put it in a body opening. In adults, large pieces of hastily eaten food often stick in the throat (esophagus), causing coughing, choking, and, if the airway is blocked, suffocation. Forceful blows to the victim's back between the shoulder blades or using the Heimlich maneuver may loosen the food. Foreign bodies in the upper throat usually cause hoarseness, wheezing, and breathlessness. A foreign body in the lower throat (trachea) may cause wheezing, a slap that can be heard, coughing, and breathing difficulty. Objects that children sometimes put in their nostrils may cause blockage, mild discomfort, or infection. Needles and hairpins swallowed by children often pass through the throat and stomach without causing problems but may become stuck at the turn of the small intestine and need to be removed by a magnet or by surgery.

foreign medical graduate (FMG), a physician trained in and graduated from a medical school outside the United States and Canada. United States citizens graduated from medical schools outside the United States and Canada are also called FMGs.

forensic medicine, a branch of medicine that deals with the legal side of health care.

forensic psychiatry, the branch of psychiatry that deals with legal issues and problems relating to mental disorders, especially that of insanity for legal purposes.

foreplay, sexual activites, as kissing and fondling, that precede sexual intercourse.

foreshortened image, an x-ray image that is smaller than the object itself. It is caused by tilting the object or lining up the x-ray tube incorrectly.

foreskin, a loose fold of skin that covers the end of the penis or clitoris. Removing it is called circumcision. Also called **prepuce.**

forest yaws, a form of American leishmaniasis, common in South and Central America. The disease is long-term, with many deep skin ulcers that sometimes spread to the nasal mucous membranes.

forewaters, the amniotic fluid between the fetus and the fetal membranes.

formaldehyde /fərmal′dəhīd/, a poisonous, colorless, foul-smelling gas that can be dissolved in water and used in that form to preserve things.

formation, a group of people that occupies and therefore defines an amount of space.

formative evaluation, judgments made about effectiveness of nursing care as it is performed.

forme fruste /fôrm′frYst′, fôrm′frŌŌst′/, **1.** an incomplete or unusual form of a disease or a disease that stops before it has run its usual course. **2.** (in genetics) a disorder that runs in families in which there is little sign of an abnormal characteristic.

formiminoglutamic acid (FIGLU) a substance formed in the urine when there is a lack of folic acid.

-formin, a combining form for phenformin-type drugs taken by mouth to decrease the amount of sugar in the blood.

formula, a simple statement, generally using numbers and other symbols, showing the contents of a chemical compound, or a method for preparing a substance.

formulary, a list of drugs. Hospitals keep formularies that list all drugs commonly stocked in the hospital pharmacy.

fornication, sexual intercourse between two people who are not married to each other. The specific legal definition varies from one area to another. In some, both persons are unmarried;

in others, one is unmarried. Sometimes the charge is adultery rather than fornication if the woman is married, regardless of whether the man is married.

Fort Bragg fever. See **pretibial fever.**

fortified milk, pasteurized milk with one or more nutrients, usually vitamin D, which has been standardized at 400 International Units per quart. Also called **fortified vitamin D milk.**

forward-leaning posture, a therapy to reduce or eliminate extra muscle activity in patients not confined to bed but with breathing difficulty. It involves walking in a slightly stooped, forward-leaning posture. For patinets who cannot walk alone, a special high walker with wheels is used.

fossa /fos′ə/, *pl.* **fossae,** a hollow or pouch, especially on the surface of the end of a bone.

Foster bed, a special bed used in the care and treatment of severely injured patients, especially those with spinal injuries. It permits horizontal turning of the patient without moving the spine. The patient can be rotated to lie in face upward or face downward positions while keeping properly rigid and keeping the injured body structures in line.

foundation, any device or material added to a remaining tooth structure to increase the stability of an overlying dental device.

fourchette /fŌŌrshet′/, a band of mucous membranes of the vagina connecting with the labia minora.

four-poster cast, a cast to keep in place the vertebrae of the neck. It contains four upright poles or posts beside the head in front and back and is placed over the shoulders. It supports the head under the chin and the back of the head. The posts prevent movement.

four-tailed bandage, a narrow piece of cloth with two ties on each end for wrapping a joint, as an elbow or knee, or a structure that sticks out, as the nose or chin.

fourth cranial nerve. See **trochlear nerve.**

fourth ventricle, a diamond-shaped hollow space of the farthest back part of the brain (hindbrain).

fovea centralis /fō′vē·ə/, an area at the center of the retina where the cells that see color (cones) are concentrated and there are no cells that detect dim light (rods).

Fowler's position, the posture taken by the patient when the head of the bed is raised 18 or 20 inches and the patient's knees are raised.

fractional anesthesia. See **continuous anesthesia.**

fractional dilatation and curettage, a technique in which each section of the uterus is examined and scraped to get samples from all parts of the uterus. It is often done using regional anesthesia in the diagnosis of cancer of the uterus.

fractionation, the giving of a dose of radiation in smaller units over a period of time rather than in a single large dose to reduce tissue damage.

fracture, an injury to a bone in which the tissue of the bone is broken. A fracture is named by the bone involved, the part of that bone, and the nature of the break.

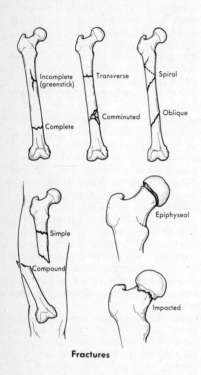

Incomplete (greenstick) — Transverse — Spiral — Comminuted — Oblique — Complete — Simple — Epiphyseal — Compound — Impacted

Fractures

fracture-dislocation, a broken bone involving the bony structures of any joint, with dislocation of the same joint.

fragilitas ossium. See **osteogenesis imperfecta.**

fragmented fracture, a broken bone that results in many bone pieces.

frambesia. See **yaws.**

franchise dentistry, the practice of dentistry under a trade name, which has been bought from another dentist or dental practice.

Frank biopsy guide, a long needle containing a hooked wire used to get samples of breast tissue for examination. The needle is inserted into the breast until its tip nearly touches abnormal tissue seen on a mammogram. The needle is withdrawn but the hooked wire remains to mark the tissue site. The surgeon cuts along the wire or otherwise approaches the hooked end of the wire and removes the tissue. See also **Kopans needle.**

frank breech, a position of the fetus in which the buttocks are at the mother's pelvic opening. The legs are straight up in front of the body,

and the feet are at the shoulders. Babies born in this position tend to hold their feet near their heads for some days after birth. Compare **complete breech, footling breech.** See also **breech birth.**

fraternal twins. See **dizygotic twins.**

freckle, a brown or tan spot on the skin usually resulting from exposure to sunlight. There is an inherited tendency to getting freckles, often seen in persons with red hair. Freckles are harmless in themselves, but people who freckle easily should avoid excess sun exposure or use protective sunscreen lotions. These individuals have a tendency to develop more serious skin changes. Compare **lentigo.**

free association, **1.** the automatic, unrestricted association of ideas, feelings, or mental images. **2.** automatic speaking of thoughts and emotions that enter the consciousness during psychoanalysis.

freebasing, a process used to increase the effect of cocaine. The resulting product is smoked.

free clinic, a clinic or health program, usually located in a neighborhood, that provides health care for walk-in patients at little or no cost.

free-floating anxiety, a general, continuous, strong fear that is not caused by any specific object, event, or source. See also **anxiety, anxiety neurosis.**

free-form foot orthosis, a brace or splint that is molded directly to a patient's foot. It requires less time and material to produce but is not as exact as other types.

free gingiva, the unattached portion of the gum that surrounds a tooth.

free nerve ending, a nerve ending that responds to specific kinds of actions (receptor) and is not enclosed in a capsule. A typical free nerve ending consists of a bare fiber (axon) that may or may not be covered by a fatty layer. It is often found in fiberlike capsules, ligaments, or synovial spaces and may react to mechanical or biochemical stimuli.

free radical, an unstable compound that reacts quickly with other molecules.

free thyroxine, the amount of the unbound thyroid hormone, thyroxine (T_4), circulating in the blood.

freeway space, the distance or separation between the facing surfaces of the upper and lower teeth when the lower jaw is in its rest position.

Freiberg's infarction, an abnormal condition characterized by breakdown of bone tissue. It most commonly affects bones of the foot.

Frei test /frī/, a test for a type of cancer (lymphogranuloma venereum).

Frejka splint /frā′kə/, a device made up of a pillow that is belted between the legs of a baby born with dislocated hips. See also **congenital dysplasia of the hips.**

fremitus /frem′itəs/, a trembling movement of the chest wall that can be heard or felt by an examining physician.

Frenkel exercises, a system of slow, repeating exercises of increasing difficulty developed by a Swiss neurologist to treat movement disorders in multiple sclerosis and similar diseases.

frenotomy /frenot′əmē/, a surgery for repairing a defective band of tissue, as the cutting or lengthening of a tongue ligament (lingual frenum) to correct tongue-tie (ankyloglossia).

frenulum linguae. See **lingual frenum.**

frenum /frē′nəm/, *pl.* **frenums, frena,** a restraining portion or structure. Also called **frenulum.**

frequency, the number of repetitions of anything within a fixed period of time, as the number of heart beats per minute.

Freudian /froi′dē·ən/, referring to Sigmund Freud (1856–1939), his psychology ideas, and rules. These ideas stress the early years of childhood as the basis for later neurotic disorders.

friction, 1. the act of rubbing one object against another. See also **attrition.** 2. a type of massage in which deeper tissues are stroked or rubbed, usually through strong circular movements of the hand. See also **massage.**

friction burn, tissue injury caused by rubbing the skin. See also **abrasion.**

friction rub, a dry, grating sound heard with a stethoscope during a medical examination. It is normal when heard over the liver and spleen. A friction rub heard over the heart sac suggests there may be swelling of the sac that surrounds the heart; a pleural friction rub over the lungs may be present in heart or lung disease.

Friedländer's bacillus /frēd′lendərz/, a bacterium linked to infection of the lungs, especially lobar pneumonia.

Friedlander's disease, a severe inflammation of the arteries. There may be swelling of the lining of the blood vessels, and the tissue cells that make up the blood vessel may grow larger. This causes obstruction of the arteries. See also **arteritis obliterans.**

Friedreich's ataxia /frēd′rīshs/, muscle weakness, loss of muscle control, weakness of the legs, and an abnormal walk. Friedreich's ataxia may be hereditary. The main feature of the disease is a breakdown of the spinal cord with possible involvement of brain nerve tracts. Friedreich's ataxia usually affects people between 5 and 20 years of age. It begins most often at puberty. Eventually, a child affected by Friedreich's ataxia may have difficulty doing simple things, as writing or handling silverware while eating. The characteristic walk of this disease is caused by a clawfoot. The walk and the posture of the affected individual are unsteady. The condition may also cause slurred speech, head trembling, and heart disorders all the signs and symptoms may increase in severity.

Friedman's test, a pregnancy test. A sample of urine from a woman is injected into a mature, unmated female rabbit. If, 2 days later, the rabbit ovaries show signs of ovulation, the test shows that the woman is pregnant.

Fried's rule, a method of estimating the dose of medication for a child by multiplying the adult dose by the child's age in months and dividing the result by 150. See also **Clark's rule, Cowling's rule.**

frigid, 1. lacking warmth of feeling, emotions, or imagination; without passion or strong feeling and stiff or formal in manner. 2. a woman who has no response to sexual advances or stimulation, or not able to have an orgasm during sexual intercourse. Compare **impotence.** See also **orgasm.** –**frigidity,** *n.*

Fröhlich's syndrome. See **adiposogenital dystrophy.**

frôlement /frôlmäN′/, 1. the rustling type of sound often heard in the chest in diseases of the heart sac (pericardium). 2. a kind of massage that uses a light brushing stroke with the hand. See also **massage.**

frontal bone, one of the bones that make up the front of the skull, located in the area of the forehead.

frontal lobe, the largest of the lobes of the brain. The frontal lobe influences personality and is linked to the higher mental activities, as planning and judgment. Compare **central lobe, occipital lobe, parietal lobe, temporal lobe.**

frontal lobe syndrome, behavior and personality changes seen following a cancer or injury of the frontal lobe of the brain. The patient may act freely, show off, and burst into a rage or become irritable. In other cases the person may become depressed, apathetic, lacking in energy, and not care about personal appearance.

frontal sinus, one of a pair of small openings (cavities) in the frontal bone of the skull. It connects to the nasal cavity. The frontal sinuses are lacking at birth, well developed between the seventh and eighth years, and reach their full size after puberty. Compare **ethmoidal air cell, maxillary sinus, sphenoidal sinus.**

frontal vein, one of a pair of surface veins of the face.

frontocortical aphasia. See **motor aphasia.**

frostbite, the effect of extreme cold on skin and other tissues. It is first noticed by the paleness of exposed skin surfaces, particularly the nose, ears, fingers, and toes. Narrowing and damage to blood vessels stops local circulation and results in oxygen starvation and tissue death. Gentle warming is first aid treatment; rubbing the affected part is avoided. Later, treatment is similar to treatment of thermal burns. Compare **chilblain, immersion foot.**

frostnip. See **frostbite.**

frottage /frôtäzh′/, sexual pleasure gotten by rubbing against the clothing of another person, as can occur in a crowd.

frotteur /frôtœr′/, a person who gets sexual pleasure from rubbing against the clothing of another person (frottage).

frozen section method, a method used in getting a tissue sample ready for a laboratory examination. The tissue is wetted down, quick-frozen, and cut into thin slices. This method is very rapid, allowing the physician to examine the sample during surgery.

fructose /fruk′tōs, frōōk-/, a form of sugar that is sweeter than sucrose. It is found in honey, several fruits, and combined in many carbohydrates. It is used as a food given in the veins. If insulin is lacking it is used up or changed in the body to glycogen. Also called **fruit sugar, levulose.**

fructosuria /frōōk′tōsōōr′ē·ə/, having the sugar fructose in the urine. This usually harmless condition is caused by the hereditary lack of the enzyme fructokinase, which normally helps break down fructose. One form of fructosuria is linked to symptoms of diabetes. Also called **levulosuria.**

fruit sugar. See **fructose.**

frustration, a feeling that results from an inability to reach one's desired goal or satisfaction.

FSH, abbreviation for **follicle stimulating hormone.**

FUDR, a trademark for an antivirus and anticancer drug (floxuridine).

fugue /fyōōg/, a mental condition marked by lack of memory (amnesia) and physical flight from an undesired situation. The person appears normal and acts as though aware of very complex activities and behavior. After it happens, the person cannot remember the actions or behavior. The condition may last for only a few days or weeks. It also may continue for several years, during which the person wanders away from home and job, gets a new job, and starts an entirely different way of life. See also **ambulatory automatism, automatism.**

fulcrum /fōōl′krəm, ful′-/, the stable point or the position on which a lever, as bones of the elbow joint, turns in moving an object. Many common movements of the body, as raising the arm and walking, are lever actions using fulcrums. The muscles provide the forces that move the bones acting as levers.

full bath, a bath in which the patient's body is placed in water up to the neck.

full diet. See **regular diet.**

full-liquid diet, a diet made up only of liquids and foods that turn to liquid at body temperature. It includes milk, milk drinks, carbonated beverages, coffee, tea, strained fruit juices, broth, strained cream soup, raw eggs, cream, infant cereals in milk, thin custards, gelatin desserts, and ice cream. The diet is given following surgery, in some infections, in some stomach disorders, and for patients too ill to chew. See also **liquid diet.**

full-lung tomography, an x-ray technique that scans both lungs to detect any hidden cancer tumors that have spread from another tumor in the body. Such tumors are hard to detect on a regular x-ray film.

fulminant hepatitis, a rare form of liver disease (hepatitis) that frequently results in death. There is a rapid worsening of the patient's condition, with brain damage, liver damage, blood-clotting disorders, kidney failure, and coma. The expected outcome for adults is generally unfavorable.

fulminating /ful′mināting/, rapid, sudden, severe, as an infection, fever, or bleeding.

Fulvicin, a trademark for an antifungus drug (griseofulvin).

fumagillin, fumigacin. See **helvolic acid.**

function, an act, process, or series of processes that serve a purpose.

functional analysis, (in psychiatry) a type of therapy that traces the sequence of events involved in producing and maintaining undesirable behavior.

functional antagonism, (in pharmacology) a situation in which two drugs produce effects that are opposite to each other.

functional bowel syndrome, See **irritable bowel syndrome.**

functional contracture. See **hypertonic contracture.**

functional disease, 1. a disease that affects function or performance rather than body tissue. 2. a condition marked by signs or symptoms of a physical disease or disorder although careful examination fails to show any sign of physical problems. The symptoms of a functional disorder are as real as those of a physical disease. Headache, lack of sexual function (impotence), certain heart problems, and constipation may be symptoms of functional disease.

functional dyspepsia, an abnormal condition marked by faulty digestion caused by a smooth muscle or nervous system problem. See also **dyspepsia.**

functional impotence. See **impotence.**

functional overlay, an emotional response to a disease. It may occur as an overreaction to an illness and is marked by symptoms that continue long after physical signs of the disease have ended.

functional progression, a sequence of rehabilitation for a musculoskeletal or similar injury. The program usually progresses from no movement while initial healing takes place, to moving the limb without resistance, to movement with resistance to increase strength and endurance.

functional psychosis, an emotional disorder with personality changes and the loss of ability to function in reality. However, there is no sign that the disorder is related to brain functions.

functional residual capacity, the amount of air still in the lungs at the end of normal breathing out.

fundal height, the height of the bottom (fundus) of the uterus. It is measured in centimeters from the top of the pubic bone joint (symphysis pubis) to the top of the uterus. Fundal height is measured at each before birth visit with calipers or with a tape measure. From the twentieth to the thirty-second weeks of pregnancy, the height in centimeters is equal to the pregnancy in weeks. Two measurements 2 weeks apart showing a variation from normal of more than 2 cm may mean that the fetus is large or small for dates or that the woman has a multiple pregnancy.

fundus /fun'dəs/, *pl.* **fundi** /fun'dī/, the base or the deepest part of an organ; the part farthest from the mouth of an organ, as the fundus of the uterus or the fundus of an eye.

funduscopy /fundus'kəpē/, the examination of the base (fundus) of the eye by means of an ophthalmoscope. **–fundoscopic, funduscopic,** *adj.*

fungal infection, any inflammation caused by a fungus. Most fungal infections are mild, but hard to get rid of. Some, particularly in older, weakened people, may become life-threatening. Some kinds of fungal infections are **aspergillosis, blastomycosis, candidiasis, coccidioidomycosis, histoplasmosis.**

fungemia /funjē'mē·ə/, having fungi in the blood. Compare **bacteremia, parasitemia, viremia.**

fungicide /fun'jisīd/, a drug that kills fungi. See also **antifungal,** def. 2. **–fungicidal,** *adj.*

fungiform papilla. See **papilla.**

-fungin, a combining form for antibiotics to treat infections caused by fungi.

fungistatic, having the effect of stopping the growth of fungi.

Fungizone, a trademark for an antifungus drug (amphotericin B).

fungus /fung'gəs/, *pl.* **fungi** /fun'jī/, a simple parasitic plant that lacks chlorophyll. It is unable to make its own food and depends on other life forms. A simple fungus reproduces by budding; many-celled fungi reproduce by making spores. Of the 100,000 known species of fungi, about 10 cause diseases in humans. See also **fungal infection. –fungal, fungous,** *adj.*

funic souffle /fyōo'nik sōo'fəl/, a soft blowing sound produced by blood rushing through the umbilical vessels in time with the sound of the fetal heart.

funiculitis /fənik'yōolī'tis/, any inflammation of a cordlike structure of the body, as the spinal cord or spermatic cord.

funiculus /fənik'yələs/, a division of the white matter of the spinal cord.

funiculus umbilicalis. See **umbilical cord.**

funis /fyōo'nis, fōo'nis/, a cordlike structure, as the umbilical cord.

funnel chest, a deformity of the chest marked by a breastbone that appears to be pushed in. It may not affect breathing, but surgery is often done for the sake of appearance. See also **pectus excavatum.**

funnel feeding, a technique in which liquids may be given by mouth to a patient who cannot move the lips or chew. A rubber tube hooked to a funnel is placed in the mouth, usually at one corner, and a liquid is poured slowly through the funnel and tube into the mouth near the back of the tongue. If the method is used for a weak or young infant, a rubber bulb or a large syringe may be used instead of a funnel. The bulb or syringe is pressed gently, slowly, and continuously to control the rate of flow and prevent choking.

funny bone, a popular name for the point at the elbow where the ulnar nerve is near the surface, causing tingling when the point is bumped.

Furacin, a trademark for a skin medication (nitrofurazone).

Furadantin, a trademark for an antibiotic (nitrofurantoin).

furcation, the part of a tooth where the roots divide.

furosemide /fyərō'səmid/, a fluid releasing drug given to treat high blood pressure, kidney failure, and fluid pooling.

Furoxone, a trademark for an anti-infection and antiprotozoa drug (furazolidone).

furrier's lung, a form of allergy that affects persons who work in the fur industry and are exposed to hair and dander of animal pelts.

furrow, a groove, as the one that separates the atria from the ventricles of the heart (atrioventricular furrow).

furuncle /fyōor'ungkəl/, a pus-making skin infection in a gland or hair gland (follicle). It is marked by pain, redness, and swelling. Tissue death in the center of the swollen area forms a core of matter that will be released, reabsorbed, or surgically removed. To prevent spread of infection it is important to avoid irritating or squeezing the sore. Treatment may include antibiotics, local moist heat, and, cutting and draining. Also called **boil. –furunculous,** *adj.*

furunculosis /fyōorung'kyōolō'sis/, a serious skin disease marked by boils or successive crops of boils.

fusiform, a structure that is tapered at both ends.

fusiform aneurysm, a ballooning of an artery in which the entire vessel is swollen. It creates a long tubelike or spindlelike swelling. Also called **Richet's aneurysm.** Compare **saccular aneurysm.**

fusimotor /fyo͞ozimō'tər/, referring to the motor nerve fibers that serve the muscle spindle.

fusion, 1. bringing together into a single thing, as in optical fusion. 2. the act of bringing together two or more bones of a joint. 3. the surgical joining together of two or more backbones.

fusion-exclusion, a mechanism by which two people can stay in close contact with each other and avoid anxiety either by excluding a third person or by focussing their energies on a third person.

fusospirochetal disease /fyo͞ozōspī'rōkē'təl/, any infection marked by seeping sores in which two kinds of bacteria, a fusiform bacillus and a spirochete, are found. Examples are trench mouth or Vincent's angina.

-fylline, a combining form for a type of drug that relaxes the air passages to improve breathing (theophylline).

F wave, a wave form recorded in nerve-conduction tests. It appears when a motor nerve is stimulated. The F wave is used in studies of motor-nerve function in the arms and legs.

G

GABA, abbreviation for **gamma-aminobutyric acid.**

GABHS, See **group A beta-hemolytic streptococcal skin disease.**

gag reflex, a normal reflex triggered by touching the soft palate or back of the throat. The response raises the palate, retracts the tongue, and contracts the throat muscles.

gait, the manner or style of walking, including rhythm and speed.

gait determinant, factor that controls the process of walking. Pelvic movements, knee and hip flexion, and knee and ankle interaction are determinants of gait.

gait disorder, an abnormality in walking, usually from arthritis, muscle disorders, or other body changes. The center of gravity may shift over the years, causing a change in how much the knee bends to keep balanced. Some muscle disorders may result in shuffling or lurching. Some gait disorders are due to medication that causes confusion or loss of coordination or an eye or ear disturbance that affects the sense of balance.

-galactia, a combining form referring to secretion of milk.

galactocele, a fluid-filled sac caused by blockage of a milk duct in the breast.

galactokinase deficiency, an inherited disorder of carbohydrate processing. Dietary galactose is not used; therefore it builds up in the blood and may cause cataracts. Food containing galactose, as milk and certain milk products, must be removed from the diet. Compare **lactase deficiency.**

galactophorous duct, a passage for milk in the lobes of the breast.

galactorrhea /gəlak'tərē'ə/, milk flow not related to childbirth or nursing. The condition may be a symptom of a pituitary gland tumor. See also **Forbes-Albright syndrome.**

galactose /gəlak'tōs/, a simple sugar found in lactose (milk sugar), nerve cell layers, sugar beets, gums, and seaweed.

galactosemia /gəlak'tōsē'mē·ə/, an inherited, disease of galactose processing, it is characterized by a lack of an enzyme. Shortly after birth, an intolerance to milk is evident. Liver and spleen enlargement, cataracts, and mental retardation develop. Because the removal of galactose from the diet ends all symptoms except mental retardation, early diagnosis and prompt therapy are required. Compare **diabetes mellitus, glycogen storage disease.** See also **galactose, inborn error of metabolism.**

galactosuria, the presence of a sugar (galactose) in the urine.

galactosyl ceramide lipidosis, an inherited disease of lipid processing, present at birth. Infants become paralyzed, blind, deaf, and increasingly retarded, and eventually die of paralysis. There is no known treatment for the disease, but it can be detected by a prenatal test (amniocentesis).

Galant reflex /gəlant'/, a normal response in the newborn to move the hips toward the side that is touched when the back is stroked along the spinal cord. The reflex disappears by about 4 weeks of age. Lack of the reflex may indicate spinal cord defect. Also called **trunk incurvation reflex.**

galea aponeurotica. See **epicranial aponeurosis.**

Galeazzi's fracture /gal'ē·at'sēz/, a fracture of the lower arm with a separation of the joint between the lower arm bones. Also called **Dupuytren's fracture.**

Galen's bandage /gā'lənz/, a bandage for the head, made up of a strip of cloth with each end divided into 3 pieces. The center of the cloth is placed on top of the head; the 2 strips in front are joined at the back of the neck; the 2 strips at the back are pulled up and fastened on the forehead; the middle strips are fastened under the chin.

gall. See **bile.**

gallbladder, a pear-shaped sac near the right lobe of the liver which holds bile. About 8 cm long and 2.5 cm wide at its thickest part, it holds about 32 cc^3 of bile. During digestion of fats, it contracts, sending bile into the first portion of the small intestine (duodenum). Blocking of the bile-carrying system may lead to liver disease (jaundice) and pain. It is a common condition in overweight, middle-aged women and may require removal.

gallbladder cancer, a cancer of the bile storage sac. Symptoms include loss of appetite, nausea, vomiting, weight loss, and severe pain near the right shoulder. Tumors of the gallbladder are often connected with gallstones. They are 3 to 4 times more common in women than in men and rarely occur before the age of 40. Physical examination shows an enlarged gallbladder in about half the cases. Complete removal of the gallbladder may cure the cancer, but partial removal of the liver also may be required.

gallstone. See **biliary calculus.**

galvanic cautery, galvanocautery. See **electrocautery.**

galvanic electric stimulation, the use of a high-voltage electric stimulator to treat muscle spasms, swelling after an injury, muscle pain, and certain other disorders. See also **transcutaneous electric nerve stimulation.**

galvanometer, a device that indicates or measures electrical current, used in certain diagnostic devices, as electrocardiographs.

Gambian trypanosomiasis, a form of African trypanosomiasis, caused by the parasite *Trypanosoma brucei gambiense*. Also called **West African sleeping sickness**. Compare **Rhodesian trypanosomiasis**. See also **African trypanosomiasis**.

gamete /gam'ēt/, 1. a mature male or female germ cell that is able to function in fertilization and that contains the haploid number of chromosomes. 2. the egg (ovum) or sperm (spermatozoon). See also **meiosis**. –**gametic**, *adj.*

gametic chromosome, any of the chromosomes contained in the sperm or egg, as opposed to those in a body cell.

gametogenesis /gam'itōjen'əsis/, the origin and growth of gametes.

gamma-aminobutyric acid (GABA), an amino acid that carries nerve messages. It is found in the brain and also in the heart, lungs, kidneys, and in certain plants.

gamma camera, a device used in nuclear medicine to scan patients who have been injected with small amounts of radioactive materials.

gamma-efferent fiber, any of the motor nerve fibers that carry impulses from the central nervous system to the fibers of the muscles. The gamma efferent fibers are responsible for deep tendon reflexes, spasms, and stiffness.

gamma globulin. See **immune gamma globulin**.

gamma-glutamyl transpeptidase, an enzyme that appears in the blood of patients with several types of liver or gallbladder disorders.

gamma radiation, a very high frequency electromagnetic emission from certain radioactive elements that comes from nuclear decay or from nuclear reactions. Gamma rays are more penetrating than alpha particles and beta radiation. Gamma radiation can injure, distort, or destroy body cells and tissue, especially cell nuclei, but controlled radiation is used to diagnose and treat various diseases. See also **radiation exposure, radiation sickness, radioactive contamination. See also alpha particles, beta rays.**

gammopathy /gamop'əthē/, an abnormal increase of gamma globulin in the blood.

gamo-, gam-, a combining form that refers to marriage or sexual union.

gamogenesis /gam'ōjen'əsis/, sexual reproduction through the joining of gametes.

gamone /gam'ōn/, a chemical substance released by the egg and sperm that is thought to attract the gametes of the opposite sex to facilitate union. Kinds of gamones are **androgamone, gynogamone.**

gampsodactyly. See **pes cavus**.

Gamulin Rh, a trademark for a passive immunizing agent, $Rh_o(D)$, immune human globulin.

ganglion /gang'glē·ən/, *pl.* **ganglia, 1.** a knot, or knotlike mass. **2.** nerve cells, collected in groups outside the central nervous system. The two types of ganglia are the sensory ganglia and the autonomic ganglia.

ganglionar neuroma, a tumor composed of nerve cell bodies and nerve fibers. It is usually found in the stomach area and occurs most often in children. The tumor is treated by chemotherapy or surgery. Also called **ganglionated neuroma, ganglionic neuroma.**

ganglionic blocking agent, a drug used to produce controlled low blood pressure as needed in certain surgical procedures. It also may be used in emergency treatment of high blood pressure. The drugs occupy receptor sites on nerve endings, stopping response of these nerves to the action of nerve impulse transmitter (acetylcholine).

ganglionic crest. See **neural crest**.

ganglionic glioma, a tumor composed of nerve cells that are nearly mature. See also **neuroblastoma.**

ganglionic neuroma. See **ganglionar neuroma**.

ganglionic ridge. See **neural crest**.

ganglionitis, an inflammation of a nerve cell.

ganglioside, a fatty substance found in the brain and other nervous system tissues. Accumulation of gangliosides because of a birth defect results in gangliosidosis or Tay-Sachs disease.

gangliosidosis type I. See **Tay-Sachs disease**.

gangliosidosis type II. See **Sandhoff's disease**.

gangrene, necrosis or death of tissue, usually the result of loss of blood supply or bacterial invasion. The arms and legs are most often affected, but gangrene can occur in the intestines, gallbladder, or other organs. Inside the body, gangrene may be a complication of hernia, appendicitis, gallbladder inflammation or blocking of the arteries to the gut. **Dry gangrene** is a problem of diabetes mellitus that has led to a thickening and hardening of the walls of the arteries (arteriosclerosis) in which the affected leg or arm becomes cold, dry, and shriveled and eventually turns black. **Moist gangrene** may follow a crushing injury or a blocking of blood flow by a clot or air bubble (embolism), tight bandages, or tourniquet. Gangrene can have an offensive odor, spread rapidly, and may result in death in a few days. In all types of gangrene, surgery is necessary to remove the dead tissue. See also **gas gangrene, open amputation.** –**gangrenous**, *adj.*

gangrenous necrosis. See **necrosis**.

gangrenous stomatitis. See **noma**.

ganja. See **cannabis**.

Gantanol, a trademark for an antibiotic (sulfamethoxazole).

Gantrisin, a trademark for an antibiotic (sulfisoxazole).

Ganzfeld effect, a sight field that is patternless, as a whitewashed surface, causing a feeling of blindness.

Garamycin, a trademark for an antibiotic (gentamicin sulfate).

Gardner-Diamond syndrome, a condition marked by large, painful, black-and-blue skin spots that appear without apparent cause but often occur with emotional upsets or abnormalities of protein processing. See also **autoerythrocyte sensitization.**

Gardner's syndrome, Bulges of tissue (polyps) on the large bowel, with fibrous dysplasia of the skull, extra teeth, tumors, and cysts. The condition is inherited.

Gardner-Wells tongs, braces attached to the skull to limit movement of patients with neck injuries. The tongs are used to apply traction to a fracture or dislocation while the patient is in a special bed, as a Stryker frame.

gargle, **1.** to hold and move a liquid at the back of the throat by tilting the head back and forcing air through the liquid. The process cleans or medicates the mouth and throat. **2.** a solution used to rinse the mouth and throat.

gargoylism. See **Hurler's syndrome.**

gas, an airlike fluid with the property of indefinite expansion. A gas has no fixed shape, and its volume is defined by temperature and pressure. Compare **liquid, solid.**

gas distention. See **flatulence.**

gas embolism, a blockage of one or more small blood vessels, especially in the muscles, tendons, and joints. It is caused by expanding bubbles of gases. Gas emboli can tear tissue and blood vessels, causing decompression sickness and death. They affect deep-sea divers who rise too quickly to the surface and are most dangerous in the central nervous system. Such embolisms are very painful. The prevention and treatment of gas embolisms involve slow decompression of gases, especially nitrogen, that are dissolved in the blood. See also **air embolism, decompression sickness, embolism.**

gas gangrene, tissue death accompanied by gas bubbles in soft tissue after surgery or injury. It is caused by anaerobic organisms, Symptoms include pain, swelling, and tenderness of the wound area, mild fever and rapid heart beat. The skin around the wound dies and ruptures, revealing dead muscle tissue. If untreated, gas gangrene is quickly fatal. Also called **anaerobic myositis.**

gasoline poisoning. See **petroleum distillate poisoning.**

gas pains. See **flatulence.**

gas therapy, the use of medical gases in respiratory therapy. Kinds of gas therapy include **carbon dioxide therapy, controlled oxygen therapy, helium therapy,** and **hyperbaric oxygenation.**

gastrectasia, an abnormal stretching of the stomach, sometimes accompanied by pain, vomiting, rapid pulse, and falling body temperature. Causes can include overeating, blocking of the exit valve of the stomach, or a hernia.

gastrectomy, surgical removal of all or, more commonly, part of the stomach. It may be done to remove a long term peptic ulcer, to stop bleeding in a punctured ulcer, or to remove a cancer. Usually, one-half to two-thirds of the stomach is removed, including the ulcer and a large area of acid-releasing mucosa. The remainder of the stomach is then joined to the middle part or the first part of the small intestine (jejunum or duodenum). If a cancer is found, the chest cavity is opened and the entire stomach is removed, along with the membrane that covers the stomach (omentum) and, usually, the spleen. The jejunum is connected to the esophagus. With the return of peristalsis, water is given by mouth. The diet gradually progresses to 6 small, bland meals a day, with 120 ml of fluid hourly between meals. See also **dumping syndrome, gastroenterostomy, G.I. series, nasogastric tube, peptic ulcer.**

gastric, referring to the stomach.

gastric analysis, examination of the contents of the stomach. It is usually done to determine the quantity of acid present and the presence of blood, bile, bacteria, and abnormal cells. A sample of gastric release is obtained via a tube passed through the nose and throat into the stomach. The total absence of hydrochloric acid is a sign of pernicious anemia. Patients with stomach ulcer and stomach cancer may release less acid than normal, while patients with duodenal ulcers release more.

gastric atrophy. See **atrophic gastritis.**

gastric cancer, a cancer of the stomach. It occurs more often in men than in women and peaks in the group 50 to 59 years of age. Symptoms include vague pains in the pit of the stomach (epigastrium), loss of appetite, weight loss, and unexplained iron-deficiency anemia. But many cases show no symptoms in the early stages and an enlarged lymph node may be the first sign of a stomach cancer. Radical subtotal gastrectomy with removal of involved tissues and rebuilding by joining the remainder of the stomach to the middle part of the small intestine (duodenum or jejunum) is usually done.

gastric dyspepsia, pain or discomfort in the stomach. See also **dyspepsia.**

gastric fistula, an abnormal passage into the stomach, usually opening on the outer surface of the abdomen. A gastric fistula may be made surgically to provide tube feeding for patients with severe disease of the esophagus.

gastric glands, glands in the stomach that produce hydrochloric acid and enzymes.

gastric inhibitory polypeptide (GIP), a hormone found in the mucous membrane of the small intestine, it is released when glucose or fatty acids enter the small intestine. The hormone causes the pancreas to release insulin and prevents the release of gastric acid.

gastric intubation, a procedure in which a tube is passed through the nose into the esophagus and stomach. It is used to feed liquids to unconscious patients or to premature or sick newborn infants. Medication can also be given in this manner. Gastric intubation is also performed to remove food from the stomach, to prevent its being sucked into the airways or the lungs, or to remove a poison and wash the stomach. See also **gastric lavage, Levin tube.**

gastric juice, digestive fluids of the gastric glands in the stomach. The acid-base balance (ph) of gastric juice is strongly acid (0.9 to 1.5). Excess release of gastric juice may lead to irritation of the stomach lining and to peptic ulcer. See also **achlorhydria, gastric analysis, gastric ulcer.**

gastric lavage, the washing out of the stomach with sterile water or a salt fluid. This is done before and after surgery to remove irritants and to remove swallowed poisons, or to prepare the stomach to have instruments placed in it. See also **irrigation.**

gastric motility, the movements of the stomach that aid in digestion, moving food through the stomach and into the first section of the small intestine (duodenum). Too much gastric motility causes pain that is usually treated with antispasm drugs. Less than normal motility is common in labor, after general anesthesia, and as a side effect of some sedative hypnotics.

gastric node, a gland linked to an organ in the abdomen or pelvis.

gastric partitioning, an operation in which part of the stomach is closed to make it hold less food. It is used to treat some types of obesity.

gastric ulcer, an erosion of the mucous layer of the stomach. It may pass through the muscle layer and break the stomach wall. The ulcer tends to return with stress and is identified by burning pain, belching, and nausea, especially when the stomach is empty or after eating certain foods. Antacid medication or milk quickly relieves the pain. Treatment includes drugs to lower the acid and spasms of the stomach and to relieve stress. If a break and bleeding occur, surgery may be necessary. Also called **peptic ulcer.**

gastrin /gas'trin/, a hormone, released by the opening to the stomach (pylorus). It causes the flow of gastric juice and causes bile and pancreatic enzyme release.

gastrinoma, a tumor found usually in the pancreas but sometimes in the small intestine. It produces digestive enzymes and often occurs with ulcers.

gastritis /gastrī'tis/, an inflammation of the lining of the stomach which occurs in two forms. **Acute gastritis** may be caused by severe burns, major surgery, aspirin, or other drugs, by food

allergens or by the presence of viral, bacterial, or chemical poisons. The symptoms — loss of appetite, nausea, vomiting, and discomfort after eating — usually go away after the cause has been removed. **Chronic gastritis** is usually a sign of underlying disease, as peptic ulcer, stomach cancer, Zollinger-Ellison syndrome, or pernicious anemia. Compare **peptic ulcer.**

gastrocamera, a small camera that can be lowered into the stomach through the throat to record images of the stomach lining.

gastrocnemius /gas'troknē'mē·əs/, a muscle in the back of the leg.

gastrocnemius gait, abnormal walking linked to a weakness of the gastrocnemius muscle.

gastrocnemius test, a test of the calf muscle (gastrocnemius). While the patient is lying face down, the examiner places fingers on the calf while the patient pulls the heel upward. If the toes curl before the heel moves, the muscle is not working correctly.

gastrocoele. See **archenteron.**

gastrocolic omentum. See **greater omentum.**

gastrocolic reflex, a wavelike movement of the colon that often occurs when food enters the stomach. When an infant is fed, this reflex may cause a bowel movement.

gastrodidymus, twins who are joined at the abdominal region. Also called **omphalodidymus.**

gastrodisciasis /gas'trōdiskī'əsis/, an infection caused by digestive tract parasites. It is common in the hog populations of Southeast Asia and is carried to humans.

gastroenteritis /gas'trō·en'tərī'tis/, inflammation of the stomach and intestines that comes with many diseases. Symptoms are loss of appetite, nausea, vomiting, abdominal pain, and diarrhea. The condition may be caused by bacterial poisons, viral invasion, chemical irritants, or to miscellaneous conditions, as lactose intolerance. The start may be slow, or abrupt and violent, with rapid loss of fluids and nutrients from vomiting and diarrhea. Low blood potassium and low blood sodium, acidosis, or alkalosis may develop. Treatment requires bed rest, sedation, intravenous replacement of nutrients, and antispasm drugs to control vomiting and diarrhea. After the serious phase, water may be given by mouth. If it produces no vomiting or diarrhea, clear fluids may be added and followed, if kept down, by a bland diet.

gastroenterostomy /gas'trō·en'təros'təmē/, surgical forming of an artificial opening between the stomach and the small intestine, usually at the middle part of the small intestine (jejunum). The operation is performed with partial stomach removal, to route food from the remainder of the stomach into the small intestine, or by itself, for perforating ulcer of the duodenum. Compare **gastrectomy.**

gastroesophageal /gas'trō·isof'əjē'əl/, referring to the stomach and the esophagus.

gastroesophageal reflux, a backflow of contents of the stomach into the esophagus. It is often the result of failure of the lower esophageal sphincter. Gastric juices are acid and produce burning pain in the esophagus. Repeated returns of reflux may cause swelling, ulcers, or narrowing of the esophagus. See also **chalasia, esophagitis, heartburn, hiatus hernia.**

gastrogavage. See **gastrostomy feeding.**

gastrohepatic omentum. See **lesser omentum.**

gastrointestinal /gas'trō-intes'tinəl/, referring to the organs of the gastrointestinal tract, from mouth to anus.

gastrointestinal allergy, an allergy to certain foods or drugs. Gastrointestinal allergy differs from food allergy, which can affect organ systems other than the digestive system. Characteristic symptoms include itching and swelling of the mouth and oral passages, nausea, vomiting, diarrhea, abdominal pain, and, if severe, allergic shock. Treatment includes identification and removal of the allergen. In childhood, gastrointestinal allergy is most often caused by cow's milk. See also **lactose intolerance.**

gastrointestinal bleeding, any bleeding from the stomach and intestines. The most common causes are peptic ulcer, diverticulitis, ulcerative colitis, and cancer. Vomiting of bright red blood or of coffee-ground colored and textured vomit indicates upper gastrointestinal bleeding, usually from the esophagus, stomach, or upper small intestine (duodenum). Tarry, black stools signs a bleeding source in the upper gastrointestinal tract; bright red blood from the rectum usually signs bleeding in the lower colon. Gastrointestinal bleeding is treated as a possible emergency. See also **coffee ground vomitus, hematochezia, melena.**

gastrointestinal gas. See **flatulence.**

gastrointestinal infection, any infection of the stomach and intestines by bacteria, viruses, parasites, or poisons. All may have symptoms of nausea, vomiting, diarrhea, and decreased appetite. Treatment usually includes bed rest, easy access to a bathroom, and food and liquids to replace lost fluids.

gastrointestinal obstruction, any blocking of the movement of intestinal contents. It may be caused by blockage or muscle failure. Blockage may be caused by bands of scar fiber that have developed from surgery, hernia, or tumor. Failure of movement may follow anesthesia, abdominal surgery, or the closing of any of the arteries to the gut. Symptoms include vomiting, abdominal pain, and abdominal bloating. Loss of fluids and exhaustion may follow. Bowel sounds are softer than normal or absent. Drugs given for pain can worsen the condition by further slowing the muscle movement of the stomach and intestines.

gastrointestinal system assessment, examination of the patient's digestive system. The patient is asked if there is or has been pain or tenderness in the mouth, gums, tongue, lips, or abdomen, or instances of belching, heartburn, nausea, vomiting, constipation, diarrhea, or painful bowel movements. Information is noted on any changes in eating, bowel habits, the color, character, frequency of stools and urine, the use of laxatives or enemas, the occurrence of hemorrhoids, and swelling of the extremities. The abdomen is examined for swelling, stiffness, rigidity, fluid accumulation, enlarged liver, visible digestive movement, and bowel sounds. The area around the anus is inspected for its general condition, color, odor, or hemorrhoids. The eyes are checked for signs of jaundice, and the skin for signs of itching and swollen blood vessels. The use of tobacco, antacids, laxatives, antidiarrheals, sedatives, tranquilizers, barbiturates, Antibiotics, and aspirin is asked about. The family medical history, especially of stomach and bowel disease, cancer, and diabetes, is an important aspect of the evaluation. Procedures that may be needed for the diagnosis include upper GI, small bowel and gallbladder series, gastric analysis, sigmoidoscopy, abdominal x-rays, and digital rectal examinations.

gastroschisis /gastros'kəsis/, a birth defect identified by incomplete closing of the abdomen wall, which causes the intestines to bulge out. Compare **omphalocele.**

gastroscopy /gastros'kəpē/, the inspection of the inside of the stomach by means of a gastroscope put in through the esophagus. See also **endoscopy, fiberoptics.** **–gastroscopic,** adj.

gastrostomy /gastros'təmē/, surgical creation of an artificial opening into the stomach through the abdominal wall. It may be performed to feed a patient with cancer of the esophagus or one who is expected to be unconscious for a long time. The front wall of the stomach is drawn forward and sewn to the abdominal wall. A tube is then inserted into an opening made in the stomach, and the opening is tightly sewn to prevent leaking of the contents of the stomach. The tube can be clamped shut, or opened to pass liquid food into the stomach.

gastrothoracopagus /gas'trōthôr'əkop'əgəs/, twins that are joined at the chest, stomach and intestines.

gastrula /gas'trŏŏlə/, a term used for a human embryo in an early stage of development.

gatch bed, a bed that has an adjustable joint that allows the knees to bend and supports the legs.

Gaucher's disease /gôshāz'/, a disease of fat processing linked to the lack of an enzyme. It is identified by liver, spleen, lymph node, and bone-marrow disorders. The death rate for this disease is high, but children with the disease who live through their teen years may live for many years. Also called **glucosyl cerebroside lipidosis.**

gauntlet bandage /gônt′lət/, a glovelike bandage that covers the hand and the fingers. See also **demigauntlet bandage.**

gauze, a see-through fabric of open weave that is usually made of cotton. It is used in surgery and for bandages and dressings. Gauze may be sterilized and soaked in an antiseptic or lotion. Kinds of gauze include **absorbable gauze, absorbent gauze, petrolatum gauze.** See also **bandage.**

gavage /gäväzh′/, the process of feeding a patient through a tube.

gavage feeding of the newborn, a method for feeding an infant in which a tube is passed through the nose or mouth into the stomach. It is used to feed a newborn with weak sucking, uncoordinated sucking and swallowing or difficulty breathing. During feeding, the infant is laid back on the mother or father's arm. The feeding tube is filled with formula and fitted with a rubber bulb or plunger (syringe). The syringe is held 6 to 8 inches above the infant's head and the flow is started by pressing on the bulb or plunger. As the formula is slowly given, the baby is stroked and is offered a pacifier to help the formula flow down, to calm the child, and to link the child's sucking and feeding reflexes. If the infant gags, spits, chokes, or vomits, flow of formula is slowed and the feeding may be stopped. To stop air from entering the stomach when the feeding is done, the tube is pinched closed as it is taken out. The infant is burped gently by patting or rubbing the back and then positioned on his or her right side in the crib. To prevent loss of the formula, the child is not moved for at least an hour after feeding.

gay, 1. any person who is homosexual. 2. referring to homosexuality.

gaze, a fixed stare or state of looking in one direction. A person with normal vision has six basic positions of gaze, each controlled by different combinations of eye muscles.

gaze palsy, a condition where the patient cannot move the eyes to all directions of gaze. A gaze palsy is often named for the affected direction of gaze, as a right gaze palsy.

g.c., *informal.* abbreviation for **gonococcus,** the organism that causes gonorrhea.

GDM, abbreviation for **gestational diabetes mellitus.**

Geiger-Müller (GM) counter /gī′gərmil′ər/, an electronic device that shows the level of radioactivity of any substance. It counts the number of electrons sent out by a substance. It cannot identify the type or energy of a particle. Also called **Geiger counter.**

gel, a substance that is firm even though it contains a large amount of liquid. It is used to soothe irritations, to stop oozing or bleeding, or to apply other drugs to an area to be treated.

gelatin film, an absorbable material used to control bleeding during surgery.

gelatiniform carcinoma. See **mucinous carcinoma.**

gelatin sponge, an absorbable material used to control bleeding in surgery and to promote healing of bed sores.

Gellhorn pessary. See **pessary.**

gemellary /jem′əler′ē/, referring to twins.

gemellipara /jem′əlip′ərə/, a woman who has given birth to twins.

gemellus, either of two small muscles connecting the hip and thigh. They turn the thigh outward.

gemellus test, a test of the gemellus muscles. The patient sits with knees bent, the examiner places one hand on the outside of the knee to hold it still, and the patient turns the thigh outward by moving the foot inward.

gemfibrozil, a drug prescribed for excess fats in the blood.

gemin-, a combining form referring to a twin, or double.

gemmation /jemä′shən/, the way a cell reproduces by budding. Also called **gemmulation.**

Gemonil, a trademark for an anticonvulsant drug (metharbital).

-gen, -gene, a combining form meaning 'that which generates.'

Genapax Tampon, a trademark for a tampon treated to fight infection (gentian violet).

gender, the particular sex of a person. See also **sex.**

gender identity, the sense of knowing to which sex one belongs. The process begins in infancy, continues during childhood, and is strengthened during the teen-age years.

gender identity disorder, a condition marked by a long-lasting feeling of discomfort over one's sex. The feeling usually begins in childhood with gender identity problems and may appear during the teen years or adulthood as asexuality, homosexuality, transvestism, or transsexualism.

gene, the physical unit that carries characteristics from parent to child. The gene is thought to be a certain nucleic acid within a DNA molecule that holds a precise area on a chromosome. It also is capable of copying itself. In man and other mammals, genes occur as pairs. They structure and regulate the way body cells and tissues develop. Kinds of genes include **dominant gene, lethal gene, mutant gene, recessive gene, sublethal gene.** See also **chromosome, cistron, DNA, operon.**

general adaptation syndrome (GAS), the defense response of the body or mind to injury or prolonged stress. It begins with a stage of shock or alarm, followed by resistance or adaptation, and ending in either a state of adjustment and healing or of exhaustion and disintegration. Also called **adaptation syndrome.** See also **posttraumatic stress disorder, stress.**

general anesthesia, the total lack of sensation and consciousness as brought on by anesthetic agents. They are usually breathed-in or injected into a vein. The kind of anesthesia used and the dose and route by which it is given depend on the reason for anesthesia. See also **anesthesia, Guedel's signs, local anesthesia, regional anesthesia.**

generalized anaphylaxis, a severe allergic reaction marked by itching, swelling caused by gathering of fluid; wheezing seizures; breathlessness; dilated pupils; a rapid, weak pulse; and falling blood pressure. It may rapidly result in shock and death. Systemic anaphylaxis, the most extreme form of allergy, may be caused by insect stings, food, or certain drugs. Penicillin injected into a vein and iodide dyes used in x-ray tests are frequent causes of anaphylactic shock. The severity of the reaction depends on the amount and route of entrance of the allergen. Generalized anaphylaxis is treated with an immediate injection of epinephrine, and the taking by mouth of an antihistamine, plus a drug to relieve bronchial spasm. See also **reagin-mediated disorder.**

generally recognized as effective (GRAE), a standard that must be met by a drug before it can be approved by the FDA as a 'new drug.' To be recognized as effective, the drug must be considered safe and effective by scientific experts. See also **generally recognized as safe.**

generally recognized as safe (GRAS), a classification by the Food and Drug Administration of food substances, especially colors, flavors, and other food additives, that are considered free of harmful effects when eaten by humans in small amounts.

general paresis, an organic mental disease resulting from long-term syphilitic infection. It is marked by decay of the brain cells; progressive insanity, trembling, and speech disturbances; muscle weakness; and, finally, paralysis. It is often linked to periods of extreme joy and of a false, exaggerated sense of self importance. Treatment requires large doses of penicillin, without which the result is almost always further decay and death. Also called **cerebral tabes, dementia paralytica, paretic dementia, syphilitic meningoencephalitis.**

general practitioner (GP), a family practice doctor. See also **family medicine.**

generation, the act or process of producing young; procreation. The period of time between the birth of one individual or organism and the birth of its offspring.

generative, referring to activity that generates new physical or mental growth.

generic, 1. a substance, product, or drug that is not protected by trademark. 2. referring to the name of a kind of drug that is also the description of the drug, as penicillin or tetracycline.

generic equivalent, a drug sold under its generic name, identical in chemical composition to one or more others sold under a trademark.

generic name, the official name assigned to a drug. A given drug is licensed under its generic name, and all manufacturers of the drug list it by its generic name. However, a drug is usually marketed under a trademark chosen by the manufacturer. See also **chemical name, established name.**

genesis, 1. the origin, generation, or developmental evolution of anything. 2. the act of producing or procreating. **–genetic,** adj.

gene splicing, the process by which a piece of DNA is attached to or inserted in a strand of DNA from another source. For example, DNA material from man and other mammals can be spliced into bacterial organisms.

genetic affinity, relationship by direct descent.

genetically significant dose (GSD), an estimate of radiation received by the genitals of the population in one year. The figure is not intended to suggest possible genetic effects from that level of radiation.

genetic code, information, carried by the DNA molecules, that decides the physical traits of an offspring, as eye color, hair color. The code fixes the pattern of amino acids that build body tissue proteins in a cell. Any error in the code results in a wrong arrangement of the amino acids in the protein, causing a birth defect. See also **anticodon, transcription, translation.**

genetic colonization, the process by which a parasite, as a virus, causes its host to make substances solely for the use of the parasite.

genetic counseling, the providing of information and advice about diseases that can be inherited. Counseling may involve a child already born, a pregnancy, or a decision to end a pregnancy or to be made sterile. Special biochemical or cytogenetic tests may be needed in genetic counseling, because many of the some 2,000 known inherited diseases have like symptoms but totally different methods of inheritance. See also **genetic screening, prenatal diagnosis.** See table on p. 340.

genetic death, the failure of an organism to survive that results from its genetic makeup.

genetic disorder. See **inherited disorder.**

genetic engineering, the process of making new DNA molecules. Enzymes are used to break the DNA molecule into pieces so that genes from another organism can be put into the chromosomes of another species. Through genetic engineering such human proteins as the growth hormone, insulin, and interferon have been produced in bacteria.

genetic equilibrium, the state within a group of like beings at which the number of times gene combinations occur does not change from gen-

Genetic diseases

Disorders of carbohydrate metabolism	Disorders of metal metabolism
Diabetes mellitus	Wilson's disease
Pentosuria	Hemochromatosis
Glycogen storage diseases	
Galactosemia	**Disorders of connective tissue, bone, and muscle**
	Familial periodic paralysis
Disorders of lipid metabolism	Muscular dystrophies
familial lipoprotein deficiency	Mucopolysaccharidoses
Familial lecithin-cholesterol acyl-transferase (L-CAT) deficiency	**Disorders of the hematopoietic system and blood**
Tay-Sachs disease	Sickle cell anemia
Gaucher's disease	Glucose 6-phosphate dehydrogenase deficiency
	Thalassemias
Disorders of protein metabolism	Hereditary spherocytosis
Familial goiter	
Phenylketonuria	**Disorders of exocrine glands**
Albinism	Cystic fibrosis
Alkaptonuria	
Tyrosinosis	
Disorders of purine and pyrimidine metabolism	
Gout	
Lesch-Nyhan syndrome	

eration to generation. The condition regularly occurs in a large group in which mating is random. See also **Hardy-Weinberg equilibrium principle.**

genetic immunity. See **natural immunity.**

genetic isolate, a group of individuals that are genetically separated by geographical, racial, social, cultural, or any other barriers that prevent them from breeding with those outside of the group.

geneticist, one who studies or applies genetics.

genetic map, a chart showing the placement of genes on a chromosome and the distance between them. Also called **linkage map.**

genetic marker, any specific gene that causes easy recognition of a genetic trait. Also called **marker gene.**

genetic population. See **deme.**

genetics, 1. the science that studies the principles and mechanics of heredity, or the means by which traits are passed from parents to offspring. 2. the total genetic makeup of a particular individual, family, group, or condition. See also **Mendel's laws.**

genetic screening, the study of a group for the purpose of finding an inherited disease. Genetic screening helps identify those in certain ethnic groups who have a high incidence of a particular disease, specifically sickle cell anemia in blacks and Tay-Sachs disease in Ashkenazic Jews. See also **genetic counseling.**

Genga's bandage. See **Theden's bandage.**

-genic, a combining form that means 'causing, forming, producing.'

geniculate neuralgia, a severe inflammation of the facial nerve, symptoms are pain, loss of the sense of taste, paralysis of the face, and a de-

crease in saliva and tears. It sometimes follows herpes zoster infection. See also **Ramsay Hunt's syndrome.**

geniohyoideus /jē′nē·ōhī·oi′dē·əs/, one of the muscles, rising from the lower jaw. It acts to draw the hyoid bone and the tongue forward.

genital herpes. See **herpes genitalis, herpes simplex.**

genitalia. See **genitals.**

genital reflex. See **sexual reflex.**

genitals, the reproductive organs. Also called **genitalia.** –**genital,** *adj.*

genital stage, the final period in the growth of sexual emotion. It begins with the teen-age years and continues through the adult years when the outer sex organs are the main source of pleasurable excitement. The important feature of this stage is the desire to build stable and meaningful sexual relations. See also **psychosexual development.**

genitourinary (GU), referring to the sexual and urinary systems of the body, either the organs, their workings, or both. Also called **urogenital.**

genogram, a diagram that shows a family tree over at least three generations.

genome /jē′nōm/, the complete set of genes in the chromosomes of each cell of a particular individual.

genotype /jē′nōtīp′/, 1. the complete set of genes of an organism or group, as determined by the combination and location of the genes on the chromosomes. 2. a group or class of organisms having the same assortment of genes. Compare **phenotype.** –**genotypic,** *adj.*

gentamicin sulfate /jen′təmī′sin/, an antibiotic given to relieve severe infections.

gentian violet /jen′shən/, A drug that attacks bacteria, infection, fungus, and intestinal worms. It is given to treat pinworms, infections of the skin, and infections of the vagina.

genu /jē'nōō/, the knee or any angular structure in the body that is shaped like the flexed knee.

genupectoral position, knee-chest position. To assume the genupectoral position, the person kneels so that the weight of the body is supported by the knees and chest. The belly is raised, the head is turned to one side and the arms are bent so that the upper part of the body can be supported in part by the elbows.

genus /jē'nəs/, *pl.* **genera,** a subdivision of a family of animals or plants. A genus usually is made up of several closely related species. The genus *Homo* has only one species, humans ("Homo sapiens"). See also **family.**

genu valgum, a deformity in which the legs are curved in so that the knees are close together, knocking as the person walks. Also called **knock-knee.**

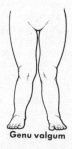
Genu valgum

genu varum, a deformity in which one or both legs are bent out at the knee. Also called **bowleg.** Compare **genu valgum.**

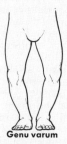
Genu varum

geo-, a combining form meaning the earth, or soil.

Geocillin, a trademark for an antibiotic (carbenicillin indanyl sodium).

geographic tongue, small white or yellowish plaques that develop on the tongue. They gradually get bigger, and shed cells in the center, leaving red patches surrounded by thickened white borders. The patches grow together, forming figures with curved outlines.

The disease may persist for months or years. It causes a burning or itching feeling, made worse by food, and is often linked to stomach and intestine problems, especially in children. Also called **benign migratory glossitis.**

Geopen, a trademark for an antibiotic (carbenicillin disodium).

geotrichosis /jē'ōtrikō'sis/, an abnormal condition, linked with a fungus, *Geotrichum candidum,* which may cause diseases of the mouth, throat, windpipe, and intestines. Geotrichosis most often occurs in people with poor disease resistance and in diabetics. Lung and windpipe problems linked to this disease may produce a cough with thick, bloody spittle. Geotrichosis has been linked to asthmatic reactions similar to allergic aspergillosis and to a type of intestinal disorder with stomach and bowel pain, diarrhea, and bleeding from the rectum. Mouth sores that may occur with this disease are usually treated with a liquid made of gentian violet: Patients having stomach and intestinal sores are given gentian violet capsules by mouth, and those having lung sores are given potassium iodide by mouth.

geriatrics /jer'ē·at'riks/, the branch of medicine dealing with aging and the diagnosis and treatment of diseases affecting the aged.

germ, **1.** any microorganism, especially one that causes disease. **2.** a unit of living matter able to develop into a self-sufficient organism, as a seed, spore, or egg. **3.** a sexual reproductive cell as a sperm or egg.

German measles. See **rubella.**

germ cell, **1.** a sexual reproductive cell in any stage of development, from the primordial embryonic form to the mature gamete. **2.** an egg or sperm or any of their preceding forms. Compare **somatic cell.**

germ disk. See **embryonic disk.**

germicide, a drug that kills disease-causing microorganisms.

germinal infection, an infection given to a child by the egg or sperm of a parent.

germinal stage, the space of time between fertilization and implantation of the zygote. During this stage the egg undergoes cell division several times, travels to the womb, and, as a blastocyst, begins to implant itself in the lining of the womb (endometrium). The germinal stage is over at about 10 days of gestation.

germinal vesicle, the nucleus of a mature oocyte before fertilization. See also **oogenesis, ovum.**

germination, the first growth and development of an organism from the time of fertilization to the forming of the embryo. **–germinate,** *v.*

germ layer, one of the three original cell layers formed during the early stages of embryo development. From these layers, the entire range of body tissue is derived. See also **ectoderm, endoderm, mesoderm.**

germ nucleus. See **pronucleus.**

germ plasm, the material of the germ cells that holds the basic reproductive and hereditary codes; the sum total of the DNA in a particular cell or organism. Compare **somatoplasm.**

-gerontic, -gerontal, a combining form meaning old age.

gerontology, the study of all aspects of aging, including the medical, mental, and other problems met by the elderly, and their effects on both the individual and society.

gerontoxon. See **arcus senilis.**

geropsychiatry, the study and treatment of mental illness in elderly persons.

Gessell Development Assessment, a program that provides information on movement, language, social, and learning development.

Gestalt psychology, a school of psychology that originated in Germany. It holds that a psychological experience is felt as a single whole, rather than as a group of separate elements. Also called **configurationism, Gestaltism.** See also **Gestalt.**

Gestalt therapy, a form of psychotherapy that stresses the unity of self-awareness, behavior, and experience. See also **Gestalt psychlogy.**

gestate, 1. to carry a growing fetus in the womb. 2. to grow and develop slowly toward maturity, as a fetus in the womb.

gestation, the period of time from the fertilization of the egg until birth. Gestation varies with the species; in humans the average length is 266 days or approximately 280 days from the beginning of the last menstrual period. See also **pregnancy.**

gestational age, the age of a fetus or a newborn, usually stated in weeks dating from the first day of the mother's last menstrual period.

gestational diabetes mellitus (GDM), a damaged ability to process carbohydrate that happens during pregnancy, and is usually caused by a lack of insulin. It disappears after delivery but, in some cases, returns years later. There are signs that destruction of insulin by the placenta plays a role in causing gestational diabetes. See also **diabetes mellitus.**

Getman visuomotor theory, a concept that the development of visual perception goes through a series of eight stages in children.

-geusia, -geustia, a combining form meaning a condition of the sense of taste.

GH, abbreviation for **growth hormone.**

ghost cells, red blood cells that have lost their hemoglobin so that only the cell covering can be seen when a urine sample is examined under a microscope. The hemoglobin is destroyed by the urine. Also called **shadow cells.**

GHRF, abbreviation for **growth hormone releasing factor.**

GI, abbreviation for **gastrointestinal.**

giant cell, an abnormally large cell. It often contains more than one nucleus and may appear as a combination of several normal cells.

giant cell arteritis. See **temporal arteritis.**

giant cell carcinoma, a cancer containing many very large primitive cells. A small percentage of lung and liver cancers contain such cells. Also called **carcinoma gigantocellulare.**

giant cell interstitial pneumonia. See **interstitial pneumonia.**

giant cell myeloma, a bone tumor of giant cells. Also called **giant cell tumor of bone.**

giant cell thyroiditis. See **de Quervain's thyroiditis.**

giant cell tumor of bone. See **giant cell myeloma.**

giant chromosome, any of the very large chromosomes found in insects and the lower animals.

giant follicular lymphoma, a white blood cell disease in which many bumps change the normal structure of a lymph node. Also called **Brill-Symmer's disease, giant follicular lymphadenopathy, Symmer's disease.**

giant hypertrophic gastritis, a disease in which large bumpy folds of tissue cover the wall of the stomach. Symptoms include loss of appetite, nausea, vomiting, and pain in the stomach and intestines. X-ray or endoscopic examination or surgery may be needed to identify this disease.

Giardia /jē·är'dē·ə/, a common type of flagellate protozoans. Many species of *Giardia* normally live in the stomach and intestines, causing swelling. See also **giardiasis.**

giardiasis /jē·ärdī'əsis/, a swelling of the intestines caused by an increase of a protozoa (*Giardia lamblia*). The source of the disease is usually water infected with *G. lamblia* cysts. Also called **traveler's diarrhea.**

gibbus /gib'əs, jib'əs/, 1. a hump, or swelling, on a body surface, usually on just one side. 2. an abnormal curving of the spine that may happen after a back bone breaks down. It may result from a broken bone or from tuberculosis of the spine.

Gibson walking splint, a kind of leg splint that allows a patient to walk.

gigantism /jigan'tizəm/, an abnormal condition marked by excess height and weight. It is most often caused by excess release of growth hormone (GH). It occurs to a lesser degree in some genetic disorders. Gigantism with normal body proportions and normal sexual development usually comes from excess GH in early childhood. Hypogonadism, by slowing puberty and closure of the growing ends of the bones, may lead to gigantism. Excessive growth often happens in males with more than one Y chromosome, and it may happen along with Klinefelter's syndrome, Marfan's syndrome, and some cases of fat disorders. Children with gigantism of the brain are mentally retarded and have a large head, large arms and legs, and a clumsy walk. They grow quickly during their first few years and then at a normal rate. Proper hormones may be given to control abnormal growth of children with hypogonadism. Gigantism is usually treated with radiation, but gland surgery may also be used. See also **acromegaly, eunuchoidism.**

Gilbert's syndrome, an inherited condition marked by excessive bile color in the blood and liver disease (jaundice). No treatment is needed. See also **hyperbilirubinemia of the newborn.**

Gilchrist's disease. See **blastomycosis.**

Gilles de la Tourette syndrome /zhēl′dəlätōōrets′/, an abnormal condition beginning in childhood, marked by face twitches, tics, and uncontrolled arm and shoulder motions. In adolescence and adulthood, the condition may get worse; the patient may grunt, snort, and shout without control. Obscene speech often develops, to the dismay of the patient and the people around him or her. There is no cure. Drug treatment is effective in many cases in controlling symptoms, showing an organic cause for this syndrome.

Gillies' operation /gil′ēz/, a surgery that reduces fractures of a skull area near the ear (zygoma and zygomatic arch) by making an incision at the hairline near the temple.

gingiva /jinjī′və/, *pl.* **gingivae,** the gum of the mouth, a mucous membrane and its supporting fiber like tissue that circles the necks of teeth. –**gingival,** *adj.*

gingival color, the color of healthy or diseased gums. It varies with the thickness of the outer layer of the gums, their natural color, and changes brought on by blood supply, pigmentation, and alterations by gum diseases.

gingival consistency, the look and feel of healthy gums. They are firm and springy to the touch. Compare **gingival color.**

gingival crevice, a normal crack between the gum and the tooth enamel.

gingival discoloration, a change in the normal color of the gums, linked to swelling, lack of blood, abnormal color, and other problems.

gingival hormonal enlargement, the swelling of the gums linked to hormone imbalance during pregnancy, puberty, and hormonal treatment.

gingival hyperplasia, a condition marked by too-fast growth of the gum tissue. It is often seen in patients treated with phenytoin for epileptic seizures.

gingival massage, the massage of the gums to clean them, improve tissue tone and blood circulation, and to harden their surface.

gingival mat, the connecting gum tissue made up of coarse, broad fibers that attach the gums to the teeth.

gingival position, the level of the gums in relation to the teeth.

gingival stippling, a series of small hollows in the surface of healthy gums. The hollows can vary in size, making the gum surface look as fine as smooth velvet, or as rough as an orange peel. See also **gingival consistency.**

gingival sulcus, any of the normal spaces between the gums and the teeth.

gingivectomy, removal of infected and diseased gum tissue, performed to stop the growth of pyorrhea. Under general anesthesia, all pockets around the teeth are scraped and overgrown tissue is removed. The exposed surface of the gum is covered with packing to prevent pain while eating and to allow new tissue to cover and fill in the areas. Bleeding and pain are associated with the procedure. The packing is removed 1 week later. Compare **gingivoplasty.**

gingivitis /jin′jivī′tis/, a condition in which the gums are red, swollen, and bleeding. Most gingivitis is the result of poor mouth care and of the buildup of bacterial plaque on the teeth. It also may be a sign of another condition, as diabetes mellitus, leukemia, or vitamin deficiency. It is common in pregnancy, usually painless, and may be sudden and serious or long-term and mild. Compare **Vincent's infection.**

gingivoplasty, the surgical shaping of the gums to maintain healthy gum tissue. Compare **gingivectomy.**

gingivostomatitis /jin′jivōstō′mətī′tis/, painful ulcers on the gums and mucous membranes of the mouth. It is the result of a herpesvirus infection. See also **herpes simplex.**

ginglymus joint. See **hinge joint.**

Giordano-Giovannetti diet /jôrdä′nōjō′vənet′ē/, a low-protein, low-fat, high-carbohydrate diet with controlled potassium and sodium intake. It is used with patients who have long-term kidney and liver failure. Protein is given only in the form of essential amino acids so that the body will use excess blood urea nitrogen to build the nonessential amino acids for tissue protein. The foods included are eggs, small amounts of milk, low-protein bread, some fruits and vegetables low in potassium, as green beans, summer squash, cabbage, pears, grapefruit, and fresh or frozen blackberries, blueberries, and boysenberries. Also called **Giovannetti diet.** See also **renal diet.**

gipoma /gipō′mə/, a tumor of the pancreas that causes changes in production of a hormone (gastric inhibitory peptide).

girdle, any curved or circular structure, as the hipline formed by the bones and tissues of the pelvis.

girdle pad, a pad that fits over the hip bone and tail bone to protect the hip in contact sports.

glabella, a flat, triangular area of bone of the forehead. It is sometimes used as a baseline for head measurements.

glabrous skin, smooth, hairless skin.

gland, an organ of specialized cells that releases material not related to its ordinary metabolism. Some glands produce fluids that smooth tissues and lessen friction; others, like the pituitary gland, produce hormones; hematopoietic glands, like the spleen, thyroid, and certain lymph nodes, take part in the production of blood.

glanders, an infection caused by a bacterium (*Pseudomonas mallei*) given to humans from horses and other domestic animals. It is marked by pus-filled swellings of the mucous membranes and the growth of skin bumps that become infected and cause an open sore. It is common in Africa, Asia, and South America but has been wiped out in Europe and North America.

gland of Montgomery. See **areolar gland.**

glands of Zeiss. See **ciliary gland.**

glandular carcinoma. See **adenocarcinoma.**

glandular fever. See **infectious mononucleosis.**

glans /glanz/, *pl.* **glandes** /glan'dēz/, **1.** a general term for a small, round mass or body. **2.** tissue that can swell and harden, as on the ends of the clitoris and the penis.

glans of clitoris, the tissue at the end of the clitoris that can swell and harden when filled with blood. It is made up of the corpora cavernosa enclosed in a dense, fiberlike membrane. Also called **glans clitoridis.**

glans penis, the cone-shaped tip of the penis that covers the end of the corpora cavernosa penis and the corpus spongiosom like a cap. The urethral opening is normally located at the center of the tip of the glans penis. The corona glandis, the widest part of the glans penis, is around the base. A fold of dark, thin, hairless skin forms the foreskin (prepuce).

Glasgow Coma Scale, a system for describing the degree of loss of consciousness in the severely ill. It is also used to predict the length and result of coma, mostly in patients with head injuries. The system involves three factors: eye opening, verbal response, and muscle response. There are four grades of eye opening, five grades of verbal response, and five grades of muscle response. The grades of eye opening range from opening the eyes when asked a question (mild loss of consciousness) to not opening the eyes at all when spoken to (severe loss of consciousness). The five grades of verbal response range from correctly answering the questions "who are you? where are you? what day and month is it?" (mild) to not responding at all to questions, or answering by

---

Glasgow coma scale

The Glasgow coma scale has been designed to quantitatively relate consciousness to motor responses, verbal responses, and eye opening. Coma is defined as no response and no eye opening. Scores of 7 or less on the Glasgow scale qualify as "coma"; all scores of 9 or more do not qualify as "coma." The examiner determines the best response the patient can make to a set of standardized stimuli. Higher points are assigned to responses that indicate increasing degrees of arousal.

1. **Best motor response.** (Examiner determines the *best* response with *either* arm.)
   a. *6 points.* Obeys simple commands. Raises arm on request or holds up specified number of fingers. Releasing a grip (not grasping, which can be reflexive) is also an appropriate test.
   b. *5 points.* Localizes noxious stimuli. Fails to obey commands but can move either arm toward a noxious cutaneous stimulus and eventually contacts it with the hand. The stimulus should be maximal and applied in various locations, i.e., sternum pressure, or trapezius pinch.
   c. *4 points.* Flexion withdrawal. Responds to noxious stimulus with arm flexion but does not localize it with the hand.
   d. *3 points.* Abnormal flexion. Adducts shoulder, flexes and pronates arm, flexes wrist, and makes a fist in response to a noxious stimulus (decorticate rigidity).
   e. *2 points.* Abnormal extension. Adducts and internally rotates shoulder, extends forearm, flexes wrist, and makes a fist in response to a noxious stimulus (decerebrate rigidity).
   f. *1 point.* No motor response. Exclude reasons for no response; for example, insufficient stimulus or spinal-cord injury.

2. **Best verbal response.** (Examiner determines the best response after arousal. Noxious stimuli are employed if necessary.) Omit this test if the patient is dysphasic, has oral injuries, or is intubated. Place a check mark after other two test category scores after totaling to indicate omission of the verbal response section.
   a. *5 points.* Oriented patient. Can converse and relate who he is, where he is, and the year and month.
   b. *4 points.* Confused patient. Is not fully oriented or demonstrates confusion.
   c. *3 points.* Verbalizes. Does not engage in sustained conversation, but uses intelligible words in an exclamation (curse) or in a disorganized manner which is nonsensical.
   d. *2 points.* Vocalizes. Makes moaning or groaning sounds that are not recognizable words.
   e. *1 point.* No vocalization. Does not make any sound even in response to noxious stimulus.

3. **Eye opening.** (Examiner determines the minimum stimulus that evokes opening of one or both eyes.) If the patient cannot realistically open the eyes because of bandages or lid edema, write "E" after the total test score to indicate omission of this component.
   a. *4 points.* Eyes open spontaneously.
   b. *3 points.* Eyes open to speech. Patient opens eyes in response to command or on being called by name.
   c. *2 points.* Eyes open to noxious stimuli.
   d. *1 point.* No eye opening in response to noxious stimuli.

From Teasdale, G., and Jennett, B.: Assessment of coma and impaired consciousness: a practical scale, Lancet 2:81-84, 1974.

making sounds that do not form words (se-vere). The grades of muscle response range from moving a hand or limb correctly when asked (mild) to no motion at all, not even simple reflex motion in arms or legs that are known not to be paralyzed (severe).

glass factor. See **factor XII.**

glaucoma /glôkō′mə, glou-/, an abnormal condition of high pressure within an eye. It is caused by a blocking of the normal flow of the watery fluid in the space between the cornea and lens of the eye (aqueous humor). **Acute (angle-closure, closed-angle, or narrow-angle) glaucoma** happens if the pupil in an eye with a narrow angle between the iris and cornea opens too wide and causes the folded iris to block the flow of aqueous humor. **Chronic (open-angle or wide-angle) glaucoma** is much more common, often occurring in both eyes; it develops slowly and is an inherited disease. Acute glaucoma happens with extreme eye pain, blurred vision, a red eye, and an abnormally wide-open pupil. Nausea and vomiting may occur. If untreated, acute glaucoma results in complete and permanent blindness within 2 to 5 days. Chronic glaucoma may show no symptoms except for gradual loss of side vision over a period of years. Sometimes headaches, blurred vision, and dull pain in the eye are present. Halos around lights and blind spots in the center of the field of vision begin to occur after the condition has developed for a while. Acute glaucoma is treated with eye drops to close the pupil and draw the iris away from the cornea, drugs that lower pressure, drugs that reduce fluid in the eye, and surgery to produce a pathway for aqueous humor. Chronic glaucoma can usually be controlled with eye drops.

★PATIENT CARE: All adults should have their eyes examined for glaucoma every three to five years. It is a good idea for patients who have glaucoma to wear a medical identification tag.

glaucomatocyclitic crisis /glôkom′ətōsiklit′ik/, a recurring increase in the internal pressure in one eye, resembling a type of suddenly occurring glaucoma (acute angle-closure glaucoma), and accompanied by signs of swelling of the iris and other parts of the eye. Also called **Posner-Schlossman syndrome.**

glenohumeral joint /glē′nōhyoo′mərəl/, the shoulder joint, formed by a cavity in the shoulder blade and the upper arm bone.

glia. See **neuroglia.**

gliadin /glī′ədin/, a protein that is obtained from wheat and rye.

gliding, 1. a smooth, continuous movement. **2.** the simplest of the 4 basic movements allowed by various joints of the skeleton. It is common to all movable joints and allows one surface to

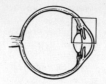

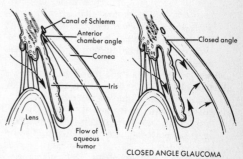

Canal of Schlemm
Anterior chamber angle
Cornea
Iris
Lens
Flow of aqueous humor
Closed angle

CLOSED ANGLE GLAUCOMA
Glaucoma

move smoothly over the next surface, no matter what shape. Compare **angular movement, circumduction, rotation.**

gliding joint, a joint in which facing bones allow only gliding movements, as in the wrist and the ankle. The ligaments or other tissues around each gliding joint limit motion. Also called **arthrodia, articulatio plana.** Compare **hinge joint, pivot joint.**

gliding zone, an area next to a joint space covered with cartilage that merges with the fibrous covering of the bone.

glipizide, a drug taken by mouth that is prescribed, along with diet and exercise, to lower blood sugar levels of patients with non-insulin-dependent diabetes.

★CAUTION: The dosage may have to be adjusted for patients taking drugs that increase blood sugar levels; elderly, weak, or undernourished patients are at risk for developing low blood sugar.

★ADVERSE EFFECTS: Among the most serious adverse reactions are nausea, heartburn, and skin allergies.

glio-, a combining form meaning the neuroglia, or a gluey substance.

glioblastoma. See **gliosarcoma.**

glioblastoma multiforme, a fast growing, pulpy cancer of the brain or the spinal cord. The tumor spreads by branching out. Also called **anaplastic astrocytoma, glioma multiforme.**

glioma /glī-ō′mə/, pl. **gliomas, gliomata,** any of the largest group of cancers of the brain, made of glial cells. Kinds of gliomas are **astrocytoma, ependymoma, glioblastoma multiforme, medulloblastoma, oligodendroglioma.**

glioma multiforme. See **gliobastoma multiforme.**

glioma sarcomatosum. See **gliosarcoma.**

glioneuroma /glī'ōnŏŏrō'mə/, *pl.* **glioneuromas, glioneuromata,** a cancer made of nerve cells and elements of their support tissue.

gliosarcoma /glī'ōsärkō'mə/, *pl.* **gliosarcomas, gliosarcomata,** a cancer made of long, thin cells in the slim, connective tissue of nerve cells. Also called **glioma, glioblastoma, spongioblastoma, spongiocytoma.**

globin, a type of protein molecule that combines with iron in the blood to form hemoglobin and myoglobin.

globule /glob'yŏŏl/, a small round mass.

globulin /glob'yŏŏlin/, one of a broad category of simple proteins. Compare **albumin.**

globus hystericus, a feeling of a lump in the throat that cannot be swallowed or coughed up. It often accompanies emotional conflict or acute anxiety.

glomangioma /glōman'jē·ō'mə/, *pl.* **glomangiomas, glomangiomatas,** a tumor that develops from a group of blood cells in the skin. Also called **angiomyoneuroma, angioneuroma.**

glomerular /glōmer'yŏŏlər/, meaning a glomerulus, especially a kidney glomerulus.

glomerular capsule. See **Bowman's capsule.**

glomerular disease, any of a group of diseases that affects the glomerulus of the kidney. There may be overgrowth, tissue death, scarring, or deposits in the kidney glomeruli. See also **glomerulonephritis.**

glomerular filtration, a process in which urine is formed when blood is filtered across small blood vessels (capillaries) in the kidney.

glomerular filtration rate (GFR), a measure of kidney function in terms of the amount of blood that can be filtered in a certain time. Aging and diseases tend to reduce the GFR.

glomerulonephritis /glōmer'yŏŏlōnəfrī'tis/, a swelling of the glomerulus of the kidney. It is marked by blood and proteins in the urine, decreased urine, and swelling. Kinds of glomerulonephritis are **acute glomerulonephritis, chronic glomerulonephritis, subacute glomerulonephritis.**

glomerulus /glōmer'yŏŏləs/, *pl.* **glomeruli, 1.** a tuft or cluster. **2.** a tuftlike structure composed of blood vessels or nerve fibers, as a kidney glomerulus.

glomus /glō'məs/, *pl.* **glomera** /glom'ərə/, a small group of tiny arteries connecting directly to veins and having a rich nerve supply.

-glossia, 1. a combining form meaning a type or condition of tongue,

glossitis /glosī'tis/, inflammation of the tongue. Severe glossitis, marked by swelling and intense pain may be felt as an ear disorder. It may develop during an infection or following a burn, bite, or other injury. Glossitis in which there is shrinking of the surface and edges of the tongue is a sign of pernicious anemia.

Long-term surface glossitis (Moeller's glossitis), in which bright red patches appear on the tip or sides of the tongue, occurs in middle-aged people, mostly women. It causes pain or a burning feeling and sensitivity to hot or spicy foods.

glossitis parasitica. See **parasitic glossitis.**

glossodynia /glos'ōdin'ē·ə/, pain in the tongue, caused by swelling, infection, or an open sore.

glossodynia exfoliativa, long term glossitis, marked by pain and sensitivity to spicy foods without any sign of disease.

glossoepiglottic /glos'ō·ep'iglot'ik/, pertaining to the tongue and the structure protecting the windpipe (epiglottis).

glossohyal /glos'ōhī'əl/, meaning the tongue and the horseshoe-shaped bone at the base of the tongue. Also called **hyoglossal.**

glossoncus /glosong'kəs/, a swelling in one spot or all over the tongue.

glossopexy /glos'əpek'sē/, when the tongue sticks to the lip.

glossopharyngeal /glos'ōfərin'jē·əl/, meaning the tongue and throat.

glossopharyngeal neuralgia, repeated attacks of severe pain in the throat, tonsils, tongue, and middle ear. It tends to affect men more than women, usually beginning after the age of 40. Attacks last from a few seconds to minutes and may be started by swallowing. The cause is not known. It is usually treated with drugs, but surgery may be needed to cut the involved nerve.

glossophytia /glos'əfit'ē·ə/, a condition of the tongue in which a black patch develops on the back. The papillae are greatly elongated and thickened like bristly hairs. The usually painless condition may be caused by heavy smoking or the use of antibiotics. See also **parasitic glossitis.**

glossoplasty /glos'ōplas'tē/, a plastic surgery on the tongue. It may be performed to correct a birth defect, repair an injury, or restore use of the tongue following removal of a cancer.

glossopyrosis /glos'ōpīrō'sis/, a burning sense in the tongue caused by a long-term swelling, by exposure to extremely hot or spicy food, or by psychogenic glossitis.

glottis, 1. a slitlike opening between the vocal cords (plica vocalis). **2.** the voice apparatus made up of the true vocal cords and the opening between them (rima glottidis). **–glottal, glottic,** *adj.*

glucagon /glŏŏ'kəgon/, a hormone, produced in the islands of Langerhans. It stimulates the changing of glycogen to glucose in the liver. Secretion of glucagon is brought on by low blood sugar and by the growth hormone. Also called **hyperglycemic-glycogenolytic factor.**

glucagonoma syndrome /glŏŏ'kəgonō'mə/, a disease associated with a tumor of the pancreas. It is marked by excess blood sugar, mouth swelling, anemia, weight loss, and a rash.

gluco-, glyco-, a combining form meaning sweetness or glucose.

glucocorticoid /gloo′kôkôr′təkoid/, a hormone that aids carbohydrate processing, acts to lessen swelling and affects many body functions. Glucocorticoids aid the release of amino acids from muscle, take fatty acids from fat stores, and increase the ability of muscles to tighten and avoid fatigue. A lack of glucocorticoids is marked by darkening of the skin, low blood sugar, weight loss, and lack of energy. An excess is linked to damaged sugar digestion, thinning of the skin, poor wound healing, infection, and overweight. Glucocorticoid release is triggered by a hormone of the pituitary. Compare **mineralocorticoid.**

gluconeogenesis, the formation of glycogen from fatty acids and proteins rather than from carbohydrates.

glucose /gloo′kōs/, a simple sugar found in certain foods, especially fruits, and a major source of energy in human and animal body fluids. Glucose, when eaten or produced by the digestion of carbohydrates, is taken into the blood from the intestines. Excess glucose in circulation is stored in the liver and muscles as glycogen and converted to glucose and released as needed. The measuring of blood glucose levels is an important test in diabetes and other disorders. See also **dextrose, glycogen.**

glucose-6-phosphate dehydrogenase (G-6-PD) deficiency, an inherited disorder in which red cells partially or completely lack an enzyme (glucose-6-phosphate dehydrogenase) needed for carbohydrate metabolism. See also **congenital nonspherocytic hemolytic anemia, favism.**

glucose-tolerance test, a test of the body's ability to process carbohydrates by giving a dose of glucose and then measuring the blood and urine for glucose. The patient usually eats a high carbohydrate diet for the three days before the test and fasts the night before. A fasting blood glucose is taken the next morning and then the patient drinks a 100-gram dose of glucose. Blood and urine are sampled for up to 6 hours after the dose. The test is used to assist in the diagnosis of diabetes or other disorders.

glucosuria /gloo′kōsoor′ē-ə/, abnormal levels of glucose in the urine from the eating of large amounts of carbohydrate or from a kidney disease, as nephrosis, or a processing disease, as diabetes mellitus. See also **glycosuria. –glucosuric,** *adj.*

glucosyl cerebroside lipidosis. See **Gaucher's disease.**

Glucotrol, a brand name for an oral drug used to treat diabetes (glipizide).

glue sniffing, the practice of breathing the vapors of toluene, a compound used as a solvent in certain glues. Intoxication and dizziness re-

sult. Long-term exposure, either accidental or knowing, may damage a number of organ systems.

glutamate /gloo′təmāt/, a salt of glutamic acid.

glutamic acid (Glu) /glootam′ik/, an amino acid occurring widely in a number of proteins. See also **amino acid, protein.**

glutamicacidemia /glootam′ikas′idē′mē-ə/, an inherited disorder in the breakdown of an amino acid (glutamic acid) resulting in high blood levels of it. The precise defect is not known, but the condition is marked by mental and physical retardation, convulsions, and fragile hair growth.

glutamic acid hydrochloride, a stomach acidifier given for low stomach acid. This drug should not be taken by patients with excess stomach acid, peptic ulcer, or a known allergy to the drug. The most serious harmful reactions to this drug are loose stools and acidosis.

glutamine (Gln), an amino acid found in many proteins in the body. It works in many reactions and helps remove ammonia from the body. See also **amino acid, protein.**

glutathione, an enzyme whose lack is often associated with anemia.

gluteal /gloo′tē-əl/, referring to the buttocks or to the muscles that form the buttocks.

gluteal gait. See **Trendelenburg gait.**

gluteal tuberosity, a ridge on the surface of the thigh bone to which is attached the gluteus maximus muscle.

gluten /gloo′tən/, a protein in wheat and other grains. It can be taken from flour by washing out the starch. It is used as an adhesive agent, and makes dough tough and elastic.

gluten enteropathy. See **celiac disease.**

glutethimide /glooteth′əmīd/, a drug that is given to soothe and quiet a patient. It is used to treat anxiety and insomnia.

gluteus /glootē′əs/, any of three muscles that form the buttocks. The gluteus maximus, the largest, straightens the hip joint. The gluteus medius rotates the thigh and moves the leg to the side. The gluteus minimus moves the leg to the side.

Gly, abbreviation for **glycine.**

glyburide, a drug taken by mouth to control diabetes. In addition to diet therapy and exercise, this drug is prescribed to lower blood glucose levels of patients with some types of diabetes. ★CAUTION: Because it is long-acting, glyburide may produce prolonged periods of low blood glucose; there is also a risk of severe low blood glucose in elderly, malnourished, or weakened patients. The dosage may need to be adjusted for patients taking other drugs that increase blood glucose levels.

★ADVERSE EFFECTS: Among the more serious adverse reactions are nausea, heartburn, and skin allergies.

-glycemia, -glycaemia, a combining form that means a 'condition of sugar in the blood.'

glycerin, a sweet, colorless, oily fluid used in drug preparations. Glycerin is used as a moistener for chapped skin, as an ingredient of suppositories for constipation, and as a sweetener for drugs. Also spelled **glycerine.**

glycerol /glis′ərôl/, an alcohol that is contained in fats. See also **glycerin.**

glycerol kinase, an enzyme in the liver and kidneys that acts in cell energy functions.

glyceryl guaiacolate. See **guaifenesin.**

glycine (Gly) /glī′sin/, an amino acid found in many animal and plant proteins. See also **amino acid, protein.**

glycobiarsol, a drug made up of mostly arsenic and bismuth, in the past used to treat intestinal amebiasis.

glycogen /glī′kəjən/, the major carbohydrate stored in animal cells. It is made from glucose and stored chiefly in the liver and, to some extent, in muscles. Glycogen is changed to glucose and released into circulation as needed by the body for energy. Also called **animal starch, hepatin, tissue dextrin.** See also **glucose.**

glycogenesis, the production of glycogen from glucose.

glycogenolysis /glī′kōjenol′isis/, the breakdown of glycogen to glucose.

glycogen storage disease, any of a group of inherited disorders of glycogen processing. An enzyme lack causes glycogen to be stored in too-large amounts in various parts of the body. Also called **glycogenosis.**

glycogen storage disease, type I. See **von Gierke's disease.**

glycogen storage disease, type II. See **Pompe's disease.**

glycogen storage disease, type III. See **Cori's disease.**

glycogen storage disease, type IV. See **Andersen's disease.**

glycogen storage disease, type V. See **McArdle's disease.**

glycogen storage disease, type VI. See **Hers' disease.**

glycolic acid, a substance in bile that aids in digestion and absorption of fats.

glycolipid, a compound made of a lipid and a carbohydrate found mostly in the tissue of the nerves.

glycolysis /glīkol′isis/, a series of reactions, occurring within cells, by which glucose and other sugars are broken down to yield acids or energy.

glycoprotein, any of the large group of protein compounds in which the nonprotein substance is a carbohydrate. These include the mucins, the mucoids, and the chondroproteins.

glycopyrrolate /glī′kōpir′əlāt/, a drug given as part of ulcer treatment.

glycoside /glī′kəsīd/, any of several carbohydrates that yield a sugar and a nonsugar when broken down. The plant *Digitalis purpurea* yields a glycoside used to treat heart disease.

glycosphingolipids /glī′kōsfing′gōlip′ids/, compounds formed from carbohydrates and a fatty substance (ceramide), found in tissues of the nervous system and also in red blood cells. Lack of an enzyme needed to break them down leads to a possibly fatal disorder of the nervous system.

glycosuria /glī′kōsŏŏr′ē·ə/, abnormal presence of a sugar, especially glucose, in the urine. It is usually linked with diabetes mellitus. **–glycosuric,** *adj.*

glycosuric acid, a compound that is made by the body as it processes tyrosine. It is found in the urine of people who have alkaptonuria.

gm, abbreviation for **gram.** Preferred is the abbreviation *g.*

-gnathia, a combining form meaning a condition of the jaw.

gnathion /nā′thē·on/, the lowest point in the lower border of the lower jaw. It is a common reference point in the diagnosis and orthodontic treatment of poor bite (malocclusion).

gnathodynamometer /nā′thōdī′nəmom′ətər/, an instrument used to measure the biting pressure of the jaws of a patient. Also called **occlusometer.**

gnathodynia /nā′thōdin′ē·ə/, a pain in the jaw, as that associated with an impacted wisdom tooth.

gnathostatic cast /nā′thōstat′ik/, a cast of the teeth.

-gnosia, a combining form meaning knowing or sensing.

goblet cell, one of the many special cells that release mucus and form glands of the lining of the stomach, the intestine, and parts of the respiratory tract. Also called **beaker cell, chalice cell.** See also **gland.**

goiter, an overgrown thyroid gland, usually seen as a swelling in the neck. The swelling may be linked to hyperthyroidism, hypothyroidism, or normal levels of thyroid function. The goiter may be cystlike or fiberlike, it may surround a large blood vessel, or a part of the swollen gland may sit beneath the sternum or in the chest hollow. Treatment may include removal, giving antithyroid drugs or radioiodine, or giving thyroid hormone. Following removal of the thyroid, the patient may need to take thyroid hormone drugs. See specific goiter. **–goitrous,** *adj.*

gold (Au), a yellowish, soft metallic element used to rebuild teeth. Gold salts, in which gold is attached to sulfur, have been used in the treatment of patients with rheumatoid arthritis but cause serious poisoning in about 10% of patients. See also **chrysotherapy.**

gold 198, a radioactive gold given for cancer of the prostate, cervix, and bladder and to lessen the fluid pooling caused by a cancer. This drug should not be taken by: patients with infected, open tumors, or unhealed wounds from surgery; pregnant or breast-feeding mothers; or persons under 18 years of age. The most serious reaction to this drug is radiation sickness.

gold compound, a drug containing gold salts, usually given with other drugs to treat rheumatoid arthritis. Gold can be poisonous and is used only under the care of a specialist in chrysotherapy.

Goldent, a trademark for a powdered gold product used in dentistry.

gold foil, pure gold that has been rolled and beaten into a very thin sheet. It is usually packed into a tooth cavity. Also called **fibrous gold.**

gold inlay, a tooth repair made of gold alloy that is melted and formed to fit a hole in the crown of a tooth.

gold knife, a dental instrument used to trim excess metal and to develop contour in tooth repairs.

Goldman-Fox knife, a dental instrument with a sharp cutting edge, for gum-tissue surgery.

gold therapy. See **chrysotherapy.**

golfer's elbow, a popular term for a condition caused by the overuse of the muscles that bend the wrist.

Golgi apparatus /gôl'jē/, one of many small structures found in the cytoplasm of most cells. It is linked to the forming of carbohydrate units of various substances. Also called **Golgi body, Golgi complex.**

Golgi-Mazzoni corpuscles /gôl'jēmatsō'nē/, a number of thin capsules that circle the nerve endings in the tissue under the skin layers of the fingers. They are special sensory end organs. Also called **Krause's terminal bulbs.** Compare **Pacini's corpuscles, Ruffini's corpuscles.**

Golgi tendon organ, a nerve ending that is sensitive to tension and stretching of a muscle.

gomphosis /gomfō'sis/, *pl.* **gomphoses,** a fiberlike joint formed by the insertion of a cone shape into a socket. An example is the root of a tooth in a hollow (alveolus) of a jaw bone. Compare **sutura, syndesmosis.**

gonad /gō'nad/, a gland that releases gametes, as an ovary or a testis. **–gonadal,** *adj.*

gonadal dose, the amount of radiation received by the genitals in an x-ray examination. It is very small for a dental or chest x-ray, more for a lower spine x-ray, and much more for a fetus from x-ray of the mother's pelvis.

gonadal dysgenesis, a variety of conditions that involve defects in the gonads. Examples include Turner's syndrome, hermaphroditism, and gonadal aplasia.

gonadal shield, a shield used to protect the gonads (testes or ovaries) of a patient from radi-

ation during an x-ray procedure. It is generally used for all patients who may be fertile, including all patients under the age of 40 and also older males.

gonadotropin, a hormone that causes the testes and the ovaries to act.

gonio-, a combining form for an angle.

goniometry /gō'nē·om'ɔtrē/, a test system for diseases that affect the sense of balance. One test uses a plank, one end of which may be raised to any height. The patient stands on the plank as one end is gradually raised. The angle where the patient can no longer hold balance is noted. **–goniometric,** *adj.*

gonioscope, an eye instrument used to examine the angle of the anterior chamber of the eye.

goniotomy /gō'nē·ot'ɔmē/, an eye operation performed to remove any obstruction to the flow of the fluid in the front chamber of the eye, usually done for glaucoma.

gono-, gon-, a combining form meaning semen or seed.

gonococcal pyomyositis, a serious swelling of a muscle caused by infection with a bacterium (*Neisseria gonorrhoeae,*). It is marked by abscess and pain. It is an unusual form of gonorrhea, and diagnosis is made by the discovery of the gonocococcal germ within the abscess.

gonococcus /gon'ɔkok'ɔs/, *pl.* **gonococci** /gon'-ɔkok'sī/, a bacterium of the species *Neisseria gonorrhoeae,* the cause of gonorrhea.

gonorrhea, a common sexually carried disease. It most often affects the sex organs, the bladder, and the kidneys and, occasionally, the throat, eye, or rectum. It is passed by contact with an infected person or by contact with body fluids containing *Neisseria gonorrhoeae.* Difficulty urinating greenish-yellow pus flow from the urethra or vagina, red or swollen urethra, and itching, burning, or pain around the vagina or urethra are symptoms. The vagina may be very swollen and red and the lower abdomen may be tense and very tender. As the infection spreads, which is more common in women than in men, nausea, vomiting, fever, and rapid heart beat may occur. Swelling of the ovaries and fallopian tubes or peritonitis can develop. Swelling of the tissues around the liver may also occur, causing pain in the upper right area of the abdomen. There may be blood stream infection with polyarthritis, tender sores on the skin of the hands and feet, and swelling of the tendons of the wrists, knees, and ankles. Gonoccocal ophthalmia can cause scars on the eyes and blindness. Gonorrhea is diagnosed by a microscopic study of a specimen of fluid. Penicillin is used to treat simple gonorrhea. It is injected into a muscle one-half hour after probenecid, a drug that acts to slow the release of the penicillin from the body, has been taken by mouth. A large, one-time dose of ampicillin is also effective. Erythromycin or tetracycline is sometimes used to treat the infection in people who are allergic to penicillin and penicillin-like drugs. The patient is tested 1 or 2 weeks later to make sure the drug was effective. The routine instillation of 1% silver nitrate in the eyes of the newborn usually prevents infection in the newborn that might result from contact with the fluids of an infected mother during vaginal delivery. It is important that the infected person's sexual contacts be treated. Before giving any antibiotic it is learned whether the person may be allergic to the antibiotic. Drugs should be available to treat any reaction that may occur. The patient is warned that until it is proven that gonorrhea is gone, the infection can be passed on, and so great care must be taken to prevent its spread. The use of condoms during sexual intercourse offers excellent protection against future venereal infection.

gonorrheal conjunctivitis, a severe, destructive form of pus-producing conjunctivitis caused by the gonococcus *(Neisseria gonorrhoeae).* Quick treatment with drugs given into the vein is needed to prevent scars on the eyes and blindness. Newborn infants receive routine instillation of 1% solution of silver nitrate or a drug ointment to prevent the disorder. See also **ophthalmia neonatorum.**

gony-, gon-, a combining form meaning a knee.

Goodell's sign /gōodelz′/, softening of the narrow opening of the womb (cervix), usually a sign of pregnancy.

Goodpasture's syndrome, long term lung bleeding. It is marked by coughing of blood, breathing difficulty, anemia, and kidney failure.

Good Samaritan legislation, laws enacted in some states to protect doctors and some other health professionals from liability in giving emergency medical aid, unless there is proven willful wrong or gross negligence.

gooseflesh. See **pilomotor reflex.**

Gordon reflex, an abnormal change in the Babinski reflex. It is made by compressing the calf muscles and results in stretching of the great toe and fanning of the other toes. The reflex is evidence of disease of the central nervous system. Compare **Chaddock reflex, Oppenheim reflex.** See also **Babinski's reflex.**

Gosselin's fracture /gôslaNz′/, a V-shaped break in the shinbone (tibia) that extends to the ankle.

goundou /gōōn′dōō/, a condition marked by bony growths of the nose and jaw bones. It occurs with yaws in people of Africa and Latin America.

gout, a disease of uric acid processing. It increases production or interferes with the passing of uric acid. Excess uric acid is converted to sodium urate crystals that settle into joints and other tissues. Men are more often affected than women. The great toe is a common site for the buildup of urate crystals. The condition can result in painful swelling of a joint, along with chills and fever. The disease is crippling and, if untreated, can lead to joint breakdown. Treatment usually includes drugs, a diet that excludes purine rich foods, as organ meats, and may include surgery. See also **chondrocalcinosis, Lesch-Nyhan syndrome, pseudogout, tophus.**

gouty arthritis. See **gout.**

Gowers' muscular dystrophy. See **distal muscular dystrophy.**

G-6-PD deficiency, abbreviation for **glucose-6-phosphate dehydrogenase deficiency.**

GP, abbreviation for **general practitioner.**

gr, abbreviation for **grain.**

graafian follicle /graf′ē·ən/, a mature ovarian bubble that breaks during ovulation to release an egg. Many primary ovarian follicles are found near the surface of the ovary. Under the influence of the follicle-triggering hormone, one ovarian follicle ripens into a graafian follicle during each menstrual cycle. The cells that form the graafian follicle are arranged in a layer 3 to 4 cells thick around a fluid. Within the follicle the egg triples in size and, when the follicle breaks, is swept into the opening of a fallopian tube. The hollow of the follicle collapses when the egg is released, and the cells lining enlarge to become the corpus luteum.

gracile /gras′il/, long, slender, and graceful.

gradation of activity, activities during therapy that are paced and changed to demand the maximum effort possible considering the patient's condition.

graded exercise test (GXT), a test given to a heart patient during recovery to predict the long-range effects of the heart attack and to determine the patient's level of function. The test is given before discharge from the hospital to set guidelines for activity programs at home and work during the recovery period. See also **exercise electrocardiogram.**

graduated bath, a bath in which the temperature of the water is slowly lowered.

graduated resistance exercise. See **progressive resistance exercise.**

GRAE, abbreviation for **generally recognized as effective.**

graft, a tissue or an organ taken from a site or a person and put into a new site or person. It is done to repair a defect in structure. The graft may be temporary, as an emergency skin transplant for burns, or permanent, as the grafted tissue growing to become a part of the body. Skin, bone, cartilage, blood vessel, nerve, muscle, cornea, and whole organs, as the kidney or the heart, may be grafted. Rejection is the major problem: fever, pain in the graft area, and loss of function 4 to 15 days later are signs of rejection. Drugs are given in large doses to prevent antibody production and rejection.

Late rejection may occur a year or more after the graft is done. Also called **transplant.** See also **allograft, autograft, isograft, skin graft, xenograft.**

graft-versus-host reaction, a rejection response of certain grafts, especially bone marrow. Rejection signs may include skin tumors with swelling, redness, open sores, scaling, and loss of hair. Such reactions may also affect the joints, the heart, and the blood cells. Also called **homologous disease.**

grain (gr), the smallest unit of mass in avoirdupois, troy, and apothecaries' weights. It is the same in all and equal to 4.79891 mg. The troy and apothecaries' ounces contain 480 grains; the avoirdupois ounce contains 437.5 grains.

grain itch, a skin condition caused by a mite that lives in grain or straw. The sore is an itchy pimple topped by a tiny blister.

gram (g, gm), a unit of mass in the metric system equal to ¹⁄₁₀₀₀ of a kilogram, 15.432 grains, and 0.0353 ounce avoirdupois.

-gram, -gramme, 1. a combining form meaning a 'drawing.' **2.** a combining form meaning '¹⁄₁₀₀₀ kilogram.'

gram calorie. See **calorie.**

gram-molecular weight, the molecule weight of a substance expressed in grams. See also **mole, molecular weight.**

gram-negative, having the pink color of a stain used in Gram's method of staining microorganisms.

gram-positive, keeping the violet color of the stain used in Gram's method of staining microorganisms.

Gram's stain, the method of staining microorganisms using a violet stain. It is followed by a counterstain. The retention of either the violet color of the stain or the pink color of the counterstain serves as a means of marking and typing bacteria. Also called **Gram's method.** See also **gram-negative, gram-positive.**

grand mal seizure, an epileptic convulsion (seizure) marked by uncontrolled muscle spasms and the stopping of breathing. When the muscle spasms are over, breathing starts again. During the fit the patient may clench the teeth, bite the tongue, and lose bladder control. After the seizure passes, the patient may fall into a deep sleep for an hour or more. Usually, the patient has no recall of the seizure on waking up. A sensory warning, or aura, usually comes before each grand mal seizure. These seizures may occur once, over a period of time, or many in a short period of time. Compare **focal seizure, petit mal seizure, psychomotor seizure.**

granular, 1. looking or feeling like sand. **2.** appearing under the microscope to have a few or many particles within or on the surface. **–granularity,** *n.*

granular conjunctivitis. See **trachoma.**

granulation tissue, soft, pink, fleshy bumps that form during the healing process of some wounds. It consists of many capillaries enclosed by fibrous tissue. Too much growth of granulation tissue results in a lump of flesh (proud flesh) growing above the skin. See also **intention, pyogenic granuloma.**

granulocyte /gran'yoŏoləsīt'/, a leukocyte containing granule in the cytoplasm. Kinds of granulocytes are **basophil, eosinophil, neutrophil.** Compare **agranulocyte.**

granulocyte transfusion, the use of specially prepared leukocytes to treat granulocytopenia. The treatment also is used to prevent serious infection in leukemic patients or those receiving cancer chemotherapy. The procedure has the same risks as a blood transfusion. Also called **buffy coat transfusion.**

granulocytic leukemia. See **acute myelocytic leukemia, chronic myelocytic leukemia.**

granulocytopenia /gran'yoŏolōsī'tōpē'nē·ə/, an abnormal condition of the blood, marked by a decrease in the normal number of granulocytes. Also called **neutropenia.** Compare **granulocytosis.** See also **leukopenia. –granulocytopenic,** *adj.*

granulocytosis /gran'yoŏolōsītō'sis/, an abnormal condition of the blood, marked by an increase in the number of granulocytes. Compare **granulocytopenia.**

granuloma /gran'yoŏolō'mə/, *pl.* **granulomas, granulomata,** a tumor of granulation tissue. It may result from swelling, injury, or infection. Granulomas may disappear without treatment, become gangrenous, spread, or remain as a center of infection. Treatment depends on the cause of the particular granuloma.

granuloma annulare, a long term skin disease of unknown cause. It consists of reddish pimples and bumps arranged in a ring.

granuloma gluteale infantum, a skin condition of the newborn marked by large, high bluish or brownish-red bumps on the buttocks. It may occur as a reaction to the use of strong steroid salves over a period of time.

granuloma inguinale, a sexually carried disease marked by open sores on the skin and the flesh under the skin of the groin and the outer sex organs. It is caused by infection with a bacterium *(Calymmatobacterium granulomatis).* Untreated, the sores spread, deepen, multiply, and become infected by other germs. All persons having granuloma inguinale are also tested for syphilis, as infection by both is common.

granulomatosis /gran'yoŏolōmətō'sis/, a condition marked by granulomas, as **berylliosis, pulmonary Wegener's granulomatosis, Wegener's granulomatosis.**

granulomatous thyroiditis. See **de Quervain's thyroiditis.**

granulosa cell tumor, a fleshy tumor with yellow streaks on an ovary. It may grow to an extremely large size and be linked to the excess production of estrogen. The tumor causes menstrual problems. Also called **folliculoma.**

granulosis, any disorder with small sandlike particles in an area of body tissue, as a skin rash marked by tiny particles beneath the surface.

-graph, 1. a combining form meaning the 'product of drawing or writing.' **2.** a combining form meaning a 'machine for making something drawn.'

graphing, the arrangement of data on a graph to show relationships between specific factors that have been measured or determined.

graphospasm. See **writer's cramp.**

GRAS, abbreviation for *generally recognized as safe.*

grasp reflex, a reflex brought on by stroking the palm or sole causing the fingers or toes to flex in a grasping motion. The reflex occurs in diseases of brain tissues. In young infants the tonic grasp reflex is normal: when one strokes the infant's palms, the stroking fingers are grasped so firmly that the child can be lifted into the air.

grass. See **cannabis.**

grass-line ligature, a fine cord composed of the fibers of a grass cloth plant. It is used in orthodontics for minor adjustments of the teeth. Its action depends on its ability to shrink when wetted by saliva.

Graves' disease, a disorder of excess thyroid hormone production. It is usually linked to an enlarged thyroid gland and bulging eyes (exophthalmos). Graves' disease, which is five times more common in women than in men, occurs most often between the ages of 20 and 40 and often follows an infection or physical or emotional stress. Typical signs are nervousness, a small tremor of the hands, weight loss, fatigue, breathlessness, palpitations, heat intolerance, and stomach and intestinal spasms. There may be an enlarged thymus, overgrowth of the lymph nodes, blurred or double vision, limited swelling, and heart and bone disorders. In patients with poorly controlled Graves' disease, infection or stress may cause a life-threatening thyroid storm. Also called **exophthalmic goiter, thyrotoxicosis, toxic goiter.**

gravid /grav′id/, pregnant; carrying fertilized eggs or a fetus. —**gravidity; gravidness,** *n.*

gravida 1 See **primigravida.**

gravida 2 See **secundigravida.**

-gravida, a combining form meaning 'pregnant woman with (specified) quantity of pregnancies.'

gravity, the heaviness or weight of an object caused by the universal effect of attraction between any object and any planetary body. The force of the gravity depends on the relative masses of the bodies and on the distance between them.

gravity-eliminated plane, a supported position in which the effect of gravity is offset. In testing of muscle strength, certain tests are run in a gravity-eliminated plane. Other tests may involve movements against the force of gravity.

gray (Gy), a measure of exposure to ionizing radiation. One gray equals 100 rad.

gray baby syndrome, a condition in premature infants, caused by a reaction to a drug (chloramphenicol). Because the baby's ability to break down and release drugs is not developed, the infant cannot process and get rid of chloramphenicol. The name of the condition comes from the typical ashen-gray skin color, which is found along with bloating of the abdomen, vomiting, difficulty breathing, and severe loss of blood circulation.

gray hepatization. See **hepatization.**

gray substance, the gray tissue that makes up the core of the spinal cord. It is arranged in two large side-by-side masses linked across the midline by a band of fibers. Each portion of the gray substance spreads out, forming the horns of the spinal cord. The horns consist mostly of cell bodies of neurons. The quantity of gray substance varies greatly at different levels of the cord. In the chest region, the gray substance is small in comparison with surrounding white substance; in the neck and the lower back regions it is larger; and in the tapered end of the cord, its proportion to the white substance is the greatest. Nuclei in the gray matter of the spinal cord function as centers for all spinal reflexes. Also called **gray matter.** Compare **white substance.** See also **spinal cord, spinal nerves.**

great auricular nerve, one of the skin branches of the cervical plexus, rising from the second and the third cranial nerves. One branch spreads to the skin of the face over the parotid gland. The other branch supplies the skin of the mastoid process and the back of the ear.

great calorie. See **calorie.**

greater omentum, a filmy, clear extension of the peritoneum. It covers the transverse colon and coils of the small intestine. The greater omentum is a movable structure that spreads into areas of injury, often sealing hernias and walling off infections that would otherwise cause peritonitis, as from a ruptured appendix. Also called **gastrocolic omentum.** Compare **lesser omentum.**

greater trochanter, a large bulge of the thigh bone (femur), to which are attached various muscles of the thigh.

greater vestibular gland. See **Bartholin's gland.**

great saphenous vein, one of the longest veins in the body. It contains 10 to 20 valves along its course through the leg and the thigh before ending in the thigh (femoral) vein. Compare **common iliac vein, femoral vein.**

great vessels, the large arteries and veins going into and coming from the heart. They include the aorta, the pulmonary arteries and veins, and the superior and inferior venae cavae.

green cancer. See **chloroma.**

greenstick fracture, a break in which the bone is bent but broken only on the outside of the bend. Children are most likely to have greenstick fractures. Keeping the bone rigid is usually effective, and healing is rapid. See also **fracture.**

-grel, a combining form for a drug that prevents clotting of platelets.

grenade-thrower's fracture, a break of the upper arm bone caused by violent muscle contractions.

Grenz rays, low-energy x-rays used to treat skin conditions. They cannot penetrate very far and are usually used by dermatologists.

Greulich-Pyle method /groi′lish-, grōō′lik-/, a test of the development of children by checking bone growth (bone age), using an x-ray of the left hand and wrist.

Grey Turner's sign, bruise of the skin of the side of the back between the ribs and hip bones in severe pancreatitis. Also called **Turner's sign.**

grid, a device used to absorb radiation scattered during an x-ray examination. A grid absorbs radiation that is not heading along straight lines from the x-ray source to the film.

grief, a pattern of physical and emotional responses to separation or loss. The effects are similar to those of fear, hunger, rage, and pain. The emotions proceed in stages from alarm to disbelief and denial, to anger and guilt, to finding a source of comfort, and, finally, to adjusting to the loss. The way in which a grieving person acts is greatly affected by the culture in which the person has been raised.

grief reaction, a group of mind and body symptoms linked to some extreme sorrow or loss, as the death of a loved one. Most serious grief reactions end after four to six weeks, although the period varies and may be much longer, especially in cases of sudden death. Also called **grief process.** See also **death, parental grief.**

grieving, anticipatory, grieving before an actual loss, as contrasted with grief in response to an actual loss. The cause is the knowledge or feeling of the coming loss of an important person in one's life, of one's well-being, or of one's personal possessions.

griffe des orteils. See **pes cavus.**

Grifulvin. a trademark for a drug that fights fungus (griseofulvin).

grinder's asthma, a breathing condition caused by breathing in fine particles put out during industrial grinding processes. See also **pneumoconiosis.**

grinder's disease. See **silicosis.**

grinding-in, a corrective grinding of one or more natural or artificial teeth to improve the surfaces.

grip and pinch strength, the ability to squeeze with the hand and fingers. It is measured by having the patient pinch on squeeze an instrument (dynamometer). Results are recorded in either pounds or kilograms of pressure.

gripes, severe spasmodic pain in the abdomen caused by an intestinal disorder. Also called **gripping.**

grippe. See **influenza.**

Grisactin, a trademark for an antifungal drug (griseofulvin).

griseofulvin /gris′ē·ōful′vin/, a drug given to treat some infections of the skin, hair, and nails. Patients with liver problems or known allergy to this drug should not take it. The most serious reactions to this drug are blood disorders. Headache, stomach and bowel problems, and rashes also may occur.

Griswald brace, a brace that controls certain types of fractures of the spine. It applies force to the front and back of the spine, relieving pressure in the area of the fracture. See also **Jewett brace.**

groin, each of two areas where the abdomen joins the thighs.

Grönblad-Strandberg syndrome /grōn′blad-strand′bərg/, an inherited disorder of connective tissue. Symptoms include premature aging and breakdown of the skin, gray or brown streaks on the retina, and blood vessel breakdown with retinal bleeding that causes loss of vision. Heart disease and high blood pressure are common. Also called **pseudoxanthoma elasticum.**

groove, a shallow furrow in various structures of the body. Grooves along the bones form channels for nerves; grooves in the bones connect the muscles to them.

gross, 1. referring to the study of tissue without magnification (macroscopic). 2. large or obese. Compare **microscopic.**

gross anatomy, the study of the organs or parts of the body large enough to be seen with the naked eye. Also called **macroscopic anatomy.**

gross sensory testing, a test of a patient's ability to sense motion at certain joints and to feel a touch on differing fingers.

ground, the background of a visual field, which can affect the ability of a patient to focus on an object.

ground itch, itching patches, pimples, and blisters of the skin caused by hookworm larvae. It occurs in warm climates and may be prevented by wearing shoes and by setting up sanitary disposal of feces. See also **hookworm.**

group, any collection of items or set of people under study. An **experimental group** is studied to determine the effect of an event, a substance, or a technique. A **control group** serves as a standard or reference for comparison with an experimental group.

group A beta-hemolytic streptococcal (GABHS) skin disease, a skin infection that affects mainly meat packers; symptoms range from mildly annoying to serious. It is probably caused by bacteria in freshly butchered meat.

group therapy, the use of psychotherapeutic techniques in a small group of persons. The group members, usually under the leadership of a psychotherapist, discuss their problems in an attempt to promote positive personal growth and change. The procedure treats a greater number of people in a shorter period of time than would be possible with individual therapy. It is used in clinics, in institutions, and in private practice. Group therapy has been found to be very effective in treating addictions. A kind of group therapy is **psychodrama.** See also **Gestalt therapy, psychotherapy, self-help group, transactional analysis.**

growing fractures, bone break that gradually separates at the edges. The cause often is pressure of soft tissues forcing the edges apart.

growing pains, 1. pains that occur in the muscles and joints of children or teenagers. They may be a result of fatigue, emotional problems, posture problems, and other causes that are not linked to growth. 2. emotional and psychological problems felt during adolescence.

growth, 1. an increase in the size of an organism or any of its parts, as measured in weight, volume, or linear dimensions. 2. the normal development of body, organs and mental powers from infancy to adulthood. In childhood, growth is measured according to approximate age at which physical changes usually appear and at which mental tasks are achieved. Such stages include the prenatal period, infancy, early childhood, middle childhood, and adolescence. There are two periods of accelerated growth. One is the first 12 months, in which the infant triples in weight, grows up to 50% of the height at birth, and rapidly develops mental, motor and social skills. The second is in the months around puberty, when the child nears adult height and secondary sexual characteristics emerge. 3. any abnormal limited increase of the size or number of cells, as in a tumor. Compare **development, differentiation, maturation.**

growth failure, a lack of normal body and mind growth. It may be a result of inherited, diet, disease, mental, or social problems. See also **failure to thrive, maternal deprivation syndrome.**

growth hormone (GH), a substance released by the pituitary gland in response to growth hormone releasing factor (GHRF) from the hypothalamus. GH promotes protein building in all cells, increases use of fatty acids for energy, and reduces use of carbohydrate. Growth effects depend on the presence of thyroid hormone, insulin, and carbohydrate. The release of GH, controlled mainly by the central nervous system, occurs in bursts. More than half the total daily amount is released during early sleep. A lack of GH causes dwarfism; an excess results in gigantism or acromegaly. Also called **somatotropic hormone, somatotropin.** See also **acromegaly, dwarfism, gigantism, somatostatin.**

growth hormone release inhibiting hormone. See **somatostatin.**

growth hormone releasing factor (GHRF), somatotropin-releasing factor released by the hypothalamus. Also called **somatoliberin.**

Grünfelder's reflex /grYn'feldərz/, an automatic curving of the great toe with a fanlike spreading of the other toes. It is caused by continued pressure on a membrane behind the ear. The reflex occurs in children who also have middle-ear disease.

grunting, abnormal, short loud breaks in breathing out. They often happen with severe chest pain. The grunt is made as the glottis briefly stops the flow of air, halting the movement of the lungs and their surrounding structures. Grunting is most often heard in a person who has pneumonia, fluid in the lungs, or broken or bruised ribs. Atelectasis in the newborn also causes grunting because of the work required for the baby to fill the lungs.

GU, abbreviation for **genitourinary.**

guaiac test, a test using a special solution (guaiac) on feces and urine to detect blood in the intestinal and urinary tracts.

guaifenesin, a white to slightly gray powder with a bitter taste and faint odor, widely used to cause coughing up of fluid. Guaifenesin increases the flow of fluid in the respiratory tract, thinning the bronchial fluids.

guanabenz acetate, a drug given for high blood pressure. Patients allergic to this drug should not take it. It can cause dizziness, sleepiness, and dry mouth.

guanadrel sulfate, a drug given for high blood pressure in patients who have not been helped by a thiazide-type diuretic. Patients who are taking certain other drugs, or who have heart trouble or allergy to this drug should not take it.

guanase. See **guanine deaminase.**

guanethidine sulfate, a drug given for mild and severe high blood pressure. Patients who are taking certain other drugs, or who have heart trouble or allergy to this drug should not take it. Among the more serious reactions are low blood pressure, salt and water buildup, slow heart beat, diarrhea, and impotence.

guanine /gwan'ēn/, a basic component of DNA and RNA. It occurs in trace amounts in most cells. See also **adenine.**

guaranine /gwərä'nin/, caffeine.

Gubbay test of motor proficiency, a screening test to identify any coordination problems according to the patient's age. It consists of eight activities, as whistling, throwing a tennis ball, and fitting shapes into appropriate slots. The results determine a clumsy from normal child.

Guedel's signs, a system for describing the stages of anesthesia during an operation.

Guérin's fracture /gãraNz'/, a fracture of the upper jaw. Also called **LeFort I fracture.**

guided imagery, a technique in which a patient focuses on mental images that help relieve pain or discomfort.

Guillain-Barré syndrome /gēyaN'bärā'/, a form of swelling of the nerves (polyneuritis). It begins between 1 and 3 weeks after a mild fever linked to a viral infection or with immunization. Pain and weakness affect the arms and legs, and paralysis may develop. The neuritis may spread to the trunk and involve the face, arms, and chest muscles. Some people may have few, mild symptoms while others may have symptoms severe enough to require critical nursing care. The disease resolves itself completely in a few weeks or a few months. Also called **acute febrile polyneuritis, acute idiopathic polyneuritis, infectious polyneuritis.**

Guinea worm infection. See **dracunculiasis.**

gullet. See **esophagus.**

gum, 1. a sticky fluid released by certain plants. **2.** See **gingiva.**

gumboil, an abscess of the gums and jawbone coming from injury, infection, or tooth decay. The gum is red, swollen, and tender. The abscess may break by itself, or it may require surgery. Also called **parulis.**

gumma /gum'ə/, *pl.* **gummas, gummata, 1.** a granuloma, caused by tertiary syphilis. It usually contains a mass of dead and swollen fiberlike tissue. Infectious syphilis germs may be found in a gumma. **2.** soft granuloma sores sometimes found with tuberculosis.

Gunning's splint, a splint used for supporting the jaws in surgery on the jaws.

gunshot fracture, a break caused by a bullet or similar missile.

Gunson method, (in radiology) an x-ray technique of the throat area during swallowing. A dark-colored shoestring is tied around the patient's throat just above the Adam's apple. The movement of the Adam's apple is then shown by the movement of the string.

Gunther's disease /gun'thərz/, an inherited disorder linked to sores brought on by sunlight. See also **porphyria.**

gurgling rale, an abnormal coarse sound heard through a stethoscope, especially over large hollows or over a windpipe nearly filled with fluids.

gurry /gur'ē/, *slang.* the body material cast off during an accident or during surgery or injury, including body fluids and tissue.

gustatory organ. See **taste bud.**

gut, 1. intestine. **2.** *informal.* stomach and bowels. **3.** thread used in surgery, made from the intestines of sheep.

Guthrie test /guth'rē/, a test for phenylketonuria. A small amount of blood is obtained from an infant and placed with a strain of a bacterium that cannot grow without phenylalanine. If phenylalanine is present, the bacteria reproduce and the test is positive. See also **phenylketonuria.**

gutta-percha, the solid, rubbery sap of various tropical trees. It is used for sealing prepared tooth cavities.

gutta-percha point, fine, tapered cylinders of gutta-percha that may be used to fill a root canal. Because they are easily seen on x-ray films, gutta-percha points are used to probe tooth hollows to measure their depth.

guttate psoriasis, a form of psoriasis made up of teardrop-shaped, red, scaly patches all over the body. A lung infection may cause this reaction in some patients. Compare **pustular psoriasis.** See also **psoriasis.**

Guyon tunnel, a tunnel formed under a ligament in the wrist through which the ulnar nerve and artery pass.

gynandrous /gīnan'drəs, jī-/, describing a man or a woman who has some of the physical characteristics usually found in the other sex, as a female pseudohermaphrodite. Compare **androgynous. –gynandry,** *n.*

gyneco-, gyn-, gyne-, gyno-, a combining form meaning a woman or the female sex.

gynecography /gīn'nə-, jin'əkog'rəfē/, an x-ray technique in which air is introduced into the abdomen to give a better picture of the female pelvic organs.

gynecoid pelvis, a type of pelvis found in women. The opening between the two pelvic bones is nearly round, the lowest bone of the spine (sacrum) is parallel to the back of the joint between the pelvic bones, the sidewalls are straight and the spines of the hip bones do not slant in. It is the ideal pelvic type for childbirth.

gynecologic examination. See **pelvic examination.**

gynecology /gī'nəkol'əjē, jī'-, jin'-/, a branch of medicine that deals with the health care of women. It is almost always studied and practiced along with obstetrics. **–gynecologic, gynecological,** *adj.*

gynecomastia /gī'nəkōmas'tē-ə, jī'-, jin'-/, an abnormal swelling of one or both breasts in men. The condition is usually temporary and harmless. It may be caused by hormonal imbalance, tumor of the testis or pituitary, drugs containing estrogen or steroids, or failure of the liver to dissolve estrogen in the bloodstream.

Gyne-Lotrimin, a trademark for a drug that fights fungus (clotrimazole).

gynephobia /gī′nəfō′bē·ə, jī′-, jin′-/, a deathly fear of women or an intense dislike of the company of women. It occurs almost always in men and may usually be traced to some frightening experience involving women that occurred in childhood.

gypsum, a mineral composed mostly of a crushed calcium compound. It is used in making plaster of Paris casts and molds for dentures. Gypsum dust may irritate the respiratory tract and the eyes.

gyrase /jī′rās/, an enzyme that enables certain DNA molecules to twist themselves into coils in order to reproduce.

-gyria, a combining form meaning the spinal twists of the brain.

gyri cerebri, the spiral twists of the outer surface of the two sides of the brain.

gyrus /jī′rəs/, *pl.* **gyri** /jī′rī/, one of the spiral twists of the surface of the brain caused by the folding in of the outer layer.

H

habit, 1. a usual way of behaving. 2. an unwilled pattern of behavior or thought. 3. the habitual use of drugs or narcotics. See also **habit spasm, habit training.**

habit spasm, an unwilled twitching or tic usually in a small muscle group of the face, neck, or shoulders that leads to movements as rapid blinking or jerking of the head to the side. The movements are often caused by emotions rather than any physical disorder. They may serve as a release for tension or worry.

habit training, the process of teaching a child how to adjust to the demands of the outside world by forming certain habits, mainly those related to eating, sleeping, elimination, and dress.

habitual abortion, abrupt ending of three pregnancies in a row before week 20. Habitual abortion can result from long-term infection, abnormal fetus, mother's hormone problems, or womb problems, as cervical incompetence. See also **cerclage, incompetent cervix.**

habitual fever. See **habitual hyperthermia.**

habitual hyperthermia, a condition of unknown cause that occurs in young females, causing body temperatures of 99° to 100.5° F regularly or off and on for years. Fatigue, sadness, vague aches and pains, loss of sleep, bowel problems, and headaches also occur. No organic cause can be found; the diagnosis is usually made only after a long period of observing the patient. No specific treatment is advised. Reassurance and psychotherapy offer the best relief. Also called **habitual fever.**

habituation, 1. psychological and emotional dependence on a drug, tobacco, or alcohol caused by repeated use, but without the addictive, physiological need to increase the dose. Compare **addiction.**

habitus /hab'itəs/, used to describe a person's looks or physique, as an athletic habitus. See also **habit.**

Haeckel's law. See **recapitulation theory.**

Haemophilus /hēmof'iləs/, disease-causing bacteria, often found in the breathing tract of humans and other animals.

Haemophilus influenzae, a bacterium found in the throats of 30% of healthy, normal people. In children and in weak older people, harmful swelling of the throat and lungs may result from infection. It can affect the heart or brain. Secondary infection by *H. influenzae* occurs with the flu and in many other lung diseases. There is an anti-*Haemophilus influenzae* serum available for protection against infection.

Hagedorn needle /hä′gedôrn/, a flat surgical needle with a cutting edge near its point and a very large eye at the other end.

Hageman factor. See **factor XII.**

Haglund's deformity, a foot disorder marked by an enlargement of the outside of the heel bone. It is a common cause of heel pain near the Achilles' tendon.

hair, a threadlike protein formed in the skin. There are three stages of hair development: **anagen,** the active growing stage; **catagen,** a short interlude between the growth and resting phases; and **telogen,** the resting, or club stage before shedding. Scalp hair grows at an average rate of 1 mm every 3 days, body and eyebrow hair at a much slower rate. Hair plucking does not stop hair growth. See also **hirsutism, lanugo.**

hair matrix carcinoma. See **basal cell carcinoma.**

hair pulling. See **trichotillomania.**

hairy-cell leukemia, a rare cancer of bloodforming tissues. Severe anemia and a very enlarged spleen, can occur. The disease occurs six times more often in men than in women. It usually appears in middle age with a gradual onset and features blood problems and sudden bruising. Removal of the spleen and chemotherapy are two treatments used. Also called **leukemic reticuloendotheliosis.**

hairy tongue, a dark, colored coating of the tongue that is a harmless and frequent side effect of some antibiotics. The condition improves with no treatment needed. See also **glossitis.**

halcinonide, a drug for use on the skin to reduce swelling.
★CAUTION: This should not be used where viral and fungal diseases of the skin, poor circulation, or known allergies to this drug or to steroid medicines exist.
★ADVERSE EFFECTS: Among the more serious side effects are skin rash and illness occurring from too long or excess use.

Halcion, a trademark for a sleeping pill (triazolam).

Haldol, a trademark for a tranquilizer (haloperidol).

half-life (t½), 1. the time needed for a radioactive substance to lose half of its activity through decay. 2. the time needed for a drug's level in the blood stream to go down to one half its beginning level. Also called **radioactive half-life. See also biologic half-life, effective half-life.**

half-sibling, one of two or more children who have at least one parent in common; a half brother or half sister. Also called **half-sib.**

halfway house, a special treatment facility, usually for mental patients who no longer need to stay in the hospital but who need some care and time to get used to living on their own.

halitosis /hal'itō'sis/, bad breath caused by poor oral hygiene, dental or mouth infections, the eating of certain foods, as garlic or alcohol, use of tobacco, or some diseases, as the odor of acetone in diabetes and ammonia in liver disease.

Hallpike caloric test, a way to check the function of the inner ear in patients with dizzy spells or hearing loss by running cool and warm water or air into the ears. See also **caloric test, nystagmus.**

hallucination, something sensed that is not caused by an outside event. It can occur in any of the senses and is so named, as auditory (hearing), gustatory (taste), olfactory (smell), tactile (feeling), or visual. Kinds of hallucinations are **hypnagogic hallucination, lilliputian hallucination, stump hallucination. –hallucinate,** *v.*

hallucinogen /həloo'sənəjen', hal'əsin'əjən, hal'yəsin'əjə/, a substance that excites the brain, causing hallucination; mood change; worry; mistakes of the senses or in judgments; loss of sense of self; increased pulse, temperature, and blood pressure; and widened pupils. Use of hallucinogens may lead to a habit, as well as possible depression or short-term insanity. Some kinds of hallucinogens are **lysergine, mescaline, peyote, phencyclidine hydrochloride,** and **psilocybin.**

hallucinosis /həloo'sinō'sis/, a diseased mental state in which one is aware mainly or only of hallucinations. A kind of hallucinosis is **alcoholic hallucinosis.**

hallux /hal'əks/, *pl.* **halluces** /hal'yoosēz/, the great toe.

hallux rigidus, a painful deformity of the great toe that limits motion at the joint where the toe joins the foot.

hallux valgus, a deformity in which the great toe is bent to the outside toward the other toes; in some cases the great toe rides over or under the other toes.

halo cast, a device used to help keep the neck and head from moving. It involves the trunk, usually with shoulder straps, and a way to fasten pins to a band around the skull. The halo cast is used to help the healing of back injuries and spine dislocations and to keep the back rigid after surgery.

halo effect, the helpful effect of a meeting, as may occur in the course of a research project or a health-care visit. The halo effect is not caused by the content of the interview or to any known act or treatment; it is the result of personal factors between the two people.

Halog, a trademark for a medicine for use on the skin to reduce swelling (halcinonide).

halogenated hydrocarbon, a general anesthetic. Nausea, vomiting, throat spasms, and soreness are less severe and frequent when this anesthesia is used. Kinds of halogenated hydrocarbons are **enflurane, halothane, isoflurane, methoxyflurane,** and **trichloroethylene.**

haloperidol /hal'ōper'ədôl/, a tranquilizer used to treat severe mental disorders and to control Gilles de la Tourette's syndrome.

haloprogin /hā'lōprō'jin/, a drug that kills bacteria and fungus, used for infections, as athlete's foot.

★CAUTION: Known allergy to this drug prevents its use.

★ADVERSE EFFECTS: Among the most serious side effects are worsening of existing sores, formation of blisters, and itching.

Halotestin, a trademark for a male hormone (fluoxymesterone).

Halotex, a trademark for an antibacterial (haloprogin).

halothane /hal'əthān/, an anesthetic that is inhaled to bring on and maintain general anesthesia.

★CAUTION: It is not advised for anesthesia during childbirth unless womb relaxation is needed.

★ADVERSE EFFECTS: Among the more serious side effects are liver cell death, heart attack, low blood pressure, nausea, and vomiting.

Halsted's forceps /hal'stedz/, **1.** also called **mosquito forceps.** A small, pointed forceps used to stop the flow of blood. **2.** a forceps with thin jaws for grasping arteries and other blood vessels.

hamamelis water. See **witch hazel,** def 2.

hamate bone /ham'āt/, a bone in the wrist, above the fourth and fifth fingers. Also called **os hamatum, unciform bone.**

Hamman-Rich syndrome. See **interstitial pneumonia.**

hammertoe, a toe permanently bent at the middle joint, causing a clawlike appearance. It may be present in more than one toe but is most common in the second toe.

hamstring muscle, any one of three muscles at the back of the thigh.

hamstring reflex, a normal, deep tendon reflex brought about by tapping one of the hamstring tendons behind the knee. This causes the tendon to contract and the knee to bend. The patient should be lying on his or her back with the knee and hip partly bent and the leg supported by the examiner's hand. See also **deep tendon reflex.**

hamstring tendon, one of the three tendons from the three hamstring muscles in the back of the thigh that connect the hamstring muscles to the knee.

hamular notch. See **pterygomaxillary notch.**

hand, the part of the upper limb below the forearm. It is the most flexible part of the skeleton and has a total of 27 bones. Also called **manus.**

handblock, a device made of a wood block several inches high with a firm handle that can be gripped by a disabled patient to give a certain amount of body support during activities, as getting into or out of a bed.

handedness, willed or unwilled preference for use of either the left or right hand. The preference is related to which side of the brain is dominant, with left-handedness occurring when the right side of the brain is dominant and vice versa. Also called **chirality, laterality.**

hand-foot syndrome. See **sickle cell crisis.**

handicapped, referring to a person who has an inborn or acquired mental or physical defect that interferes with normal functions of the body or the ability to be self-sufficient in modern society. Compare **disability.**

hangman's fracture, a break in the lower neckbones.

hangnail, a piece of partly disconnected skin of the cuticle or nail fold. Tearing the piece of skin causes a red, painful, easily infected sore. ("Hang" is not related to the verb but is an old English word for pain.) Early treatment is to trim the hangnail close with nail clippers. For red, sore cases an antibiotic ointment and protective bandage are used.

Hanot's disease /hanōz'/, gallbladder disease. See also **biliary cirrhosis.**

Hansen's disease. See **leprosy.**

haploid /hap'loid/, having a single set of chromosomes, as in sex cells. Also called **monoploid.** –**haploidy,** *n.*

haptics, the science concerned with studying the sense of touch. –**haptic,** *adj.*

haptoglobin /hap'tōglō'bin/, a blood protein. The quantity of haptoglobin is increased in certain long-term diseases and swelling disorders and is decreased or absent in some kinds of anemia. Compare **transferrin.** See also **hemoglobinemia, hemoglobinuria.**

hard data, information about a patient that is obtained by observation and measurement, including laboratory data, as opposed to information collected by talking to the patient.

hardening of the arteries, a disease in which arteries thicken and become less elastic (arteriosclerosis).

hard fibroma, a tumor composed of fiberlike tissue in which there are few cells. Also called **fibroma durum.**

hardness of x-rays, the relative penetrating power of x-rays. In general, the shorter the wavelength, the harder the radiation. Also called **hard radiation.** Compare **soft radiation.**

hard palate, the bony part of the roof of the mouth, behind the soft palate and bounded in front and on the sides by the gums and teeth. Compare **soft palate.**

hard radiation. See **hardness of x-rays.**

harelip. See **cleft lip.**

hare's eye. See **lagophthalmos.**

harlequin color, a short-term flushing of the skin on the lower side of the body with paleness of the upward side. Commonly seen in normal young infants, it disappears as the child matures.

harlequin fetus, an infant whose skin at birth is completely covered with thick, horny scales that look like armor and are divided by deep red splits. The condition is the most severe form of bony outgrowth of the newborn. The infant is stillborn or dies within a few days of birth. Also called **ichthyosis fetus.**

Harmonyl, a trademark for a high blood pressure medicine (deserpidine).

Harris tube, a tube used to remove pressure from the stomach and intestines. It contains mercury and is passed through the nose and carried through the digestive tract by gravity.

Hartmann's curet, a spoon shaped knife to remove adenoids. See also **curet.**

Hartnup's disease, an inborn disorder affecting the skin and mental state. Common symptoms of the disease are dry, scaly skin sores; irritation of tongue and stomach, diarrhea; mental problems; and allergy to the sun. Brief exposure to the sun may cause redness, swelling, and blisters. Treatment focuses on diet.

Harvard pump, a small pump that can be adjusted to give small amounts of liquid medicine through the vein. It is commonly used with drugs to bring on labor. Compare **Abbot pump.**

harvest fever. See **leptospirosis.**

harvest mite. See **chigger.**

Hashimoto's disease /hä'shimō'tōz/, a disease of the immune system that attacks the thyroid gland. The disease seems to be inherited, but it is 20 times more common in women than in men. It occurs most frequently between 30 and 50 years of age but may arise in young children. The thyroid develops a goiter which can cause difficult swallowing and a feeling of local pressure. Therapy with thyroid hormone is advised for patients with low thyroid levels and can prevent further growth of the goiter. Also called **Hashimoto's struma, Hashimoto's thyroiditis, lymphocytic thyroiditis, struma lymphomatosa.**

hashish. See **cannabis.**

Haverhill fever /hā'vəril/, a fever caused by infection with *Streptobacillus moniliformis*, carried by the bite of a rat. The bacterium is normally present in rat saliva. Usually the wound from the bite heals, but within 10 days fever, chills, vomiting, headache, muscle and joint pain, and a rash appear. Treatment with antibiotics is effective. Also called **streptobacillary ratbite fever.**

haversian canal /havur'shən/, one of the many tiny lengthwise canals in bone tissue. Each contains blood vessels, connective tissue, nerve fibers, and, sometimes, lymph vessels. The canals are connected to each other and are part of a complex network. See also **haversian canaliculus, haversian system, Volkmann's canal.**

haversian canaliculus, any one of the many tiny passages leading from the pits of bone tissue to larger haversian canals. See also **haversian canal, haversian system.**

haversian system, a circular section of bone tissue, consisting of plates in the bone around a central canal. See also **haversian canal, haversian canaliculus, Volkmann's canal.**

Hawthorne effect, a general, unintentional, but usually helpful effect on a person, a group of people, or the function of the system being studied. The Hawthorne effect is the effect of an encounter, as with a researcher or healthcare provider, or of a change in a program or facility, as by painting an office or changing the lighting system. The Hawthorne effect is likely to confuse the results of a study, because it is usually present and difficult to define.

hay fever, *informal.* an acute seasonal allergic irritation of the nose and sinuses caused by tree, grass, or weed pollens. Also called **pollinosis.** See also **allergic rhinitis, organic dust.**

hazard, a situation or thing that increases the chance of a loss from some danger that may cause injury or illness. **–hazardous,** *adj.*

Hb, abbreviation for **hemoglobin.**

HB, abbreviation for **hepatitis B.**

HCG radioreceptor assay, a urine test to detect pregnancy or missed abortion. The test is negative (within 2 hours) if the patient is not pregnant and positive (within 1 hour) if the patient is pregnant. Also called **pregnancy test.**

HCl, an abbreviation for *hydrochloride.*

headache, a pain in the head from any cause. Kinds of headaches include **functional headache, migraine headache, organic headache, sinus headache,** and **tension headache.** Also called **cephalalgia.**

head and neck cancer, any cancerous tumors of the upper breathing and eating tract, facial features, and organs in the neck, appearing as lumps or sores that usually produce early symptoms. Tumors of the mouth, lips, and tongue usually begin as a swelling or nonhealing sore that occur in men over 60 years of age. Long-term alcoholism, heavy use of tobacco, poor oral hygiene, syphilis, and Plummer-Vinson syndrome may help bring on these cancers. Cancers of the nose cause bleeding, blockage in breathing, and facial and dental pain. Upper throat tumors can involve nasal blockage, middle-ear problems, and hearing loss. Middle-throat tumors cause difficulty swallowing and breathing, pain, and lockjaw. Most lower-throat tumors cause hoarseness, difficulty swallowing and breathing, cough, and swollen glands. Other cancers can attack the salivary glands, jaw, and ear. Cancers of the tear glands, parathyroid, and eyes are all rare. Surgery and radiation are the main treatments, but their use may cause problems with swallowing and speaking. Chemotherapy is less effective because of the poor nutritional state of many patients with head or neck tumors. Plastic surgery and artificial parts are often needed to correct deformities and restore functions in patients who have had surgery or radiation on a head or neck tumor. See also specific cancer.

head, eye, ear, nose, and throat (HEENT), a specialty in medicine concerned with the structure, functions, and diseases of the head, eyes, ears, nose, and throat and with the diagnosis and treatment of disorders of those structures.

head injury, any damage to the head resulting from piercing the skull or from the brain knocking too fast against the skull. Blood vessels, nerves, and membranes enclosing the brain are torn; bleeding, pooling of fluid, and blockage of blood flow may result. Infection of the brain's enclosing membranes is a serious result that often follows breaking the bones of the cavities behind the nose. See also **concussion.**

head kidney. See **pronephros.**

head nurse, the manager of the personnel, including nurses working on a floor, ward, or unit.

head process, a strand of cells in the early stages of the embryo's development in animals with backbones (vertebrates). It is the group of cells around which the embryo develops. Also called **notochordal plate.**

Heaf test /hēf/, a tuberculin skin test using a method of several skin punctures. See also **tuberculin test.**

healing, the act or process in which the normal, healthy structures and functions are restored to parts of the body that were diseased, damaged, or not functioning. See also **intention, wound repair.**

health, a state of physical, mental, and social well-being and the absence of disease or other abnormal condition. It is a condition that involves constant change and adaptation to stress. See also **high-level wellness, homeostasis.**

health assessment, evaluating the health status of a patient by performing a physical examination after obtaining a health history. Various laboratory tests may also be ordered. A major part of care after the health assessment is counseling and education that may explain body functioning and that advises the patient on a healthful way of life. The techniques of the health assessment include feeling (palpation), tapping (percussion), listening (auscultation), and looking (observation).

health behavior, an action taken by a person to maintain, attain, or regain good health and to prevent illness. Health behavior comes from a person's health beliefs. Some common health behaviors are regular exercise, eating a balanced diet, and getting vaccinations on schedule.

health care consumer, any actual or potential receiver of health care, as a patient in a hospital, a client in a community mental health center, or a member of a prepaid health-maintenance organization.

health care industry, the complex of services provided by hospitals and other institutions, nurses, doctors, dentists, government agencies, voluntary agencies, clinics, drug and medical equipment companies, and health insurance companies.

health care system, the complete network of agencies, facilities, and all providers of health care in a certain geographic area. Nurses form the largest number of providers in a health care system.

health certificate, a statement signed by a health-care provider that tells the state of health of a person.

health consumer. See **health care consumer.**

health culture, a system that tries to explain and treat sickness and to maintain health. Health cultures are part of the larger culture or tradition of a people. It may be a popular or folk system, or it may be a technical or scientific one.

health economics, a social system that studies the supply and demand of health care resources and the impact of health services on a population.

health education, an educational program, directed to the general public, that attempts to improve, maintain, and safeguard the health of the community.

health history, (in nursing and medicine) a collection of information obtained from the patient and from other sources concerning the patient's physical status and psychological, social, and sexual functions. The history provides the basis for the diagnosis, treatment, care, and follow-up of the patient. The first part of the history describes the present illness (PI) and any factors or behaviors that make the symptoms better or worse. The patient's own words often serve as the best description and may be quoted. The second part of the history gives an account of previous illnesses, conditions, allergies, transfusions, immunizations, screening tests, and hospitalizations. A work history, describing the patient's work and exposure to stress, poisons, radiation, or other work hazards, may be included. The effect of the current illness on the patient's work is also

noted. A social history is taken in which the patient's social, cultural, and family settings are outlined, focusing on aspects that might have an effect on the current illness. In some cases a sexual history may be relevant. Kinds of history include **complete health history, episodic health history,** and **interval health history.** Also called **medical history.** See also **occupational history, review of systems, sexual history.**

health maintenance, a program planned to prevent illness, to maintain the best level of function, and to promote health. It is central to health care, especially to nursing care at all levels.

health maintenance, alterations in, a nursing diagnosis that describes the condition in which the patient is unable to identify, manage, or seek help to maintain health. The causes of the problem include the lack of or major changes in written, verbal, or other communication skills; mental damage or the inability to make careful and thoughtful judgments; damage to or lack of motor skills; lack of money; or the inability to cope. The defining features include a proven lack of knowledge about basic health practices or the inability to take responsibility for meeting those needs, the inability to adapt to changes around one, a lack of money or other resources or means of support, a history of the lack of health seeking behavior, or an increased interest in improving health behavior. See also **nursing diagnosis.**

Health Maintenance Organization (HMO), a type of group health care practice that provides health maintenance and treatment services to members who pay a flat, regular fee that is set without regard to the amount or kind of services received. Some of the first HMOs, Kaiser-Permanente among them, have shown that high-quality medical care can often be provided at less expense by such a system than by other health care systems. In addition to diagnostic and treatment services, including hospitalization and surgery, an HMO often offers extra services, as dental, mental, and eye care, and prescription drugs. Federal financial support for setting up HMOs was provided under Title XIII of the 1973 U.S. Public Health Service Act.

health physicist, a health scientist concerned with the potential hazards, to patients and health care providers, of using certain equipment and materials, as radioactive materials.

health physics, the study of the effects of radiation on the body and the methods for protecting people from the side effects of the radiation. Health physics is concerned with discovering new ways to protect people from these untoward effects. Also called **medical physics.**

health policy, 1. a statement about a goal in health care and a plan for reaching that goal; for example, to prevent an epidemic, a program for vaccinating a population is developed and put into practice.

health professional, any person who has completed a course of study in a field of health, as a registered nurse, physical therapist, or physician. The person is usually licensed by a government agency or certified by a professional organization.

health provider, any individual who provides health services to health care consumers.

health-related services, services other than medical care, given by a hospital or clinic, that may contribute directly or indirectly to the physical or mental health and well-being of patients. These may include personal or social services.

health resources, all materials, personnel, facilities, funds, and anything else that can be used for providing health care and services.

health risk, a factor that increases one's chances for illness or death. These factors may include social or income levels, certain individual behaviors, family and individual histories, and certain physical changes.

health risk appraisal, a process of determining the likelihood that a person may develop prematurely a health problem having a high illness and death rate.

health screening, a program designed to evaluate the health state and potential of an individual. In the process it may be found that a person has a certain disease or condition or is at greater than normal risk of developing it. Health screening may include taking a personal and family health history and performing a physical examination, laboratory tests, and x-ray tests. These may be followed by counseling, education, referral, or further testing.

health service area, a geographic region organized under the National Health Planning and Resources Development Act of 1974, for the effective planning and development of health services.

health supervision, health teaching, counseling, or keeping track of the state of the patient's health. This does not include actual physical care. Such supervision occurs in health care agencies, clinics, doctor's offices, or the patient's home. Compare **care of the sick.**

health systems agency (HSA), an agency established under the terms of the National Health Planning and Resources Development Act of 1974. Health planning agencies are intended to provide health planning and fund raising services in each of several health service areas established by the Act. Health systems agencies are nonprofit and include private organizations, public regional planning bodies, or local government agencies and consumers. See also **health systems plan.**

health systems plan, a plan in which the long-range health goals of a health services area are specified. Health systems plans are prepared by health systems agencies. See also **health policy.**

hearing, the special sense that allows sound to be perceived. It is the major function of the ear. Hearing loss can range from mild damage to complete deafness. See also **deafness.**

hearing aid, an electronic device that increases the volume of sound for persons with damaged hearing. The device consists of a microphone, a battery power supply, an amplifier, and a receiver. The microphone receives sound waves, the sound waves are changed to electric impulses that are amplified with the aid of the power supply, and the receiver converts the electric impulses back into sound vibrations. The receiver is designed, depending on the cause of the hearing loss, to send sound through the outer ear canal or through the skull. See also **cochlear implants.**

heart, the muscular, cone-shaped organ, about the size of a clenched fist, that pumps blood throughout the body. It beats normally about 70 times per minute by balanced nerve impulses and muscle squeezes. The organ is about 12 cm long, 8 cm wide at its broadest part, and 6 cm thick. The weight of the heart in men averages between 280 and 340 g and in women, between 230 and 280 g. The layers of the heart, starting from the outside, are the epicardium, the myocardium, and the endocardium. The chambers of the heart include two ventricles with thick muscular walls, making up most of the organ, and two atria with thin muscular walls. An inner wall (septum) separates the ventricles and extends between the atria, dividing the heart into the right and the left sides. The left side of the heart pumps blood with oxygen from the lung veins into the aorta and on to all parts of the body. The right side of the heart pumps blood from which the oxygen has been removed into the lung arteries. Both atria contract almost at the same time, followed quickly by the con traction of the ventricles. Factors affecting the pulse rate are emotion, exercise, hormones, temperature, pain, and stress.

heart block, an interference with the normal travel of electric impulses that control activity of the heart muscle. The delay or block can occur in a number of different locations in the heart. See also **atrioventricular block, bundle branch block, cardiac conduction defect, infranodal block, intraatrial block, intraventricular block, sinoatrial block.**

heartburn, a painful burning sensation in the throat (esophagus) just below the breastbone. Heartburn is usually caused by stomach contents flowing back into the esophagus but may be caused by too much acid in the stomach or

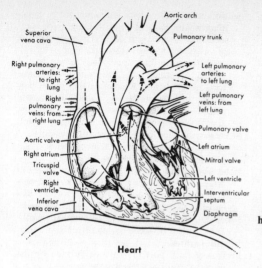

Aortic arch
Superior vena cava
Pulmonary trunk
Right pulmonary arteries: to right lung
Left pulmonary arteries: to left lung
Right pulmonary veins: from right lung
Left pulmonary veins: from left lung
Pulmonary valve
Aortic valve
Left atrium
Right atrium
Mitral valve
Tricuspid valve
Left ventricle
Right ventricle
Interventricular septum
Inferior vena cava
Diaphragm

Heart

peptic ulcer. Antacids relieve the symptoms but do not cure the heartburn. Also called **pyrosis.** See also **gastroesophageal reflux, hiatus hernia.**

heart failure, a condition in which the heart cannot pump enough blood to meet the metabolic needs of body tissues. Extreme exertion may cause heart failure in patients with normal hearts if there is a mismatch between the needs of the body and the volume of blood pumped by the heart. Many patients develop heart failure from more than one cause. Many of the symptoms linked to heart failure are caused by the malfunction of organs other than the heart, especially the lungs, kidneys, and liver. Heart failure is closely linked to many forms of heart disease and is commonly diagnosed only after the diagnosis of heart disease. Most kinds of heart disease first affect the left side of the heart, and clinicians commonly divide heart failures into left-sided heart failure and right-sided heart failure. Swelling of hands and feet occurs with right-sided heart failure and difficulty in breathing with left-sided heart failure. Current studies indicate that heart failure in infants and children is usually the result of inherited heart disease. The common causes of heart failure after 40 years of age are coronary hardening of the arteries with coagulation of blood inside the heart, high blood pressure, disease of the heart valves, lung disease, and general damage to the heart muscle. Some individuals may suffer heart failure caused by a combination of inherited heart disease and acquired disease. Some of the factors that may cause heart failure in heart-disease patients without symptoms are sudden strenuous effort, increased work load, too much salt in the diet, sudden emotional upset, and the giving of ex-

cessive volumes of fluids by vein. The treatment for heart failure commonly involves reducing the workload of the heart, giving certain drugs, as digitalis, to increase heart-muscle strength, salt-free diets, diuretics, and surgery. Many patients with heart failure, especially elderly patients, become constipated and require laxatives, as mineral oil, milk of magnesia, and cascara sagrada. The sudden onset of fluid in the lungs linked to some cases of heart failure is a life-threatening condition requiring immediate treatment. This condition of fluid in the lungs (acute pulmonary edema) may sometimes be confused with bronchial asthma, and caution is required in the giving of appropriate drugs. See also **compensated heart failure, congestive heart failure.**

heart-lung machine, a machine that takes over the functions of the heart and lungs, especially during heart surgery. The blood is detoured from the veins through an oxygenator, where oxygen is added to the blood, and returned to the arteries.

heart massage. See **cardiac massage.**

heart murmur. See **cardiac murmur.**

heart rate, the pulse, figured by counting the number of contractions of the heart per unit of time. Tachycardia is a heart rate of more than 100 beats per minute; bradycardia is a heart rate of fewer than 60 beats per minute. See also **pulse.**

heart scan, an image of the heart, obtained after injecting a radioactive material into a vein. It is used for determining the size, shape, and location of the heart, for diagnosing pericarditis, and for viewing the chambers of the heart. See also **cardiography, echocardiogram.**

heart sound, a normal noise produced within the heart during the heart-beat cycle that may reveal abnormal heart structure or function.

heart surgery, any surgery involving the heart. It may be done to correct acquired or inherited defects, to replace diseased valves, to open or bypass blocked vessels, or to put an artificial part or a transplant in place. Two major types of heart surgery are performed—closed and open. The closed technique is done through a small cut, without using the heart-lung machine. In the open technique the heart chambers are open and fully visible, and blood is detoured around the area by the heart-lung machine. The mortality rate is highest during the first 48 hours after surgery. Kinds of heart surgery include **Blalock-Taussig procedure, coronary bypass,** and **endarterectomy.** See also **arrhythmia, fibrillation, heart-lung machine, hypothermia, pulmonary edema.**

heart valve, one of the four structures in the heart that control the flow of blood by opening and closing with each heart beat. The valves permit the flow of blood in only one direction, and any one of the valves may become defective, permitting the backflow linked to heart murmurs. Also called **cardiac valve**. See also **heart, semilunar valve, tricuspid valve**.

heat cramp, any cramp in the arm, leg, or stomach caused by too little water and salt in the body because of heat exhaustion. It usually occurs after vigorous physical exertion in very hot weather or under other conditions that cause heavy sweating and use up body fluids and salts. Also called **cane-cutter's cramp, fireman's cramp, miner's cramp, stoker's cramp**. See also **heat exhaustion**.

heated nebulization, a method of breathing therapy using a heating device that makes a spray with a higher water content than that of a cold atomizer. The mist may be given through a mask or in a tent. Croup in infancy is often treated with a heated nebulizer.

heat exhaustion, an abnormal condition marked by weakness, dizziness, nausea, muscle cramps, and fainting. It is caused by low levels of body fluid and salts resulting from exposure to intense heat or the inability to adjust to heat. Body temperature is near normal; blood pressure may drop but usually returns to normal as the person is placed in a lying-down position; the skin is cool, damp, and pale. The person usually recovers with rest and replacement of water and salt. Compare **heat hyperpyrexia**. See also **heat cramp**.

heat hyperpyrexia, a severe and sometimes fatal condition that results from the failure of the body to regulate its temperature. This is caused by prolonged exposure to the sun or to high temperatures. Lessening or lack of sweating is an early symptom. Body temperature of 105° F or higher, fast pulse rate, hot and dry skin, headache, confusion, blackouts, and convulsions may occur. Treatment includes cooling, resting, and fluid replacement. Also called **heatstroke, siriasis, sunstroke**. See also **hyperpyrexia**. Compare **heat exhaustion**.

heat labile. See **thermolabile**.

heat rash, a pimpling or blistery reddening of the skin that results from excess exposure to heat and high humidity. Tingling and prickling sensations are common. Prevention and treatment include cool, dry temperatures, a good flow of air, and absorbent powders. See also **miliaria**.

heatstroke. See **heat hyperpyrexia**.

heaves, 1. a long-term breathing disease of horses, similar to emphysema. The symptoms are wheezing, coughing, and difficult breathing on exertion. The causes of the condition are unknown. **2.** *informal.* vomiting and retching.

heavy metal, a metallic element with a specific gravity five or more times that of water. The heavy metals are antimony, arsenic, bismuth, cadmium, cerium, chromium, cobalt, copper, gallium, gold, iron, lead, manganese, mercury, nickel, platinum, silver, tellurium, thallium,

tin, uranium, vanadium, and zinc. Small amounts of many of these elements are common and necessary in the diet. Large amounts of any of them may cause poisoning.

heavy metal poisoning, poisoning caused by the eating, breathing, or absorption of various toxic heavy metals. Kinds of heavy metal poisoning include **antimony poisoning, arsenic poisoning, cadmium poisoning, lead poisoning,** and **mercury poisoning**. See also **heavy metal**.

heavy vaginal bleeding. See **vaginal bleeding**.

hebephrenia, hebephrenic schizophrenia. See **disorganized schizophrenia**.

Heberden's node /hē'bərdənz/, an abnormal enlargement of bone or cartilage in a joint of a finger. This most often occurs in wasting diseases of the joints. Compare **Bouchard's node**.

hebetude /heb'itood'/, a state of dullness or lethargy, typical of some forms of schizophrenia.

heboid paranoia. See **paranoid schizophrenia**.

heel, the back part of the foot, formed by the largest tarsal bone, the calcaneus.

heel-knee test, a way to check coordination of movements of the legs. In the test the patient, lying face down, is asked to touch the knee of one leg with the heel of the other.

heel-shin test, a way to check coordination of movements of the legs. In the test the patient, lying face down, is asked to pass the heel of one leg slowly down the shin of the other leg from the knee to the ankle.

HEENT, abbreviation for **head, eyes, ears, nose, and throat**.

Hegar's sign /hā'gärz/, a softening of the uterine cervix early in pregnancy. It is a probable sign of pregnancy.

height, the measurement of a structure, organ, or other object from bottom to top, when it is placed or viewed in an upright position.

Heimlich maneuver /hīm'lik/, an emergency technique for dislodging a piece of food or other object lodged in the windpipe to prevent suffocation. The choking person is grasped from behind by the rescuer whose fist, thumb side in, is placed just below the victim's breastbone with the other hand placed firmly over

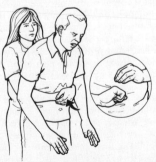

Heimlich maneuver

the fist. The rescuer then pulls the fist firmly and abruptly into the top of the stomach, forcing the blockage up the windpipe. If repeated attempts do not free the airway, an emergency incision in the windpipe (tracheotomy) may be necessary. See also **cardiopulmonary resuscitation.**

Heinz bodies /hīnts/, oddly shaped bits of altered hemoglobin found in the red blood cells of persons who are allergic to certain chemicals.

Heliodorus' bandage. See **T bandage.**

helium therapy, the use of helium gas mixtures to treat patients with blocked airways. Because it is a lighter gas than nitrogen, less pressure is needed to drive the helium past the obstruction.

helix, a coiled, spiral-like formation typical of many organic molecules, as deoxyribonucleic acid (DNA).

Heller's test, a laboratory test for protein in the urine. The urine is spread on nitric acid. If a ring appears between the two fluids, protein is present.

helminth /hel'minth/, a worm, especially one of the disease-causing parasites of the division Metazoa fluke. These include flukes, tapeworms, and roundworms.

helminthiasis /hel'minthī'əsis/, a disease caused by invasion of the body by worms (helminths) that may be in the skin, muscles or intestines. Ascariasis, bilharziasis, filariasis, hookworm, and trichinosis are common forms of the disease.

helper T cell. See **T cell.**

helper virus, a virus that must be present if another defective virus is to successfully copy itself.

helplessness, a feeling of a loss of control, usually after repeated failures, of being unable to move or frozen by circumstances beyond one's control, with the result that one is unable to make decisions.

helvolic acid /helvol'ik/, an antibiotic, made from the mold *Aspergillus fumigatus.* Also called **fumagillin, fumigacin.**

hemadsorption /hē'madsôrp'shən, hem'-/, a process in which a substance or an agent, as certain viruses, sticks to the surface of a red blood cell. The process occurs naturally, or it may be brought about for laboratory study of bacteriological specimens.

hemagglutination /hē'məgloo'tinā'shən, hem'-/, a reaction between germs and the body's defenses that causes red cells to clump together. See **ABO blood groups.**

hemagglutinin, a kind of antibody that causes red blood cells to clump together.

hemangioblastoma /hēman'jē-ōblastō'mə/, *pl.* **hemangioblastomas, hemangioblastomata,** a brain tumor made up of an excess growth of small blood vessels and vessel-forming cells.

hemangioendothelioma /hēman'jē-ō·en'dōthē'-lē·ō'mə/, *pl.* **hemangioendotheliomas, hemangioendotheliomata, 1.** also called **angioendothelioma.** A tumor that grows around an artery or a vein. The harmless form is seen in children and is usually cured by simple removal. It rarely becomes cancerous. **2.** cancerous hemangioendothelioma. See also **angiosarcoma.**

hemangioma /hēman'jē-ō'mə/, *pl.* **hemangiomas, hemangiomata,** a harmless tumor made up of a mass of blood vessels. Kinds of hemangiomas include **capillary hemangioma, cavernous hemangioma,** and **nevus flammeus.**

hemangioma simplex. See **capillary hemangioma.**

hemangiosarcoma. See **angiosarcoma.**

hematemesis /hē'mətem'əsis, hem'-/, vomiting of bright red blood, indicating rapid bleeding of the upper digestive tract. It is often linked to enlarged veins in the gullet or peptic ulcer. See also **gastrointestinal bleeding.**

hematocele /hem'ətōsēl'/, a blood-filled sac in part of the scrotum. It is usually caused by injury and may require surgery.

hematochezia, the passage of red blood through the rectum. The cause is usually bleeding in the colon or rectum, but it can result from the loss of blood higher in the digestive tract. Blood passed from the stomach or small intestine generally loses its red color because of contact with enzymes. Cancer, colitis, and ulcers are among causes of hematochezia. Compare **melena.**

hematocrit /himat'ōkrit/, a measure of the number of red cells found in the blood, stated as a percentage of the total blood volume. The normal range is between 43% and 49% in men, and between 37% and 43% in women. See also **complete blood count, differential white blood cell count.**

hematogenic shock, a condition of shock caused by the loss of blood or plasma.

hematogenous /hēmətoj'ənəs/, coming from or carried in the blood.

hematologic death syndrome, a group of symptoms of radiation damage to the blood cells, marked by nausea, vomiting, fever, diarrhea, infections, anemia, bleeding, and a decrease in the number of white blood cells. The average survival time for someone with this condition is between 10 and 60 days.

hematologic effect, (in radiology) the response of blood cells to radiation. In general, all types of blood cells are destroyed by radiation, the more the radiation, the more the destruction. However, white blood cells are affected first and reduced in number within minutes or hours after exposure to radiation. Red blood cells are less sensitive and may not show radiation effects for several weeks.

hematologist /hē'mətol'əjist, hem'-/, a physician who specializes in the study of blood and its diseases (hematology).

hematology /hē'mətol'əjē, hem'-/, the scientific medical study of blood and blood-forming tissues. **-hematologic, hematological,** *adj.*

hematoma /hē'mətō'mə, hem'-/, *pl.* **hematomas, hematomata,** a collection of blood that has escaped from the vessels and becomes trapped in the tissues of the skin or in an organ. This can result from injury or surgery. First, there is frank bleeding into the space; if the space is limited, pressure slows and eventually stops the flow of blood. The blood clots, the clot hardens, and the mass can be felt by the examiner and is often painful to the patient. A hematoma may be drained early in the process and bleeding stopped with pressure. If necessary, the bleeding may be stopped by surgically tying off the bleeding vessel. Much blood may be lost, and infection is a serious complication. Also called **blood blister.**

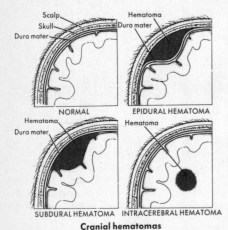

Cranial hematomas

-hematoma, a combining form meaning a 'swelling containing blood.'

hematomyelia, the appearance of blood in the fluid of the spinal cord.

hematopoiesis /hē'mətōpō·ē'sis, hem'-/, the normal formation and development of blood cells in the bone marrow. In severe anemia and other blood disorders, cells may be produced in organs outside the marrow (extramedullary hematopoiesis). See also **erythropoiesis.** **-hematopoietic,** *adj.*

hematopoietic syndrome, a group of symptoms linked with the effects of radiation on the blood and lymph tissues. It is marked by nausea and vomiting, loss of appetite, tiredness, destruction of blood cells and bone marrow, and a decrease in size of the spleen and lymph nodes.

hematospermia, the presence of blood in the semen. Causes may include infection, interrup-

tion of sexual intercourse, frequent sex, or lack of sex. The condition is rarely serious and may respond to antibiotics.

hematuria /hē'mətōōr'ē·ə, hem'-/, abnormal presence of blood in the urine. Hematuria can be caused by many kidney diseases and disorders of the genital and urinary systems. **-hematuric,** *adj.*

heme /hēm/, the colored, nonprotein part of the hemoglobin molecule in the blood that contains iron. Heme carries oxygen in the red blood cells, releasing it to tissues that give off excess amounts of carbon dioxide (CO_2). See also **hemoglobin, porphobilinogen, protoporphyrin.**

hemeralopia /hem'ərəlō'pē·ə/, an abnormal visual condition in which bright light causes blurring of vision. Hemeralopia is an unpleasant side effect of certain medications used to prevent convulsions (anticonvulsants), as in treating children affected with petit mal epilepsy. Also called **day blindness, night sight. -hemeralopic,** *adj.*

-hemia. See **-emia.**

hemiacephalus, a deformed fetus in which the brain and most of the skull are lacking. See also **anencephaly.**

hemianesthesia, a loss of feeling on one side of the body.

hemianopia, defective vision or blindness in one half of the visual field.

hemiarthroplasty /hem'ē·är'thrəplas'tē/, surgery for the repair of an injured or diseased hip joint. It involves the replacement of the top of the thigh bone (head of the femur) without replacement of the hip socket.

hemiataxia, a loss of muscle control affecting one side of the body, usually from a stroke or injury to the part of the brain that controls movement (cerebellum). It can be on the same side or the opposite side from the injury.

hemiazygous vein /hem'ē·əzī'gəs/, a vein in the trunk of the body.

hemiballismus. See **ballismus.**

hemicellulose /hem'ēsel'yŏŏlōs/, a type of carbohydrate that makes up most of the stiff portion of the cell walls of plants. It resembles cellulose but is easier to dissolve and to digest. See also **dietary fiber.**

hemicephalia, a birth defect consisting of the absence of one side of the top layer of the brain. It is caused by the halt of brain growth in the fetus.

hemicephalus, a deformed fetus lacking one half of the upper brain.

hemicrania, 1. a headache, usually migraine, that affects only one side of the head. **2.** a birth defect in which one half of the skull in the fetus is missing.

hemidiaphragm, either the left or right side of the diaphragm. Although the diaphragm is a single structure, the right and left halves are supplied by separate nerves, and each side can function separately from the other.

hemiectromelia, a birth defect in which the limbs on one side of the body are not fully formed. **–hemiectromelus,** *n.*

hemignathia /hem′ēnā′thē·ə/, **1.** a birth defect in which the lower jaw on one side of the face is not fully formed. **2.** a condition of having only one jaw. **–hemignathus,** *n.*

hemihyperplasia, overdevelopment or excessive growth of one-half of a specific organ or body part, or of all the organs and parts on one side of the body.

hemihypoplasia, partial or incomplete development of one-half of a specific organ or body part, or of all the organs and parts on one side of the body.

hemikaryon /hem′ēker′ē·on/, a cell nucleus that contains the halved (haploid) number of chromosomes, or one-half of the diploid number, as that of the sex cells. Compare **amphikaryon.** **–hemikaryotic,** *adj.*

hemimelia, a growth disorder marked by the absence or extreme shortening of the lower portion of one or more of the limbs. The condition may involve either or both of the bones of the lower arm or leg and is named for whichever is absent or defective, as fibular, radial, tibial, or ulnar hemimelia. See also **ectromelia, phocomelia.**

hemipagus /hemip′əgəs/, evenly joined twins who are united at the chest.

hemiparesis, muscular weakness of one-half of the body.

hemiplegia /hem′iplē′jə/, paralysis of one side of the body. Kinds of hemiplegia are **cerebral hemiplegia, facial hemiplegia, infantile hemiplegia,** and **spastic hemiplegia.** Also called **unilateral paralysis.** Compare **diplegia, paraplegia, quadriplegia. –hemiplegic,** *adj.*

hemisomus /hem′isō′məs/, a fetus or patient in which one side of the body is malformed, defective, or absent.

hemisphere, 1. one-half of a sphere or globe. **2.** the lateral half of the brain. **–hemispheric, hemispherical,** *adj.*

hemiteras /hem′ēter′əs/, *pl.* **hemiterata,** any patient with a birth defect that is not so severe or disabling as to be called a monstrous (teratic) condition. **–hemiteratic,** *adj.*

hemivertebra, an abnormal birth defect in which a backbone (vertebra) fails to develop completely. As a result of the growth defect of the spine, a wedge-shaped vertebra develops, and neighboring vertebrae expand or tilt to fit the deformity. A singular hemivertebra may pose few if any signs and symptoms. Depending on the degree of curvature of the spine involved, any related deformity may become more apparent with growth.

hemoblastic leukemia. See **stem cell leukemia.**

hemochromatosis /hē′mōkrō′mətō′sis, hem′-/, a rare disease in which iron deposits build up throughout the body. Enlarged liver, skin discoloration, diabetes mellitus, and heart failure may occur. The disease most often develops in men over 40 years of age and as a result of some anemias requiring multiple blood transfusions. Compare **hemosiderosis.** See also **iron metabolism, siderosis, thalassemia.**

hemoconcentration, an increase in the number of red blood cells resulting either from a decrease in the liquid content of blood or increased production of red cells.

hemocytoblastic leukemia. See **stem cell leukemia.**

hemodiafiltration, a technique similar to hemofiltration used to remove waste products, especially uric acid, from the blood.

hemodialysis /hē′mōdī·al′isis, hem′-/, a procedure in which impurities or wastes are removed from the blood. It is used in treating kidney failure and to remove poison from the blood. The patient's blood is run from the body through a machine to be filtered and is then returned to the patient's blood vessels. See also **arteriovenous fistula, external shunt.** ★METHOD: The bloodstream is dialyzed by means of tubes or needles put into a large vein and a large artery. The procedure takes from 3 to 8 hours and may be needed daily in serious situations or two or three times a week in longterm kidney failure.

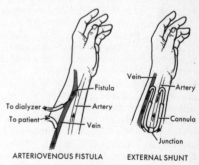

ARTERIOVENOUS FISTULA   EXTERNAL SHUNT
Hemodialysis

hemodialysis technician, a registered nurse who has received special training in the operation of hemodialysis equipment and treatment of patients with kidney disorders.

hemodialyzer. See **dialyzer.**

hemodynamics, the study of factors affecting the force and flow of circulating blood.

Hemofil, a trademark for a human antibleeding medication.

hemofiltration, a type of hemodialysis used to remove waste products, especially uric acid, from the blood.

hemoglobin (Hb) /hē'məglō'bən/, a complex protein-iron compound in the blood that carries oxygen to the cells from the lungs and carbon dioxide away from the cells to the lungs. Each red blood cell contains 200 to 300 molecules of hemoglobin. Each molecule of hemoglobin contains several molecules of heme, each of which can carry one molecule of oxygen. See also **carboxyhemoglobin, complete blood count, differential white blood cell count, erythrocyte, erythropoiesis, heme, hemoglobinopathy, hemolysin, oxyhemoglobin,** and see specific hemoglobins.

hemoglobin A (Hb A), a normal hemoglobin. Also called **adult hemoglobin.** Compare **hemoglobin F.** See also **hemoglobinopathy, hemoglobin variant.**

hemoglobin C (Hb C) disease, an inherited blood disorder involving mild but long-term destruction of red blood cells. It is related to the presence of hemoglobin C, an abnormal form of the red cell-coloring substance. See also **hemoglobin variant.**

hemoglobin electrophoresis, a test to identify various abnormal hemoglobins in the blood, including certain inherited disorders, as sickle cell anemia.

hemoglobinemia /hē'mōglō'binē'mē·ə, hem'-/, presence of free hemoglobin in the blood plasma.

hemoglobin F (Hb F), the normal hemoglobin of the fetus, most of which is broken down in the first days after birth and replaced by hemoglobin A. It can carry more oxygen and is present in increased amounts in some diseases, including sickle cell anemia, aplastic anemia, and leukemia. Small amounts are produced throughout life.

hemoglobinopathy /hē'mōglō'binop'əthē, hem'-/, any of a group of inherited disorders known by changes in the structure of the hemoglobin molecule. Kinds of hemoglobinopathies include **hemoglobin C disease, hemoglobin S-C disease,** and **sickle cell anemia.** Compare **thalassemia.** See also **hemoglobin, hemoglobin A, sickle cell thalassemia, sickle cell trait.**

hemoglobin S (Hb S), an abnormal type of hemoglobin that causes sickle cell anemia, a disorder in which the blood cells tend to become sickle-shaped, to move slowly, to clump together, and to break down. See also **hemoglobin variant, sickle cell anemia, sickle cell crisis, sickle cell trait.**

hemoglobinuria, an abnormal presence in the urine of hemoglobin that is unattached to red blood cells. Hemoglobinuria can result from various diseases of the body's defense system or certain blood disorders. Kinds of hemoglobinuria include **cold hemoglobinuria, march hemoglobinuria,** and **nocturnal hemoglobinuria.**

hemoglobin variant, any type of hemoglobin other than hemoglobin A, the normal hemoglobin. These variations are determined in the genes and, depending on the kind and extent of change, result in changed physical and chemical function of the red blood cells. See also **hemoglobinopathy, hemoglobin S, sickle cell thalassemia.**

hemogram, a written record or graph of a count of the solid components of the blood. See also **complete blood count.**

hemolysin /himol'əsin/, any one of the many substances that dissolve red blood cells. Hemolysins are produced by many kinds of bacteria, including some of the staph and strep germs. They are also found in venoms and in certain vegetables. Hemolysins appear to aid the bacteria in invading blood cells. See also **hemoglobin, hemolysis.**

hemolysis /himol'isis/, the breakdown of red blood cells and the release of hemoglobin. It occurs normally at the end of the life span of a red cell. However, it may occur under many other circumstances, as when fighting off disease or as a side effect of hemodialysis or artificial heart aids, as pacemakers. Adding excessive liquid to the blood by vein can also cause hemolysis. See also **hemolysin, hemolytic anemia, transfusion reaction.** –**hemolytic,** *adj.*

hemolytic anemia, a disorder involving the premature destruction of red blood cells. Anemia may be slight or absent if the bone marrow is able to increase production of red blood cells. The condition may occur with some infectious diseases, with certain inherited red cell disorders, or as a response to drugs or other poisonous agents. Compare **aplastic anemia, congenital nonspherocytic hemolytic anemia, iron deficiency anemia, myelophthisic anemia, nonspherocytic anemia.** See also **anemia, hemolysis, spherocytosis.**

hemolytic jaundice, a yellowish discoloration of the skin caused by a breakdown of red blood cells.

hemolytic uremia syndrome, a rare kidney disorder, the cause of which is unknown, that usually occurs in infancy.

hemopericardium, a buildup of blood within the sac surrounding the heart.

hemoperitoneum, a buildup of blood surrounding the organs in the trunk of the body.

hemophilia /hē'mōfē'lyə, hem'-/, a group of hereditary bleeding disorders in which there is a lack of one of the factors needed to clot the blood. The severity of the disorder varies greatly with the extent of the lack. Greater-than-usual loss of blood during dental work, nosebleeds, blood blisters, and bleeding into the joints are common problems in hemophilia. Severe internal bleeding is less common. See **von Willebrand's disease,** specific blood factors. **–hemophiliac,** *n.,* **hemophilic,** *adj.*

Defective gene is found on X chromosome. When faulty X chromosome is present in a male, the male will be a hemophiliac.

Ⓧ Y

When faulty X chromosome is present in a female, she will be a carrier of hemophilia.

Ⓧ X

In conception between a normal male and a carrier female, four possibilities arise:

Ⓧ X ——— XY

Ⓧ Y
Hemophiliac son (mother's carrier X)

XY
Normal son (mother's good X chromosome)

Ⓧ X
Carrier daughter (mother's carrier X and father's X)

XX
Normal daughter (mother's good X and father's X)

XX ——— Ⓧ Y

XY   Ⓧ x

In conception between a hemophiliac male and a normal female, son will be normal but daughter will be carrier.

Hemophilia inheritance pattern

hemophilia A, a hereditary blood disorder, considered the classic type of hemophilia in contrast to hemophilia B and hemophilia C, which may be less severe. See also **coagulation factor, hemophilia.**

hemophilia B, a hereditary blood disorder, similar to but less severe than hemophilia A. Also called **Christmas disease.** See **coagulation factor, hemophilia.**

hemophilia C, a hereditary blood disorder, similar to but less severe than hemophilia A. Also called **Rosenthal's syndrome.** See also **coagulation factor, hemophilia.**

hemopoietic /hē'mōpō-et'ik, hem'-/, related to the production and growth of various types of blood cells.

hemoptysis /himop'tisis/, coughing up of blood from the respiratory tract. Blood-streaked spit often occurs in minor infections of the upper breathing tract or in bronchitis. Heavier bleeding may indicate *Aspergillus* infection, lung abcess, tuberculosis, or cancer. Treatment includes watching the patient for signs of shock, preventing suffocation, and stopping the bleeding. Antibiotics and cough medicines may be given. Sedatives and tranquilizers are not given because they tend to make breathing shallower. Compare **hematemesis.**

hemorrhage, a loss of a large amount of blood in a short period of time, either outside or inside the body. Hemorrhage may be from arteries, veins, or capillaries.

★DIAGNOSIS: Symptoms are related to shock:

rapid pulse, thirst, cold and clammy skin, sighing breaths, dizziness; fainting, paleness, apprehension, restlessness, and low blood pressure. If bleeding is within a cavity or joint, pain will develop as the cavity is stretched by the rapidly expanding amount of blood.

★TREATMENT: All effort is made to stop the bleeding. If hemorrhage is external, pressure is applied directly to the wound or to the proper points. The part of the body that is wounded may be raised. Ice, applied directly to the wound, may slow bleeding by shrinking the blood vessels. Body temperature may be maintained by keeping the person covered and flat. If an arm or leg is wounded, and if the bleeding is severe, a tourniquet may be applied near the wound.

★PATIENT CARE: A tourniquet is not applied if there is any other way to stop the flow, because the risk is great that the limb will not survive the loss of oxygen caused by blocking the supply of blood. The tourniquet is not removed until surgical repair of the wound is possible. Internal bleeding requires prompt medical attention. The patient is kept warm and quiet. **–hemorrhagic,** *adj.*

hemorrhagic diathesis, an inherited high risk for any one of a number of abnormalities marked by heavy bleeding. See also **Fanconi's syndrome, hemophilia, von Willebrand's disease.**

hemorrhagic disease of newborn, a bleeding disorder of newborns usually caused by a lack of vitamin K.

hemorrhagic familial angiomatosis. See **Osler-Weber-Rendu disease.**

hemorrhagic fever, an infection, marked by fever, chills, headache, sadness, and breathing or digestive symptom. These are followed by capillary bleeding and, in severe infection, dangerously reduced urine output, kidney failure, low blood pressure, and, possibly, death. Many forms of the disease occur in specific geographic areas. Some kinds of hemorrhagic fever are **Argentine hemorrhagic fever, dengue fever,** and **Far Eastern hemorrhagic fever.**

hemorrhagic gastritis, a form of serious stomach irritation usually caused by a toxic agent, as alcohol, aspirin or other drugs, or bacterial poisons that irritate the lining of the stomach. If bleeding is heavy, drugs to shrink the blood vessels and ice-water bathing of the stomach may be necessary. Nausea, vomiting, and heartburn may persist after the irritant is removed.

hemorrhagic lung. See **congestive atelectasis.**

hemorrhagic scurvy. See **infantile scurvy.**

hemorrhagic shock, a state of physical collapse and helplessness caused by the sudden and rapid loss of significant amounts of blood. Severe injuries often cause such blood losses, which, in turn, produce low blood pressure. Death occurs within a relatively short time unless transfusion is quickly given to restore normal blood volume. Hemorrhagic shock often occurs with secondary shock. Compare **primary shock.**

hemorrhoid, an enlarged vein in the lower rectum or anus caused by blockage in the veins of the area.

★DIAGNOSIS: Internal hemorrhoids begin above the internal opening of the anus. If they become large enough to protrude from the anus, they become squeezed and painful. Small internal hemorrhoids may bleed with bowel movements. External hemorrhoids appear outside the anal opening. They are usually not painful, and bleeding does not occur unless a hemorrhoidal vein breaks or becomes blocked.

★TREATMENT: Treatment includes the use of surface medication to lubricate, kill the pain, and shrink the hemorrhoid; sitz baths and cold or hot packs are also soothing. The hemorrhoids may need to be hardened by injection, tied off, or removed by a surgical procedure. Tying off is increasingly the preferred treatment. It is simple, effective, and does not require anesthesia. The hemorrhoid is grasped with a forceps and a rubber band is slipped over the enlarged part, causing the tissue to die and the hemorrhoid to fall off, usually within 1 week.

★PATIENT CARE: Straining to defecate, constipation, and too-much sitting cause hemorrhoids. Because pregnancy can help bring on hemorrhoids, the pregnant woman is advised to avoid constipation.

hemosiderin /hē′mōsid′ərin/, an iron-rich colored substance that is a product of red cell breakdown. Iron is often stored in this form.

hemosiderosis /hē′mōsid′ərō′sis, hem′-/, an increased deposit of iron in a variety of tissues, usually without tissue damage. It is often linked to diseases involving long-term, extensive destruction of red blood cells, as thalassemia major. Compare **hemochromatosis, sideroblastic anemia.** See also **ferritin, iron transport, siderosis, thalassemia, transferrin.**

hemostasis /himos′təsis, hē′məstā′sis/, the stopping of bleeding by mechanic or chemical means or by the complex clotting process of the body. Compare **blood clotting.** See also **platelet, thrombus, vasoconstriction.**

hemostat. See **Halsted's forceps.**

hemostatic, having to do with a procedure, device, or substance that stops the flow of blood. Direct pressure, tourniquets, and surgical clamps are mechanical hemostatic measures. Cold packs are hemostatic and include the use of an ice bag on the stomach to halt womb bleeding and washing out the stomach with an iced solution to check stomach bleeding.

hemostatic forceps. See **artery forceps.**

hemothorax /hē′mōthôr′aks, hem′-/, a buildup of blood and fluid in the chest cavity, usually because of injury. Hemothorax may also be caused by small blood vessels that break as a result of swelling from pneumonia, tuberculosis, or tumors. Shock from hemorrhage, pain, and breathing failure follows if emergency care is not available.

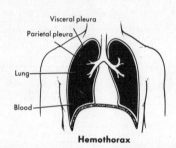

Hemothorax

hemotroph /hē′mətrof/, the food substances that go to the embryo from the mother's bloodstream after the development of the placenta. Also spelled **hemotrophe.** Also called **hemotrophic nutrition.** Compare **embryotroph.** –**hemotrophic,** *adj.*

Henle's fissure /hen′lēz/, one of many patches of connective tissue between the muscle fibers of the heart.

Henle's loop, a U-shaped portion of the tubes of the kidneys.

Henoch-Schönlein purpura /hen′ôkhshœn′līn/, a short-term allergic disorder of blood vessels, chiefly found in children. It is marked by wet skin sores that appear mainly on the lower stomach, buttocks, and legs, and usually pain in the knees and ankles. Other joint pain, stomach bleeding, and blood in the urine are also common findings. The disease lasts up to 6 weeks and has no long-term effects if kidney involvement is not severe. Also called **anaphylactoid purpura, Schönlein-Henoch purpura.**

Hensen's knot, Hensen's node. See **primitive node.**

hen worker's lung. See **pigeon breeder's lung.**

heparin /hep′ərin/, a naturally occurring substance that acts in the body to prevent clotting in the veins. It is produced in the connective tissue surrounding capillaries, particularly in the lungs and liver. See also **heparin sodium.**

heparin sodium, a drug to prevent blood clotting, given for a variety of blood vessel disorders.

★CAUTION: Known allergy to this drug forbids its use. It is given only when the patient's blood can be monitored frequently.

★ADVERSE EFFECTS: The most serious side

effect is rapid bleeding. Disorders involving blood vessel spasms may occur.

hepatic /hipat'ik/, having to do with the liver.

hepatic adenoma, a rapidly growing liver tumor that may become very large and may break, causing deadly internal bleeding. It is sometimes called a "pill tumor" because it is often linked to patients who use birth-control pills.

hepatic amebiasis, enlargement and tenderness of the liver that often occurs with amebic dysentery. The swelling results from infection with *Entamoeba histolytica.* See also **amebiasis, amebic dysentery,** *Entamoeba histolytica.*

hepatic coma, a mental side effect of serious liver damage caused by long-term or sudden liver disease. Either waste that is poisonous to the brain is not removed in the liver before being sent back into the blood flowing to the far ends of the body, or substances that the brain requires are not made in the liver and, therefore, are not available to the brain. Symptoms include variable consciousness, weakness, slowness, and coma, trembling of the hands, personality change, memory loss, and rapid breathing. Convulsions and death may occur. The outcome varies depending on the seriousness of the condition and the treatment. Treatment in most cases includes cleansing enemas, low-protein diet, and specific treatment for the underlying cause. Also called **portal-systemic encephalopathy.** See also **cirrhosis, hepatitis.**

hepatic fistula, an abnormal passage from the liver to another organ or body structure.

hepatic node, a lump in one of three groups of lymph glands found in the lower trunk and the pelvic organs supplied by branches of the celiac artery. Compare **gastric node, pancreaticolienal node.**

hepatic porphyria. See **porphyria.**

hepatic vein catheterization, the insertion of a long, fine tube (catheter) into a liver vein to record vein pressure within the liver. The catheter is inserted through a vein in the arm and is passed through the heart and down into the small hepatic vessel.

hepatin. See **glycogen.**

hepatitis /hep'əti'tis/, an inflammation of the liver, involving yellowing of the skin, enlarged liver, loss of appetite, stomach discomfort, abnormal liver function, clay-colored stools, and dark urine. The condition may be caused by bacterial or viral infection, worms or other parasites, alcohol, drugs, poison, or transfusion of the wrong type of blood. It may be mild and brief or severe, intense, and life-threatening. The liver usually is able to grow back its tissue, but severe hepatitis may lead to permanent damage. Compare **anicteric hepatitis.** See also **viral hepatitis.**

hepatitis A, a form of infectious hepatitis caused by the hepatitis A virus, and having slow onset of signs and symptoms. The virus may be spread by direct contact or through fecal-infected food or water. The infection most often occurs in young adults and is usually followed by complete recovery. Also called **acute infective hepatitis.** See **viral hepatitis.**

hepatitis B, a form of hepatitis caused by the hepatitis B virus and having rapid onset of sudden symptoms and signs. The virus can be carried in blood products used for transfusion or by the use of unsterile needles and instruments. The infection may be severe and result in prolonged illness, destruction of liver cells, cirrhosis, or death. Also called **serum hepatitis.** See **viral hepatitis.**

hepatitis B immune globulin (HBIG), a drug to protect one against infection by the hepatitis B virus.

★CAUTION: Known allergy to the drug or to gamma globulin prohibits its use.

★ADVERSE EFFECTS: Among the most serious side effects are severe allergic reactions. Pain and swelling at the site of injection also may occur.

hepatitis B surface antigen. See **Australia antigen.**

hepatization, the changing of lung tissue into a solid mass looking like the liver, as in early pneumonia in which the gathering of red blood cells in the air sacs produce **red hepatization.** In later stages of pneumonia, when white blood cells fill the air sacs, the process becomes **gray hepatization,** or **yellow hepatization** when fat deposits join the process.

hepatocarcinoma, hepatocellular carcinoma. See **malignant hepatoma.**

hepatocyte, the most basic liver cell that performs all the functions of the liver.

hepatoduodenal ligament /hep'ətōdoo·ədē'nəl, -doo·od'inəl/, a fold in the abdominal cavity between the liver and the small intestine, containing the hepatic artery, the common bile duct, the portal vein, lymphatics, and the hepatic plexus of nerves. These organs are enclosed within a fiberlike capsule between the two layers of the ligament. Compare **hepatogastric ligament.**

hepatogastric ligament /hep'ətōgas'trik/, the portion of a fold in the abdominal cavity between the liver and the stomach. Compare **hepatoduodenal ligament.**

hepatojugular reflux /hep'ətōjug'yoolər/, an increase of pressure in the jugular vein when pressure is applied for 30 to 60 seconds over the stomach, suggestive of right-sided heart failure.

hepatolenticular degeneration /həpat'ōlentik'yoolər/, an abnormal condition related to a problem with processing copper in the body. Patients with this condition develop a buildup of copper in the body that can cause cirrhosis of the liver, deep coloring of the cornea of the eye, and serious breakdown of the brain and spinal cord nerves. Also called **Wilson's disease.**

hepatoma /hep'ətō'mə/, *pl.* **hepatomas, hepatomata,** a cancerous tumor of the liver causing enlargement of the liver, pain, low blood pressure, loss of appetite and weight, and fluid buildup in the abdominal cavity. It is most often found together with hepatitis or cirrhosis of the liver.

hepatomegaly /hep'ətōmeg'əlē/, abnormal enlargement of the liver, usually a sign of liver disease. It is often found by tapping and feeling the area as part of a physical examination. The liver can easily be felt below the ribs and is tender to the touch. Hepatomegaly may be caused by hepatitis or other infection, alcoholism, obstruction of bile ducts, or cancer.

hepatopancreatic ampulla, the widening formed where the pancreatic and bile ducts open into the small intestine. Also called **ampulla of the bile duct, ampulla of Vater.**

hepatotoxic, something that may destroy liver cells.

hepatotoxicity /hep'ətōtoksis'itē/, the tendency of a substance, usually a drug or alcohol, to have a harmful effect on the liver.

heptachlor poisoning /hep'təklôr'/, a form of insecticide poisoning.

heptaploid. See **polyploid.**

herald patch. See **pityriasis rosea.**

herb bath, a medicinal bath taken in water containing aromatic herbs.

herbicide poisoning, a poisoning caused by eating, breathing, or skin contact with a substance intended for use as a weed killer. Many of the commonly used farming weed killers can produce symptoms ranging from skin irritation to low blood pressure, liver and kidney damage, and coma or fits. Death can result from a dose as small as 1 to 10 g. If eaten, vomiting or cleansing of the stomach should be induced. Some herbicides can be extremely poisonous, causing burning stomach or throat pain, diarrhea, or other severe symptoms.

hereditability, the degree to which a given trait is inherited.

hereditary, having to do with a feature, condition, or disease passed down from parent to offspring; inborn; inherited. Compare **acquired, congenital, familial.**

hereditary ataxia, one of a group of inherited destructive diseases of the spinal cord, brain, and nerves causing tremor, spasm, wasting of muscle, bone change, and sensory problems leading to poor movement control. Kinds of hereditary ataxia include **ataxia telangiectasia and Friedreich's ataxia.**

hereditary brown enamel. See amelogenesis imperfecta.

hereditary deforming chondroplasia. See **diaphyseal aclasis.**

hereditary disorder. See **inherited disorder.**

hereditary elliptocytosis. See **elliptocytosis.**

hereditary enamel hypoplasia. See **amelogenesis imperfecta.**

hereditary essential tremor. See **essential tremor.**

hereditary hemorrhagic telangiectasia. See **Osler-Weber-Rendu disease.**

hereditary hyperuricemia. See **Lesch-Nyhan syndrome.**

hereditary multiple exostoses, a rare disease running in families in which bony outgrowths form on the shafts of the long bones and eventually develop into caps of cartilage covering the ends of the bones. The affected joints lose their ease of movement, and the bones stop growing. The disease begins in childhood and has no cure. Very rarely, the cap of an exostosis may become cancerous. See also **Ollier's dyschondroplasia.**

hereditary opalescent dentin. See **dentinogenesis imperfecta.**

hereditary oral disease, any abnormal, inborn defects of the mouth and its parts, as deformed teeth, tongue, gums, or cleft palate. Many hereditary oral diseases are part of other inherited diseases.

hereditary protoporphyria. See **porphyria.**

hereditary spherocytosis. See **spherocytic anemia.**

hereditary tyrosinemia. See **tyrosinemia.**

heredity, 1. the process by which particular traits or conditions are passed along from parents to offspring, causing resemblance of individuals related by blood. It involves the division and rejoining of genes during cell division and fertilization. Heredity is affected by events that occur during the development of the embryo. 2. the total genetic makeup of an individual; the sum of the features inherited from ancestors and the possibilities of passing on these qualities to offspring.

heredofamilial tremor. See **essential tremor.**

Hering-Breuer reflexes, controlling signals sent by the nerves that maintain the rhythm of breathing and prevent the overfilling of the air sacs in the lungs. Hering-Breuer reflexes are well developed at birth. They are brought on by filling up of the airway, increased pressures in the windpipe, or inflation of the lungs. The inflation reflex stops breathing in and stimulates breathing out; the deflation reflex stops breathing out and begins breathing in. These reflexes are overactive when there is not enough air to breathe.

hermaphroditism /hərmaf'rədītiz'əm/, a rare condition in which both male and female sex organs exist in the same person. The condition results from a chromosomal abnormality. Also called **hermaphrodism.** Compare **pseudohermaphroditism.**

hernia, a breakthrough of an organ through a tear in the muscle wall that surrounds it. A hernia may be present at birth, may come from the failure of certain structures to close after birth, or may be acquired later in life because of overweight, muscular weakness, surgery, or illness. Kinds of hernia include **abdominal hernia, diaphragmatic hernia, femoral hernia, hiatus hernia, inguinal hernia,** and **umbilical hernia.** See also **herniorrhaphy.**

herniated disk, a break in the cartilage surrounding a disk in the spine, releasing the fluid that cushions the back bones above and below. The resultant pressure on spinal nerve roots may cause considerable pain and damage the nerves. The condition most occurs in the lower back. Also called **herniated nucleus pulposus, ruptured intervertebral disk, slipped disk.**

herniated intervertebral disk. See **herniated disk.**

herniation, a breakthrough of a body organ or part of an organ through a tear in a membrane, muscle, or other tissue. See also **hernia, hiatus.**

herniorrhaphy, the surgical repair of a hernia.

heroin, a morphinelike drug with no currently acceptable medical use in the United States. Heroin is controlled by law in the Comprehensive Drug Abuse Prevention and Control Act of 1970. According to this law, it may not be prescribed to patients but only used for research and teaching use or for chemical analysis by permission from the Drug Enforcement Administration of the Department of Justice. Heroin, like other opium products, can produce relief from pain, slowing of breathing, spasms in the digestive system, and physical dependence. Its major effects are on the brain and spinal cord, the bowel, and the hormone functions and nervous reflexes. Illegally-gotten heroin is commonly used by persons who become addicted and suffer from higher death rate than nonaddicts of similar age. Some studies conducted in the United States and England have shown that the majority of heroin users are relatively young people who have been introduced to the drug by friends, first start using heroin out of curiosity, but continue because of its pleasant-feeling effects. Such persons commonly show similar patterns of behavior, social problems, and disease. Heroin use in the United States reached epidemic proportions during the 1960s and in 1971 became a major cause of death in New York City among males between 15 and 35 years of age. The problem decreased somewhat during the 1970s but has apparently increased and spread from the larger cities to the smaller communities across the country. Street use of the drug commonly begins with sniffing powdered heroin, which is absorbed through the moist lining of the nose, throat and breathing tract. Other methods of taking the drug include injecting it under the skin or into a vein. Heroin, which loses much of its pain-killing power when taken by mouth, is more powerful than morphine and acts more rapidly. It is changed into morphine by the body and builds up in the organs, bones, and brain. Heroin taken in the vein is felt almost immediately and produces reactions that last from 3 to 6 hours. Many users compare the initial feeling to a sexual orgasm. Heroin addicts may easily spend as much as $300 or more daily for the drug and inject themselves every 3 to 6 hours. Repeated use of this drug causes a gradual decrease in the effects felt (tolerance). Physical dependence develops along with tolerance. Withdrawal from heroin after using it even a few times commonly causes severe symptoms. Withdrawal signs usually come shortly before the next planned dose and include anxiety, restlessness, irritability, and craving for another dose. Other withdrawal signs that may appear 8 to 15 hours after the last dose include watery eyes, perspiration, yawning, and restless sleep. On awakening from such sleep the severely addicted heroin user may experience further withdrawal signs, as vomiting, pain in the bones, diarrhea, convulsions, and heart attack. Withdrawal signs usually peak at between 36 and 48 hours and gradually fade during the following 10 days. Anxiety and depression related to use of the drug may persist for months in many heroin addicts under treatment. Most authorities consider such addiction a complex disease caused by imbalances in body chemistry brought on by the heroin, together with deep psychological and social factors. A variety of liquid substances, as quinine, are used to dissolve street heroin for injection. Impure states of such liquids, together with dirty needles and other unhealthy factors are responsible for more than half the deaths related to the illegal use of heroin. The most frequent disorders related to injections of impure heroin are tetanus, skin abscesses, infection, and swollen veins. Heroin-connected lung complications may include pneumonia, internal bleeding, and tuberculosis. Many nerve disorders may result from the use of street heroin. Women heroin addicts who become pregnant often give birth to premature babies who easily get blood poisoning and may well be addicted to heroin at birth. Heroin addicts frequently return to use of the drug during withdrawal treatment. Withdrawal symptoms, as altered blood pressure and pulse rate, anxiety, and depression, may last for months. Methadone is commonly used as a substitute drug in the treatment of heroin addiction. Also being studied is the effectiveness of methadone alcohol, which can have the same effects as heroin that last for 72 hours. Numerous outpatient programs staffed by former opiate users seek to give psychological and helpful support for addicts trying to break their drug habits. Some of these programs are Synanon, Daytop Village, and Phoenix House. Research and community-supported mental-health projects continue to seek more effective treatment methods for addicts, many of whom are successfully cured. Denying heroin to addicts in prisons has been much less effective in curing addicts, and most authorities believe that gradual withdrawal under medical care, with counseling, is the most promising approach. Also called **diacetylmorphine.**

herpangina /hur'panjī'nə/, a viral infection, usually of young children, marked by sore throat, headache, loss of appetite, and pain in the stomach, neck, and arms and legs. Feverish fits and vomiting may occur in infants. Pimples or blisters may form in the throat and on the tongue, the roof of the mouth, or the tonsils. These turn into shallow sores that heal by themselves. The disease usually runs its course in less than 1 week. Treatment aims to relieve symptoms.

herpes genitalis, an infection caused by Type 2 herpes simplex virus (HSV2), usually passed along by sexual contact, that causes painful blisters on the skin and moist lining of the sex organs of males and females. When acquired during pregnancy, the virus may be passed from the mother's blood to the fetus or to the newborn by direct contact with infected tissue during birth.

★DIAGNOSIS: In the male, herpes genitalis infections may resemble penile ulcers. A small group of blisters surrounded by redness of the skin may occur on the tip or foreskin. These turn into surface sores that often heal in 5 to 7 days, although they also may become infected. The sores are painful and often give a burning sensation, urinary problems, fever, illness, and swelling of the lymph nodes in the groin area. The female patient may have the same or similar problems, and members of both sexes may complain of painful sexual intercourse. In the female, herpes genitalis lesions are likely to appear as groups of surface sores on the surfaces of the cervix, vagina, or perineum. There may be a discharge from the cervix. Vaginal blisters may appear as mucous open sores. This herpes virus tends to cause repeated attacks.

★TREATMENT: Treatment of herpes genitalis sores is with the antibiotic acyclovir. Untreated, an attack of the disease will generally go away by itself in time. Sores may be cleansed with soap and water, where possible, to prevent secondary infections, and drying medications may be applied to sores that rupture or ooze. Secondary infections are treated with appropriate antibiotics. Except for experimental antiviral drugs, there are no specific cures or vaccines for the control of recurrent herpes infections.

★PATIENT CARE: Extreme caution must be taken in contacts with infected patients. Smears for laboratory analysis are obtained by cleansing fresh blisters with alcohol and removing fluid from the base of lesions with a cotton swab or wooden applicator. Rubber gloves are worn and the hands washed after contact to prevent transfer of virus particles from blisters to other skin or mucous membranes of the patient or other individuals. Transfer of the virus to the eye results in swelling of the cornea. Infections that develop in pregnant women may progress to viruses in the blood and a danger of death and illness in the fetus. An attack of herpes within 3 weeks of delivery usually requires that the infant be delivered by cesarean section to avoid dangerous herpesvirus infection of the newborn.

herpes gestationis, a generalized itching or blistering rash appearing in the last 3 to 6 months of pregnancy and disappearing several weeks after delivery. The sores often come back with later pregnancies and are often linked with premature birth and increased fetal death.

herpes labialis. See **herpes simplex.**

herpes simplex, an infection caused by a herpes simplex virus (HSV), which attacks the skin and nervous system and usually produces small, short-lasting, irritating, and sometimes painful fluid-filled blisters on the skin and mucous membranes. HSV1 (oral herpes, herpes labialis) infections tend to occur in the facial area, particularly around the mouth and nose; HSV2 (herpes genitalis) infections are usually limited to the genital area.

★DIAGNOSIS: The first symptoms of a herpes simplex infection usually include burning, tingling, or itching sensations around the edges of the lips or nose within 1 or 2 weeks after contact with an infected person. Several hours later, small red pimples develop in the irritated area, followed by the formation of small fever blisters filled with fluid. Several small blisters may merge to form a larger blister. The blisters generally cause itching, pain, or similar discomfort. Other effects often include a mild fever and enlargement of the lymph nodes in the neck. Within 1 week after the onset of symptoms, thin yellow crusts form on the blisters as healing begins. In skin areas that are moist or protected or in severe cases, healing may be delayed. Genital herpes infections in adolescence can increase the risk of cervical cancer in adulthood.

★TREATMENT: Treatment of herpes simplex is to relieve symptoms. The sores may be washed gently with soap and water to reduce the risk of secondary infection. Application to the skin of drying medications, as alcohol solutions, may speed healing, but they are very painful. Where secondary infections have begun, antibiotics are prescribed.

★PATIENT CARE: Because herpes viruses are extremely contagious, extreme care should be taken in contacts with patients to avoid catching the infection and carrying it to other per sons. Washing the hands and wearing rubber gloves while working about the mouth of a patient help prevent passing along the virus. Once acquired, the virus tends to rest without symptoms in the skin or tissues of the nervous system and may be stimulated into an active attack by things like fever, physical or emotional stress, exposure to sunlight, or certain foods or drugs. Sunscreen lotions offer some protection against exposure to the sun, and patients are advised to avoid those things which bring about an attack. The complications of herpetic infections may include swelling of the brain, swelling of the cornea of the eye, and swollen gums. In cases involving other complications, antibiotics, blood transfusions, IV solutions, and other therapy may be required. In uncomplicated cases, the herpes attack usually runs its course in 3 weeks or less.

herpesvirus /hur′pēzvī′rəs/, any of five related viruses including herpes simplex viruses 1 and 2, varicellazoster virus, Epstein-Barr virus, and cytomegalovirus.

herpesvirus hominis. See **herpes simplex.**

herpes zoster, a severe infection caused by the varicellazoster virus (VZV), affecting mainly adults. It causes painful skin blisters that follow the underlying route of brain or spinal nerves infected by the virus. ★DIAGNOSIS: The pain and blisters usually occur on only one side of the body and any sensory nerve may be affected. The pain, which may be constant or off and on, surface or deep, usually comes before other effects and may mimic other disorders, as appendicitis or pleurisy. Early symptoms may include digestive system disturbances, vague discomfort, fever, and headache. The blisters usually evolve from small red bumps along the path of a nerve, and the skin of the area is overly sensitive. All of the sores may appear within a period of hours, but they most often develop gradually over a period of several days. The bumps swell and, after about 3 days, become thickened with dead cell material. Usually, at the end of the first week, the bumps develop crusts. The symptoms may persist for 3 to 5 weeks, but in most cases they lessen after 2 weeks. ★TREATMENT: Treatment is mainly to relieve symptoms and includes calamine lotion or similar medications to relieve itching and aspirin or pain-killers for pain symptoms. Cool compresses may be applied to the affected skin areas. Skin medicines that prevent swelling may be given for severe cases and for elderly patients who may experience jabbing pain along a nerve following a herpes attack. Surgery to remove an affected nerve may be ad-

vised in cases of severe pain that fail to respond to more conservative treatment. ★PATIENT CARE: Bed rest is encouraged during the early stages of zoster infection, when fever and other overall effects occur. Irritation of the blisters may be worsened by contact with clothing or bed linen. The use of nonstick dressings and of cradles to prevent direct contact of affected skin areas with irritating fabrics relieves discomfort. Older patients have greatest risk of complications, as exhaustion and jabbing pain (neuralgia) may last for several months after the skin sores have cleared. Other complications are geniculate zoster, with involvement of the ear, face, and soft palate, and ophthalmic herpes zoster, which can result in corneal damage in the eye. An attack of herpes zoster does not make one immune to further attacks, but most patients recover without permanent effects except for occasional scarring at sites of especially bad blistering. Evidence indicates VZV remains at rest, without symptoms in the body of a person once infected, and a person lacking varicella immunity can catch chickenpox from a herpes zoster patient. Also called **shingles.** See also **herpes simplex, varicellazoster virus.**

herpes zoster oticus, a herpes zoster infection causing severe pain in the outer ear structures and pain or paralysis along the facial nerve. The disease may also result in hearing loss and dizziness. The dizziness is usually short-lived, but the hearing loss and facial paralysis may be permanent. There may be blisters along the outer ear canal and flesh of the ear. Treatment is generally to relieve symptoms, with diazepam (a sedative) given for dizziness, aspirin for pain, and anti-swelling medicines for other symptoms.

herpes zoster virus. See **chickenpox.**

herpetiform /hərpet′ifôrm′/, having clusters of blisters; resembling the skin sores of some herpesvirus infections.

Herplex, a trademark for an antiviral drug (idoxuridine).

Hers' disease, an uncommon condition in which the body is unable to store starch correctly. It features an enlarged liver and a buildup of abnormally large amounts of starch in the liver as a result of its inability to break down starch. The condition is inherited as a recessive trait. There is no known treatment. Also called **glycogen storage disease, type VI.** See also **glycogen storage disease.**

hertz (Hz), a unit of measurement of wave frequency equal to one cycle per second (cps).

Herxheimer's reaction /harks′hī′mərz/, an increase in symptoms after a drug is given. The reaction was first seen in penicillin treatment of syphilis, but has been found to occur in other diseases as well.

hesperidin /hesper′idin/, a sugar substance occurring in most citrus fruits, especially in the spongy casing of oranges and lemons.

hetastarch, a substance to increase the volume of blood plasma, given to help treat shock and leukophoresis.

★CAUTION: Severe bleeding, severe heart or kidney problems with excessive or insufficient urination, or known allergy to this drug prohibits its use.

★ADVERSE EFFECTS: Among the more serious side effects are influenza-like symptoms, muscle pain, fluid retention, and extreme allergic reaction.

heterauxesis. See **allometric growth.**

hetero-, heter-, a combining form meaning 'pertaining to another': *heteroalbumose, heterochronia, heterogamy.*

heteroallele /het′ərō·əlēl′/, one of a set of genes located at a specific place on similar chromosomes that differs from the other of the pair, resulting in a mutation. **–heteroallelic,** *adj.*

heteroblastic, developing from different germ layers or kinds of tissue rather than from a single type. Compare **homoblastic.**

heterocephalus, a malformed fetus that has two heads of unequal size. **–heterocephalous, heterocephalic,** *adj.*

heterochromatin, that portion of chromosome material that plays no role in the expression of inborn traits, but may function in controlling various bodily processes. Compare **euchromatin.** See also **chromatin** **–heterchromatic,** *adj.*

heterochromatinization, the process that changes euchromatin into heterochromatin; the inactivation of one of the X chromosomes in the mammalian female during the early stages of the embryo's growth. See also **Lyon hypothesis.**

heterochromosome, a sex chromosome. See also **heterotypical chromosomes. –heterochromosomal,** *adj.*

heterodidymus /het′ərōdid′iməs/, a joined twin fetus in which the incomplete twin consists of a head, neck, and chest attached to the chest wall of the completely formed twin. Also called **heterodymus.**

heteroeroticism, sexual feeling or activity directed toward another individual. Also called **alloeroticism, heteroerotism.** Compare **autoeroticism.**

heterogamete, a sex cell that differs considerably in size and structure from the one with which it unites, specifically referring to those of humans and mammals as opposed to those of lower plants and animals. Compare **anisogamete, isogamete.**

heterogamy /het′ərog′əmē/, **1.** sexual reproduction in which there is joining of dissimilar sex cells, usually differing in size and structure. The word primarily refers to the reproductive processes of humans and mammals as opposed to certain lower plants and animals. Compare

anisogamy, isogamy. **–heterogamous,** *adj.*

heterogeneous, 1. consisting of unlike elements or parts. **2.** not having a uniform quality throughout. Compare **homogeneous. –heterogeneity,** *adj.*

heterogenous /het′əroj′ənəs/, derived or developed from another source or from two different sources.

heterograft. See **xenograft.**

heterologous. See **xenogeneic.**

heterologous insemination. See **artificial insemination-donor.**

heterologous tumor, a tumor consisting of tissue different from that around it.

heterologous twins. See **dizygotic twins.**

heterophil antibody test, a test for the presence of heterophil antibodies in the blood of patients suspected of having infectious mononucleosis. This antibody eventually appears in the blood of more than 80% of the patients with mononucleosis; so it is a good way to diagnose the disease. See also **Epstein-Barr virus.**

heteroploid /het′ərəploid′/, **1.** used to describe an individual, organism, strain, or cell that has fewer or more whole chromosomes in its body cells than is normal for its species. **2.** such an individual, organism, strain, or cell. See also **aneuploid, euploid.**

heteroploidy /het′ərəploi′dē/, the state or condition of having an abnormal number of chromosomes.

heterosexual, 1. a person whose sexual desire or preference is for people of the opposite sex. **2.** used to describe sexual desire or preference for people of the opposite sex. **–heterosexuality,** *n.*

heterosexual panic, a sudden attack of anxiety resulting in the frantic pursuit of heterosexual activity in response to unconscious or unrecognized homosexual impulses. Compare **homosexual panic.**

heterosis /het′ərō′sis/, the advantage or improvement that comes from crossbreeding plants or animals. Also called **hybrid vigor.**

heterotopic ossification, a noncancerous overgrowth of bone, often occurring after a break in the bone, that is sometimes confused with certain bone tumors when seen on x-ray film. Also called **exuberant callus, myositis ossificans.**

heterotypic chromosomes, any unmatched pair of chromosomes, specifically the sex chromosomes.

heterozygosis /het′ərōzīgō′sis/, **1.** the formation of a fertilized egg by the union of two sex cells that have dissimilar pairs of genes. **2.** the production of hybrids through crossbreeding. **–heterozygotic,** *adj.*

heterozygous /het′ərəzī′gəs/, having two different genes at the same place on matched chromosomes. An individual who is heterozygous for a particular trait has inherited a gene for that trait from one parent and the alternative gene from the other parent. A person heterozygous for a genetic disease caused by a dominant gene, as Huntington's chorea, will show the disease. An individual heterozygous for a hereditary disorder produced by a recessive gene, as sickle cell anemia, will not show the disease, or will have a milder form of it. The offspring of a heterozygous carrier of a genetic disorder have a 50% chance of inheriting the gene dominant for the trait. Compare **homozygous.**

hexachlorophene, a cleanser and antiseptic for external use. It may also be used as an antiseptic scrub and as a disinfectant for nonliving things.

★CAUTION: Known allergy to this drug prohibits its use. It can be absorbed into the system when used on burns, broken skin, mucous membranes, and infant skin, leading to blood poisoning. The skin should be rinsed thoroughly to prevent absorption of the drug into the bloodstream.

★ADVERSE EFFECTS: Among the more serious side effects are skin rash and nervous disorders.

Hexadrol, a trademark for a hormone that affects starch processing in the body (dexamethasone).

hexafluorenium bromide, a drug used in anesthesia to prolong skeletal muscle relaxation.

★CAUTION: Known allergy to this drug or to bromides prohibits its use.

★ADVERSE EFFECTS: Among the more serious side effects are muscle relaxation that lasts too long and resultant stopping of breathing, allergic reactions, and low blood pressure.

hexamethylenamine. See **methenamine.**

hexamethylmelamine, an experimental antitumor drug that has been used to treat cancers of the lungs, cervix, and ovaries.

hexanoic acid. See **caproic acid.**

hexaploid. See **polyploid.**

hexenmilch. See **witch's milk.**

hexocyclium methylsulfate, a drug prescribed to help treat ulcers.

★CAUTION: Narrow-angle glaucoma, asthma, blockage of the genital, urinary, or digestive

tract, ulcerative inflammation of the colon, or known allergy to this drug prohibits its use.

★ADVERSE EFFECTS: Among the more serious side effects are blurred vision, brain and nervous system effects, rapid heart rate, dry mouth, decreased sweating, and allergic reactions.

hexylcaine hydrochloride, a local anesthetic for use on unbroken mucous membranes of the breathing, digestive, and urinary tracts.

HHS, abbreviation for **Department of Health and Human Services.**

hiatus /hī·ā′təs/, a usually normal opening in a membrane or other body tissue. **–hiatal,** *adj.*

hiatus hernia, breakthrough of a portion of the stomach upward through the diaphragm. The condition occurs in about 40% of the population, and most people display few, if any, symptoms. The worst symptom is the backflow of the acid contents of the stomach into the throat (known also as heartburn). Diagnosis is made easily on x-ray films. Surgical treatment is usually unnecessary, and efforts should be directed toward relieving the discomfort caused by stomach contents backflow. See also **diaphragmatic hernia, gastroesophageal reflux, heartburn.**

hibakusha /hē′bäkōō′shä/, persons who have been exposed to atomic bomb explosions. In 1985, some 370,000 hibakusha still lived in Hiroshima and Nagasaki, more than 40 years after the World War II atomic bomb attacks. Their average age was over 60.

hibernoma /hī′bərnō′mə/, *pl.* **hibernomas, hibernomata,** a noncancerous tumor, usually on the hips or the back, composed of fat cells that are partly or entirely left over from the fetal stage of growth. Also called **fat cell lipoma, fetal lipoma.**

hiccup, a sound that is produced by the unintentional squeezing of the diaphragm, followed by rapid closure of the vocal cords. Hiccups have a variety of causes, including indigestion, rapid eating, certain types of surgery, and epidemic inflammation of the brain. Most attacks of hiccups do not last longer than a few minutes, but long-lasting or repeated attacks sometimes oc-

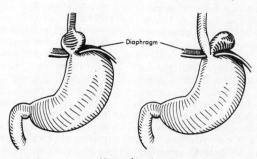

Hiatus hernia

cur. The condition is most often seen in men. Sedatives are used in extreme cases. Also spelled **hiccough. Also called singultus.**

hickory stick fracture. See **greenstick fracture.**

hidradenitis. See **hydradenitis.**

hidrosis /hidrō'sis, hī-/, to sweat. Compare **anhidrosis, dyshidrosis, hyperhidrosis. –hidrotic,** *adj.*

high blood pressure. See **hypertension.**

high-density lipoprotein (HDL), a protein in blood plasma involved in carrying cholesterol and other fats from the blood to the tissues. See also **low-density lipoprotein, very low-density lipoprotein.**

high-energy phosphate compound, a chemical compound that fuels muscle contraction, active transport of substances across cell membranes, and the production of many substances in the body.

highest intercostal vein, one of a pair of veins that drain the blood from the upper chest.

high forceps, a childbirth operation in which forceps are used to deliver a baby whose head has not entered the birth canal. The procedure is considered hazardous and is generally condemned. Compare **low forceps, mid forceps.** See also **forceps delivery, obstetric forceps.**

high-Fowler's position, placement of the patient in a near-sitting position by raising the head of the bed at more than a 45-degree angle.

high-level wellness, a concept of health that stresses the working together of body, mind, and environment to ensure the highest level of functioning of an individual.

high-potassium diet, a diet that contains foods rich in potassium, including all leafy green vegetables, Brussels sprouts, citrus fruits, bananas, dates, raisins, beans, meats, and whole grains. It is advised for any condition resulting in the loss of fluid, as acute diarrhea, high blood pressure, and diabetic coma. It is also advised for patients receiving thiazide or corticosteroid therapy.

high-protein diet, a diet that contains large amounts of protein, consisting largely of meats, fish, milk, beans, and nuts. It may be advised in protein loss from any cause, to strengthen a patient prior to surgery, in kidney syndromes, or in liver disorders. It is not advised in cases of liver failure or when function of the kidneys is so weakened that added protein could result in harmful levels of urea and other acids in the body.

high-risk infant, any newborn, regardless of birth weight, size, or length of time in the womb, who, because of conditions or circumstances that interfere with the normal birth process or postbirth growth and development, has a greater-than-average chance of sickness or death, especially within the first 28 days of life. See also **neonatal period, premature infant.**

high-vitamin diet, a diet that includes a variety of foods that contain healthful amounts of all of the vitamins necessary for the processes of the body. It is often ordered in combination with other prescribed diets containing larger-than-usual amounts of protein or calories, especially when treating severe or long-lasting infection, malnutrition, or vitamin deficiency.

hilus /hī'ləs/, *pl.* **hili,** a depression or pit at that part of an organ where vessels and nerves enter.

hindgut, the lower end of the embryonic digestive tract. It is formed by the development of the tail fold and eventually becomes part of the small and large intestines, rectum, bladder, and urogenital openings. Compare **foregut, midgut.** See also **cloaca.**

hind kidney. See **metanephros.**

hinge axis-orbital plane, a plane that is usually determined by marking three points on the face of the patient. Two of the points, one on each side of the face, are located on the line where the upper and lower jaws are joined. The third point is located on the face at the level of the eye socket just beneath the eye. The hinge axis-orbital plane is used to diagnose and treat misaligned teeth.

hinge joint, a fluid-filled joint in which bone surfaces are closely molded together in a manner that permits extensive motion in one plane. The joints of the fingers are hinge joints. Also called **ginglymus joint.** Compare **gliding joint, pivot joint.**

hip. See **coxa.**

hip bath. See **sitz bath.**

hipbone. See **innominate bone.**

hip joint. See **coxal articulation.**

hippocampal commissure, a thin, triangular layer of crosswise fibers that connects the middle edges of the two sides of the hippocampus, a structure in the lower brain.

hippocampal fissure, a division reaching from the lowest point of the corpus callosum to the tip of the temporal lobe of the brain.

hippocampus, *pl.* **hippocampi,** a structure of the brain that functions as an important part of the limbic system. Also called **Ammon's horn, hippocampus major.**

hippocampus minor. See **calcar avis.**

Hippocrates /hipok'rətēz/, a Greek physician born about 460 BC on the island of Cos, a center for the worship of Æsculapius. Called the "Father of Medicine," Hippocrates introduced a scientific approach to healing by seeking physical causes for disease rather than magic or mythic relationships believed in by members of the Æsculapian cults of the time. He also gathered case records of illnesses, including results of treatments given, and developed the art of ethical bedside care. See also **Æsculapius, Hippocratic oath.**

Hippocrates' bandage. See **capeline bandage.**

Hippocratic oath /hip'əkrat'ik/, an oath, thought to have come from Hippocrates, that serves as an ethical guide for the medical profession. It is traditionally part of the graduation ceremonies of medical colleges and reads as follows:

I swear by Apollo the physician, by Æsculapius, Hygeia, and Panacea, and I take to witness all the gods, and all the goddesses, to keep according to my ability and my judgment the following Oath:

To consider dear to me as my parents him who taught me this art; to live in common with him and if necessary to share my goods with him; to look upon his children as my own brothers, to teach them this art if they so desire without fee or written promise; to impart to my sons and the sons of the master who taught me and the disciples who have enrolled themselves and have agreed to the rules of the profession, but to these alone, the precepts and the instruction. I will prescribe regimen for the good of my patients according to my ability and my judgment and never do harm to anyone. To please no one will I prescribe a deadly drug, nor give advice which may cause his death. Nor will I give a woman a pessary to procure abortion. But I will preserve the purity of my life and my art. I will not cut for stone, even for patients in whom the disease is manifest; I will leave this operation to be performed by practitioners (specialists in this art). In every house where I come I will enter only for the good of my patients, keeping myself far from all intentional ill-doing and all seduction, and especially from the pleasures of love with women or with men, be they free or slaves. All that may come to my knowledge in the exercise of my profession or outside of my profession or in daily commerce with men, which ought not to be spread abroad, I will keep secret and will never reveal. If I keep this oath faithfully, may I enjoy my life and practice my art, respected by all men and in all times; but if I swerve from it or violate it, may the reverse be my lot. See also **Æsculapius, Hippocrates.**

hip replacement, an operation to replace the hip joint with an artificial ball and socket joint. This is performed to relieve a constantly painful and stiff hip in serious cases of arthritis, an improperly healed break, or destruction of the joint. Antibiotics are given before the operation, and the patient is taught to walk with crutches. Surgery is done under general anesthesia. After the operation, the patient is placed in traction. The most frequent complications are infection requiring removal of the new joint, or its dislocation. Movement begins gradually, with frequent short walks. Sitting for more than 1 hour is to be avoided, and hip bending beyond 90 degrees may cause dislocation of the new joint. The patient continues an exercise program after release from the hospital to keep the hip moving freely and to strengthen the muscles.

Hiprex, a trademark for a urinary antibacterial (methenamine hippurate).

Hirschfeld's method, a toothbrushing technique in which the bristles are placed against the outer surfaces of the teeth at a slight angle and in contact with the teeth and gums, then vigorously rotated in very small circles.

Hirschsprung's disease /hirsh'sprŏongz/, the inborn absence of nerves in the smooth muscle wall of the colon, resulting in poor or absent squeezing motion in the affected part of the colon, buildup of feces, and widening of the bowel (megacolon). Symptoms include vomiting, diarrhea, and constipation. The stomach may stretch to several times its normal size. The condition is usually diagnosed in infancy, but it may not be recognized until much later in childhood, when there is loss of appetite, lack of urge to defecate, bloating of the stomach, and poor health. Surgical repair in early childhood is usually successful. The colon is temporarily rerouted to a new opening in the surface of the body (colostomy) and the portion of the bowel lacking nerves is removed. The colostomy is almost always reversed a few months later. Also called **aganglionic megacolon, congenital megacolon.**

hirsutism /hur'sŏotiz'əm/, excessive body hair in a masculine pattern as a result of heredity, hormonal imbalance, porphyria, or medication. Treatment of the specific cause will usually stop growth of more hair. Excess hair may be removed by scraping, electrolysis, chemical removal, shaving, plucking, or rubbing with pumice. Fine facial hair may be most effectively minimized by bleaching. Also called **hypertrichosis.** –**hirsute,** *adj.,* **hirsuteness,** *n.*

hirsutoid papilloma of the penis /hur'sŏotoid/, a condition marked by clusters of small, white bumps on the surrounding edge of the end of the penis. Also called **papillomatosis coronae penis, pearly penile papules.**

His. See **histidine.**

His bundle. See **bundle of His.**

His-Purkinje system, a nerve system in the heart tissues that leads from the bundle of His to the Purkinje fibers.

Hispril, a trademark for an antihistamine (diphenylpyraline hydrochloride).

histamine /his'təmēn, -min/, a compound, found in all cells, produced by the breakdown of histidine. It is released in allergic reactions and causes widening of capillaries, decreased blood pressure, increased release of gastric juice, and tightening of smooth muscles of the bronchi and uterus.

histamine headache, a headache related to the release of histamine from the body tissues and marked by symptoms of dilated carotid arteries, fluid accumulation under the eyes, tearing or watery eyes, and runny nose. Symptoms include sudden sharp pain on one side of the head, involving the facial area from the neck to the temple. Treatment includes the use of antihistamines and ergot that help tighten the arteries. Also called **cluster headache, Horton's histamine cephalalgia.** See also **cephalalgia.**

histidine (His), a basic amino acid found in many proteins and the substance from which histamine is produced. It is an essential amino acid in infants. See also **amino acid, protein.**

histiocyte. See **macrophage.**

histiocytic leukemia. See **monocytic leukemia.**

histiocytic malignant lymphoma, a tumor on a lymph gland. Also called **clasmocytic lymphoma, reticulum cell sarcoma.**

histocompatibility antigens, a group of antigens on the surface of many cells. Histocompatibility antigens are the cause of most graft rejections that occur in organ transplants. See also **isoantigen, histocompatibility locus.**

histography /histog′rəfē/, the process of describing or creating pictures of tissues and cells. **–histographer,** *n.,* **histographic,** *adj.,* **histographically,** *adv.*

histoid neoplasm, a growth that resembles the tissues in which it originates. Compare **organoid neoplasm.**

histologist /histol′əjist/, a medical scientist who specializes in the study of histology. See also **histology.**

histology /histol′əjē/, **1.** the science dealing with the microscopic identification of cells and tissue. **2.** the structure of organ tissues, including the makeup of cells and their organization into various body tissues. **–histologic, histological,** *adj.,* **histologically,** *adv.*

histone /his′tōn/, any of a group of proteins, found in the cell nucleus, especially of glandular tissue. They help to regulate gene activity. Histones also interfere with clotting of the blood and have been found in the urine of patients with leukemia and fevers.

histoplasma agglutinin, an antibody against fungal lung infections.

Histoplasma capsulatum, a fungus that causes histoplasmosis, common in the Mississippi River Valley. The fungus, spread by airborne spores from soil infected with the droppings of infected birds, acts as a parasite on the cells of the body's defense system.

histoplasmosis /his′tōplazmō′sis/, an infection caused by breathing in spores of the fungus *Histoplasma capsulatum.* **Primary histoplasmosis** features fever, discomfort, cough, and swollen glands. Recovery without treatment is usual; small hard areas remain in the lungs and affected lymph glands. **Progressive histoplasmosis,** the sometimes fatal form of the infection, is known by open sores in the mouth and

nose, enlargement of the spleen, liver, and lymph nodes, and severe and widespread infection of the lungs. Infection makes one immune; a histoplasmin skin test may be performed to identify people who may safely work with infected soil. The disease is most common in the Mississippi and Ohio valleys.

history, **1.** a record of past events. **2.** a systematic account of the medical and other occurrences in a patient's life and of factors in family, ancestors, and environment that may have a bearing on the patient's condition.

history of present illness, an account obtained during the interview with the patient of the beginning, duration, and features of the present illness, as well as of any acts or factors that make the symptoms better or worse. The patient is asked what is believed to be the cause of the symptoms and whether a similar condition has occurred in the past.

histotoxin, any substance that is poisonous to the body tissues. It is usually produced within the body rather than coming from outside. **–histotoxic,** *adj.*

histotroph, histotrophe, histotrophic nutrition. See **embryotroph.**

histrionic personality, a personality that features overblown, emotionally unstable, overly dramatic, and self-centered behavior patterns as a means of attracting attention, consciously or unconsciously. Also called **hysteric personality.** See also **histrionic personality disorder.**

histrionic personality disorder, a disorder having dramatic and intensely exaggerated behavior, which is typically self-centered and results in severe disturbance in the patient's relationships with others. This can lead to psychosomatic disorders, depression, alcoholism, and drug dependency. Symptoms include emotional excitability, such as irrational angry outbursts or tantrums; abnormal craving for activity and excitement; overreaction to minor events; self-serving threats and gestures; self-centeredness, inconsiderateness; inconsistency; and continuous demand for reassurance because of feelings of helplessness and dependency. A person having this disorder is seen by others as vain, demanding, shallow, self-centered, and self-pampering. The disorder is more common in women than in men and is treated by various psychotherapies, depending on the individual and the severity of the condition. See also **narcissistic personality disorder.**

HIV, abbreviation for *human immunodeficiency virus.*

hives. See **urticaria.**

HMO, abbreviation for **Health Maintenance Organization.**

HMS Liquifilm, a trademark for an eye solution containing an anti-inflammatory hormone (medrysone).

H₂O, symbol for **water.**

Hodgkin's disease /hoj'kinz/, a cancerous disorder with painless, steady enlargement of lymph glands, usually first in the neck; enlarged spleen; and the presence of Reed-Sternberg cells, which are large, unusual white cells. Symptoms include loss of appetite, weight loss, generalized itching, low-grade fever, night sweats, a decrease of red blood cells, and increase of white blood cells. The disease is diagnosed in about 7,100 Americans annually, causes approximately 1,700 deaths a year, affects twice as many males as females, and usually develops between 15 and 35 years of age. Radiation of lymph nodes, using a covering mantle to protect other organs, is the usual treatment for early stages of the disease. Combination chemotherapy is the treatment for advanced disease. In more than one-half of the patients treated, the symptoms go away for long periods of time, and 60% to 90% of those with limited spreading of the disease may be cured. It is widely held that Hodgkin's disease may start as a swelling or infection and then develop into a tumor. According to another theory it may be a disorder of the immune system. Clusters of cases have been reported, but there is no definite evidence of an infectious agent, and the cause of the disease remains a mystery.

Hoffmann's atrophy. See **Werdnig-Hoffmann disease.**

Hoffmann's reflex, an abnormal reflex brought about by sudden, forceful striking of the nail of the index, middle, or ring finger, resulting in bending of the thumb and of the middle and end joints of one of the other fingers. It is a possible sign of motor nerve disease. Also called **Hoffmann's sign.**

holandric /holan'drik/, **1.** referring to genes located on the base of the Y chromosome. **2.** of or pertaining to traits or conditions passed on only from the father (the paternal line). Compare **hologynic.**

holandric inheritance, the inheritance of traits or conditions only from the father (the paternal line), passed on by genes carried on the Y chromosome. Compare **hologynic inheritance.**

holistic /hōlis'tik/, having to do with the whole; considering all factors, as holistic medicine. Also **wholistic.**

holistic counseling, a form of therapy that focuses on the whole person (mind, body, and spirit) and health; the goal is growth of the whole person.

holistic health care, a system of total patient care that considers the physical, emotional, social, economic, and spiritual needs of the patient. It also considers the patient's response to the illness and the impact of the illness on the patient's ability to meet self-care needs. Holis-

tic nursing is the modern nursing practice that expresses this philosophy of care. Also called **comprehensive care.**

Hollenback condenser. See **pneumatic condenser.**

holoacardius /hō'lō·əkär'dē·əs/, a separate, grossly defective identical-twin fetus. It is usually composed of a shapeless, nonformed mass in which the heart is absent and the circulation in the womb is provided totally by the heart of the healthy twin through a rerouted blood vessel.

holoacardius acephalus, a grossly defective separate twin fetus that lacks a heart, a head, and most of the upper portion of the body.

holoacardius acormus, a grossly defective, separate twin fetus in which the trunk is malformed and little more than the head is recognizable.

holoacardius amorphus, a malformed separate twin fetus in which there are no recognizable or formed parts.

holocephalic /hō'lōsifal'ik/, a malformed fetus in which several parts are lacking although the head is complete.

holodiastolic. See **pandiastolic.**

hologynic /hol'ōjin'ik/, **1.** designating genes located on attached X chromosomes. **2.** of or pertaining to traits or conditions passed on only from the mother (the maternal line). Compare **holandric.**

hologynic inheritance, the inheritance of traits or conditions only from the mother (the maternal line), passed on by genes located on attached X chromosomes. The phenomenon is not known to occur in humans. Compare **holandric inheritance.**

holoprosencephaly /hol'ōpros'ensef'əlē/, a birth defect caused by the failure of the forebrain to divide into halves during embryonic development. It is known by many midline facial defects, including the development of only one eye in severe cases. It can also be caused by an extra chromosome, being just one of many developmental defects. See also **trisomy 13.** –**holoprosencephalic, holoprosencephalous,** *adj.*

holorachischisis. See **complete rachischisis.**

holosystolic. See **pansystolic.**

Holtzman inkblot technique, a version of the Rorschach test in which many more pictures of inkblots are used, the subject is allowed only one answer to each design, and the scoring is mainly objective rather than subjective.

Homan's sign, pain in the calf that occurs with bending the foot back, indicating blood clots or swollen veins due to clots (thrombophlebitis).

home care, a health service provided in the patient's home for the purpose of promoting, maintaining, or restoring health or minimizing the effects of illness and disability. Service may include medical, dental, or nursing care, speech or physical therapy, the homemaking services of a home health aide, or transportation service. Nursing may be provided by a registered nurse, licensed practical nurse, or a home health aide. Some hospitals have homecare services that include regular visits by a nurse and a physician to patients in their homes.

home health agency, an organization that provides health care in the home. Medicare certification for a home health agency depends on the providing of skilled-nursing services and of at least one additional therapeutic service.

home maintenance management: impaired, a nursing diagnosis that describes the situation in which a person is unable to maintain a safe, healthy home environment without help. See also **nursing diagnosis.**

homeodynamics, the constantly changing body functions while keeping an overall balance of systems and health.

Homeopathic Pharmacopoeia of the United States, one of the three official drug lists specified in the Federal Food, Drug, and Cosmetic Act. See also **compendium, National Formulary, United States Pharmacopoeia.**

homeopathist /hō′mē·op′əthist/, a physician who practices homeopathy.

homeopathy /hō′mē·op′əthē/, a system of healing based on the theory that "like cures like." The theory was advanced in the late 18th century by Dr. Samuel Hahnemann, who believed that a large amount of a particular drug may cause symptoms of a disease and a mild dose may reduce those symptoms; thus, some disease symptoms could be treated by very small doses of medicine. In practice, homeopathists dilute drugs with milk sugar in ratios of 1 to 10 to achieve the smallest dose of a drug that seems necessary to control the symptoms in a patient. They also prescribe only one medication at a time. Compare **allopathy. –homeopathic,** *adj.*

homeostasis /hō′mē·əstā′sis/, a relatively constant state within the body, naturally maintained. Various sensing, feedback, and control systems bring about this steady state, especially the reticular formation in the brainstem and the hormone-producing glands. Some of the functions controlled by homeostatic mechanisms are the heart beat, blood production, blood pressure, body temperature, salt balance, breathing, and glandular secretion. **–homeostatic,** *adj.*

homicide, the death of one human being caused by another human. Homicide is usually intentional and often violent.

hominal physiology, the study of the specific physical and chemical processes involved in the normal functioning of humans; human physiology.

homiothermal. See **warm-blooded.**

homiothermic, referring to the ability of warm-blooded animals to keep a relatively stable body temperature regardless of the temperature of the environment. This ability is not fully developed in newborn humans.

homo-, **1.** a combining form meaning 'the same': *homocentric, homodont, homolysis.*

homoblastic, developing from a single type of tissue. Compare **heteroblastic.**

homochronous inheritance, the appearance of traits or conditions in the offspring at the same age as they appeared in the parents.

homocystinuria /hō′mōsis′tinŏŏr′ē·ə/, a rare disease known by the abnormal presence of homocystine, an amino acid, in the blood and urine. The disease is inherited and symptoms include mental retardation, softening of the bones leading to skeletal abnormalities, dislocated lenses, and blood clots in the veins. Treatment may include a diet low in methionine, and large doses of vitamin B_6. Long-term results of treatment are not available. **–homocystinuric,** *adj.*

homogeneous, **1.** consisting of similar elements or parts. **2.** having a uniform quality throughout. Compare **heterogeneous. –homogeneity,** *adj.*

homogenesis, reproduction by the same process in succeeding generations so that offspring are similar to the parents. Compare **heterogenesis.**

homogenetic, **1.** of or pertaining to homogenesis. **2.** homogenous, def. 2.

homogenized milk /hōmoj′ənīzd/, pasteurized milk that has been mechanically treated to reduce and spread the fat evenly throughout so that the cream cannot separate and the protein is more digestible.

homogenous /hōmoj′ənəs/, **1.** homogeneous. **2.** having a likeness in form or structure because of a common ancestral origin. Compare **heterogenous. 3.** homoplasty.

homogentisic acid. See **glycosuric acid.**

homogeny /hōmoj′ənē/, **1.** homogenesis. **2.** a likeness in structure or form because of a common ancestral origin. Compare **homoplasty.**

homograft. See **allograft.**

homolateral, pertaining to the same side of the body.

homolog /hom′əlog/, any organ corresponding in function, origin, and structure to another organ, as the flippers of a seal that correspond to human hands. Also spelled **homologue.** Compare **analog. –homologous,** *adj.*

homologous chromosomes, any two chromosomes in the doubled set of the body cell that are identical in size, shape, and gene placement. In humans there are 22 pairs of homologous chromosomes and one pair of sex chromosomes, with one member of each pair coming from the mother and the other from the father. Any difference in the size, number, or genetic makeup of the chromosomes leads to defects or disorders from mild to severe in the affected individual.

homologous disease. See **graft-versus-host reaction.**

homologous insemination. See **artificial insemination-husband.**

homologous tumor, a tumor made up of cells resembling those of the tissue in which it is growing.

homonymous hemianopia, blindness or defective vision in the right or left halves of the visual fields of both eyes. This condition is frequently seen in people who have suffered a stroke.

homoplasty, having a likeness in form or structure because of similar environmental conditions or parallel evolution rather than because of common ancestral origin. Compare **homogeny.** –**homoplastic,** *adj.*

homosexual, 1. of, pertaining to, or denoting the same sex. **2.** a person who is sexually attracted to members of the same sex. Compare **heterosexual.** See also **lesbian.**

homosexual panic, a sudden attack of anxiety based on possible unconscious desires and a conscious fear of being homosexual. Compare **heterosexual panic.**

homothermal. See **warm-blooded.**

homozygosis /hō′mōzīgō′sis/, **1.** the fertilization of an egg by the union of two sex cells that have one or more pairs of identical genes. **2.** the production of purebred organisms or strains through the process of inbreeding.

homozygous /hō′məzī′gəs/, having two identical genes at the same place on matched chromosomes. An individual who is homozygous for a particular characteristic has inherited from each parent one of two identical genes for that characteristic. A person homozygous for a genetic disease caused by a pair of recessive genes, as sickle cell anemia, shows the disorder, and his or her offspring have a 100% chance of inheriting the gene for the disease. Compare **heterozygous.**

homunculus /hōmung′kyələs/, *pl.* **homunculi, 1.** a dwarf in which all the body parts are in proportion and in which there is no deformity or abnormality. **2.** (in early theories of development), a minute and complete human being contained in each of the eggs (germ cells) that after fertilization grows from the microscopic to normal size; the term was also applied to the human fetus. **3.** (in psychiatry) a little man, created by the imagination, who possesses magical powers.

hookworm, a common name for a roundworm of the genera *Ancylostoma, Necator,* or *Uncinaria.* Most hookworm infections in the Western Hemisphere are caused by the species *Necator americanus.*

hopelessness, a psychological condition in which one believes that all efforts to change one's life situation will be fruitless.

hordeolum /hôrdē′ələm/, a boil on the edge of the eyelid formed in the root of an eyelash. Treatment includes hot compresses and antibiotic eye medicines; it occasionally requires opening and drainage. Also called **sty.** Compare **chalazion.**

horizon, a specific stage of development of the human embryo based on the appearance and final development of certain body parts. There are 23 horizons, each lasting 2 to 3 days, beginning with the fertilization of the egg and ending 7 to 9 weeks later with the beginning of the fetal period of development in the womb.

horizontal fissure of the right lung, the break between the upper and middle lobes of the right lung.

horizontal resorption, a pattern of bone loss in disease of the tissues surrounding the teeth. Compare **vertical resorption.** See also **resorption.**

horizontal transmission, the spread of an infectious germ from one person or group to another, usually through contact with contaminated material, such as spit or feces.

hormone, a complex chemical substance produced in one part or organ of the body that starts or runs the activity of an organ or a group of cells in another part of the body. Hormones from the endocrine glands are carried through the bloodstream to the target organ. Release of these hormones is regulated by other hormones, by nerve signals, and by a signal from the target organ indicates a decreased need for the stimulating hormone. This is the basic principle of birth-control pills. A steady supply of female hormones in the pills causes a lowered release of the hormones that ordinarily cause the ovary to develop and release the egg, along with the same female hormones (estrogen and progesterone). Other hormones are released by organs for specific reasons, most commonly in the digestive tract.

Horner's syndrome, a nerve condition involving narrowed pupils, drooping eyelids, and unusual facial dryness resulting from an injury to the spinal cord, with damage to a neck nerve. In the case of accidental, sudden injury, the person is carried flat with as little movement as possible.

horny layer. See **stratum corneum.**

horripilation. See **pilomotor reflex.**

horse serum, any vaccine prepared from the blood of a horse, especially tetanus antitoxin. Because many people are allergic to horse serum, a skin test for allergy is usually performed before the vaccine is given. Human tetanus serum is preferred.

horseshoe fistula, an abnormal, semicircular passage in the area around the anus with both openings on the surface of the skin.

Hortega cells. See **microglia.**

Horton's arteritis. See **temporal arteritis.**

Horton's headache. See **migrainous cranial neuralgia.**

Horton's histamine cephalalgia. See **histamine headache.**

hospice /hos'pis/, a system of family-centered care designed to assist the patient with a long-term illness to be comfortable and to maintain a satisfactory life style through the last phases of dying. Hospice care includes home visits, professional medical help available on call, teaching and emotional support of the family, and physical care of the patient. Some hospice programs provide care in a center, as well as in the home. See also **emotional care of the dying patient, stages of dying.**

hospital-acquired infection. See **nosocomial infection.**

hospitalism, the physical or mental effects of hospitalization or institutionalization on patients, especially infants and children who show this condition through social withdrawal, personality disorders, and stunted growth. See also **anaclitic depression.**

host, 1. an organism that is a victim of parasitic invasion. A **primary** or **definitive host** is one in which the adult parasite lives and reproduces. A **secondary** or **intermediate host** is one in which the parasite exists in its nonsexual, larval stage. A **reservoir host** is a primary animal host for organisms that are sometimes parasitic in humans and from which humans may become infected. **2.** the recipient of a transplanted organ or tissue. Compare **donor.**

hostility, the tendency of an organism to threaten harm to another or to itself. The hostility may be expressed passively and actively.

hot bath, a bath in which the temperature of the water is gradually raised to about 106° F.

hot flash, a short-lasting feeling of warmth experienced by some women during or after menopause. Hot flashes result from blood flow disturbances caused by hormone changes. The exact cause is not known. Most menopausal women do not experience hot flashes; among those who do, the frequency, length, and strength of flashes vary widely. Though physically harmless, the symptom may be extremely disturbing or, rarely, disabling. Hot flashes may be relieved by the taking of the hormone estrogen in cycles. Also called **hot flush.**

hot line, a means of contacting a trained counselor or specific agency for help with a particular problem, as a rape hot line or a battered-child hot line. The person needing help calls a telephone number and speaks to a counselor who remains nameless and who offers emotional support, advice for action, and referral to other medical, social, or community services. Such services are usually staffed by volunteers who answer phones 24 hours a day, 7 days a week.

hour glass uterus, a womb with a segment of circular muscle fibers that contract during labor, causing lack of progress in the birth despite adequate labor contractions. The baby is pushed back in rather than out during contractions.

housemaid's knee, a long lasting swelling of the fluid sac in front of the kneecap, with redness. It is caused by long and repeated pressure of the knee on a hard surface.

house physician, a physician on call and immediately available in a hospital or other health-care facility.

house surgeon, a surgeon on call and immediately available on the premises of a hospital.

housewives' eczema, a common term for skin irritation of the hands caused and worsened by their frequent soaking in water and by the use of soaps and detergents.

Houston's valves. See **plicae transversales recti.**

Howell-Jolly bodies, round, grainy particles in the red blood cells, visible in blood samples under a microscope. They are most commonly seen in people who have blood diseases, as anemia and leukemia, or no spleen, either from birth or because of surgical removal.

HPV, 1. an abbreviation for **human papilloma virus. 2.** abbreviaton for **human parvovirus.**

h.s., (in prescriptions) abbreviation for *hora somni,* a Latin phrase meaning "bedtime."

HSA, abbreviation for **health systems agency.**

HSV, abbreviation for *herpes simplex virus.* See **herpes genitalis, herpes simplex.**

Hubbard tank, a large tank in which a patient may be placed to perform underwater exercise. It heats the water and is generally used for exercising the trunk and legs. See also **whirlpool bath.**

Huhn's gland, a gland embedded in tissues on the underneath surface of the tongue.

human bite, a wound caused by the piercing of skin by human teeth. Bacteria are usually present, and serious infection often follows. The area is treated by being thoroughly washed, using an antiseptic, and rinsing well. The wound is examined often and antibiotics given, if necessary.

human chorionic gonadotropin. See **chorionic gonadotropin.**

human chorionic somatomammotropin (HCS), a hormone produced during pregnancy. It regulates carbohydrate and protein processing in the mother to ensure that the fetus receives glucose for energy and protein for growth. HCS may also cause diabeteslike symptoms in the mother.

human immunodeficiency virus, the virus that causes AIDS. Infection with this virus severely weakens the immune system so that the patient is susceptible to many diseases. The most common are various infections and cancers. A person may be infected with the virus but not show symptoms for many years. The virus may be transmitted through sexual contact, infected blood (either through transfusions or sharing needles), or from mother to child during pregnancy or breast feeding. The drug zidovudine (AZT) may be used to slow the progression of the disease, but there is no cure.

human ecology, the study of how individuals and their environments, as well as individuals within the environment, interact.

human insulin, a product manufactured from two forms of bacteria found naturally in the human digestive tract (*Escherichia coli*) by genetic engineering. Human insulin does not cause the allergic reactions that animal insulins do, especially in patients who only require insulin on a short-term basis. See also **insulin, def. 2.**

human investigations committee, a committee set up in a hospital, school, or university to judge applications for research involving human subjects. Its purpose is to protect the rights of the people to be studied. Also called **human subjects review committee.**

humanistic existential therapy, a kind of mental therapy that promotes self-awareness and personal growth. It achieves this by stressing current reality and by discovering and changing the patient's usual actions to help make the most of a person's potential. This process may be made easier in a group setting, where problems are revealed through interaction with others. Kinds of humanistic existential psychotherapy are **client-oriented therapy, existential therapy, Gestalt therapy.** Also called **existential humanistic psychotherapy.**

human leukocyte antigen (HLA), a system of four genetic markers on chromosome 6. Each marker is linked to certain diseases or conditions. The HLA system is used to judge the similarity of the tissues of different persons. Perfect tissue compatibility exists only between identical twins.

human natural killer cells, white blood cells that are able to burst tumor cells and cells infected by viruses as part of the body's natural defense against disease.

human papilloma virus (HPV), a virus that is the cause of common warts of the hands and feet, as well as sores in the mouth and around the anus and genitals. More than 50 types of HPV have been identified, some of which are linked to cancerous conditions. The virus can be spread through sexual contact and is often found in women with cancer of the cervix. There is no specific cure for an HPV infection, but the virus can often be controlled by drugs such as podophyllin or interferon. Warts can be removed by freezing, laser treatment, or surgery.

human parvovirus (HPV), a small virus particle that has been linked to several diseases, including some anemias in which the red blood cells are destroyed. Parvoviruses of various types also infect wild animals and pets.

human placental lactogen (HPL), a hormone produced in the placenta that may be lacking in certain abnormalities of pregnancy.

human protein C, an agent that stops blood clotting. It is made by bacteria that have been altered genetically (genetic engineering).

human subjects investigation committee. See **human investigations committee.**

Humatin, a trademark for a drug that fights amebic infections (paromomycin sulfate).

humeral. See **humerus.**

humeral articulation. See **shoulder joint.**

humerus /hyo͞o'mərəs/, *pl.* **humeri,** the largest bone of the upper arm. The lower end has several grooves that connect with the two bones in the lower arm (radius and ulna). Also called **arm bone.** –**humeral,** *adj.*

humidifier lung, a type of allergic lung condition common among workers involved with refrigeration and air-conditioning equipment. The allergy is to two kinds of fungus, *Micropolyspora* and *Thermoactinomyces.* Symptoms of the short-term form of the disease include chills, cough, fever, difficult breathing, loss of appetite, nausea, and vomiting. The long-term form of the disease is known by fatigue, cough, weight loss, and difficult breathing during exercise. Also called **air conditioner lung.** See also **pneumonitis.**

humoral immunity /hyo͞o'mərəl/, one of the two forms of immunity against invaders, as bacteria and foreign tissue. Humoral immunity is the result of the development and the continuing presence of circulating antibodies which are produced by the body's defense system. Compare **cellular immunity.**

humoral response, one of a broad category of allergic reactions. Compare **cell-mediated immunity.**

Humorsol, a trademark for a drug used to treat glaucoma and crossed eyes. (demecarium bromide).

hung-up reflex, a deep tendon reflex in which, after a stimulus is given and the reflex action takes place, there is a slow return of the limb to its neutral position. This delayed return is typical of the reflexes in patients with underactive thyroid. See also **deep tendon reflex.**

Hunner's ulcer. See **interstitial cystitis.**

Hunter's canal. See **adductor canal.**

Hunter's syndrome, an inborn defect affecting only males, resulting in dwarfism, hunchback, gargoylelike features (Hurler's syndrome), and mental retardation. It is passed along as an X-linked recessive trait. Females who carry the gene can be identified by biochemical tests, and known carriers may choose to abort if amniocentesis reveals a male fetus. Males born of women who carry the trait have a 50% chance of having the syndrome. Also called **MPS II.** See also **mucopolysaccharidosis.**

Huntington's chorea, a rare, abnormal inherited condition known by gradual decline and mental breakdown that ends in insanity. An individual with the condition usually shows the first signs after age 50 and dies about 15 years later. Also called **chronic chorea, degenerative chorea.**

Hurler's syndrome, an inherited abnormality that causes severe mental retardation. The symptoms of Hurler's syndrome begin within the first few months of life. Usual signs of the disease are enlargement of the liver and the spleen, often with heart involvement. Facial features of individuals affected by Hurler's syndrome include a low forehead and an enlarged head, sometimes resulting from water on the brain. Clouding of the eyes is common, and the neck is short. There is hunchback, and the hands and the fingers are short and broad. Rigidly bent limbs are common with this disease. Hurler's syndrome usually results in death during childhood from heart or lung failures. Also called **gargoylism, MPS I.** See also **mucopolysaccharidosis.**

Hürthle cell adenoma, a noncancerous tumor of the thyroid gland composed of large cells (Hürthle cells). Compare **Hürthle cell carcinoma.**

Hürthle cell carcinoma, a cancerous tumor of the thyroid gland composed of large cells (Hürthle cells). Tumors of this kind occur more often in women than in men. See also **Hürthle cell adenoma.**

Hürthle cell tumor, a tumor of the thyroid gland composed of large cells (Hürthle cells); it may be harmless (Hürthle cell adenoma) or cancerous (Hürthle cell carcinoma).

husband-coached childbirth. See **Bradley method.**

Hutchinson's disease. See **angioma serpiginosum.**

Hutchinson's freckle, a tan patch on the skin that grows slowly, becoming mottled, dark, thick, and bumpy. The spot is usually seen on one side of the face of an elderly person. Removal is recommended because it often becomes cancerous. Also called **lentigo maligna.** See also **melanoma.**

Hutchinson's teeth, a feature of inherited syphilis in which the permanent incisor teeth are peg-shaped, widely spaced, and notched at the end with a centrally placed crescent-shaped deformity. See also **syphilis.**

Hutchinson's triad, the clouding of the cornea, notched teeth, and deafness characteristic of inherited syphilis. See also **syphilis.**

Hutchison-type neuroblastoma, a nerve cancer that has spread to the brain.

hyaline cartilage, the gristly, elastic connective tissue that thinly covers the moving ends of bones, connects the ribs to the breastbone, and supports the nose, windpipe, and part of the voicebox. It tends to harden in advanced age. Compare **yellow cartilage, white fibrocartilage.**

hyaline cast, a transparent cast composed of mucoprotein.

hyaline membrane disease. See **acute respiratory distress syndrome of the newborn.**

hyaline thrombus, a clear, colorless mass consisting of broken-down red blood cells.

hyaloid artery /hī'əloid/, a blood vessel in the embryo that branches to supply the inside of the eye and develops part of the blood supply to the eye lens. The hyaloid artery disappears from the fetus in the ninth month of pregnancy, leaving a leftover, hyaloid canal, which remains in the adult as a narrow passage through the eye.

hybrid, 1. an offspring produced from mating plants or animals from different species, varieties, or genotypes. 2. of or pertaining to such a plant or animal.

hybridization, 1. the process of producing hybrids by crossbreeding.

hybrid vigor. See **heterosis.**

Hycodan, a trademark for a drug used for cough relief.

Hycomine, a trademark for a drug used to treat coughs.

hydantoin /hīdan'tō·in/, any one of a group of medications, similar to the barbiturates, that act to limit epileptic seizures and reduce the spread of the abnormal electric excitation from the point where the seizure starts. The most common hydantoin in current use is phenytoin. Serious adverse effects of the drug include heart collapse and slowing down of brain activity when too much is given through the vein, as may occur in the emergency treatment of epileptic seizure. Long-term harmful effects are related to the dose and the route through which the drug is given. Phenytoin is sometimes also prescribed in the treatment of shooting pain in a facial nerve and heart beat irregularities.

hydatid /hī'dətid/, a cyst or cystlike structure that usually is filled with fluid, especially the cyst formed around the developing dog tapeworm *Echinococcus granulosus.* Humans and sheep can become hosts to the worm by eating the eggs. Hydatid cysts may be discovered by feeling around the area of the liver, where they most often occur. A sudden allergic reaction may occur if the cyst ruptures. See also **hydatid cyst, hydatid mole, hydatidosis. –hydatidiform,** *adj.*

hydatid cyst, a cyst in the liver that contains larvae of the tapeworm *Echinococcus granulosus,* whose eggs are carried from the intestinal tract to the liver through the blood. Patients generally lack symptoms, except for a swollen liver and a dull ache over the right upper quarter of the stomach. X-ray tests are used in diagnosis, and because no medical treatment is available, surgical removal of the cyst is required. Compare **hydatid mole.**

hydatid disease. See **echinococcosis.**

hydatid mole, a tumor-like mass in the uterus occurring in approximately one in 1,500 pregnancies in the United States and eight times more frequently in some Oriental countries. It is more common in older and younger women than in those between 20 and 40 years of age. The cause of the disorder is not known; it may be the result of defective ovulation, a womb abnormality, or inadequate diet. Typical signs of the condition are extreme nausea, uterine bleeding, anemia, overactive thyroid, an unusually large womb for the length of pregnancy, absence of fetal heart sounds, fluid buildup, and high blood pressure. In most cases the mole is discovered when abortion is threatened or in progress. Oxytocin may be used to bring on the passing of a mole that is not naturally aborted, and scraping is usually performed several days later to be certain that no molar tissue remains in the uterus. It is important that pregnancy be avoided for at least 1 year and that the patient be watched for signs of cancer. Also called **hydatidiform mole.** See also **trophoblastic disease.**

hydatidosis /hī'dətidō'sis/, infection with the tapeworm *Echinococcus granulosus.* See also **hydatid cyst.**

Hydeltrasol, a trademark for an anti-swelling drug (prednisolone sodium phosphate).

Hydeltra TBA, a trademark for an anti-swelling drug (prednisolone tebutate).

Hydergine, a trademark for a drug used to treat peripheral vein disease.

hydradenitis /hī'dradəni'tis/, an infection or swelling of the sweat glands. Also spelled **hidradenitis.**

hydralazine /hīdral'əzēn/, a drug prescribed in the treatment of high blood pressure.

★CAUTION: Coronary artery disease, rheumatic heart disease, or known allergy to this drug prohibits its use.

★ADVERSE EFFECTS: Among the most serious side effects are chest pains, rapid or irregular heart beat, loss of appetite, tremors, blood disorders, depression, nausea, and irritation of the nerves.

hydralazine hydrochloride, a drug prescribed in the treatment of high blood pressure.

★CAUTION: Coronary artery disease, rheumatic heart disease, or known allergy to this drug prohibits its use.

★ADVERSE EFFECTS: Among the more serious side effects are headache, loss of appetite, rapid heart beat, digestive tract disturbances, and a syndrome resembling the skin disease lupus erythematosus.

hydramnios /hīdram'nē-əs/, an abnormal condition of pregnancy known by an excess of fluid surrounding the fetus. It occurs in less than 1% of pregnancies and is diagnosed by feeling, ultrasound, or x-ray examination. It is linked to maternal disorders, including blood poisoning of pregnancy and diabetes mellitus. Some fetal disorders may interfere with normal exchange of amniotic fluid, resulting in hydramnios. The chances of premature breaking of the water sac, premature labor, and stillbirth are increased. Periodic drawing off of fluid may be necessary. Also called **hydramnion, polyhydramnios.** Compare **acute hydramnios, oligohydramnios.**

hydrargyrism. See **mercury poisoning.**

Hydrea, a trademark for an antitumor drug (hydroxyurea).

hydremic ascites, an abnormal accumulation of fluid within the cavity of the trunk, with dilution of the blood as in protein calorie malnutrition. See also **ascites.**

hydroa /hīdrō'ə/, an unusual blistering skin condition of childhood that comes each summer after exposure to sunlight, sometimes accompanied by itching and thickening of the skin. Hydroa usually disappears soon after puberty. Treatment includes use of sunscreen lotions and the avoidance of exposure to sunlight.

hydrocarbon, any one of a large group of chemical compounds found in living things, the molecules of which are made up of hydrogen and carbon, many of which are derived from petroleum.

hydrocele /hī'drōsēl'/, an accumulation of fluid in any saclike cavity or duct, specifically in the membrane surrounding the testicles or along the spermatic cord. The condition is caused by swelling of the sex organs or by obstruction in the cord. Inborn hydrocele is caused by failure of the canal between the trunk cavity and the scrotum to close completely during prenatal development. In some newborn infants the defect may correct itself. Treatment for lasting hydrocele is surgery. Drawing off of fluid is only a temporary measure and may cause infection. See also **inguinal hernia.**

hydrocephalus, a disease state marked by an abnormal amount of spinal fluid, usually under high pressure, in the head causing widening of the ventricles. Interference with the normal flow of cerebrospinal fluid may be caused by increased release of fluid, blockage in the ventricular system, or reabsorption from a cerebral space. These may result from developmental problems, infection, trauma, or brain tumors. Also called **hydrocephaly. –hydrocephalic,** *adj., n.*

★OBSERVATIONS: The condition may be inborn with rapid onset of symptoms or it may progress slowly so that neurological signs do not come until early to late childhood or even until early adulthood. In infants, the head grows at an abnormal rate with separation of the sutures, bulging softspots, and dilated scalp veins. The face becomes relatively small and the eyes seem sunk in the sockets. Typical behavior includes irritability with lethargy and vomiting, leg spasticity, and failure of normal reflex actions. If the condition progresses, lower brain-stem function is disrupted, the skull becomes enormous, the cortex is destroyed, and the infant displays sleepiness, seizures, and heart and lung blockage, often not surviving the neonatal period. At later onset, after the cranial sutures have fused and the skull has formed, symptoms are primarily neurological and include headache, swelling of the optic disc, and loss of muscular coordination. Hydrocephalus in infants is suspected when head growth is above the normal rate. In all age groups diagnosis is confirmed by such procedures as spinal fluid examination, air encephalography, arteriography, and echoencephalography.

★TREATMENT: Treatment is usually surgery to correct the ventricular blockage, reduce the making of spinal fluid, or shunt the excess fluid to the heart or peritoneal cavity. Surgically treated hydrocephalus with continued neurosurgical and medical management has a survival rate of approximately 80%, but prognosis depends largely on the cause of the condition. Hydrocephalus is often found with myelomeningocele, in which case there is a less favorable prognosis.

★PATIENT CONSIDERATIONS: Primary care of the child with hydrocephalus consists of good nutrition and proper positioning and support to prevent extra strain on the neck. Parents need to know the signs of shunt malfunction or infection and how to pump the shunt.

hydrochloric acid, a compound of hydrogen and chlorine. Hydrochloric acid is secreted in the stomach. It is a main part of gastric juice.

hydrochlorothiazide, a diuretic used to treat hypertension and swelling (edema).

★CAUTION: Anuria or allergy to this drug, to other thiazide medication, or to sulfonamide derivatives prevents its use.

★ADVERSE EFFECTS: Among the more serious side effects are low or high blood sugar, high uric acid, and allergic reactions.

hydrocholeretics, drugs that stimulate the making of bile with a low specific gravity or with a minimal proportion of solid constituents.

Hydrocil, a trademark for a laxative (psyllium hydrophilic muciloid).

hydrocodone bitartrate, a narcotic given to treat cough.

★CAUTION: Drug dependence or allergy to this drug prevents its use.

★ADVERSE EFFECTS: Among the more serious side effects are drug dependence and respiratory and circulatory depression.

hydrocortisone, hydrocortisone acetate, hydrocortisone cyclopentylpropionate, hydrocortisone sodium succinate. See **cortisol.**

hydrocortisone valerate, a steroid. used topically as an anti-inflammatory agent.

★CAUTION: Viral and fungal skin diseases that occur where circulation is slowed or allergy to steroids prevents its use.

★ADVERSE REACTIONS: Among the more serious side effects are various systemic effects that may occur from long or great use. Local irritation of the skin may occur.

Hydrocortone, a trademark for a glucocorticoid (hydrocortisone acetate).

HydroDIURIL, a trademark for a diuretic (hydrochlorothiazide).

hydroflumethiazide, a diuretic used to treat hypertension and swelling.

★CAUTION: Anuria or allergy to this drug, to other thiazide medication, or to sulfonamide derivatives prevents its use.

★ADVERSE EFFECTS: Among the more serious side effects are blood disorders, low blood pressure, high blood calcium, high blood sugar, high uric acid, and allergic reactions.

hydrogen (H), a gaseous element, normally a colorless, odorless, highly inflammable gas. As part of water, hydrogen is crucial in the interaction of acids, bases, and salts in the body and in the fluid balance needed for the body to survive. Hydrogen enables water to dissolve the different substances on which the body depends, as oxygen and food substances.

hydrogenation. See **reduction.**

hydrogen peroxide, a topical anti-infective. It is used to cleanse open wounds, as a mouthwash, and to aid in removing earwax.

★CAUTION: Irritations to skin or mucous membranes or allergy to this agent prevent its use.

★ADVERSE EFFECTS: There are no known side effects.

hydromorphone hydrochloride, a narcotic used to treat moderate to severe pain.

★CAUTION: It is used with caution in many cases, including head injuries, asthma, impaired kidney or liver function, or unstable heart. Allergy to this drug prevents its use.

★ADVERSE EFFECTS: Among the most serious side effects are drowsiness, dizziness, nausea, constipation, slowed breathing and blood flow, and drug addiction.

hydronephrosis /hī'drōnefrō'sis/, swelling of the pelvis by urine that cannot flow past a blockage in a ureter. Ureteral obstruction may be caused by a tumor, a stone lodged in the ureter, inflammation of the prostate gland, or a urinary-tract infection. The person may have pain in the flank. Surgery to remove the blockage may be needed. Prolonged hydronephrosis will result in eventual loss of kidney function. See also **urinary calculi. –hydro-nephrotic,** *adj.*

hydropenia, lack of water in the body tissues.

hydrophobia, 1. *nontechnical.* rabies. **2.** a morbid, extreme fear of water.

hydrophthalmos. See **congenital glaucoma.**

Hydropres, a trademark for a drug containing a diuretic (hydrochlorothiazide) and an antihypertensive (reserpine).

hydrops /hī′drops/, an abnormal amount of clear, watery fluid in a body tissue or cavity, as a joint, a fallopian tube, the middle ear, or the gallbladder. Hydrops in the entire body may occur in infants born with thalassemia or severe Rh sensitization. Formerly called **dropsy.**

hydrops fetalis, massive edema in the fetus or newborn, usually along with severe erythroblastosis fetalis. Severe anemia occurs. The condition often leads to death, even with immediate exchange transfusions after delivery. Also called **fetal hydrops.**

hydroquinone /hī′drōkwin′ōn/, a bleaching agent. It is given to reduce pigmentation in certain skin conditions in which an excess of melanin causes hyperpigmentation.

★CAUTION: Sunburn, prickly heat, other skin irritation, or allergy to this drug prevents its use.

★ADVERSE EFFECTS: Among the more serious side effects are tingling, redness, burning, and severe swelling of the skin.

hydrosalpinx /hī′drōsal′pingks/, an abnormal state of the fallopian tube in which the tube is cystically enlarged and filled with clear fluid. It results from infection that has previously blocked the tube at both ends.

hydrotherapy, the use of water to treat mental and physical problems. Hydrotherapy may include continuous tub baths, wet sheet packs, or shower sprays.

hydrothorax, a nonswelling buildup of serum in one or both plural cavities.

hydroxyamphetamine hydrobromide, a drug used to dilate the pupil for eye tests and as a diagnostic aid in Horner's syndrome.

★CAUTION: Narrow-angle glaucoma or allergy to this drug prevents its use.

★ADVERSE EFFECTS: Among the more serious side effects are high inner eye pressure and photophobia.

hydroxyandrosterone, a sex hormone released by the testes and adrenal glands.

hydroxybenzene. See carbolic acid.

hydroxychloroquine sulfate, an antiprotozoal, antirheumatic drug. It suppresses lupus erythematosus and polymorphous light eruption. It is used to stop malaria and liver amebas.

★CAUTION: Concurrent use of other 4-aminoquinolones or gold salts or allergy to this drug or to other 4-aminoquinolones prevents its use. It is used with caution in people with alcoholism, blood disease, severe nerve disor-

der, retinal or visual field damage, psoriasis, or porphyria. The drug is not usually recommended in pregnancy because it has been associated with damage to the central nervous system of the fetus.

★ADVERSE EFFECTS: Among the many severe side effects are retinopathy, eye clouding, polyneuritis, seizure, agranulocytosis, and hepatitis. The incidence and severity of these and many other side effects increase with the dose and prolonged duration of treatment.

17-hydroxycorticosteroid, any of the hormones, as cortisol, released by adrenal glands, measured in the urine to test adrenal function and diagnose hypoadrenalism or hyperadrenalism.

11-hydroxyetiocholanolone, a sex hormone released by the testes and adrenal glands.

5-hydroxyindoleacetic acid, an acid measured in the blood and urine to diagnose some tumors. It commonly rises above normal levels in whole blood in association with asthma, diarrhea, rapid heart beat, and other symptoms and is elevated in the urine of patients with carcinoid syndrome.

hydroxyprogesterone caproate, a steroid given to treat advanced adenocarcinoma of the uterine corpus, amenorrhea, and abnormal uterine bleeding caused by hormonal imbalance in the absence of organic disease.

★CAUTION: Badly impaired liver function, breast cancer, undiagnosed abnormal genital bleeding, near abortion, thromboembolitic disorders, or allergy to this drug prevents its use.

★ADVERSE EFFECTS: Among the most serious side effects are thrombophlebitis, blood clots in the lungs, stroke, tumors of the eye, loss of appetite, swelling, high blood pressure, jaundice, and depression.

hydroxyproline, an amino acid that is raised in the urine in bone diseases and some genetic disorders, as Marfan's syndrome.

5-hydroxytryptamine. See serotonin.

hydroxyurea /hīdrok′siyoŏrē′ə/, a drug used to treat tumors.

★CAUTION: Bone-marrow depression or allergy to this drug prevents its use. It is not to be given to women who are or might become pregnant.

★ADVERSE EFFECTS: The most serious side effect is bone-marrow depression. GI disturbances and dermatitis may occur.

hydroxyzine hydrochloride /hīdrok′səzēn/, a minor tranquilizer. It is given to relieve anxiety, nervous tension, hyperkinesis, and motion sickness.

★CAUTION: Allergy to this drug is the only caution.

★ADVERSE EFFECTS: No serious side effects have been observed. Decreased mental alertness is sometimes seen.

Hygroton, a trademark for a diuretic (chlorthalidone).

Hylorel, a trademark for a high blood pressure drug (guanadrel sulfate).

hymen /hī'mən/, a fold of mucous membrane, skin, and fibrous tissue at the vagina entrance. It may be absent, small, thin and pliant, or, rarely, tough and dense, completely blocking the entrance. When the hymen is broken, small rounded elevations remain. See also **carunculae hymenales.**

hymenal tag /hī'mənəl/, normal hymenal tissue protruding from the floor of the vagina during the first weeks after birth. It disappears without treatment.

Hymenolepis /hī'minol'əpis/, a genus of intestinal tapeworms infesting humans. Heavy infestation of some may cause intestinal pain, bloody stools, and nervous system disorders, especially in children. Contaminated food spreads the disease, which is endemic in the United States. Quinacrine hydrochloride or hexylresorcinol is used to treat the infestation.

hymenotomy /hī'mənot'əmē/, the surgical cutting of the hymen.

hyoglossal. See **glossohyal.**

hyoscine hydrobromide. See **scopolamine hydrobromide.**

hyoscyamine /hī'əsī'əmēn/, a drug used to treat hypermotility of the GI and the lower urinary tracts.

★CAUTION: Narrow-angle glaucoma, asthma, blockage of the urinary or digestive tracts, severe ulcerative colitis, or allergy to this drug prevents its use.

★ADVERSE EFFECTS: Among the more serious side effects are blurred vision, central nervous system effects, rapid heart rate, dry mouth, decreased sweating, and allergic reactions.

hypalgesia, the sense of a painful stimulus to a degree that varies widely from a normal perception of the same stimulus.

Hyperab, a trademark for a passive immunizing agent (rabies immune globulin).

hyperacidity, too much acidity, as in the stomach. See also **hyperchlorhydria.**

hyperactivity, any abnormally increased activity either of the entire organism or of certain organ, as the heart or thyroid. Compare **hypoactivity.** See also **attention deficit disorder.**

hyperadrenalism. See **Cushing's disease.**

hyperadrenocorticism. See **Cushing's syndrome.**

hyperaldosteronism. See **aldosteronism.**

hyperalimentation, 1. overfeeding or the eating of too great an amount of nutrients. 2. See **total parenteral nutrition.**

hyperammonemia /hī'pəram'ōnē'mē·ə/, too much ammonia in the blood. Ammonia is produced in the intestine, absorbed into the blood, and detoxified in the liver. If there is over-production of ammonia or a decreased ability to detoxify it, levels in the blood may increase. Untreated, the condition leads to vomiting, lethargy, coma, and death.

hyperbaric oxygenation, giving oxygen at high atmospheric pressure. The procedure is done in special chambers that permit the delivery of pure oxygen at atmospheric pressure that is three times normal. Hyperbaric oxygenation has been used to treat carbon monoxide poisoning, air embolism, smoke inhalation, acute cyanide poisoning, and decompression sickness. It is also used in certain cases of blood loss or anemia in which increased oxygen may help compensate for the hemoglobin deficiency.

hyperbetalipoproteinemia /hī'pərbā'təlip'ōprō'tēnē'mē·ə/, type II hyperlipoproteinemia. It is a genetic disorder of lipid metabolism, in which there are too high levels of blood cholesterol, and a yellow plaque appears on the tendons of the heels, knees, and fingers. There is a marked tendency to develop atherosclerosis and early heart attack, especially among males. Treatment attempts to reduce blood cholesterol levels. The patient is usually counseled to avoid most meats, eggs, milk products, and all saturated fats. He is encouraged to eat fish, grains, fruits, vegetables, lean poultry, and unsaturated fats. Exercise may be recommended, and drugs may be prescribed in some cases. See also **cholesterolemia.**

hyperbilirubinemia /hī'pərbil'iroō'binē'mē·ə/, too much of the bile pigment bilirubin in the blood. It is often characterized by jaundice, anorexia, and malaise. Hyperbilirubinemia is most often linked to liver disease or obstruction of bile. But it also occurs when there is too much destruction of red blood cells. Treatment is specific to the underlying condition. When bilirubin levels are high, treatment includes light ray therapy and hydration. See also **jaundice.**

hyperbilirubinemia of the newborn, an excess of bilirubin in the blood of the newborn. It is caused by poor liver function. Also called **neonatal hyperbilirubinemia.** See also **breast milk jaundice, cholestasis, Crigler-Najjar syndrome, Dubin-Johnson syndrome, erythroblastosis fetalis, Gilbert's syndrome, kernicterus, phototherapy in the newborn, Rotor syndrome.**

★OBSERVATIONS: Blood bilirubin levels are up in the normal newborn because infants have a low ability to excrete bilirubin, owing to a low albumin concentration and a lack of intestinal bacteria. Clinically observable jaundice or bilirubin levels exceeding 5 mg/100 ml within the first 24 hours of life are abnormal and indicate a pathological cause. Severely affected infants also show signs of anemia, which quickly worsen, causing decreased oxygen-carrying capacity that may lead to heart failure and shock. Kernicterus is also possible in severe cases. Early symptoms of it are lethargy, poor feeding, and vomiting, severe excitation or depression, including tremors, twitching, convulsion, a high-pitched cry, diminished deep tendon reflexes, and the absence of sucking reflexes. The mortality may reach 50%. After effects of kernicterus include mental retardation, cerebral palsy, delayed or abnormal motor development, hearing loss, perceptual problems, and behavioral disorders.

★TREATMENT: Infants with mild jaundice require no treatment, only observation. Light ray therapy is the usual treatment for severe or increasing hyperbilirubinemia.

hypercalcemia /hī'pərkalsē'mē·ə/, too much calcium in the blood. It most often results from excessive bone loss and release of calcium, as occurs in hyperparathyroidism, spreading bone tumors, Paget's disease, and osteoporosis. Patients with hypercalcemia are confused and have belly pain, muscle pain, and weakness. Extremely high levels of blood calcium may result in shock, kidney failure, and death. Hypercalciuria is also found in most patients with elevated blood calcium. Prednisone, diuretics, isotonic saline, and other drugs may be used in treatment. **–hypercalcemic,** *adj.*

hypercalciuria /hī'pərkal'sēyŏŏr'ē·ə/, too much calcium in the urine, resulting from conditions such as sarcoid, hyperparathyroidism, or certain types of arthritis, marked by large amounts of bone loss. Immobilized patients are often hypercalciuric. Some people absorb more calcium than is normal and therefore excrete large amounts into their urine. Concentrated amounts of calcium in the urinary tract may form kidney stones. Treatment is to correct any underlying disease condition and limit consumption of calcium. Also called **hypercalcinuria.** Compare **hypercalcemia. –hypercalciuric,** *adj.*

hypercapnia /hī'pərkap'nē·ə/, too much carbon dioxide in the blood. Also called **hypercarbia.**

hyperchloremia, too much chloride in the blood.

hyperchlorhydria, too great a release of hydrochloric acid by cells lining the stomach. See also **hyperacidity.**

hypercholesterolemia, too much cholesterol present in the blood. High levels of cholesterol and other lipids may lead to the development of hardening of the arteries. Hypercholesterolemia may be reduced or prevented by avoiding saturated fats, which are found in red meats, eggs, and dairy products.

hypercholesterolemic xanthomatosis. See **familial hypercholesterolemia.**

hyperchromic, having a greater density of color or pigment.

hyperchylomicronemia, type I hyperlipoproteinemia. It is a rare inborn deficiency of an enzyme essential to fat metabolism. Fat builds up in the blood as chylomicrons. The condition affects children and young adults. They develop fatty deposits in the skin, enlarged liver, and abdominal pain. Strict limitation of dietary fat

may allow the person to avoid discomfort and complications. Also called **familial lipoprotein lipase deficiency.** See also **chylomicron.**

hypercoagulability, a tendency of the blood to coagulate too rapidly.

hyperdactyly. See **polydactyly.**

hyperdiploid. See **hyperploid.**

hyperdynamic syndrome, a cluster of symptoms that signal the onset of shock from germs. It often includes a shaking chill, rapid rise in temperature, flushing of the skin, galloping pulse, and alternating rise and fall of the blood pressure. This is a medical emergency that requires expert medical support in a hospital. Emergency measures include keeping the patient warm and elevating the feet to assist blood return. Usually, nothing is given by mouth. See also **septic shock.**

hyperemesis gravidarum /hī'pərem'isis/, an abnormal condition of pregnancy marked by long-term vomiting, weight loss, and fluid and electrolyte imbalance. If the condition is severe, brain damage, liver and kidney failure, and death may result. Effective therapy stops vomiting and gives enough fluids and foods and stable emotions. Women are placed at bed rest. Antiemetics safe for the fetus are given. Fluids, electrolytes, nutrients, and vitamins are given through the veins if the woman is unable to retain fluids by mouth. The fetal heart rate is measured frequently. Psychiatric consultation and therapy are sometimes beneficial. Termination of pregnancy will cure the problem, but is almost never required.

hyperemia /hī'pərē'mē·ə/, increased blood in part of the body. It is caused by increased blood flow, as in the inflammatory response, local relaxation of arterioles, or blockage of the outflow of blood from an area. Skin in a hyperemic area usually becomes reddened and warm. **–hyperemic,** *adj.*

hyperextension, (of a joint) a position of maximum extension.

hyperextension suspension, a bone procedure used in the positioning of hip muscles after an operation. The procedure uses traction equipment, including metal frames, ropes, and pulleys. These relieve the weight of the lower limbs and properly position the muscles of the hip, without applying traction to the lower limbs involved. The ropes used to suspend the lower limbs are attached by rings to long leg casts. Compare **balanced suspension, lower extremity suspension, upper extremity suspension.**

hyperflexia, the forcible over-bending of a limb.

hyperfunction, increased function of any organ or system.

hypergenesis, too much growth; overdevelopment. The condition may involve the entire body, as in gigantism, or any particular part. It may even result in the formation of extra parts, as the development of additional fingers or toes. **–hypergenetic,** *adj.*

hypergenetic teratism, an inborn condition in which there is excessive growth of a part or organ or the entire body, as in gigantism.

hyperglycemia /hī′pərglīsē′mē·ə/, too much glucose in the blood. Most often linked to diabetes mellitus. The condition may occur in newborns, after the giving of certain hormones, and with an excess infusion of intravenous solutions containing glucose. Compare **hypoglycemia.**

hyperglycemic-glycogenolytic factor. See **glucagon.**

hyperglycemic-hyperosmolar nonketotic coma, a diabetic coma in which the level of ketone bodies is normal. It is often a consequence of overtreatment with hyperosmolar solutions.

hyperhidrosis /hī′pərhīdrō′sis, -hidrō′sis/, too much sweating. It is often caused by heat, overactive thyroid, strong emotion, menopause, or infection. Therapy usually includes antiperspirants. It may involve surgery to remove axillary sweat glands.

hyperimmune, having an unusual abundance of antibodies, producing a greater-than-normal immunity.

hyperinsulinism, too much insulin in the body, as may occur when a greater-than-required dose is given.

hyperkalemia /hī′pərkəlē′mē·ə/, too much potassium in the blood. This condition is seen frequently in kidney failure. Early signs are nausea, diarrhea, and muscle weakness. Heart irregularlies also result. Treatment of severe hyperkalemia includes the intravenous giving of sodium bicarbonate, calcium salts, and dextrose. Hemodialysis is used if these measures fail.

hyperkalemic periodic paralysis. See **adynamia episodica hereditaria.**

hyperkeratosis /hī′pərker′ətō′sis/, formation of skin overgrowth. See also **callus, corn.**

hyperkinesis. See **attention deficit disorder.**

hyperlipidemia, an excess of lipids in the blood. See also **antilipidemic.**

hyperlipoproteinemia /hī′pərlip′ōprō′tēnē′mē·ə/, any of a large group of disorders of lipoprotein metabolism marked by too much of certain protein-bound lipids and other fatty substances in the blood. The treatment includes diet to control obesity and reduce lipoprotein levels in the blood.

hypermagnesemia /hī′pərmag′nisē′mē·ə/, too much magnesium in the blood. Found in people with kidney failure and in those who use a large quantity of drugs containing magnesium, as antacids. Irregular heart beat and depression of deep tendon reflexes and breathing result. Treatment often includes intravenous fluids, a diuretic, and hemodialysis.

hypermenorrhea. See **menorrhagia.**

hypermetria /hī′pərmē′trē·ə/, a form of dysmetria, marked by lessened power to control the range of muscular action, causing movements that overreach the intended goal of the affected individual. Compare **hypometria.**

hypermetropia, hypermetropy, See **hyperopia.**

hypermorph /hī′pərmôrf′/, **1.** a person whose arms and legs are too long in relation to the trunk, and whose sitting height is disproportionate to the standing height. **2.** (in genetics) a mutant gene that shows increased activity in the expression of a trait. Compare **amorph, antimorph, hypomorph.**

hypernatremia /hī′pərnatrē′mē·ə/, overconcentration of sodium in the blood, caused by an excess loss of water and electrolytes resulting from diarrhea, excessive sweating, or inadequate water intake. When water loss is caused by kidney dysfunction, urine is profuse and dilute. If water loss is not through the kidneys, as in diarrhea and excess sweating, the urine is scanty and highly concentrated. People with hypernatremia may become mentally confused, have seizures, and lapse into coma. The treatment is restoration of fluid and electrolyte balance by mouth or by slow injections into the veins. Care must be taken to restore water balance slowly, or more electrolyte imbalances may occur. See also **diabetes insipidus.**

hyperopia /hī′pərō′pē·ə/, farsightedness. A state caused by an error of refraction in which rays of light entering the eye are brought into focus behind the retina. Also called **hypermetropia, hypermetropy.** Compare **myopia.**

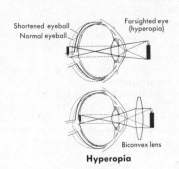

Shortened eyeball
Normal eyeball
Farsighted eye (hyperopia)
Biconvex lens

Hyperopia

hyperosmia, an abnormally high sensitivity to odors. Compare **anosmia.**

hyperosmolarity, a state of abnormally high osmolarity. **–hyperosmolar,** *adj.*

hyperoxia, a condition in which oxygen pressure in the blood is too high.

hyperparathyroidism, overactivity of one or more of the four parathyroid glands. Too much parathyroid hormone (PTH) is made. Calcium is drawn from the bones and much of it is then absorbed by the kidneys, stomach, and intestines.

, ★PATIENT CONSIDERATIONS: During treatment, the amounts of calcium, phosphorus, potassium, and magnesium in the blood are regularly measured. Bones break easily, so care must be taken to avoid any accidents. Water may be given through the veins to dilute the calcium build-up. The lungs are regularly listened to and tapped to detect any fluid buildup in them. Jerky muscle movements (tetany) are a warning sign of severe lowering of blood sugar (hypoglycemia). Mild exercise is painful but promotes healing of bones.

hyperphenylalaninemia /hī′pərfen′ilal′əninē′mē·ə/, an abnormally high amount of phenylalanine in the blood. This symptom may be the result of one of several defects in the process of breaking down phenylalanine. See also **phenylketonuria.**

hyperphoria /hī′pərfôr′ē·ə/, the tendency of an eye to deviate upward.

hyperpigmentation, unusual darkening of the skin. Causes include heredity, drugs, exposure to the sun, and too little adrenaline. Compare **hypopigmentation.** See also **chloasma, melanocyte stimulating hormone.**

hyperplasia /hī′pərplā′zhə/, an increase in the number of cells of a body part. Compare **hypertrophy, hypoplasia.**

hyperploid /hī′pərploid/, **1.** of or referring to a person, organism, strain, or cell that has one or more chromosomes in excess of the basic number or of an exact multiple of the basic number characteristic of the species. The result is unbalanced sets of chromosomes, which are referred to as hyperdiploid, hypertriploid, hypertetraploid, and so on, depending on the number of multiples of the basic number of chromosomes they contain. **2.** such an individual, organism, strain, or cell. Compare **hypoploid.** See also **trisomy.**

hyperploidy /hī′pərploi′dē/, any increase in chromosome number that involves individual chromosomes rather than entire sets, resulting in more than the normal number characteristic of the species, as in Down's syndrome. Compare **hypoploidy.**

hyperpnea /hī′pərpnē′ə/, a deep, rapid, or labored breathing. It occurs normally with exercise, and abnormally with pain, fever, hysteria, or any condition in which the supply of oxygen is inadequate, as heart disease and lung disease. Also spelled **hyperpnoea. Compare dyspnea, hypopnea, orthopnea.** See also **respiratory rate. –hyperpneic, hyperpnoic,** adj.

hyperprolactinemia, too much prolactin in the blood. The condition is caused by a hypothalamic-pituitary problem. In women it is usual ly linked to breast problems; in men it may be a factor in decreased sexual interest and impotence. It may be a result of endocrine side effects related to certain tranquilizers.

hyperptyalism. See **ptyalism.**

hyperpyrexia /hī′pərpīrek′sē·ə/, an extremely high temperature sometimes occurring in serious infectious diseases, especially in young children. Cancerous hyperpyrexia, marked by a rapid rise in temperature, rapid heart beat rapid breathing, sweating, rigidity, and blotchy blue discoloring of the skin and mucous membranes occasionally occurs in patients under general anesthesia. A high temperature may be reduced by sponging the body with tepid water and alcohol, by giving a tepid tub bath, or by giving aspirin or acetaminophen. See also **fever. –hyperpyretic,** adj.

hyperreflection, a drive to pay great attention to oneself.

hyperreflexia, a neurological condition marked by increased reflex reactions.

hypersensitivity, an abnormal condition marked by an over-reaction to a particular stimulus. See also **allergy. –hypersensitive,** adj.

hypersensitivity pneumonitis. See **extrinsic allergic alveolitis.**

hypersensitivity reaction, an unusual and excessive response of the immune system to a sensitizing antigen. The antigenic stimulant is an allergen. Several factors fix the strength of an allergic response: the responsiveness of the host to the allergen, the amount of allergen, the kind of allergen, its way into the body, the timing of the exposures, and the site of the allergen-immune mediator reaction.

hypersomnia /hī′pərsom′nē·ə/, **1.** very deep or long sleep, usually caused by psychological rather than physical factors and marked by confusion on waking. **2.** great drowsiness, often with lethargy. Compare **narcolepsy.**

hyperspadias. See **epispadias.**

hypersplenism /hī′pərsplē′nizəm/, a syndrome consisting of a large spleen and a lack of one or more types of blood cells. The numerous causes of this syndrome include tumors, anemia, malaria, tuberculosis, and various connective tissue and inflammatory diseases. Patients complain of stomach pain on the left side and often feel full after very little food, because the large spleen is pressing on the stomach. On physical examination the enlarged spleen is felt and abnormal bruits (vascular sounds) are heard with a stethoscope over the stomach area. Treatment of the cause may cure the syndrome. The spleen is removed (splenectomy) only in certain cases. See also **splenectomy.**

Hyperstat, a trademark for a drug that dilates blood vessels.

hypertelorism /hī′pərtel′əriz′əm/, a developmental defect marked by an abnormally wide space between two organs or parts. A kind of hypertelorism is **ocular hypertelorism.** Compare **hypotelorism.**

hypertension, a common disorder, often without symptoms marked by high blood pressure persistently exceeding 140/90. Essential hypertension, the most frequent kind, has no one known cause, but the risk of it is increased by overweight, a high sodium level in the blood, a high cholesterol level, and a family history of high blood pressure. Known causes of hypertension include adrenal problems, over-active thyroid gland, certain pregnancies and kidney disorders. Hypertension is more common in men than in women and is twice as great in blacks as in whites. Persons with mild or moderate hypertension may have no symptoms or may experience headaches, especially on rising, ringing in the ears, lightheadedness, easy fatigability, and the feeling that their heart is beating wildly. With sustained hypertension, artery walls become thickened and resistant to blood flow, and, as a result, the blood supply to the heart may be reduced causing angina or heart attack. High blood pressure is often accompanied by anxiety attacks, rapid or irregular heart beat, profuse sweating, pallor, nausea, and, in some cases, fluid in the lungs. Malignant hypertension, marked by a diastolic pressure higher than 120, severe headaches, blurred vision, and confusion, may result in heart attack or stroke. Drugs used to treat hypertension include diuretics, as thiazide derivatives; vasodilators, as hydralazine and prazosin; sympathetic nervous system (SNS) depressants, as rauwolfia alkaloids; SNS inhibitors, as guanethidine and methyldopa; and ganglionic blocking agents, as clonidine and propranolol. Patients with high blood pressure are advised to follow a low-sodium, low-saturated-fat diet, to reduce calories to control obesity, to exercise, to avoid stress, and to take adequate rest. Kinds of hypertension are **essential hypertension, malignant hypertension, and secondary hypertension.** See also **blood pressure.**

hypertensive crisis, a sudden severe increase in blood pressure to a level exceeding 200/120, occurring most often in untreated hypertension and in patients who have stopped taking prescribed antihypertensive medication.

★PATIENT CONSIDERATIONS: A major concern for patients who have suffered a hypertensive crisis is observing and reporting of any sign of lower-than-normal pressure. Upon discharge the patient must watch for symptoms of any dramatic increase or decrease in blood pressure, adhere to the prescribed diet and medication, and avoid fatigue, heavy lifting, smoking, and stressful situations.

hypertensive encephalopathy, a set of symptoms, including headache, convulsions, and coma, associated with a certain type of kidney disease (glomerulonephritis).

hypertetraploid. See **hyperploid.**

hyperthermia /hī′pərthur′mē·ə/, **1.** a much higher than normal body temperature produced by the patient's physician as treatment or accidently as a byproduct of treatment.

hyperthyroidism, a condition marked by hyperactivity of the thyroid gland. The gland is usually swollen, releasing greater-than-normal amounts of thyroid hormones, and the body processes are accelerated. Nervousness, abnormal bulging of the eyeballs, tremor, constant hunger, weight loss, fatigue, heat intolerance, rapid and irregular heart beat, and diarrhea may develop. Antithyroid drugs are usually prescribed. Radioactive iodine may be given in certain cases. Surgical removal of the gland is sometimes necessary. Untreated hyperthyroidism may lead to death because of heart failure. See also **thyroid storm.**

hypertonic contracture, long-term muscle contraction as a result of constant nerve stimulation in some paralysis. Anesthetics or sleep eliminates this condition. Also called **functional contracture.**

hypertrichosis. See **hirsutism.**

hypertriglyceridemia. See **hyperchylomicronemia.**

hypertriploid. See **hyperploid.**

hypertrophic angioma. See **hemangioendothelioma.**

hypertrophic catarrh, a chronic condition marked by inflammation and discharge from a mucous membrane, with thickening of the mucous and submucous tissue. Compare **atrophic catarrh.** See also **catarrh.**

hypertrophic gastritis, an inflamed state of the stomach by pain, nausea, vomiting, and bloating. It is distinguished from other forms of gastritis by the presence of prominent folds, enlarged glands, and lumps on the wall of the stomach. This condition often occurs with peptic ulcer, Zollinger-Ellison syndrome, or excessive production of stomach fluids.

hypertrophic gingivitis. See **gingivitis.**

hypertrophic obstructive cardiomyopathy. See **idiopathic hypertrophic subaortic stenosis.**

hypertrophy /hīpur′trəfē/, an increase in the size of an organ caused by an increase in the size of the cells rather than the number of cells. Kinds of hypertrophy include **adaptive hypertrophy, compensatory hypertrophy, Marie's hypertrophy, physiologic hypertrophy,** and **unilateral hypertrophy.** Compare **atrophy, hyperplasia.** –**hypertrophic,** adj.

hyperuricemia. See **gout.**

hyperventilation, a breathing rate that is greater than that necessary for the exchange of oxygen and carbon dioxide. It is the result of an increased frequency of breathing, an increased volume, or a combination of both. It causes excess intake of oxygen and the blowing off of carbon dioxide. Chest pain, dizziness, faintness, numbness of the fingers and toes, and psychomotor impairment occur as a result. Causes of hyperventilation include asthma or early emphysema; increased metabolism because of exercise, fever, hyperthyroidism, or infections; damage to the central nervous system, as in cerebral thrombosis, encephalitis, head injuries, or meningitis; certain hormones and drugs, difficulties with mechanical respirators; and mental factors, as high anxiety or pain. Compare **hypoventilation.** See also **respiratory center.**

hypervitaminosis, an abnormal condition resulting from intake of dangerous amounts of one or more vitamins, especially over a long period of time. Serious effects may result from overdoses of vitamins A, D, E, or K, but rarely with the water-soluble B and C vitamins. Compare **avitaminosis.** See also specific vitamins.

hypervolemia, an increase in the amount of fluid outside the cells, particularly in the volume of circulating blood.

hypesthesia /hī′pəristhē′zhə/, abnormally low level of feeling in response to stimulation of the sensory nerves. Touch, pain, heat, and cold are poorly perceived. Also called **hypoesthesia.** –**hypesthetic,** *adj.*

hyphema /hīfē′mə/, a bleeding into the forward chamber of the eye, usually caused by a blow to the eye. Bedrest is required. The patient should be treated by an ophthalmologist who can decide the need for removing the blood, and the need for medication. Glaucoma may result from recurrent bleeding. Also called **hyphemia** /hīfē′mē·ə/ .

hypnagogic hallucination, one that occurs in the period between wakefulness and sleep. See also **hallucination.**

hypnagogue /hip′nəgog/, an agent or substance that tends to induce sleep or the feeling of dreamy sleepiness, as occurs before falling asleep. See also **hypnotic.** –**hypnagogic,** *adj.*

hypnoanalysis, the use of hypnosis along with other techniques in psychoanalysis.

hypnosis, a passive, trancelike state that resembles normal sleep during which perception and memory are changed, resulting in increased responsiveness to suggestion. The condition is usually caused by the monotonous repetition of words and gestures while the subject is completely relaxed. Susceptibility to hypnosis varies from person to person. Hypnosis is used in some forms of psychotherapy and psychoanalysis to gain access to the subconscious, in behavior changing programs to help a person stop overeating or smoking or to end other unwanted behavior, or in medicine to reduce pain and aid relaxation.

hypnotherapy, the use of hypnosis along with other techniques in psychotherapy.

hypnotics, a class of drugs often used as sedatives.

hypnotic trance, an artificially induced sleeplike state, as in hypnosis.

hypnotism, the study or practice of producing hypnosis.

hypnotist, one who practices hypnotism.

hypnotize, 1. to put into a state of hypnosis. 2. to fascinate, entrance, or control through personal charm.

hypoacidity, a lack of acid.

hypoactivity, any abnormally low activity of the body or its organs, as lowered heart output, thyroid gland or intestinal activity. Compare **hyperactivity,** def. 1.

hypoadrenalism. See **Addison's disease.**

hypoalimentation, a condition of insufficient or inadequate nourishment.

hypobetalipoproteinemia /hī′pōbā′təlip′ōprō′-tēnē′mē·ə/, an inherited condition in which there are less-than-normal amounts of water-soluble fats in the blood. Blood lipids and cholesterol are present at less than the expected levels regardless of how much fat is eaten. There are no symptoms, and treatment is unnecessary. Compare **hyperbetalipoproteinemia.**

hypocalcemia /hī′pōkalsē′mē·ə/, too little calcium in the blood that may be caused by hypoparathyroidism, too little vitamin D consumption, kidney failure, severe inflammation of the pancreas, or too little magnesium and protein in the blood. Mild hypocalcemia has no symptoms. Severe hypocalcemia is marked by irregular heart beat, muscle spasms, and burning or prickling feelings of the hands, feet, lips, and tongue. The underlying disorder is diagnosed and treated, and calcium is given by mouth or through the veins. Hypocalcemia is also seen in immature newborn babies, in infants born of mothers with diabetes, or in normal babies delivered by normal mothers after a long or hard labor and delivery. It is marked by vomiting, twitching of arms and legs, poor muscle tone, high-pitched crying, and difficulty in breathing. See also **tetany.** –**hypocalcemic,** *adj.*

hypochloremia, a decrease in the chloride level in the blood. The condition may occur as a result of long-term use of a stomach pump.

hypochloremic alkalosis, an increase in the body's alkalinity resulting from increased blood bicarbonate and loss of chloride from the body.

hypochlorhydria, too low a level of hydrochloric acid in the stomach.

hypochlorous acid, a greenish-yellow liquid taken from a water solution of lime. An unstable compound that breaks down to hydrochloric acid and water, hypochlorous acid is used as a bleaching agent and disinfectant.

hypochondria, hypochondriac neurosis. See **hypochondriasis.**

hypochondriac region, the part of the upper belly on both sides and beneath the lower ribs. Also called **hypochondrium.** See also **abdominal regions.**

hypochondriasis /hī'pōkəndrī'əsis/, **1.** also called **hypochondria.** a recurring and abnormal concern about the health of the body. **2.** also called **hypochondriac neurosis.** A condition marked by extreme anxiety, depression, and the belief that certain real or imagined physical symptoms are signs of a serious illness or disease despite rational medical evidence that this is not the case. The condition is caused by some unsolved mental problem and may involve a specific organ, as the heart, lungs, or eyes, or several body systems at various times or at the same time. In severe cases, the distorted body-mind relationship is so strong that actual symptoms and disease may develop. Treatment usually consists of psychotherapy to uncover the underlying emotional conflict. –**hypochondriac** /hī'pōkon'drē·ak/, *adj., n.,* **hypochondriac** /hī'pōkəndrī'ak/, **hypochondriacal,** *adj.*

hypochondrium. See **hypochondriac region.**

hypochromic /hī'pōkrō'mik/, having less than normal color, usually describing a red blood cell and characterizing anemias linked to decreased manufacture of hemoglobin. Compare **normochromic.** See also **hypochromic anemia, red cell indices.**

hypochromic anemia, any of a large group of anemias marked by decreased hemoglobin in the red blood cells. See also **anemia, red cell indices.**

hypocytic leukemia. See **aleukemic leukemia.**

hypodermatoclysis. See **hypodermoclysis.**

hypodermic, of or pertaining to the area below the skin, as a hypodermic injection.

hypodermic needle, a short, thin, hollow needle that attaches to a syringe for injecting a drug under the skin or into vessels or for withdrawing a fluid, as blood, for examination.

hypodermoclysis /hī'pōdərmok'lisis/, the injection of a solution beneath the skin tissue to supply the patient with a continuous and large amount of fluid, nutrients and other important substances. The procedure is used to replace the loss or too little intake of water and salt during illness or surgery or after shock or excessive bleeding and is performed only when the patient is unable to take fluids through the veins, mouth, or rectum. The process takes a long time. Also called **hypoder matoclysis, interstitial infusion, subcutaneous infusion.**

hypodiploid. See **hypoploid.**

hypoesthesia. See **hypesthesia.**

hypofibrinogenemia, too little fibrinogen, a blood-clotting factor, in the blood. The condition may occur as a side effect of early detachment of the placenta in pregnancy.

hypogammaglobulinemia, a less-than-normal concentration of gamma globulin in the blood, usually the result of increased protein breakdown or the loss of protein through urination. The condition is associated with a decreased resistance to infection. Compare **agammaglobulinemia.**

hypogastric artery. See **internal iliac artery.**

hypogastrium. See **pubic region.**

hypogenitalism, a condition of retarded sexual development caused by a defect in male or female hormone production in the testicles or ovaries.

hypogeusia, reduced taste.

hypoglossal nerve, either of a pair of nerves in the head needed for swallowing and for moving the tongue. Also called **nervus hypoglossus, twelfth nerve.**

hypoglycemia /hī'pōglīsē'mē·ə/, a less-than-normal amount of sugar in the blood, usually caused by being given too much insulin, excessive release of insulin by the pancreas, or low food intake. The condition may result in weakness, headache, hunger, problems with vision, loss of muscle coordination, anxiety, personality changes, and, if untreated, delirium, coma, and death. The treatment is the giving of sugar in orange juice by mouth if the person is conscious or through the veins if the person is unconscious. Compare **diabetic coma.**

hypoglycemic agent, any of a large group of quite different drugs, including insulin, prescribed to decrease the amount of sugar in the blood. One of these, phenformin, has been recently removed from the market in the United States, primarily because of its tendency to cause an excess of lactic acid.

hypoglycemic shock treatment. See **insulin shock treatment.**

hypokalemia /hī'pōkəlē'mē·ə/, a condition in which too little potassium is found in the bloodstream. Hypokalemia is marked by abnormal ECG, weakness, and non-rigid paralysis and may be caused by starvation, treatment of diabetes, or adrenal tumor, or by taking diuretics. Mild hypokalemia may go away when the underlying condition is corrected. Severe hypokalemia may be treated by giving potassium chloride, orally or by injection, and by a diet high in potassium. Compare **hyperkalemia.** See also **electrolyte balance.**

hypokalemic alkalosis, an unhealthy condition resulting from the accumulation of alkalinity or the loss of acid from the body associated with a low level of potassium in the blood. See also **hypokalemia.**

hypolipemia. See **hypolipoproteinemia.**

hypolipoproteinemia /hī′pōlip′ōprō′tēnē′mē·ə/, a group of defects in fatty protein (lipoprotein) that result in varying signs. Primary, or hereditary, hypolipoproteinemia factors include abnormal transport of triglycerides in the blood, low levels of high-density lipoproteins, high levels of low-density lipoproteins, and abnormal depositing of fats in the body, especially in the kidneys and the liver. In some of the cases eye, intestinal, and nerve effects are also present. The condition may also accompany anemia, intestinal troubles or malnutrition. Kinds of hypolipoproteinemias are **abetalipoproteinemia, hypobetalipoproteinemia, lecithin-cholesterol acyltransferase deficiency,** and **Tangier disease.**

hypomagnesemia /hī′pōmag′nisē′mē·ə/, abnormally low magnesium in the blood, resulting in nausea, vomiting, muscle weakness, tremors, muscle spasms, and lethargy. Mild hypomagnesemia is usually the result of too-little absorption of magnesium in the kidney or intestine, although it is also seen after long-term feeding by injection and during nursing. A more severe form is associated with intestinal problems, protein malnutrition, and parathyroid disease. Magnesium salts to correct the condition may be given orally or through the veins.

hypomania, a mentally unhealthy state characterized by optimism, excitability, a marked hyperactivity and talkativeness, heightened sexual interest, quick anger and irritability, and a decreased need for sleep. **–hypomaniac, n., hypomanic,** adj.

hypometria /hī′pōmē′trē·ə/, an abnormal condition marked by inability to control the range of muscular action, resulting in movements that fall short of the intended goals of the affected person. Compare **hypermetria.**

hypomorph, 1. a person whose legs are too short in relation to the trunk and whose sitting height is too great a fraction of his or her standing height. 2. (in genetics) a mutant gene that has a reduced effect on the expression of a trait but at a level too low to result in abnormal development. Also called **leaky gene.** Compare **amorph, antimorph, hypermorph.**

hyponatremia /hī′pōnatrē′mē·ə/, less than the normal amount of sodium in the blood, caused by too little excretion of water or by too much water in the bloodstream. In a severe case, the person may develop water intoxication, with confusion and lethargy, leading to muscle spasms, convulsions, and coma. Treatment may be by injecting a balanced solution into the veins.

hypoparathyroidism, a condition of lowered parathyroid function, which can be caused by a problem in the gland itself or by raised blood calcium levels.

hypopharyngeal, 1. of, referring to or involving the hypopharynx. 2. situated below the pharynx.

hypophosphatasia /hī′pōfos′fətā′zhə/, inherited absence of alkaline phosphatase, an enzyme essential to the buildup of calcium in bone tissue. Affected newborns vomit, grow slowly, and often die in infancy. Children who survive have many skeletal abnormalities and are dwarfs. There is no known treatment.

hypophosphatemic rickets /hī′pōfos′fətē′mik/, a rare condition occurring in certain families in which there is poor resorption of phosphate in the kidneys and poor absorption of calcium in the small intestine, resulting in softening of the bones, retarded growth, skeletal deformities, and pain. Treatment includes taking phosphate and vitamin D by mouth.

hypophyseal cachexia. See **panhypopituitarism.**

hypophyseal dwarf. See **pituitary dwarf.**

hypophysectomy /hīpof′əsek′təmē/, surgical removal of the pituitary gland. It may be done to slow the growth and spread of endocrine-dependent cancerous tumors of the breast, ovary, or prostate gland, to halt the break down of the retina in diabetes, or to remove a pituitary tumor. The gland is removed only if other treatment, as x-ray therapy, radioactive implants, or freezing fails to destroy all pituitary tissue. General anesthesia is given, the skull is opened, and the gland is completely removed. **–hypophysectomize,** v.

hypophysis cerebri. See **pituitary gland.**

hypopigmentation, unusual lack of skin color, seen, e.g., in albinos. Compare **hyperpigmentation.**

hypopituitarism, an abnormal condition caused by diminished activity of the pituitary gland and marked by large deposits of fat and by adolescent characteristics.

hypoplasia /hī′pōplā′zhə/, incomplete or under-developed organ or tissue, usually the result of a decrease in the number of cells. Kinds of hypoplasia are **cartilage-hair hypoplasia** and **enamel hypoplasia.** Also called **hypoplasty.** Compare **aplasia, hyperplasia.** See also **oligomeganephronia, osteogenesis imperfecta. –hypoplastic,** adj.

hypoplasia of the mesenchyme. See **osteogenesis imperfecta.**

hypoplastic anemia, a broad class of anemias marked by low production of red blood cells. Compare **aplastic anemia, polycythemia.** See also **anemia.**

hypoplastic dwarf. See **primordial dwarf.**

hypoploid /hī′pəploid/, 1. also **hypoploidic.** Of or pertaining to a person, organism, strain, or cell that has fewer than the basic number or an exact multiple of the basic number of chromosomes characteristic of the species. The result is unbalanced sets of chromosomes, which are referred to as hypodiploid, hypotriploid, hypotetraploid, and so on, depending on the number of multiples of the basic number of chromosomes they contain. **2.** such an individual, organism, strain, or cell. Compare **hyperploid.** See also **monosomy.**

hypoploidy /hī′pōploi′dē/, any decrease in chromosome number that involves individual chromosomes rather than entire sets, resulting in fewer than the normal number characteristic of the species, as in Turner's syndrome. Compare **hyperploidy.**

hypopnea /hīpop′nē·ə, hī′pōnē′ə/, shallow or slow breathing. In well-conditioned athletes, it is normal and is accompanied by a slow pulse; otherwise, it is common in damage to the brain stem, in which case it is accompanied by a rapid, weak pulse and is a grave sign. See also **respiratory rate.**

hypopotassemia, too-little potassium in the blood.

hypoproteinemia /hī′pōprō′tēnē′mē·ə/, a condition marked by a decrease in the amount of protein in the blood to an abnormally low level, accompanied by swelling of the tissues, nausea, vomiting, diarrhea, and abdominal pain. It may be caused by too-little protein in the diet, by certain intestinal diseases, or by kidney failure. Also called **intestinal lymphangiectasia.**

hypoprothrombinemia /hī′pōprōthrom′binē′mē·ə/, an abnormal reduction in the amount of prothrombin (factor II) in the blood, marked by poor clot formation, longer bleeding time, and possibly by uncontrolled bleeding. The condition is usually the result of inadequate production of prothrombin in the liver, most often the result of a low vitamin K level caused by severe liver disease or by anticoagulant therapy with the drug dicumarol. See also **blood clotting.**

hypoptyalism /hī′pōtī′əliz′əm/, a condition in which there is a decrease in the amount of saliva released by the salivary glands. See also **hyposalivation, ptyalism.**

hypopyon, a gathering of pus in the front chamber of an eye, appearing as a gray fluid between the cornea and the iris. It may occur as a side effect of conjunctivitis, herpetic keratitis, or corneal ulcer.

hyporeflexia, a nerve condition marked by weakened reflex reactions.

hyposalivation, a low rate of saliva flow that may be associated with excess loss of body fluids, radiation therapy of the salivary gland regions, anxiety, the use of drugs, as atropine and antihistamines, vitamin deficiency, various forms of parotitis, or various syndromes, as Plummer-Vinson syndrome. Also called **xerostomia, asialorrhea.** ＼

hyposensitization. See **immunotherapy.**

hypospadias /hī′pəspā′dē·əs/, an inherited defect in which the urinary opening is on the underside of the penis. Incontinence does not occur because nothing else is defective. Surgical correction is performed as necessary for cosmetic, urological, or reproductive purposes. A corresponding defect in women is rare but recognized by the location of the urinary opening in the vagina. Compare **epispadias.**

hypostatic pneumonia, a type of pneumomia linked to elderly or weak persons who remain in the same position for long periods. Gravity tends to accelerate fluid congestion in one area of the lungs, increasing the likelihood of infection.

hypotelorism /hī′pōtel′əriz′əm/, a condition marked by an abnormally decreased distance between two organs or parts. A kind of hypotelorism is **ocular hypotelorism.** Compare **hypertelorism.**

hypotension, an abnormal condition in which the blood pressure is too low for normal functioning.

hypotensive anesthesia. See **deliberate hypotension.**

hypotetraploid. See **hypoploid.**

hypothalamic amenorrhea, stopping of menstruation caused by conditions that inhibit the hypothalamus from starting the cycle of interactions of the brain, pituitary, and ovary necessary for ovulation and menstruation. Examples of causes are stress, anxiety, and acute weight loss. See **amenorrhea.**

hypothalamus /hī′pōthal′əməs/, a portion of the brain, forming the floor and part of the side wall of the third ventricle. It activates, controls, and integrates part of the nervous system, the endocrine processes, and many bodily functions, as temperature, sleep, and appetite. Compare **epithalamus, metathalamus, subthalamus, thalamus.** –**hypothalamic,** *adj.*

hypothenar, the fleshy raised part of the palm just below the little finger.

hypothermia /hī′pōthur′mē·ə/, **1.** an abnormal and dangerous condition in which the temperature of the body is below 95° F (35° C). It is usually caused by prolonged exposure to cold. Breathing is shallow and slow, and the heart rate is faint and slow. The person is very pale and may appear to be dead. People who are very old or very young, people who have heart or circulation problems, and people who are hungry, tired, or under the influence of alcohol are most likely to get hypothermia. Treatment includes slowly warming the person. Hospitalization is necessary. **2.** purposely lowering body temperature with cooling mattresses or ice to prepare for surgery.

hypothermia blanket, a covering used to promote heat loss from the body of a patient with a high temperature.

hypothermia therapy, lowering a patient's body temperature to counteract long term high fever caused by certain diseases, or, less frequently, as an aid to anesthesia in heart or brain surgery.

★METHOD: Hypothermia may be produced by placing crushed ice around the patient, or by placing the body in ice water. It may also be done by circulating the blood through coils submerged in a refrigerant. Most commonly it is done by applying cooling blankets or vinyl pads containing coils through which cold water and alcohol are pumped. At the termination of hypothermia, the cooling blanket is replaced by regular blankets and the patient usually warms at his or her own rate. As the patient's temperature approaches normal, the warming blankets are removed.

hypothesis /hīpoth'isis/, (in research) a statement derived from a theory that predicts the relation among certain things or events. Kinds of hypotheses include **causal hypothesis, null hypothesis,** and **predictive hypothesis.**

hypothyroid dwarf. See **cretin dwarf.**

hypothyroidism, a condition marked by decreased activity of the thyroid gland. It is sometimes caused by surgical removal of all or part of the gland. An overdose of antithyroid medicine, release of thyroid stimulating hormone by the pituitary gland, or atrophy of the thyroid gland itself can also be responsible. Weight gain, sluggishness, dryness of the skin, constipation, arthritis, and slowing of the processes of the body may occur. Untreated, hypothyroidism leads to severe facial swelling, coma, and death. Treatment is by giving the deficient hormone. Dosage is adjusted to maintain normal levels of thyroid hormones.

hypotriploid. See **hypoploid.**

hypoventilation, an abnormal condition of the lungs, marked by the patient's turning blue, clubbing of the fingers, increase in red cell mass in the blood, and increased carbon dioxide pressure in the arteries. Lowered breathing rate also results. It occurs when the amount of air that enters the lungs and takes part in gas exchanges is not adequate for the needs of the body. Hypoventilation may be caused by uneven distribution of air breathed in, (as in bronchitis), obesity, disease of the bone structure, nerves or muscles affecting the chest, decreased response of the breathing center to carbon dioxide, and reduced functional lung tissue, as in emphysema. Treatment includes weight reduction in cases of obesity, artificial respiration, and surgically opening the trachea. Compare **hyperventilation.** See also **respiratory center.**

hypovitaminosis. See **avitaminosis.**

hypovolemia, an abnormally low circulating blood volume.

hypovolemic shock, a state of physical collapse caused by massive blood loss, circulatory failure, and too-little blood to the tissues. The loss of about one-fifth of total blood volume in the affected person can produce this condition. The common signs include low blood pressure, feeble pulse, clammy skin, too-rapid heart beat, rapid breathing, and reduced urinary output. The associated blood losses may stem from bleeding from the stomach or intestines, internal bleeding, external bleeding, or excessive reduction of blood volume in the vessels, and body fluids. Disorders that may cause hypovolemic shock are liquid loss from too-much perspiration, severe diarrhea, long-term vomiting, intestinal blockage, certain inflammations in the belly, and severe burns, which deplete body fluids. Effects may include severe kidney or brain damage. Treatment focuses on replacing blood and fluid volumes, locating of bleeding sites, and the control of bleeding. Without fast treatment there is further collapse that can cause death. Compare **cardiogenic shock.** See also **electric shock, shock.**

hypoxemia /hī'poksē'mē·ə/, an abnormal lack of oxygen in the blood in the arteries. Symptoms of acute hypoxemia are the patient turning blue, restlessness, stupor, coma, increased blood pressure, too-rapid heart beat, and an initial increase in heart output that later falls, resulting in low blood pressure and irregular heart beat or heart stoppage. Chronic hypoxemia stimulates red blood cell production by the bone marrow, leading to an excess of red cells. Hypoxemia caused by decreased oxygen pressure in the blood or too little oxygen intake improves with oxygen therapy. Hypoxemia resulting from shunting of blood from the right side of the heart to the left side of the heart without exchange of gases in the lungs is treated with bronchial hygiene and breathing therapy. Compare **hypoxia. See also anoxia, asphyxia.**

hypoxia, too-little oxygen in the cells characterized by the patient turning blue, a too-rapid heart rate, high blood pressure, contractions of blood vessels, dizziness, and mental confusion. Mild hypoxia increases heart and respiratory rates. However, the central mechanisms that regulate breathing fail in severe hypoxia, leading to irregular breathing, failure to breathe, and heart failure. Increased sensitivity to the effect of certain drugs in reducing breathing is common in chronic hypoxia, resulting in severe depression or failure of breathing when relatively small doses of opiates are taken. The tissues most sensitive to hypoxia are the brain, heart, vessels of the lungs, and liver. Treatment may include heart and lung stimulant drugs, oxygen therapy, mechanic ventilation, and frequent analysis of blood gases. Compare **hypoxemia.** See also **anoxia, chemoreceptor, hyperventilation, respiratory center.**

hypsibrachycephaly /hips'ibrakisef'əlē/, having a skull that is high with a broad forehead. See

also **brachycephaly, oxycephaly. –hypsi-
brachycephalic,** *adj., n.*

hypsicephaly. See **oxycephaly.**

hysterectomy, removal of the uterus by surgery, performed to remove tumors of the uterus or to treat chronic pelvic inflammation, uterine bleeding, and precancerous and cancerous conditions of the uterus. Types of hysterectomy include **total hysterectomy,** in which the uterus and cervix are removed, and **radical hysterectomy,** in which ovaries, oviducts, lymph nodes and lymph channels are removed with the uterus and cervix. Menstruation ceases after either type is performed. First, a vaginal douche may be given. Under general or spinal anesthesia the uterus is removed. One or both ovaries and oviducts may be removed at the same time. After the operation, food and oral fluids are restricted to prevent swelling. Toe-to-knee elastic stockings or bandages are reapplied twice a day to give snug, even support and to prevent circulation problems. The lower half of the bed is kept flat, and the patient is instructed to avoid sharply flexing the thighs or knees, because inflammation of the blood vessels of the pelvis and upper thigh is a frequent complication. Low back pain or scanty urine may indicate a blocked ureter. A kind of hysterectomy is **cesarean hysterectomy.** Compare **hysterosalpingo-oophorectomy. –hysterectomize,** *v.*

hysteria, 1. a state of tension or excitement in a person or group, marked by unmanageable fear and short term loss of control over the emotions.

hysteric amaurosis, blindness, most often after emotional shock, lasting for hours, days, or months.

hysteric apepsia. See **anorexia nervosa.**

hysteric fever, an abnormal rise in body temperature without general symptoms, often seen in hysteric neurosis.

hysteric lethargy, a sleep caused by hypnosis. See also **hypnosis, lethargy.**

hysteric mania, a mood problem marked by symptoms of hysteria and mania.

hysteric neurosis, a form of neurosis in which extreme excitability and anxiety caused by an emotional conflict are changed into physical symptoms having no organic basis or into states of changed consciousness or identity. Kinds of hysteric neurosis are **conversion disorder and dissociative disorder.**

hysteric personality. See **histrionic personality.**

hysteric trance, a sleepwalking state that is a symptom of hysteric neurosis.

hysterogram, the x-ray record of a uterus made after injecting a contrast medium in the uterine cavity. See also **hysterosalpingogram.**

hysterolaparotomy /his′tərōlap′ərot′əmē/, abdominal hysterectomy or hysterotomy.

hysterosalpingogram /his′tərōsalping′gōgram′/, an x-ray film of the uterus and the fallopian tubes to see the cavity of the uterus and the passageway of the tubes. A blockage of a structure is shown on the film because the radiopaque substance cannot pass to the further structures and leave the ends of the tubes into the peritoneal cavity. Serial hysterosalpingograms are useful in the diagnosis of the cause of infertility.

hysterosalpingo-oophorectomy, surgery to remove one or both ovaries and oviducts along with the uterus, done often to treat malignant neoplastic disease of the reproductive tract and chronic endometriosis. To avoid the severe symptoms of sudden menopause, a portion of one ovary is left, unless there is cancer. Under general anesthesia, the uterus, one or both oviducts, and one or both ovaries are removed. If both ovaries are removed and there is no cancer, estrogen replacement therapy is often begun right away. Elastic stockings or bandages are used on the legs twice a day to prevent circulatory stasis because inflammation of the blood vessels of the pelvis or thigh is a frequent complication. The lower half of the bed is kept flat, and the patient is instructed to avoid sharply flexing the thighs or knees. Low back pain or scanty urine may indicate a blocked ureter. Compare **hysterectomy.**

hysteroscopy, direct visual inspection of the cervical canal and uterine cavity through a hysteroscope, performed to examine the endometrium, to secure a specimen for biopsy, to remove an intrauterine device, or to remove cervical polyps. Under spinal anesthesia, the endoscope is passed through the vagina and into the uterus. The surrounding tissues are examined. The nurse keeps the patient flat in bed for the next 8 hours. The procedure is not performed during pregnancy, acute pelvic inflammation, chronic upper genital tract infection, recent uterine perforation, and known or suspected cervical cancer. **–hysteroscope,** *n.,* **hysteroscopic,** *adj.*

hysterotomy, surgical cutting of the uterus, done as a method of abortion in a pregnancy beyond the first trimester. Under general or spinal anesthesia, the lower segment of the uterus is cut, and the products of conception are withdrawn. Later care includes close observation for too much vaginal bleeding.

Hytone, a trademark for a steroid (hydrocortisone), used in a topical ointment for the relief of inflammation of the skin.

I

I, **1.** symbol for **inspired gas. 2.** symbol for **iodine.**

iatrogenic /ī'atrōjen'ik, yat-/, caused by treatment or diagnostic procedures. An iatrogenic disorder is a condition caused by medical personnel or procedures or through exposure to the environment of a health-care facility. See also **nosocomial.** —**iatrogenesis,** *n.*

ibuprofen /ībyoō'prəfin/, a nonsteroidal anti-inflammatory agent prescribed in the treatment of rheumatoid and osteoarthritis conditions.

★CAUTION: Kidney dysfunction, stomach or intestinal disorders, or known allergy to this drug, to other nonsteroid anti-inflammatory drugs, or to aspirin prohibits its use.

★ADVERSE EFFECTS: Among the more serious side effects are stomach trouble, gastric or duodenal ulceration, dizziness, skin rash, and ringing in the ear. Ibuprofen may interact with other drugs.

IC, abbreviation for **inspiratory capacity.**

-icam, a combining form for drugs of the isoxicam group that reduce inflammation.

ichthammol /ik'thəmôl/, a local anti-infective to treat some skin diseases.

ichthyosis /ik'thē·ō'sis/, any of several inherited skin conditions in which the skin is dry and cracked, like fish scales. It usually appears at or shortly after birth and may be part of one of several rare syndromes. Some types respond temporarily to bath oils. A rare, acquired variety occurs in adult life with some tumors. Also called **fish skin disease, xeroderma.**

ichthyosis congenita, ichthyosis fetalis. See **lamellar exfoliation of the newborn.**

ichthyosis fetus. See **harlequin fetus.**

ichthyosis vulgaris, an inherited skin problem marked by large, dry, dark scales that cover the face, neck, scalp, ears, and back. It appears several months to 1 year after birth. Treatment is by softening creams to aid removal of scales. Also called **ichthyosis simplex.** See also **sex-linked ichthyosis.**

ICP, abbreviation for **intracranial pressure.**

ICSH, abbreviation for **interstitial cell-stimulating hormone.** See **luteinizing hormone.**

ictal, referring to a sudden, sharp onset, as convulsions of an epileptic seizure.

icterus. See **jaundice.**

icterus index, a liver function test in which the blood serum is compared in intensity of color with that of potassium dichromate, normal being recorded in a numeric range of 3 to 5. When too much bilirubin is present and liver disease shows up, the index is usually 15 or higher; subnormal values are found with various anemias.

icterus neonatorum, a liver condition in a newborn infant.

ictus /ik'təs/, *pl.* **ictuses, ictus,** a seizure. —**ictal, ictic,** *adj.*

ICU, abbreviation for **intensive care unit.**

id, (in psychoanalysis) the part of the psyche working in the unconscious that is the source of instinctive energy, impulses, and drives. It is based on the pleasure principle and has strong tendencies to self-preservation. Compare **ego, superego.**

ID, abbreviation for **infectious disease.**

IDDM, abbreviation for **insulin-dependent diabetes mellitus.**

idea, thought, concept, intention, or impression that is in the mind as a result of awareness, understanding, etc. Kinds of ideas include **autochthonous idea, compulsive idea, dominant idea, fixed idea, idea of influence, idea of persecution,** and **idea of reference.**

idealized image, the self-image of a person with a compulsion to be perfect and to be admired. It results in high, unreachable goals. The person tries to live up to his or her ideal and to have others agree that the person and the image are one and the same.

idea of influence, an obsessive delusion, often seen in paranoid disorders, that external forces or persons are controlling one's thoughts, actions, and feelings.

idea of persecution, an obsessive delusion, often in paranoid disorders, that one is threatened, discriminated against, or mistreated by others or by outside forces.

idea of reference, an obsessive delusion that the statements or actions of others refer to oneself, usually viewed as negative, often seen in paranoid disorders. Also called **delusion of reference, referential idea.**

ideational apraxia, a condition in which the conceptual process is lost, often because of a brain injury. The patient cannot form a plan of movement and does not know the right use of an object because of not knowing its purpose. There is no loss of motor movement, but the reason for the movement is confused. Also called **sensory apraxia.** See also **apraxia.**

idée fixe. See **fixed idea.**

identical twins. See **monozygotic twins.**

identification, an unconscious defense mechanism by which a person patterns his or her personality on that of another person, assuming the person's nature and actions. The process is a normal function of personality growth and learning. It adds to the gaining of interests and ideals. Kinds of identification are **competitive identification** and **positive identification.**

identity, the concept of having a conscious understanding of being oneself, separate and distinct from others. **Identity confusion** refers to a state in which one does not have a clear and consistent image of a separate and distinct self. **Identity diffusion** is a confusion about one's perception of oneself, causing a high level of anxiety.

identity crisis, a time of being confused about one's sense of self and role in society, occurring most often in the change from one stage of life to the next. Identity crises are most common during adolescence. Then a quick rise in the strength of internal drives, with greater peer pressure and parents' or society's expectations of more mature behavior, often leads to conflicts. The youngster may be confused about personal worth, abilities, values, goals, choice of career, and place in the world. The erosion of family life, mobility of the population, and changes in the relation between the sexes all cause a higher rate of identity crises. Although confusion regarding one's identity is usually considered an adolescent problem, it also is common among old people who lose their status in the community and their place as head of a family.

ideomotor apraxia, the inability to put an idea into motion, caused by some interference with the transmission of the right impulses from the brain to the motor centers. There is no loss of ability to do an action automatically, as tying shoelaces, but the action cannot be done on request. The condition is often caused by a brain disease. Also called **classic apraxia, ideokinetic apraxia, limb-kinetic apraxia, transcortical apraxia.** See also **apraxia.**

ideophobia /ī'dē·ō-/, an anxiety disorder marked by the irrational fear or distrust of ideas or reason. See also **phobia.**

idiomere. See **chromomere.**

idiopathic /id'ē·ōpath'ik/, without a known cause.

idiopathic disease, a disease that develops without an apparent or known cause although it may have a recognizable pattern of signs and symptoms and may be curable.

idiopathic hypertrophic subaortic stenosis, a disorder of the heart, usually involving the left ventricle, that obstructs emptying. Also called **hypertrophic obstructive cardiomyopathy.**

idiopathic multiple pigmented hemorrhagic sarcoma. See **Kaposi's sarcoma.**

idiopathic respiratory distress syndrome. See **hyaline membrane disease.**

idiopathic scoliosis, an abnormal condition marked by sideways curving of the spine. It is the most common type of scoliosis, evident in 70% of all patients with scoliosis and up to 80% of those with structural scoliosis. It may occur at any age, but three types mostly occur in certain age groups. The infantile type affects 1- to 3-year-olds. The juvenile type affects 3- to 10-year-olds. The adolescent type affects preadolescents and adolescents. The most common type is the adolescent type. Early diagnosis is hard because the associated curvature is often hidden by clothes. Many states have started scoliosis screening programs to catch this condition early. The signs of scoliosis include unlevel shoulders, a prominent shoulder blade, a prominent breast, a prominent flank area, an unlevel or a prominent hip, poor posture, and obvious curvature. During diagnosis it is necessary to view the patient from the front and from the back and while the patient is bending. Other signs that may be linked to idiopathic scoliosis are occasional pain and fatigue and decreased lung function. X-ray films of the spine in the bending position are important in learning the flexibility of the curvature and the chance of natural correction. Neurological deficits are commonly associated with severe curvature and vary according to how much the curvature has pushed on the spinal cord. Some signs of such pushing are reflex, sensation, and motor changes of the lower extremities. Nonsurgical treatment commonly employs observation, exercise, and a Milwaukee brace. Observation and exercise often suffice, the observation consisting of physical examinations and X-ray monitoring of the progress of the curvature. Great degrees of curvature usually require the use of a Milwaukee brace in addition to observation and exercise. The Milwaukee brace, which is usually worn 23 hours a day, is used to control the progress of the curvature. The exercise program is used when the adolescent is out of the brace. Extra exercises are done in the brace. Surgery may be required to prevent progress of the deformity. Preoperative traction may also be used. Some physicians apply a preoperative cast to their patients, especially if surgery must be postponed. Blood may be replaced after surgery.

idiopathic thrombocytopenic purpura (ITP), bleeding into the skin and other organs caused by a lack of platelets. **Acute ITP** is a disease of children that may follow a viral infection, lasts a few weeks to a few months, and usually has no residual effects. **Chronic ITP** is more common in adolescents and adults, begins less obviously, and lasts longer. Antibodies to platelets are found in patients with ITP. The condition may be passed to the fetus if a pregnant woman has it. Treatment includes steroids and removal of the spleen. See also **thrombocytopenia, thrombocytopenic purpura.**

idiopathy /id'ē·op'əthē/, any primary disease with no apparent cause. **–idiopathic,** *adj.*

idiosyncrasy /id'ē·ōsin'krəsē/, **1.** a physical or behavioral feature unique to an individual or group. **2.** an person's unique allergy to a drug, food, etc. Also called **idiocrasy** /id′ē·ok′rəsē/. See also **allergy. –idiosyncratic,** *adj.*

idiot, an old term for a very retarded person with an IQ below 20, unable to develop past the mental age of 3 or 4 years. Compare **imbecile, moron.** See also **mental retardation. –idiocy,** *n.,* **idiotic,** *adj.*

idiot savant /idē·ō′ savänt′/, *pl.* **idiot savants, idiots savants,** a person with severe mental retardation who is able to perform some unusual mental feats, primarily those involving music, puzzle-solving, or the manipulation of numbers.

idoxuridine /ī′doksyŏŏr′ədēn/, an ophthalmic antiviral given for herpes simplex keratitis.
★CAUTION: Deep ulceration of the cornea or known allergy to this drug prohibits its use.
★ADVERSE EFFECTS: Among the more serious side effects are visual problems and eye discomfort.

id reaction, the allergy caused by a fungal infection that causes very itchy skin and blisters. These blisters are usually distant from the primary fungus infection.

I:E ratio, (in respiratory therapy) the length of breathing in (inspiration) as compared to breathing out (expiration). In the normal adult, inspiration takes about half as long as expiration. An increased ratio (longer inspiration) can cause problems in blood flow. A decreased ratio (shorter expiration) is safer.

-ifene, a combining form for drugs of the clomifene and tamoxifen group that decrease the effects of estrogen.

Ig, abbreviation for **immunoglobulin.**

IgA, abbreviation for **immunoglobulin A.**

IgA deficiency, a selective lack of immunoglobulin A, the most common type of immunoglobulin deficiency, appearing in about 1 in 400 individuals. Immunoglobulin A is a major protein antibody in the saliva and the mucous membranes of the intestines and the bronchi. It protects against bacterial and viral infections. The IgA deficiency is common in patients with rheumatoid arthritis.
★OBSERVATIONS: Symptoms of IgA deficiency are often lacking in patients whose immune systems may be compensating for low IgA with extra amounts of IgM to assure adequate defenses. Common symptoms are allergies linked to chronic lung infection, stomach and intestinal diseases, autoimmune diseases, as rheumatoid arthritis, systemic lupus erythematosus, and chronic hepatitis, and malignant tumors. The age of onset varies. Some children with IgA deficiency may begin to make the immunoglobulin spontaneously when their recurrent infections wane and their conditions improve. Diagnoses of IgA-deficient patients depend on the results of tests that commonly show normal

IgE and IgM levels while IgA levels are low.
★INTERVENTION: There is no known cure for selective IgA deficiency; treatment usually involves the effort to control associated diseases.
★PATIENT CONSIDERATIONS: The patient with IgA deficiency should not receive gamma globulin. When the IgA deficient patient needs a blood transfusion, the risk of harmful reaction can be reduced by using washed red blood cells. Using the crossmatched blood of an IgA-deficient donor in such a transfusion is considered safer and completely avoids the risk of a side effect. The IgA deficiency is lifelong, and patients with this are commonly told to watch for symptoms and to seek treatment promptly.

IgD, abbreviation for **immunoglobulin D.**

IgE, abbreviation for **immunoglobulin E.**

IgG, abbreviation for **immunoglobulin G.**

IgM, abbreviation for **immunoglobulin M.**

IGT, abbreviation for **impaired glucose tolerance.**

Ikwa fever. See **trench fever.**

Ile, abbreviation for **isoleucine.**

ileal conduit, a way to route urine through intestinal tissue. Tubes are put in a piece of detached intestine, which is then sewed to a hole in the abdominal wall where a collecting device is fixed.

ileitis /il′ē·ī′tis/, swelling of the lowest part of the small intestine. See also **Crohn's disease.**

ileoanal anastomosis /il′ē·ō·ā′nəl/, surgery in which the colon and rectum are removed and the anus is attached to the small intestine. The operation is a treatment for ulcerative colitis.

ileocecal valve, the valve between the lowest part of the small intestine and the start of the large intestine. The valve has two flaps that project into the large intestine, allowing the contents of the intestine to pass only in a forward direction.

ileocecostomy. See **cecolieostomy.**

ileocystoplasty, surgery in which the bladder is rebuilt with a piece of intestine.

ileostomate /il′ē·os′təmāt/, a person who had an ileostomy.

ileostomy /il′ē·os′təmē/, surgery to form an opening of the ileum onto the surface of the abdomen, through which fecal matter is emptied. The operation is used for severe or recurrent ulcerative colitis, Crohn's disease, or cancer of the large bowel. A low-residue diet is given before surgery and is reduced to fluids 24 hours before surgery to decrease intestinal residue. Intestinal antibiotics are given to lessen bacteria. The diseased portion of the large bowel is removed in a permanent ileostomy; sometimes segments of bowel may be reconnected after healing. A pouch may be made with part of the intestine. After surgery, the patient wears a temporary disposable bag to collect the semiliquid fecal matter. Because the secretions contain enzymes that can ulcerate the skin, the nurse makes sure nothing leaks from the bag. If a pouch is present, it is irrigated or drained three or four times a day. Compare **colostomy.** See also **enterostomy, ostomy irrigation, stoma.**

ileum /il′ē·əm/, *pl.* **ilea,** a portion of the small intestine. It opens into the large intestine. —**ileac, ileal,** *adj.*

ileus /il′ē·əs/, a blockage of the intestines. It is caused by immobility of the bowel, or by the intestine being blocked by mechanic means.

iliac region. See **inguinal region.**

illicit, referring to an act that is against the law or not allowed.

illness, an abnormal state in which the social, physical, emotional, or mental function of a person is reduced, compared with that person's previous state.

illness behavior, the manner in which people watch their own bodies, interpret symptoms, take action, and make use of health-care facilities.

illness experience, the process of being ill, of five stages: phase I, noticing a symptom; phase II, taking on a sick role; phase III, making contact for health care; phase IV, being dependent (a patient); and phase V, getting well or being rehabilitated. Each stage is marked by certain decisions, behaviors, and end points. During phase I, the person decides something is wrong and tries to improve it. Phase I ends with the person accepting the reality of the symptom, no longer delaying any act to find help or denying the symptom. During phase II the person decides that the illness is real and that care is needed. Advice is sought. This gives the person permission to act sick and to be excused from usual duties. The outcome of this phase is acceptance of the role—or denial of its necessity. In phase III professional advice is sought; authoritative declarations identify and validate the illness and legitimize the sick role. The person usually asks for help and treatment. Denial may still occur, and the patient may "shop" more for medical care or may accept the illness, the medical authority, and the plan for treatment. In phase IV professional treatment is accepted by the person, who is now seen as a patient. At any time during this phase the dependent patient may develop mixed feelings and decide to reject treatment, the care giver, and the illness. More often, care is accepted with mixed feelings. The patient needs to be informed and given emotional support during this phase. During phase V, the patient gives up the sick role. The usual tasks and roles are resumed as much as possible. Some people do not willingly give up the sick role, becoming, in their own eyes, chronically ill, or they malinger, acting sick. Most people accept the recovery and work toward rehabilitation.

illness prevention, A system of health-education programs and activities designed to protect patients from health threats, decreasing risk factors and promoting healthy behavior.

illumination, the lighting of a part of the body or of an object under a microscope for the purpose of looking closely. —**illuminate,** *v.*

illusion, a false understanding of an external sensory stimulus, usually visual or auditory, as a mirage in the desert or voices on the wind. Compare **delusion, hallucination.**

Ilopan, a trademark for a precursor of coenzyme A (dexpanthenol).

Ilosone, a trademark for an antibacterial (erythromycin estolate).

image, **1.** a visual reproduction of the likeness of someone or something, as a painting, photograph, or sculpture. **2.** an optic representation of an object, as that made by refraction or reflection. **3.** a person or thing that looks like another. **4.** a mental picture, idea, or concept of an objective reality. **5.** (in psychology) a mental representation of something seen before and later changed by other events. Kinds of images include **body image, eidetic image, memory image, mental image, motor image,** and **tactile image.**

image foreshortening, (in radiology) an x-ray image that is smaller than the object itself. It is caused by the object or x-ray tube being in the wrong position.

image format, (in computed tomography) the way in which an image is stored, as on a floppy disk, magnetic tape, or film.

imagery, (in psychiatry) the forming of mental concepts, figures, ideas; any product of the imagination. In mentally ill persons these images are often bizarre and delusional.

imagination, **1.** the ability to form, or the act or process of forming mental images or concepts of things that are not directly available to the senses. **2.** (in psychology) the ability to reproduce images or ideas in the memory by the suggestion of related ideas or to regroup former ideas and concepts to form new images and ideas concerned with a goal or problem. See also **fantasy.**

imaging, the forming of a mental picture of someone or something using imagination. See also **fantasy.**

imago /imā′gō/, (in analytic psychology) an unconscious, usually idealized mental image of an important person as one's mother, in a person's youth. See also **identification.**

imbalance, **1.** lack of balance between opposing muscle groups. **2.** an abnormal balance of fluid and electrolytes in the body tissues. **3.** an unequal distribution of subjects in a population group, as an only girl in a large family of boys. **4.** a person with mental abilities that are remarkable in one area but lacking in others, as an idiot savant.

imbecile, *obsolete.* a moderately retarded person having an I.Q. of 20 to 49, unable to develop past a mental age of 7 or 8 years. Compare **idiot, moron.** See also **mental retardation.** **–imbecile, imbecilic,** *adj.,* **imbecility,** *n.*

imbricate /im′brikāt/, to build a surface with overlapping layers of material. Surgeons may imbricate with layers of tissue when closing a wound or other opening in a body part. **–imbrication,** *n.*

Imferon, a trademark for an injectable hematinic (iron dextran).

iminoglycinuria, a benign familial condition marked by the abnormal urinary release of certain amino acids.

imipramine hydrochloride, a tricyclic antidepressant that is slow to start acting. It is given to treat mental depression.
★CAUTION: This should not be used by patients who are also taking monoamine oxidase inhibitors, have had recent heart trouble or seizures, or known allergy to other tricyclic drugs.
★ADVERSE EFFECTS: Among the more serious side effects are sedation, stomach or intestinal troubles, and heart and neurological reactions. It should not be stopped quickly. This drug interacts with many other drugs.

immature baby, a term sometimes used for an infant weighing less than 1,134 g (2.5 lb) and who is quite underdeveloped at birth.

immediate auscultation, a method of checking a patient by placing an ear or stethoscope on the skin directly over the body part being studied.

immediate hypersensitivity, an allergic reaction that occurs within minutes after exposure to an allergen.

immediate percussion. See **percussion.**

immediate posttraumatic automatism, a posttraumatic state in which a person acts spontaneously and automatically without any memory of the behavior.

immersion, the placing of a body or an object into water or other liquid so that it is completely covered by the liquid. **–immerse,** *v.*

immersion foot, an abnormal state of the feet marked by damage to the muscles, nerves, skin and blood vessels. It is caused by long exposure to dampness or by long immersion in cold water. See also **frostbite.**

imminent abortion. See **inevitable abortion.**

immiscible /imis′əbəl/, incapable of being mixed, as oil and water. Compare **miscible.**

immune complex hypersensitivity, an IgG- or IgM-dependent, sudden allergy to certain substances. A skin test results in redness and swelling in 3 to 8 hours. It is seen in serum sickness, Arthus reaction, and glomerulonephritis. Also called **type III hypersensitivity.** Compare **anaphylactic hypersensitivity, cell-mediated immune response, cytotoxic hypersensitivity.**

immune gamma globulin, passive immunizing agents obtained from pooled human plasma. Also called **immune globulin.** See also **immunoglobulin G.** It is given for immunization against measles, poliomyelitis, chickenpox, serum hepatitis after transfusion, hepatitis A, agammaglobulinemia, and hypogammaglobulinemia.
★CAUTION: Known allergy to gamma globulins prohibits its use.
★ADVERSE EFFECTS: Among the more serious side effects are pain and inflammation at the site of injection and allergic reactions.

immune globulin. See **immune gamma globulin.**

immune human globulin, a sterile solution of globulins that comes from adult human blood; used to immunize.

immune response, a defense of the body that makes antibodies to kill invading antigens and cancer. Main parts of the immune system and response are immunoglobulins, lymphocytes, phagocytes, complement properdin, the migratory inhibitory factor, and interferon. The kinds of immune response are humoral immune response, and cell-mediated immune response. The groups of immunoglobulins are M, G, A, E, and D. Immunoglobulin M is the main antibody made after first contact with an antigen. Some cells help end tissue inflammation. They also fight fungi, viruses, and tumors and try to reject organ transplants. In transplant surgery, certain drugs and radiation stop transplant rejection. Immune response protects the body from bacterial and viral infections. Immune response may start right away with antigen contact or may delay for 48 hours. One protein of the immune response is interferon. It is made by body cells after a virus invades. It fights and may slow the growth of cancer cells. Immunity can be natural or acquired. Natural immunity, or inherited resistance to certain infectious organisms can be affected by diet, mental health, surroundings, metabolism, and the strength of invading pathogens.

immune serum. See **antiserum.**

immune serum globulin. See **chickenpox, immune human globulin, immunoglobulin antibody.**

immune system, a complex that protects the body from disease organisms and other foreign bodies. The system includes the humoral immune response and the cell-mediated response. The immune system also protects the body from invasion by making local barriers and inflammation. The humoral response and the cell-mediated response develop if these first defenses fail to protect the body. The humoral immune response is especially effective against bacterial and viral invasions. The main organs of the immune response system are the bone marrow, the thymus, and the lymphoid tissues. The system uses other organs, too, as the lymph nodes, the spleen, and the lymphatic vessels. The response may start as soon as the antigen invades or start as long as 48 hours later.

immunity, 1. (in civil law) exemption from a duty required by law, as an exemption from tax or penalty for crime, or protection against suit. 2. the quality of being insusceptible to or unaffected by a certain disease or state. Kinds of immunity are **active immunity** and **passive immunity.** –**immune,** *adj.*

immunization, a process by which resistance to an infectious disease is induced or augmented.

immunodeficient, referring to an abnormal state of the immune system in which immunity is too low and resistance to infection is decreased. Kinds of immunodeficient states are **hypogammaglobulinemia** and **lymphoid aplasia.**

immunodiagnosis. See **serologic diagnosis.**

immunodiagnostic, of a diagnosis based on an antigen-antibody reaction. In many cases, a tumor releases antigenic substance into the blood; finding of a particular antigen can give a sign of the tumor associated with that antigen.

immunogen /immyōo′nəjən/, any agent or substance able to provoke an immune response or cause immunity. –**immunogenic,** *adj.*

immunoglobulin, any of five structurally and antigenically distinct antibodies in the serum and external secretions of the body. In response to certain antigens, immunoglobulins are formed in the bone marrow, spleen, and all lymphoid tissue of the body except the thymus. Kinds of immunoglobulins are **IgA, IgD, IgE, IgG,** and **IgM.** Also called **immune serum globulin.** See also **antibody, antigen, immunity.**

immunoglobulin A (IgA), one of the five classes of antibodies made by the body and one of the most common. It is found in all secretions of the body and is the major antibody in the mucous membrane of the intestines, bronchi, saliva, and tears. IgA combines with protein in the mucosa and defends body surfaces against invading microorganisms. Research indicates that it protects body tissues by seeking out foreign microorganisms and starting an antigen-antibody reaction. The normal concentrations of IgA in serum are 50 to 250 mg/dl. Compare **immunoglobulin D, immunoglobulin E, immunoglobulin G, immunoglobulin M.**

immunoglobulin D (IgD), one of the five classes of antibodies produced by the body. It is a specialized protein found in small amounts in serum tissue. The precise function of IgD is not known, but it increases in quantity during allergic reactions to milk, insulin, penicillin, and various toxins. The normal concentrations of IgD in serum are 0.5 to 3 mg/dl. Compare **immunoglobulin A, immunoglobulin E, immunoglobulin G, immunoglobulin M.**

immunoglobulin E (IgE), one of the five classes of fluid antibodies produced by the human body. It is concentrated in the lung, the skin, and the cells of mucous membranes. It provides the main defense against antigens from the environment and is believed to be stimulated by immunoglobulin A. IgE reacts with certain antigens to release certain chemicals that cause reddening of the skin. The normal concentrations of IgE in the blood are 0.01 to 0.04 mg/dl. Compare **immunoglobulin A, immunoglobulin D, immunoglobulin G, immunoglobulin M.**

immunoglobulin G (IgG), one of the five classes of fluid antibodies, produced by the human body. It is a specialized protein produced by the body in response to invasions by bacteria, fungi, and viruses. In pregnancy IgG crosses the placenta to the fetus and protects against red cell antigens and white cell antigens. The normal concentrations of IgG in the blood are 800 to 1,600 mg/dl. Compare **immunoglobulin A, immunoglobulin D, immunoglobulin E, immunoglobulin M.**

immunoglobulin M (IgM), one of the five classes of fluid antibodies produced by the human body. It is the largest in molecular structure. It is the first immunoglobulin the body produces when challenged by antigens and is found in circulating fluids. IgM triggers the increased production of immunoglobulin G and the important complexes required for effective antibody response. The normal concentrations of IgM in the blood are 40 to 120 mg/dl. Compare **immunoglobulin A, immunoglobulin D, immunoglobulin E, immunoglobulin G.**

immunohematology, the study of antigen-antibody reactions and their effects on blood.

immunologic tests, tests based on the principles of antigen-antibody reactions.

immunologic theory of aging, the belief that normal cells are not recognized as such by the body's immune system, thereby triggering immune reactions within the person's own body.

immunologist, a specialist in immunology.

immunology, the study of the reaction of tissues of the immune system of the body to stimulation by antigens.

immunomodulator, a substance that acts to change the body's immune response by increasing or decreasing the ability of the immune system to produce modified blood antibodies or cells that recognize and react with the antigen that caused their production. Some immunomodulating substances are naturally present in the body. Some of these are available in various prescription drugs. –**immunomodulation,** *n.*

immunopotency, the ability of an antigen to cause an immune response.

immunosuppression, 1. the giving of agents that reduce the ability of the immune system to respond to stimulation by antigens. Immunosuppression may be deliberate, as when preparing for bone marrow or other transplants to prevent rejection of the donor tissue, or an accidental byproduct, as often results from chemotherapy for the treatment of cancer. **2.** an abnormal condition of the immune system characterized by markedly lowered ability to respond to stimulation by antigens. –**immunosuppressed,** *adj.*

immunosuppressive, **1.** of or pertaining to a substance or procedure that lessens or prevents an immune response. **2.** an immunosuppressive agent.

immunotherapy, a special treatment for allergies. Increasingly large doses of the offending allergens are given to gradually develop immunity. Immunotherapy is based on the premise that low doses of the offending allergen will bind with IgG to prevent an allergic reaction, slowing the action of IgE by promoting the synthesis of the blocking IgG antibody. The person exposed to the offending allergen develops more blocking antibody the more he or she is exposed. The blocking antibody binds to the circulating antigen and seems to decrease the allergic response, or it eliminates it by producing a tolerance toward the antigen. In immunotherapy low doses of the offending allergen are gradually increased throughout the year or during a 3- to 6-month period before the allergy season starts; it usually continues until the patient shows no allergic response for 2 to 5 years. Also called **hyposensitization.** –**immunotherapeutic,** *adj.*

immunotoxin (IT), a poison from a plant or animal that is bound to an antibody and used to destroy specific target cells. For example, the plant toxin ricin bound to an antibody will guide the ricin molecules to tumor cells. The ricin prevents the target cells from producing proteins, and the cells die.

Imodium, a trademark for drug (loperamide hydrochloride) used as an antidiarrheal agent.

Imovax, a trademark for a rabies virus vaccine (rabies human diploid cell vaccine).

impacted, tightly or firmly wedged in too limited a space. –**impact,** *v.,* **impaction,** *n.*

impacted fracture, a bone break in which the adjacent ends of the fractured bone are wedged together.

impacted tooth, a tooth so positioned against another tooth, bone, or soft tissue that its full emergence is impossible or unlikely. Compare **embedded tooth.**

impaction, **1.** the poor positioning or blockage of a tooth that prevents it from breaking through the gum. **2.** the presence of a large, hard mass of feces in the rectum or colon.

impaired glucose tolerance (IGT), a condition in which blood glucose levels after fasting are higher than normal but lower than those for diabetes. In some patients this represents a stage in the natural history of diabetes, but in a substantial number of persons IGT either does not progress or reverts to normal. See also **diabetes mellitus.**

impairment, any disorder in structure or function resulting from abnormalities that interfere with normal activities.

impedance audiometry. See **audiometry.**

imperative conception, a thought or impression that appears in the mind without known cause and cannot be eliminated, as an obsession.

imperative idea. See **compulsive idea.**

imperforate /impur′fərit/, lacking a normal opening in a body organ or passageway. An infant may be born with an imperforate anus. Compare **perforate.**

imperforate anus, any of several inborn defects of the anus. The common form is anal agenesis, in which the rectal pouch ends before reaching the surface. An abnormal canal to the surface is present in 80% to 90% of cases. Other forms include anal stenosis, in which the anal opening is small, and anal membrane atresia, in which the anal membrane covers the opening creating an obstruction.

★OBSERVATIONS: The defect is often found at birth. Inspection reveals an absence of the anus or the presence of a thin membrane covering it. An x-ray examination is made with an opaque marker placed at the usual site of the anus. The infant is held upside down. Air moving through the intestines into the bowel or the rectum is seen on the x-ray film. Anal stenosis is treated with daily insertion of a finger begun in the hospital and continued at home by the parents. An imperforate anal membrane is removed, and a finger is inserted daily as the skin heals. Surgical reconstruction is done to treat anal agenesis in infants in whom the pouch is too low. An anus is made surgically. Anal atresia in which the pouch at the end of the bowel is too high may require a colostomy.

★PATIENT CARE: Often it is the nurse who finds the problem because the thermometer cannot be inserted in taking the newborn's temperature. A newborn who does not pass any stool in the first 24 hours requires examination for the defect. Care of the newborn treated surgically for any of these conditions requires close attention.

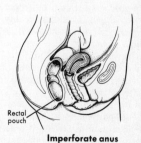

Rectal pouch

Imperforate anus

impermeable, (of a tissue, membrane, or film) preventing the passage of a substance through it.

impetigo /im′pəti′gō/, an infection of the skin beginning as a redness and progressing to itching blisters, breakdown of the skin, and honey-colored crusts. Lesions usually form on the face and spread locally. The disorder is highly contagious by contact with the discharge from the lesions. Acute kidney trouble is an occasional complication. Treatment includes thorough cleansing with antibacterial soap and water, compresses of Burow's solution, removal of crusts, and use of systemic antibiotics. Treatment is essential to prevent spread of infection. Use of individual washcloths and linens, and careful and frequent hand washing are needed. **–impetiginous,** *adj.*

implant, 1. (in radiotherapy) a radioactive substance embedded in tissue for therapy. Seeds containing iodine 125 may be implanted permanently in prostate and chest tumors. Seeds of iridium 192 in ribbons or wire may be embedded temporarily in head and neck cancers. Sealed sources of cesium 137 or radium 226 may be implanted in the body cavity temporarily in the treatment of cancers of the female organs. Strontium 90 in sealed sources may be embedded for a brief period (usually less than 2 minutes) in treating eye tumors. Needles containing radium 226 may be used as temporary implants. Patients with radioactive implants tend to be isolated from other patients. 2. (in surgery) material inserted or grafted into an organ or structure of the body. The implant may be of tissue, as in a blood vessel graft, or of an artificial substance, as an artificial hip, a pacemaker, or a container of radioactive material.

implantation dermoid cyst, a tumor derived from embryo tissues, caused by an injury that forces part of the outer germ layer of the embryo into the embryo's body.

implant restoration, a one-tooth crown or many-tooth crown or bridge that replaces a missing tooth or teeth.

implosion, 1. a bursting inward. 2. a psychiatric treatment for people disabled by fear and anxiety in which the person is made immune to anxiety-producing stimuli by repeated intense exposure in imagination or reality, until the stimuli are no longer stressful. Also called **flooding. –implode,** *v.*

implosive therapy. See **flooding.**

impotence, 1. weakness. 2. inability of the adult male to achieve erection or, less commonly, to ejaculate having achieved an erection. Several forms are recognized. **Functional impotence** has a psychological basis. **Anatomic impotence** results from faulty genitals. **Atonic impotence** involves disturbed neuromuscular function.

Poor health, age, drugs, and fatigue can inhibit normal sexual function. Also called **impotency. –impotent,** *adj.*

impregnate, 1. to make pregnant; to fertilize. 2. to saturate or mix with another substance. **–impregnable,** *adj.,* **impregnation,** *n.*

impression, 1. (in dentistry and prosthetic medicine) a mold of a part of the mouth or other part of the body from which a replacement part may be formed. 2. (in the medical record) the examiner's diagnosis or assessment of a problem, disease, or condition. 3. a strong sensation or effect on the mind or feelings.

imprinting, (in ethology) a special type of learning that occurs at critical points during the early stages of development in animals. One kind is behavior shaping. Another is the formation of social attachments. The new behavior is quickly acquired and cannot be lost. It is usually species-specific, but animals exposed to members of a different species during this short period may become attached to and copy that particular species instead of their own. The degree to which imprinting occurs in human development has not been determined. See also **bonding.**

impulse, 1. (in psychology) a sudden, strong, often irrational drive, urge, desire, or action resulting from a particular feeling or mental state. 2. also called **nerve impulse, neural impulse.** (in physiology) the electrochemical process by which messages are sent along the nerves. **–impulsive,** *adj.*

impulsion, an abnormal, irrational urge to commit an illegal or out-of-place act.

Imutran, a trademark for an immunosuppressive (azathioprine).

IMV, abbreviation for **intermittent mandatory ventilation.**

In, symbol for **indium.**

inactivation, a reversible change in the physical properties of a protein caused by heat or chemicals.

inactive colon, decreased tone of the bowel resulting in fewer contractions and propelling movements. It causes delay in the normal 12-hour time it takes the contents to pass through the intestine and colon. Colon inactivity may be caused by oversized colon, aging, depression, faulty habits of elimination, inadequate fluid intake, lack of exercise, a low-residue or starvation diet, prolonged bed rest, or a neurological disease. Normal function of the colon is frequently reduced by the continued use of laxatives. Acquired megacolon, characterized by a too-large, inactive bowel and chronic constipation, is common in retarded children and adults with chronic mental illness. In congenital megacolon (Hirschsprung's disease), congenital absence of reflex activity in the colon results in loss of function. It causes massive dilatation of the proximal segment of the large bowel and extreme constipation. The disorder is more common in males than females and in severe cases retards growth. Treatment of inactive colon includes a training program to establish regular bowel habits, the use of stool softeners to increase fecal bulk, and a diet containing adequate roughage.

inadequate personality, a personality marked by a lack of physical stamina, immature emotions, social instability, poor judgment, reduced drive, ineptness—especially in interpersonal relationships—and an inability to adapt or react well to new or stressful situations.

inanimate, not alive; lacking signs of life.

inanition /in'ənish'ən/, **1.** an exhausted condition from lack of food and water or a defect in digestion; starvation. **2.** a state of lethargy marked by a loss of vitality or vigor.

inanition fever, a temporary, mild fever in the newborn in the first few days after birth, usually caused by water loss.

inborn, innate; acquired or occurring during life in the uterus. See also **congenital, hereditary, inborn error of metabolism.**

inborn error of metabolism, one of many abnormal metabolic conditions caused by an inherited defect of an enzyme or other protein. People with such diseases are each defective in only protein. But they generally display a large number of physical signs characteristic of the genetic trait. The diseases are rare. Kinds of inborn errors of metabolism include **phenylketonuria, Tay-Sachs disease, Lesch-Nyhan syndrome, galactosemia,** and **glucose-6-phosphate dehydrogenase deficiency.**

inborn reflex. See **unconditioned response.**

inbreeding, the production of offspring by the mating of closely related persons, organisms, or plants. Self-fertilization is the most extreme form. It normally occurs in certain plants and lower animals. The practice provides a greater chance for both desirable and undesirable recessive traits to show up in the offspring. In humans, the amount of inbreeding in a specific population is largely controlled by tradition and cultural practices. In plants and animals, inbreeding is a standard method for developing desirable types and pure lines. Compare **outbreeding.**

incarcerate, to trap, imprison, or confine, as a loop of intestine in a hernia. See also **hernia.**

incest, sexual intercourse between members of the same family. Intercourse with distant relatives does not count. Intercourse is incest only when those participating could not legally marry. **–incestuous,** *adj.*

incidence, 1. the number of times an event occurs. **2.** (in epidemiology) the number of new cases in a particular period of time. Incidence is often expressed as a ratio. The number of cases is often expressed as a ratio. The number of cases is divided by the population at risk. See also **rate.**

incidental additives, food additives caused by pesticides, herbicides, or chemicals used in food processing.

incident report, a report, usually confidential, describing an accident or a break in policies or orders involving a patient, employee, visitor, or student in a health-care facility.

incineration, the burning of waste materials.

incipient, coming into existence; at an initial stage; beginning to appear, as a symptom or disease.

incipient dental caries, a dental condition in which tooth decay can first be seen.

incision, 1. a cut made surgically by a sharp instrument creating an opening into an organ or space in the body. **2.** the act of making an incision.

incisor, one of the eight front teeth, four in each dental arch. They first appear as milk teeth during infancy. They are replaced by permanent incisors during childhood. They last until old age. The crown of the incisor is chisel-shaped and has a sharp cutting edge. Its front surface is convex, smooth, and highly polished. Its inner surface is concave and, in many individuals, is marked by an inverted V-shaped ridge near the gum of the upper arch. The neck of the incisor is constricted. The root is single, long, and conic. The upper incisors are larger and stronger than the lower and are directed at a slant downward and forward. Compare **canine tooth, molar, premolar.**

inclusion, 1. the act of enclosing or the state of being enclosed. **2.** a structure within another, as inclusions inside of the cells.

inclusion bodies, microscopic objects of various shapes and sizes observed in the blood cells or other tissue cells, depending on the type of disease.

inclusion conjunctivitis, an acute, pus-filled infection caused by *Chlamydia* organisms. It occurs in two forms: one in infants marked by redness and pus discharge, and one in the adult that is less severe, and discharges less pus. Local use of antibiotics is effective treatment. Also called **swimming pool conjunctivitis.**

inclusion dermoid cyst, a tumor derived from embryo tissues, caused by a foreign tissue being enclosed when a developed cleft closes.

inclusiveness principle, a rule that response to objects in the environment is proportional to the stimulus provided by each object.

incoherent, 1. disordered; without logical connection; disjointed; lacking relevance. **2.** unable to express one's ideas in an orderly, clear way, usually as a result of emotional stress.

incompatible, unable to coexist. A tissue transplant may be rejected because recipient and donor antibody factors are incompatible.

incompetence, lack of ability. Body organs that do not function adequately may be described as incompetent. Kinds of incompetence include **aortic incompetence,** and **valvular incompetence.** –**incompetent,** *adj.*

incompetency, the legal status of a person said to be unable to provide for his or her own needs and protection. The status must be proved in a special court hearing, as a result of which the person can lose certain civil rights. The ruling of incompetency can be dropped if another court hearing finds the same person competent.

incompetent cervix, (in obstetrics) a condition marked by opening of the mouth of the uterus before term without labor or contractions of the uterus. Miscarriage or premature delivery may result. Incompetent cervix is treated by a procedure in which the uterus is held closed by a surgically implanted suture.

incomplete abortion, termination of pregnancy in which the products of conception are not entirely expelled or removed. It often causes bleeding that may require surgical cleaning by curettage, uterine stimulation, and blood replacement. Infection is also a frequent side effect of incomplete abortion. Compare **complete abortion.**

incomplete fistula. See **blind fistula.**

incomplete fracture, a bone break in which the crack in the bone tissue does not completely traverse the width of the affected bone.

incongruent communication, a pattern in which the sender says one thing with words but another with his or her body language. The listener does not know which message to accept. See also **double bind.**

incontinence, the inability to control urination or defecation, common in the aged. Treatment includes bladder retraining, implanting of an artificial sphincter, and the use of internal or external drainage devices. Stress incontinence is caused by coughing, straining, or heavy lifting. It occurs more often in women than in men. Mild cases may be treated by exercises or they may respond to drug therapy. Severe cases may require surgery to correct the defect. Bowel incontinence may result from relaxation of the anal sphincter or by central nervous system or spinal cord disorders and may be treated by a program of bowel training. See also **bowel training.** –**incontinent,** *adj.*

increment, 1. an increase or gain. 2. the act of growing or increasing. 3. the amount of an increase or gain in pressure in the uterus as contractions begin in labor. –**incremental,** *adj.*

incrustation, hardened fluid discharge, scale, or scab.

incubation period, 1. the time between exposure to a disease-causing organism and the onset of symptoms of a disease. 2. the time required for the growth of an embryo in an egg or for the growth and reproduction of tissue cells or microorganisms being grown in a special laboratory environment. 3. the time allowed for a chemical reaction or process to proceed.

incubator, an apparatus used to provide a controlled environment, especially a certain temperature. Other environmental factors, as darkness, light, oxygen, moisture, or dryness, may also be provided. An incubator for cultivating eggs or microorganisms in a laboratory and an incubator for premature infants are examples.

incudectomy /in′kyo͞odek′təmē/, surgical removal of the "anvil" of the ear. This is done to treat deafness resulting from decay of the tip of the anvil. Local or general anesthesia is used. The defective anvil is removed and replaced with a bone chip graft so that sound vibrations are again transmitted. After the operation, the patient must change position slowly to avoid dizziness, avoid blowing the nose and sneezing, and report any fever, headache, dizziness or pain in the ear.

incus /ing′kəs/, *pl.* **incudes** /inko͞o′dēz/, also called the anvil, one of the three ossicles in the middle ear. It communicates sound vibrations. Compare **malleus, stapes.** See also **middle ear.**

indandione derivative, an oral anticoagulant designed for long-term therapeutic use in patients who cannot tolerate most oral anticoagulants. The indandiones are difficult to control and may cause grave adverse effects, including severe kidney and liver problems. For this reason, coumarin derivatives are preferred. Extreme fatigue, sore throat, chills, and fever are signs of impending toxicity and require discontinuation of the drug. Compare **coumarin.**

indentation, a notch, pit, or depression in the surface of an object, as toothmarks on the tongue or skin. –**indent,** *v.*

Inderal, a trademark for a beta-adrenergic blocking agent (propranolol).

indeterminate cleavage, division of a fertilized ovum into two parts that have similar developmental potential; each of which, if isolated, can give rise to a complete individual embryo. Also called **regulative cleavage.** Compare **determinate cleavage.** See also **regulative development.**

index case, (in epidemiology) the first case of a disease by contrast with subsequent cases. See also **propositus.**

index myopia, a kind of nearsightedness caused by a change in physical properties of the media of the eye.

Indian tick fever. See **Marseilles fever.**

indican, a substance (potassium indoxyl sulfate) produced in the intestine by the breakdown of tryptophan, absorbed by the intestinal wall, and passed in the urine. It may be high in the urine of patients on high-protein diets or those suffering from disease of the stomach and intestines.

indication, a reason to prescribe a medication or perform a treatment, as a bacterial infection may be an indication for prescribing a specific antibiotic or as appendicitis is an indication for appendectomy. **–indicate,** *v.*

indigenous /indij'ənəs/, native to or found naturally in a specified area or environment, as certain species of bacteria in the human digestive tract.

indigestion. See **dyspepsia.**

indirect anaphylaxis, a strong reaction to a person's own antigen that occurs because the antigen has been altered in some way.

indirect division. See **mitosis.**

indirect nursing care functions, nursing activities used to solve problems with a client who is responsible for putting into effect any recommended changes.

indirect percussion. See **percussion.**

indirect restorative method, the technique for making a new tooth on a cast of the original, as the indirect construction of an inlay. After a die is made from an impression of the prepared tooth, a wax pattern is formed and inverted. The cast inlay is then fitted and finished on the die, and fused to the tooth.

indirect retainer, a part of a removable partial denture that resists movement of an extension away from its tissue supported by means of lever action.

individual immunity, a form of natural immunity not shared by most other members of the race and species. It is rare and probably occurs because the person had an infection that went unnoticed. Compare **racial immunity, species immunity.**

individual psychology, a modified system of psychoanalysis, developed by Alfred Adler, that views poor adaptive behavior and personality disorders as resulting from conflict between the desire to dominate and feelings of inferiority. See also **inferiority complex.**

Indocin, a trademark for an agent (indomethacin) for reducing inflammation.

indomethacin, a nonsteroid agent for reducing inflammation. It is given to treat arthritis and certain other inflammatory conditions.

induce, to cause or stimulate the start of an activity, as an enzyme induces a metabolic activity. See also **induced fever. –inducer, induction,** *n.*

induced abortion, an intentional ending of a pregnancy before the fetus has developed enough to live if born. Twenty to 50% of pregnancies are ended deliberately, at the request of the mother or for medical reasons. Ending of a pregnancy by a trained person under proper conditions is safe. Unskilled abortions can be extremely hazardous because of the danger of infection and damage to the uterus. Infection and excessive bleeding after criminal abortion have been leading causes of maternal death. Compare **spontaneous abortion.** See also **criminal abortion, septic abortion, therapeutic abortion.**

induced fever, a deliberate raising of body temperature by heat or by inoculating with a fever-producing organism in order to kill heat-sensitive germs.

induced hypotension. See **deliberate hypotension.**

induced lethargy, a trancelike state produced during hypnosis. See also **hypnosis, lethargy.**

induced trance, a state like sleepwalking resulting from a hysteric neurosis or from hypnotism.

induction of anesthesia, all parts of the anesthetic process that occur before the patient reaches the desired level of anesthesia, including giving a sedative, tranquilizer, or hypnosis beforehand, giving oxygen, and giving the anesthetic itself.

induction of labor, an obstetric procedure in which labor is initiated artificially by rupturing the fetal membranes or giving a drug to start contractions. It is performed electively or because the condition of the fetus or mother requires it. Elective induction is carried out for the convenience of the mother or the obstetrician, often to avoid the possibility of delivery outside of the hospital when labor is coming soon and the mother is expecting to have an unusually rapid birth. Elective inductions are done less often now than in the past. Elective induction requires a full-term pregnancy, a fetal weight of at least 2,500 g (5½ lbs.), a cervix judged ready to dilate, and other favorable factors. Errors in estimating fetal age and weight may result in the delivery of an unexpectedly immature or low-birthweight infant. Induction is performed for medical reasons when the risk of induction is judged to be less than that of continuing the pregnancy. This is often done in such conditions as premature rupture of the membranes, severe maternal diabetes, and intractable preeclampsia. Surgical induction is effected by rupturing the fetal membranes, often with stripping of the membranes and stretching of the cervix with the fingers. It is very often carried out in conjunction with medical induction. Medical induction is achieved through the giving of appropriate drugs. Electronic fetal and uterine monitoring is usually done during induction of labor to avoid overstimulating the uterus and causing fetal distress. Ideally, induced labor mimics natural labor, but in practice this is not usually achieved. Longer and harder contractions commonly occur. In addition to unexpected fetal immaturity, complications of induction of labor are numerous. Also, if the induction fails to produce effective labor, cesarean section is often required. For this reason, induction of labor is usually not attempted unless delivery must be hastened to avoid severe fetal or maternal problems.

induction phase, the period of time during which a normal cell changes into a cancerous cell.

induration, hardening of a tissue, particularly the skin, because of excess fluid retention, inflammation, or growth of a tumor. **–indurated,** *adj.*

industrial psychology, the application of psychological principles and techniques to the problems of business and industry. It includes the selection of personnel, the motivation of workers, and the development of training programs.

indwelling catheter, any catheter designed to be left in place for a prolonged period. See also **self-retaining catheter.**

inert, **1.** not moving or acting, as inert matter. **2.** (of a chemical substance) not taking part in a chemical reaction or acting as a catalyst, as neon or an inert gas. **3.** (of a medical ingredient) not medically active; serving only as a bulking, binding, or sweetening agent or other nonmedical function in a medication.

inert gas, a chemically inactive gaseous element. The inert gases are argon, helium, krypton, neon, radon, and xenon. Also called **noble gas.**

inertia, **1.** the tendency of a body at rest or in motion to remain at rest or in motion in the same direction unless acted on by an outside force. **2.** an abnormal state marked by a general inactivity or sluggishness, as colonic inertia or uterine inertia.

inevitable abortion, a condition of pregnancy in which sudden miscarriage cannot be prevented. It is marked by bleeding, uterine cramping, dilatation of the cervix, and other symptoms. If heavy bleeding occurs, immediate emptying of the uterus may be required. The point at which an inevitable abortion becomes an incomplete abortion is of legal interest because of the statutory difference between spontaneous and induced abortion. In clinical practice, precise differentiation is seldom practicable. Compare **incomplete abortion, imminent abortion, threatened abortion.**

infant, **1.** a child who is in the earliest stage of extrauterine life. Infancy covers the time extending from birth to about 12 months of age, when the baby is able to assume an erect posture. Some extend the period to 24 months of age. **2.** (in law) a person not of full legal age; a minor. **3.** of or pertaining to infancy; in an early stage of development. **–infantile,** *adj.*

infant botulism, a condition of poisoning that occurs in children less than 6 months of age. It is marked by severe loss of tone in all muscles, constipation, lethargy, and feeding difficulties, and it may lead to inability to breathe. Treat-

ment includes optimal management of fluids, electrolytes, and nutrition. Help in breathing may also be necessary.

infant death, the death of a live-born infant before 1 year of age.

infant feeder, a device for feeding small or weak infants who cannot suck hard enough to nurse from the breast or to get milk from a bottle. The feeder resembles a bulb syringe with a long, soft nipple on the end. The bulb is squeezed slowly and gently. It permits the baby to suck and swallow without great effort and prevents the escape of fluid into the infant's trachea.

infant feeding. See **bottle feeding, breast feeding.**

infanticide /infan'tisīde/, **1.** the killing of an infant or young child. The act is often a psychotic reaction associated with severe depression. Infanticide may become a neurotic obsession in mothers who do not want the baby or who do not feel physically, mentally, or emotionally capable of caring for or coping with it. **2.** one who takes the life of an infant or young child. **–infanticidal,** *adj.*

infantile, **1.** of, relating to, or typical of infants or infancy. **2.** lacking maturity, sophistication, or reasonableness. **3.** affected with infantilism. **4.** being in a very early stage of development.

infantile amnesia, (in psychology) the inability to remember events from early childhood. It is explained by a theory that a memory for skills develops earlier than a memory for facts, which may not develop until the third year. Thus a person may learn skills without remembering how they were learned.

infantile arteritis, a disorder in infants and young children marked by inflammation of many arteries.

infantile autism, a condition marked by abnormal emotional, social, and speech development in a child. It may result from an organic brain problem, in which case it occurs before 3 years of age. It may be associated with childhood schizophrenia, in which case the autism occurs later, but before adolescence. The autistic child remains fixed at one of the stages a normal infant passes through as it develops. If the condition is caused by organic brain disease, the child appears unable to proceed beyond the current stage of development, though there is no regression to an earlier stage. If the condition accompanies schizophrenia in later childhood, regression occurs. Treatment includes psychotherapy, often accompanied by play therapy.

infantile celiac disease. See **celiac disease.**

infantile cerebral sphingolipidosis. See **Tay-Sachs disease.**

infantile dwarf, a person whose mental and physical development is greatly retarded.

infantile eczema. See **atopic dermatitis.**

infantile hemiplegia, paralysis of one side of the body in an infant. It may occur at birth from brain bleeding, in utero from lack of oxygen, or from a fever in infancy.

infantile paralysis. See **poliomyelitis.**

infantile pellagra. See **kwashiorkor.**

infantile scurvy, a nutritional disease caused by too-little vitamin C in the diet. It most commonly occurs because cow's milk, unfortified with vitamin C, is the principal food in an infant's diet. Families are counseled to feed their children foods rich in vitamin C or to use a formula supplemented with this vitamin. Also called **Barlow's disease, hemorrhagic scurvy.** See also **ascorbic acid, citric acid, scurvy.**

infantile spinal muscular atrophy. See **Werdnig-Hoffmann disease.**

infantile uterus, a uterus that has failed to attain adult form.

infantilism /in'fəntəliz'əm/, **1.** a condition in which various anatomic, physiological, and psychological traits of childhood persist in the adult. It is marked by mental retardation, underdeveloped sex organs, and, usually, small stature. Compare **progeria. 2.** a condition, usually of psychological rather than organic origin, marked by speech and voice patterns in an older child or adult that are typical of very young children.

infant mortality, the statistic rate of infant death during the first year after live birth. It is expressed as the number of such births per 1,000 live births in a given geographical area in a given period of time. Neonatal mortality accounts for 70% of infant mortality.

infant of addicted mother, a newborn infant showing withdrawal symptoms, usually within the first 24 hours of life. Most commonly these are caused by maternal dependence on heroin, methadone, diazepam, phenobarbital, or alcohol. See also **fetal alcohol syndrome.**
★OBSERVATIONS: Typical symptoms include tremors, irritability, hyperactive reflexes, increased muscle tone, twitching, increased mucus production, nasal congestion, breathing distress, excessing sweating, high temperature, vomiting, diarrhea, and excess water loss. The infants cry shrilly, often sneeze, frantically suck their fists, but feed poorly. They often yawn but have trouble falling asleep. They are usually pale, and are often born with nose and knee abrasions. They are subject to convulsions.
★INTERVENTION: The infant is kept warm, snugly swaddled in a padded crib, and exposed to minimal light, sound, and tactile stimulation. The baby is handled only when necessary and is then held firmly, close to the body. Fluid and drugs are introduced directly into the blood. Small, frequent feedings of concentrated formula are usual. Before each feeding

the infant's nasopharynx is suctioned. If the buttocks becomes inflammed because of diarrhea, a paste of zinc oxide and karaya powder is applied. If the infant's flailing about is likely to cause abrasions, bony parts of the body may be protected with light padding and the hands with the mitts of the infant shirt.
★PATIENT CONSIDERATIONS: These high-risk infants require special attention. It is important for the mother to be encouraged to participate in her baby's care as soon as possible. The nurse may help to promote parent-child bonding.

infant psychiatry, the branch of psychiatry that specializes in the diagnosis and treatment of the psychologically abnormal syndromes and symptoms of infants. Such conditions are associated with early abnormalities of several sorts. These include poor infant-parent attachment, infantile autism, avoidance reaction, persistent stranger and separation anxiety, early signs of aggression, hyperactivity, cyclic vomiting, and disturbances in sleeping, eating, and elimination.

infarct /infärkt'/, a localized area of decay in a tissue, vessel, organ, of part resulting from an interruption in the blood supply to the area, or, less frequently, by the blockage of a vein that ordinarily carries blood away from the area. An infarct may resemble a red swollen bruise, because of bleeding and an accumulation of blood in the area. Some infarcts are pale and white, caused by a lack of blood to the area. Kinds of infarct include **anemic infarct, calcareous infarct, cicatrized infarct, hemorrhagic infarct,** and **uric acid infarct.** –infarcted, *adj.*

infarct extension, a decay in heart tissue that has spread beyond the original area, usually as a result of the death of neighboring cells.

infarction, 1. the development and formation of an infarct. **2.** an infarct. Kinds of infarction include **myocardial infarction** and **pulmonary infarction.**

infect, to transmit a germ that may cause an infectious disease in another person.

infected abortion, abortion of an immature pregnancy in which the products of conception have become infected. Fever is present, and antibiotic therapy and emptying of the uterus are required. Compare **septic abortion.**

infection, 1. the invasion of the body by germs that reproduce and multiply, causing disease by local cell injury, release of poisons, or germ-antibody reaction in the cells. **2.** a disease caused by the invasion of the body by germs. Compare **infestation.**

infectious, 1. capable of causing an infection. **2.** caused by an infection.

infectious hepatitis. See **hepatitis A.**

infectious mononucleosis, an acute herpesvirus infection caused by the Epstein-Barr virus

(EBV). It is marked by fever, sore throat, swollen lymph glands, abnormal liver function, and bruising. The disease is usually transmitted by droplet infection but is not highly contagious. Young people are most often affected. In childhood, the disease is mild and usually unnoticed. The older the person, the more severe the symptoms are likely to be. Infection gives permanent immunity. Treatment is primarily of the symptoms. Bed rest is required to prevent serious complications of the liver or spleen, analgesics to control pain, and salt gargles for throat discomfort. Rupture of the spleen may occur, requiring immediate surgery and blood transfusion. See also **Epstein-Barr virus, viral infection.**

infectious myringitis, an inflammatory, contagious condition of the eardrum caused by infection. It is marked by the development of painful blisters on the eardrum. Also called **bullous myringitis.**

infectious nucleic acid, DNA or, more commonly, viral RNA that is able to infect the cell and to induce it to produce viruses.

infectious parotitis. See **mumps.**

infectious polyneuritis. See **Guillain-Barré syndrome.**

infective tubulointerstitial nephritis, an acute inflammation of the kidneys caused by an infection by certain germs. The condition is marked by chills, fever, nausea and vomiting, flank pain, and other symptoms. The kidney may become enlarged, and portions of the renal cortex destroyed.

infectivity, the ability of a germ to spread rapidly from one host to another.

inferior, 1. below a given point of reference, as the feet are inferior to the legs. 2. of poorer quality or value. Compare **superior.**

inferior aperture of minor pelvis, an irregular opening in the bone structure at the rear of the pelvis.

inferior aperture of thorax, an irregular opening in the bone structure at the center of the front of the chest.

inferior conjunctival fornix, a space in the fold of the thin membrane lining the eyelid. It is created by the reflection of the membrane covering the eyeball and the lining of the lower eyelid. Compare **superior conjunctival fornix.**

inferior gastric node, a node in one of two groups of stomach lymph nodes, lying near the greater curvature of the stomach. Compare **hepatic node, superior gastric node.**

inferiority complex, 1. a feeling of fear and resentment resulting from a sense of being physically inadequate. It is marked by a variety of abnormal behaviors. 2. (in psychoanalysis) a complex marked by striving for unrealistic goals because of an unresolved Oedipus complex. 3. *informal,* a feeling of being inferior.

inferior maxillary bone. See **mandible.**

inferior mesenteric node, a node in one of the three groups of lymph glands serving the viscera of the belly and the pelvis. The inferior mesenteric nodes are linked with the branches of the inferior mesenteric artery. They are divided into a group of small nodes along the branches of the left colic and sigmoid arteries, another group in the colon, and a group touching the muscular coat of the rectum. The inferior mesenteric nodes drain the descending colon, the iliac and sigmoid parts of the colon, and the upper part of the rectum. Compare **gastric node, superior mesenteric node.**

inferior mesenteric vein, the vein in the lower body that returns the blood from the rectum and the colon. Compare **superior mesenteric vein.**

inferior orbital fissure, a groove in the wall of the eye socket that contains certain nerves and vessels.

inferior phrenic artery, a small branch of the abdominal aorta, arising from the aorta itself, the renal artery, or the main abdominal artery. It supplies the diaphragm with blood.

inferior radioulnar joint. See **distal radioulnar articulation.**

inferior sagittal sinus, a channel draining blood from the brain into the internal jugular vein. Compare **straight sinus, superior sagittal sinus, transverse sinus.**

inferior subscapular nerve /subskap'yŏŏlər/, a small nerve in the back. Compare **superior subscapular nerve.**

inferior thyroid vein, a vein that arises in the venous plexus on the thyroid gland and forms a plexus ventral to the trachea. The inferior thyroid veins contain valves at their terminations. They receive veins from the esophagus, the trachea, and the larynx.

inferior ulnar collateral artery, one of a number of branches of arteries in the arm, arising near the elbow, passing inward to form an arch with the deep brachial artery, and carrying blood to the muscles of the forearm. Compare **superior ulnar collateral artery.**

inferior vena cava, the large vein that returns blood to the heart from parts of the body below the diaphragm. The vessel receives blood from the two common iliacs, the lumbar veins, and the veins from the testicles. Compare **superior vena cava.**

inferolateral /in'fərōlat'ərəl/, below and to the side.

inferomedial, below and toward the center.

infertile, not being able to produce offspring. This condition may be present in one or both sex partners. It may be temporary and reversible. The cause may be physical, including immature sex organs, abnormalities of the reproductive system, hormone imbalance, and trouble in other organ systems. It may result from psychological or emotional problems.

The condition is classified as primary if pregnancy has never occurred, and secondary when there have been one or more pregnancies. Compare **sterile.** **–infertility,** *n.*

infest, to attack, invade, and live on the skin or in the organs of the body. Compare **infect.**

infestation, the presence of animal parasites in the environment, on the skin, or in the hair.

infiltration, the process whereby a fluid passes into the tissues, as when an intravenous fluid catheter comes out of the vein.

inflammation, the response of the tissues of the body to irritation or injury. Inflammation may be acute or chronic. Its chief signs are redness, heat, swelling, and pain, accompanied by loss of function. The severity, timing, and local character of any particular inflammation depend on the cause, the area affected, and the condition of the person.

inflammatory bowel disease. See **ulcerative colitis.**

inflammatory fracture, a fracture of bone tissue weakened by inflammation.

inflatable pessary. See **pessary.**

influenza, a highly contagious infection, usually of the lungs, caused by a virus and transmitted by airborne particles. It occurs in isolated cases and epidemics. Symptoms include sore throat, cough, fever, muscular pains, and weakness. The incubation period is brief (from 1 to 3 days), and the onset is usually sudden, with chills, fever, and general discomfort. Treatment is of symptoms and usually involves bed rest, aspirin, and drinking of fluids. Fever and nonlocal symptoms distinguish influenza from the common cold. Complete recovery in from 3 to 10 days is the rule. However, bacterial pneumonia may occur among high-risk patients, as the elderly, the very young, and people who have chronic diseases of the lungs. Yearly vaccination with the currently prevalent strain of influenza virus is recommended for elderly or debilitated persons. Also called **grippe, la grippe,** *(informal)* **flu.**

influenza-virus vaccine, an active immunizing agent, prescribed for immunization against influenza. Acute infection or allergy to eggs prohibits its use.

informal admission, a type of admission to a psychiatric hospital in which there is no formal or written application and the patient is free to leave at any time. See also **involuntary patient.**

informed consent, permission obtained from a patient to perform a specific test or procedure. Informed consent is required before performing surgery and before admitting a patient to a research study. The document used must be written in a language understood by the patient. It must be dated and signed by the patient and at least one witness. Included in the document are clear, rational statements that describe the procedure or test. They must also

clarify the risk to the patient, the expected benefits to the patient, the expected consequences of not allowing the test or procedure, and the other procedures or diagnostic aids that are available. Also required is a statement that care will not be withheld if the patient does not consent. Informed consent is voluntary. By law, informed consent must be obtained more than some specified number of days or hours before certain procedures, including therapeutic abortion and sterilization. It must always be obtained when the patient is fully competent.

infraction fracture, a bone fracture marked by a small line that shows up in X-ray examination. It is most commonly associated with a disorder of metabolism. See also **greenstick fracture.**

infranodal block /in′frənōdəl/, a type of block in the heart. An impairment of the stimulatory mechanism of the heart causes blockage of the impulse in certain bundles of fibers. The condition is most often seen in older patients. Symptoms include frequent episodes of fainting and a pulse rate of between 20 and 50 beats per minute. The usual therapy is the implantation of a pacemaker. Compare **bundle branch block, intraventricular block.** See also **Adams-Stokes syndrome, atrioventricular block, cardiac conduction defect, heart block, intraatrial block, sinoatrial block.**

infrapatellar fat pad, an area of soft tissue in front of the knee just below the knee cap.

infraradian rhythm, a rhythm in the body that repeats in patterns greater than 24-hour periods.

infrared therapy, treatment by exposure to various wavelengths of infrared radiation (radiant heat).

infusate, a fluid given through the veins over a period of time.

infusion, **1.** the introduction of a substance, as a fluid, nutrient, or drug, directly into a vein by means of gravity flow. Compare **injection, instillation, insufflation. 2.** the substance introduced into the body by infusion. **3.** the steeping of a substance, as an herb, in order to extract its medicinal properties. **4.** the extract obtained by the steeping process. **–infuse,** *v.*

infusion pump, an apparatus that delivers measured amounts of a drug through injection over a period of time. Some kinds of infusion pumps can be implanted surgically.

ingrown hair, a hair that fails to follow the normal channel to the surface. The free end becomes embedded in the skin. The hair then acts like a foreign body. Inflammation and pus formation follow.

ingrown toenail, a toenail whose top edge grows or is pressed into the skin of the toe, causing an inflammation. Infection is common. Treatment includes wider shoes, proper trimming of the nail, and surgery to narrow the nail.

inguinal /ing'gwinəl/, of or pertaining to the groin.

inguinal canal, the tubular passage through the lower layers of the belly wall. It is a common site for hernias.

inguinal falx, The tendons of some muscles going to the pubic bone. It is inserted into the crest of the pubis, and strengthens that part of the front wall of the groin. The width and the strength of the inguinal falx vary. Also called **conjoined tendon.**

inguinal hernia, a hernia in which a loop of intestine enters the inguinal canal, sometimes filling, in a male, the entire scrotal sac. An inguinal hernia is usually repaired surgically, to prevent its blocking passage of waste through the bowel. Of all hernias, 75% to 80% are inguinal hernias. See also **hernia.**

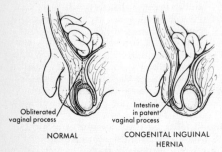

Obliterated vaginal process

Intestine in patent vaginal process

NORMAL   CONGENITAL INGUINAL
                                   HERNIA

Inguinal hernia

inguinal node, a lymph node in the upper thigh. Compare **anterior tibial node, popliteal node.**

inguinal region, the part of the groin surrounding the inguinal canal, in the lower zone on both sides of the pubic organ. Also called **iliac region.** See also **abdominal regions.**

inguinal ring, either of the two openings of the inguinal canal.

INH. See **isoniazid.**

inhalant, a substance that is breathed into the body. It may be medication, as an aerosol, given in respiratory therapy, or a chemical, as in glue sniffing.

inhalation administration of medication, giving a drug by inhalation of the vapor released from a small, fragile glass container packed in a fine mesh that is crushed for immediate use. Amyl nitrate and ammonia act quickly and are often used in this way. The medication is absorbed into the blood through the mucous membrane of the nasal passages. Vaporized medication is also given by inhalation. See also **inhalation therapy.**

inhalation analgesia, the occasional giving of anesthetic gas during the second stage of labor to reduce pain. Consciousness is retained to allow the woman to follow instructions and to avoid the unwelcome effects of general anesthesia.

inhalation anesthesia, giving of an anesthetic gas or a volatile anesthetic liquid via a carrier gas. General anesthesia by gas inhalation has been used to permit surgical operations for more than a century. But the mechanism by which these anesthetics dull the pain centers of the brain is not yet understood. Giving an inhalation anesthetic is usually preceded by a short-acting sedative or hypnotic drug, often a barbiturate directly into the veins or muscles.

inhalation therapy, a treatment in which a substance is introduced into the lungs by breathing. Oxygen, water, and various drugs may be given using techniques of inhalation therapy. The goals of treatment are varied. They include improved strength of breathing in a bedridden patient, reducing bronchial swelling in an asthmatic, or loosening of mucus in a person with chronic lung disease.

inhale, to breathe in or to draw in with the breath. **–inhalation,** *n.*

inherent, inborn, innate; natural to an environment. Compare **indigenous.**

inherent rate, the rate of impulse formation caused by a given pacemaker location in the heart.

inheritance, **1.** the acquiring by an offspring of genetic material from its parents. Traits or conditions are transmitted in this way from one generation to the next. **2.** the sum total of the genetic qualities or traits transmitted from parents to offspring; the total genetic makeup of the fertilized ovum. Kinds of inheritance include **alternative inheritance, amphigenous inheritance, autosomal inheritance, blending inheritance, codominant inheritance, complemental inheritance, crisscross inheritance, cytoplasmic inheritance, holandric inheritance, hologynic inheritance, homochronous inheritance, maternal inheritance, mendelism, monofactorial inheritance, multifactorial inheritance, supplemental inheritance,** and **x-linked inheritance. –inherited,** *adj.* **inherit,** *v.*

inherited disorder, any disease or condition that is genetically determined. Also called **genetic disorder, hereditary disorder.**

inhibin, a hormone that inhibits the activity of another hormone (follicle stimulating hormone).

inhibiting hormone. See **hormone.**

inhibition, **1.** the act or state of inhibiting or of being inhibited, restrained, prevented, or held back. **2.** (in psychology) the unconscious restraint of a certain behavior, usually resulting from the social or cultural forces; the condition inducing this restraint. **3.** (in psychoanalysis) the process in which the superego prevents the conscious expression of an unconscious instinctual drive, thought, or urge. **4.** (in physiology) restraining, checking, or arresting the action of an organ or cell. Also the reducing of a physiological activity by a negative stimulation. **5.** (in chemistry) the stopping or slowing down of the rate of a chemical reaction.

inhibitor, a drug or other chemical that prevents or lessens a certain action.

inhibitory, tending to stop or slow a process, as a neuron that lowers the intensity of a nerve impulse. Compare **induce.**

inion /in′ē·on/, the most prominent point of the back of the head, where the occipital bone protrudes the farthest.

initial contact stance stage, one of the five stages in the stance phase of walking or gait. It is the moment when the foot touches the ground or floor, and the leg prepares to accept the weight of the body. The initial contact stance stage figures in the diagnoses of many abnormal orthopedic conditions. It is often correlated with studies of the muscles used in walking. Compare **loading response stance stage, midstance, preswing stance stage, terminal stance.** See also **swing phase of gait.**

initiator, a substance that causes a change in a normal cell and can cause it to grow uncontrollably. Examples include radiation, aflatoxins, urethane, and nitrosamines.

injection, 1. the act of forcing a liquid into the body with a syringe. Injections are named according to where they are given; the most common are into the arteries (intraarterial), into the skin (intradermal), into the muscles (intramuscular), into the veins (intravenous), and under the skin (subcutaneous). Compare **infusion, instillation, insufflate. 2.** the substance injected. **3.** redness and swelling observed in the physical examination of a part of the body, caused by enlargement of the blood vessels from inflammation or infection. –**inject,** *v.*

injection cap, a piece of rubber stretched over a plastic cap. Needles can be inserted through the rubber into a catheter or glass tube.

injection technique. See **intradermal injection, intramuscular injection, intrathecal injection, intravenous injection, subcutaneous injection,** and see other specific injection techniques.

injury: potential for, a nursing diagnosis of a greater-than-normal likelihood of injury. The cause of the condition may be internal or external. The internal factors may be biological, chemical, physiological, psychological, or developmental. The external factors may be biological, chemical, physiological, psychological, or interpersonal. The defining characteristics of a somatic potential for injury include abnormal sensory function, malnutrition, abnormal condition of the blood, broken skin, developmental abnormality, or psychological problems. The defining characteristics of an environmental potential for injury include lack of immunization; presence of germs, chemical

pollutants, poisons, alcohol, nicotine, or food additives; modes of transportation; physical aspects of the community, buildings, equipment, or facilities; nonavailability of assistance; and various psychological factors. See also **nursing diagnosis.**

inlay splint, a casting for fixing or supporting one or more adjacent teeth. It is composed of two or more inlays soldered together or a single casting.

inlet, a passage leading into a cavity, as a pelvic inlet that marks the brim of the pelvic cavity.

inlet contraction. See **contraction.**

in loco parentis /inlō′kō pəren′tis/, a Latin phrase meaning "in the place of the parent": the taking on by a person or institution of the parental obligations of caring for a child without adoption.

innate, 1. existing in or belonging to a person from birth; inborn; heriditary; congenital. **2.** referring to a natural and essential trait of something or someone; inherent. **3.** originating in or produced by the intellect or the mind.

innate immunity. See **natural immunity.**

inner cell mass, a cluster of cells localized around a central part of a fertilized ovum. The embryo develops from it. See also **trophoblast.**

inner ear. See **internal ear.**

innervation, the distribution or supply of nerve fibers or nerve impulses to a part of the body.

innervation apraxia. See **motor apraxia.**

innidation. See **nidation.**

innocent, benign, or healthy; not malignant, as an innocent heart murmur.

innominate artery, one of the three arteries that branch from the arch of the aorta. It divides into the right common carotid and the right subclavian arteries. Also called **brachicephalic artery, brachiocephalic trunk.**

innominate bone, the hipbone. It consists of the ilium, ischium, and pubis. It joins with the sacrum and coccyx to form the pelvis. Also called **os coxae.**

innominate vein, a large vein on either side of the neck. It is formed by the union of the internal jugular and subclavian veins. The two veins drain blood from the head, neck, and upper extremities and unite to form the superior vena cava. Also called **brachiocephalic vein.**

Inocor, a brand name for a drug that strengthens the heart beat (amrinone lactate).

inoculate, to introduce a substance into the body to produce or increase immunity to a disease or condition. It is introduced by making multiple scratches in the skin after placing a drop of the substance on the skin, by puncture of the skin with an implement bearing multiple short tines, or by injection.

inoculum /inok′yooləm/, *pl.* **inocula,** a substance introduced into the body to cause or to increase immunity to a given disease or condition. Also called **inoculant.** See also **immune system.**

inorganic dust, dry, finely powdered particles of an inorganic substance, especially dust. When inhaled it can cause abnormal conditions of the lungs. See also **anthracosis, asbestosis, berylliosis, pneumoconiosis, silicosis.**

inorganic phosphorus, phosphorus that may be measured in the blood as phosphate ions. Its increased concentration may indicate bone, kidney, or glandular diseases; decreased concentration may be associated with alcoholism, vitamin deficiency, and other problems. Normal concentrations in the blood of adults are 1.8 to 2.6 mEq/L. See also **phosphorus.**

inosine /in'əsēn, -sīn/, a substance derived from animal tissue, especially intestines, originally used in food processing and flavoring. It has also been used in the treatment of heart disorders and is now under investigation in studies of cancer and virus chemotherapy. See also **inosiplex.**

inosiplex, a form of inosine that acts as a stimulator of the immune system. It is currently under investigation for use in cancer therapy and in the treatment of virus infections. Also called **methisoprinol.**

inotropic, pertaining to the force of muscle contractions, particularly contractions of the heart muscle. An inotropic agent increases the ability of the heart tissue to contract easily.

inpatient, 1. a patient who has been admitted to a hospital or other health-care facility for at least an overnight stay. 2. of or pertaining to the treatment or care of such a patient. Also of or pertaining to a health-care facility to which a patient may be admitted for 24-hour care. Compare **outpatient.**

input, the information or material that enters a system.

insanity, *informal.* a severe mental disorder or defect. It is used more in legal and social than in medical terminology. It refers to those mental illnesses that are so serious as to interfere with one's ability to function within the legal limits of society and to look after one's personal affairs. When a person is classified as insane, various legal actions can ensue, as commitment to an institution, appointment of a guardian, or dissolution of a contract. See also **psychosis.**

insect bite, the bite of an arthropod, not necessarily just of an insect properly speaking. Louse, flea, mite, tick, and spider bites all qualify. Many arthropods inject venom that produces poisoning or severe local reaction. Others inject saliva that may contain viruses, or substances that produce mild irritation. The degree of irritation of an insect's bite is affected by the design and shape of its mouthparts. A horsefly, for example, makes a short lateral and coarse wound, while a tick takes

hold with its backward curved teeth, making its removal difficult. Spiders inflict a sharp pinprick bite that may remain unnoticed until the injected venom has begun to produce a painful reaction. Treatment of a bite depends on the species of insect, the reaction to the bite, and the risk of further trouble developing from it. First-aid treatment is generally symptomatic and includes ice or cold packs, careful cleaning of the wound, and antihistamines or specific antivenin as necessary.

insecticide poisoning. See **chlorinated organic insecticide poisoning.**

insemination, the injection of semen into the uterus, either artificially or through sexual intercourse.

insensible perspiration, the loss of fluid from the body by evaporation, as normally occurs during breathing. A small amount of perspiration is continually released by the sweat glands in the skin. The portion that evaporates before it may be observed also contributes to insensible perspiration. Also called **insensible water loss.**

insertion, (in anatomy) the place of attachment, as of a muscle to the bone it moves.

insertion forceps. See **point forceps.**

insertion site, the point in a vein where a needle or catheter is inserted.

insidious /insid'ē-əs/, describing a change that is gradual, subtle, or imperceptible. Certain chronic diseases, as glaucoma, can develop insidiously. Their symptoms are not detected by the patient until the disorder is established. Compare **acute.**

insight, 1. the capacity of grasping the true nature of a situation or a deep truth. 2. an instance of penetrating or comprehending a deep truth, primarily through intuitive understanding. 3. (in psychology) a type of self-understanding covering rational and emotional awareness of the unconscious nature, origin, and mechanisms of one's attitudes, feelings, and behavior. Insight is one of the most important goals of psychotherapy. Along with integration, it leads to change in faulty behavior. See also **integration.**

in situ /in si'too, sit'oo/, 1. in the natural or usual place. 2. describing a cancer that has not spread or invaded neighboring tissues, as carcinoma in situ.

insomnia, chronic inability to sleep or to remain asleep through the night; wakefulness; sleeplessness. The condition is caused by a variety of physical and psychological factors. These include emotional stress, physical pain and discomfort, disturbances in brain function, drug abuse and drug dependence, neuroses, psychoses, and psychological problems that produce anxiety, irrational fears, and tensions. Treatment may include giving sedatives, tranquilizers or hypnotics, psychotherapy, and exercise.

insomniac, 1. a person with insomnia. 2. referring to insomnia. 3. typical of or occurring during a period of sleeplessness.

inspiration, the act of drawing air into the lungs in order to exchange oxygen for carbon dioxide; breathing in. The major muscle of inspiration is the diaphragm, the contraction of which creates a low pressure in the chest, causing the lungs to expand and air to flow inward. Since expiration is usually a passive process, these muscles of inspiration alone perform normal breathing. Lungs at maximal inspiration have an average total capacity of 5,500 to 6,000 ml of air. Compare **expiration.** See also **inspiratory reserve volume.**

inspiratory, of or pertaining to inspiration.

inspiratory capacity (IC), the maximum volume of air that can be inhaled into the lungs from the normal resting position after exhaling. It is measured with a spirometer.

inspiratory reserve volume, the maximum volume of air that can be further inspired from the normal resting position after inhaling.

instillation, 1. a procedure in which a fluid is slowly introduced into a cavity of the body and allowed to remain for a specific length of time before being withdrawn. It is done to expose the tissues of the area to the solution, to warmth or cold, or to a drug or substance in the solution. 2. a solution so introduced. Compare **infusion, injection, insufflate. –instill,** v.

instinct, an inborn response to a need, as life instincts of hunger, thirst, and sex or the destructive and aggressive death instincts.

instinctive reflex. See **unconditioned response.**

institutionalism syndrome, a condition marked by withdrawal, submissiveness, and lack of energy and initiative. The person may resist leaving a hospital, even when the surroundings are barely adequate, because the setting is familiar and predictable, with few demands.

instrument, a surgical tool or device designed to perform a specific function, as cutting, dissecting, grasping, holding, retracting, or suturing. Surgical instruments are usually made of steel. They are specially treated to be durable, heat-resistant, rust-resistant, and stain-proof. Proper care of surgical instruments is essential. It includes correct use, careful handling, inspection for defects, adequate and appropriate sterilization, and proper labeling, dating, and storage. Some kinds of instruments are **clamp, needle holder, retractor,** and **speculum.**

instrumental conditioning. See **operant conditioning.**

instrumentation, the use of instruments for treatment and diagnosis.

insufficiency, inability of an organ or other body part to perform a necessary function adequately. Some kinds of insufficiency are **adre-** **nal insufficiency, aortic insuffiency, ileocecal insufficiency, pulmonary insufficiency,** and **valvular insufficiency.**

insufflate /insuf'lāt/, to blow a gas or powder into a tube, cavity, or organ. It is done to allow visual examination, to remove an obstruction, or to apply medication. See also. **Rubin's test. –insufflation,** n.

insulation, a substance that offers a barrier to the passage of heat or electricity.

insulin, 1. a naturally occurring hormone released by the pancreas in response to increased levels of sugar in the blood. The hormone acts to regulate the metabolism of sugar and some of the processes necessary for the metabolism of fats, carbohydrates, and proteins. Insulin lowers blood sugar levels and promotes transport and entry of sugar into the muscle cells and other tissues. Inadequate secretion of insulin results in hyperglycemia, and in the characteristic signs of diabetes mellitus, including lethargy and weight loss. Uncorrected severe deficiency of insulin is incompatible with life. 2. a pharmacological preparation of the hormone given in treating diabetes mellitus. The preparations of insulin available for prescription vary in promptness, intensity, and duration of action. They are termed rapid-acting, intermediate-acting, and long-acting. Most forms of insulin drugs are given by subcutaneous injection in individualized dosage schedules. Many drugs interact with insulin, among them the monoamine oxidase inhibitors, corticosteroids, salicylates, thiazide diuretics, and phenytoin. Fever, stress, infection, pregnancy, surgery, and hyperthyroidism may significantly increase insulin requirements. Liver disease, hypothyroidism, vomiting, and renal disease may decrease them. See also **human insulin.**

insulin-dependent diabetes mellitus (IDDM), an inability of the body to process carbohydrate caused by an overt insulin deficiency. It occurs in children and is marked by loss of weight, diminished strength, and marked irritability. The onset is usually rapid, but about one-third of the patients have a remission within 3 months. This stage may continue for days or years, but diabetes then progresses quickly to a state of total dependence on insulin. Occasionally, the disease is without symptoms and is discovered only by tests for postprandial hyperglycemia or glucose tolerance. Insulin-dependent diabetes mellitus tends to be unstable and hard to control. The patients are quite sensitive to insulin and physical activity and liable to develop ketoacidosis. Recent evidence suggests that insulin-dependent diabetes mellitus may be caused by environmental factors, as a virus. Previously called brittle diabetes, juvenile diabetes, juvenile-onset diabetes, JOD, juvenile-onset-type diabetes, ketosis-prone diabetes. Compare **non-insulin-dependent diabetes mellitus.** See also **diabetes mellitus.**

insulin injection, the use of a hypodermic needle to give insulin, either under the skin (subcutaneous) or into a vein (intravenous).

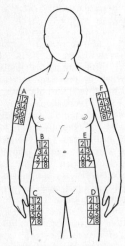

Insulin injection sites

insulin kinase, an enzyme, assumed to be present in the liver, that activates insulin.

insulinogenic, promoting the production and release of insulin by the pancreas.

insulinoma /in′soōolinō′mə/, pl. **insulinomas, insulinomata,** a benign tumor of the insulin-secreting cells of the pancreas. Surgical removal of the tumor may be possible, thus limiting the development of hypoglycemia. Also called **insuloma, islet cell adenoma.** Compare **islet cell tumor.**

insulin reaction, the ill effects caused by too high levels of circulating insulin. See **hyperinsulinism.**

insulin resistance, a complication of diabetes marked by a need for a high dose of insulin, more than 200 units per day, to control the high blood sugar and blood ketone levels. The cause is certain antibodies that reduce the effect of insulin. Insulin resistance also may occur with such diseases as acanthosis nigrans, Werner's syndrome, ataxia telangiectasia, Älstrom syndrome, pineal hyperplasia syndrome, and various lipodystrophic disorders.

insulin shock, hypoglycemic shock caused by an overdose of insulin, a decreased intake of food, or too much exercise. It is characterized by sweating, trembling, chilliness, nervousness, irritability, hunger, hallucination, numbness, and pallor. Uncorrected, it will progress to convulsions, coma, and death. Treatment requires an immediate dose of glucose (sugar). Compare **ketoacidosis.**

insulin shock treatment, the injection of large, convulsion-producing doses of insulin. It is given as a therapeutic measure in psychoses, especially schizophrenia.. Electric shock therapy is currently given more commonly than insulin shock. It is used chiefly for manic-depressive psychosis. Also called **hypoglycemic shock treatment.**

insulin tolerance test, a test of the body's ability to use insulin. Insulin is given and blood glucose is measured at regular intervals. Thirty minutes after the insulin is given, blood glucose is usually lower but not less than half of the fasting glucose level. Glucose levels usually return to normal after about 90 minutes. In people with hypoglycemia, the glucose levels may drop lower and be slower to return to normal.

insuloma. See **insulinoma.**

Intal, a trademark for an antiasthmatic (cromolyn sodium).

intangible elements, psychological factors, as reasoning ability, knowledge, emotions, and attitudes.

integral dose, (in radiotherapy) the total amount of energy absorbed by a patient or object during exposure to radiation. Also called **volume dose.**

integrating dose meter, (in radiotherapy) a meter, usually designed to be placed on the patient's skin, with a system for determining the total radiation given during an exposure. A device may be included to stop the exposure when the desired value is reached.

integration, 1. the act or process of unifying or bringing together. 2. (in psychology) the organization of all elements of the personality into a coordinated, functional, adapted whole; one of the primary goals in psychotherapy. It involves assimilating insight and coordinating new and old experiences and emotional reactions so an effective change can occur in behavior, thinking, or feeling. See also **insight.** –**integrate,** v.

integration of self, one of the factors in high-level health. It is necessary for maturity and is marked by the integration of mind, body, and spirit into one smoothly working unit.

integument /integ′yoōmənt/, a covering or skin. –**integumentary,** adj.

integumentary system, the skin and its extensions, hair, nails, and sweat and sebaceous glands. See also the **Color Atlas of Human Anatomy, integument.**

integumentary system assessment, an evaluation of the general condition of a patient's skin and of factors that may contribute to the presence of a skin disorder.

intellect, 1. the power and ability of the mind to know and understand. Intellect is contrasted with feeling or with willing. 2. a person having a great capacity for thought and knowledge. –**intellectual,** *adj., n.*

intellectualization, (in psychiatry) a defense mechanism in which reasoning is used to block a confronting and unconscious conflict and the emotional stress linked to it.

intelligence, 1. the ability to acquire, retain, and apply experience, understanding, knowledge, reasoning, and judgment in coping with new experiences. 2. the use of such ability. See also **intelligence quotient.** –**intelligent,** *adj.*

intelligence quotient (IQ), a numeric expression of one's intellectual level as measured against the average of one's own group. On several of the usual scales it is found by dividing mental age, derived through psychological testing, by the chronological age and multiplying the result by 100. Average IQ is considered to be 100. See also **mental retardation.**

intelligence test, any test standardized to determine a person's mental age by measuring capacity to absorb information and to solve problems. These tests are used by the medical profession to diagnose mental retardation and determine degrees of it. They also aid in the planning of therapeutic programs for such persons. Two kinds of intelligence tests are **Stanford-Binet** and **Wechsler-Bellevue scale.** Compare **achievement test, aptitude test, personality test, psychologic test.**

intensive care, constant, complex, health care as given for various acute life-threatening conditions, as multiple trauma, severe burns, or heart attack; also after certain kinds of surgery. Care is most often given in an intensive care unit. Such units are usually equipped with various advanced machines and devices for treating and monitoring the patient. Also called **critical care.**

intensive care unit (ICU), a hospital unit in which parents needing close monitoring and intensive care are housed for as long as needed. An ICU contains highly technical monitoring devices and equipment. The staff in the unit is trained to give critical care as needed by the patients. See also **coronary care unit, neonatal care unit.**

intention, a kind of healing process. Healing by **first intention** is the union of the edges of a wound to complete healing without scar formation or granulation. Healing by **second intention** is wound closure in which the edges are separated, granulation develops to fill the gap, and, finally, tissue quickly grows in over the granulations, producing a thin scar. Healing by **third intention** is wound closure in which granulation fills the gap with tissue growing over the granulation at a slower rate and producing a larger scar.

interactional model, a type of family therapy that views the family as a communication system of interlocking subsets of family members. Family problems occur when the rules of interaction become vague. The goal of the therapy is to help the family set clear rules for family relationships.

interaction coaching, an attempt to change disturbed mother-infant interactions. The goal is to improve the "fit" between mother and child.

interactionist theory, a theory about aging that views age-related changes as resulting from the interaction of individual characteristics of the person, the society, and the history of that person's interactions with the society.

interarticular fibrocartilage, one of four kinds of fibrocartilage, consisting of flattened plates between the articular cartilage of the most active joints, at the wrist, and knee joints. The plates absorb shocks and increase mobility. Compare **circumferential fibrocartilage, connecting fibrocartilage, stratiform fibrocartilage.**

intercapillary glomerulosclerosis, an abnormal condition marked by degeneration of certain capillaries in the kidney (the renal glomeruli). It is associated with diabetes. It often produces hypertension. Also called **Kimmelstiel-Wilson disease.**

intercellular, between or among cells.

interchange. See **reciprocal translocation.**

interconceptional gynecologic care, health care of a woman during her reproductive years, except during pregnancies, and within 6 weeks after delivery. Testing for cervical cancer, breast and pelvic examinations, and evaluation of general health, are routine aspects of interconceptual care. Testing and treatment for pelvic, vaginal, or genital infections may be required. A contraceptive method may also be discussed, taught, prescribed, or provided. The basic examination is usually performed annually. The method of contraception may be adjusted or changed. Infections or other complaints are investigated, diagnosed, and treated as symptoms appear. Interconceptional care is increasingly given by nurse practitioners or nurse midwives. These nurses follow rules for treatment and referral drawn up in consultation with a gynecologist.

intercondylar fracture /in'tərkon'dilər/, a fracture of the tissue between the round lumps at the end of a bone (condyles).

intercostal, of or pertaining to the space between two ribs.

intercostal bulging, the visible bulging of the soft tissues of the intercostal spaces that occurs when it is harder to exhale, as in asthma, cystic fibrosis, or blocking of a breath passage by a foreign body. Compare **retraction of the chest.**

intercostal muscles, the muscles that connect the ribs to each other. They are called external and internal, and they function as breathing muscles when needed.

intercostal node, a node in one of three groups of lymph nodes near the dorsal parts of the intercostal spaces. Such nodes are associated with lymphatic vessels that drain the rear sides of the chest. Compare **diaphragmatic node, sternal node.** See also **lymphatic system, lymph node.**

intercourse, *informal.* sexual intercourse. See **coitus.**

intercurrent disease, a disease that develops in and may alter the course of another disease.

interdental canal, any of the nutrient channels that pass upward to the teeth through the lower jaw. Also called **nutrient canal.**

interdental gingiva, the soft supporting tissue that normally fills the space between two adjacent teeth.

interdental groove, a linear, vertical depression on the gum between two teeth.

interdental spillway, the space between two adjacent teeth.

interferon, a natural protein found in cells when they are exposed to a virus or other foreign materials. It stimulates production of a protein in neighboring cells that stops the growth of the virus, thus protecting them from infection.

interferon nomenclature, a system (recommended by the International Interferon Nomenclature Committee) for naming types of interferon. For a specific product, "interferon" is the first word of the name. It is followed by a Greek letter, spelled out, and a number and a lowercase letter attached by a dash. An example is interferon alpha-2a.

interfibrillar mass of Flemming, interfilar mass. See **hyaloplasm.**

interior mesenteric artery, a branch of the abdominal aorta. It arises just above the division into the common iliacs and supplies much of the colon and rectum.

interlace mode, (in radiology) a process that uses a conventional TV camera tube to enhance the quality of a projected image.

interleukin-1 (IL-1), a protein of the immune system that activates resting T cells and macrophage cells. It causes inflammation, and helps produce other substances in the immune system. It can also cause fever, sleep, release of the hormone ACTH, and some resistance to infection.

interleukin-2 (IL-2), a protein of the immune system that causes activated T cells to divide. IL-2 is used in the laboratory to grow identical duplicates of T cells (clones) with specific immune functions.

interleukin-3 (IL-3), a protein of the immune system that supports the growth of bone marrow cells and causes mast cells to grow.

interleukin-4 (IL-4) , an immune system protein that causes the growth of activated B cells, resting T cells, and mast cells. See also **B cell stimulating factor-1.**

interlobular duct, any duct connecting or draining the small lobes of a gland.

interlocked twins, identical twins so positioned in the uterus that their necks become entwined, making vaginal delivery impossible. Also called **interlocking twins.**

intermediate-acting insulin, a preparation extracted from beef pancreas or pork pancreas and then chemically modified. It has an intermediate range of action. See also **insulin.** Compare **long-acting insulin, short-acting insulin.**

intermediate care, a level of medical care for certain chronically ill or disabled individuals. Room and board are provided but skilled nursing care is not.

intermediate care facility, a health facility that provides intermediate care. Medical-related services are offered to persons with a variety of conditions requiring institutional facilities. The degree of care is less than what is provided by a hospital or skilled-nursing facility. An example is a health-care facility for mentally retarded persons.

intermediate cell mass. See **nephrotome.**

intermediate cuneiform bone, the smallest of the three cuneiform bones of the foot. It is located between the medial and the lateral cuneiform bones. It has six surfaces and is attached to various ligaments. Also called **middle cuneiform bone, second cuneiform bone.**

intermediate host, any animal in which the larval (intermediate) stages of a parasite develop. Humans are intermediate hosts for malaria parasites. Also called **secondary host.** Compare **dead-end host, definitive host, reservoir host.** See also **host,** def. 1.

intermediate mesoderm. See **nephrotome.**

intermenstrual, of or pertaining to the time between menstrual periods.

intermenstrual fever, the normal, slight rise in temperature that marks ovulation. It usually occurs about 14 days before the onset of menstruation.

intermittent, alternating between periods of activity and inactivity, as rheumatoid arthritis, which is marked by periods of symptoms and periods of remission.

intermittent assisted ventilation (IAV), (in respiratory therapy) a system in which a respirator is used but only when the breathing of the patient falls below a certain level. Also called **intermittent demand ventilation (IDV).**

intermittent claudication. See **claudication.**

intermittent fever, a fever that recurs in cycles, as in malaria. Kinds of intermittent fever include **bidoutertian malaria, double quartan malaria,** and **quartan malaria.**

intermittent mandatory ventilation (IMV), a method of breathing therapy in which the patient is allowed to breathe independently and then, at certain intervals, a ventilation machine forces him to take a breath under pressure. Compare **continuous positive pressure breathing, intermittent positive pressure breathing.** See also **respiratory therapy.**

intermittent positive pressure breathing. See **IPPB.**

intermittent positive pressure breathing unit. See **IPPB unit.**

intermittent positive pressure ventilation. See **IPPB.**

intern, a doctor in the first postgraduate year, learning medical practice under supervision before starting a residency. Also spelled **interne.**

internal, within or outside. –**internally,** *adv.*

internal cuneiform bone. See **medial cuneiform bone.**

internal ear, the complex inner structure of the ear, communicating directly with the acoustic nerve. It passes sound vibrations from the middle ear through the fluid-filled network of canals joining at a vestibule connected to the cochlea. Also called **inner ear, labyrinth.** Compare **external ear, middle ear.**

internal fertilization, the union of gametes within the body of the female after insemination. See also **artificial insemination.**

internal fistula, an abnormal passage between two internal organs or structures.

internal fixation, any method of holding together pieces of fractured bone without using appliances outside the skin. After open reduction of the fracture, smooth or threaded pins, Kirschner wires, screws, plates attached by screws, or medullary nails may be used to stabilize the fragments. Sometimes the device is removed at a later operation, or it may just remain. Compare **external pin fixation.**

internalization, the process of adopting, either unconsciously or consciously through learning and socialization, the attitudes, beliefs, values, and standards of someone else or, more generally, of the society or group to which one belongs. See also **socialization.**

internal jugular vein, one of a pair of veins in the neck. Each vein collects blood from one side of the brain, the face, and the neck. At the base of the skull, in some people, the vein forms a jugular bulb. Compare **external jugular vein.**

internal mammary artery bypass, surgery to clear a coronary artery blockage.

internal medicine, the branch of medicine concerned with study of the physiology and pathology of internal organs and with medical diagnosis and treatment of disorders of organs.

internal oblique muscle. See **obliquus internus abdominis.**

internal podalic version and total breech extraction. See **version and extraction.**

internal pterygoid muscle. See **pterygoideus medialis.**

internal respiratory nerve of Bell. See **phrenic nerve.**

International Commission on Radiation Protection (ICRP), a nongovernmental organization founded in England in 1928 to provide general guidance on the safe use of radiation sources, including measures and codes to practice medical radiology. It was originally set up as a source of information about the hazards of x-rays in medicine but was changed in 1950 to include effects of nuclear energy.

International Red Cross Society, an international charity organization, based in Geneva, Switzerland. It provides humane treatment to victims of war and disaster. It assures neutral hospitals and medical personnel during war. See **American Red Cross.**

International System of Units, the standardization of measurement of substances, including some antibiotics, vitamins, enzymes, and hormones. An International Unit (I.U.) of substance is the amount that produces a specific biological result. Each I.U. of a substance has the same strength and action as another unit of the same substance. See also **centimetergram-second system, CIPM.**

International Unit (IU, I.U.), a unit of measure in the International System of Units. See also **SI units.**

internist, a doctor specializing in internal medicine.

interocclusal record, a record of the positional relation of opposing teeth or jaws to each other, made on surfaces of occlusal rims or teeth with a plastic that hardens, as plaster of Paris, wax, or zinc.

interoceptive /in'tərōsep'tiv/, referring to stimuli from within the body regarding the function of internal organs or to receptors they activate. Compare **exteroceptive, proprioception.**

interoceptor, any sensory nerve ending in cells in the viscera that responds to stimuli from within the body regarding the function of the internal organs, as digestion, excretion, and blood pressure. Compare **exteroceptor, proprioceptor.**

interparietal fissure. See **intraparietal sulcus.**

interperiosteal fracture /in'tərper'ē·os'tē·əl/, a fracture in which the periosteum is not disrupted.

interpersonal psychiatry, a theory of psychiatry, introduced by Sullivan, that stresses relationships with others as the most important factor in personality development.

interpersonal therapy, psychotherapy that views faulty communications, interactions, and inter-relationships as basic factors in maladaptive behavior. One kind of interpersonal therapy is **transactional analysis.**

interphase, the stage in the cell cycle when the cell is not dividing, the chromosomes are not individually distinguishable, and such activities as DNA synthesis occur. See also **anaphase, interkinesis, metaphase, mitosis, prophase, telophase.**

interproximal film. See **bite-wing film.**

intersex, any person with body features of both sexes or whose external genitals are ambiguous or different from the normal male or female. See also **hermaphrodite, intersexuality, pseudohermaphrodite.**

intersexuality, the state in which a person has male and female body features to varying degrees or in which the appearance of the external genitals is ambiguous or differs from the gonadal or genetic sex. See also **hermaphroditism, pseudohermaphroditism.** –**intersexual,** *adj.*

★DIAGNOSIS: Conditions marked by ambiguous or inappropriate genitals are seen at birth, but other may not be seen until later as resulting from delayed development or infertility. There are conditions producing ambiguous genitals in newborns requiring prompt care: the masculinized female, of which the common type is congenital adrenal hyperplasia, caused by an inherited deficiency in certain enzymes; the incompletely masculinized male, produced as an inherited X-linked recessive or autosomal dominant trait and caused by a deficiency in certain enzymes or the unresponsiveness of genital structures to testosterone; the true hermaphrodite, which is rare; and mixed gonadal dysgenesis. In cases of sexual ambiguity at birth, several tests are done to assign gender. These include a buccal smear, gonadal biopsy, chromosomal analysis, endoscopic and x-ray studies to show the presence, absence, or nature of internal genitals, and biochemical tests.

★METHOD: Sex determination should be made as soon as possible after birth to minimize medical, social, and psychological problems. The main criterion for gender choice is the infant's anatomy rather than genetic sex, although diagnostic tests are done to help in gender selection. Usually, female pseudohermaphrodites are reared as females with early genital reconstruction and hormone treatment throughout life. Male intersex conditions caused by developmental abnormalities are often treated surgically to establish male genital appearance and function. In cases of ambiguous genitals, it is suggested the infant be reared as female because the outcome of surgical and medical treatment is likely to be better.

★PATIENT CONSIDERATIONS: Gender determination of an infant whose sex is doubtful is more a psychological and social problem than a medical emergency. Such cases are always highly emotional for parents, who feel guilt and shame, and much support and encouragement are needed. Of special importance is educating the family about the abnormality, mostly what can be done now and in the long term. The parents should set realistic goals for the child, depending on the severity of the condition and treatment possible.

interstitial /in'tərstish'əl/, referring to the space between tissues.

interstitial cystitis, a bladder inflammation, thought to be associated with an autoimmune or allergic response. The bladder wall becomes inflamed, ulcerated, and scarred, causing frequent, painful urination. Treatment may include distention of the bladder and cauterization of the ulcers or weekly lavage of the bladder until the inflammation clears. Both are done under anesthesia. Corticosteroids are often given to control inflammation. The problem is mostly in women of middle age and may look like the early stages of bladder cancer. Cystoscopy and biopsy are needed for diagnosis. Also called **Hunner's ulcer.**

interstitial emphysema, a form of emphysema in which air or gas escapes into the interstitial tissues of the lung after a penetrating injury or a rupture in an alveolar wall. As the alveoli must be decompressed, there is danger that the pleura will be torn, resulting in a pneumothorax. The state is diagnosed by chest x-ray films. See also **emphysema, pneumothorax.**

interstitial growth, an increased in size by hyperplasia or hypertrophy inside a part or structure already formed. Compare **appositional growth.**

interstitial hypertrophic neuropathy. See **Dejerine-Sottas disease.**

interstitial infusion. See **hypodermoclysis.**

interstitial keratitis, an uncommon inflammation in the layers of the cornea. The first symptom is a diffuse haziness. Blood vessels may grow into the area and cause permanent opacities. Its causes are syphilis, tuberculosis, leprosy, and vascular allergy.

interstitial lung disease, a breathing disorder marked by a dry cough and shortness of breath during exercise. The patient may have swallowing disorders or joint and muscle pain and may have been exposed on the job to dusts, as asbestos or silica. X-rays usually show fiberlike deposits, usually in the lower parts of the lungs. The scarring of lung tissue is often the result of the immune system's response to an inhaled substance. Interstitial lung disease may also come from viral, bacterial, or other types of infections, cancers, inherited disorders or those present from birth, and circulation problems. The condition may progress to breathing failure and heart failure or it may go away without treatment.

interstitial myositis. See **myositis.**

interstitial nephritis, inflammation of the interstitial tissue of the kidney. It may be acute or chronic. **Acute interstitial nephritis** is an allergic reaction to some drugs, often sulfonamide or methicillin. Acute renal failure, fever, and rash are common in this condition. Most people regain normal kidney function when the offending drug is stopped. **Chronic interstitial nephritis** is a syndrome of interstitial inflammation and structural changes, sometimes found with such conditions as ureteral obstruction, exposure of the kidney to toxin, or rejection of a transplant. Gradually, renal failure, nausea, vomiting, weight loss, fatigue, and anemia develop. The nurse watches carefully for signs of electrolyte imbalance, dehydration, and hypovolemia, especially if there is frequent vomiting. Fluids and electrolytes may be replaced by vein. Treatment includes correction of the underlying cause. If the cause is obstruction of the urinary tract, rapid recovery may follow removal of the obstruction; in other cases hemodialysis and kidney transplant may be needed.

interstitial plasma cell pneumonia. See **pneumocystosis.**

interstitial pneumonia, a diffuse, chronic inflammation of the lungs. The symptoms of this state are progressive dyspnea, clubbing of the fingers, cyanosis, and fever. The disease may be caused by allergy to certain drugs. Interstitial pneumonia may also be an autoimmune reaction, since it often accompanies celiac disease, rheumatoid arthritis, Sjögren's syndrome, and systemic sclerosis. X-ray films of the lungs show patchy shadows and mottling, as in bronchopneumonia. Later stages of the disease reveal bronchiectasis, dilatation of the bronchi, and shrinkage of the lungs. Treatment includes bed rest, oxygen therapy, and corticosteroids. Most patients die in 6 months to a few years, usually from cardiac or respiratory failure. Also called **diffuse fibrosing alveolitis, giant cell interstitial pneumonia, Hamman-Rich syndrome.** Compare **bronchopneumonia.**

interstitial pregnancy. See **ectopic pregnancy.**

interstitial therapy, radiotherapy in which needles or wires that contain radioactive material are put in tumor areas.

interstitial tubal pregnancy, a kind of tubal pregnancy in which implantation occurs in the interstitial portion of a fallopian tube. See also **tubal pregnancy.**

intertrigo /in'tərtrī'gō/, an irritation of opposing skin surfaces caused by friction. Common sites are the axillae, the folds beneath large breasts, and the inner thighs. Infection may occur if the area is also warm and moist. Prevention is by weight reduction, powdering, cleansing, and antifungal topical medication when necessary. –**intertriginous,** *adj.*

intertrochanteric fracture, a fracture marked by a crack in the tissue of the proximal femur between the greater and the lesser trochanters.

intervention, any act to prevent harm to a patient or to improve the mental, emotional, or physical function of a patient. See also **nursing intervention.**

intervertebral /in'tərvur'təbrəl/, referring to the space between any two vertebrae, as the fibrocartilaginous disks.

intervertebral disk, one of the fibrous disks found between spinal vertebrae. The disks vary in size, shape, thickness, and number depending on location in the back and on which vertebrae they separate.

intervertebral fibrocartilage. See **intervertebral disk.**

interview, a communication with a patient to gather specific information. A **problem-seeking interview** focuses on gathering information to identify a patient's problems. A **problem-solving interview** focuses on problems that have been defined by the patient or a health-care professional.

intestinal amebiasis. See **amebic dysentery.**

intestinal angina, chronic vascular insufficiency of the mesentery caused by atherosclerosis and resulting ischemia of the smooth muscle of the small bowel. Stomach pain or cramping after eating, constipation, and weight loss are characteristic of the condition. Also called **chronic intestinal ischemia.**

intestinal apoplexy, the sudden blockage of one of the three main arteries to the intestines by an embolism or a thrombus. This state leads rapidly to death of intestinal tissue and is often fatal. Treatment is often surgery. The blockage is removed, and often, the affected portion of the bowel is resected. See also **atherosclerosis.**

intestinal dyspepsia, an abnormal state marked by faulty digestion found with a problem originating in the intestines. See also **dyspepsia.**

intestinal fistula, an abnormal passage from the intestine to an external abdominal opening or stoma, usually created surgically for the exit of feces after removal of a malignant or severely ulcerated segment of the bowel. See also **colostomy.**

intestinal infarction. See **intestinal strangulation.**

intestinal flu, a viral gastroenteritis, often caused by infection. It is marked by stomach cramps, diarrhea, nausea, and vomiting. Outbreaks may be sporadic or epidemic, and the disease usually is mild. Treatment is symptomatic. Diarrhea may be controlled by antidiarrheal medicine and a diet of clear fluids. See also **enteric infection, gastroenteritis.**

intestinal juices, the secretions of glands lining the intestine.

intestinal lymphangiectasia. See **hypoproteinemia.**

intestinal obstruction, any blockage that causes failure of the intestine contents to pass through the bowel. The most common cause is a mechanic blockage resulting from adhesions, impacted feces, tumor of the bowel, hernia, and inflammatory bowel disease. Small bowel blockage may cause severe pain, vomiting of fecal matter, dehydration, and eventually a drop in blood pressure. Colon blockage causes less severe pain, marked stomach swelling, and constipation. X-ray test shows the level of obstruction and its cause. Treatment includes the emptying of intestinal contents by an intestinal tube. Surgery is sometimes needed. Fluid balance and electrolyte balance are restored by intravenous infusion. Nonnarcotic analgesics are often given to avoid the decrease in intestinal motility that often accompanies the giving of narcotic analgesics. Also called *(informal)* **ileus.** See also **hernia, intussusception, volvulus.**

intestinal strangulation, stopping of blood flow to the bowel, causing swelling, cyanosis, and gangrene of the affected loop of bowel. This state is often caused by a hernia, intussusception, or volvulus. Early signs of intestinal strangulation are like those of intestinal obstruction, but peritonitis, shock, and the presence of a tender mass in the abdomen are important in making a differential diagnosis. Besides surgery, treatment includes the immediate correction of fluid and electrolyte imbalance. Also called **intestinal infarction.**

intestine, the portion of the food canal from the stomach to the anus. it includes the small and large intestines. **–intestinal,** *adj.*

intoe. See **metatarsus varus.**

intolerance, a state marked by an inability to absorb or metabolize a nutrient or medicine. Exposure to the substance may cause an adverse reaction, as in lactose intolerance. Compare **allergy, atopic.**

intoxication, 1. the state of being poisoned by a drug or other toxic substance. 2. the state of being drunk because of drinking too much alcohol. 3. a state of mental or emotional hyperexcitability, usually happiness.

intoxication amaurosis, loss of vision without an apparent ophthalmic lesion, caused by a systemic poison, as alcohol or tobacco.

intraabdomial pressure, the pressure within the belly.

intraaortic balloon pump, a device that assists in the management of refractory left ventricular failure. The balloon is attached to a catheter inserted in the aorta and is automatically inflated during diastole and deflated during systole. See also **counterpulsation.**

intraarterial, referring to a structure or action inside an artery.

intraarticular, in a joint.

intraarticular fracture, a fracture involving the articular surfaces of a joint.

intraarticular injection, the injection of medicine into a joint space, usually to reduce inflammation, as in bursitis or fibromyositis. With the same technique, fluid may be drawn from the joint space if there is too much fluid in a joint, caused by trauma or inflammation.

intraatrial, in an atrium in the heart.

intraatrial block, delayed or abnormal conduction within the atria, identified on an electrocardiogram. See also **atrioventricular block, heart block, intraventricular block, sinoatrial block.**

intracanalicular fibroma /in'trəkan'əlik'yoōlər/, a tumor with glandular epithelium and fibrous tissue, in the breast.

intracanicular papilloma /in'trəkənik'yoōlər/, a benign warty growth in certain glands, especially the breast.

intracapsular fracture /in'trəkap'soōlər/, a fracture in the capsule of a joint.

intracardiac catheter. See **cardiac catheter.**

intracardiac lead, 1. an electrocardiographic conductor in which the exploring electrode is placed in a heart chamber. 2. *informal.* a tracing made by such a lead on an electrocardiograph.

intracartilaginous ossification. See **ossification.**

intracatheter, a thin, flexible plastic catheter put in a blood vessel to give blood, fluid, or medication. Also called *(informal)* **intracath.**

intracavitary /in'trəkav'itər'ē/, referring to the space within a body cavity.

intracavitary therapy, a kind of radiotherapy in which radioactive sources are put in a body cavity to irradiate the walls of the cavity or nearby tissues.

intracellular fluid, a fluid in cell membranes in most of the body, with dissolved solutes essential to electrolyte balance and healthy metabolism. Also called **intracellular water (ICW).** Compare **extracellular fluid, interstitial fluid, lymph, plasma.**

intracerebral, in the brain tissue, inside the bony skull.

intracoronal retainer, 1. a tooth retainer. The tooth cavity and cast restoration lie largely within the tooth crown, as an inlay. 2. a direct retainer used in making removable partial dentures.

intracranial aneurysm, any aneurysm of the cerebral arteries. Rupture of an intracranial aneurysm results in mortality approaching 50%. There is high risk of recurrence in survivors. Signs are sudden severe headache, stiff neck, nausea, vomiting, and, sometimes, fainting. Some forms may be treated surgically. Kinds of intracranial aneurysms include **berry aneurysm, fusiform aneurysm,** and **mycotic aneurysm.**

intracranial electroencephalography. See **electroencephalography.**

intracranial pressure, pressure in the cranium.

intractable, having no relief, as a symptom or disease that is not helped by treatment.

intracutaneous, in the layers of the skin.

intracystic papilloma, a benign epithelial tumor formed with a cystic adenoma.

intradermal test, a procedure to identify suspected allergens by injecting the patient with extracts of the allergens. The injections are at spaced intervals, often in the forearm or in scapular region. The patient is also given the diluent alone as a control. The test is positive if, in 15 to 30 minutes, the injection of extract produces a wheal surrounded by redness and the control injection causes no symptoms. The intradermal test starts with highly dilute solutions, and, if the first test is negative, the process is repeated with stronger solutions. This gradual method is to prevent a systemic reaction, which is more of a risk with intradermal testing than with other kinds of allergy testing, as the scratch test. Intradermal testing tends to be more accurate than the scratch test and is often done if scratch test results are negative or unclear. Intradermal testing limits to from 20 to 30 the number of suspected allergens that can be tested at once on one patient. Also called **subcutaneous test.** Compare **patch test, scratch test.** See also **conjunctival test, use test.**

intradermal injection, the inserting of a hypodermic needle into the skin to leave a substance, as a serum or vaccine.

intraductal carcinoma, an often large growth found often in the breast.

intradural lipoma, a fatty tumor of the spine or sacrum, causing pain and dysfunction.

intraepidermal carcinoma, a growth of skin cells that often is at many sites at the same time. The lesions grow slowly without healing at the center. They resist chemotherapy and radiation. Also called **Bowen's disease, Bowen's precancerous dermatosis, precancerous dermatitis.**

intraepidermal vesicle, a fluid-filled blisterlike sac within the outermost layer of the skin. It is usually less than one-half inch in diameter.

intraepithelial carcinoma. See **carcinoma in situ.**

intrafusal muscle, the tissue within a skeletal muscle that monitors the tension in a muscle.

intramembranous ossification. See **ossification.**

intramuscular injection, putting a hypodermic needle in a muscle to give a medicine.

★METHOD: The site is first cleaned with alcohol or acetone. The needle is put in with a quick thrust. The solution is slowly introduced by pushing the plunger of the syringe, the needle is withdrawn quickly, and the site is massaged.

★OUTCOME: Infection may result from nonaseptic technique. Some medications can cause tissue death if put in the subcutaneous

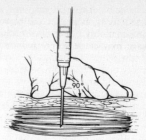

Intramuscular injection

tissues. Often, the medication may leave a knot in the muscle that is not painful and that leaves slowly over several weeks or months. The lump should not grow larger or more painful. If it does, probably an abscess has formed.

intraocular, referring to the eyball.

intraocular pressure, the internal pressure of the eye, regulated via the fine sieve of the trabecular meshwork. In older persons, the meshwork may be blocked, causing higher intraocular pressure. See also **glaucoma.**

intraoperative, referring to the period of time during surgery.

intraoperative hyperthermia, heat delivered to internal sites that have been exposed by surgery. After heating the patient is "closed."

intraoperative ultrasound, a technique that uses a portable ultrasound device to scan the spinal cord during spinal surgery. The method helps surgeons locate and see the size of tumors of the central nervous system that may not be found by other techniques.

intraoral orthodontic appliance, an orthodontic device in the mouth to correct poor tooth contact.

intrapartal care, care of a pregnant woman from the start of labor to the end of the third stage of labor with the release of the placenta. See also **antepartal care, newborn intrapartal care, postpartal care.**

★METHOD: Uterine contractions come more often, for longer, and stronger. Pressure of the fetus causes dilation of the cervix, causing a bloody discharge called "bloody show." An examination of the mother is done, and urine is measured regularly through labor and tested. The position of the fetus is found by feeling the belly. The cervical dilatation is determined by vaginal examination, using careful aseptic technique. The fetal heart rate is counted, and variations are noted in relation to the timing and strength of contractions. See also **emergency childbirth.** The nurse gives emotional support and aids physical comfort throughout labor and delivery. After delivery of the infant, the mother is watched for bleeding. The uterine fundus may need to be massaged to cause it to contract. The placenta is weighed and examined for completeness. The episiotomy, if done, or any tear is usually repaired after delivery of the placenta. Depending on the mother's choice and condition and the policy of the maternity service, the infant may be placed in a warmer or on the mother's abdomen. The mother and infant are watched for a while in the delivery area before being moved to the postpartum unit.

★OUTCOME: During labor and delivery, several danger signs alert the observer to problems. These signs include strong, continuous uterine contractions; marked change of the fetal heart rate; sudden, excessive fetal movement; continuous stomach pain with increased fundal height; vaginal bleeding; protruding umbilical cord; a large amount of amniotic fluid; or an elevation or drop in the mother's temperature, pulse, or blood pressure. Normal delivery of a healthy baby from a healthy mother is the usual outcome.

intrapartal period, the time spanning labor and birth.

intrapartum, referring to the period of labor and delivery.

intraperiosteal fracture /in′trəper′ē·os′tē·əl/, a fracture that does not rupture the bone cover.

intrapsychic conflict, emotional conflict within oneself. See also **conflict.**

intrapulmonary shunt, (in respiratory therapy) a condition in which blood is routed to a part of the lung that does not have good air exchange. The blood passes through this region without picking up much oxygen. The condition may occur during collapse of a part of the lung (atelectasis), pneumonia, water in the lung (pulmonary edema), and adult respiratory distress syndrome (ARDS).

intrarenal hemodynamics, the pattern of blood flow in the kidney. Normally the outer layers of the kidney receive most of the blood flow.

intrathecal /in′trəthē′kəl/, referring to a structure, process, or substance in a sheath, as the spinal fluid in the theca of the spinal canal.

intrathecal injection, putting a hypodermic needle in the subarachnoid space for the purpose of leaving a substance to spread through the spinal fluid.

intrathoracic goiter, an enlargement of the thyroid gland that protrudes into the thoracic cavity.

intrauterine device (IUD) /in′trəyoo̅′tərin/, a birth-control device consisting of a bent strip of plastic or other material that is put in the uterus to prevent pregnancy. It is not known how it works. It is put in during or just after menstruation when the cervix is slightly open and menstruation assures that a pregnancy does not exist. The tail string of the IUD hangs from the cervix. By feeling the string with her finger from time to time, the wearer can be sure the device is in place. The string also gives a way to remove the IUD. The rate of failure for the IUD method of contraception is about two to four unplanned pregnancies in 100 women with the device for 1 year. IUDs can cause problems. Infection is the most serious. Such infections in pregnancy may be lethal; so the IUD is removed if pregnancy is suspected. Some other complications are cervicitis, perforation of the uterus, salpingitis causing sterility, ectopic pregnancy, abortion, embedding of the device in the wall of the uterus, endometritis, bleeding, pain, cramping, undetected expulsion, and irritation of the penis. Women without problems using an IUD are commonly able to retain the device safely for several years, or indefinitely. Also called **intrauterine contraceptive device (IUCD),** (informal) **coil,** (informal) **loop.**

intrauterine fracture, a fracture during fetal life.

intrauterine growth curve, a line on a graph showing the mean weight for gestational age through pregnancy to term. It classifies infants by maturity and development.

intrauterine growth retardation, an abnormal process in which the development and maturation of the fetus is delayed by genetic factors, maternal disease, or fetal malnutrition caused by placental insufficiency. See also **small for gestational age infant.**

intravascular coagulation test, a test for finding internal blood clotting.

intravenous (IV), referring to the inside of a vein, as of a thrombus or an injection, infusion, or catheter.

intravenous alimentation. See **total parenteral nutrition.**

intravenous bolus, a large dose of medication given in the vein, usually within 1 to 30 minutes. The IV bolus is often used when medicine is needed quickly, as in an emergency, when drugs are given that cannot be diluted, as many cancer chemotherapeutic drugs, and when a peak drug level is needed in the bloodstream of the patient. The IV bolus is not used when the medicine must be diluted or when the rapid giving of the medicine, as potassium chloride, could cause death. The IV bolus is normally not used for patients with decreased cardiac outputs, decreased urinary outputs, pulmonary congestion, or systemic edema. Such patients have lower tolerance to medicine, so these must be diluted more than usual and given slower. The IV bolus site is prepared with an antiseptic. If a primary IV line is already in, the IV bolus is given by mixing the prescribed drug with the right amount of diluent, after first learning if the drug is compatible with the primary IV solution. Also called **intravenous push.**

intravenous cholangiography, (in diagnostic radiology) a procedure for outlining the major bile ducts. A material is injected, and x-ray films are taken. See also **cholangiography.**

intravenous controller, any device that automatically delivers IV fluid at selectable flow rates, usually between one and 69 drops per minute. The controller commonly has with a rate selector, drop sensor, drop indicator, and drop alarm. When the infusion does not flow at the right rate, the drop alarm gives a signal. The controller cannot give the pressure of a true pump and should not be used for highly viscous fluid or keeping an artery open. Compare **intravenous peristaltic pump, intravenous piston pump, intravenous syringe pump.**

intravenous DSA (IV-DSA), a form of angiography in which dye is in a vein, rather than an artery.

intravenous fat emulsion, a preparation of 10% fat given by vein to keep up the weight or growth of patients. Such fat emulsions are made from soybean oil and egg-yolk. IV emulsions are not administered to patients suffering from abnormal fat metabolism, severe hepatic diseases, some blood-clotting defects, lung diseases, lipoid nephrosis, hepatocellular damage, or bone marrow dyscrasia, or to patients treated with anabolic inhibitory drugs. If possible, the IV fat emulsion is administered during daytime so the patient may eat normally with rest during the night and a lower night urinary flow. The patient's fluid intake and output are regularly measured during the delivery of the emulsion, and daily blood studies are conducted to find the level of free-floating triglycerides. Hepatic function tests are done if the patient receives IV fat emulsion infusions over a long period of time. Immediate side effects or those that may occur up to 2½ hours after the onset of the infusion may include temperature rise, flushing, sweating, pressure sensations over the eyes, nausea, vomiting, headache, chest and back pains, dyspnea, and cyanosis. Delayed side effects or those that may occur within 10 days of the onset of such infusions may include hepatomegaly, splenomegaly, thrombocytopenia, focal seizures, hyperlipemia, hepatic damage, jaundice, hemorrhagic diathesis, and gastroduodenal ulcer.

intravenous feeding, the giving of nutrients through a vein.

intravenous infusion, 1. a solution given in a vein through an infusion set that has a vacuum bottle or bag with the solution and tubing connecting the bottle to a catheter or needle in the patient's vein. **2.** the process of giving a solution in a vein. Swelling of the limb near the site of entry may mean the catheter or needle is in subcutaneous tissue, not in the vein. The fluid may be infiltrating the tissue spaces. It should be withdrawn and the limb raised. Redness, swelling, heat, and pain around the vein at the site of injection may

indicate thrombophlebitis. The infusion should be stopped and the inflammation treated. The infusion is often restarted elsewhere. See also **venipuncture.**

intravenous injection, a hypodermic injection in a vein to give a single dose of medicine, inject a contrast medium, or begin an IV infusion of blood, medication, or fluid solution, as saline or dextrose in water. See also **venipuncture.**

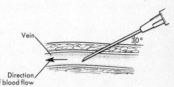

Intravenous injection (note bevel direction of needle)

intravenous peristaltic pump, any of several devices for giving IV fluids by pressure on the IV tubing rather than on the fluid itself. This device has a drop sensor, rate selector, power-switch indicator lamp, and drop indicator and alarm. The drop alarm sounds when the infusion does not flow at the right rate. Compare **intravenous controller, intravenous piston pump, intravenous syringe pump.**

intravenous piston pump, any of several devices that control the infusion of IV fluids by piston action. IV piston pumps are commonly equipped with indicators that show flow rates, dose limits, and cumulative fluid volumes. Such pumps are equipped with infiltration and flow alarms. The pump reduces the delivery rate to a keep-vein-open rate if the proper flow rate or dose limit is exceeded. The pump stops the IV fluid if the IV line is clogged or if infiltration is detected. Compare **intravenous controller, intravenous peristaltic pump, intravenous syringe pump.**

intravenous push. See **intravenous bolus.**

intravenous pyelography (IVP), a technique in radiology for evaluating the urinary system. A contrast medium is put in a vein, and x-ray films are taken as the medium is cleared from the blood. The renal calyces, renal pelvis, ureters, and urinary bladder are all visible on the x-ray films. Tumors, cysts, stones, and many structural and functional abnormalities may be seen using this technique. A cathartic or an enema is usually given the day before the procedure. The person is given nothing by mouth from midnight before the test to induce some dehydration. The patient may be asked to void right before injection of the dye. Also called **descending urography, excretory urography.**

intravenous syringe pump, any of several devices that automatically compress a syringe plunger at a certain rate. Such devices are used with disposable syringes that can deliver blood, medications, or nutrients by IV, arterial, or subcutaneous routes. IV syringe pumps are often used to treat infants and ambulatory patients. Compare **intravenous controller, intravenous peristaltic pump, intravenous piston pump.**

intravenous therapy, the administration of fluids or drugs in the general circulation through a venipuncture.

intravenous urography. See **intravenous pyelography.**

intraventricular /in′trəventrik′yoolər/, referring to the space in a ventricle.

intraventricular block, the slowed conduction or stoppage of the cardiac excitatory impulse in the ventricles. The block is seen on an electrocardiogram. The block can be caused by coronary artery disease, valvular heart disease, ventricular hypertrophy and fibrosis, cardiomyopathy, or idiopathic degeneration of the conduction system. Outcome depends on the basic heart condition. Kinds of intraventricular block include **bundle branch block** and **infranodal block.** See also **heart block, intraatrial block, Purkinje's network, sinoatrial block.**

intraventricular hydrocephalus. See **hydrocephalus.**

intrinsic, 1. natural or inherent. **2.** coming from or in an organ or tissue.

intrinsic asthma, a nonseasonal, nonallergic form of asthma usually starting later in life than allergic asthma. It tends to be chronic and long-lasting rather than episodic. The trigger factors include breathing irritating pollutants, as dust particles, smoke, aerosols, strong cooking odors, paint fumes, and other volatile substances. Bronchospasm may also occur in cold, damp weather, after sudden breathing of cold, dry air, and after exercise or violent coughing or laughing. Breathing infections, as the common cold, and mental factors, as anxiety, may also cause attacks. Compare **allergic asthma.** See also **asthma.**

intrinsic factor, a substance released by the gastric mucosa, essential for intestinal absorption of cyanocobalamin (vitamin B_{12}). A lack of intrinsic factor, caused by gastrectomy, myxedema, or atrophy of the gastric mucosa, causes pernicious anemia. See also **pernicious anemia.**

intrinsic minus hand deformity, an abnormality resulting from damage to some of the nerves at the wrist. This results in curling of the fingers and overextension of the joints between the hand and the fingers.

introjection, an unconscious mechanism in which someone builds into his or her own ego structure the qualities of someone else.

Intron A, a brand name for an anticancer drug given by injection (interferon alpha-2b, recombinant).

Intropin, a trademark for an adrenergic (dopamine hydrochloride).

introspection, 1. the act of examining one's own thoughts and emotions by focusing on the inner self. **2.** a tendency to look inward at the inner self. **–introspective,** *adj.*

introversion, 1. the tendency to direct one's interests, thoughts, and energies inward or to things concerned only with the self. **2.** the state of being mainly concerned with one's own inner experience. Also spelled **intraversion.** Compare **extroversion.**

introvert, 1. a person whose interests are directed inward and who is shy, withdrawn, emotionally reserved, and self-absorbed. **2.** to turn inward or to direct one's interests and thoughts to oneself. Compare **extrovert.** See also **egocentric.**

intubation, passing a tube into a body aperture, as putting a breathing tube through the mouth or nose or into the trachea to provide an airway for anesthetic gas or oxygen. **Blind intubation** is putting a breathing tube in without using a laryngoscope. Kinds of intubation are **endotracheal intubation, nasogastric intubation.**

intussusception /in′təsəsep′shən/, the sinking of one part of the bowel into the next, like a telescope effect. Such intestinal blockage may involve the small intestine, colon, or ileum. Intussusception occurs most often in infants and small children. It is marked by intestinal pain, vomiting, and bloody mucus in the stool. Barium enema is used to confirm the diagnosis, and surgery is often needed to clear the blockage. See also **intestinal obstruction.**

inulin /in′yoolin/, a fructose-derived substance used in kidney function tests.

inulin clearance, a test of the rate of filtration of a starch, inulin, in the glomerulus of the kidney. Inulin is given by mouth.

inunction, 1. the rubbing of a drug mixed with oil or fat into the skin, with absorption of the active agent. **2.** any compound so applied.

inundation fever. See **scrub typhus.**

in utero /yoo′tərō/, inside the uterus.

invagination, 1. a state in which one part of a structure telescopes into another, as the intestine during peristalsis. If the invagination is extensive or involves a tumor or polyps, it may cause intestinal blockage. Then surgery is needed. **2.** surgery to fix a hernia by replacing the contents of the hernial sac in the abdominal cavity. Anesthesia may be used. No upper respiratory infection, chronic cough, or allergy with sneezing can be present, for it will weaken the repair. See also **hernia, intestinal obstruction, peristalsis. –invaginate,** *v.*

invariable behavior, behavior that results from physical response to a stimulus and is not changed by individual experience, as a reflex. Compare **variable behavior.**

invasion, the process by which cancer cells move into deeper tissue and into blood vessels and lymph channels.

invasive, marked by a tendency to spread.

invasive carcinoma, a cancerous growth with cells that destroy surrounding tissues.

invasive mole. See **chorioadenoma destruens.**

invasive thermometry, measurement of tissue temperature using probes directly in the tissue.

inverse anaphylaxis, a strong allergic reaction caused by an antibody rather than an antigen. Also called **reverse anaphylaxis.**

inverse relationship. See **negative relationship.**

Inversine, a trademark for a nerve-blocking drug (mecamylamine hydrochloride).

inversion, 1. an abnormal state in which an organ is turned inside out, as a uterine inversion. **2.** a chromosomal defect in which two or more parts of a chromosome break off and separate. They rejoin the chromosome in the wrong order.

invert, 1. a homosexual. **2.** to turn something upside down or inside out.

investigational device exemption (I.D.E.), an agreement through which the federal government permits testing of new medical devices.

investigational new drug (IND), a drug not yet approved by the Food and Drug Administration, only for use in experiments to see its safety and effectiveness. The use of an investigational new drug in human subjects requires approval by the Food and Drug Administration of an application that has reports of animal toxicity tests, descriptions of proposed clinical trials, and a list of the investigators and their qualifications.

in vitro /in vē′trō/, (of a biological reaction) occurring in laboratory apparatus. Compare **in vivo.**

in vivo /in vē′vō/, (of a biological reaction) occurring in a living organism. Compare **in vitro.**

in vivo tracer study, (in nuclear medicine) a diagnostic procedure in which a series of radiograms of a given radioactive tracer show structures or processes.

involuntary, without conscious control or direction. See also **autonomy.**

involuntary muscle. See **smooth muscle.**

involuntary nervous system. See **visceral nervous system.**

involuntary patient, a patient admitted to a psychiatric hospital without his or her consent through a legal process of commitment. See also **informal admission.**

involution, a normal process marked by decreasing size of an organ, as involution of the uterus after birth.

involutional melancholia, a state of depression during menopause. The problem starts slowly and is marked by pessimism, irritability, insomnia, loss of appetite, feelings of anxiety, and an increase in motor activity, ranging from mere restlessness to extreme agitation. In the rare cases where treatment is needed antidepressant drugs, electroshock treatment, and psychotherapy may be used. Also called **climacteric melancholia, involutional depression, involutional psychosis.** See also **depression.**

inward aggression, destructive behavior against oneself. See also **aggression, masochism.**

iodine (I), An essential trace element, almost 80% of the iodine present in the body is in the thyroid gland. A lack of iodine can result in goiter or cretinism. Iodine is found in seafoods, iodized salt, and some dairy products. Radioisotopes of iodine are used to treat thyroid cancer.

iodism, a state caused by too much iodine. It is marked by increased salivation, rhinitis, weakness, and skin eruption. See also **ioderma.**

iodize, to treat or impregnate with iodine. Table salt is iodized to prevent goiter in areas with too little iodine in the drinking water or food.

iodochlorhydroxyquin /ī·ō′dōklôrhīdrok′səkwin/, a drug given to treat eczema, athete's foot, and other fungal infections.

★CAUTION: Tuberculosis or viral skin conditions or allergy to this drug or to iodine prohibits its use.

★ADVERSE EFFECTS: The most serious side effect is irritation to sensitive skin.

iododerma /ī·ō′dōdur′mə/, a skin rash caused by an allergy to ingested iodides. Treatment is removing iodides from the diet.

iodoform, a surface anti-infective used as an antiseptic.

iodophor, an antiseptic or disinfectant that combined iodine with something else, as a detergent.

iodoquinol, drug to treat intestinal amebas.

★CAUTION: Liver disease and allergy to iodine or 8-hydroxyquinolines prohibits its use.

★ADVERSE EFFECTS: Among the most serious side effects are dizziness, swollen thyroid gland, optic neuropathy, eye wasting, and peripheral neuropathy.

ion /ī′ən, ī′on/, an atom or group of atoms with an electric charge.

Ionamin, a trademark for an anorectic (phentermine).

ionic bonding, a force that holds atoms together by the actual transfer of one part of an atom (electron) to another atom. Many salts are held together in solid form by ionic bonds. In the case of potassium chloride, an electron is transferred from potassium to chloride, forming the bond. In water, ionic compounds do not stay together but separate into individual ions (dissolve).

inoic dissociation, the process by which individual atoms in an ionic compound separate from each other (dissolve) when placed in water.

ionization, the process in which a neutral atom or molecule gains or loses electrons. Ionizing radiation causes ionization as it passes through body tissue. Ionization can cause cell death or change.

ionizing radiation, electromagnetic and particulate rays (as x-rays and beta rays) that break substances in their paths into ions. Ionizing radiation kills cells or slows their growth. It causes gene changes and chromosome breaks.

iontophoretic pilocarpine test, a sweat test for cystic fibrosis. Pilocarpine iontophoresis causes sweat, which is absorbed from the forearm in a weighed gauze pad. The sweat sample is then analyzed for sodium and chloride electrolytes.

ipecac, a drug to cause vomiting in some poisonings and drug overdoses.

★CAUTION: Allergy to this drug prohibits its use. It is not for unconscious patients or for poisoning by petroleum distillates, strong alkalis, acids, or strychnine.

★ADVERSE EFFECTS:
The most serious side effect is heart poisoning if vomiting does not occur and the drug is retained. If vomiting does not occur, the ipecac is removed by gastric lavage.

ipomea /ipəmē'ə/, a resin made from dried root of *Ipomoea orizabensis,* formerly used as a cathartic.

IPPB (intermittent positive pressure breathing), a form of respiration assisted by a ventilator in which compressed gas is delivered to the person's airways until a preset pressure is reached. Passive exhalation is allowed through a valve, and the cycle starts again. Also called **(IPPV) intermittent positive pressure ventilation.** The nurse sees that the patient closes the lips on the mouthpiece and does not allow air to escape from the nose or mouth during inspiration. The patient should let the lungs be filled by the machine and should not touch the controls. Ventilation may be improved by the use of the IPPB unit. Secretions may be thinned and cleared, and the passages may be humidified.

IPPB unit, a ventilator to put air in the lungs at a preset pressure. It promotes full lung expansion, improves oxygenation, and puts medicine in the breathing channels.

IQ, abbreviation for **intelligence quotient.**

iridectomy, surgery to remove part of the iris of the eye, often to restore drainage of the humor in glaucoma or to remove a foreign body or tumor. General anesthesia is used. After surgery the patient is watched for hemorrhage or excessive pain.

iridotomy, a cut in the iris of the eye to relieve blockage of the pupil, to enlarge the pupil in cataract extraction, or to treat postoperative glaucoma. Anesthesia is used. Atropine and an antibiotic are given. A dressing and shield are applied. Afterward, the dressing is watched for drainage. Great pain is abnormal. See also **iridectomy, iris.**

iris, a circular, contracting disc suspended between the cornea and the crystalline lens of the eye. Dark pigment under the translucent tissue of the iris are arranged in different people to produce different colored irises. Albinos have no pigment. In blue eyes the pigment cells are only on the back surface of the iris, but in gray eyes, brown eyes, and black eyes the pigment cells appear in the front layer. See also **dilatator pupillae, sphincter pupillae.** –**iridic,** *adj.*

iritis, an inflammatory condition of the iris of the eye characterized by pain, tearing, photophobia, and, if severe, lessened visual sharpness. On examination the eye looks cloudy, the iris bulges, and the pupil is contracted. The cause is often unknown. The pupil is dilated, and a steroid may be given to reduce inflammation. If the inflammation is allowed to continue and the pupil is left constricted, permanent scarring may occur, lowering vision.

iron (Fe), a common metallic element needed to make hemoglobin.

iron deficiency anemia, anemia caused by too little iron in the hemoglobin, marked by pallor, fatigue, and weakness. Iron deficiency may be caused by too little dietary iron, poor absorption of iron, or chronic bleeding. Iron can be replaced by ferrous sulfate; the oral form is best, if tolerated. The anemia should be gone in 2 months, but therapy lasts another 4 months to replace tissue stores. Compare **hemolytic anemia, hypoplastic anemia.** See also **anemia, iron metabolism, nutritional anemia, red cell indices.**

iron dextran, a drug to treat iron deficiency anemia not helped by oral iron therapy.

★CAUTION: Early pregnancy, anemias other than iron deficiency anemia, or allergy to this drug prohibits its use.

★ADVERSE EFFECTS: Among the more serious side effects are severe allergic reactions, including fatal anaphylaxis. Inflammation or phlebitis at the site of injection, arthralgia, headache, GI distress, fever, and lesser allergic reactions may occur.

iron lung. See **Drinker respirator.**

iron metabolism, processes involved in the entry of iron in the body through its absorption, its transport and storage, its formation of hemoglobin, and its eventual excretion. The normal iron distribution in a 70 kg adult (male) totals approximately 3.7 g with more than 65% of this in circulating hemoglobin. Another 27% is found in the storage pool. The body normally saves iron so well that loss, usually only through the feces, is normally limited to about

1 mg/day. This amount is easily provided by a dietary intake of only 10 mg/day. Iron deficiency may follow long intervals of inadequate iron intake (especially in women) or after great blood loss. Iron overload can occur in disorders in which normal regulation of iron absorption is faulty. It is also caused by injecting large doses of iron or blood for therapy. See also **anemia, hemochromatosis, iron deficiency anemia, iron transport.**

iron-rich food, any nutrient with a lot of iron. The best source of dietary iron is liver, with oysters, clams, heart, kidney, lean meat, and tongue as second choices. Leafy green vegetables are the best plant sources. See also **iron, iron deficiency anemia.**

iron salts poisoning, poisoning caused by overdose of ferric or ferrous salts, marked by vomiting, bloody diarrhea, blue skin, and stomach pain. Therapy includes gastric lavage, emetics, deferoxamine, and supportive therapy.

iron saturation, the capacity of iron to saturate transferrin, measured in the blood to detect iron excess or deficiency. The normal iron saturation capacity in serum is 20% to 55%. See also **total iron.**

irradiation, exposure to radiant energy like heat, light, or x-ray. Radioactive sources of radiant energy, such as x-rays or isotopes of iodine or cobalt, are used to examine internal body structures. Radioactivity destroys microorganisms or cells that are cancerous. Infrared or ultraviolet light produces heat in tissues to relieve pain and soreness or to treat acne, psoriasis, or other skin ailments. Ultraviolet light is also used to identify some bacteria and toxic molds. See also **radiation sickness, radioactivity, ultraviolet. –irradiate,** *v.*

irreducible, unable to be returned to the normal position or state, as an irreducible hernia. See also **incarcerate.**

irrelevance, (in psychiatry) any response, action, or statement not pertinent to the existing situation or condition that signifies a neurotic or psychotic condition.

irreversible coma. See **brain death.**

irrigate, to clean by squirting fluid onto an area, usually with a slow steady pressure on a syringe plunger. It may be done to cleanse a wound or to clear tubing.

irrigation, the process of washing out a body cavity or wounded area with a stream of water or other fluid. It is also used to cleanse a tube or drain in the body, as an indwelling catheter. The process is often done with water, saline, aminoacetic acid, or antiseptic solutions on the eye, ear, throat, vagina, and urinary tract. Gentle pressure is used in starting the fluid, except in the cleaning of wounds. The solution is removed from internal cavities through suction or by drainage. See also **lavage. –irrigate,** *v.*

irrigator, an apparatus with a flexible tube for flushing or washing out a body cavity.

irritable bowel syndrome, abnormally increased motility of the small and large intestines, often with emotional stress. Mostly young adults are affected. They complain of diarrhea and, sometimes, pain in the lower abdomen. The pain is often stopped by moving the bowels. In diagnosing irritable bowel syndrome, other more serious conditions, as dysentery, lactose intolerance, and the inflammatory bowel disease, must be ruled out. Because there is no organic disease in irritable bowel syndrome, no specific treatment is needed. Many persons benefit from the use of bulk-producing agents in the diet. Antidiarrheal drugs help lower the frequency of stool. Although this is a functional disorder, patients experience pain and discomfort and need emotional support. Mild tranquilizers or antidepressants are sometimes given to relieve anxiety or depression. Also called **mucous colitis, spastic colon.**

irritation fibroma, a local peripheral, tumor-like swelling of connective tissue caused by prolonged irritation. It commonly develops on or near the gums.

ischemia /iskē′mē-ə/, poor blood supply to an organ or part, often marked by pain and organ dysfunction, as in ischemic heart disease. Some causes of ischemia are arterial embolism, atherosclerosis, thrombosis, and vasoconstriction. Compare **infarction. –ischemic,** *adj.*

ischemic contracture, See **Volkmann's contracture.**

ischemic heart disease, a state caused by lack of oxygen to tissue cells.

ischemic lumbago, a pain in the lower back and buttocks caused by vascular insufficiency, as in blockage of the abdominal aorta.

ischemic pain, the unpleasant, often very painful feeling associated with ischemia, caused by peripheral vascular disease, from decreased blood flow caused by constricting orthopedic casts, or from poor blood flow caused by surgical trauma or accidental injury. Ischemic pain caused by occlusive arterial disease is often severe and may not be relieved, even with narcotics. The individual with peripheral vessel disease may experience ischemic pain only while exercising because the demands for oxygen cannot be met by the low blood flow. The ischemic pain of partial vessel blockage is not as severe as the abrupt pain of a completely blocked artery, as by an embolism. The ischemic pain caused by the pressure of a cast is difficult to distinguish from the sharp pain caused by surgical intervention, because both types of pain may be local rather than spread out, as is the pain caused by trauma. See also **pain intervention, pain mechanism.**

ischial spines /is′kē-əl/, two bony projections that

are part of the ischial bones of the hip that form the lower border of the pelvis.

Ishihara color test /ish′ēhä′rə/, a test of color vision using a series of plates on which are printed round dots in many colors and patterns. People with normal color vision can discern specific numbers or patterns on the plates; the inability to pick out a given number or shape means a specific lack in color perception.

island fever. See **scrub typhus.**

islands of Langerhans /lang′gərhanz/, pancreas cells that make insulin, glucagon, and pancreatic polypeptide. Their secretions are important regulators of sugar metabolism. Also called **islets of Langerhans.**

islet cell adenoma. See **insulinoma.**

islet cell antibody, an immunoglobulin that reacts with all pancreatic islet cells. These antibodies are in about 60% to 70% of newly diagnosed, insulin-dependent diabetic patients. The presence of the antibody is temporary.

islet cell tumor, any tumor of the islands of Langerhans.

islets of Langerhans. See **islands of Langerhans.**

Ismelin, a trademark for a high blood pressure drug (guanethidine sulfate).

isocapnic, referring to steady levels of carbon dioxide in the tissues even though breathing rates change.

isocarboxazid, a drug to treat mental depression.
★CAUTION: Liver or kidney dysfunction, congestive heart failure, pheochromocytoma, use of a nervous system drug or foods high in tryptophan or tyramine, or allergy to this drug prohibits its use.
★ADVERSE EFFECTS: Among the more serious side effects are hyperactivity, irregular heart beat, low blood pressure, vertigo, dry mouth, constipation, and blurred vision. Monoamine oxidase inhibitors cause many bad drug interactions.

isodose chart, (in radiotherapy) a graph of the distribution of radiation in a medium. Isodose charts are made for x-rays traversing the body, and for work areas where x-rays or radionuclides are used.

isoelectric electroencephalogram. See **flat electroencephalogram.**

isoetharine, isoetharine hydrochloride. See **isoetharine mesylate.**

isoetharine mesylate, a drug for bronchial asthma, bronchitis, and emphysema.
★CAUTION: A history of irregular heart beat or allergy to this drug or to sympathomimetic drugs prohibits its use.
★ADVERSE EFFECTS: Among the more serious side effects are irregular or rapid heart rate, dizziness, nervousness, and headache.

isoimmunization, the development of antibodies in a species with antigens from the same species, as the development of anti-Rh antibodies in an Rh-negative person.

isoflurophate, a drug for open-angle glaucoma and esotropia.
★CAUTION: Uveal inflammation or allergy to this drug or to other like drugs prohibits its use.
★ADVERSE EFFECTS: Among the more serious side effects are nervous system effects, sight problems, a puzzling rise in inner eye pressure, and, with long-term use, growth of cataracts.

isofosfamide. See **isophosphamide.**

isogamete /īsōgam′ēt/, a reproductive cell of the same size and structure as the one with which it unites. Compare **anisogamete, heterogamete.** –**isogametic,** *adj.*

isogamy /īsog′əmē/, sexual reproduction in which there is fusion of gametes of the same size and structure, as in certain algae, fungi, and protozoa. Compare **anisogamy, heterogamy.** –**isogamous,** *adj.*

isogeneic. See **syngeneic.**

isogenesis, development from a common origin and according to similar processes. Also called **isogeny** /īsoj′ənē/. –**isogenetic, isogenic,** *adj.*

isograft, transplant of compatible tissue from genetically identical individuals, as between a patient and identical twin or between animals of a highly inbred strain. Compare **allograft, autograft, xenograft.** See also **graft.**

isohemagglutinin. See **isoagglutinin.**

isohydric shift, reactions in red blood cells in which carbon dioxide is taken and oxygen is let go, making no excess hydrogen ions.

isolation, the separation of a seriously ill patient from others to stop the spread of infection or protect the patient from irritating factors. A patient given radiation implant therapy may be isolated to reduce exposing hospital workers to radioactivity.

isolation incubator, an incubator bed kept for premature or other infants who require isolation.

Isolette, a trademark for a self-contained incubator that has a controlled heat, humidity, and oxygen area for the isolation and care of premature and low weight newborns. It is of clear plastic with a large door and portholes for access to the child with minimum heat and oxygen loss. A mechanism monitors the child's temperature and controls heat in the unit.

isoleucine (Ile) /ī′sōloo′sēn/, an amino acid in most dietary proteins. It is needed for proper growth in infants and nitrogen balance in adults. See also **amino acid, maple syrup urine disease, protein.**

isomers /ī′səmərz/, molecules with the same weight and formula but different arrangements, so that they act differently.

isometheptene hydrochloride, a drug in some fixed-combination drugs for migraine.

isometric exercise, a form of active exercise that raises muscle tension by putting pressure against stable resistance. This may be done by opposing different muscles in the same person, as by pressing the hands together or by making a limb push or pull against an immovable object. There is no joint movement and the muscle length is the same, but muscle strength and tone are maintained or improved. Compare **isotonic exercise.** See also **exercise.**

isometric growth, an increase in size of different organs or parts of an organism at the same rate. Compare **allometric growth.**

isoniazid /īsəni′əzid/, also called **INH (isonicotinic acid hydrazide).** It is used to treat tuberculosis caused by mycobacteria sensitive to the drug.

★CAUTION: Liver disease, a previous history of a negative reaction to isoniazid, or allergy to this drug prohibits its use.

★ADVERSE EFFECTS: Among the more serious side effects in long-term treatment are liver disease and nervous system disorders. Rashes, fever, and central nervous system effects often occur.

isophane insulin suspension, a modified form of protamine zinc insulin suspension. It is an insulin often prescribed. Also called **NPH insulin.**

isophosphamide, an antitumor drug that is taken from cyclophosphamide and used like cyclophosphamide. Also called **isofosfamide.** See also **cyclophosphamide.**

isoprenaline. See **isoproterenol hydrochloride.**

isopropamide iodide, a drug used to treat ulcers.

★CAUTION: Narrow-angle glaucoma, asthma, obstruction of the genitourinary or intestinal tract, ulcerative colitis, or allergy to this drug prohibits its use.

★ADVERSE EFFECTS: Among the more serious side effects are blurred vision, central nervous system effects, rapid heart rate, dry mouth, lower sweating, and allergic reactions.

isopropanol. See **isopropyl alcohol.**

isopropyl alcohol /īsōprō′pil/, a clear, colorless, bitter aromatic liquid that can be mixed with water, ether, chloroform, and ethyl alcohol. A solution of 70% isopropyl alcohol in water is used as a rubbing compound. Also called **avantin, dimethyl carbinol, isopropanol.** See also **alcohol.**

isopropylaminoacetic acid. See **valine.**

isoproterenol hydrochloride /īsōprəter′ənol/, a bronchodilator and a cardiac stimulant.

★CAUTION: Irregular heart beat or allergy to this drug prohibits its use.

★ADVERSE EFFECTS: Among the more serious side effects are heart problems, low blood pressure, and worsening chest pain.

Isoptin, a trademark for a slow channel blocker or calcium ion antagonist (verapamil).

Isopto Atropine, a trademark for a nervous system drug (atropine sulfate).

Isopto Carbachol, a trademark for a nervous system drug (carbachol).

Isopto Carpine, a trademark for a nervous system drug (pilocarpine hydrochloride).

Isopto Cetamide, a trademark for an antibacterial (sulfacetamide sodium).

Isopto Homatropine, a trademark for a nervous system drug (homatropine hydrobromide).

Isopto Hyoscine, a trademark for a nervous system drug (scopolamine hydrobromide).

Isordil, a trademark for a drug used to stop chest pain (isosorbide dinitrate).

isosmotic. See **isotonic.**

isosorbide dinitrate, a drug used to stop chest pain. It is used as a coronary vasodilator in the treatment of certain heart problems.

★CAUTION: Known allergy to this drug prohibits its use.

★ADVERSE EFFECTS: The most serious side effect is occasional marked low blood pressure. Flushing, headache, and dizziness also may occur.

isotones, atoms with the same number of neutrons but different numbers of protons.

isotonic /īsəton′ik/, (of a solution) having the same concentration of solute as another solution. Also **isosmotic.** Compare **hypertonic, hypotonic.**

isotonic exercise, a form of exercise in which the muscle contracts and causes movement. Throughout the procedure there is little change in the resistance so the force of the contraction remains constant. Such exercise greatly improves joint mobility. It also helps to improve muscle strength and tone. Compare **isometric exercise.** See also **exercise.**

isotope /ī′sətōp/, one of two or more forms of a chemical element having almost the same properties. Radioactive isotopes are used in many diagnostic and therapeutic procedures.

isotopic tracer /ī′sətop′ik/, an isotope or isotopes of an element put into a sample to permit observation of the course of the element through a chemical, physical, or biological process.

isotretinoin, an antiacne drug given for cystic acne.

isoxsuprine hydrochloride, a drug to relieve symptoms of brain blood vessel problems and to improve blood flow in hardening of the arteries, Raynaud's disease, and Buerger's disease.

★CAUTION: Allergy to this drug is the only constraint.

★ADVERSE EFFECTS: Among the more serious side effects are rapid heart rate, low blood pressure, and skin problems.

Isuprel, a trademark for a beta-adrenergic stimulant (isoproterenol).

IT, abbreviation for immunotoxin.

itch, **1.** to feel a sensation, usually on the skin, that makes one want to scratch. **2.** a tingling, annoying feeling on the skin that makes one want to scratch it, as may be caused in some people by rhus dermatitis, a mosquito bite, or an allergic reaction. **3.** the pruritic skin caused by infestation with the parasitic mite *Sarcoptes scabiei.* **–itchy,** *adj.*

IU, I.U., abbreviation for **International Unit.**

IUCD, abbreviation for **intrauterine contraceptive device.** See **intrauterine device.**

IUD, abbreviation for **intrauterine device.**

IV, **1.** abbreviation for **intravenous. 2.** *informal.* a bottle of fluid, infusion set with tubing, and an intracatheter, used in intravenous therapy. **3.** giving of fluids or drugs by injection in a vein.

ivory bones. See **osteopetrosis.**

IV push, a technique in which a large amount of drug or IV fluid is given rapidly via IV injection or infusion. Methergine may be given this way to cause rapid contraction of the uterus in postpartum bleeding. See also **intravenous injection.**

IV-type traction frame, a metal support that holds traction equipment consisting of two metal uprights, one at each end of the bed, which support an overhead metal bar. Each upright is clamped to a horizontal bar that fits in holders inserting at the corners of the bed. Compare **claw-type traction frame.** See also **traction frame.**

Ixodes /iksō'dēz/, parasitic, hard-shelled ticks that carry infections, as Rocky Mountain spotted fever.

ixodid /iksod'id, iksō'did/, of or pertaining to certain hard ticks.

J

Jaccoud's dissociated fever /zhäkōōz'/, a form of meningitis with a slow pulse rate.

jacket, a garment to support the torso. Some kinds of jackets are **Minerva jacket** and **Sayre's jacket.**

jacket restraint, an orthopedic device to hold the patient's trunk still in traction and to keep the patient from sitting up in bed. The restraint is attached to both sides of the bedspring frame by buckled webbing straps sewn into the side seams of the restraint. The jacket restraint may be used with most kinds of traction. Compare **diaper restraint, sling restraint.**

jackknife position, position in which the patient is placed on the back in a semisitting position, with the shoulders elevated and the thighs flexed at right angles to the abdomen. Examination and instrumentation of the male urethra is aided by this position.

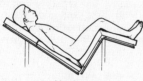

Jackknife position

Jackson crib, a removable orthodontic appliance kept in position by crib-shaped wires.

jacksonian seizure. See **focal seizure.**

Jacquemier's sign /zhäkmē·äz'/, a deepening of the color of the vaginal mucosa just below the urethral orifice. It may be noted after the fourth week of pregnancy, but it is not a reliable sign of pregnancy.

jail fever. See **epidemic typhus.**

Jakob-Creutzfeldt disease. See **Creutzfeldt-Jakob disease.**

jamais vu /zhämävY', -vē, -vōō'/, the feeling of being a stranger with a person one knows or when in a familiar place. It occurs sometimes in normal people but more often in people who have temporal lobe epilepsy. The French phrase means "never seen." Compare **déjà vu.**

Janeway lesion, a small erythematous or hemorrhagic macule on the palms or soles. It is sometimes a sign of subacute bacterial endocarditis.

janiceps /jan'əseps/, a joined twin fetus with the heads fused, the faces looking in opposite directions. The faces and bodies of both twins may be fully formed or one member may be only partially formed and act as a parasite on the more fully developed fetus.

Jansen's disease. See **metaphyseal dysostosis.**

Japanese encephalitis, a severe epidemic infection of brain tissue seen in East Asia and the South Pacific, including Australia and New Zealand. It is marked by shaking chills, paralysis, and weight loss, and caused by a group of B arboviruses carried by mosquitos. Mortality may be as high as 33%. Various neurological and psychiatrical sequelae are common. There is no specific treatment. Also called **Japanese B encephalitis.**

Japanese flood fever, Japanese river fever. See **scrub tyhus.**

JAPHA /jaf'ə, jä'ä'pē'äch'ä'/, abbreviation for *Journal of the American Public Health Association.*

Jarisch-Herxheimer reaction /jä'risherks'hīmər/, a sudden passing fever and worsening of skin lesions seen a few hours after the giving of penicillin or other antibiotics to treat spirosis, or relapsing fever. It lasts less than 24 hours and needs no treatment.

Jarvik-7, an artificial heart designed by R. K. Jarvik for use in humans. The Jarvik-7 was an early model depending on air pressure to drive the ventricles. See also **electrohydraulic heart.**

Jarotzky's treatment /jərot'skēz/, treating gastric ulcer by a bland diet of egg whites, fresh butter, bread, milk, and noodles.

jaundice, a yellow discoloring of the skin, mucous membranes, and eyes, caused by too much bilirubin in the blood. Persons with jaundice may also have nausea, vomiting, and stomach pain and may pass dark urine. Jaundice is a symptom of many disorders, including liver diseases, biliary obstruction, and the hemolytic anemias. Newborns often develop physiological jaundice, which leaves after a few days. Rarer disorders causing jaundice are Crigler-Najjar syndrome and Gilbert's syndrome. Useful diagnostic procedures include tests of liver function, visualization on x-ray films, CAT scan, ultrasound, endoscopy or exploratory surgery, and biopsy. Also called **icterus** /ik'tərəs/ . See also **anicteric hepatitis, hyperbilirubinemia.** **–jaundiced,** *adj.*

jaw, a common term used to describe the maxillae and the mandible and the soft tissue that covers these structures. See also **jaw relation.**

jaw reflex, an abnormal reflex elicited by tapping the chin with a rubber hammer while the mouth is half open and the jaw muscles are relaxed. A quick snapping shut of the jaw implies damage to part of the area of cerebral cortex. Also called **chin reflex, jaw jerk, mandibular reflex.**

jaw relation, any relation of the mandible to the maxillae.

Jefferson fracture, a fracture marked by bursting of the atlas ring.

jejunal feeding tube /jijōō′nəl/, a hollow tube inserted into the small intestine through the stomach wall for giving liquified foods.

jejunoileitis. See **Crohn's disease.**

jejunostomy /jij′ōōnos′təmē/, an operation to make an artificial opening to the small intestine through the stomach wall. It may be a permanent or temporary opening.

jejunum /jijōō′nəm/, *pl.* **jejuna,** one of the three portions of the small intestine, connecting with the duodenum and the ileum. The jejunum has a slightly larger diameter, a deeper color, and a thicker wall than the ileum. It has heavy, circular folds that are not in the lower part of the ileum. Compare **ileum.** –**jejunal,** *adj.*

jellyfish sting, a wound caused by skin contact with a jellyfish, a sea animal with a bell-shaped, jellylike body and many long tentacles with stingers. In most cases a tender, red welt forms on the affected skin. In some cases, depending on the sensitivity of the person and the species of jellyfish, there may be severe local pain and nausea, weakness, nasal discharge, muscle spasm, and sweating. To treat, carefully remove tentacles and apply a compress of alcohol, aromatic spirits of ammonia, or Dakin's solution. Calcium gluconate may be given to stop muscle spasms.

Jendrassik's maneuver /yendrä′shiks/, (in neurology) a diagnostic procedure in which the patient hooks the flexed fingers of the two hands together and tries to pull them apart. While this tension is being exerted, the lower extremity reflexes are tested.

jet humidifier, a humidifier that breaks the water into small droplets of vapor. Air passes through a small opening after entering the humidifier, forming bubbles of water and air. The vapor produced by the unit has a maximum amount of water vapor and a minimum of liquid water particles.

jet lag, a condition marked by fatigue, sleeplessness, and sluggish body functions caused by disruption of the normal circadian rhythm caused by air travel across several time zones.

Jeune's syndrome /zhoenz, zhōōnz/ an inherited form of short-limbed dwarfism with narrowing of the upper chest and, occasionally, more than the normal number of fingers or toes. Also called **asphyxiating thoracic dysplasia.**

jigger. See **chigoe.**

jock itch. See **tinea cruris.**

Jod-Basedow phenomenon, thyrotoxicosis when dietary iodine is given to a patient with endemic goiter in an area of environmental iodine deficiency. It is presumed that iodine deficiency protects some patients with endemic goiter from thyrotoxicosis. The phenomenon may also occur when large doses of iodine are given to patients with nontoxic multinodular goiter in areas with enough environmental iodine. There is a danger of inducing the phenomenon if iodine-containing drugs, as x-ray contrast media, are given to elderly patients with nontoxic multinodular goiter.

jogger's heel, a painful problem common among joggers and distance runners. It is marked by bruising, bursitis, fasciitis, or calcaneal spurs, caused by repetitive and forceful strikes of the heel on the ground. Wise choice of well-fitting running shoes and avoidance of running on hard surfaces help avoid recurrence. Rest, heat, or corticosteroid medication or aspirin may be used.

Johnson's method, (in dentistry) a technique for filling root canals. A plastic material is forced into the root canal until it is sealed.

joint, any of the connections between bones. Each is classified according to structure and movability as fibrous, cartilaginous, or synovial. Fibrous joints are immovable, cartilaginous joints slightly movable, and synovial joints freely movable. Typical immovable joints connect most of the bones of the skull with a sutural ligament. Typical slightly movable joints connect the vertebrae and the pubic bones. Most of the joints in the body are freely movable. Also called **articulation.** See also **cartilaginous joint, fibrous joint, synovial joint.**

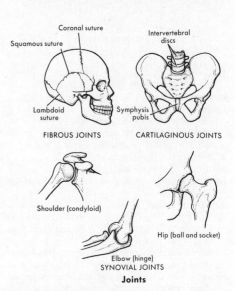

FIBROUS JOINTS   CARTILAGINOUS JOINTS

SYNOVIAL JOINTS

Joints

joint and several liability, (in law) a state in which several persons share the liability for a plaintiff's injury and may be found liable individually or as a group.

joint appointment, 1. a faculty appointment to two institutions in a university or system, as to the schools of nursing and medicine. **2.** (in academic nursing) the appointment of the faculty of a university to a clinical service of an associated service institution. A psychiatric nurse might hold appointment in a university as an assistant professor and be a clinical nurse specialist in a service institution. See also **unification model.**

joint chondroma, a cartilaginous mass that develops in the synovial membrane of a joint.

joint fracture, a break in the articular surfaces of the bony structures of a joint.

joint instability, an abnormal increase in joint movement.

joint mouse, a small, movable stone in or near a joint, usually a knee.

joint practice, 1. the practice of a physician and nurse practitioner, usually private, who work as a team, sharing responsibility for a group of patients. **2.** (in inpatient nursing) the practice of making joint decisions about patient care by committees of physicians and nurses working on a division.

Jones criteria, standard guidelines for diagnosis of rheumatic fever, as recommended by the American Heart Association. See also **rheumatic fever.**

joystick, a stick or lever that can be moved to control a computer or the direction of an electric wheelchair. See also **mouse, trackball.**

J-pouch, a holding area for feces that is formed by folding over the lower end of the small intestine in an operation in which the colon and rectum are removed but the anus is left intact.

Judd method, (in radiology) a way to position a patient for x-rays of the two vertebrae in the neck (atlas and odontoid).

judgment, (in psychiatry) seeing the relation of ideas and forming right conclusions from them and experience.

judgment call, *slang.* a decision based on experience, especially a judgment that solves a serious problem in which the data are inconclusive.

jugu-, a combining form meaning 'throat or neck.'

jugular fossa, a deep depression on the inside of one of the large bones forming the lower head (petrosa of the temporal bone).

jugular process, a portion of the cuplike bone (occipital bone) at the back of the skull.

jugular pulse, a pulse in the jugular vein.

jugular venous pressure (JVP), blood pressure in the jugular vein, which reflects the blood volume and pressure in the right side of the heart. JVP is estimated by tilting the patient's head and observing the neck veins. With a high JVP the neck veins may be swollen as high as the angle of the jaw.

juice, any fluid secreted by the tissues of animals or plants. In humans, the word often refers to

juice of the digestive glands. Kinds of juices include **gastric juice, intestinal juice,** and **pancreatic juice.**

jumentous, having a strong animal smell, especially that of a horse. It is used to describe the urine smell in some disease conditions.

junctional tachycardia, an automatic heart rhythm of greater than 100 beats/minute, emanating from the AV junction. It is often caused by digitalis toxicity.

junction nevus, a hairless, flat or slightly raised, brown skin blemish. A junction nevus may be found anywhere on the body. All nevi of the palms and soles and all pigmented nevi in early childhood are of this type. Cancerous change may be signaled by increase in size, hardness or darkening, bleeding, or the appearance of darkening around the nevus. Junction nevi with these changes and lesions found in areas subject to trauma should be removed.

junctura cartilaginea. See **cartilaginous joint.**

junctura fibrosa. See **fibrous joint.**

junctura synovialis. See **synovial joint.**

jungian psychology. See **analytic psychology.**

Junin fever. See **Argentine hemorrhagic fever.**

junk, *slang.* heroin.

juvenile, 1. a young person; child. **2.** referring to, or suitable for a young person; youthful. **3.** physiologically immature. **4.** denoting psychological or intellectual immaturity; childish.

juvenile alveolar rhabdomyosarcoma, a quickly growing muscle tumor with a grave prognosis, in children and adolescents, chiefly in the extremities.

juvenile angiofibroma. See **nasopharyngeal angiofibroma.**

juvenile delinquency, antisocial or illegal acts by children or adolescents that cannot be controlled by parents, endanger others, and concern law enforcement agencies. Such behavior is marked by aggression, destruction, hostility, and cruelty. It occurs more often in boys than girls. Causes are poor parent-child relations, especially parental rejection and apathy, and an unstable family life where discipline is lax, erratic, or overly strict, or involves harsh physical punishment. Punitive treatments, mainly jails and reform schools, usually worsen the situation. Foster home placement, work and recreational programs, and counseling have been more successful. Behavior therapy and other forms of psychotherapy, often with the parents and the child, are also used. See also **antisocial personality disorder, behavior disorder.**

juvenile delinquent, a person who acts illegally and who is not old enough to be treated as an adult under the laws of the community. Also called **juvenile offender.**

juvenile diabetes. See **insulin-dependent diabetes mellitus.**

juvenile kyphosis. See **Scheuermann's disease.**

juvenile lentigo. See **lentigo.**

juvenile-onset diabetes. See **insulin-dependent diabetes mellitus.**

juvenile periodontitis, an abnormal state that may affect the dental alveoli, especially in children and adolescents. It is marked by severe pocketing and bone loss. Formerly called **periodontosis.**

juvenile rheumatoid arthritis, a form of rheumatoid arthritis, usually affecting the larger joints of children under 16 years of age. Skeletal development may be impaired. Treatments are analgesia, anti-inflammatory drugs, and rest. The recovery rate in this form is better than in the adult forms of rheumatoid arthritis. Also called **Still's disease.**

juvenile spinal muscular atrophy, a disorder beginning in childhood causing muscle wasting. It usually begins in the legs and pelvis. Also called **Wohlfart-Kugelberg-Welander disease.**

juvenile xanthogranuloma, a skin problem marked by groups of yellow, red, or brown papules or nodules on the arms and legs, and in some cases on the eyeball, meninges, and testes. The lesions often appear in infancy or early childhood and disappear in a few years.

juxtaposition, the placement of objects end to end or side by side.

K

K, symbol for **potassium.**

-kacin, a combining form for antibiotics from a certain bacterium *(Streptomyces kanamyceticus).*

Kahn test, 1. a blood test for syphilis. A blood sample from a patient stands overnight in a mixture with a test chemical. If a white substance settles out, it shows a positive sign for syphilis. **2.** a test for the presence of cancer by measuring the amount of a protein in a blood sample.

kakke disease. See **beriberi.**

kala-azar /kä′lə-əär′/, a disease carried to humans, particularly children, by the bite of the sand fly. Kala-azar occurs primarily in Asia, parts of Africa, the U.S.S.R., several South and Central American countries, and the Mediterranean region. Symptoms include anemia, enlarged liver and spleen, fever, and weight loss. Patients with kala-azar are likely to develop other infections. Untreated, the disease has an extremely high death rate. Treatment includes drugs, blood transfusions for anemia, bed rest, and adequate nutrition. Also called **Assam fever, black fever, dumdum fever, ponos, visceral leishmaniasis.** See also **leishmaniasis.**

kalemia, the presence of potassium in the blood.

kaliuresis /kal′iyŏŏrē′sis/, the excretion of potassium in the urine

Kallmann's syndrome, a condition characterized by the absence of the sense of smell and by poorly developed reproductive glands.

kanamycin sulfate, an antibiotic given to treat certain severe infections and infections resistant to other antibiotics.

★CAUTION: Known allergy to this drug or to other related antibiotics prohibits its use. Drugs that can cause damage to the ears may interact. It is used with caution in patients having impaired kidney function and in the elderly.

★ADVERSE EFFECTS: Among the more serious side effects are kidney disorders, loss of hearing and sense of balance, paralysis, and allergic reactions.

Kanner's syndrome, a form of a mental disorder (psychosis) affecting infants and children that begins in the first 30 months of life. It is marked by abnormal emotional, social, and speech development (infantile autism). The child avoids eye contact and generally fails to develop social relations. He or she develops many rituals, repeating the same acts or movements over and over. There may be mental retardation and language disorders. Treat-

ment may include psychotherapy and special education, depending on the child's intelligence.

Kantrex, a trademark for an antibiotic (kanamycin sulfate).

Kanulase, a trademark for a drug that reduces intestinal gas.

Kaochlor, a trademark for a mineral replacement remedy (potassium chloride).

kaodzera. See **Rhodesian trypanosomiasis.**

kaolin /kā′əlin/, a fine white clay taken orally to treat diarrhea, often in combination with a softening agent, pectin. Kaolin in an ointment base is also used on the skin as an adsorbent and protective cream.

Kaon, a trademark for a mineral replacement remedy (potassium chloride).

Kaopectate, a trademark for a drug to treat diarrhea containing an adsorbent (kaolin) and a softening agent (pectin).

Kaposi's sarcoma /kap′əsēz/, a cancer that begins as soft, brownish or purple pimples on the feet and slowly spreads through the skin to the lymph nodes and abdominal organs. It occurs most often in men and is occasionally associated with AIDS (aquired immune deficiency syndrome), diabetes, lymph cancer, or other disorders. Radiation therapy and drugs are used to treat the cancer. Also called **idiopathic multiple pigmented hemorrhagic sarcoma, multiple idiopathic hemorrhagic sarcoma.**

Kaposi's varicelliform eruption. See **eczema herpeticum.**

karaya powder, a dried form of a gummy plant secretion used as a bulk laxative. Symptoms, such as pain, are reduced in patients with irritable bowel disease or with other intestinal problems. Because of its ability to absorb water, karaya powder may also be used in treating acute diarrhea. Also used as a drying agent in preparing the skin for dressings around decubitus ulcers.

karyenchyma. See **karyolymph.**

karyogamy /ker′ē-og′əmē/, the fusion of cell nuclei, as in fertilization. **–karyogamic,** *adj.*

karyogenesis /ker′ē-ōjen′əsis/, the formation and development of the cell nucleus. **–karyogenetic,** *adj.*

karyolymph /ker′ē-əlimf′/, the clear, fluid substance of the nucleus. Also called **karyenchyma.**

karyolysis /ker′ē-ol′isis/, the dissolution of the cell nucleus. It occurs normally, both as a form of cell death and during the generation of new cells.

karyometry, the measurement of the nucleus of a cell. **–karyometric,** *adj.*

karyomorphism, the shape or form of a cell nucleus, especially that of the leukocyte (white blood cell). **–karyomorphic,** *adj.*

karyon /ker'ē·on/, the nucleus of a cell.

karyophage /ker'ē·ōfāj'/, a parasite within a cell that destroys the nucleus of the cell it infects.

karyopyknosis /ker'ē·ōpiknō'sis/, the state of a cell in which the nucleus has shrunk and the genetic material has condensed into solid masses, as in skin cells.

karyosome /ker'ē·əsōm'/, a dense, irregular mass of genetic material in the cell nucleus that may be confused with the nucleolus. Also called **chromatin nucleolus, chromocenter, false nucleolus, prochromosome.**

karyospherical /ker'ē·ōfer'ikə/, pertaining to a spherically shaped nucleus.

karyostasis /ker'ē·os'təsis/, the resting stage of the nucleus between cell division. See also **interphase. –karyostatic,** *adj.*

karyotheca /ker'ē·əthē'kə/, the membrane that encloses a cell nucleus. **–karyothecal,** *adj.*

karyotype /ker'ē·ətīp'/, **1.** the total portrait of the chromosomes in a body cell of an individual or species, as photographed through a microscope lens. It shows the number, form, size, and arrangement of chromosomes within the nucleus. **2.** a diagram of the chromosomes in a body cell of an individual or species, arranged in pairs in descending order of size. See also **chromosome, Denver classification. –karyotypic,** *adj.*

Kasabach method /Kas'əbak/, (in radiology) a way to position a patient for an x-ray of the top of the second vertebra in the neck (odontoid process).

katadidymus /kat'ədid'əməs/, twins whose bodies are joined in the lower portion of the body and separated at the top.

Kawasaki disease. See **mucocutaneous lymph node syndrome.**

KayCiel, a trademark for a mineral replacement drug (potassium chloride).

Kayser-Fleischer ring /kī'zərfli'shər/, a gray-green to red-gold colored ring at the outer margin of the cornea of the eye. It is a sign of Wilson's disease, a rare disorder caused by a defect in the body's use of copper. See also **Wilson's disease.**

K cell. See **null cell.**

kefir /kef'ər/, a slightly bubbly acid beverage prepared from the milk of cows, sheep, or goats through fermentation. It is an important source of the bacteria necessary in the gastrointestinal tract to synthesize vitamin K. Also spelled **kephir.**

Keflex, a trademark for an antibiotic (cephalexin).

Kefzol, a trademark for an antibiotic (cefazolin sodium).

Kegel exercises, a system of exercises in which a woman strengthens the muscles of her pelvic diaphragm and pubic area, particularly after childbirth. The exercises involve the familiar muscular squeezing action required to stop the urinary stream while voiding. The action is performed in a systematic way to increase her ability to contract the muscles of the vaginal opening or to improve retention of urine. When the woman can cause the contraction, she is asked to hold it for 6 to 10 seconds, and then allow the muscles to relax completely. Performance of the next step requires four or five repetitions of the exercise in a series three to four times a day. The rapidity with which a woman can, during voiding, close off the urinary stream is taken as a measure of the strength and tone of her pelvic muscles. Ideally, she should be able to perform the action completely and almost instantly. Also called **pubococcygeus exercises.**

Keith-Flack node. See **sinoatrial node.**

Keith-Wegener-Barker classification system, a method for classifying high blood pressure (hypertension) by observing changes in the retina of the eye. The stages are classified into four groups; group 4 is the most severe.

Kellgren's syndrome /kel'grinz/, a form of osteoarthritis affecting the joints of the hands, feet, knees, and spine. Also called **erosive osteoarthritis.**

keloid /kē'loid/, overgrowth of scar tissue at the site of a wound of the skin. The new tissue is elevated, rounded, and firm, with irregular, clawlike margins. Young women and blacks are particularly liable to develop keloids. Most keloids flatten and become less noticeable over a period of years. Treatment may include solid carbon dioxide, liquid nitrogen, hormone injections, radiation, and surgery. Also spelled **cheloid.**

keloidosis /kē'loidō'sis/, habitual or multiple formation of keloids. Also spelled **cheloidosis.**

Kelvin scale (K), an absolute temperature scale calculated from the point at which molecules appear to stop moving, $-273°C$. To convert Celcius degrees to Kelvin, add 273.

Kemadrin, a trademark for a skeletal muscle relaxant (procyclidine hydrochloride).

Kempner rice-fruit diet. See **rice diet.**

Kenalog, a trademark for an adrenal hormone (triamcinolone acetonide).

Kennedy classification, a method of classifying conditions of missing teeth and partial dentures, based on the position of the spaces between the remaining teeth.

Kenny treatment. See **Sister Kenny's treatment.**

kenophobia /kē'nō-/, an abnormal fear of large and open spaces. Also called **agoraphobia.**

Kenya fever. See **Marseilles fever.**

kerasin, a substance in brain tissue that consists of a fatty acid, a sugar, and a type of alcohol (sphingosine).

keratectomy, surgical removal of a portion of the cornea of the eye. The tissue is cut out using local anesthesia. An antibiotic and a light dressing are then applied. New corneal tissue grows rapidly, filling a small cut area in about 60 hours.

keratic /kərat′ik/, pertaining to the cornea.

keratic precipitate, a group of cells that form on the surface of the cornea after injury or inflammation, sometimes obscuring vision.

keratin /ker′ətin/, a fibrous, sulfur-containing protein, the primary component of human skin, hair, nails, and tooth enamel. Gastric juice of the stomach does not dissolve the protein. For this reason it is often used as a coating for pills that must pass through the stomach unchanged to be dissolved in the intestines.

keratinization, a process by which skin cells exposed to the environment lose their moisture and are replaced by horny tissue.

keratinocyte, a cell of the outer layer of the skin (epidermis) that produces keratin and other proteins. These cells constitute 95% of the epidermis.

keratitis /ker′ətī′tis/, any inflammation of the cornea of the eye.

keratoacanthoma /ker′ətō·ak′anthō′mə/, *pl.* **keratoacanthomas, keratoacanthomata,** a rapidly growing, noncancerous, flesh-colored pimple with a central plug of keratin. The lesion usually occurs on the face or the back of hands and arms. It disappears spontaneously in 4 to 6 months, leaving a slightly depressed scar.

keratoconjunctivitis /ker′ətōkənjungk′tivī′tis/, inflammation of the cornea and the conjunctiva (mucous membrane lining the eyelid).

keratoconjunctivitis sicca, dryness of the cornea because of a lack of tear secretions. The corneal surface appears dull and rough, and the eye feels gritty and irritated.

keratoconus /ker′ətōkō′nəs/, a conelike bulge on the cornea of the eye. More common in females, it may result in severe astigmatism. Contact lenses usually restore visual acuity.

keratoderma blennorrhagica, the development of callus and cornlike lesions of the palms, soles, and nails. It occurs in some patients with Reiter's syndrome.

keratohyalin, a substance in the epidermis (outer layer of skin) that contributes to the functional maturity of keratin in skin, hair, and nails. See also **keratin.**

keratolysis /ker′ətol′sis/, an abnormal loosening and shedding of the outer layer of the skin, which usually involves the palms of the hands or soles of the feet. It may occur as a birth defect in which the skin is shed at periodic intervals. –**keratolytic,** *adj.*

keratomalacia /ker′ətōmələ′shə/, an eye condition characterized by dryness and ulceration of the cornea, resulting from severe vitamin A deficiency. Diseases such as ulcerative colitis or cystic fibrosis may cause the deficiency. Infants and children who are given diluted bottle-feeding formula, or who are fed skimmed milk because of an allergy, are also likely to develop the eye disorder. Symptoms include night blindness, sensitivity to light, and swelling and redness of the eyelids. Without adequate treatment, the cornea eventually softens and develops holes, resulting in blindness. Treatment consists of vitamin A supplements. An adequate diet containing whole milk and foods rich in vitamin A prevents the condition. See also **vitamin A.**

keratomycosis linguae. See **parasitic glossitis.**

keratopathy /ker′ətop′əthē/, any noninflammatory disease of the cornea. Compare **keratitis.**

keratoplasty, eye surgery in which a cloudy portion of the cornea is removed.

keratosis /ker′ətō′sis/, any skin condition in which there is overgrowth and thickening of the outer skin layers. Kinds of keratosis include **actinic keratosis, keratosis senilis,** and **seborrheic keratosis.** –**keratotic,** *adj.*

keratosis follicularis, a skin disorder characterized by pimples that merge to form dark, crusted, wartlike patches. These growths may spread widely, ulcerate, and become covered with pus. Treatment includes large oral doses of vitamin A, vitamin A acid skin cream, and adrenal hormone drugs. Also called **Darier's disease.**

kerion /kir′ē·on/, an inflamed, boggy tumor that develops as a reaction to a fungus infection of the skin. It may accompany ringworm of the scalp. The lesion heals within a short time without treatment.

Kerley lines, (in radiology) lines that appear on chest x-rays and are associated with certain disease conditions, as congestive heart failure. They are several centimeters in length and may point in many directions.

kernicterus, an abnormal accumulation in central nervous system tissues of bilirubin, a yellowish pigment normally present in bile. The cause is an excessive amount of the pigment circulating in blood. See also **hyperbilirubinemia of the newborn.**

Kernig's sign, a diagnostic sign for meningitis, an inflammation of the brain or spinal cord. An attempt by the patient to extend the leg completely after the knee has been bent causes pain in back of the leg.

kerosene poisoning, the effects of swallowing kerosene or breathing its fumes. Symptoms after swallowing kerosene include drowsiness, fever, a rapid heart beat, and trembling. Vomiting should not be induced. Severe lung inflammation will occur if the fluid is inhaled. Treatment to retard absorption of kerosene in the stomach usually includes 1 or 2 ounces of vegetable oil. A physician should flush out the stomach with a catheter, using several quarts of water. A salt water cathartic follows. Treatment for poisoning by inhalation includes fresh air, oxygen, and emergency resuscitation if necessary. See also **petroleum distillate poisoning.**

ketamine hydrochloride /kē'təmēn/, a general anesthetic administered by injection. It can be useful for brief, minor surgery and to relax the patient before general inhalation anesthesia. However, its use can lead to psychic disorders following surgery.

ketoacidosis /kē'tō·as'idō'sis/, acidosis, an excessive level of acid in the blood, accompanied by ketosis, an increase of ketones in blood. Ketones are substances normally processed by the liver from fats. The condition may occur as a complication of diabetes mellitus. Symptoms are a fruity odor of the breath, mental confusion, breathing distress, nausea, vomiting, dehydration, weight loss, and, if untreated, coma. Emergency treatment includes administrating insulin, intravenous fluids, and correcting the body's acid-base balance. Compare **insulin shock.** See also **diabetes mellitus, ketosis.** **–ketoacidotic,** *adj.*

ketoaciduria /kē'tō·as'idōōr'ē·ə/, presence in the urine of excessive amounts of ketones, substances processed by the liver from fats. It results from uncontrolled diabetes mellitus, starvation, or any other condition in which fats are consumed as body fuel instead of carbohydrates. Also called **ketonuria.** See also **Acetest, ketosis. –ketoaciduric,** *adj.*

ketoconazole, an antifungal agent prescribed for the treatment of candidiasis, coccidioidomycosis, histoplasmosis, and other fungal diseases.
★CAUTION: Known allergy to this drug prohibits its use. It should not be used for fungal meningitis.
★ADVERSE EFFECTS: The most serious side effects are liver disorders.

ketogenic diet /kē'tojen'ik/, a diet that is high in fats and low in carbohydrates.

ketone bodies, a group name for ketones, substances produced in the body through a normal change fats undergo in the liver. They are used as fuel in muscles. Excessive production of these bodies leads to their excretion in urine, as in diabetes mellitus. Also called **acetone bodies.**

ketonemia, the presence of substances produced by the liver (ketones) in the blood. It causes a fruity breath odor.

ketosis /kitō'sis/, an abnormal accumulation of ketones in body tissues and fluid. This condition occurs in starvation, occasionally in pregnancy, and, most frequently, in diabetes mellitus. Symptoms are ketones in urine, loss of potassium in urine, and a fruity odor on the breath. Untreated, ketosis may progress to ketoacidosis, coma, and death. See also **diabetes**

mellitus, ketoacidosis, ketone bodies, starvation. **–ketotic,** *adj.*

17-ketosteroid, an adrenal gland hormone commonly measured in the blood and urine to help diagnose Addison's disease, Cushing's syndrome, stress, and endocrine problems associated with precocious puberty, feminization in men, and excessive hair growth.

Kew Gardens spotted fever. See **rickettsialpox.**

key points of control, areas of the body that can be handled by a physical therapist to reduce spasms throughout the body and to guide the patient's active movements. The key points are the shoulder and the hips.

kg, abbreviation for **kilogram.**

kidney, one of a pair of bean-shaped urinary organs in the back of the abdomen on each side of the spine. The tops of the kidneys are on a level with the border of the lowest ribs. In most individuals, the right kidney is slightly lower on the right side of the body than on the left because of the location of the liver above it. Each kidney is about 11 cm long, 6 cm wide, and 2.5 cm thick. In men, each kidney weighs from 125 to 170 g; in women, each kidney weighs from 115 to 155 g. In the newborn, the kidneys are about three times as large in proportion to the body weight as in the adult. The kidneys produce and eliminate urine through a complex system with more than 2 million tiny filters (nephrons). The nephrons filter blood under high pressure, removing urea, salts, and other soluble wastes. These wastes are then sent from the body as urine. The kidneys return the purified fluid to the blood, thus helping to maintain the water balance of the body. More than 2,500 pints of blood pass through the kidneys every day, entering the kidneys through arteries and leaving through the veins. All of the blood in the body passes through the kidneys about 20 times every hour but only about one-fifth is filtered by the nephrons during that period. Hormones control the function of the kidneys in regulating the water content of the body. The pituitary gland produces the most important, the antidiuretic hormone (ADH). ADH stimulates the reabsorption of water into the blood. If water intake is not enough to make up for the water lost in perspiration and in breathing, the pituitary gland releases more ADH, thus reducing the amount of water released in urine. If the blood is too dilute, the pituitary gland reduces the secretion of ADH, causing a larger flow of water into urine.

kidney cancer, a cancer of the filtration tissue of the kidney or of the renal pelvis, the urine-collecting system attached to the kidney. Cancer of the filtration tissue accounts for 80% of kidney tumors, occurring twice as frequently in men as in women. Cancers of the renal pelvis are equally frequent in men and women.

Causes identified with the disease are exposure to chemicals such as benzene, tobacco smoke, and the use of drugs containing phenacetin. Characteristic symptoms include bloody urine, back pain, and fever. Diagnosis may be made from urinalysis, ultrasound imaging, x-ray examination, and microscopic studies of cells. Surgery to remove the cancerous kidney is the usual treatment. Neighboring tissues that are no longer needed, such as the tubes leading to the bladder, may also be taken out. The remaining kidney, if healthy, can generally make up for the loss. Following surgery, radiation and anticancer drugs may be used to destroy any cancer cells remaining. See also **ultrasound imaging, Wilms' tumor.**

kidney dialysis. See **hemodialysis.**

kidney disease, any of a large group of conditions including infectious, inflammatory, obstructive, circulatory, and cancerous disorders of the kidney. Characteristics of kidney disease are bloody urine, persistent protein in urine, pus in urine, edema, difficult urination, and pain in the back. Specific symptoms vary with the type of disorder. For example, bloody urine with severe, colicky pain suggests obstruction by a kidney stone. Bloody urine without pain may indicate kidney cancer. Protein in urine is generally a sign of disease in the filtration units of the kidney. Pus in urine indicates infectious disease. Laboratory tests and other procedures are necessary to diagnose the specific kidney disease. Treatment depends on the type of kidney disease diagnosed. Some forms may lead to kidney failure, coma, and death unless hemodialysis is started. See also **glomerulonephritis, hemodialysis, nephrotic syndrome, renal failure, urinary calculus.**

kidney failure, *informal.* renal failure.

kidney machine. See **hemodialysis.**

kidney stone. See **renal calculus.**

Kielland rotation, an obstetric operation in which forceps are used in turning the head of the fetus to a position that will make childbirth easier, especially when the active stage of labor has been interrupted. Because Kielland rotation may increase the chance of harm to the mother and to the baby, cesarean section is often preferred. See also **forceps delivery, obstetric forceps.**

Kiesselbach's plexus /kē'səlbäkhs', -bäks'/, an intersection of small, fragile arteries and veins located in the skin on top of the wall dividing the nostrils (nasal septum).

killer cell. See **null cell.**

kilo-, a combining form meaning 'one thousand,' as in kilocalorie or kilogram.

kilogram (kg) /kil'əgram/, a unit for the measurement of mass in the metric system. One kilogram is equal to 1,000 grams or to 2.2046 pounds avoirdupois.

kilogram calorie. See **calorie.**

Kimmelstiel-Wilson's disease. See **intercapillaryglomerulosclerosis.**

kind firmness, (in psychology) a direct, clear, and confident approach to a patient in which rules and regulations are calmly stated in response to misbehavior and requests.

kinematics /kin'əmat'iks, kī-'/, the study of the motion of the body without regard to the forces acting to produce the motion. Kinematics considers the motions of all body parts relative to the part involved in the motion. For example, the movements of the fingers are considered in relation to the midline of the hand, not the midline of the body. The most common types of motions studied in kinematics are flexion, extension, rotation, and contraction and relaxation of muscles. Kinematics is especially important in the diagnosis and treatment of joint disorders. Also spelled **cinematics.** Compare **kinetics.**

kinesic behavior, movements or actions used for communication that serve to achieve or maintain bonds of attachment between people.

kinesics /kinē'siks/, the study of body position and movement in communication between people. It is used especially in mental-health examinations. See also **body language.**

kinesiologic electromyography /kinē'sē·ōloj'ik/, the study of muscle activity involved in body movements.

kinesiology /kinē'sē·ol'əjē, kī-/, the scientific study of muscular activity and of the anatomy, physiology, and mechanics of body movement.

kinesthesia /kin'esthē'zhə, the awareness of one's own body parts, weight, and movement.

kinesthetic memory, the mental recollection of movement, weight, resistance, and position of the body or its parts.

kinetics /kinet'iks, kī-/, the study of the forces that produce, stop, or modify motions of the body. Newton's first and third laws of inertia are especially applicable to kinetics. Newton's first law states that bodies at rest tend to stay at rest and that bodies in motion tend to keep moving. Newton's third law states that action and reaction are equal in magnitude but opposite in direction. These two laws are applied to forces produced by muscles that act on body joints. The reaction forces of the muscles contribute to the balance and motion of the body. Compare **kinematics.**

kinetotherapeutic bath /kinet'ōthur'əpyoo'tik/, a bath in which underwater exercises are performed to strengthen weak or partially paralyzed muscles.

kin group, family members, whether related by blood or marriage.

Kirklin staging system, a system for predicting the outcome of colon cancer, based on how far the tumor has spread into the bowel area. See also **cancer staging, Duke's classification, TNM.**

Kirschner's wire /kursh'nərz/, a threaded or smooth metallic wire used in mending fractures or for skeletal traction.

Kite method, (in radiology) a technique for positioning the leg of a patient born with a clubfoot for x-ray examination.

kiting, *informal.* illegal altering of a drug prescription to indicate that more of a drug was prescribed than actually ordered by a physician. Kiting may be done by a patient seeking greater quantities of drugs, especially narcotics, or may be done by a pharmacist to increase reimbursement from a third party, such as an involved insurance company.

Klebsiella /kleb'zē·el'ə/, a kind of bacteria that causes several respiratory diseases, including bronchitis, sinusitis, and some forms of pneumonia.

kleeblattschädel deformity syndrome. See **cloverleaf skull deformity.**

Kleine-Levin syndrome /klīn'ləvən'/, a disorder often associated with psychotic conditions, characterized by abnormal drowsiness, hunger, and excessive activity. Episodes of sleep may last for several hours or days and are followed by confusion on awakening. There is no specific treatment. Compare **narcolepsy.**

kleptolagnia /klep'tōlag'nē·ə/, sexual excitement or satisfaction produced by stealing.

kleptomania, a neurosis characterized by an abnormal, uncontrollable, and repeated urge to steal. Objects are not taken for their monetary value, immediate need, or use but for their symbolic meaning, which may be associated with an emotional conflict. The objects are usually given away, returned secretly, or kept and hidden. People who have the condition experience an increased sense of tension before committing the theft and intense satisfaction during the act. Afterward, they show signs of depression, guilt, and anxiety over the possibility of being arrested. In less severe cases, the impulse is expressed by a continuous borrowing of objects and not returning them. Treatment consists of psychotherapy to find the basic emotional problems. Also spelled **cleptomania. –kleptomaniac,** *n.*

Klinefelter's syndrome /klīn'feltərz/, an abnormal condition of male sexual characteristics in which the body cells contain one or more extra X chromosomes (female sex chromosomes). Characteristics include small, firm testicles; long legs; femalelike breasts, and varicose veins. The severity of the abnormalities increases with greater numbers of X chromosomes. The most common abnormality is a 47 XXY karyotype. The man may appear generally normal, although infertile. Men with the karyotype XXXXY have severe physical mal-

formations and mental retardation. See also **karyotype.**

Klippel-Feil syndrome. See **congenital short neck syndrome.**

K-Lor, a trademark for a mineral replacement drug (potassium chloride).

Klorvess, a trademark for a mineral supplement (potassium chloride).

Klumpke's palsy /kloomp'kēz/, a wasting and paralysis of the forearm that is present at birth. The condition may be accompanied by other disorders due to involvement of nerves that regulate body functions that are not consciously controlled. Also called *Dejerine-Klumpke's paralysis.*

K-Lyte/Cl, a trademark for a mineral replacement drug (potassium chloride).

kneading, a grasping, rolling, and pressing movement used in massaging the muscles. See also **massage.**

knee, a joint with a group of parts that connects the thigh with the lower leg. It consists of three rounded bone surfaces (condyloid joints), 12 bands of fibrous tissue (ligaments), 13 fluid-filled sacs (bursae), and the kneecap (patella). The largest bursa is the prepatellar (kneecap) bursa between the patellar ligament and the skin. The painful condition 'housemaid's knee' is caused by inflammation of the prepatellar bursa. The knee may easily be injured by blows, sudden stops, and turns because of the lack of protection from surrounding muscles. Torn ligaments of the knee joint are common among athletes and produce a variety of signs and symptoms. These include fluid surrounding the knee joint, differences in shape, tenderness on touching, black-and-blue spots, weakness of the joint, and crackling noises. Although x-ray examination may reveal abnormal bone positions resulting from torn ligaments, the most serious knee ligament injuries are not visible on x-ray films. Treatment involves suctioning excessive joint fluid, compressing the joint to control swelling, and using tape, or splints. Surgery may be necessary to repair severely torn ligaments. Torn cartilege joint cushions (menisci) are also common sports injuries and can cause severe pain, swelling, and greatly reduced motion. Surgery may be required. Arthritis commonly affects the knee, especially in elderly individuals, and requires special care. See also **ligamental tears.**

knee-ankle interaction, one of the major factors that controls leg motion in walking. It helps to minimize the change in the body's center of gravity during walking. The diagnosis and treatment of various bone and joint diseases often includes observing knee-ankle interaction. Compare **knee-hip flexion, lateral pelvic displacement, pelvic rotation, pelvic tilt.**

kneecap. See **patella.**

knee-chest position. See **genupectoral position.**

knee-hip flexion, a body movement that allows the passage of body weight over the supporting leg during walking. Knee-hip flexion may be used in the diagnosis and treatment of various bone and joint diseases. Compare **knee-ankle interaction, lateral pelvic displacement, pelvic rotation, pelvic tilt.**

knee-jerk reflex. See **patellar reflex.**

knee joint, the complex, hinged joint at the knee that, with its ligaments, permits flexion, extension, and, in certain positions, rotation of the leg. It is a common site for sprains and dislocations. Also called **articulatio genus.** See also **knee.**

knee replacement, the surgical insertion of a hinged artificial joint. It relieves pain and restores motion to a knee affected by arthritis or injury. The diseased bone surfaces are removed and a two-piece metallic hinge is cemented into the cavities of the upper and lower leg bones (femur and tibia). After surgery, the knee is held in position, usually with a plaster cast. Physical therapy includes exercise and whirlpool baths. The mobility and range of motion of the joint increase slowly. See also **arthroplasty, hip replacement, osteoarthritis, plastic surgery.**

knee sling, a leg support in sling form used under the knee in conjunction with a traction device for holding, positioning, and lining up the lower legs (Russell's traction).

knife needle, a surgical knife with a needle point, used to remove a cataract and in other eye operations, as glaucoma surgery.

knock-knee. See **genu valgum.**

Knoop hardness test, a method of measuring tooth surface hardness by resistance of the tooth to a tool made of diamond.

knot, lacing together the surgical ligature or suture ends so that the material used, such as silk or wire, remains in place.

Koch's postulates /kōks/, the conditions for establishing that a microorganism (bacteria or virus) causes a particular disease. They are: (1) the microorganism must be observed in all cases of the disease; (2) the microorganism must be isolated and grown in a pure culture medium; (3) microorganisms from the pure culture must reproduce the disease when inoculated in a test animal; (4) the same kind of microorganism must be recovered from the experimentally diseased animal. See also **medium.**

Koebner phenomenon /kōb'nər/, skin lesions that develop at the site of an injury resulting in psoriasis, or a similar kind of skin disease. See also **psoriasis.**

koilonychia /koi'lōnik'ē·ə/, spoon nails; a condition in which fingernails are thin and curved inwardly from side to side. Usually inherited, it may also occur with blood disorders, such as iron deficiency anemia and Raynaud's phenomenon.

Kopan's needle, a long needle used to locate the position of a breast tumor on an x-ray. The needle is inserted into the approximate location of the tumor and is left in place while x-rays are taken so that it can be moved if necessary. In some cases the location of the tumor is further identified for the surgeon by injecting a colored dye.

Koplik's spots /kop'liks/, small red spots with bluish-white centers found on the inside of the mouth of persons with measles. The rash of measles usually erupts 1 or 2 days after the appearance of Koplik's spots.

Korotkoff sounds /kôrot'kôf/, sounds heard during a blood pressure reading with a sphygmomanometer (blood pressure gauge) and stethoscope. As air is released from the gauge cuff, pressure on the artery is reduced. Blood can then be heard pulsing through the artery. See also **blood pressure, diastole, sphygmomanometer, systole.**

Korsakoff's psychosis /kôr'səkôfs/, a form of memory loss often seen in chronic alcoholics. The person is usually disoriented and gives false information to conceal the condition. The cause can often be traced to a deficiency of B complex vitamins, especially thiamine and B_{12}. Compare **Wernicke's encephalopathy.**

kosher /kō'shər/, conforming to or prepared in accordance with the dietary or ceremonial laws of Judaism.

Krabbe's disease. See **galactosyl ceramide lipidosis.**

Kraske position /kras'kə/, a position used for rectal or kidney surgery in which the patient lies face down with hips elevated.

kraurosis /krôrō'sis/, a thickening and shriveling of the skin. See also **kraurosis vulvae.**

kraurosis vulvae, a skin disease of aged women characterized by dryness, itching, and atrophy of the vulva. The condition often leads to cancer. See also **lichen sclerosis et atrophicus.**

Krause's corpuscles, nerve endings that are sensitive to temperature. They are found in the outer lining of the eye, mucous membranes of the lips and tongue, the penis and clitoris, and membranes of certain joints.

Krebs' citric acid cycle /krebz/, a series of enzyme reactions in which the body uses carbohydrates, proteins, and fats to yield carbon dioxide, water, and energy for organ functions. Also called **tricarboxylic acid cycle.** See also **acetylcoenzyme A.**

Krukenberg's tumor /krōō'kənbərgz/, a tumor of the ovary that has spread from cancer cells of the stomach or intestines. Also called **carcinoma mucocellulare.**

KS, abbreviation for *Kaposi's sarcoma*

Kuchendorf method, (in radiology) a technique for positioning a patient for x-rays of the knee-cap (patella).

Kulchitsky cell carcinoma. See **carcinoid.**

Kulchitsky's cell. See **argentaffin cell.**

Küntscher nail /kōōnt′shər/, a stainless steel nail used in bone surgery to repair fractures of the long bones, especially the femur, the long bone of the thigh. Also called **Küntscher intramedullary nail.**

Kupffer's cells /kŏōp′fərz/, liver cells that filter bacteria and other small, foreign proteins out of the blood.

kuru /kōō′rōō/, a slow, fatal viral infection of the central nervous system seen only in natives of the New Guinea Highlands. Symptoms, which include loss of mental ability, speech and vision problems, and paralysis, may not appear for 30 or more years after contact with the virus. Death usually occurs within months after the first symptoms. The disease is believed to be the result of cannibalism. Incidence of the disease has decreased with the reduction of cannibalism.

Kussmaul breathing /kōōs′moul/, abnormally deep, very rapid breathing with sighing. It occurs in diabetic acidosis, a condition of too-much acid in the blood.

Kussmaul's sign, 1. a pulse that rises in rate when exhaling and falls when inhaling. It occurs in certain heart and chest disorders. **2.** convulsions and coma associated with a disorder of the stomach and intestines caused by swallowing a poison.

kwashiorkor /kwä′shē·ôr′kôr/, an early childhood malnutrition disease caused by severe protein deficiency and found mostly in Africa. Because calorie-rich starches such as breadfruit are available, the child may not lose weight. Eventually the following symptoms occur: retarded growth, changes in skin and hair pigmentation, diarrhea, loss of appetite, fluid accumulation, anemia, liver failure, and abnormal fiber growth in body tissues. A skimmed milk formula must be used in treating kwashiorkor. Fats are difficult for the child to digest. Additional foods are then given until a full, well-balanced diet is achieved. Also called **infantile pellagra, malignant malnutrition.** See also **marasmic kwashiorkor, marasmus.**

Kwell, a trademark for a drug that destroys lice and mites (gamma benzene hexachloride).

Kyasanur forest disease, a virus infection transmitted to humans by the bite of a tick that lives on animals in western India. Symptoms include fever, headache, muscle ache, cough, and abdominal and eye pain. Treatment is limited to relieving symptoms.

kymography /kēmog′rəfē/, a method for recording motion pictures of body organs, as the heart and large blood vessels.

kyphoscoliosis /kī′fŏskō′lē·ō′sis/, a forward and to-the-side, humplike curvature of the spine, often associated with cor pulmonale, a heart disorder. Compare **kyphosis, scoliosis. –kyphoscoliotic,** *adj.*

kyphosis /kīfō′sis/, a forward, humplike curvature of the spine. Kyphosis may be caused by rickets or tuberculosis of the spine. If the curvature progresses there may be moderate back pain. Treatment includes spine-stretching exercises and sleeping without a pillow, with a board under the mattress. A back brace may be used for severe kyphosis, or surgery may be required. **–kyphotic,** *adj.*

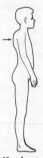

Kyphosis

L

L, symbol for **liter.**

label, a substance, usually radioactive, with a special attraction for a specific organ, tissue, or cell, in which it may become deposited. The radioactivity gives a signal that can be followed through various body processes, making it useful in diagnosis, as in locating a tumor.

labeling, providing information on a drug, food, device, or cosmetic to the purchaser or user. The information may be given as printing on a carton, adhesive label, or package insert. Regulations for labeling are decided by the Food and Drug Administration. The label must contain directions for use, unless such directions are exempted by regulation, as well as warnings. It may not contain false or misleading information.

labeltalol hydrochloride, a drug used to treat high blood pressure.

★CAUTION: Should not be given to patients with asthma or emphysema. It should be used with caution in patients with diabetes because it may mask symptoms of low blood sugar, especially abnormally fast heart beat.

★ADVERSE EFFECTS: Among the most serious adverse reactions are unusually low blood pressure that occurs when standing up after sitting or lying down (orthostatic hypotension), fatigue, headache, skin rashes, numbness or tingling of the scalp, nausea, vomiting, and constipation.

labia, *sing.* **labium,** the fleshy, liplike edges of an organ or tissue, as the folds of skin at the opening of the vagina.

labial bar, a dental device that joins parts of a removable partial denture.

labial flange, the part of a denture rim that occupies the lip side of the gums.

labia majora /majôr'ə/, *sing.* **labium majus** /mã'jəs/, two long lips of skin, one on each side of the vaginal opening, that form the border of the vulva. Each labium contains connective tissue, fat, and a thin layer of muscle. In some women the outer surface of each lip may be covered with coarse pubic hair. The labia majora and the pouch of skin (scrotum) containing the male testes are derived from the same tissues of the embryo.

labia minora /minôr'ə/, *sing.* **labium minus** /mē'nəs/, two folds of skin between the labia majora, extending from the clitoris backward on both sides of the vaginal opening. Each labium divides into an upper and a lower division.

labile /lā'bil/, **1.** unstable; characterized by a tendency to change or to be easily altered. **2.** de-

scribing a personality with rapidly shifting or changing emotions.

labiolingual fixed orthodontic appliance, an orthodontic device for correcting or improving malocclusion, as when the upper and lower teeth do not come together properly. The device includes anchor bands attached to the first permanent molars of both jaws.

labor, the time and processes that occur during childbirth from the beginning of cervical dilatation to the delivery of the placenta, or afterbirth. See illustration on p. 450. See also **birth, cardinal movements of labor, station.**

laboratory, a facility, room, or building in which scientific research, experimentation, or testing are carried out.

laboratory error, any error made by the personnel in a clinical laboratory in performing a test, in interpreting the results, or in reporting or recording the results. Laboratory error must always be considered a possible explanation for findings that disagree with the condition of the patient.

laboratory medicine, the branch of medicine in which specimens of tissue, fluid, or other body substance are examined in the laboratory.

laboratory test, a procedure, usually conducted in a laboratory, that is intended to detect, identify, or measure one or more important substances, evaluate organ functions, or establish the nature of a disease. Laboratory tests range from quite simple to extremely sophisticated. In modern medical practice, they are commonly used to help establish or confirm a diagnosis and often aid in managing a disease.

labor coach, a person who assists a woman in labor and delivery. The coach, often the father of the baby, encourages the woman to use properly the breathing patterns, body positions, massage, and other techniques that were taught in a program of preparation for childbirth. The goal of a labor coach is to minimize the need for drugs for relieving pain. See also **monitrice.**

labored breathing, abnormal respiration characterized by increased effort, including use of the muscles of the chest wall, noisy breathing, grunting, or flaring of the nostrils.

labyrinth. See **internal ear.**

labyrinthitis, inflammation of the fluid-filled canals of the inner ear, resulting in dizziness.

laceration, a torn, jagged wound. **–lacerate,** *v.,* **lacerated,** *adj.*

lacrimal /lak'riməl/, pertaining to tears. Also spelled **lachrymal.**

lacrimal apparatus, a network of structures of the eye that secrete tears and drain them from

449

the surface of the eyeball. These parts include the lacrimal glands, the lacrimal ducts, the lacrimal sacs, and the nasolacrimal ducts.

lacrimal bone, one of the smallest and most fragile bones of the face, located at the front of the inner wall of the eye socket.

lacrimal caruncle, the small, reddish bulge of tissue that fills the space between the inner margins of the upper and the lower eyelids. It contains oil and sweat glands and secretes a whitish substance that collects in the corner of the eye.

lacrimal duct, one of two channels through which tears pass from the inner corner of the eye to the lacrimal sac. Also called **lacrimal canaliculi.** See also **lacrimal sac.**

lacrimal fistula, an abnormal channel from a tear duct to the surface of the eye or eyelid.

lacrimal gland, one of a pair of oval-shaped glands about the size of an almond situated above the eye. The gland has about 10 ducts that run beneath the membrane lining the upper eyelid and open along its edge. The watery secretion from the gland consists of the tears, slightly alkaline and salty, that moisten the eye.

lacrimal papilla, the small elevation on the margin of each eyelid, through which tears emerge from the lacrimal gland.

lacrimal sac, one of two sacs lodged in a deep groove formed by the face bones between the inner corners of the eyes and the nose. Tears from the eyes fill the sacs, and drain down small tubes (nasolacrimal ducts) into the cavity of the nose.

lacrimation /lak′rimā′shən/, **1.** the normal continuous secretion of tears by the lacrimal glands above the eyes. **2.** an excessive amount of tear production, as in crying or weeping. Also spelled **lachrymation.**

lactalbumin /lak′təlbyo͞o′min/, a highly nutritious protein found in milk. It is similar to serum albumin. See also **albumin, serum albumin.**

lactase, an enzyme that increases the rate of the conversion of milk sugar (lactose) to glucose and galactose, carbohydrates needed by the body for energy. Lactase is concentrated in the kidney, liver, and intestinal lining. Also called **beta-galactosidase.**

lactase deficiency, an abnormality in which the amount of the enzyme lactase is deficient, resulting in the inability to digest milk sugar (lactose). The deficiency may be inherited, and occurs in infancy in severe form, persisting throughout life. Persons of Asiatic and African heritage acquire the disorder more frequently. Lactase deficiency may also result from intes-

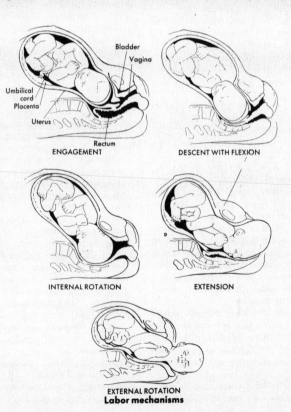

ENGAGEMENT

Bladder
Vagina
Umbilical cord
Placenta
Uterus
Rectum

DESCENT WITH FLEXION

INTERNAL ROTATION

EXTENSION

EXTERNAL ROTATION
Labor mechanisms

tinal surgery, any disease of the small intestine in which structural changes occur, malnutrition, or appear as a natural process of aging. See also **lactose intolerance.**

lactation, the process of the synthesis and secretion of milk from the breasts for the nourishment of an infant. See also **breast feeding.**

lacteal /lak′tē·əl/, pertaining to milk.

lacteal fistula, an abnormal passage opening into a milk duct in the breast.

lacteal gland, one of the many lymph capillaries in the fingerlike projections (villi) of the small intestine wall. The capillary is filled with a fluid (chyle) that turns milky white during the absorption of fat.

lactic, referring to milk and milk products. See also **lactic acid, lactose.**

lactic acid, an organic acid normally present in tissue. One form of lactic acid in muscle and blood is a product of the transformation of the carbohydrates, glucose and glycogen, to energy during strenuous physical exercise. Lactic acid is also found in the stomach, in sour milk, and in certain other foods, as sauerkraut. Also called **alpha-hydroxypropionic acid.** See also **glycolysis.**

lactic acidosis, a disorder characterized by an accumulation of lactic acid in the blood that causes oxygen starvation in tissues. It may occur after vigorous exercise, or from liver impairment, respiratory failure, tumors, or heart and blood vessel diseases.

lactiferous duct. See **mammary duct.**

Lactinex, a trademark for a drug containing bacteria, *Lactobacillus,* used for gastrointestinal disorders.

Lactobacillus, any of a group of rod-shaped bacteria that produce lactic acid from carbohydrates. Some species are normally found in the human intestinal tract and vagina.

lactogen /lak′təjən/, a drug or other agent that stimulates the production and secretion of milk. **–lactogenic,** *adj.*

lacto-ovovegetarian, one whose diet consists primarily of foods of vegetable origin and also includes eggs (*ovo*), milk, and cheese (*lacto*), but no meat, fish, or poultry. Also called **ovolactovegetarian.**

lactose, a sugar found in the milk of all mammals. Lactose is used as a laxative or a diuretic, and in some formulas for infant feeding. Also called **lactin, milk sugar.** See also **sugar.**

lactose intolerance, a disorder resulting in the inability to digest milk sugar (lactose) because of an enzyme, lactase, deficiency. Symptoms include bloating, intestinal gas, nausea, diarrhea, and abdominal cramps. The diet must be adjusted to restrict such foods as milk, cheese, butter, margarine, and any other products containing milk. See also **lactase deficiency.**

lactosuria, the presence of milk sugar (lactose) in the urine, a condition that may occur in late pregnancy or during breast milk production (lactation).

lactovegetarian, one whose diet consists of milk and milk products (*lacto*) in addition to foods of vegetable origin but does not include eggs, meat, fish, or poultry.

lactulose, a nonabsorbable synthetic sugar used as a laxative in chronic constipation. Its ability to increase fecal water content, however, may also cause diarrhea.

lacuna /ləkyōō′nə/, *pl.* **lacunae,** a small cavity within a structure, especially bony tissue.

Laënnec's catarrh /lā′əneks′/, a form of bronchial asthma characterized by the discharge of small, round, beadlike bodies of sputum called **Laënnec's pearls.**

Laetrile /lā′ətril/, a substance composed primarily of amygdalin, a cyanide-producing chemical derived from apricot pits. Laetrile has been offered as a cancer medication despite clinical studies by the National Cancer Institute that failed to show benefits from its use. It is claimed that amygdalin is converted by enzymes in cancer cells to substances (benzaldehyde and hydrogen cyanide) that kill the cancer cells. Also called **vitamin B_{17}.**

lagophthalmos /lag′əfthal′məs/, an abnormal condition in which an eye cannot be fully closed because of a nervous system or muscle disorder. Also called **hare's eye.**

la grippe. See **influenza.**

LAK, abbreviation for **lymphokine-activated killer cells.**

laked blood /lākt/, blood in which degeneration of the red blood cells has occurred, as may happen in poisoning or severe burns.

laliophobia /lā′lē·ō-/, a dread of talking caused by fear and anxiety that one will stammer or stutter.

lallation /lalā′shən/, **1.** babbling, repetitive, unintelligible speech, like the babbling of an infant. **2.** a speech disorder characterized by a defective pronunciation of words containing the sound "l" or by the use of the sound "l" in place of the sound "r."

Lamaze method /ləmäz′/, a system of preparation for childbirth developed in the 1950s by a French obstetrician, Fernand Lamaze. It is based on experiments with psychological conditioning in Russia. The Lamaze method has become the most often used means of teaching natural childbirth, without the use of drugs. It requires classes, practice at home, and coaching during labor and delivery, often by a trained coach called a 'monitrice.' The classes, given during pregnancy, teach the physiology of pregnancy and childbirth, exercises to develop strength and control in the abdominal muscles and those of the vaginal area, and techniques of breathing and relaxation. The woman is conditioned by repetition and practice to concentrate on a focal point she chooses, consciously relax all muscles, and to breathe in a special way at a particular rate—thereby training herself to ignore the sensations associated with labor. The kind and rate of breathing changes with the advancing stages of labor. During the early part of the first stage of labor, when the uterine cervix is dilated less than 5 cm (2 inches) and the contractions occur every 2 to 4 minutes, last 40 to 60 seconds, and are of mild to moderate strength, the mother does slow chest breathing during contractions. She may use rhythmic fingertip massage on her lower abdomen. The rate of respiration increases from about 10 to 12 breaths per minute as labor intensifies. A deep "cleansing breath" is taken before and after each contraction. During the active part of the first stage of labor up to the transition to the second stage, the cervix continues dilating. The interval between contractions decreases and the intensity and duration increase as labor progresses. During contractions, the mother breathes quietly and shallowly in her chest. The rate of her breathing varies with the strength of the contractions, increasing during a contraction to as fast as once a second at the peak and slowing to every 6 seconds as the uterus relaxes. She continues to concentrate on the focal point she selected, to perform the massage of her abdomen, to relax her vaginal muscles, and to take a cleansing breath at the beginning and end of each contraction. At the end of the first stage of labor, when the cervix is almost completely dilated and the contractions are strong, occurring about every 2 minutes and lasting 60 to 90 seconds, the mother begins to feel the urge to bear down and push during contractions. She avoids pushing before full dilation by combining several light, shallow breaths in the chest with short puffing exhalations as the urge increases during the contractions. During the second stage of labor, the cervix is fully dilated and contractions are strong, frequent, and expulsive. During contractions, the mother draws her legs back, flexing the thighs against the abdomen, holding them with her hands. With her chin tucked on her chest, she blocks the air from escaping from her lungs, and she bears down forcibly. Depending on the length of the contraction, several pushes of 15 or more seconds may be possible during the contraction. As the baby's head becomes visible in the vagina (crowns), she pants lightly so that the head may be delivered slowly. The advantages of the method include the need for little or no pain-relieving drugs. Compare **Bradley method, Read method.**

lambda, **1.** the Greek letter represented by the letter L or 1. **2.** a space between the bones of the back of an infant's skull covered by tough membranes.

lamella /ləmel'ə/, *pl.* **lamellae, 1.** a thin leaf or plate, as of bone. **2.** a medicated disk, prepared from glycerin for insertion under the eyelid, where it dissolves and is absorbed.

lamellar exfoliation of the newborn, a congenital skin disorder in which a scaly membrane that covers the fetus peels off within 24 hours of birth. Complete healing or a less severe process of reforming and shedding of the scales then occurs. Also called **ichthyosis congenita, ichthyosis fetalis, lamellar desquamation of the newborn, lamellar ichthyosis of the newborn.**

lamina /lam'inə/, *pl.* **laminae,** a thin, flat plate or layer, such as the lamina of the thyroid cartilage that overlays the structure on each side.

lamina propria, a layer of connective tissue that lies just under the surface of the mucous membrane.

laminaria tent, a cone of dried seaweed that swells as it absorbs water and therefore is sometimes used to dilate the cervix in preparation for induced abortion or induced labor.

laminated thrombus, a blood clot made up of a collection of blood platelets, clotting factors, and cellular elements, arranged in layers apparently formed at different times.

laminectomy, the surgical chipping away of the thin bony arches (laminae) of one or more vertebrae, performed to relieve compression of the spinal cord, as caused by a bone displaced in an injury or the result of degeneration of a cartilage disk. Fusion of some vertebrae may be necessary for stability of the spine if several laminae are removed. Walking may begin 3 to 5 days after surgery. **–laminectomize,** *v.*

lance, to puncture a pus-forming lesion to release accumulated matter. After application of a local anesthetic, the lesion is opened, and the pus drained. A deep infection may require insertion of a drainage tube. If a boil is on the face, an antibiotic is given to prevent infection from spreading into the brain. Infected matter from the lesion must be kept off surrounding skin to prevent a recurrence.

Lancereaux's diabetes /lan'sərōz/, a chronic disease of the transformation (metabolism) of carbohydrates to energy characterized by extreme loss of body weight. See also **diabetes mellitus.**

lancet, a short, pointed blade used to obtain a drop of blood for a blood sample. It has a guard above the blade that prevents deep incision.

lancinating /lan'sinā'ting/, pertaining to a sensation that is sharply piercing or tearing, as a pain may be.

Landau reflex /lan'dou/, a normal response of

infants when lying on the back to maintain an arc with the head raised and the legs slightly flexed. The reflex is poor in those with floppy infant syndrome and exaggerated in certain other disorders.

landmark position, the correct position of the hands on the chest in cardiopulmonary resuscitation. See also **cardiopulmonary resuscitation.**

Landsteiner's classification /land'stī'nərz/, the classification of human blood into groups A, B, AB, and O used for identification in blood transfusions.

lanolin, a fatlike substance from the wool of sheep. It contains about 25% water as a water-in-oil emulsion and is used as an ointment base and a softening agent for the skin. Also called **hydrous wool fat.**

Lanoxin, a trademark for a heart tonic (digoxin).

lanugo /lanyo͞o'gō/, **1.** the soft, downy hair covering a normal fetus, beginning with the fifth month of life in the uterus and almost entirely shed by the ninth month. **2.** the fine, soft hair covering all parts of the body except palms, soles, and areas where other types of hair are normally found. Also called **vellus hair.**

laparoscope /lap'ərəskōp'/, an instrument consisting of a lighted tube with magnifying lenses that is inserted through the abdominal wall for examining the abdominal cavity. Also called **celioscope, peritoneoscope.**

laparoscopy /lap'əros'kəpē/, the examination of the abdominal cavity with a laparoscope through a small incision in the abdominal wall. The procedure is also used for examining the ovaries and fallopian tubes. Also called **abdominoscopy.**

laparotomy /lap'ərot'əmē/, a surgical incision into a cavity of the abdomen, usually performed using general or regional anesthesia, often on an exploratory basis. Some kinds of laparotomy are **appendectomy, cholecystectomy, colostomy. –laparotomize,** v.

large calorie. See **calorie.**

large for gestational age (LGA) infant, an infant whose size and weight at birth fall above the 90th percentile (upper 10%) of appropriate for gestational age infants, whether delivered prematurely, at term, or later than term. Maternal diabetes mellitus is a cause of rapid fetal growth. LGA infants born of diabetic mothers are generally obese, with very pink skin and red, shiny cheeks. They are often listless and limp, feed poorly, and have low blood sugar (hypoglycemia) within the first few hours. Often these infants develop breathing problems (respiratory distress syndrome) caused by poor lung maturation.

large intestine, the portion of the digestive tract comprising the cecum, appendix, the ascending, transverse, and descending colons, and the rectum. The ileocecal valve separates the cecum from the ileum, preventing a reverse flow into the small intestine.

Larodopa, a trademark for an antiparkinsonian drug (levodopa).

laryngeal cancer, a malignant tumor arising from the lining of the voicebox (larynx). Laryngeal tumors are almost 20 times more common in men than in women and occur most frequently between 50 and 70 years of age. Chronic alcoholism and heavy use of tobacco increase the risk of developing the cancer. Persistent hoarseness is usually the first sign. Advanced lesions may cause a sore throat, breathing and swallowing difficulties, and swelling of the lymph glands in the neck. Treatment for small lesions is usually radiation. Surgical removal (laryngectomy), often combined with radiation, is indicated for extensive lesions. Following the operation, many persons with laryngectomies learn esophageal speech, some use an electric voicebox, and a few undergo surgical reconstruction. See also **laryngectomy.**

laryngeal catheterization, inserting a tube (catheter) into the voicebox (larynx) to remove secretions or introduce gases.

laryngeal prominence. See **Adam's apple.**

laryngectomy, surgical removal of the voicebox (larynx) to treat cancer. Before surgery, the patient usually meets with a speech specialist to learn about devices and methods for talking without a larynx. During the operation, an opening called a tracheostomy is made from the outside of the throat to the windpipe (trachea) to ensure an adequate airway for breathing. In a partial laryngectomy only the vocal cords are removed, and the tracheostomy is closed within several days. If the cancer is extensive, the entire larynx, the Adam's apple, and a tissue flap (epiglottis) that closes the windpipe when a person swallows are all removed. The tracheostomy becomes permanent after surgery. A laryngectomy tube, which remains in the throat for about 1 month, is inserted. A humidifier or vaporizer may be used to decrease coughing and the production of mucus. Intake of fluids by mouth begin after 1 week. A magic slate or notepad may be used by the patient for communication. **–laryngectomize,** v.

laryngismus /ler'injiz'məs/, a condition of uncontrolled spasms of the voicebox (larynx). The patient makes a crowing sound on taking a breath. The skin may become bluish from a lack of oxygen. The condition occurs in inflammation of the larynx and with rickets. The relatively small larynx of the infant and young child is particularly affected by spasms when infected or irritated and may become partially or totally obstructed.

laryngitis, inflammation of the mucous membrane lining the voicebox (larynx), accompanied by swelling of the vocal cords with hoarseness or loss of voice. It may be caused by a cold, irritating fumes, or sudden temperature changes. Chronic laryngitis may result from excessive use of the voice or heavy smoking. In acute laryngitis, there may be a cough, and the throat usually feels scratchy and painful. The patient should remain in an environment with an even temperature, avoid talking, exposure to tobacco smoke, and inhale steam containing menthol, oil of pine, or similar aromatic vapors. Acute laryngitis may cause serious breathing problems in children under 5 years of age. The child may develop a hoarse, barking cough, noisy breathing, become restless, and gasp for air. Treatment includes providing large amounts of vaporized cool mist. Chronic laryngitis may be treated by removing irritants, avoiding smoking, voice rest, correcting faulty voice habits, cough medication, steam inhalations, and spraying the throat with medications recommended by the physician. See also **laryngismus.**

laryngocele /ləring'gōsēl/, an abnormal cavity containing air that is connected to the small cavity (ventricle) of the voicebox. It is caused by the protrusion of the mucous membrane of the ventricle and may move and enlarge the false vocal cord, resulting in hoarseness and breathing difficulties. Because it is also a possible site for infection, it is usually removed.

laryngopharyngitis /ləring'gōfer'injī'tis/, inflammation of both the voicebox (larynx) and throat (pharynx). See also **laryngitis, pharyngitis.**

laryngopharyngography /lering'gōfer'ingog'rəfē/, the x-ray examination of the voicebox (larynx) and the throat (pharynx). Also called **laryngography.**

laryngopharynx /lering'gōfer'ingks/, one of the three regions of the throat, extending from the hyoid bone at the base of the tongue to the esophagus. **–laryngopharyngeal** /lering'gōferin'jē·əl/, adj.

laryngoscope, an instrument with a light and magnifying lenses for examining the larynx.

laryngospasm, a sudden, temporary closure of the larynx. See also **laryngismus.**

laryngotracheobronchitis (LTB) /lering'gōtrā'kē·ōbrongkī'tis/, an inflammation of the throat and bronchial tubes leading to the lungs. Symptoms are hoarseness, a dry cough, and breathing difficulty. Among the causes are infection by certain viruses, and the bacteria associated with bronchitis, influenza, and diptheria. Treatment includes steam inhalations, cough suppressants, and, for bacterial infections, appropriate antibiotics. See also **croup.**

larynx /ler'ingks/, the voicebox that is part of the air passage connecting the throat with the windpipe (trachea) leading toward the lungs. It produces a large bump in the neck called the Adam's apple, which remains the same size in both sexes until puberty, and then becomes larger in men than in women. The larynx, lined with mucous membrane, forms the bottom portion of the front wall of the throat. It is composed of rings of cartilages, all connected together by ligaments and moved by various muscles. **–laryngeal,** adj.

LAS, abbreviation for **lymphadenopathy syndrome.**

Lasan, a trademark for an ointment (anthralin) to treat a skin disease, psoriasis.

laser, acronym for *light amplification by stimulated emission of radiation,* a source of intense radiation of the visible, ultraviolet, or infrared portions of the light spectrum. Lasers are used in surgery to divide or weld tissues or to destroy tissue cells. Also called **optical maser.**

Lasix, a trademark for a water pill or diuretic (furosemide).

Lassa fever /lä'sə/, a highly contagious disease caused by a virus found mainly in Africa, and named for a village in Nigeria, Lassa, where the disease was first reported. Symptoms are fever, throat inflammation, swallowing difficulty, and bleeding under the skin. Escape of fluid from lung membranes, edema and kidney failure, and death from heart failure often re-

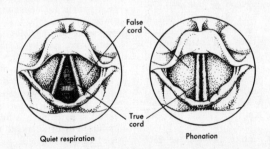

False cord

True cord

Quiet respiration   Phonation

Larynx

sult. Strict precautions are taken against the spread of infection.

latency stage, a period in psychosexual development occurring between early childhood and puberty.

latent, pertaining to a condition that is inactive or existing as a potential problem, as tuberculosis may be latent for a long period of time and then become active under certain conditions.

latent heart failure, an abnormal condition characterized by a heart disease that does not cause problems during rest but produces pain or other symptoms under conditions of increased stress, such as during exercise, fever, and emotional excitement. During stress situations, the heart affected by latent failure is unable to pump enough blood to meet the needs of body tissues and structures.

latent period, an interval between the time of exposure to an injurious dose of radiation and the response of the body tissues to the radiation.

latent phase, the early stage of childbirth that is characterized by irregular, infrequent, and mild contractions of the uterus and little or no dilation of the cervix or descent of the fetus. Also called **prodromal labor.**

latent schizophrenia, a form of schizophrenia characterized by the presence of mild symptoms of the disease in a person with no previous history of psychotic behavior. Also called **borderline schizophrenia, pseudoneurotic schizophrenia, pseudopsychopathic schizophrenia.**

lateral, 1. on the side. 2. away from the middle of the body or body part or organ.

lateral abdominal region. See **lateral region.**

lateral aortic node, a lymph node in any of three clusters of lymph nodes serving the pelvis and abdomen.

lateral cerebral sulcus, a deep furrow or cleft marking the division of the temporal, frontal, and parietal lobes of the brain. Also called **fissure of Sylvius.**

lateral condensation method, a technique for filling and sealing tooth root canals. A small cone of gutta-percha, a rubberlike substance, is sealed into the root tip; other cones are forced into the root until the canal is filled.

lateral humeral epicondylitis. See **tennis elbow.**

lateralization, the tendency for certain processes to be more highly developed on one side of the brain than the other, as development of spatial and musical thoughts in the right side of the brain and verbal and logical processes in the left side of the brain in most persons.

lateral pelvic displacement, one of the major leg muscle actions produced by the horizontal shift of the pelvis, and that helps to synchronize the movements of walking. It is often a factor in the diagnosis and treatment of various bone or joint diseases, deformities, and abnormal conditions.

lateral recumbent position, the posture assumed by a person lying on the left side with the right thigh and knee drawn up. Also called **English position, obstetric position.**

lateral region, the part of the abdomen on both sides of the navel. Also called **external abdominal region, lateral abdominal region, lumbar region.** See also **abdominal regions.**

lateral rocking, a sideways rocking of the body used to move the body forward or backward when normal muscle action is not possible. The technique is used by some disabled persons to move to or from the edge of a chair or to a different sitting position on a bed. The rocking is performed while leaning the trunk forward with the arms in front.

lateral rotation, a turning away from the midline of the body, as when twisting to the left or right.

latex fixation test, a blood test used in the diagnosis of rheumatoid arthritis.

latissimus dorsi, one of a pair of large triangular muscles of the back. The base of the triangle is at the level of the lower four ribs. The fibers of the muscle converge at the top of the humerus, the long bone of the upper arm. The latissimus dorsi moves the arm, draws the shoulder back and down, and helps draw the body up when climbing.

latitude, the ability of an x-ray system to produce acceptable images over a range of exposures.

Lauenstein method, (in radiology) a technique for positioning a patient in order to x-ray the hip joint. The knee of the leg to be x-rayed is bent, and the thigh is drawn up to nearly a right angle. Also called **frog leg position.**

laughing gas, *informal.* nitrous oxide, a side effect of which is laughter or giggling when administered in less than anesthetizing amounts.

lavage /ləväzh′/, the process of washing out an organ, usually the bladder, bowel, sinuses, or stomach for therapeutic purposes, as when a poison has been swallowed. Kinds of lavage are **blood lavage, gastric lavage, peritoneal dialysis.** See also **irrigation.**

law, a rule, standard, or principle that states a fact or a relationship between factors.

Law method, (in radiology) any of several techniques for positioning a patient for x-rays of the bones of the face, sinuses, and relationship of the teeth to the jaw bones.

lax, a condition of relaxation or looseness.

laxative, 1. pertaining to a substance that causes evacuation of the bowel by a mild action. 2. a laxative agent that promotes bowel evacuation by increasing the bulk of the feces, by softening the stool, or by lubricating the intestinal wall. Compare **cathartic.**

lazy colon. See **atonia constipation.**

lazy leukocyte syndrome, a disease affecting children in which immunity is low and resistance to infection is decreased. It is characterized by recurring mouth inflammation, gum problems (gingivitis), ear infections, and low-grade fever with a severe drop in the white blood cells in the blood. The condition is treated with normal human serum.

LBW, abbreviation for **low birth weight.**

LD, abbreviation for *lethal dose.*

LD50, the size of a dose of a particular substance that would kill one-half of the population of people or animals receiving such a dose.

L-dopa. See **levodopa.**

LDL, abbreviation for **low density lipoprotein.**

LE, abbreviation for **lupus erythematosus.** See **systemic lupus erythematosus.**

lead /lēd/, an electric connection attached to the body to record electric activity, especially of the heart or brain. See also **electrocardiograph, electroencephalograph.**

lead pipe fracture /led/, a fracture that compresses the bony tissue at the point of impact and creates a straight line (linear) fracture on the opposite side of the same bone.

lead poisoning /led/, an abnormal condition caused by swallowing or breathing substances containing lead. Many children have developed the condition as a result of eating flakes of lead paint peeling from walls or furniture. Poisoning also occurs from drinking water carried in lead pipes, lead salts in certain foods and wines, the use of pewter or earthenware dishes covered with lead glaze, and the use of leaded gasoline. Breathing of lead fumes is common in industry. Symptoms of chronic lead poisoning are extreme irritability, loss of appetite, and anemia. This condition may progress to the acute form. Symptoms of the acute form of lead poisoning are a burning sensation in the mouth and esophagus, colic, constipation, or diarrhea, mental disturbances, and paralysis of the arms and legs, followed in severe cases by convulsions and muscular collapse. If lead is swallowed, treatment includes washing out the stomach with magnesium or sodium sulfate. Brain disease must be anticipated in children with lead poisoning.

lead shielding, the use of aprons and other devices containing lead as protection against x-rays. A layer of lead 1 mm thick should offer adequate protection.

leakage radiation, radiation that leaks from x-ray equipment used in radiation therapy.

learned helplessness, a type of behavior and personality trait of a person who believes he or she is powerless, with no control over the environment, and that answers are useless.

learning disability, an abnormal condition often affecting children of normal or above-average intelligence, characterized by difficulty in learning such fundamental procedures as reading, writing, and arithmetic. The condition may result from medical and psychological causes.

leather bottle stomach, a thickening of the wall of the stomach, resulting in a rigid, shrunken, inelastic organ. The layer of connective tissue of the stomach becomes fibrous and thick. Causes of this condition include cancer, syphilis, and Crohn's disease involving the stomach. Also called **linitis plastica.**

Leber's congenital amaurosis /lā'bərz/, a kind of blindness or severely impaired vision that occurs at birth or shortly thereafter. The eyes appear normal externally, but reaction of the pupils to light is sluggish or absent. The eye disorder may be associated with mental retardation and epilepsy. One kind of Leber's amaurosis results in complete blindness, but with a second kind the patient has very slight vision. Also called **amaurosis congenita of Leber.**

Leboyer method of delivery /ləboiyā'/, a method of childbirth developed by the French obstetrician, Charles Leboyer. It has four basic features, including: (1) a gentle, controlled delivery in a quiet, dimly lit room; (2) avoiding pulling on the infant's head; (3) avoiding overstimulating the infant's nervous system; and (4) encouraging maternal-infant bonding. The goal of the method is to minimize the shock of birth by gently and pleasantly introducing the newborn to life outside of the womb. Unnecessary intervention in the process of birth is avoided. Following delivery, the baby is gently laid on the mother's abdomen. The infant's back is massaged as the umbilical cord stops pulsating, and, when regular spontaneous breathing is established, the baby is gently supported in a warm tub of water. Many birth centers and obstetric services have found no side effects from this method. Some studies have claimed superior psychological, social, and intellectual development in children delivered by this method. Compare **Bradley method, Lamaze method, Read method.**

lecithin /les'ithin/, any of a group of phosphorus-rich fats common in plants and animals. Lecithins are found in the liver, nerve tissue, semen, bile, and blood. They are essential for transforming fats in the body. Rich dietary sources are soybeans, egg yolk, and corn. Deficiency leads to liver and kidney disorders, high serum cholesterol levels, atherosclerosis, and arteriosclerosis.

lecithin/sphingomyelin ratio, the ratio of two components of amniotic fluid from the bag of waters holding the fetus in a pregnant woman. The measurement is used for predicting fetal lung maturity.

Ledercillin VK, a trademark for an antibiotic (penicillin V potassium).

Lee-Davidsohn test, a test for infectious mononucleosis using red blood cells from a horse. See also **heterophil antibody test.**

Lee-White, a method of determining the length of time required for a clot to form in a test tube of blood. It is often used as a test during treatment for a blood clot, or frostbite.

left common carotid artery, the longer of the two common carotid arteries, the main blood supply to the head and neck.

left coronary artery, an artery supplying both ventricles and the left atrium of the heart. Compare **right coronary artery.**

left-handedness, a natural tendency by some persons to favor the use of the left hand in performing certain tasks. Also called **sinistrality.**

left-heart failure, a heart condition characterized by reduced ability of the left side of the heart to pump blood to the arteries of the heart. Left-heart failure is usually related to right-heart failure, because both sides of the heart are part of a circuit. The impairment of one side will eventually affect the other.

left hepatic duct, the duct that drains the bile from the left lobe of the liver.

left pulmonary artery, the shorter and smaller of two arteries conveying blood from the heart to the lungs.

left ventricle, the thick-walled chamber of the heart that pumps blood through the aorta, the arteries, and capillaries to the body's tissues. It has walls about three times thicker than those of the right ventricle, and is longer and more conic. See also **heart.**

left ventricular assist device (LVAD), a mechanical pump that is used to aid artificially the natural pumping action of the left ventricle of the heart.

left ventricular failure, heart failure in which the left ventricle, the chamber that pumps blood to the body's tissues, fails to contract forcefully enough to maintain a normal output of blood. Fluid accumlates in the lungs because of the weakened blood flow. The heart usually becomes enlarged and develops a sound called a gallop. Other signs include breathlessness, pale skin, sweating, and often high blood pressure. Treatment consists of drugs for sedation, water pills (diuretics), a heart tonic (digitalis), and rest.

leg cylinder cast, a device of plaster of Paris or fiberglass to immobilize the leg in treating fractures in the legs from the ankle to the upper thigh. The foot is not encased. The leg cylinder cast is especially used for knee disorders, as fractures and dislocations, soft tissue injury, positioning and immobilization after surgery, and for correction of deformities.

Legionnaires' disease, an acute bacterial pneumonia caused by infection with *Legionella pneumophila* and characterized by an influenza-like illness followed within 1 week by high fever, chills, muscle aches, and headache. Symptoms may include dry cough, inflammation of the membrane covering the lungs (pleurisy), and sometimes diarrhea. Usually the disease is self-limited, but the death rate has been 15% to 20% in a few localized epidemics. Contaminated air-conditioning cooling towers and moist soil may be a source of organisms. Person-to-person contagion has not occurred. The risk of infection is increased by the presence of other conditions, as heart and lung diseases. Treatment includes supportive care of the symptoms and antibiotics. Also called **legionellosis.**

leiomyofibroma /lī′ōmī′ōfībrō′mə/, a tumor of smooth muscle cells and fibrous connective tissue, commonly occurring in the uterus in middle-aged women. See also **fibroid.**

leiomyoma /lī′ōmī·ō′mə/, *pl.* **leiomyomas, leiomyomata,** a noncancerous smooth muscle tumor most commonly occurring in the stomach, esophagus, or small intestine. Surgery is necessary if the tumor causes sudden and possibly severe bleeding.

leiomyoma cutis, a tumor of the smooth muscles that raise the hair. The lesion is characterized by many small, tender, red masses of tissue.

leiomyoma uteri, a noncancerous tumor of the smooth muscle of the uterus. It appears firm, round, and gray-white. Multiple tumors of this kind develop most often in the wall of the uterus and occur most frequently in women between 30 and 50 years of age. Also called **fibromyoma uteri, myoma previum,** *(informal)* **fibroids.**

leishmaniasis /lēsh′mənī′əsis/, infection with a protozoan parasite of the *Leishmania* group that is transmitted to humans by sand flies. The diseases caused by these microorganisms may involve the skin or abdominal organs, causing ulcers or a skin disorder that resembles leprosy. Kinds of leishmaniasis are **American leishmaniasis, kala-azar, oriental sore.**

length of stay (LOS), the period of time a patient remains in a hospital or other health-care facility as an inpatient.

lens capsule, the clear, thin, elastic membrane that surrounds the lens of the eye.

lens implant, an artifical eye lens of clear plastic that is usually put in an eye at the time a clouded or opaque lens (cataract) is removed. It may also be used for patients with extreme nearsightedness or other visual abnormalities. The operation may be performed with a local anesthetic, but general anesthesia is used more often. Following removal of the cataract, the lens is inserted through an incision in the cornea. There are several ways to hold the artificial lens in place. With extremely fine stitches, it may be sewn to the iris inside the front chamber of the eye. The plastic lens may also be put in the sac from which the natural lens was removed. With this method, a medicated eye drop must be used regularly afterward to prevent the iris from opening too widely, which would allow the plastic lens to slip. The artificial lens does not cause the problems associated with cataract spectacles, which cause a greater-than-normal enlargement of images. However, a high rate of complications is reported in the surgery, and the procedure is not performed for patients with diabetes mellitus or certain eye disorders.

Lente Insulin, a trademark for an antidiabetic agent (insulin zinc suspension).

lentigo /lentī′gō/, *pl.* **lentigines** /lentij′ənēz/, a tan or brown spot on the skin brought on by sun exposure, usually in a middle-aged or older person. Another variety, called **juvenile lentigo** and unrelated to sunlight, appears in children 2 to 5 years of age. The colored material in a lentigo is at a deeper level of the skin than in a freckle. Both types are noncancerous, and no treatment is necessary. Compare **freckle.**

lentigo maligna melanoma, a tumor developing from a frecklelike lesion on the face or other exposed surfaces of the skin in elderly patients. Flat, tan or brown, with irregular darker spots, it causes no symptoms. One of the three major types of pigmented tumor (melanoma), it occurs in about 10% to 15% of melanoma patients.

lentivirus, a member of a subfamily of retroviruses that includes the AIDS virus. Lentiviruses are usually slow viruses. Symptoms often do not appear until several years after exposure.

lepromin test /leprō′min/, a skin sensitivity test used to distinguish between two forms of leprosy.

leprosy, a chronic disease, caused by *Mycobacterium leprae,* that may take either of two forms. **Tuberculoid leprosy,** seen in those with high resistance to the disease-causing bacteria, appears as a thickening of nerves of the skin with saucer-shaped skin lesions. **Lepromatous leprosy,** seen in those with little resistance, involves many systems of the body, with widespread skin lesions, eye inflammation, destruction of nose cartilage and bone, and atrophy of the testicles. Blindness may result. Death from leprosy is rare unless tuberculosis or another disease occurs at the same time. Contrary to common belief, leprosy is not very contagious. Prolonged, intimate contact is required for it to be spread between individuals. Children are more susceptible than adults. Treatment with sulfa drugs for several years usually results in improvement of skin lesions, but recovery from nerve impairment is limited. Plastic surgery, physical therapy, and psychotherapy are often necessary. The disease is found mostly in undeveloped tropical and subtropical countries. In the United States, pa-

tients may be sent to the U.S. Public Health Service leprosarium in Carville, Louisiana. A vaccine may protect against leprosy. Also called **Hansen's disease.**

leptocyte. See **target cell.**

leptocytosis /lep′tōsītō′sis/, a blood condition in which abnormal red blood cells that resemble "bull's eye" targets are present in the blood. A form of anemia (thalassemia), some kinds of liver disease, and absence of the spleen are associated with leptocytosis.

leptospirosis /lep′tōspīrō′sis/, an acute infectious disease caused by a microorganism, *Leptospira interrogans,* transmitted in the urine of infected animals, especially rodents or dogs. Human infections arise from direct contact with the urine or tissues of the infected animal or indirectly from contact with contaminated water or soil. Symptoms may include jaundice, bleeding into the skin, fever, chills, and muscular pain. Treatment with antibiotics may be effective if given during the first few days of the disease. Severe infections can damage the kidneys and the liver. The most serious form of the disease is called **Weil's disease.** Also called **autumn fever.**

Leriche's syndrome /lərēshs′/, a blood vessel disorder marked by gradual obstruction of the abdominal aorta, the artery that supplies blood to the stomach, liver, and spleen. Symptoms include pain in buttocks, thighs, or calves, absence of pulsation in leg arteries, pallor and coldness of the legs, gangrene of the toes, and impotence in men. Treatment may include removal of the obstruction or surgery to install a synthetic bypass graft.

lesbian, **1.** a female homosexual. **2.** referring to the sexual preference or desire of one woman for another. **–lesbianism,** *n.*

Lesch-Nyhan syndrome /lesh′nī′han/, a hereditary disorder affecting males, in which there is an excess production of uric acid, normally present in blood and urine. The syndrome includes mental retardation, self-mutilation of the fingers and lips by biting, impaired kidney function, and abnormal physical development.

lesion, **1.** a wound, injury, or other destructive change in body tissue. **2.** any visible, local abnormality of the tissues of the skin, as a wound, sore, rash, or boil. A lesion may be described as benign (noncancerous), malignant (cancerous), gross (visible), occult (of unknown cause), or primary (first). See table on pp. 459-460.

lesser occipital nerve, one of a pair of nerves that runs along the side of the head behind the ear.

lesser omentum, an extension of the membrane (peritoneum) lining the abdominal wall from the layers covering the surfaces of the stomach and the first part of the small intestine.

Types of skin lesions

Observed skin changes	Differentiation	Term	Example	
Change in color or texture				
Spot	Circumscribed, flat, color change	Macule	Freckle	
Discoloration, (reddish-purple)	Bleeding beneath the surface, injury to tissue	Contusion	Bruise	**Macule**
Soft whitening	Caused by repeated wetting of skin	Maceration	Between toes after soaking	
Flake	Dry cells of surface	Scale	Dandruff	
Roughness from dried fluid	Dry exudate over lesions	Crust	Eczema, impetigo	
Roughness from cells	Leathery thickening of outer skin layer	Lichenification	Callus on foot	
Silvery scale	Buildup of scale	Plaque	Psoriasis	
Change in shape				
Solid mass, *cellular* growth	Less than 5 mm	Papule	Small mole, raised rash	
	5 mm to 2 cm	Nodule	Enlarged lymph node	
	Greater than 2 cm	Tumor	Benign or malignant tumor	
	Excess connective tissue over scar	Keloid	Overgrown scar	

Papule **Nodule** **Tumor**

Observed skin changes	Differentiation	Term	Example
Fluid-filled lesions	Less than 1 cm, clear fluid	Vesicle	Blister, chickenpox
	Greater than 1 cm, clear fluid	Bulla	Large blister, pemphigus
	Small, thick yellowish fluid (pus)	Pustule	Acne
	Semisolid	Cyst	Sebaceous cyst

Vesicle **Bulla**

continued.

Types of skin lesions — cont'd

Observed skin changes	Differentiation	Term	Example
Swelling of tissue	Generalized swelling; fluid between cells	Edema	Inflammation, swelling of feet
	Circumscribed surface edema, transient, some itching	Wheal	Allergic reaction

Wheal

Breaks in skin surfaces Oozing, scraped surface	Loss of superficial surface of skin	Abrasion	"Floor burn," scrape
Linear crack or cleft	Slit or splitting of skin layers	Fissure	Athlete's foot

Fissure

Scooped-out depression	Loss of deeper layers of skin	Ulcer	Decubitus, stasis ulcer

Ulcer

Superficial linear skin breaks	Scratch marks, frequently by fingernails	Excoriations	Scratching
Jagged cut	Tearing of skin surface	Laceration	Accidental cut by blunt object
Linear cut, edges approximated	Cutting by sharp instrument	Incision	Knife cut
Vascular lesions Small, flat, round, purplish-red spot	Intradermal or submucous hemorrhage	Petechia	Bleeding tendency, vitamin C deficiency
Spiderlike, red, small	Dilatation of capillaries, arterioles, or venules	Telangiectasis	Liver disease, vitamin B deficiency, sun-damaged skin
Discoloration, reddish-purple	Escape of blood into tissue	Ecchymosis	Trauma to blood vessels

let-down, a sensation in the breasts of women who are breast feeding an infant, it often occurs as the milk flows into the ducts.

lethal, capable of causing death.

lethal gene, any gene that produces an effect causing death of the organism at some stage of development from fertilization of the egg to adulthood. In humans, examples of diseases caused by lethal genes are Huntington's chorea and sickle cell anemia.

lethargy, **1.** the state or quality of being indifferent or sluggish. **2.** stupor or coma resulting from disease or hypnosis.

lethality, the probability that a person threatening suicide will succeed, based on the method intended, how specific the plan is, and the availability of the means.

leucine (Leu) /lōō′sēn/, a white, crystalline amino acid essential for optimal growth in infants and nitrogen balance in adults. It cannot be synthesized by the body and is obtained by the conversion of protein during digestion. An inherited inability of the body to use leucine properly is called maple syrup urine disease. See also **amino acid, maple syrup urine disease.**

leucocyte. See **leukocyte.**

leucovorin calcium, an antianemic drug given to treat an overdose of a folic acid antagonist, as methotrexate drugs, and certain other types of anemia.

★CAUTION: Anemia caused by vitamin B_{12} or known allergy to this drug prohibits its use.

★ADVERSE EFFECTS: Allergic reactions may occur.

leukapheresis, a process by which blood is withdrawn from a vein, white blood cells are selectively removed, and the remaining blood is recycled back into the donor. The white cells may be used for treating patients with blood deficiencies.

leukemia, a cancer of blood-forming organs characterized by the replacement of bone marrow with immature white blood cells (leukocytes), and the presence of abnormal numbers and forms of immature white cells in circulation. Approximately 20,500 new cases in adults and 2,500 in children are diagnosed annually in the United States alone, and the disease causes about 15,900 deaths a year. Males are affected twice as frequently as females. The cause of leukemia is not clear, but it may result from exposure to radiation, benzene, or other chemicals that are toxic to bone marrow. The risk of the disease is increased in individuals with other diseases, as Down's syndrome. The risk is also higher in an identical twin of a leukemia patient. Leukemia is classified according to the kinds of abnormal cells, the course of the disease, and the duration of disease. Acute leukemia usually begins suddenly. It rapidly progresses from early signs, as fatigue, pale skin, weight loss, and easy bruising, to fever, bleeding, extreme weakness, bone or joint pain, and repeated infections. Chronic leukemia develops slowly. Signs similar to those of the acute form of the disease may not appear for years. Diagnoses of acute and chronic forms are made by blood tests and bone marrow studies. The most effective treatment includes intensive chemotherapy, using antibiotics to prevent infections, and blood transfusions.

leukemia cutis, a condition, usually affecting the skin of the face, in which yellowish, red, or purple lesions and large accumulations of white (leukemic) blood cells develop. Also called **lymphoderma perniciosa.**

leukemoid reaction, an abnormal condition resembling leukemia in which the white blood cell count rises in response to an allergy, inflammatory disease, infection, poison, hemorrhage, burn, or other causes of severe physical stress. Compare **leukemia.**

Leukeran, a trademark for an anticancer drug (chlorambucil).

-leukin, a combining form for certain protein products, which are active in the immune system (interleukin-2).

leukocyte /lōō′kəsīt/, a white blood cell. There are five types of leukocytes, classified by the presence or absence of small particles (granules) in the cytoplasm, the main substance of the cell. The agranulocytes, or those without granules, are lymphocytes and monocytes. The granulocytes, white cells with granules, are called neutrophils, basophils, and eosinophils. White cells are able to squeeze through spaces between cells and migrate by amebalike movements. Leukocytes are larger than red blood cells (erythrocytes). A cubic millimeter of normal blood usually contains 5,000 to 10,000 leukocytes. Among the most important functions of the leukocytes are the destruction of bacteria, fungi, and viruses, and rendering harmless poisonous substances that may result from allergic reactions and cellular injury. Also called **leucocyte, white blood cell, white corpuscle.**

leukocyte alkaline phosphatase, an enzyme that is abnormally abundant in various diseases, as cirrhosis of the liver and certain infections.

leukocytosis /lōō′kōsītō′sis/, an abnormal increase in the number of circulating white blood cells. This often accompanies bacterial, but not usually viral, infections. The normal range is 5,000 to 10,000 white cells per cubic millimeter of blood. Leukemia may be associated with a white blood cell count as high as 500,000 to 1 million per cubic millimeter of blood.

leukoderma /lōōkōdur′mə/, loss of skin pigment, especially in patches, caused by a number of disorders. Compare **vitiligo.**

leukoerythroblastic anemia /lōō′kō·erith′rōblas′-tik/, an abnormal condition in which there are large numbers of immature white and red blood cells. It is characteristic of some anemias that result from a tumor in bone marrow.

leukonychia /loo'kōnik'ē·ə/, a harmless condition in which white patches appear under the nails. Injury or infection can cause white spots or streaks on nails. A common cause is the presence of air bubbles under the nails.

leukopenia /loo'kōpē'nē·ə/, an abnormal decrease in the number of white blood cells to fewer than 5,000 cells per cubic millimeter. It may be caused by an adverse drug reaction, radiation poisoning, or other abnormal conditions and may affect one or all kinds of white blood cells.

leukophoresis /loo'kōfərē'sis/, a laboratory procedure in which white blood cells are separated for identifying and evaluating the types of white cells and their amounts.

leukoplakia /loo'kōplā'kē·ə/, a precancerous, slowly developing change in the normal tissue of a mucous membrane. Thickened, white patches that are slightly raised appear. They may occur on the penis or vulva. Those on the lips and inside surface of the cheeks are associated with pipe smoking.

leukopoiesis /loo'kōpō·ē'sis/, the process by which white blood cells form and develop in bone marrow or in lymph tissue. See also **leukocyte.**

leukorrhea /loo'kərē'ə/, a white discharge from the vagina. Normally, vaginal discharge occurs in varying amounts during the course of the menstrual cycle. A greater-than-usual amount is normal in pregnancy and a decrease is to be expected after childbirth and after menopause. A heavy, irritating, foul-smelling, green or yellow discharge may indicate vaginal or uterine infection or other disease. Leukorrhea is the most common reason for women to seek gynecological care. See also **vaginal discharge.**

leukotoxin /loo'kətok'sin/, a substance that can inactivate or destroy white blood cells. **–leukotoxic,** *adj.*

leukotrienes, a group of chemical compounds that occur naturally in white blood cells (leukocytes). They are able to produce allergic and inflammatory reactions, and may take part in the development of asthma and rheumatoid arthritis.

levamisole, a drug used against a wide variety of tiny parasitic worms (nematodes). It has also been used in the treatment of bacterial and viral infections.

levator /livā'tər/, *pl.* **levatores** /lev'ətôr'ēz/, a muscle that raises a structure of the body.

levator ani, one of a pair of muscles of the pelvis that stretches across the bottom of the pelvic cavity like a hammock, supporting the pelvic organs.

levator palpebrae superioris, one of the three muscles of the upper eyelid, also considered a muscle of the eye. It raises the eyelid.

levator scapulae, a muscle of the back and sides of the neck. It acts to raise the scapula of the shoulder.

LeVeen shunt, a tube (shunt) that is surgically implanted to drain an accumulation of fluid in the abdominal cavity in cirrhosis of the liver, right-sided heart failure, or cancer of the abdomen. Using general anesthesia, the surgeon inserts a silicone-rubber tube into a blood vessel (superior vena cava) leading to the heart. When the patient inhales, the fluid pressure in the abdominal cavity rises, while that in the blood vessel falls. The difference in pressure allows fluid to enter the shunt.

lever, any bone and associated joint of the body that act together so that force applied to one end of the bone will lift a weight at another point. An example is the action of muscles that move the forearm at the elbow joint.

Levin tube /lev'in/, a plastic catheter that is inserted through the nose and throat and into the stomach. See also **gastric intubation.**

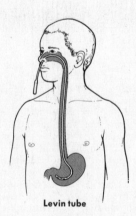

Levin tube

levitation, a hallucination that one is floating or rising in the air. The sensation may also occur in dreams. **–levitate,** *v.*

levodopa /lē'vōdō'pə/, a drug prescribed in the treatment of Parkinson's disease, juvenile forms of Huntington's disease, and chronic manganese poisoning.

Levo-Dromoran, a trademark for a narcotic painkiller (levorphanol tartrate).

Levophed Bitartrate, a trademark for a drug used to raise blood pressure (norepinephrine bitartrate).

levorphanol tartrate, a narcotic analgesic drug prescribed for pain relief, particularly before an operation.

★CAUTION: Alcoholism, asthma, depressed

SKELETAL SYSTEM

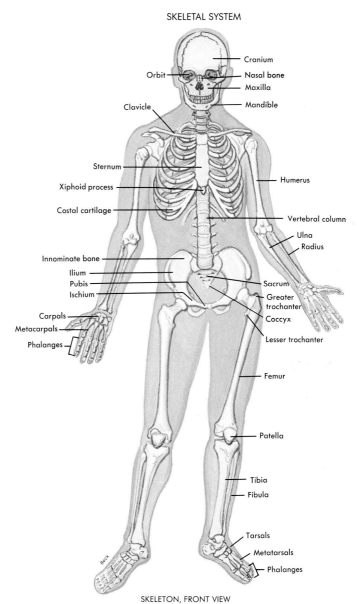

Cranium

Orbit

Nasal bone

Maxilla

Mandible

Clavicle

Sternum

Xiphoid process

Costal cartilage

Humerus

Vertebral column

Ulna

Radius

Innominate bone

Ilium

Pubis

Ischium

Sacrum

Greater trochanter

Coccyx

Lesser trochanter

Carpals

Metacarpals

Phalanges

Femur

Patella

Tibia

Fibula

Tarsals

Metatarsals

Phalanges

Beck

SKELETON, FRONT VIEW

Axial skeleton is shown in blue. Appendicular system is bone colored.

SKELETAL SYSTEM

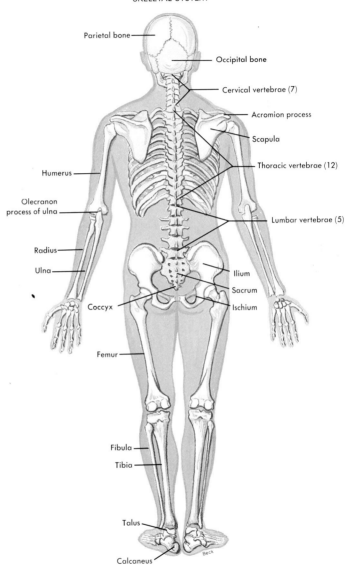

Parietal bone

Occipital bone

Cervical vertebrae (7)

Acromion process

Scapula

Thoracic vertebrae (12)

Humerus

Olecranon
process of ulna

Lumbar vertebrae (5)

Radius

Ulna

Ilium

Sacrum

Coccyx

Ischium

Femur

Fibula

Tibia

Talus

Calcaneus

Beck

SKELETON, REAR VIEW
Axial skeleton is shown in blue. Appendicular system is bone colored.

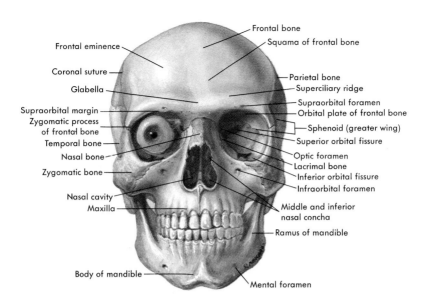

Frontal eminence

Coronal suture

Glabella

Supraorbital margin

Zygomatic process
of frontal bone

Temporal bone

Nasal bone

Zygomatic bone

Nasal cavity

Maxilla

Body of mandible

Frontal bone

Squama of frontal bone

Parietal bone

Superciliary ridge

Supraorbital foramen

Orbital plate of frontal bone

Sphenoid (greater wing)

Superior orbital fissure

Optic foramen

Lacrimal bone

Inferior orbital fissure

Infraorbital foramen

Middle and inferior
nasal concha

Ramus of mandible

Mental foramen

FRONT AND SIDE VIEWS OF SKULL

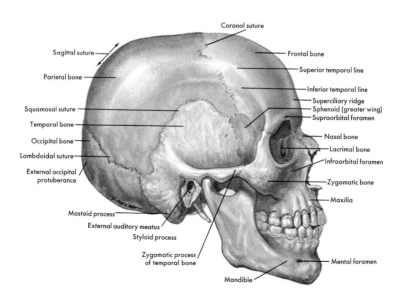

Coronal suture

Sagittal suture

Parietal bone

Squamosal suture

Temporal bone

Occipital bone

Lambdoidal suture

External occipital
protuberance

Mastoid process

External auditory meatus

Styloid process

Zygomatic process
of temporal bone

Mandible

Frontal bone

Superior temporal line

Inferior temporal line

Superciliary ridge

Sphenoid (greater wing)

Supraorbital foramen

Nasal bone

Lacrimal bone

Infraorbital foramen

Zygomatic bone

Maxilla

Mental foramen

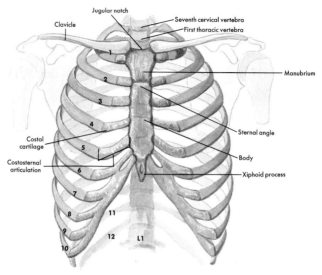

Jugular notch

Clavicle

Seventh cervical vertebra

First thoracic vertebra

Manubrium

Sternal angle

Costal cartilage

Costosternal articulation

Body

Xiphoid process

THORAX AND RIBS

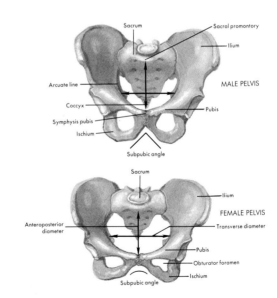

Sacrum

Sacral promontory

Ilium

Arcuate line

MALE PELVIS

Coccyx

Pubis

Symphysis pubis

Ischium

Subpubic angle

Sacrum

Ilium

FEMALE PELVIS

Anteroposterior diameter

Transverse diameter

Pubis

Obturator foramen

Ischium

Subpubic angle

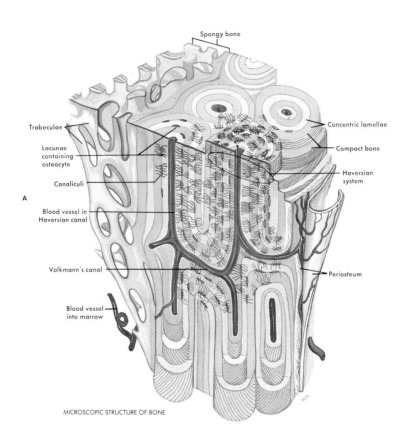

Spongy bone

Trabeculae

Lacunae
containing
osteocyte

Canaliculi

A

Blood vessel in
Haversian canal

Volkmann's canal

Blood vessel
into marrow

Concentric lamellae

Compact bone

Haversian
system

Periosteum

MICROSCOPIC STRUCTURE OF BONE

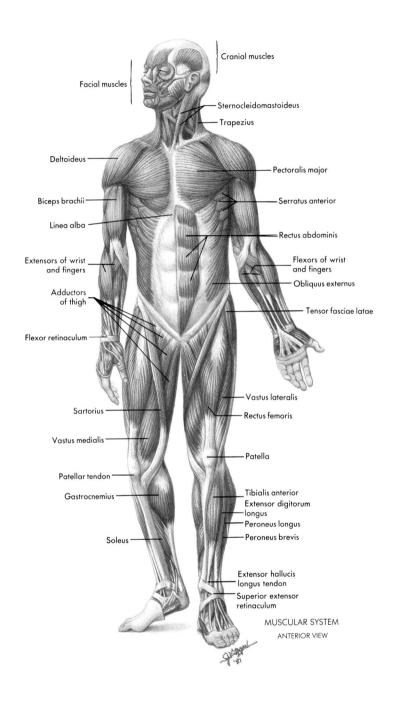

Cranial muscles

Facial muscles

Sternocleidomastoideus

Trapezius

Deltoideus

Pectoralis major

Biceps brachii

Serratus anterior

Linea alba

Rectus abdominis

Extensors of wrist
and fingers

Flexors of wrist
and fingers

Adductors
of thigh

Obliquus externus

Tensor fasciae latae

Flexor retinaculum

Vastus lateralis

Sartorius

Rectus femoris

Vastus medialis

Patella

Patellar tendon

Tibialis anterior

Gastrocnemius

Extensor digitorum
longus

Peroneus longus

Peroneus brevis

Soleus

Extensor hallucis
longus tendon

Superior extensor
retinaculum

MUSCULAR SYSTEM

ANTERIOR VIEW

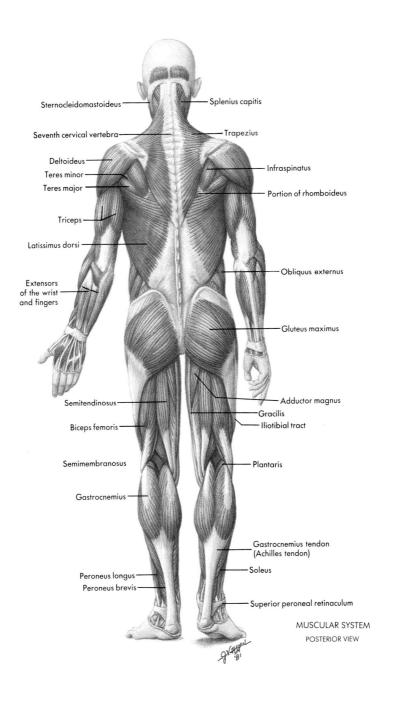

Sternocleidomastoideus

Seventh cervical vertebra

Deltoideus

Teres minor

Teres major

Triceps

Latissimus dorsi

Extensors
of the wrist
and fingers

Semitendinosus

Biceps femoris

Semimembranosus

Gastrocnemius

Peroneus longus
Peroneus brevis

Splenius capitis

Trapezius

Infraspinatus

Portion of rhomboideus

Obliquus externus

Gluteus maximus

Adductor magnus

Gracilis

Iliotibial tract

Plantaris

Gastrocnemius tendon
(Achilles tendon)

Soleus

Superior peroneal retinaculum

MUSCULAR SYSTEM

POSTERIOR VIEW

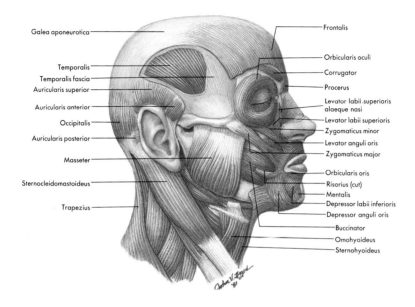

Galea aponeurotica

Temporalis
Temporalis fascia
Auricularis superior

Auricularis anterior

Occipitalis

Auricularis posterior

Masseter

Sternocleidomastoideus

Trapezius

Frontalis

Orbicularis oculi
Corrugator
Procerus
Levator labii superioris
alaeque nasi
Levator labii superioris
Zygomaticus minor
Levator anguli oris
Zygomaticus major

Orbicularis oris
Risorius (cut)
Mentalis
Depressor labii inferioris
Depressor anguli oris
Buccinator
Omohyoideus
Sternohyoideus

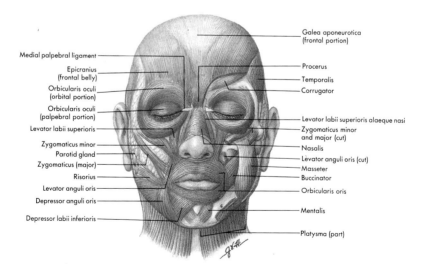

Medial palpebral ligament

Epicranius
(frontal belly)
Orbicularis oculi
(orbital portion)
Orbicularis oculi
(palpebral portion)
Levator labii superioris

Zygomaticus minor
Parotid gland
Zygomaticus (major)
Risorius
Levator anguli oris
Depressor anguli oris

Depressor labii inferioris

Galea aponeurotica
(frontal portion)

Procerus
Temporalis
Corrugator

Levator labii superioris alaeque nasi
Zygomaticus minor
and major (cut)
Nasalis
Levator anguli oris (cut)
Masseter
Buccinator
Orbicularis oris

Mentalis

Platysma (part)

SIDE AND FRONT VIEWS OF MUSCLES OF THE FACE, HEAD, AND JAW

PRINCIPAL VEINS AND ARTERIES

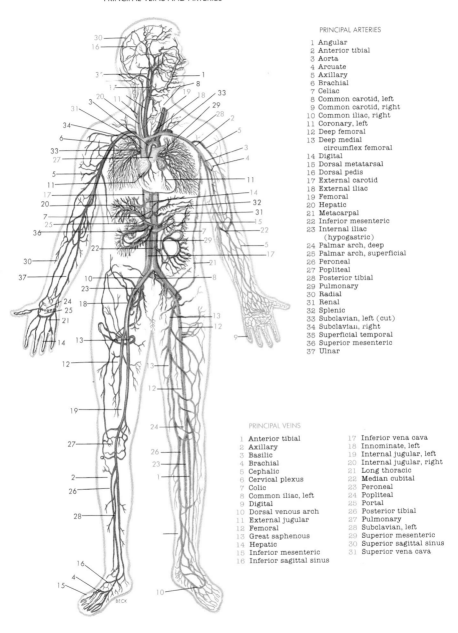

PRINCIPAL ARTERIES

1 Angular
2 Anterior tibial
3 Aorta
4 Arcuate
5 Axillary
6 Brachial
7 Celiac
8 Common carotid, left
9 Common carotid, right
10 Common iliac, right
11 Coronary, left
12 Deep femoral
13 Deep medial
   circumflex femoral
14 Digital
15 Dorsal metatarsal
16 Dorsal pedis
17 External carotid
18 External iliac
19 Femoral
20 Hepatic
21 Metacarpal
22 Inferior mesenteric
23 Internal iliac
   (hypogastric)
24 Palmar arch, deep
25 Palmar arch, superficial
26 Peroneal
27 Popliteal
28 Posterior tibial
29 Pulmonary
30 Radial
31 Renal
32 Splenic
33 Subclavian, left (cut)
34 Subclavian, right
35 Superficial temporal
36 Superior mesenteric
37 Ulnar

PRINCIPAL VEINS

1 Anterior tibial
2 Axillary
3 Basilic
4 Brachial
5 Cephalic
6 Cervical plexus
7 Colic
8 Common iliac, left
9 Digital
10 Dorsal venous arch
11 External jugular
12 Femoral
13 Great saphenous
14 Hepatic
15 Inferior mesenteric
16 Inferior sagittal sinus
17 Inferior vena cava
18 Innominate, left
19 Internal jugular, left
20 Internal jugular, right
21 Long thoracic
22 Median cubital
23 Peroneal
24 Popliteal
25 Portal
26 Posterior tibial
27 Pulmonary
28 Subclavian, left
29 Superior mesenteric
30 Superior sagittal sinus
31 Superior vena cava

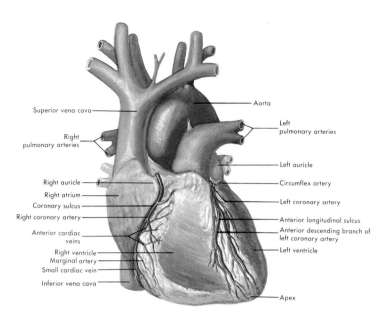

Superior vena cava —

Right
pulmonary arteries

Right auricle —
Right atrium —
Coronary sulcus —
Right coronary artery —
Anterior cardiac
veins

Right ventricle —
Marginal artery —
Small cardiac vein —
Inferior vena cava —

—— Aorta

Left
pulmonary arteries

—— Left auricle
—— Circumflex artery
—— Left coronary artery
—— Anterior longitudinal sulcus
—— Anterior descending branch of
left coronary artery
—— Left ventricle

—— Apex

CORONARY VESSELS (FRONTAL VIEW)

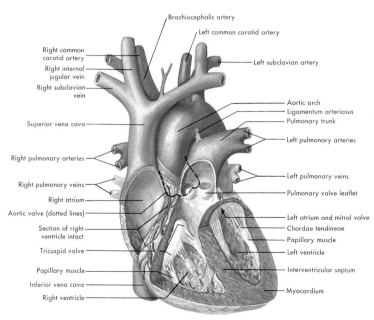

Brachiocephalic artery

Left common carotid artery

Right common
carotid artery
Right internal
jugular vein
Right subclavian
vein

Superior vena cava —

Right pulmonary arteries —

Right pulmonary veins —
Right atrium —
Aortic valve (dotted lines) —
Section of right
ventricle intact
Tricuspid valve —

Papillary muscle —
Inferior vena cava —
Right ventricle —

—— Left subclavian artery

—— Aortic arch
—— Ligamentum arteriosus
—— Pulmonary trunk
—— Left pulmonary arteries

—— Left pulmonary veins
—— Pulmonary valve leaflet

—— Left atrium and mitral valve
—— Chordae tendineae
—— Papillary muscle
—— Left ventricle
—— Interventricular septum

—— Myocardium

HUMAN HEART IN FRONTAL SECTION

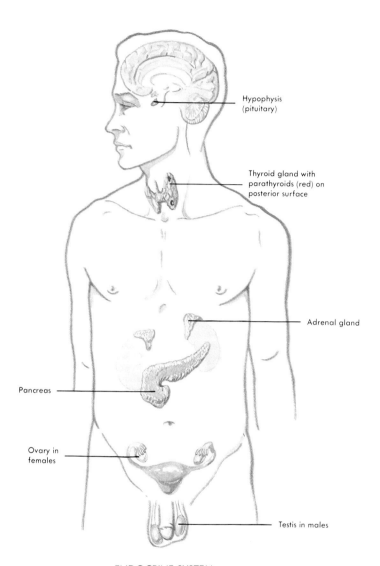

Hypophysis
(pituitary)

Thyroid gland with
parathyroids (red) on
posterior surface

Adrenal gland

Pancreas

Ovary in
females

Testis in males

ENDOCRINE SYSTEM

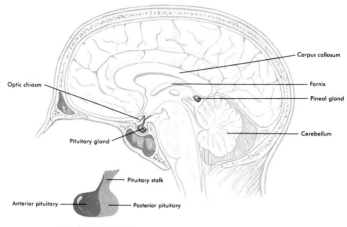

Optic chiasm

Corpus callosum

Fornix

Pineal gland

Cerebellum

Pituitary gland

Pituitary stalk

Anterior pituitary

Posterior pituitary

DETAIL OF PITUITARY GLAND

LOCATION OF THE PITUITARY AND PINEAL GLANDS

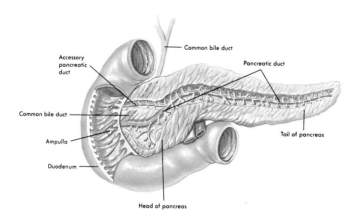

Accessory
pancreatic
duct

Common bile duct

Pancreatic duct

Common bile duct

Ampulla

Tail of pancreas

Duodenum

Head of pancreas

THE PANCREAS

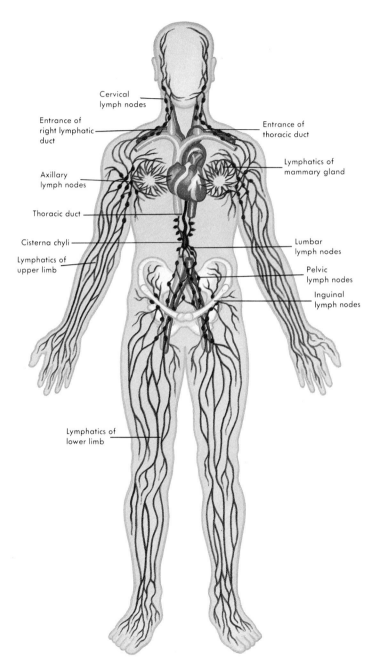

Cervical
lymph nodes

Entrance of
right lymphatic
duct

Entrance of
thoracic duct

Lymphatics of
mammary gland

Axillary
lymph nodes

Thoracic duct

Cisterna chyli

Lumbar
lymph nodes

Lymphatics of
upper limb

Pelvic
lymph nodes

Inguinal
lymph nodes

Lymphatics of
lower limb

LYMPHATIC SYSTEM

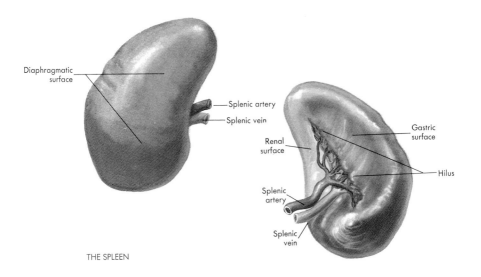

Diaphragmatic
surface

Splenic artery

Splenic vein

Renal
surface

Gastric
surface

Hilus

Splenic
artery

Splenic
vein

THE SPLEEN

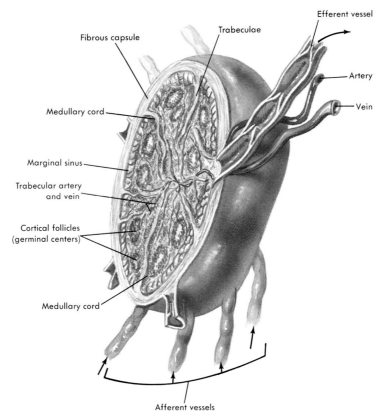

Fibrous capsule

Trabeculae

Efferent vessel

Artery

Vein

Medullary cord

Marginal sinus

Trabecular artery
and vein

Cortical follicles
(germinal centers)

Medullary cord

Afferent vessels

SCHEMATIC SECTION OF A LYMPH NODE

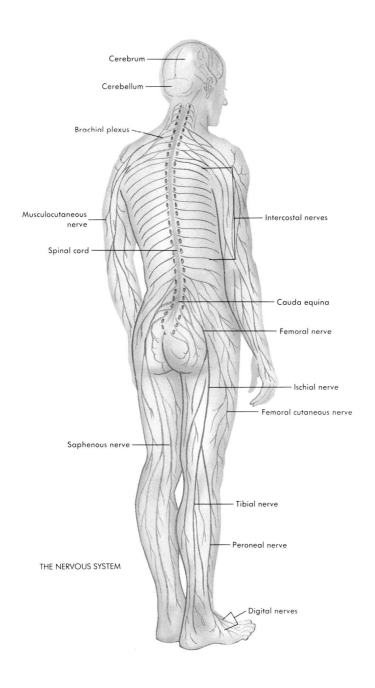

Cerebrum

Cerebellum

Brachial plexus

Musculocutaneous
nerve

Spinal cord

Intercostal nerves

Cauda equina

Femoral nerve

Ischial nerve

Femoral cutaneous nerve

Saphenous nerve

Tibial nerve

Peroneal nerve

THE NERVOUS SYSTEM

Digital nerves

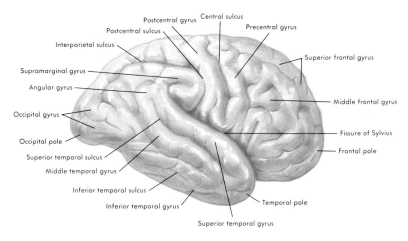

Postcentral gyrus
Central sulcus
Postcentral sulcus
Precentral gyrus
Interparietal sulcus
Supramarginal gyrus
Angular gyrus
Superior frontal gyrus
Occipital gyrus
Middle frontal gyrus
Occipital pole
Fissure of Sylvius
Superior temporal sulcus
Frontal pole
Middle temporal gyrus
Inferior temporal sulcus
Inferior temporal gyrus
Temporal pole
Superior temporal gyrus

SURFACE ANATOMY OF CEREBRAL CORTEX

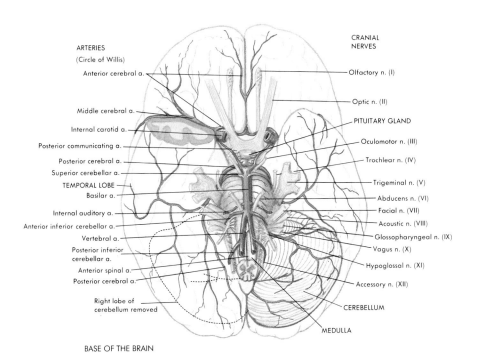

ARTERIES
(Circle of Willis)

CRANIAL
NERVES

Anterior cerebral a.
Olfactory n. (I)

Optic n. (II)

Middle cerebral a.
PITUITARY GLAND

Internal carotid a.
Oculomotor n. (III)

Posterior communicating a.
Trochlear n. (IV)

Posterior cerebral a.
Superior cerebellar a.
Trigeminal n. (V)

TEMPORAL LOBE
Abducens n. (VI)

Basilar a.
Facial n. (VII)

Internal auditory a.
Acoustic n. (VIII)

Anterior inferior cerebellar a.
Glossopharyngeal n. (IX)

Vertebral a.
Vagus n. (X)

Posterior inferior
cerebellar a.
Hypoglossal n. (XI)

Anterior spinal a.
Accessory n. (XII)

Posterior cerebral a.

Right lobe of
cerebellum removed
CEREBELLUM

MEDULLA

BASE OF THE BRAIN

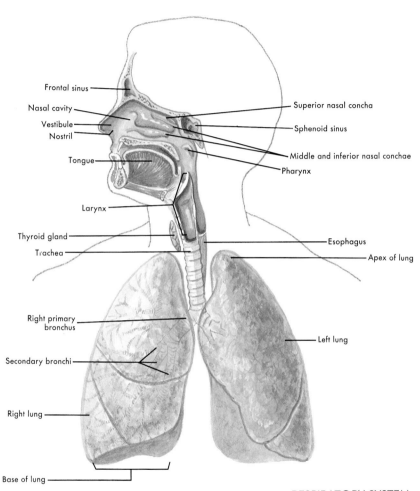

Frontal sinus

Nasal cavity

Vestibule

Nostril

Tongue

Larynx

Thyroid gland

Trachea

Right primary bronchus

Secondary bronchi

Right lung

Base of lung

Superior nasal concha

Sphenoid sinus

Middle and inferior nasal conchae

Pharynx

Esophagus

Apex of lung

Left lung

RESPIRATORY SYSTEM

STRUCTURES OF THE NASAL PASSAGES AND THE THROAT

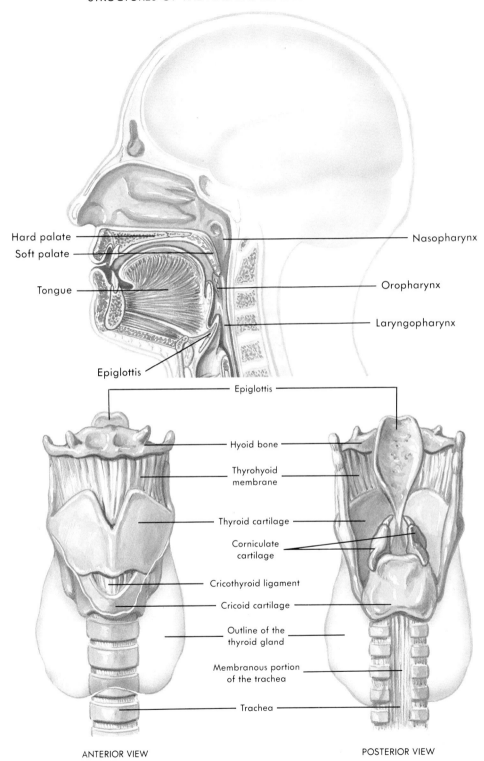

Hard palate

Soft palate

Tongue

Epiglottis

Nasopharynx

Oropharynx

Laryngopharynx

Epiglottis

Hyoid bone

Thyrohyoid membrane

Thyroid cartilage

Corniculate cartilage

Cricothyroid ligament

Cricoid cartilage

Outline of the thyroid gland

Membranous portion of the trachea

Trachea

ANTERIOR VIEW

POSTERIOR VIEW

STRUCTURE OF THE LARYNX AND UPPER TRACHEA

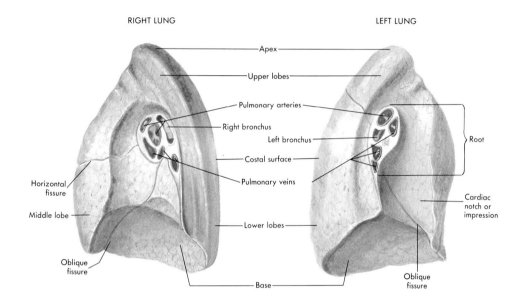

RIGHT LUNG   LEFT LUNG

Apex

Upper lobes

Pulmonary arteries

Right bronchus

Left bronchus   Root

Costal surface

Horizontal
fissure   Cardiac
                                                                           notch or
Middle lobe   impression

                              Lower lobes

Oblique
fissure   Oblique
                                                                      fissure
                              Base

Pulmonary veins

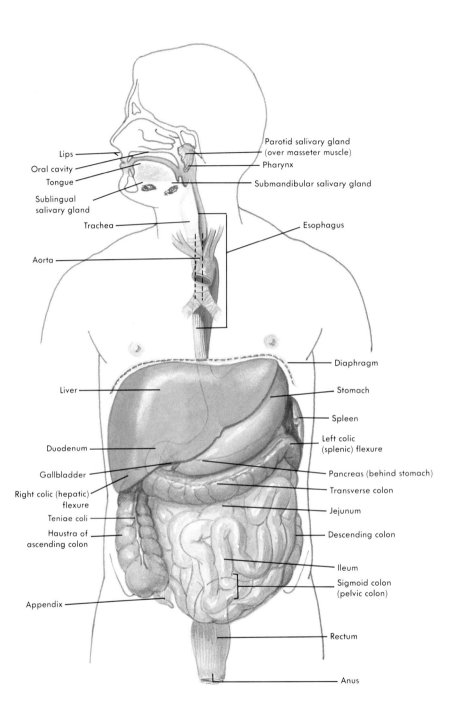

Lips

Oral cavity

Tongue

Sublingual
salivary gland

Trachea

Aorta

Parotid salivary gland
(over masseter muscle)

Pharynx

Submandibular salivary gland

Esophagus

Diaphragm

Liver

Stomach

Spleen

Duodenum

Left colic
(splenic) flexure

Gallbladder

Pancreas (behind stomach)

Right colic (hepatic)
flexure

Transverse colon

Teniae coli

Jejunum

Haustra of
ascending colon

Descending colon

Ileum

Sigmoid colon
(pelvic colon)

Appendix

Rectum

Anus

DIGESTIVE SYSTEM

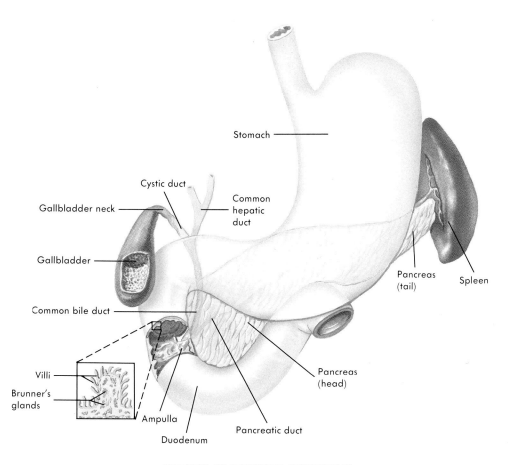

Stomach

Cystic duct

Common
hepatic
duct

Gallbladder neck

Gallbladder

Common bile duct

Villi

Brunner's
glands

Ampulla

Duodenum

Pancreatic duct

Pancreas
(head)

Pancreas
(tail)

Spleen

SOURCES OF INTESTINAL SECRETIONS

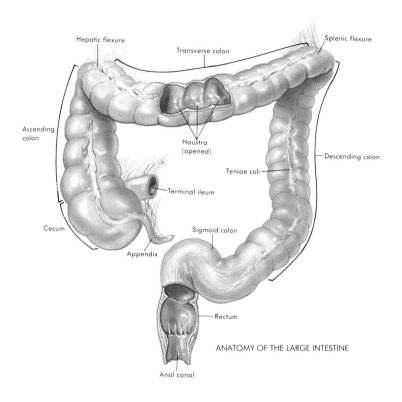

Hepatic flexure

Transverse colon

Splenic flexure

Ascending colon

Haustra (opened)

Descending colon

Teniae coli

Terminal ileum

Cecum

Sigmoid colon

Appendix

Rectum

ANATOMY OF THE LARGE INTESTINE

Anal canal

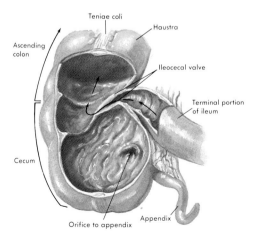

Teniae coli

Haustra

Ascending colon

Ileocecal valve

Terminal portion of ileum

Cecum

Orifice to appendix

Appendix

ENLARGED DETAIL OF THE CECUM AND TERMINAL ILEUM

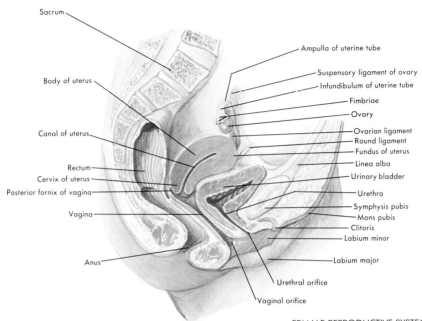

Sacrum

Ampulla of uterine tube

Suspensory ligament of ovary

Infundibulum of uterine tube

Body of uterus

Fimbriae

Ovary

Ovarian ligament

Round ligament

Canal of uterus

Fundus of uterus

Linea alba

Rectum

Urinary bladder

Cervix of uterus

Posterior fornix of vagina

Urethra

Symphysis pubis

Vagina

Mons pubis

Clitoris

Labium minor

Anus

Labium major

Urethral orifice

Vaginal orifice

FEMALE REPRODUCTIVE SYSTEM

MEDIAN SAGITTAL SECTION

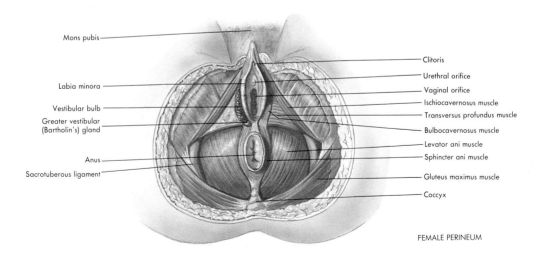

Mons pubis

Clitoris

Urethral orifice

Labia minora

Vaginal orifice

Ischiocavernosus muscle

Vestibular bulb

Transversus profundus muscle

Greater vestibular
(Bartholin's) gland

Bulbocavernosus muscle

Levator ani muscle

Anus

Sphincter ani muscle

Sacrotuberous ligament

Gluteus maximus muscle

Coccyx

FEMALE PERINEUM

LYMPHATIC DRAINAGE OF THE FEMALE BREAST

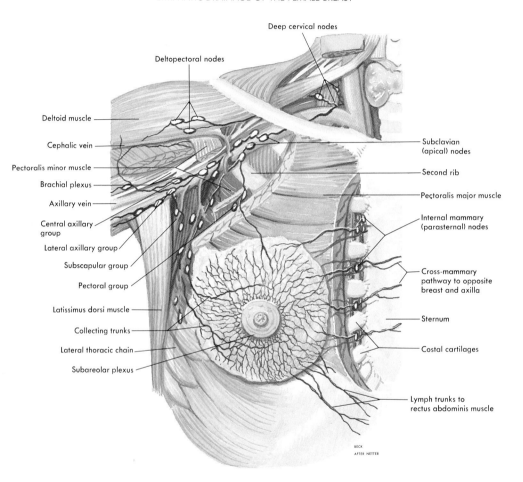

Deep cervical nodes

Deltopectoral nodes

Deltoid muscle

Cephalic vein

Pectoralis minor muscle

Brachial plexus

Axillary vein

Central axillary group

Lateral axillary group

Subscapular group

Pectoral group

Latissimus dorsi muscle

Collecting trunks

Lateral thoracic chain

Subareolar plexus

Subclavian (apical) nodes

Second rib

Pectoralis major muscle

Internal mammary (parasternal) nodes

Cross-mammary pathway to opposite breast and axilla

Sternum

Costal cartilages

Lymph trunks to rectus abdominis muscle

BECK
AFTER NETTER

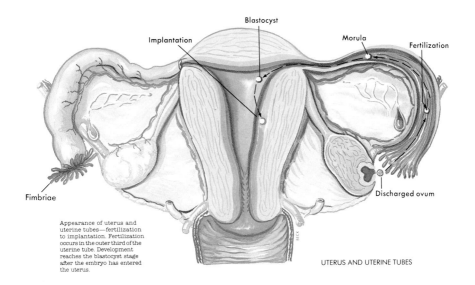

Implantation

Blastocyst

Morula

Fertilization

Fimbriae

Discharged ovum

Appearance of uterus and
uterine tubes—fertilization
to implantation. Fertilization
occurs in the outer third of the
uterine tube. Development
reaches the blastocyst stage
after the embryo has entered
the uterus.

UTERUS AND UTERINE TUBES

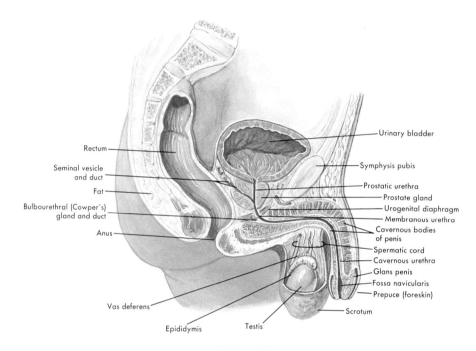

Rectum

Seminal vesicle
and duct

Fat

Bulbourethral (Cowper's)
gland and duct

Anus

Vas deferens

Epididymis

Testis

Urinary bladder

Symphysis pubis

Prostatic urethra

Prostate gland

Urogenital diaphragm

Membranous urethra

Cavernous bodies
of penis

Spermatic cord

Cavernous urethra

Glans penis

Fossa navicularis

Prepuce (foreskin)

Scrotum

Median sagittal section

MALE REPRODUCTIVE SYSTEM

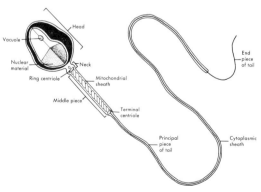

Vacuole

Nuclear
material

Ring centriole

Middle piece

Head

Neck

Mitochondrial
sheath

Terminal
centriole

Principal
piece
of tail

End
piece
of tail

Cytoplasmic
sheath

ANATOMY OF A SPERM

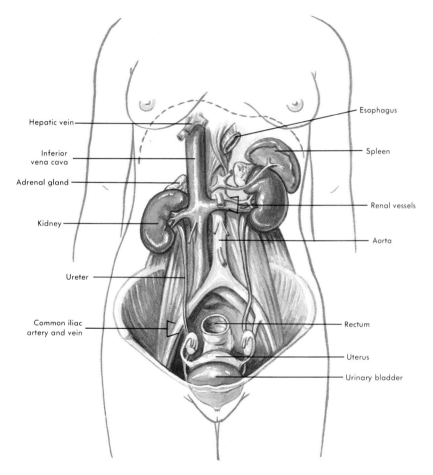

Hepatic vein

Inferior
vena cava

Adrenal gland

Kidney

Ureter

Common iliac
artery and vein

Esophagus

Spleen

Renal vessels

Aorta

Rectum

Uterus

Urinary bladder

URINARY SYSTEM

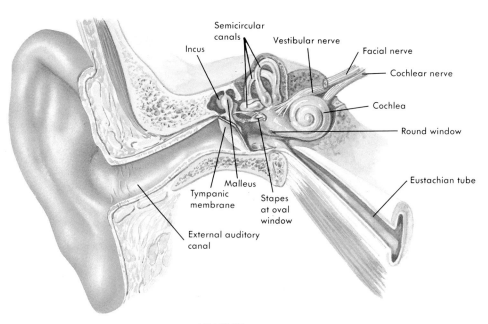

Semicircular
canals

Vestibular nerve

Facial nerve

Incus

Cochlear nerve

Cochlea

Round window

Eustachian tube

Malleus

Tympanic
membrane

Stapes
at oval
window

External auditory
canal

HEARING

GROSS ANATOMY OF THE EAR—FRONTAL SECTION

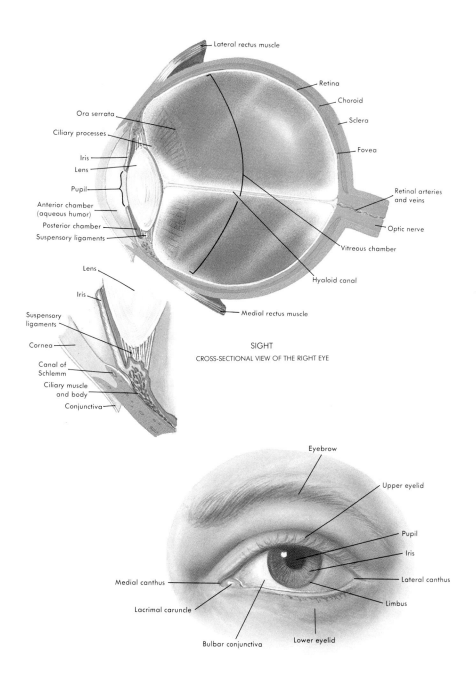

Lateral rectus muscle

Retina

Choroid

Sclera

Fovea

Ora serrata

Ciliary processes

Iris

Lens

Pupil

Retinal arteries and veins

Anterior chamber (aqueous humor)

Posterior chamber

Suspensory ligaments

Optic nerve

Vitreous chamber

Hyaloid canal

Lens

Iris

Suspensory ligaments

Cornea

Canal of Schlemm

Ciliary muscle and body

Conjunctiva

Medial rectus muscle

SIGHT

CROSS-SECTIONAL VIEW OF THE RIGHT EYE

Eyebrow

Upper eyelid

Pupil

Iris

Medial canthus

Lateral canthus

Lacrimal caruncle

Limbus

Bulbar conjunctiva

Lower eyelid

NORMAL ANATOMY

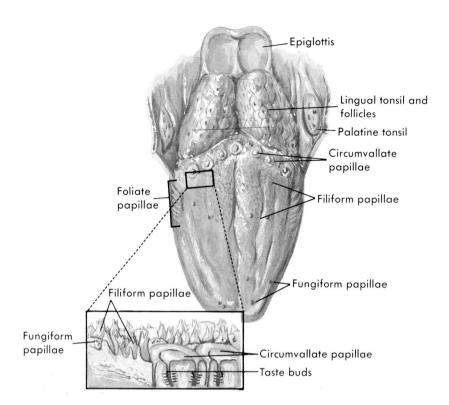

Epiglottis

Lingual tonsil and follicles

Palatine tonsil

Circumvallate papillae

Filiform papillae

Fungiform papillae

Foliate papillae

Filiform papillae

Fungiform papillae

Circumvallate papillae

Taste buds

TASTE

PAPILLAE ON THE TONGUE AND LOCATION OF THE TASTE BUDS

OLFACTORY NERVE DISTRIBUTION TO MUCOSA OF NASAL CAVITY

Frontal sinus

Cribriform plate of ethmoid bone

Internal nasal branches of anterior ethmoidal nerve

Olfactory tract

Olfactory bulb

Superior nasal concha

Sphenoid sinus

Nasal bone

Olfactory nerves

BECK

SMELL

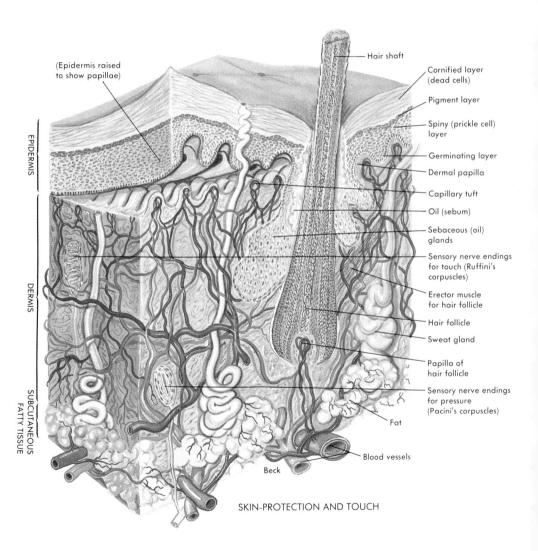

Hair shaft

(Epidermis raised
to show papillae)

Cornified layer
(dead cells)

Pigment layer

Spiny (prickle cell)
layer

Germinating layer

Dermal papilla

Capillary tuft

Oil (sebum)

Sebaceous (oil)
glands

Sensory nerve endings
for touch (Ruffini's
corpuscles)

Erector muscle
for hair follicle

Hair follicle

Sweat gland

Papilla of
hair follicle

Sensory nerve endings
for pressure
(Pacini's corpuscles)

Fat

Blood vessels

Beck

EPIDERMIS

DERMIS

SUBCUTANEOUS
FATTY TISSUE

SKIN-PROTECTION AND TOUCH

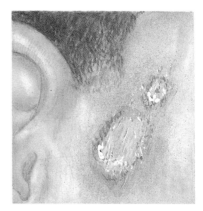

Tinea corporis
(ringworm)

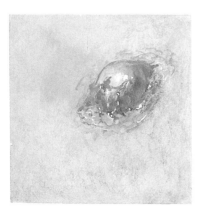

Squamous cell
carcinoma

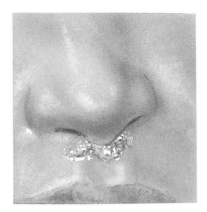

Impetigo contagiosa

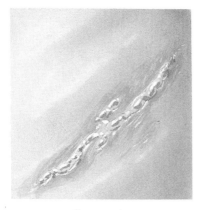

Herpes zoster
(shingles)

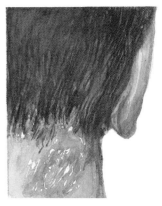

Dermatitis

COMMON SKIN DISORDERS

breathing, oxygen deficiency, or known allergy to this drug prohibits its use.

★ADVERSE EFFECTS: Among the more serious side effects are drug dependence, falling blood pressure, heart beat irregularities, and retention of urine.

Levsinex, a trademark for a peptic ulcer drug (hyoscyamine sulfate).

levulose. See **fructose.**

Leydig cells /lī′dig/, cells of the testes that secrete testosterone, a male sex hormone.

Leydig cell tumor, a generally noncancerous tumor of the interstitial cells of a testis. It may cause breast development in men and premature sexual development if the lesion occurs before puberty.

LGA, abbreviation for **large for gestational age.**

LGV, abbreviation for **lymphogranuloma venereum,** a sexually transmitted disease.

Lhermitte's sign /ler′mits/, sudden, temporary, electricitylike shocks spreading down the body when the head is flexed forward. It occurs chiefly in multiple sclerosis but also in compression disorders of the spinal cord in the neck.

liberation, 1. the process of drug release into a body organ or system from the dosage given. 2. the activation of an enzyme or chemical reaction.

libidinal development. See **psychosexual development.**

libidinous, pertaining to the libido, sexual desire. Also **libidinal.** –**libidinize,** *v.*

libido /libē′dō, libī′dō/, the psychic energy or instinctual drive associated with sexual desire, pleasure, or creativity.

Libman-Sacks endocarditis /lib′mənsaks′/, an abnormal condition of the heart. It is characterized by wartlike lesions that develop near the heart valves but rarely affect valve function. Also called **Libman-Sacks disease, Libman-Sacks syndrome.**

Librax, a trademark for a gastrointestinal drug containing a sedative (chlordiazepoxide hydrochloride).

Libritabs, a trademark for an antianxiety agent (chlordiazepoxide hydrochloride).

Librium, a trademark for an antianxiety agent (chlordiazepoxide hydrochloride).

licensed practical nurse (LPN), *U.S.* a person trained in basic nursing techniques and direct patient care who practices under the supervision of a registered nurse. The course of training usually lasts 1 year. In Canada an LPN is called a nursing assistant. Also called *U.S.* **licensed vocational nurse.**

licensed psychologist, a person who has earned a Ph.D. in psychology from an accredited graduate school and has completed 2 to 3 years of postgraduate training with special emphasis on the diagnosis and treatment of psychological disorders. Also called **clinical psychologist.** See also **psychotherapist.**

lichenification /līken′ifikā′shən/, a thickening and hardening of the skin, often resulting from irritation caused by repeated scratching of an itching lesion. –**lichenified,** *adj.*

lichen nitidus /lī′kən/, a skin disorder in which numerous small, flat, pale, glistening pimples form. Also called **Pinkus' disease.**

lichen planus, a noncancerous, chronic, itching skin disease of unknown cause, characterized by small, flat, purplish pimples or patches with fine, gray lines on the surface. Common sites are surfaces of wrists, forearms, ankles, abdomen, and lower back. On mucous membranes the lesions appear gray and lacy. Nails may have ridges running lengthwise. Compare **leukoplakia.**

lichen sclerosis et atrophicus, a chronic skin disease characterized by white, flat pimples with a red outer ring and black, hard plugs. In advanced cases, the pimples tend to merge into large, white patches of thin, itching skin. Lesions often occur on the trunk of the body and, frequently, in the anogenital regions.

lichen simplex chronicus, a skin disease in which a patch of itching pimples forms. Emotional factors and injury, such as scratching of lesions, prolong the symptoms. Treatment may include applying corticosteroid drugs on the skin to relieve the itching.

Lidex, a trademark for an adrenal gland hormone (fluocinonide).

lidocaine hydrochloride /lī′dəkān/, a local anesthetic agent prescribed for skin or mucous membranes and also used internally as an antiarrhythmic agent.

lid poppers, *slang.* amphetamines.

lie, the relationship between the head-to-foot position of the fetus in the uterus and that of the mother. In a longitudinal lie, the fetus is lying vertically, or up and down in the uterus. In a transverse lie, the fetus is positioned horizontally, across the opening of the cervix, making delivery difficult.

lie detector, an electronic instrument used to detect suspected lying or anxiety in regard to specific questions. A commonly used lie detector is the polygraph recorder that records pulse, breathing rate, blood pressure, and perspiration. Some experts believe that certain patterns of polygraph recordings indicate anxiety, guilt, or fear—emotions that are likely to occur when the subject is lying.

lienal vein /lē·ē′nəl/, a large vein of the lower body that is important in circulating blood from the spleen. Also called **splenic vein.**

lienography /lē′ənog′rəfē/, the x-ray examination of the spleen after is has been injected with a dye.

life island, a plastic bubble enclosing a bed, used to provide a germ-free environment for a patient.

life review, 1. (in psychiatry) a progressive return to conscious awareness of past experiences. 2. reminiscences that occur in old age as a result of the realization that death is inevitable.

lifesaving measure, any type of nursing action taken when a patient's physical or mental status is seriously threatened.

life science, the study of the laws and properties of living matter. Some kinds of life science are **anatomy, bacteriology, biology.** Compare **physical science.**

life space, a term used by American psychologists to describe all of the influences existing at the same time that may affect individual behavior. The total of the influences make up the life space.

lifestyle-induced health problems, diseases with histories that include known exposure to certain health-threatening or risk factors. An example is heart disease associated with cigarette smoking, poor eating habits, lack of exercise, and psychological stress.

lifetime reserve, a lifetime total of days of inpatient hospitalization benefits that may be drawn on by a patient who has exhausted the maximum benefits allowed under Medicare for a single spell of illness.

ligament, 1. a white, shiny, flexible band of fibrous tissue binding joints together and connecting various bones and cartilages. Such ligaments are slightly elastic and composed of parallel bundles of connective tissue. When part of a joint membrane, they are covered with fibrous tissue that blends with surrounding connective tissue. Yellow elastic ligaments connect certain parts of adjoining vertebrae. Compare **tendon.** 2. a layer of membrane with little or no stretching ability, extending from one abdominal organ to another. See also **broad ligament.**

ligamenta flava, the bands of yellow elastic tissue connecting adjacent vertebrae from the neck to the sacrum between the hipbones. They are thin, broad, and long in the neck region, thicker in the chest region, and thickest in the lower back region. They help to hold the body erect.

ligamental tear, a complete or a partial tear of the fibers of a ligament connecting and surrounding the bones of a joint. An injury to the joint, such as from a sudden twisting motion or a forceful blow, causes torn ligaments. This may occur at any joint but is most common in the knees, especially in young adults, and is often associated with sports injuries. Usually, the injury involves more than one structure because of the way in which they connect with and support each other. Treatment depends on the severity of the injury. A mild injury may cause little damage with tenderness, swelling, and pain with stress. Rest, compression, applications of heat and cold, elevation, and early use are usually recommended. An anti-inflammatory agent may be injected. In addition to these measures, treatment for a moderate injury in which few fibers have been completely torn requires removing any fluid accumulation and supporting the joint. Treatment for a severe, complete tear may require preventing movement, followed by physical therapy, or if necessary, surgical repair. Good physical condition may help prevent many injuries. Proper care during healing prevents permanent disability, such as instability, stiffness, or recurrent pain in the joint.

ligation /līgā'shən/, tying off a blood vessel or duct with a suture or wire to stop or prevent bleeding during surgery, to stop hemorrhage from an injury, or to prevent passage of material through a duct, as in ligation of the fallopian tubes to sterilize a woman. In treating varicose veins, the longest vein (saphenous) of the leg is tied off (ligated) above the swollen portion. See also **ligature, saphenous vein, tubal ligation, varicose veins.**

ligature, 1. a suture. 2. a wire, such as used in orthodontia to straighten teeth.

light, radiant energy of the wavelength and frequency that stimulate visual receptor cells in the retina of the eye to produce nerve impulses that are perceived in the brain as vision.

light bath, the exposure of the patient's uncovered skin to the sun or to ultraviolet light rays from an artificial source for healing purposes.

light chain disease, a type of bone marrow cancer in which plasma cell tumors produce only identical light chain proteins. Persons with light chain disease may develop bone lesions in which the bone decomposes, excessive calcium in the blood (hypercalcemia), impaired kidney function, and buildup of a waxy, starchy protein in tissues and organs (amyloidosis). The increase in light chain proteins tends to overwhelm the kidney, causing damage. See also **gammapathy, heavy chain disease, multiple myeloma.**

light diet, a diet suitable for convalescent or bedridden patients taking little or no exercise. It consists of simple, moderate quantities of soft-cooked and easily digested foods, including meats, potatoes, rice, eggs, pasta, some fruits, refined cereals, and breads. It avoids all highly seasoned and fried foods.

lightening, a sensation reported by many women late in pregnancy as the fetus settles lower in the pelvis, leaving more space in the upper abdomen. The diaphragm, no longer restricted by pressure of the uterus beneath it, can move down more fully, allowing deeper breaths to be taken. The stomach, also less compressed, can comfortably hold more food at each meal. The profile of the abdomen changes with lightening, because the round, full uterus is visibly lower. The fetus is then said to have 'dropped.'

light reflex, the mechanism by which the pupil of the eye reacts to changes in light and darkness. Also called **pupillary reflex.**

lignin /lig'nin/, a type of cellulose that forms the cell walls of plants. It provides bulk in the diet necessary for proper functioning of the stomach and intestines. See also **dietary fiber.**

lilliputian hallucination /lil'ipyoo'shən/, a false mental image in which things seem smaller than they actually are. See also **hallucination.**

limb, a body part, such as an arm or leg, or a branch of an internal organ.

limb-girdle muscular dystrophy, a form of muscular dystrophy in which weakness and atrophy of the muscles begins in the shoulder or in the pelvis. The condition is progressive, spreading to other body areas, regardless of the area in which it begins. See also **muscular dystrophy.**

limbic system, a group of related nervous system structures within the midbrain that are associated with various emotions and feelings, as anger, fear, sexual arousal, pleasure, and sadness. Unless the limbic system is regulated by other brain areas, attacks of uncontrollable rage may occur in some individuals. The function of the system is poorly understood.

limited fluctuation method of dosing, a method of drug administration in which the dose is not allowed to rise or fall beyond certain maximum and minimum limits.

limp, an abnormal pattern of walking, often favoring one leg.

Lincocin, a trademark for an antibiotic drug (lincomycin).

lincomycin hydrochloride, an antibiotic drug prescribed in the treatment of certain infections.

★CAUTION: Known allergy to this drug or to similar drugs prohibits its use.

★ADVERSE EFFECTS: Among the more common side effects are blood disorders, diarrhea, and the development of gastrointestinal infections.

lindane /lin'dān/, a drug prescribed in the treatment of pediculosis and scabies, skin diseases caused by lice and mites.

★CAUTION: It is not usually given to infants or pregnant women and is not applied to the face. Known allergy to this drug prohibits its use.

★ADVERSE EFFECTS: Among the most serious side effects are nerve damage and anemia. Irritation of eyes, skin, and mucous tissues may occur.

Lindbergh pump, a device used to preserve an organ of the body, usually during transport from a donor to a recipient for an organ transplant. The pump forces oxygen and other essential nutrients into the organ's tissues. Also called **Carrel-Lindbergh pump.**

line, a stripe, streak, or narrow ridge, often imaginary, that connects areas of the body or that separates various parts of the body, as the hair line or nipple line. Also called **linea.**

linea alba /lin'ē·ə/, a seam that runs along the middle line of the abdomen beneath the skin, formed by the fusion of three sheets of tissue fibers into a single tendon extending from the breastbone to the pubic area. It contains the navel.

linea albicantes. See **stretch mark.**

linea nigra, a dark line appearing on the abdomen of a pregnant woman during the latter part of the pregnancy. It usually extends from the pubic area to the navel.

linear fracture, a fracture that runs along the length of a bone.

linear grid. See **grid.**

line compensator, an electrical device that monitors electric power for medical devices, as x-ray equipment, and makes automatic adjustments for changes in voltage.

lingual artery, one of a pair of arteries that branch along the sides of the neck and head to supply the tongue and surrounding muscles.

lingual crib, an orthodontic device consisting of a wire frame suspended on the inner surface of the upper front teeth. It discourages undesirable thumb and tongue habits that can produce malocclusions in children.

lingual frenum, a band of tissue that extends from the floor of the mouth to the underside of the tongue and causes tongue-tie, a speech impediment. Also called **frenulum linguae.**

lingual goiter, a tumor at the back of the tongue formed by an enlarged or misplaced thyroid gland.

lingual rest, a metal extension onto the tongue side of a front tooth to provide support for a removable partial denture.

lingual tonsil, a mass of small lymph nodes (nodules) that form part of the mucous membrane near the root of the tongue. The lingual tonsil is part of the body's defense system against infection.

liniment, a remedy, usually containing an alcoholic, oily, or soapy substance, that is rubbed on the skin as a counterirritant, producing an inflammatory reaction to reduce one elsewhere.

linitis /lini'tis/, inflammation of the stomach lining.

linitis plastica. See **leather bottle stomach.**

linkage, the location of two or more genes on the same chromosome so that they tend to be transmitted together as a unit. The closer the genes are to each other, the more likely they are to be inherited as a group and associated with a specific trait.

linoleic acid /lin'əlē'ik/, a colorless to straw-colored essential fatty acid that occurs in linseed and safflower oils. Linoleic acid is used in margarine, animal feeds, emulsifying agents, soaps, and drugs.

linolenic acid, an unsaturated fatty acid essential for normal human nutrition. It occurs in compounds of linseed and other vegetable oils.

Lioresal, a trademark for an antispastic and muscle-relaxant agent (baclofen).

liothyronine sodium /lī′ōthī′rənēn/, a synthetic thyroid hormone prescribed in the treatment of thyroid deficiency, simple goiter, or cretinism.

★CAUTION: Excessive thyroid hormone, heart disorders, or known allergy to this drug prohibits its use. It is used with caution in patients with diabetes mellitus.

★ADVERSE EFFECTS: Among the serious side effects, usually caused by overdosage, are thyroid toxicity, nausea, vomiting, high blood pressure, nervousness, and loss of weight.

liotrix /lī′ətriks/, a uniform mixture of the thyroid hormones T_3 and T_4 prescribed in the treatment of hypothyroid conditions.

★CAUTION: Most diseases, abnormal conditions of the heart, or known allergy to this drug prohibits its use.

★ADVERSE EFFECTS: Among the more serious side effects are rapid heart beat, nervousness, insomnia, and fever.

lip, 1. either the upper or lower fleshy structure surrounding the opening of the mouth. 2. any rimlike structure bordering a cavity or groove.

lipase /lī′pās, lip′ās/, any of several digestive system enzymes that increase the breakdown of fats (lipids).

lipectomy /lipek′təmē/, surgical removal of fat beneath the skin, as from the abdominal wall. Also called **adipectomy.**

lipedema /lip′ədē′mə/, a condition in which fat deposits accumulate in the legs, from the hips to the ankles, accompanied by tenderness in the affected areas. Treatment involves changes in diet.

lipemia /lipē′mē·ə/, a condition in which increased amounts of fats are present in the blood, a normal occurrence after eating.

lipid, any of the various fats or fatlike substances in plant or animal tissues. Lipids are insoluble in water but soluble in alcohol, chloroform, ether, and other organic solvents. They are stored in the body and serve as an energy reserve but may be elevated in certain diseases, such as atherosclerosis. Kinds of lipids are **cholesterol, fatty acids, neutral fat, phospholipids, phospholipid as phosphorus, triglycerides.**

lipidosis /lip′idō′sis/, any disorder that involves the accumulation of abnormal levels of certain fats (lipids) in the body. Kinds of lipidoses are **Gaucher's disease, Krabbe's disease, Niemann-Pick disease, Tay-Sachs disease.**

lipiduria /lip′idoŏr′ē·ə/, the presence of fat bodies (lipids) in the urine.

lipoatrophic diabetes /lip′ō·atrof′ik/, an inherited disease characterized by insulin-resistant diabetes mellitus, loss of body fat, a skin disease marked by dark-colored, wartlike areas in body folds (acanthosis nigricans), and enlarged muscles. It is associated with a disorder of a portion of the brain (hypothalamus) resulting in excessive amounts of certain hormones in the blood.

lipoatrophy /lip′ō·at′rəfē/, a breakdown of fat below the skin at the site of an insulin injection. In usually occurs after several injections at the same site. Compare **lipohypertrophy.**

lipochrome /lip′əkrōm/, any fat-soluble pigment that gives the natural yellow color to fatty tissues or foods, such as butter, egg yolk, and yellow corn. See also **carotenoid.**

lipodystrophia progressiva, an abnormal accumulation of fat around the buttocks and thighs with a progressive disappearance of fat beneath the skin from areas above the waist. It affects mainly young girls. Also called **lipomatosis atrophicans.**

lipodystrophy /lip′ōdis′trəfē/, any abnormality in the transformation (metabolism) of fats, particularly one in which the fat deposits under the skin are affected.

lip of hip fracture, a fracture of the lip of the hip socket, often associated with hip displacement.

lipofuscin /lip′əfus′in/, a group of fats found in abundance in the cells of adults. Studies suggest that lipofuscins contribute to the aging process in a cell.

lipohypertrophy /lip′ōhīpur′trəfē/, a buildup of fat tissue under the skin at the site of an insulin injection. Compare **lipoatrophy.**

lipoid /lip′oid/, any substance that resembles a fat.

lipolysis /lipol′isis/, the breakdown or destruction of fats.

lipoma /lipō′mə/, pl. **lipomas, lipomata,** a tumor consisting of fat cells. Also called **adipose tumor.** See also **multiple lipomatosis.** –**lipomatous,** adj.

lipoma annulare colli, an accumulation of fat around the neck; it is not a true fat tumor. Also called **Madelung's neck.**

lipoma arborescens, a fatty tumor of a joint, with a treelike distribution of fat cells.

lipoma capsulare, a tumor of fat cells in the capsule of an organ, such as the capsule or sheath covering the kidney.

lipoma fibrosum, a fatty tumor containing masses of fibrous tissue.

lipomatosis /lip′ōmətō′sis/, abnormal tumorlike accumulations of fat in body tissues.

lipomatosis dolorosa, abnormal accumulations of painful or tender fat deposits. Also called **lipoma dolorosa.**

lipomatous myxoma, a tumor containing fatty tissue that begins in connective tissue.

lipomatous nephritis, a rare condition in which the kidney filtration units are replaced by fatty tissue. Kidney failure may result. Also called **lipoma diffusum renis, lipomatosis renis.**

lipoprotein /lip'ōprō'tēn/, a protein in which fats (lipids) form a part of the molecule. Practically all of the lipids in human blood are present as lipoproteins. Kinds of lipoproteins are **chylomicrons, high density lipoproteins (HDL), low density lipoproteins (LDL), very low density lipoproteins (VLDL).**

liposarcoma /lip'ōsärkō'mə/, pl. **liposarcomas, liposarcomata,** a cancerous growth of fat cells.

liposuction, a technique for removing fatty tissue from overweight patients with a suction-pump device. It is used primarily to remove or reduce areas of fat around the stomach, breasts, legs, face, and upper arms where the skin will tighten and regain a normal appearance. Also called **suction lipectomy.**

Liquaemin Sodium, a trademark for a blood anticoagulant (heparin sodium).

liquefaction, the process in which a solid or a gas is made liquid.

liquid, a state of matter, intermediate between solid and gas, in which the substance flows freely with little application of force and assumes the shape of the vessel in which it is contained.

liquid diet, a diet consisting of foods that can be served in liquid or strained form plus custard, ice cream, pudding, tapioca, and soft-cooked eggs. It is prescribed in acute infections, in acute inflammatory conditions of the gastrointestinal tract, and for patients unable to consume soft or semifluid foods, usually following surgery. See also **full liquid diet.**

liquid glucose, a thick, syrupy, odorless, colorless, or yellowish liquid used as a food, chiefly in treating dehydration.

liquor, any fluid or liquid, as the amniotic fluid in a pregnant woman's uterus (liquor amnii).

liquor amnii. See **amniotic fluid.**

liquorice, a dried root of gummy texture from a plant used as a flavoring agent in medicines, especially in cough syrups and laxatives. Also spelled **licorice.**

Lisfranc's fracture /lisfrangks'/, a fracture dislocation of the foot in which one or all of the toe bones are displaced.

lisping, the faulty pronunciation of one or more related consonant sounds, usually /s/ and /z/.

Listeria monocytogenes /mon'ōsītoj'inēz/, a common species of bacteria that causes listeriosis.

listeriosis /listir'ē·ō'sis/, a disease caused by a type of bacteria that infects shellfish, birds, spiders, and mammals in all areas of the world. It is transmitted to humans by direct contact with infected animals, by inhalation of dust, or contact with sewage or soil contaminated with the organism. All secretions from an infected person may contain the organism. The signs of infection are circulatory collapse, shock, heart inflammation, enlarged liver and spleen, and a

dark, red rash over the trunk and the legs. The signs and severity of the disease vary according to the site of infection and the age and condition of the patient. Newborns and debilitated older patients are more vulnerable. Pregnant women may experience a mild, brief episode of illness but fetal infection acquired through the placenta is usually fatal. If infection is suspected in a pregnant woman, treatment is begun immediately. Infection in the newborn apparently results from exposure to the organism in the birth canal of an infected mother. Meningitis and brain inflammation occur in 75% of cases. Treatment may include antibiotics given by injection. Also spelled **listerosis.**

Lithane, a trademark for an antimanic drug (lithium carbonate) for use in manic-depressive psychosis.

lithiasis /lithī'əsis/, the formation of stones (calculi) from mineral salts in the hollow organs or ducts of the body. Stone formation occurs most commonly in the gallbladder, kidney, and lower urinary tract. Lithiasis may produce no symptoms. More often the condition irritates, inflames, or obstructs the organ, and is extremely painful. Surgery may be necessary if the stones cannot be excreted spontaneously. Lower urinary tract stones often can be dissolved.

lithium (Li), a silvery-white alkali metal occurring in various compounds. Lithium carbonate is a salt of lithium commonly used for psychiatric treatment in the United States. It has been effective in preventing recurrent attacks of manic-depressive illnesses and has helped to correct sleep disorders in manic patients.

lithium carbonate, an antimanic agent prescribed in the treatment of manic episodes of manic-depressive disorder.
★CAUTION: It is used with caution in the presence of kidney or heart disease and is not recommended for children under 12 years of age. Known allergy to this drug prohibits its use.
★ADVERSE EFFECTS: Among the most serious side effects are kidney damage, excessive thirst and urination, and impairment of mental and physical abilities. Retention of sodium and fluid in the body tissues may occur.

lithopedion /lith'əpē'dē·ən/, a fetus that has died in the uterus and has become hardened or bonelike. Also called **lithopedium, calcified fetus, ostembryon, osteopedion.**

lithotomy /lithot'əmē/, the surgical removal of a stone (calculus), especially one from the urinary tract.

lithotomy position, a bodily posture on an examining table in which the patient lies on the back with the hips and knees fully flexed. For obstetric procedures, the buttocks are at the edge of the table and the feet are held in stirrups. Also called **dorsosacral position.** See illustration on p. 468.

lithotrite /lith'ətrīt/, an instrument for crushing a

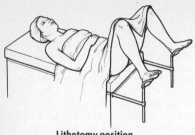

Lithotomy position

stone in the urinary bladder. Also called **lithotriptor.** –**lithotrity,** *n.*

litmus paper, absorbent paper coated with litmus, a blue dye, that is used to determine acidity or alkalinity in body fluids, such as urine. Acid substances or solutions turn blue litmus to red. Alkaline substances or solutions do not cause a color change in blue litmus.

litter, a stretcher.

live birth, the birth of an infant that exhibits any sign of life, such as breathing, heart beat, umbilical cord pulsation, or movement of voluntary muscles. Length of pregnancy of the mother is not considered. A live birth is not always one in which the infant is capable of continuing life (viable).

livedo /livē′dō/, a blue or reddish mottling or blotching of the skin. It worsens in cold weather and probably is caused by a spasm of small arteries (arterioles).

livedo reticularis, a disorder of constricted blood vessels, aggravated by exposure to cold. It causes a reddish-blue mottling of the skin with a typical "fishnet" appearance that can involve an entire leg and, less often, an arm.

liver, the largest gland of the body and one of its most complex organs. Located in the upper right portion of the abdominal cavity, the liver attaches to the diaphragm by two ligaments. During deep breathing, the liver rolls forward and downward, and can be felt through the abdominal wall. It is completely covered by a membrane (peritoneum) except along the line of attachment to another of the ligaments holding it in place. The liver is divided into four lobes, with the right lobe much larger than the others. It contains as many as 100,000 smaller lobes (lobules) amd is served by two separate blood supplies. The hepatic artery conveys oxygenated blood from the heart to the liver. The hepatic portal vein conveys nutrient-filled blood from the stomach and the intestines. At any given moment the liver holds about 1 pint of blood or approximately 13% of the total blood supply of the body. Dark reddish-brown in color, it has a soft, solid consistency and is shaped like an irregular hemisphere. The adult liver in men weighs about

1.8 kg (3.9 pounds); in women, about 1.3 kg (2.8 pounds). More than 500 of its functions have been identified. Some of its major functions are producing bile by liver cells; processing glucose, proteins, vitamins, fats, and most of the other compounds used by the body; producing hemoglobin for vital use of its iron content in red blood cells; and converting poisonous ammonia to urea. Bile from the liver is stored in the gallbladder, in the hepatic duct, and in numerous blood vessels. The liver cells produce about 1 pint of bile daily. They also render harmless numerous substances, such as alcohol, nicotine, and other poisons, as well as various harmful substances produced by the intestine. See also **gallbladder.**

liver biopsy, a diagnostic procedure in which a special needle is introduced into the liver using local anesthesia to obtain a specimen for laboratory examination.

liver cancer, a malignant tumor of the liver, occurring most frequently by the spread of cells from another cancer in the body. Primary liver cancer (one that originates in the liver) is common in Africa and Southeast Asia but relatively uncommon in the United States. Primary tumors are six to 10 times more prevalent in men than in women, develop most often in the sixth decade of life, and are associated with cirrhosis of the liver in 70% of the cases. Other risk factors include an excess of iron in the liver, schistosomiasis infection from the fluke parasite, exposure to chemicals such as vinyl chloride or arsenic, and possibly nutritional deficiencies. Although alcoholism may be a factor, nonalcoholic cirrhosis is a greater risk than alcoholic cirrhosis. Aflatoxins, cancer-causing substances produced by fungus in moldy grain and peanuts, appear to be linked to high rates of liver cancer in tropical areas. Characteristics of liver cancer are abdominal bloating, loss of appetite, weakness, a dull upper abdominal pain, fluid accumulation, mild jaundice, and a tender enlarged liver. Primary liver cancers spread to the portal vein and lymphatic vessels, and migrate to lymph nodes, the lungs, brain, and other sites. Total surgical removal of a liver lobe is the preferred treatment for primary tumors. Because the liver is able to regenerate itself, 80% of it may be removed. Anticancer drugs may result in temporary tumor regression. Irradiation is very destructive to all liver cells and is not a recommended treatment.

liver disease, any of a group of liver disorders. The most important diseases in this group are cirrhosis, bile problems (cholestasis), and hepatitis. Characteristics of liver disease are jaundice, loss of appetite, liver enlargement, fluid accumulation, and impaired consciousness. See also **cholestasis, cirrhosis, hepatitis.**

liver flap. See **asterixis.**

liver function test, a test used to evaluate various functions of the liver, such as metabolism, storage, filtration, and excretion.

liver scan, a technique of visualizing the size, shape, and consistency of the liver by injecting into a vein a radioactively labeled compound that is taken up and trapped in the cells of the liver. The radiation emitted by the compound is recorded by a radiation detector and can be photographed with a special camera or filmed with x-rays. Liver scans are most useful for locating abscesses or tumors. See also **label.**

liver spot, *nontechnical.* a brown or black slightly raised lesion seen on older persons.

living-in unit, a room provided in some hospitals for mothers who want to assume immediate care of their newborn infants under the supervision of nursing personnel.

living will, a written agreement between a patient and physician to withhold heroic measures if the patient's condition is found to be terminal.

livor mortis /lī'vər/, the purple discoloration of the skin of some body areas after death as a result of blood cell destruction.

lizard bite, bites of the large Gila monster of Arizona, New Mexico, and Utah, and the beaded lizard of Mexico. They are the only lizards known to be venomous. The symptoms of their bites and the recommended treatment are similar to those of the bites from moderately poisonous snakes.

L.M.D., abbreviation for **local medical doctor,** used by house staff or others to distinguish a patient's primary physician from medical school professors, attending specialists, house staff, or physicians. Also called **P.M.D.**

LMP, abbreviation for *last menstrual period.*

loads, *slang.* a combination of a sedative hypnotic (glutethimide) and a major narcotic analgesic (codeine). The medications are taken orally by drug abusers for an effect reported to be similar to that produced by heroin. An overdose may cause rolling eye movements, slurred speech, breathing difficulty, seizures, coma, and death.

lobar pneumonia, a severe infection of one or more of the lobes of the lungs. *Streptococcus pneumoniae* bacteria usually cause the disease but other bacteria can also produce it. Signs of infection are fever, chills, cough with bloody sputum, rapid shallow breathing, bluish skin coloration, nausea, vomiting, and inflammation of the membrane covering the lungs (pleurisy). With an early diagnosis, appropriate antibiotic therapy is highly successful. Complications include lung abscess, lung collapse, pus accumulation, and inflammation of the membrane surrounding the heart (pericarditis). Precautions against spread of the contagious disease are important. Because the fatality rate in the el-

derly and those with other diseases is high, a preventive injection of pneumococcal vaccine is recommended for them. Compare **bronchopneumonia.**

lobe, **1.** a roundish projection of any structure. **2.** a semidetached portion of any organ, outlined by clefts, furrows, or connective tissue, as the lobes of the brain, liver, and lungs. **–lobar, lobular,** *adj.*

lobectomy, a type of chest surgery in which a lobe of a lung is removed. A lobectomy may be performed to remove a cancer and to treat uncontrolled bronchial inflammation, an injury with hemorrhage, or tuberculosis. Before surgery, any respiratory infection is cleared and smoking is forbidden. The chest cavity is entered through a long back-to-front incision to remove the diseased lobe. During the first 24 hours after surgery, oxygen is given. The remaining lung tissue overexpands to fill the new space. **–lobectomize,** *v.*

lobotomy, brain surgery in which nerve fibers in the frontal lobe of the brain are severed. Severe, difficult-to-treat depression and pain are among the reasons for the operation. The procedure was overused in the treatment of mental patients in the past. It is rarely performed now because it has many unpredictable and undesirable effects, including loss of blader and bowel control, personality change, aggressiveness or apathy, and socially unacceptable behavior. Also called **leukotomy.**

lobster-claw deformity. See **bidactyly.**

lobular carcinoma, a tumor that often forms a widely spread mass and accounts for a small percentage of breast tumors.

lobule /lob'yo͞ol/, a small lobe, as the ear lobe.

local, **1.** pertaining to a small, defined area of the body. **2.** pertaining to a treatment or drug applied locally to a small area, as a local anesthetic.

local adaption syndrome (LAS), the response of a specific tissue, organ, or body system that occurs as a reaction to stress. See also **general adaption syndrome.**

local anesthesia, the direct administration of a local anesthetic agent to cause the loss of feeling in a small area of the body. Brief surgical or dental procedures are the most common reasons for using local anesthesia. The anesthetic may be applied to the surface of the skin or membrane or injected through or under the skin. Principal drawbacks to using local anesthesia are allergic reactions to certain anesthetics and occasional difficulty in deadening the local nerves. The advantage is that a conscious patient can cooperate and does not require breathing support. To avoid general anesthesia, some major surgical procedures are occasionally performed using local anesthesia. The tissues are anesthetized layer by layer, as the surgeon approaches the deeper structures of the body. Regional anesthesia has largely replaced this procedure. In all cases, the recommended dosage of any anesthetic agent is the smallest possible to achieve the desired loss of pain, because side effects are directly related to the total amount of drug given. Each anesthetic agent carries a recommended maximum allowable dose that is not safely exceeded. Compare **general anesthesia, regional anesthesia, topical anesthesia.**

local anesthetic, a substance used to reduce or eliminate nerve sensation, specifically pain, in a limited area of the body. Local anesthetics act by blocking transmission of nerve impulses. More than 100 drugs are available for local anesthesia. Any substance potent enough to induce local anesthesia can also cause adverse side effects, ranging from easily reversible skin disorders to fatal sensitivity reactions or both lung and heart arrest.

local cerebral blood flow (LCBF), (in positron emission tomography) the image of blood flow through the brain. It is expressed in units per milliliters of blood flow per minute.

local cerebral metabolic rate of glucose utilization (LCMRG), (in positron emission tomography) an image of the brain expressed in units of milligrams of sugar (glucose) metabolism per minute per 100g of brain tissue.

local control, the arrest of cancer growth at a site of treatment.

local hypothermia, heating a local area of tissue to beneficial temperatures that usually destroy disease organisms.

localization film, an x-ray film taken to confirm a treatment effect or to view the position of a radioactive implant, especially for computing the dose delivered.

localizer image, (in computed tomography) an image used to locate a specific body part.

lochia /lō'kē·ə/, the discharge that flows from the vagina following childbirth. During the first few days, the lochia is red and consists of blood, discarded cells from the uterus and placental tissue, and fetal body matter, such as hair or fat from the skin covering. After the third day, the amount of blood lessens, the lochia becomes darker and thinner, and then watery as evacuation of solid material is completed. During the second week, white blood cells and bacteria appear in large numbers along with fatty material, causing the lochia to appear yellow. During and after the third week, the amount of lochia decreases markedly. Cessation of the flow of lochia at about 6 weeks is usual. –**lochial,** *adj.*

locking point, a point on the body at which light pressure can be applied to help a weak or debilitated person maintain a certain posture or position. A basic locking point is the body's center of gravity, at the level of the sacral vertebra in the lower back area, where mild pressure can assist a person in standing or walking erect.

lockjaw. See tetanus.

locum tenens /lō'kəm ten'ənz/, a temporary substitute for a physician who is away from the practice. It is derived from Latin words meaning "holding someone's place."

locus, a specific place or position, as the locus of a particular gene on a chromosome, or the locus of infection, a site in the body where an infection originates.

Loestrin, a trademark for a birth-control pill containing an estrogen (ethinyl estradiol) and a progestin (norethindrone acetate).

Lofenalac, a trademark for a commercial milk-substitute formula that is low in an amino acid, phenylalamine, and used for infants with phenylketonuria. It is made from a milk protein (casein) and supplemented with an amino acid, tyrosine, and fortified with added fat, carbohydrate, minerals, and vitamins to balance the formula. See also **phenylketonuria.**

Löffler's syndrome /lef'lərz/, a disorder marked by loss of appetite, breathlessness, cough, fever, and weight loss. Recovery is spontaneous and prompt.

log-roll, a maneuver used to turn a bedridden person from one side to the other or completely over without flexing the spinal column. The arms of the patient are folded across the chest and the legs are extended. A draw sheet under the person is manipulated to make the procedure easier.

loiasis /lō·ī'əsis/, a worm infestation (filariasis) caused by a round worm *Loa loa,* which may migrate for 10 to 15 years under the skin producing localized inflammations known as Calabar swellings. Occasionally, the migrating worms may be visible beneath the eyelids. The disease is acquired through the bite of an infected African deer fly. A similar disease occurs in Asia.

loin, a part of the body on each side of the spinal column between the lowest ribs and the hip bones.

Lomotil, a trademark for an antidiarrheal drug.

lomustine, an anticancer agent prescribed in the treatment of a variety of malignant tumor diseases.

★CAUTION: Known allergy to this drug prohibits its use.

★ADVERSE EFFECTS: Among the more serious side effects are bone marrow disorders, nausea, and vomiting.

Lonalac, a trademark for a low sodium, nutritional supplement.

long-acting drug, a remedy with a prolonged effect. It may result from the slow release of the drug or depend on a gradual absorption of small amounts of the drug over an extended period of time.

long-acting insulin, a preparation of beef or pork pancreas modified by the presence of zinc. An injection of the preparation takes effect within 8 hours, reaches a peak of action in 16 to 24 hours, and lasts more than 36 hours. Also called **slow-acting insulin, ultralente insulin.**

long-acting thyroid stimulator (LATS), a natural substance, probably an antibody, that causes prolonged stimulation of the thyroid gland. Rapid growth of the gland and excess activity of thyroid function results in hyperthyroidism. It is found in the blood of 50% of patients affected with Graves' disease.

long-arm cast, an orthopedic cast that immobilizes the arm from the hand to the upper arm. It is used in the treatment of fractures of the arm, for postoperative positioning of the arm, and to correct deformities of the lower arm, wrist, or elbow. Compare **short-arm cast.**

long bones, the bones that contribute to the height or length of an arm or leg.

longitudinal, 1. referring to a measurement in the direction of the long axis of an organ, object, or body, such as an imaginary line from head to toe. 2. referring to a scientific study that is conducted over a long period of time.

long-leg cast, an orthopedic cast that immobilizes the leg from the toes to the upper thigh. It is used in treating fractures and dislocations of the knee, for postoperative positioning and immobilization of the knee, lower leg, and ankle, and for correction of deformities of the foot, lower leg, and knee. Compare **short-leg cast.**

long-leg cast with walker, an orthopedic cast that immobilizes the leg from the toes to the upper thigh and used in treating certain fractures of the leg. This type of cast is the same as the long-leg cast but with the addition of a rubber walker. The patient can walk, wearing the cast, when weight-bearing on the foot is allowed.

long-term memory, the ability to recall sensations, events, ideas, and other information for long periods of time without apparent effort.

long-term care, the provision of medical care services on a repeated or continuing basis to persons with chronic physical or mental disorders. The care may be provided in various settings ranging from institutions to private homes.

long tract signs, signs of nervous system disorders, such as repeated involuntary muscle contractions or loss of bladder control. They usually indicate a lesion in the middle or upper portions of the spinal cord or in the brain, disrupting nerve impulses normally transmitted over long nerve tracts.

Loniten, a trademark for a high blood pressure drug (minoxidil).

loop. See **intrauterine device.**

loop colostomy, a type of temporary intestinal opening (colostomy) on the surface of the abdomen made as part of the surgical repair of Hirschsprung's disease, a congenital disorder of the colon. A segment of large intestine (colon) is brought through an abdominal incision, formed into a loop, and sewn onto the skin of the abdomen. An opening is then made on the outside surface of the loop. After complete healing of the surgical repair of the colon, usually within a few months to 1 year, the colostomy is closed.

loop of Henle /hen′lē/, the U-shaped portion of a kidney filtration tubule.

loosening, a psychological disturbance in which the association of ideas and thought patterns become so vague, diffuse, and unfocused as to lack any logical sequences or relationship to any preceding concepts or themes. The condition is frequently a symptom of schizophrenia.

Lo/Ovral, a trademark for a birth-control pill containing an estrogen (ethinyl estradiol) and a progestin (norgestrel).

loperamide hydrochloride, a drug prescribed in the treatment of diarrhea.

★CAUTION: Known allergy to this drug prohibits its use. It is not given to patients in whom constipation must be avoided.

★ADVERSE EFFECTS: Among the most serious reactions are abdominal pain, constipation, nausea, and vomiting.

Lopid, a trademark for a fat metabolism regulating agent (gemfibrozil).

Lopressor, a trademark for a drug used to treat high blood pressure (metoprolol tartrate).

Loprox, a trademark for a drug used to treat fungus infections (ciclopirox olamine).

lordosis /lôrdō′sis/, an abnormal, increased degree of forward curvature of any part of the spine.

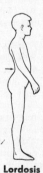

Lordosis

Lorelco, a trademark for a cholesterol reducing drug (probucol).

lotion, a liquid preparation applied to protect the skin or to treat a skin disorder.

Lotrimin, a trademark for a drug used to treat fungus infections (clotrimazole).

Lotusate, a trademark for a barbiturate sedative (talbutal).

Lou Gehrig's disease. See **amyotrophic lateral sclerosis.**

Louis-Bar syndrome. See **ataxia-telangiectasia.**

loupe /lo͞op/, a magnifying lens mounted in a frame worn on the head by an examining physician, and used to examine the eyes.

louse bite, a tiny puncture wound produced by a louse, a small, wingless insect. Diseases such as typhus, trench fever, and relapsing fever may be transmitted by lice. Head and body lice are common parasites and are frequently found among schoolchildren. The bite may cause intense itching, resulting in infection from scratching. Bathing, applying an approved insecticide, and cleaning clothes and bed linens are recommended procedures for treatment and prevention against the spread of lice.

low back pain, pain at the base of the spine that may be caused by a muscle sprain or strain, arthritis, a tumor, or a ruptured cartilage disk between vertebrae. Other causes are poor posture, obesity, enlarged prostate gland, sagging abdominal muscles, sitting for prolonged periods of time, or excessive physical effort involving the back muscles. The pain may be accompanied by muscle weakness or spasms. It may radiate down the back of one or both legs, as in sciatica. It may be started or increased by coughing, sneezing, rising from a seated position, lifting, stretching, bending, or turning. To guard against the pain, the patient may decrease the range of motion of the spine. The low back pain patient should sleep on a firm mattress with the knees flexed and supported. Pain killers, muscle relaxants, and tranquilizers may help, as may applying dry or moist heat. When the pain subsides, the patient may increase activity if fatigue is avoided. A corset or back brace may be required. The patient should use a straight-backed chair and not cross or extend the legs.

low birth weight (LBW) infant, an infant whose weight at birth is less than 2,500 grams (5.5 pounds). These babies are at risk for developing oxygen starvation during labor, low blood sugar after birth, and growth retardation in childhood, especially if the low birth weight is the result of a prolonged deficiency before birth, maternal malnutrition, or the mother's drug or alcohol addiction. Many low birth weight infants have no problems and develop normally, their smallness being inherited or the problem that caused their slowed growth being mild or brief.

low calcium diet, a diet that restricts the use of calcium and eliminates most of the dairy foods, all breads made with milk, fresh or dry, and deep-green leafy vegetables. It is prescribed for patients who form kidney stones. Meats, including beef, lamb, pork, veal, and poultry; fish; vegetables; legumes; and fruits are recommended.

low caloric diet, a diet that limits the intake of calories, usually to cause a reduction in body weight. Such diets may be designated as 800 calorie, 1,000 calorie, or other specific numbers of calories. Exchange lists may be used to allow patients to select foods they like from groups of foods that are sources of carbohydrates, proteins, and fats.

low cervical cesarean section, a method for surgically delivering a baby through a sideways (horizontal) incision in the thin lower part of the uterus. This incision bleeds less during surgery and heals with a stronger scar than the higher up-and-down (vertical) scar of the traditional cesarean section. See also **cesarean section.**

low cholesterol diet, a diet that restricts foods containing animal fats, such as egg yolk, cream, butter, milk, muscle and organ meats, and shellfish and recommends poultry, fish, vegetables, fruits, cottage cheese, and fats from plant sources (polyunsaturated). The diet is for patients with high serum cholesterol levels, heart disorders, obesity, and excessive blood fats. Also called **low saturated fat diet.**

low density lipoprotein (LDL), a blood substance containing large amounts of cholesterol and triglycerides. The high cholesterol content is a potential cause of heart disease. See also **cholesterol, triglyceride.**

lower extremity suspension, a procedure used in the treatment of bone fractures and the correction of abnormalities of the legs. Traction equipment, including metal frames, ropes, and pulleys, relieves the weight of the leg.

lower motor neuron paralysis, an injury to or lesion in the spinal cord. There is decreased muscle tone, diminished or absent reflexes, local twitching of muscle groups, and progressive wasting of the muscles.

lower respiratory tract, a division of the respiratory system that includes the left and the right bronchi and the alveoli where the exchange of oxygen and carbon dioxide occurs during the breathing cycle. The bronchi, which are branches of the trachea, or windpipe, divide into smaller bronchioles in the lung tissue; the bronchioles divide into alveolar ducts; the ducts into alveolar sacs; and the sacs into alveoli. The alveolar sacs and the alveoli present a total lung surface of about 850 square feet for the exchange of oxygen and carbon dioxide. The exchange occurs between the cells lining the alveoli and the tiny capillaries in the alveolar walls. The lower respiratory tract is a common site of infections, obstructive conditions, and lung cancer. See also **lung, upper respiratory tract.**

low fat diet, a diet containing limited amounts of fat and consisting chiefly of easily digestible foods with a high carbohydrate content. Included are all vegetables, lean meats, fish, fowl, pasta, cereals, and whole-wheat or enriched bread. Egg yolk and fatty meats are restricted. Cream, fried foods, foods prepared in oil, gravy, cheese, peanut butter, and olives are also omitted. The diet may be recommended for gallbladder disease and malabsorption syndromes.

low fat milk, milk containing 1% to 2% fat, intermediate in fat content between whole and skimmed milk.

low forceps, an obstetrical operation in which forceps are used to deliver a baby whose head is on the pelvic floor, near the outlet. The procedure is performed most often to shorten normal labor and to control delivery. It is commonly required for mothers whose strength has been weakened by drugs or fatigue. Also called **outlet forceps, prophylactic forceps.** See also **forceps delivery, obstetric forceps.**

low-grade fever, a temperature that is above 98.6° F (37° C) but lower than 100.4° F (38° C) for 24 hours.

Lown-Ganong-Levine syndrome (LGL) /lōn′-genôN′ləvēn′/, a disorder of the impulse of the muscle contraction signal of the heart (atrioventricular (AV) conduction system). Treatments include the use of antiarrhythmic drugs and implantation of a pacemaker. See also **atrioventricular (AV) block.**

low residue diet, a diet that will leave a minimal residue of feces in the lower intestinal tract after digestion and absorption. It consists of tender meats, poultry, fish, eggs, white bread, pasta, simple desserts, clear soups, tea, and coffee. Omitted are highly seasoned or fried foods, all fruits and fruit juices, raw vegetables, whole-grain cereals and bread, nuts, jams, and, usually, milk. The diet is prescribed in cases of pouchlike formations in the intestinal wall (diverticulosis) and inflammation of the pouches (diverticulitis) and before and after gastrointestinal surgery. Because it is lacking in calcium, iron, and vitamins, the diet should be used only for a limited period of time.

low salt diet. See **low sodium diet.**

low saturated fat diet. See **low cholesterol diet.**

low sodium diet, a diet that restricts the use of table salt (sodium chloride) plus other compounds containing sodium, as baking powder or soda, and certain food additives such asmonosodium glutamate, sodium citrate, sodium propionate, and sodium sulfate. It is prescribed for high blood pressure, fluid accumulation in tissues (edema), especially when associated with heart, kidney, or liver disease, and during treatment with steroid hormones. The degree of sodium restriction depends on the severity of the condition. Included in the diet are eggs, skimmed milk, beef, poultry, lamb, pork, veal, fish, potatoes, green beans, broccoli, asparagus, peas, salad ingredients, and fresh fruits. Many flavoring extracts, spices, and herbs are used to add taste to the diet. Foods avoided include fresh or canned shellfish, ham, bacon, frankfurters, luncheon meats, sausage, cheese, salted butter or margarine, any breads or cereals made with salt, beets, carrots, celery, sauerkraut, spinach, and most canned or frozen foods—unless prepared without sodium. Also to be avoided are many drugs, as laxatives, sedatives, and alkalizers, which contain sodium, and drinking water from a source using a water softener that adds sodium to replace calcium in the water. Also called **low salt diet, salt-free diet, sodium-restricted diet.**

loxapine, a tranquilizer given to treat a severe mental disorder (schizophrenia).

★CAUTION: Parkinson's disease, administration of sedatives or tranquilizers at the same time, liver or kidney dysfunction, low blood pressure, or known allergy to this drug prohibits its use.

★ADVERSE EFFECTS: Among the more serious side effects are low blood pressure, liver impairment, and a variety of nervous system and allergic reactions.

Loxitane, a trademark for a tranquilizer (loxapine succinate).

lozenge. See **troche.**

LPN, abbreviation for **licensed practical nurse.**

LPS Act, a California law named for sponsors of the legislation (Lanterman, Petris, and Short) that provides for the protection and treatment of persons judged to be "gravely disabled" and, thus, unable to provide food, clothing, or shelter for themselves. The legislation was designed to safeguard the constitutional rights of patients threatened with involuntary commitment on the basis of a psychiatric diagnosis. The LPS Act was considered a progressive measure in that it made "ability to function" the standard for determining the need for establishing guardianships for senior citizens or other individuals who might appear to be mentally disordered.

LSD, abbreviation for **lysergic acid diethylamide.** See **lysergide.**

lucid /loo′sid/, clear, rational, and able to be understood.

lucid interval, a period of relative mental clarity between periods of irrationality, especially in organic brain disorders, as delirium or dementia.

lucid lethargy, a mental state characterized by a loss of will and an inability to act, even though the patient is conscious and has normal thinking function. See also **lethargy.**

Ludiomil, a trademark for an antidepressant drug (maprotiline hydrochloride).

Ludwig's angina /lōōd'vigz/, an acute streptococcal infection of the floor of the mouth and parts of the neck. It causes the tongue to become swollen, thereby blocking the airway to the lungs. It is treated with penicillin.

lues. See **syphilis.**

-luetic, -luic, a combining form pertaining to syphilis.

Lufyllin, a trademark for a smooth muscle relaxant (dyphylline).

lukewarm bath, a bath in which the temperature of the water is between 90° F (32.2° C) and 96° F (35.5° C).

lumbago /lumbā'gō/, pain in the lower back (lumbar region) caused by muscle strain, rheumatoid arthritis, osteoarthritis, or a ruptured spinal disk. Ischemic lumbago, characterized by pain in the lower back and buttocks, is caused by poor blood circulation to the area.

lumbar /lum'bər, lum'bär/, pertaining to the part of the body between the chest and the pelvis, particularly the lower back area.

lumbar nerves, the five pairs of spinal nerves in the lumbar region.

lumbar node, a lymph node in one of the seven groups serving the abdomen and the pelvis.

lumbar plexus, a network of nerves formed by divisions of the first three and part of the fourth lumbar nerves. It is located on the inside of the back abdominal wall.

lumbar puncture (LP), introducing a hollow needle into the lumbar portion of the spinal canal. It is performed in various therapeutic and diagnostic procedures that include obtaining cerebrospinal fluid for laboratory analysis; evaluating the canal for the presence of a tumor; and injecting a dye for x-ray visualization of the structures of the nervous system, including the spinal canal and brain. Therapeutic reasons for lumbar puncture include removing blood or pus from the canal space; injecting drugs; withdrawing cerebrospinal fluid to reduce pressure in the skull; introducing an anesthetic to induce spinal anesthesia; and placing a small amount of the patient's blood in the space to form a clot to patch a cut or hole in the spinal membrane. Lumbar puncture is not performed if a brain tumor is suspected, if there are signs of infection at the site of puncture, or if other cerebrospinal procedures are planned in the near future. Infection, leakage of cerebrospinal fluid, headache, nausea, vomiting, urination difficulty, or signs of meningitis occur in approximately 25% of patients.

lumbar subarachnoid peritoneostomy, a surgical procedure for draining cerebrospinal fluid (CSF) in hydrocephalus, usually in the new-

born. The procedure may be used when a temporary shunt is needed. See also **hydrocephalus.**

lumbar subarachnoid ureterostomy, a surgical procedure for draining excess cerebrospinal fluid (CSF) though the ureter to the bladder in hydrocephalus, usually in the newborn. See also **hydrocephalus.**

lumbar veins, four pairs of veins that collect blood by dorsal tributaries from the loins and by abdominal tributaries from the walls of the abdomen.

lumbar vertebra, one of the five largest segments of the movable part of the spinal column. The lubar vertebrae are larger and heavier than verterbrae higher in the spinal column because they must support more weight. The body of each lumbar vertebra is flattened or slightly concave. The bony spine at the back of each vertebra is thick, broad, and shorter than vertebrae at the level of the chest. The body of the fifth lumbar vertebra is defective in some individuals, tending to weaken the spinal column.

lumbosacral plexus /lum'bōsā'krəl/, a combination of lumbar, sacral, and coccygeal nerves that supply the legs and pelvic area.

lumen /lōō'mən/, pl. **lumina, lumens,** a cavity or the channel within any organ or structure of the body.

lumpectomy /lumpek'təmē/, surgical removal of a breast tumor without removing large amounts of surrounding tissue or adjacent lymph nodes. See also **breast cancer.**

lunar month, a period of 4 weeks or 28 days, approximately the time required for the moon to revolve about the earth. Some biological rhythms follow the lunar month, as the average menstrual cycle.

lunate bone, one of the bones of the wrist.

Lundh test, a test of the pancreas in which it is stimulated by a formula diet, and an enzyme (lipase) is measured in samples taken from the small intestine.

lung, one of a pair of light, spongy organs in the chest. The highly elastic lungs are the main part of the body's breathing system. They provide the mechanisms for inhaling air from which oxygen is extracted and for exhaling carbon dioxide, a waste product of the body. The lungs are served by two artery systems. The pulmonary arteries bring deoxygenated blood to the lungs where the oxygen is replaced. The bronchial arteries supply blood to nourish the lung tissues. Most of the blood brought to the lungs by the two artery systems returns to the heart through the pulmonary veins. The surfaces of the lungs cradle the heart. Each lung is cone-shaped and has a peak, a base, three borders, and two surfaces. The peak is rounded and extends into the root of the neck about 4 cm above the first rib. The base of the lung is broad and curved, rests on the surface of the diaphragm, and moves with the diaphragm, down during inhaling and up during exhaling. The quantity of air that can be exhaled from the lungs after the deepest breath averages 3,700 cc, about 4 quarts. The lungs are composed of lobes that are smooth and shiny on their surface. The right lung contains three lobes; the left lung, two lobes. Each lung is covered with a thin, moist (pleural) membrane. An inner coat contains many elastic fibers lining the entire surface of the organ. Within this fibrous layer are secondary small lobes (lobules) divided into primary lobules, each of which consists of blood vessels, lymph vessels, nerves, and a duct (alveolar) connecting with air spaces. The color of the lungs at birth is pinkish-white, and darkens in later life. The coloring comes from carbon granules that are inhaled from the atmosphere. The carbon deposits increase with age and are more abundant in men than women. The lungs of men are usually heavier and have a greater capacity than the lungs of women.

lung cancer, a respiratory disorder attributable to cigarette smoking in 75% of cases. Other causes are exposure to asbestos, arsenic, beryllium, chromium, coal products, ionizing radiation, iron oxide, nickel, petroleum, uranium, and various other chemicals. Lung cancer develops most often in scarred or chronically diseased lungs, and is usually far advanced when detected. Symptoms of lung cancer include persistent cough, breathing difficulty, pus or blood-streaked sputum, chest pain, and repeated attacks of bronchitis or pneumonia. Lung cancers spread widely to other organs. Oat-cell carcinomas, which resemble tiny oat seeds, usually invade bone marrow, whereas large-cell lung cancers spread to lymph nodes in the chest and the gastrointestinal system. Surgery is the most effective treatment, but only one-half of the cases can be treated by surgery by the time the disease is detected. Surgery is not performed if cancer cells are found in nearby lymph nodes. Radiation is used to treat localized lesions and cancers untreatable by surgery. Chemotherapy is especially prescribed for oat-cell carcinoma. Bacillus Calmette-Guérin vaccine, an antituberculosis drug that stimulates the natural resistance to disease (immune system), is administered to some patients with early stage lung cancer.

lung capacities, lung volumes that consist of two or more of the four primary (not overlapping) volumes. These are expiratory reserve volume (the largest amount of air that can be forced out of the lungs after normal breathing out); inspiratory reserve volume (the largest amount of air that can be inhaled after normal breathing in); residual volume (the amount of air left in the lungs after completely exhaling); and tidal volume (the amount of air inhaled and exhaled during normal breathing). Functional residual capacity is the sum of the tidal volume and inspiratory reserve volume. Inpiratory capacity is the sum of the tidal volume and inspiratory reserve volume. Total lung capacity is the sum of the expiratory reserve volume, the tidal volume, and the inspiratory reserve volume. Total lung capacity, at the end of complete inhaling, is the sum of the functional residual capacity and the inspiratory capacity.

lung scan, a radiographic examination of a lung and its function. See also **radiography.**

lunula, *pl.* **lunulae,** the crescent-shaped pale area at the base of a fingernail or toenail.

lupus, *nontechnical.* lupus erythematosus.

lupus erythematosus. See **systemic lupus erythematosus.**

lupus erythematosus preparation (LE prep), a laboratory test for lupus erythematosus in which white blood cells are mixed with a specimen of the patient's blood serum. Large, spheric granules appear within the white cells if the patient has lupus erythematosus.

lupus vulgaris, a form of skin tuberculosis in which areas of the skin become ulcerated and heal slowly, leaving deeply scarred tissue. The disease is not related to lupus erythematosus.

Luride, a trademark for a chemical (sodium fluoride) that reduces tooth decay and cavities.

luteal /lōō'tē·əl/, pertaining to the corpus luteum of the female ovary or its functions or effects.

luteinizing hormone (LH), a hormone produced by the pituitary gland. In men, it stimulates the secretion of testosterone, the male sex hormone, by the interstitial cells of the testes. Testosterone, together with follicle stimulating hormone (FSH), stimulates the testes to produce sperm. In females, luteinizing hormone, working together with FSH, stimulates the tiny cavities (follicles) containing ova, or egg cells, in the ovary to secrete estrogen, the female sex hormone. High concentrations of estrogen cause a surge of LH, which stimulates the release (ovulation) of an egg cell from the ovary. LH then induces the change of the ovum follicle into the corpus luteum, which becomes a temporary sex hormone gland that continues to secrete estrogen and progesterone hormones.

luxated joint, the condition of being completely out of joint, in which no parts of the joint meet each other.

LVN, abbreviation for **licensed vocational nurse.** See **licensed practical nurse.**

lycopene /lī'kəpin/, a red chemical that is the carotenoid pigment in tomatoes and various berries and fruits. It is considered the primary substance from which all natural carotenoid pigments are derived. See also **carotenoid.**

lying-in, **1.** designating the time before, during, and after childbirth. **2.** designating a hospital that provides care for women in childbirth.

Lyme arthritis. See **Lyme disease.**

Lyme disease, an acute inflammatory disease, involving one or more joints, believed to be transmitted by a tickborne disease organism. The condition was originally described in Lyme, Connecticut, but has also been reported in other parts of the United States and, sporadically, in other countries. Knees, other large joints, and jaw (temperomandibular) joints are most commonly involved, with local inflammation and swelling. Chills, fever, headache, discomfort, and a skin eruption often precede the joint manifestations. Occasionally heart conduction abnormalities, a form of meningitis, or Bell's palsy may be associated conditions. Symptoms appear in episodes lasting about 1 week, but recur at intervals of from 1 to several weeks, then decline in severity over a 2- or 3-year period. There is no important permanent joint damage. Treatment includes pain killers for joint symptoms and corticosteroid hormones to reduce heart and nervous system symptoms.

lymph, a thin, clear, slightly yellow fluid originating in many organs and tissues of the body. It circulates through the lymphatic vessels and is filtered by the lymph nodes. Lymph enters the bloodstream at the junction of the internal jugular and subclavian veins at the base of the neck. Its composition varies depending on the organ or tissue it is in, but generally contains about 95% water, a few red blood cells, and variable numbers of white blood cells. It is similar to blood plasma except for a lower amount of protein material. See also **chyle.**

lymphadenitis /limfad'ini'tis, lim'fəd-/, an inflammatory condition of the lymph nodes, usually the result of circulating cancer cells, a bacterial infection, or other inflammatory condition. The nodes may be swollen, hard, smooth or irregular, red, and may feel hot. The location of the affected node is usually related to the site or origin of disease.

lymphadenopathy /limfad'inop'əthe/, any disorder of the lymph nodes or lymph vessels.

lymphadenopathy syndrome (LAS), a persistent swelling of the lymph nodes, which is often part of the AIDS-related complex.

lymphangiectasia /limfan'jē·ektā'zhə/, a dilation of the smaller lymphatic vessels. It usually results from obstruction in the larger vessels, such as occurs in pelvic tuberculosis and certain infectious diseases.

lymphangiography, the x-ray examination of lymph glands and lymphatic vessels after an injection of a dye. Also called **lymphography.**

lymphangioma /limfan'jē·ō'mə/, *pl.* **lymphangiomas, lymphangiomata,** a yellowish-tan tumor on the skin, composed of a mass of dilated lymph vessels. It is often removed by surgery or a form of surgery using an electric current (electrocoagulation) for cosmetic reasons. Also called **angioma lymphaticum.**

lymphangioma cavernosum, a tumor formed by dilated lymphatic vessels and filled with lymph that is often mixed with coagulated blood. The lesion may cause extensive enlargement of the affected tissue, especially of the tongue and lips. Also called **cavernous lymphangioma.**

lymphangioma circumscriptum, a skin lesion that develops from enlarged lymph vessels. Most commonly seen in young children, it may be pink or yellow and may grow to several centimeters in diameter.

lymphangitis /lim'fanji'tis/, an inflammation of one or more lymphatic vessels, often resulting from an acute streptococcal infection caused by an insect or animal bite in an arm or leg. Fine red streaks may extend from the infected area to the armpit or groin. Other signs are fever, chills, headache, and muscle ache. The infection may spread to the bloodstream. Antibiotics and hot soaks are usually prescribed as treatment.

lymphatic /limfat'ik/, pertaining to the lymphatic system of the body.

lymphatic capillary plexus, one of the networks of small lymphatic vessels that collect lymph from the lakes of fluid that ooze from tissue cells. The plexuses are especially abundant in the skin but also lace many other areas, such as the mucous membranes of the respiratory and digestive systems, testes, ovaries, liver, kidneys, and heart. See also **lymphatic system.**

lymphatic system, a vast, complex network of capillaries, thin vessels, valves, ducts, nodes, and organs. It helps to protect and maintain the fluid environment of the body by producing, filtering, and conveying lymph and by producing various blood cells. The lymphatic network transports fats, proteins, and other substances to the blood system. It also restores 60% of the fluid that leaks out of the blood capillaries and cells into spaces between cells during normal metabolism. Small valves throughout the lymphatic network help to control the flow of lymph. At the junction with the blood vein system, the valves prevent blood from flowing into the lymphatic vessels. The lymph collected throughout the body drains into the blood through two ducts situated in the neck. Various body movements, such as lung pressure changes, muscular contractions, and movements of organs surrounding lymphatic vessels combine to squeeze the lymph through the lymphatic system. The thoracic duct on the left side of the neck is the major vessel of the lymphatic system and conveys lymph from the whole body, except for the upper right side, which is served by the right lymphatic duct. Lymphatic vessels resemble veins but have more valves, thinner walls, and contain lymph nodes. The lymphatic capillaries, which are the beginning of the system, form a continuous network over the entire body, except for the cornea of the eye. The system also includes specialized lymphatic organs, such as the tonsils, thymus, and spleen. The lymphatics of the intestine contain a special milky substance called chyle. Lymph flows into the general circulation at a average rate of about 125 ml per hour. The rate may jump to as high as 1,800 ml per hour during vigorous exercise. See also **chyle, lymph, lymph node, spleen, thymus.**

lymphedema /lim'fĭdē'mə/, a disorder in which lymph accumulates in soft tissue with swelling caused by inflammation, obstruction, or removal of lymph vessels. Congenital lymphedema (Milroy's disease) is a hereditary disorder characterized by obstruction of the lymph vessels. Lymphedema praecox occurs in adolescence, chiefly in women, and causes swelling of the lower limbs, apparently because of an overgrowth of lymph vessels. Secondary lymphedema may follow surgical removal of lymph channels with the breast in mastectomy, obstruction of lymph drainage caused by tumors, or the infestation of lymph vessels with worm parasites. Lymphedema of the lower limbs begins with mild swelling of the foot and gradually extends to the entire leg. Prolonged standing, pregnancy, obesity, warm weather, and the menstrual period aggravate the condition. There is no cure for the disorder, but lymph drainage from the leg can be improved if the patient sleeps with the foot of the bed slightly elevated, wears elastic stockings, and takes moderate exercise regularly. Light massage in the direction of the lymph flow and diuretics may be prescribed; constricting clothing and salty or spicy foods that increase thirst are avoided. Surgery may be performed to remove enlarged lymph channels that disfigure tissue.

lymph node, one of many small oval structures that filter the lymph, fight infection, and in which there are formed white blood cells and blood plasma cells. Lymph nodes are of different sizes, some as small as pinheads, others as large as beans. Each node is enclosed in a fibrous capsule, is composed of a lighter-colored outer portion and a darker inner portion, and consists of closely packed white cells (lymphocytes), connective tissue, and lymph pathways. Lymph flows into the node through lymphatic vessels that open into the internal pathways. Lymphocytes are added to the lymph within the node before it flows out. Most lymph nodes are clustered in specific areas, as the mouth, neck, lower arm, armpit, and groin. The lymphatic network and nodes of the breast are especially crucial in the diag-

nosis and treatment of breast cancer in women. Cancer cells from a "primary" breast tumor often spread through the lymphatic system to other parts of the body. Also called **lymph gland.**

lymphocyte /lim'fəsīt/, one of two kinds of small white blood cells (leukocytes). Lymphocytes normally include 25% of the total white blood cell count but increase in number in response to infection. They occur in two forms: **B cells** and **T cells.** Each develops uniquely, and each has its own function. The function of the B cell is to search out, identify, and bind with specific intruders (allergens or antigens). B cells create antibodies for insertion into their own cell membranes. They reproduce by simple division. Each of the clones display identical antibodies on their surface membranes. When exposed to a specific allergen or antigen, the B cell is activated. It travels to the spleen or to the lymph nodes, and rapidly produces **plasma cells** and **memory cells.** Plasma cells create and secrete large amounts of antibody. Memory cells do not secrete antibodies, but if reexposure to the specific intruder occurs, they develop into antibody-secreting plasma cells. T cells are lymphocytes that have circulated through the thymus gland and have become thymocytes. When exposed to an antigen, they divide rapidly and produce large numbers of new T cells sensitized to that antigen. T cells are often called 'killer cells' because they secrete special chemical compounds and assist B cells in destroying foreign protein. T cells also appear to play a significant role in the body's resistance to the growth and spread of cancer cells.

lymphocytic choriomeningitis, a virus infection of the brain and spinal cord membranes and the cerebrospinal fluid. It is characterized by fever, headache, and stiff neck. The infection occurs primarily in young adults, most often in the fall and winter. Recovery usually takes place within 2 weeks.

lymphocytopenia /lim'fōsī'təpē'nē-ə/, a smaller-than-normal number of white cells (lymphocytes) in the blood circulation, occurring as a blood disorder or in association with nutritional deficiency, cancer, or infectious mononucleosis.

lymphocytosis /lim'fōsītō'sis/, a rapid reproduction of certain white blood cells (lymphocytes), as occurs in certain chronic diseases and during recovery from acute infections.

lymphogranuloma venereum (LGV), a sexually transmitted disease caused by a strain of the bacterium *Chlamydia trachomatis*. Signs are ulcerative genital lesions, marked swelling of the lymph nodes in the groin, headache, and fever. Ulcerations of the rectum occur less commonly. Antibiotics are usually prescribed for the patient and for any person with whom there has been sexual contact. Also called **lymphopathia venereum.** See also *Chlamydia.*

lymphokine /lim'fōkīn/, a chemical factor produced and released by T-lymphocytes (thymocytes). It attracts bacteria-destroying cells (macrophages) to the site of infection or inflammation and prepares them for attack. See also **lymphocyte.**

lymphokine-activiated killer (LAK) cells, cells that attack organisms foreign to the human body. They are produced in the presence of one protein (interleukin-2) and in the absence of another (an antigen) that causes the formation of antibodies for infection control. These cells are different from human killer cells (peripheral T lymphocytes or memory cytotoxic thymus-derived lymphocytes). Patients with low amounts of the immune system agent gamma globulin (hypogammaglobulinemia) have too few LAK cells. These patients are also at much-greater-than-average risk of developing cancer.

lymphoma /limfō'mə/, *pl.* **lymphomas, lymphomata,** a tumor of lymphoid tissue that is usually cancerous, but in some cases may not be. Lymphoid tissue is netlike and holds lymphocytes, a type of white blood cell, in its spaces. The various lymphomas differ in degree of cellular structure and content, but their effects are similar. The appearance of a painless, enlarged lymph node or nodes in the neck is followed by weakness, fever, weight loss, and anemia. With widespread involvement of lymphoid tissue, the spleen and liver usually enlarge. Gastrointestinal disturbances and bone lesions frequently develop. Men are more likely than women to develop lymphoid tumors. Treatment for lymphoma includes radiation and drugs.

lymphoma staging, a system for classifying lymphomas according to the stage of the disease for the purpose of appropriate treatment. Stage I involves a single lymph node region. Stage II includes two or more lymph node regions on the same side of the diaphragm. In Stage III, lymph nodes on both sides of the diaphragm are affected. There may be involvement of the spleen or of another organ or site. Stage IV is typified by widespread involvement of one or more body organs or sites with or without lymph node involvement.

lymphopathia venereum. See **lymphogranuloma venereum.**

lymphosarcoma cell leukemia, a cancer of blood-forming tissues. Many lymphoma cancer cells in the blood circulation infiltrate surrounding tissues. The disease may accompany lymphoma or exist as a separate entity with more bone marrow involvement than is found in lymphoma.

Lyon hypothesis, a theory that only one of the two X chromosomes normally found in female tissue cells is functional, the other having become inactive early in development. Female body cells contain some X chromosomes from her father, and some from her mother. Sex-linked genes may therefore appear on some of her cells and not on others.

Lyon's ring, a type of inherited disorder of the female urethra in which narrowing of the upper or lower portions of the urethra leads to involuntary loss of urine, pain in urinating, and repeated infections. The disorder is treated surgically.

lypressin /līpres'in/, an antidiuretic nasal spray prescribed in diabetes insipidus to decrease urinary water loss.
★CAUTION: Blood vessel disease or known allergy to this drug prohibits its use.
★ADVERSE EFFECTS: Among thé most serious side effects are chest pains in patients with heart disease, nausea, and cramping.

lysergide /līsur'jīd/, a semisynthetic hallucinogenic drug derived from ergot, a fungus of cereal grains. It acts at many sites in the central nervous system from the brain to the spinal cord. In susceptible individuals, as little as 20 to 25 micrograms of the potent drug may cause eye pupil dilation, increased blood pressure, tremors, muscle weakness, and increased body temperature. Larger doses also produce dizziness, drowsiness, numbness or tingling sensations, euphoria or discomfort, and mind alterations. Colors may be heard, sounds visualized, and time is felt to pass slowly. It has been proposed, but not approved, to treat alcoholism, and to relieve pain in terminal cancer patients. Also called **LSD, lysergic acid diethylamide,** *(slang)* **acid.** See also **hallucinogen.**

Lysholm method, (in radiology) any of several techniques for positioning a patient for x-ray examination of the bottom of the skull, two parts of the skull surrounding the ear, and the bones between the eye sockets and nose.

lysine (Lys) /lī'sēn, lī'sin/, an essential amino acid needed for proper growth in infants and for maintenance of nitrogen balance in adults. See also **amino acid, protein.**

lysinemia /lī'sinē'mē·ə/, a condition caused by an inborn error of metabolism, resulting in the inability to use the essential amino acid lysine. It is characterized by muscle weakness and mental retardation. Treatment consists of a diet that controls the intake of lysine by reducing proteins rich in lysine, such as milk and meats, and including more fruits, vegetables, and rice. See also **metabolism.**

lysis /lī'sis/, destruction or dissolution of a cell or molecule through the action of a specific agent, such as an enzyme or antibody.

lysis of adhesions, surgery performed to free binding scar tissue (adhesions).

Lysodren, a trademark for an anticancer drug (mitotane).

lysosome /lī′səsōm/, a particle in a cell that contains enzymes capable of destroying the cell. Lysosomes are found in most cells but are particularly prominent in white blood cells and in the cells of the liver and kidney. If their enzymes are released into the cell, they cause self-digestion of the cell. It is believed that lysosomes may play an important role in certain self-destructive diseases in which the wasting of tissue occurs, as muscular dystrophy.

lysozyme, an enzyme with antiseptic actions that destroys some foreign organisms. It is found in white blood cells and is normally present in saliva, sweat, breast milk, and tears.

lytes /līts/, *informal.* electrolytes, especially minerals such as potassium, sodium, phosphorus, magnesium, and calcium in the blood.

lytic cocktail /lit′ik/, *informal.* an anesthetic compound of chlorpromazine, meperidine, and promethazine that blocks the autonomic nervous system, depresses the circulatory system, and induces paralysis of nerve activity.

Lytren, a trademark for a nutritional supplement containing various electrolytes.

M

m, abbreviation for **meter.**

macerate /mas'ərāt/, to soften something solid by soaking. **–maceration,** *n.*

maceration, the softening and breaking down of the skin from prolonged exposure to moisture. It may be caused by prolonged exposure to amniotic fluid in the mother's uterus in the case of a baby that is past due or a dead fetus.

machismo, (in psychology) a concept of the male that includes both the culturally desirable traits of courage and fearlessness and the detrimental behaviors of heavy drinking, seduction of women, and domineering and abusive spouse behavior.

macrencephaly /mak'rənsef'əlē/, an inborn disorder marked by an abnormally large brain. Also called **macroencephaly.**

macro-, a combining form meaning 'large, or abnormal size.'

macrocephaly /mak'rōsef'əlē/, a birth defect marked by a head and brain that are too large in relation to the body. It is linked to some degree of mental defect and slowed growth. The head is much larger than the average size for age, sex, and race. The face is usually normal. Macrocephaly is different from hydrocephalus, in which the growth of the head is caused by too-much fluid of the brain and spine, usually under increased pressure. Tests may be needed to tell the two conditions apart. Also spelled **macrocephalia.** Also called **megalocephaly.** See also **hydrocephalus.**

macrocyte /mak'rəsīt/, an unusually large, mature red blood cell. See also **macrocytic anemia.**

macrocytic anemia, a disorder of the blood marked by blocked blood cells and abnormal, large, fragile, red blood cells. Macrocytic anemia most often results from a lack of folic acid and vitamin B$_{12}$.

Macrodantin, a trademark for an antibiotic (nitrofurantoin).

Macrodex, a trademark for a blood plasma expander (dextran).

macrogenitosomia /mak'rōjen'itōsō'mē·ə/, a condition in which the sex organs are prematurely large. It results from an excess of a male sex hormone (androgen) during fetal growth. It is marked in boys by enlarged outer genitals and in girls by some outer male genital appearance (pseudohermaphroditism).

macroglossia /mak'rōglos'ē·ə/, a birth defect marked by the large size of the tongue, as seen in Down's syndrome.

macrognathia /mak'rōnā'thē·ə/, an abnormally large growth of the jaw. Compare **micrognathia.** **–macrognathic,** *adj.*

macrolide, any group of antibiotics produced by bacteria that grow without oxygen (actinomycetes) and hold a violet color when stained (gram-positive). They include erythromycin and troleanodomycin. Macrolides are generally used against gram-positive bacteria and in patients allergic to penicillins.

macromolecule, a very large molecule, like those found in proteins or certain carbohydrates.

macronutrient, a chemical element needed in large amounts for the body. Macronutrients include carbon, hydrogen, oxygen, nitrogen, potassium, sodium, calcium, chloride, magnesium, phosphorus, and sulfur. Also called **macroelement, major element.** Compare **micronutrient.**

macrophage /mak'rəfāj/, any large cell that can surround and digest foreign substances in the body, as protozoa or bacteria. They are found in the liver, spleen, and in the loose connective tissue. See also **phagocyte, reticuloendothelial system.**

macula /mak'yo͞olə/, *pl.* **maculae,** a small colored area or a spot, as a freckle of a measles rash, that is separate or different from the surrounding tissue. It may be permanent. Also called **macule.**

macula lutea, a small, oval, yellow area of the retina of the eye. Near the optic nerve, it has special cones at its center. Accurate sight occurs when an image is focused on this special part of the macula lutea. Also called *(informal)* **macula.**

Madelung's neck. See **lipoma annulare colli.**

mad hatter's disease. See **mercury poisoning.**

Madura foot /maj'o͞orə/, a destructive, tropical fungal infection of the foot. It is named for a district in India. Also called **maduromycosis.**

mafenide acetate, a drug given to treat burns. It prevents infections.
★CAUTION: Allergy to this drug or to sulfonamide prohibits its use.
★ADVERSE EFFECTS: Among the more serious side effects are allergic reactions and new infections, particularly by *Candida albicans.*

magaldrate, an antacid given for stomach upset linked to heartburn, sour stomach, or acid indigestion.
★CAUTION: It may change absorption of other drugs, as tetracyclines.
★ADVERSE EFFECTS: There may be a change in bowel function.

magical thinking, (in psychology) a belief that merely thinking about an event in the outside world can cause it to occur. It is regarded as a form of return to an early stage of development.

magic-bullet approach, the use of a specific drug to cure or relieve the symptoms of a given disease or condition.

magnesemia, the presence of magnesium in the blood.

magnesium (Mg), a silver-white mineral. Magnesium is a plentiful mineral in the cell fluids of the body and is needed for many chemical activities. It also is important for nerves and muscles. About 50% of the body's magnesium is in the bones.

magnesium sulfate, a salt of magnesium given by injection to prevent seizures, especially in preeclampsia of pregnancy. It is also given by mouth to treat constipation and heartburn and to correct a lack of magnesium in the body. Also called **Epsom salts.**
★CAUTION: It is used with care in kidney disease or if the patient is allergic to the drug. Difficulty in breathing, severe heart problems, or symptoms of appendicitis or constipation prohibits its use.
★ADVERSE EFFECTS: The most serious side effect is a shutdown of the blood flow from too-much magnesium in the blood. Difficulty in breathing, confusion, and muscle weakness also may happen.

magnetic resonance imaging (MRI). See **nuclear magnetic resonance.**

magnification, (in psychology) mental distortion in which the effects of one's behavior are increased. See also **minimization.**

main en griffe. See **clawhand.**

maintenance dose, the amount of drug needed to keep a desired amount of the drug in the tissues. A part of a drug is lost through the body's normal processes, as excretion.

Majocchi's granuloma, a ringworm that affects mainly the lower legs. It is caused by the fungus *Trichophyton.* This fungus infects the hairs of the affected site and raises spongy tumors. The tumors last for 3 to 4 months and are slowly absorbed. They may also decay, often leaving deep scars. Also called **trichophytic granuloma.**

major depressive episode. See **endogenous depression.**

major element. See **macronutrient.**

major medical insurance, insurance coverage developed to offset the costs of lengthy or major illness and injury. Most major medical insurance policies are written to pay a certain amount of costs up to a certain figure, beyond which payment is made in full up to a maximum amount. After the maximum amount, payment stops. Many policies require the insured to pay a deductible.

major surgery, any surgery that needs general anesthesia or help in breathing or both. Compare **minor surgery.**

major mental disorder, any of a group of mental diseases marked by unnatural emotional behavior, by mood changes and confused thoughts, and by other symptoms seen with either depressed or manic diseases. The disturbances may occur as separate incidents but may be continuous or occur in repeating patterns. It is not caused by any physical disease of the brain.

mal /mal, mäl/, *French.* an illness or disease, as grand mal or petit mal.

mal-, a combining form meaning abnormal, as in maladjustment, malalignment, malignant.

malabsorption, a failure of the intestines to absorb nutrients. It occurs in celiac disease, sprue, dysentery, and diarrhea. It may result from a birth defect involving the digestion or from malnutrition. It may also result from any abnormal chemical or physical condition of the digestive system that prevents needed food elements from being absorbed. See **inborn error of metabolism, malnutrition.**

malabsorption syndrome, a group of symptoms resulting from disorders in the intestines' ability to absorb nutrients from foods eaten. It may lead to loss of appetite, weight loss, swollen abdomen, muscle cramps, bone pain, and fat in the feces. Anemia, weakness, and tiredness can occur because iron, folic acid, and vitamin B_{12} are not absorbed in right amounts. Among the many conditions causing this syndrome are stomach or small bowel surgery, celiac disease, tropical sprue, cystic fibrosis, Whipple's disease, and intestinal lymphangiectasia, a disease involving the grouping of the lymph ducts in the intestines. Treatment and its result depend on the specific condition. See also **celiac disease, cystic fibrosis, hypoproteinemia, tropical sprue.**

malacia /məlā′shə/, an abnormal softening or a sponginess in any part or any tissue of the body.

malaise, a vague feeling of body weakness or discomfort, often indicating the beginning of disease.

malalignment, a failure of parts of the body to line up normally, as teeth that do not conform to the dental arch.

malaria /məler′ē·ə/, a serious infection caused by one or more of at least four different species of the protozoan organism *Plasmodium,* carried by a mosquito bite. It leads to chills, fever, anemia, and a large spleen. Malaria tends to become a lifelong disease. The disease is usually carried from human to human by a bite from an infected *Anopheles* mosquito. Malaria can also be spread by blood transfusion or by the use of an infected needle. The disease is mostly to be found in the tropical areas of South and Central America, Africa, and Asia. However, a number of new cases are brought to North America by refugees, military personnel, and travelers. *Plasmodium* parasites enter the red blood cells of the infected human, where they mature, reproduce, and burst out every so often. Malaria attacks (paroxysms) occur at regular intervals. They go together with the growth of new parasites in the body. Because the life cycle of the infecting parasite changes with the species, the patterns of chills and fever differ, as do the length and seriousness of the disease. Bouts of malaria usually last from 1 to 4 weeks. Attacks occur less often as the disease continues. It is common for malaria to recur. The disease can last for years. Chloroquine, given by mouth or by injection into the muscle, is the drug given for all but those strains of *Plasmodium* immune to chloroquine. They are treated with a combination of quinine, pyrimethamine, and one of the sulfa drugs. Through the use of insecticides and destruction of swamps, the disease has disappeared from many parts of the world. Worldwide destruction of the disease has not been possible. Insecticide-immune mosquitoes and drug-immune protozoa have developed. Prevention with antimalarial drugs is important for those visiting areas where infection is possible. The use of netting and mosquito repellent is advised. See also **antimalaria, biduotertian fever, blackwater fever, falciparum malaria, quartan malaria,** *Plasmodium,* **tertian malaria.** –**malarial,** *adj.*

Malassezia, a type of fungus. *Malassezia furfur* causes a disease that makes brownish patches on the skin (tinea versicolor). *M. ovalis* is an organism that does not cause a disease, but is found in areas of oil glands and is linked to dandruff.

malathion poisoning, a toxic condition caused by swallowing malathion or by absorbing it through the skin. Malathion is an organophosphorus insecticide. It is a chemical cousin of military nerve gas. Symptoms of poisoning include vomiting, nausea, stomach cramps, headache, dizziness, weakness, confusion, convulsions, and breathing problems. Treatment includes immediately giving atropine by injection, an insecticide antidote, flushing the stomach with water, giving a salt-water enema, help in breathing, and oxygen. Malathion is much less toxic than parathion, an agricultural insecticide. Parathion is the only organophosphorus insecticide approved for household use.

Malayan pit viper venom. See **ancrod.**

mal del pinto. See **pinta.**

male, 1. referring to the sex that produces sperm cells and fertilizes the female to have offspring; masculine. 2. a male person.

male reproductive system assessment, an evaluation of the condition of the patient's sex organs, past and present genital or urinary infections and disorders, and reproductive history. The man is questioned about his children, and sexual activity. Other questions concern the frequency, or difficulty in urinating, discharge from the penis, hernia, genital sores, discomfort or pain in the groin, lower back, or legs, and past treatment for an inflammation (epididymitis), gonorrhea, genital herpes, swollen scrotum (hydrocele), nonspecific disease of the urethra (urethritis), undescended testicle (orchitis), disease of the prostate (prostatitis), syphilis, and varicose testicular veins (varicocele). The examiner, while inspecting the genitals, wears rubber gloves to prevent infection. The penis is examined for swelling and small tumors, as herpes blisters, or a syphilitic sore, chancre, or scar. Conditions that may be noted include failed closure of the urethra during fetal growth (hypospadias or epispadias), lengthening of the foreskin narrowing the urinary meatus, or swelling of the penis caused by a retracted, tight foreskin. The urethral opening is inspected for pus or a bloody discharge. The scrotum is observed for symmetry and shape. In elderly or weakened men the scrotum may be long and flat. The normally smooth testicles, epididymides, and spermatic cords are examined by hand for the presence of nodes, varicose veins, and the size, location, and consistency of any mass in the scrotum. Fluid felt around the testicles may be seen by darkening the room and shining a flashlight on the scrotum. The patient is asked to cough or bear down to reveal a hernia. The abdomen is felt above the pubic bones to see if the bladder is filled with fluid. The lymph nodes in the groin are felt. The amount and appearance of pubic hair is observed. The prostate may be examined with the patient bent at a right angle over a table. The examiner's well-oiled gloved forefinger reaches into the rectum and feels the lobes and middle line of the gland. The size, consistency, and any lump suggesting a tumor of the normally smooth, firm prostate are carefully noted. If additional studies are needed, a microscope slide is prepared from the first urine passed following massage of the prostate. If prostate cancer is suspected, a diagnosis is usually based on a laboratory test of tissue (biopsy), or examination of a sample of the prostate tissue. The male reproductive system assessment includes laboratory studies of discharge from the penis. A microscope slide sample usually shows or rules out a diagnosis of gonorrhea. Tests may be needed to see if nonspecific urethritis is caused by *Escherichia coli, Pseudomonas, Staphylococcus, Streptococcus,* or other bacteria. Syphilis may be diagnosed by a blood test. If infertility is a problem, examinations of many semen samples are carried out. Each specimen taken after 3 days of avoiding sexual intercourse is inspected in the laboratory to see if the amount of the semen is close to the normal (3.5 ml average). It is also determined whether the semen has an average amount of acid (pH of 7.7) and a sperm count of 60 million to 150 million per ml.

male sexual dysfunction, impaired or inadequate ability of a man to carry on his sex life to his own satisfaction. Symptoms are often psychological in origin. They include difficulties in starting and maintaining an erection, ejaculating too soon, inability to ejaculate, and even loss of desire. Men are often ashamed of the problem and ask the physician to treat a "prostate problem," they hope that the physician will understand the message. Compare **female sexual dysfunction.** See also **impotence, premature ejaculation, sexual dysfunction.**

malformation, an abnormal structure in the body. See also **birth defect, congenital anomaly.**

malignant /məlig′nənt/, **1.** tending to become worse and possibly cause death. **2.** describing a tumor that is cancerous, involving many organs, and spreading. **–malignancy,** *n.*

malignant hepatoma, a cancerous tumor of the liver. Primary liver cancer is less common in the United States than in Africa and the Far East. The only useful treatment is to remove the tumor. This is often not possible, because the tumors grow rapidly and spread through both lobes of the liver. The outcome is poor. Also called **hepatocarcinoma, hepatocellular carcinoma, liver cell carcinoma.**

malignant hypertension, the most life-threatening form of high blood pressure (hypertension). It is marked by very high blood pressure that may damage the tissues of small vessels, the brain, the eyes (retinas), heart, and kidneys. It affects more blacks than whites. It may be caused by a variety of factors, as stress, a family history of the disease, being overweight, tobacco, birth control pills, high intake of table salt (sodium chloride), an inactive life style, and aging. Many patients with this condition have signs of low blood potassium, blood that is alkaline, and the release of high levels of an adrenal gland hormone (aldosterone). See also **essential hypertension.**

malignant hyperthermia (MH), an inherited disorder marked by often fatal high body temperature, with rigid muscles occurring in affected patients exposed to certain anesthetic drugs. Treatment includes giving a skeletal muscle relaxant (dantrolene) or 100% oxygen, cooling procedures, and correcting blood acid levels and excess blood potassium. Patients who have malignant hyperthermia are informed of their condition and told that many of their close relatives are likely to have the same chance of getting the disorder.

malignant malnutrition. See **kwashiorkor.**

malignant neoplasm, a tumor that tends to grow, invade nearby tissues, and spread through the bloodstream. It usually has an irregular shape and is made up of imperfectly developed cells.

If untreated it may result in the death of the patient. Its malignancy varies with the kind of tumor and the condition of the patient.

malignant neuroma. See **neurosarcoma.**

malignant pustule. See **anthrax.**

malingering, a conscious faking of the symptoms of a disease or injury to gain some desired end.

malleolus /məle′ələs/, *pl.* **malleoli,** a rounded bony structure, as the bump on each side of the ankle.

malleus /mal′ē·əs/, one of the three tiny bones (ossicles) in the middle ear, resembling a hammer or mallet. It is connected to the eardrum and carries sound vibrations to the anvil (incus), which interacts with the stirrup (stapes). The stapes carries the vibrations to the inner ear. See also **incus, middle ear, stapes.**

Mallory-Weiss syndrome, a condition in which heavy bleeding follows a break in the mucous membrane of the esophagus at its connection with the stomach. The break is usually caused by repeated vomiting. This happens often to alcoholics or to persons whose opening (pylorus) between the stomach and intestine is blocked. Surgery is usually necessary to stop the bleeding. After repair, the chance for recovery is excellent.

malnutrition, any disorder concerning nutrition. It may result from an unbalanced diet or from eating too-little or too-much food. It may also result from improper body use of foods. Compare **deficiency disease.**

malocclusion /mal′əkloo′zhən/, abnormal contact of the teeth of the upper jaw with the teeth of the lower jaw. See also **occlusion.**

malpighian corpuscle, one of the small, round, deep red bodies in the outer tissues (cortex) of the kidney. The corpuscles are thought to be part of a filter system through which nonprotein substances in blood plasma enter small tubes (tubules) in the kidney for urination. Also called **Malpighian body, renal corpuscle.**

malpractice, professional mistake that is a direct cause of injury or harm to a patient. It may result from a lack of professional knowledge, experience, or skill that can be expected in others in the profession. It may also result from a failure to use reasonable care or judgment in applying professional knowledge, experience, or skill.

Malta fever. See **brucellosis.**

malt worker's lung, a breathing disorder acquired by exposure to fungus particles in moldy barley grain or malt. See also **organic dust.**

mammary gland, one of two half-sphere-shaped glands on the chest of mature females. It is also seen in simple form in children and in males. Gland tissue forms a ring of lobes with small sacs (alveoli). Each lobe has a system of ducts for the passage of milk from the alveoli to the nipple. The inner portion of the breast is filled with gland tissue. The outer portion is made up mostly of fatty tissue. The left breast is usually larger than the right. Also called **breast, mamma.** See also **lactation.**

mammogram, an x-ray film of the soft tissues of the breast made to identify various lumps (cysts or tumors).

mammoplasty, surgical reshaping of the breasts. It is done to reduce or lift large or sagging breasts, to enlarge small breasts, or to reconstruct a breast after removal of a tumor. To reduce the size of the breasts and raise them, excess tissue is removed from the bottom of the breasts. The breast is then lifted. The nipple is brought through an opening in an overhanging skin flap. To enlarge a breast, a thin plastic sac of silicone fluid may be inserted in a pouch formed beneath the breast on the chest wall. The complications after surgery are infection and, with the use of implants, rejection by tissues of the foreign body.

mammothermography, a procedure in which a special test (infrared thermography) is used for examining the breast to detect abnormal growths. It is done by outlining hot and cold tissue areas. Compare **mammography.** See also **thermography.**

Mandelamine, a trademark for an antibiotic (methenamine mandelate).

mandible /man'dibəl/, a large bone forming the lower jaw. It consists of a horizontal part that has the lower teeth and two vertical parts that join the body at almost right angles. The body of the mandible is curved, looking somewhat like a horseshoe. The vertical parts form a joint with the upper jaw (maxilla).

mandibular sling, the connection between the lower jaw (mandible) and the upper jaw (maxilla), formed by the two face muscles. The mouth is opened and closed as the mandible moves with the help of the mandibular sling.

Mandol, a trademark for an antibiotic (cefamandole nafate).

maneuver, in obstetrics, moving the fetus to aid in childbirth.

mania, a mood disorder with too-much excitement, excess elation, overactivity, nervousness, talking too much, flight of ideas, and not paying attention. Violent, destructive, or self-destructive behavior occurs at times. It is seen in the major mental disorders, as the manic phase of bipolar disorder, and in certain organic brain diseases, as dementia. Kinds of mania include **Bell's mania, dancing mania, epileptic mania, hysteric mania, periodic mania, puerperal mania, religious mania.** –maniac, *n., adj.,* maniacal, *adj.*

-maniac, a combining form meaning a patient with a type of psychosis.

-manic, a combining form meaning a specific psychosis.

manic depressive, a patient with or showing the symptoms of bipolar disorder.

manipulation, the skillful use of the hands in therapy or diagnosis, as feeling with the hands, resetting a dislocation, turning the unborn, or some treatments in physical therapy and bone therapy (osteopathy). See also **massage.**

mannitol, a medication composed of sugar. It is given to cause urination, and to reduce pressure in the brain and eyeball. Other uses are to cause the release of poisons and other toxic wastes, and to check kidney function.
★CAUTION: Fluid in the lungs, dehydration, or known allergy to this drug prohibits its use.
★ADVERSE EFFECTS: Among the more serious side effects are fluid in the lungs, heart failure, headache, vomiting, and confusion.

manometer /mənom'ətər/, a device for measuring the pressure of a fluid. It has a tube marked with a scale. The tube contains a fluid, as mercury, that is difficult to compress. The level of the fluid in the tube varies with the pressure of the fluid being measured. A kind of manometer (sphygmomanometer) is used to measure blood pressure.

Mantadil, a trademark for a skin cream with an adrenal hormone (hydrocortisone acetate) and an antihistamine (chlorcyclizine hydrochloride).

Mantoux test /mantoo'/, a tuberculosis skin test, it consists of an injection of a pure form of the tuberclosis bacterium. A hardened, raised red area appearing 24 to 72 hours after injection is a positive reaction. See also **tuberculin test.**

manual rotation, a maneuver in which a baby's head is turned by the hand of a physician in the birth canal to make childbirth easier. Compare **forceps rotation.**

manus. See **hand.**

many-tailed bandage, a broad, evenly shaped bandage with both ends split into strips of equal size and number. As the bandage is placed on the stomach, chest, or limb, the ends may be overlapped and the cut ends tied together.

MAO inhibitor. See **monoamine oxidase inhibitor.**

Maolate, a trademark for a skeletal muscle relaxant (chlorphenesin carbamate).

maple bark disease, a type of lung disease (pneumonitis) caused by a mold *Cryptostroma corticale,* found in the bark of maple trees. In a sensitive patient the condition may be sudden, with fever, cough, and vomiting. It also may be long-term, with weakness, weight loss, uncomfortable breathing when exercising, and coughing up sputum.

maple syrup urine disease, an inherited disorder in which an enzyme needed for the breakdown of three amino acids (valine, leucine, and isoleucine) is lacking. The disease is usually discovered in infancy. It is recognized by the typical maple syrup odor of the urine and by unnatural reflexes. Stress, fever, infection, and taking in lysine, leucine, or isoleucine make the condition worse. Treatment includes a diet avoiding these amino acids. Kidney dialysis or blood transfusion are seldom given. Also called **branched chain ketoaciduria.**

maprotiline hydrochloride, an antidepressant similar to the tricyclics. It is given for the treatment of depression.

marasmus /mərazˈməs/, a condition of excess malnutrition and wasting, mostly in young children. It is marked by step-by-step wasting of skin tissue and muscle. It results from a lack of enough calories and proteins. Marasmus is seen in children with failure to thrive and in starvation. Less commonly, it occurs as a result of an inability to absorb or use protein. Care of the marasmic child involves restoring the fluid and mineral balance. It is followed by the slow and gradual addition of regular foods as they are tolerated. Stimulation that is right for the developmental age should be given. As much of the care of the child as possible is given by one person, if the child has also been emotionally starved. See also **failure to thrive, kwashiorkor.**

Marax, a trademark for a respiratory drug containing a smooth muscle relaxant (theophylline), a stimulant (ephedrine sulfate), and a tranquilizer (hydroxyzine hydrochloride).

marble bones. See **osteopetrosis.**

Marburg-Ebola virus disease /märˈbərgebˈələ/, a serious disease with fever, rash and severe stomach and intestinal bleeding. An epidemic in Marburg, Germany, in 1967, was traced to imported African green monkeys. In 1976, in the Ebola River District of Zaire and Sudan, an explosive epidemic occurred with a death rate of 85%. There is no effective treatment. Also called **hemorrhagic fever.**

Marcaine Hydrochloride, a trademark for a local anesthetic (bupivacaine hydrochloride).

march foot, an abnormal condition of the foot. It is caused by excess use, as in a long march. The forefoot is swollen and painful. One or more of the foot bones may be broken. See also **stress fracture.**

march hemoglobinuria, a rare, abnormal condition, marked by blood hemoglobin in the urine, that occurs after excess physical exercise or prolonged exercise, as marching or long-distance running.

Marchiafava-Micheli disease /märˈkyəfäˈvəmikäˈ-lē/, a disorder of unknown cause marked by episodes of bloody urine. It occurs usually, but not always, at night.

Marcus Gunn pupil sign, a test for disease of the optic nerve or retina of the eye. In a dark room a beam of light is moved from one eye to the other. Normal narrowing of the pupil of an affected eye occurs when the beam is directed

at the opposite eye. As the light is moved to the abnormal eye, the direct reaction to light is weaker and both pupils appear to widen. It indicates poor conduction by the optic nerve fibers. Also called **swinging light test.**

Marezine, a trademark for a motion-sickness drug (cyclizine hydrochloride) that can be injected.

Marfan's syndrome /märfäNzˈ/, an inherited condition with excess length of the bones, often linked with problems of the eyes, heart, and circulation. The disease causes major muscle and bone disorders, as underdeveloped muscles, weak ligaments, excess joint movements, and long bones. Changes of the heart and the circulation include breaking of the elastic fibers in the walls of the major heart artery (aorta), which may lead to a break in the major artery. Visual changes include many disorders, as dislocation of the lens of the eye. The disease affects men and women equally. It lengthens the legs so that most adult patients with the disease are over 6 feet tall. The arms and legs of patients with Marfan's syndrome are very long and spiderlike. The fingers and toes are greatly lengthened. The skulls of Marfan's syndrome patients are usually uneven in shape or size. A curved spine may develop and increase during adolescence. No specific treatment is known for Marfan's syndrome. Many of the problems may be treated with surgery.

marginal placenta previa, a placenta that becomes stuck in the lower part of the uterus. Its edges touch or spread to some degree over the opening of the uterine cervix. During labor, as the cervix widens, bleeding may occur from the separation of the placenta from the uterus beneath it. Bleeding may be so light as to pose no serious problem. In some cases heavy bleeding may occur, but the pressure of the fetus is often enough to act as a plug, stopping the bleeding. Cesarean section is not usually necessary. See also **placenta previa.**

Marie's hypertrophy, a long-term swelling of the joints. It is caused by a swelling of the membrane covering the bones. Also called **hypertrophic pulmonary osteopathy.**

Marie-Strümpell disease. See **ankylosing spondylitis.**

marijuana. See **cannabis.**

mark, any birthmark (nevus).

Marplan, a trademark for an antidepressant (isocarboxazid).

marrow. See **bone marrow.**

Marseilles fever, a disease commonly found around the Mediterranean, in Africa, the Crimea, and India. It is caused by *Rickettsia conorii* carried by a brown tick. Symptoms are chills, fever, an ulcer covered with a black crust at the site of the tick bite, and a rash appearing on the second to fourth day. Also called **bou-**

tonneuse fever, Bruch's disease, Conor's disease, escharonodulaire, Indian tick fever, Kenya fever.

Marshall-Marchetti operation, surgery done to correct the inability to urinate. The surgery puts the urethra and bladder into their normal position. Also called **Marshall-Marchetti-Krantz operation.**

masculine, having the physical characteristics of a male. –**masculinize,** v.

masculinization, the normal development of male sex properties. See also **virilization.**

mask, 1. to hide, as a treatment that may mask the development of a disease. **2.** to cover, as a skin-toned cosmetic that may mask a colored mole. **3.** a cover worn over the nose and mouth to prevent breathing in toxic or irritating materials, to control delivery of oxygen or anesthetic gas, or to protect a patient from germs exhaled by medical personnel.

masking, 1. concealing a disorder by a second condition, as when a person begins a weight-loss diet while an undiagnosed wasting disease, as cancer, has developed. The loss of body weight is considered to be the result of the diet. The disease is not noted. This delays diagnosis and treatment. **2.** the unconscious display of a personality trait that hides a behavior disorder.

masking agent, a cosmetic preparation for covering moles, surgical scars, and other marks. Masking agents are generally made up of a flesh-colored dye in a lotion or cream base.

mask of pregnancy. See **chloasma.**

masochism /mas'ōkiz'əm/, pleasure gotten from receiving physical, mental, or emotional abuse. The abuse may be given by another person or by oneself. Compare **sadism.** Also called **passive algolagnia.**

mass, 1. the physical condition of matter that gives it weight and inertia. **2.** a group of cells clumped together as a tumor. Compare **weight.** See also **inertia.**

massage, the manipulation of the soft tissue of the body through stroking, rubbing, kneading, or tapping. The purpose is to increase circulation, to improve muscle tone, and to relax the patient. It is done either with bare hands or through mechanical means, as a vibrator. The most common sites for massage are the back, knees, elbows, and heels. Care is taken not to massage inflamed areas (particularly of the legs, because of the danger of loosening blood clots), open wounds and areas of rash, or tumors. Massage is done with the patient lying face down or on the side, in a comfortable position. Lotion or cream is put on the area to be massaged.

masseter /masē'tər/, the thick, rectangular muscle in the cheek that closes the jaw. It is one of four muscles used in chewing.

mass reflex, an abnormal condition, seen in patients with a cut spinal cord. It is marked by a large nerve discharge. This results in muscle spasms, involuntary urination and defecation, high blood pressure, and heavy sweating. A mass reflex may be caused by scratching or other painful stimulation of the skin, a bloated bladder or intestines, cold weather, sitting for too long, or emotional stress. Muscle spasms may be so violent as to throw the patient off a bed or stretcher. Drugs to reduce mass reflexes and exercises in warm water help. Surgery on the brain and nerves may be necessary.

mastalgia /mastal'jə/, pain in the breast caused by clogging or "caking" during milk release, an infection, a breast disease including lumps (cysts), especially during or before menstruation, or advanced cancer. The early stages of breast cancer are seldom painful. –**mastalgic,** adj.

mast cell, a part of the connective tissue containing large grains made up of histamine and other substances that are freed from the mast cell because of an injury and infection.

mastectomy /mastek'təmē/, removing through surgery one or both breasts. It is done to treat a cancer. In a simple mastectomy, only breast tissue is removed. In a radical mastectomy, some of the muscles of the chest are removed with the breast and with all lymph nodes in the armpit. In a modified radical mastectomy, the large muscles of the chest that move the arm are saved. After surgery the patient is encouraged to take deep breaths and to cough often. The affected arm is set with the hand pointed up or on pillows so that the hand is higher than the lower arm. The lower arm is above heart level. Hand and wrist movements and movements of the elbow are begun within 24 hours and done often. No outward (external) rotation of the upper arm is allowed before the 10th day. An elastic bandage and, later, an elastic sleeve are used to reduce the amount of fluid in the arm. The patient is fitted with an artificial breast (prosthesis) when the wound is completely healed. Emotional support and counseling are necessary. See chart on p. 487. See also **breast cancer, modified radical mastectomy, radical mastectomy, simple mastectomy.** –**mastectomize,** v.

mastication, chewing, tearing, or grinding food with the teeth while it becomes mixed with saliva. See also **bolus, digestion, ptyalin.**

masticatory system, the group of organs, structures, and nerves used in chewing. It includes the jaws, the teeth and their supporting structures, the hinge (temporomandibular) joints, the tongue, lips, and cheeks. Also called masticatory apparatus.

mastitis /mastī'tis/, an inflamed breast. It is usually caused by bacterial infection. **Acute mastitis** is most common in the first 2 months

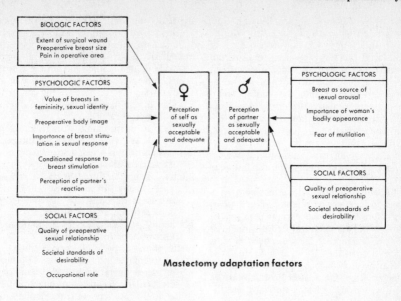

Mastectomy adaptation factors

of breast feeding. It is marked by pain, swelling, redness, lymph gland disorders, and fever. If not properly treated, sores may form. Antibiotics, rest, painkillers, and warm soaks are usually prescribed. Usually breast feeding may continue. **Chronic tuberculous mastitis** is rare. When it occurs it is the spread of tuberculosis from the lungs and ribs beneath the breast.

mastoid /mas'toid/, referring to a portion (mastoid) of the temporal bone of the skull.

mastoidectomy, removing with surgery a portion of the mastoid bone at the side of the skull. It may be done to treat long-term pus-forming, middle ear infection (otitis media) or mastoid bone inflammation (mastoiditis) when antibiotics are not useful. Entry is made through the ear canal or from behind the ear. In a simple mastoidectomy, infected bone cells are removed. The eardrum is cut to drain the middle ear. Antibiotics are then put in the ear. In a radical procedure, the eardrum and most middle ear structures are removed. After surgery a hearing aid may be used. In a modified radical procedure, the eardrum and the middle ear structures are saved. The patient will hear better than after a radical mastoidectomy. Dizziness is common after a mastoidectomy and may be expected to last for several days.

mastoiditis /mas'toidi'tis/, an infection of one of the mastoid bones, usually an extension of a middle ear infection. It is marked by earache, fever, headache, and discomfort. The infection is difficult to treat. It often needs antibiotics given by injection for several days. Children are most often affected. Some hearing loss may follow the infection.

mastoid process, the projection of a portion of the temporal bone at the side of the skull that is the attachment for various muscles. A hollow section of the mastoid process has air cells. They are the site of infections that spread from the ear. See also **temporal bone.**

masturbation, sexual activity in which the penis or clitoris is stimulated by means other than sexual intercourse. It leads usually to an orgasm. It is done, at least once in a while, by most people. It is considered to be normal and harmless. Also called, in men, **onanism.**

materia medica, 1. the study of drugs and other substances used in medicine, their origins, preparation, uses, and effects. 2. a substance or a drug used in medicine.

Materna, a trademark for a multivitamin supplement with calcium and iron for pregnant women.

maternal and child health (MCH) services, various services and programs organized for the purpose of giving medical and social services for mothers and children. Medical services include care before and after birth, family planning care, and child care in infancy.

maternal death, the death of a woman during the child bearing cycle.

maternal deprivation syndrome, a condition in which slowed growth occurs as a result of a lack of physical or emotional stimulation. It is seen most often in infants. Symptoms include a lack of physical growth, with weight abnormally low for age and size, malnutrition, excess withdrawal, silence, and irritability. The child also has an unnatural stiffness and rigidity with a slow response to others. Causes of the syndrome involve factors as parents not caring, emotional unstableness or insecurity of the mother, or lack of or too-slow development of mother-child bonding. Other factors are unreal expectations and disappointment about the sex or appearance of the child, and unfavorable conditions within the family. Treatment may require hospitalization, especially in cases of severe malnutrition. Emotionally deprived children often are slow in intellectual development, fail to learn normal social behavior, and are unable to form trusting, meaningful relationships with others. See also **failure to thrive.**

maternal-infant bonding, the attachment of a mother to her newborn baby. The process starts before birth as the parents plan for the pregnancy and then discover that the mother is pregnant. The mother feels the baby moving. She then accepts the baby as an individual, and makes plans for the baby after birth. In the first minutes and hours after birth, a sensitive period occurs during which the baby and the mother become intimate. The mother touches the baby and holds it to get eye-to-eye contact. The infant looks back eye-to-eye. The mother speaks in a quiet, high-pitched voice. The mother and the baby react to the voice and sounds of the other (entrainment). The infant's movements are a response to the mother's voice. She is encouraged to continue the process. The release of oxytocin and prolactin hormones by the mother's pituitary gland is begun by the baby's sucking or licking of the mother's breasts. The mother gives her body heat for the baby's warmth and comfort. Thus, the extended contact in the newborn period satisfies the physical and emotional needs of the mother and baby. After the baby is born, silver nitrate drops are not placed in the baby's eyes until the mother and the baby have had time to be together for eye contact because the drops cause a film to form over the eyes, dimming vision. During the first hour after birth the parents and the infant are not separated. They are given as much privacy as possible. Skin-to-skin contact is encouraged. Various methods may be used to keep the baby's temperature normal. In the maternity ward, the mother and the baby are kept together for at least 5 hours a day. Ideally, they are together for 24 hours a day in a 24-hour rooming-in unit.

maternal mortality, 1. the death of a woman as a result of bearing children. 2. the number of maternal deaths per 100,000 births.

maternity cycle, the prebirth (antepartal), birth (intrapartal), and postbirth (postpartal) periods of pregnancy and the return of reproductive organs to normal (puerperium). The cycle lasts from conception to 6 weeks after birth.

maternity nursing, nursing care of women and their babies during pregnancy, birth, and the first days after birth.

matrifocal family /mat'rifō'kəl/, a family unit made up of a mother and her children. Biological fathers have a temporary place in the family during the first years of the children's lives. They have a more permanent position in their own original families.

matrix, 1. a substance found between tissue cells. 2. also called **ground substance.** a basic substance from which a specific organ or kind of tissue develops.

matter, 1. anything that has mass and occupies space. 2. any substance not otherwise identified as to its parts, as gray matter, pus, or blood serum oozing from a wound.

Matulane, a trademark for an anticancer drug (procarbazine hydrochloride).

maturation, 1. the process or condition of coming to complete development. In humans, the full development of physical, emotional, and intellectual capacities that enable a person to be at a higher level of competence and ability to adapt. 2. the final stages in the formation of germ cells (ova or spermatazoa) in which the number of chromosomes in each cell is reduced to the number needed for reproduction. See also **meiosis, oogenesis, spermatogenesis.**

maturational crisis, a transistional or developmental period within a person's life, as puberty, when his or her psychological balance is upset.

mature, to become fully developed; to ripen.

mature cell leukemia. See **polymorphocytic leukemia.**

maturity, 1. a state of complete growth or development, usually the period of life between adolescence and old age. 2. the stage at which an organism can reproduce.

maturity onset diabetes. See **noninsulin dependent diabetes mellitus**

maxilla /maksil'ə/, pl. **maxillae,** one of a pair of large bones that form the upper jaw.

-maxilla, a combining form meaning the 'upper jaw or the bones composing it.'

maxillary sinus, one of the pair of large air cells forming a hole in the body of the upper jaw. The mucous membrane lining the sinus is next to the nasal cavity. Compare **ethmoidal air cell, frontal sinus, sphenoidal sinus.**

maxillofacial prosthesis, an artificial replacement for part, or all, of the upper jaw, nose, or cheek. It is applied when plastic surgery using normal body tissue is not adequate.

maximal breathing capacity (MBC), the amount of oxygen and carbon dioxide that can be exchanged per minute at the greatest rate and depth of breathing by a person.

maximal midexpiratory flow rate, the average amount of air flow during the middle half (in terms of volume) of a forced exhaling after the largest possible amount of air has been inhaled. It is used in testing the lungs to detect and evaluate continuous, widespread lung diseases as bronchitis, emphysema, and asthma.

maximal voluntary ventilation, the largest amount of air that a person can breathe by voluntary effort (per unit of time) breathing as quickly and deeply as possible. It is used in testing the lungs. The results are expressed in volume units per minute.

maximal expiratory flow rate (MEFR), the rate of the most rapid flow of carbon dioxide from the lungs possible when a person exhales or breathes out.

maximum oxygen uptake, the greatest amount of oxygen that can be moved by the bloodstream from the lungs to the working muscle tissue. Also called **aerobic capacity.**

maximum permissible dose (MPD), the estimated greatest amount of radiation (such as x-ray) to which a person may be exposed with the least risk of experiencing disease of the white blood cells (leukemia), cancer, or genetic defects. The MPD for the general population is 500 mrems (milli roentgen equivalent man, a unit of measure for radiation) per year, a figure that is 10% of the whole-body MPD of 5,000 mrems per year for radiation workers. Other MPDs range from 50 mrems for the fetal growing period of a pregnant woman to 75 rems in any one year, or 15 rems in a 3-month period for the hands of persons who are exposed to radiation in their occupation. Also called **allowable dose, tolerance dose.** See also **accumulated dose equivalent.**

maximum permissible dose equivalent, the most radiation that a person or a specific body part can receive in a given period.

May-Hegglin anomaly, an inherited blood disorder that is usually harmless. It may be linked to a decreased ability of the blood to clot.

mazindol /mă′zindōl/, a drug used to decrease the appetite. It is given to reduce food intake in the case of overweight caused by overeating. ★CAUTION: An eye disease (glaucoma), history of drug abuse, use of a monoamine oxidase inhibitor at the same time, or known allergy to this drug prohibits its use. ★ADVERSE EFFECTS: Among the more serious side effects are inability to sleep, irregular heart beats, dizziness, dry mouth, rapid heart beat, and allergic reactions.

McArdle's disease /məkär′dəlz/, an inherited disease marked by large amounts of body starch (glycogen) in skeletal muscle. It is milder than other glycogen-storage diseases. It leads only to muscle weakness and cramping after exercise. There is no known treatment. Also called **glycogen storage disease, type V.** See also **glycogen storage disease.**

McBurney's point, a place on the stomach that is very sensitive in acute appendicitis, placed in the normal area of the appendix about 2 inches from the edge of the right hipbone on a line between that bone and the navel. See also **appendicitis.**

McBurney's sign, a severe pain and extreme tenderness when McBurney's point is touched. Such a reaction may show that the patient has appendicitis.

mcg, abbreviation for **microgram.**

McMurray's sign, a click heard when moving the lower leg bone (tibia) on the upper leg bone (femur), showing injury to cartilage in the kneecap.

M.D., abbreviation for *Doctor of Medicine.* See **physician.**

Meals on Wheels, a program that takes hot meals to elderly, physically disabled, or other persons who cannot give themselves nutritionally adequate warm meals daily.

mean marrow dose (MMD), an arbitrary measure of the estimated average annual body radiation received by the population of the United States. The figure is 77 mrad (milli radiation absorbed dose) and includes both persons exposed to radiation and persons not exposed during the period. It is expressed in terms of bone marrow because radiation exposure to that tissue is assumed to be a cause of leukemia.

measles, an acute, highly contagious, viral disease that occurs foremost in young children who have not been vaccinated. Measles is carried by direct contact with droplets spread from the nose, throat, and mouth of infected patients, usually in the early stage of the disease. Indirect spreading by uninfected persons or by infected articles is unusual. An inactive period of 7 to 14 days is followed by the beginning stage of the disease. It is marked by fever, discomfort, runny nose, cough, eye irritation, sensitivity to light, and loss of appetite. Diagnosis is based on laboratory tests or on identifying small red spots (Koplik spots) inside of the cheeks, which appear 1 to 2 days before the appearance of the rash. Throat swelling develops. The temperature may rise to 103° F or 104° F. The rash first appears as irregular brownish-pink spots around the hairline, the ears, and the neck. It spreads rapidly, within 24 to 48 hours, to the body, arms, and legs. The red and dense patches give the skin a blotchy appearance. Within 3 to 5 days, the fever decreases, the spots flatten, turn a brownish color, and begin to fade. Routine treatment consists of bed rest, antifever drugs, antibiotics to control bacterial infection. If necessary, calamine lotion, corn starch solution, or cool water are used to relieve itching. Preventive measures include vaccinating with measles virus vaccine after the child is 1 year of age. Passive immunization with immune serum globulin is advised for unvaccinated individuals exposed to the disease. One attack of the disease means the patient will never have the disease again. Complications occur sometimes. The most common are middle ear infection (otitis media), pneumonia, swelling of the bronchial tubes, loss of speech (laryngitis), and, occasionally, brain swelling (encephalitis) and appendicitis. Also called **morbilli, rubeola.** See also **roseola infantum, rubella.**

measles and rubella virus vaccine live, an active immunizing agent. It is given to prevent measles and rubella.
★CAUTION: Suppressed natural resistance, use of costeroid drugs at the same time, tuberculosis, known or suspected pregnancy, and allergy to neomycin prohibit its use. Tumors of the lymphatic system or bone marrow, or active disease infection also prohibits its use. It should not be given for 3 months after use of whole blood, plasma, or immune serum globulin. It also should not be given for 1 month before or after vaccination with other live virus vaccines, except mumps vaccine.
★ADVERSE EFFECTS: The most serious side effect is a strong allergic reaction.

measles, mumps, and rubella virus vaccine live (MMR), an active immunizing agent. It is given for simultaneous vaccination against measles, mumps, and rubella.
★CAUTION: Suppressed natural resistance, simultaneous use of steroid drugs, tuberculosis, and allergy to neomycin prohibits its use. Tumors of the lymph system or bone marrow, known or suspected pregnancy, or severe infection also prohibits its use. It is not given for 3 months after use of whole blood, plasma, or immune serum globulin. It is also not given for 1 month before or after vaccination with other live virus vaccines.
★ADVERSE EFFECTS: The most serious side effect is a strong allergic reaction.

meatorrhaphy /mē'ətôr'əfē/, suturing the cut end of the urethra to the penis after surgery to enlarge the opening (urethral meatus).

meatus /mē·ā'təs/, an opening or tunnel through any part of the body, as the external acoustic meatus that leads from the outer ear to the eardrum (tympanic membrane).

Mebaral, a trademark for an anticonvulsant and sedative drug (mephobarbital).

mebendazole, an antiworm (anthelmintic) drug given to treat pinworm, whipworm, roundworm, and hookworm infestations.
★CAUTION: Pregnancy or known allergy to this drug prohibits its use.
★ADVERSE EFFECTS: Among the most serious side effects are intestinal pain and diarrhea.

MEC, abbreviation for *minimum effective concentration,* or the smallest amount needed for a drug to work. The drug is effective at any level above this value.

mechanism, 1. an instrument of process by which something is done, results, or comes into being. **2.** a machine or machinelike system. **3.** a stimulus-response system. **4.** a habit or drive.

mechanoreceptor, any sensory nerve ending that responds to mechanical stimulation, as touch, pressure, sound, and muscle contractions. See also **proprioceptor.**

mechlorethamine hydrochloride, an anticancer drug given to treat a variety of tumors. Also called **nitrogen mustard.**
★CAUTION: Bone marrow disorders, pregnancy, infection, or known allergy to this drug prohibits its use.
★ADVERSE EFFECTS: Among the most serious side effects are bone marrow problems and swelling at the injection site. Nausea, vomiting, and hair loss also may occur.

Meckel's diverticulum, a sac pushing through the wall of the small intestine. It results from the incomplete closing of the embryonic yolk stalk before birth. It occurs in 1% to 2% of the general population. The diverticulum usually causes no symptoms, but it may cause signs of appendicitis in infancy, sudden and painless bleeding, usually in childhood, or symptoms of blocked intestines. Surgery is advised to avoid swelling of the intestines. Blockage and blood loss may occur. Many Meckel's diverticula are discovered during surgery for other causes.

Meclan, a trademark for an antibiotic (meclocycline sulfosalicylate).

meclizine hydrochloride, an antihistamine given to prevent and treat motion sickness.
★CAUTION: Newborn infants and nursing mothers are not given this drug. Asthma or known allergy to this drug prohibits its use.
★ADVERSE EFFECTS: Among the more serious side effects are drowsiness, skin rash, allergic reactions, dry mouth, rapid heart beat, and nervousness.

meclofenamate sodium, an anti-inflammatory drug given in the treatment of rheumatoid arthritis and osteoarthritis.

Meclomen, a trademark for an antiinflammatory drug (meclofenamate sodium).

meconium /mikō'nē·əm/, a material that collects in the intestines of a fetus. It forms the first stool of a newborn. Thick and sticky, it is usually greenish to black in color. Meconium is composed of secretions of the intestinal glands, some amniotic fluid, and debris, as bile dyes, fatty acids, skin cells, mucus, fine hair, and blood. With drinking breast milk or formula and good bowel function, the color, texture, and number of the stools per day change by the third or fourth day after the start of feedings. Meconium in the amniotic fluid during labor may mean the baby is in distress.

meconium aspiration, the breathing in of meconium by the baby, as from the amniotic fluid. It can block the air passages and result in failure of the lungs to expand or cause other breathing problems, as pneumonia.

meconium ileus, blockage of the small intestine in the newborn caused by a concentration of thick, dry meconium. Symptoms include a swollen abdomen, vomiting, failure to pass meconium within the first 24 to 48 hours after birth, and rapid loss of fluids. It is caused by lack of pancreatic enzymes and is the earliest sign of cystic fibrosis. In simple cases, the blockage may be dislodged by giving enemas. Fluid loss is replaced by injection to prevent dehydration. If two to three enemas do not dislodge the blockage, surgery is necessary. See also **cystic fibrosis, meconium plug syndrome.**

meconium plug syndrome, blockage of the large intestine in the newborn. It is caused by thick, rubbery meconium that may fill the whole colon and part of the small intestine. Symptoms include failure to pass meconium within the first 24 to 48 hours following birth, a swollen abdomen, and vomiting if complete intestinal blockage occurs. A barium enema will reveal the plug and in most cases will dislodge it from the bowel wall. Additional gentle saltwater (saline) enemas may be needed to expel the plug. The condition may be a sign of Hirschsprung's disease or cystic fibrosis. See also **meconium ileus.**

medcard, a small card with the name, dose, and schedule of doses of each patient's drugs. It is used in giving drugs to each patient.

MEDEX, a physician's assistant who has gained medical experience during military service and further training in a physician's assistant program.

medial, placed near the middle of the body.

medial cuneiform bone, the largest of the wedge-shaped (cuneiform) bones of the foot. It links the toes to the ankle bones.

medial rotation, a turning toward the middle of the body. Compare **lateral rotation.** See also **rotation.**

median effective dose (ED$_{50}$), the dose of a drug that causes a specific effect in one-half of the patients to whom it is given.

median lethal dose (MLD), the amount of radiation that will kill 50% of the individuals in a large group of animals or organisms within a certain period of time. Also called **LD$_{50}$.**

median nerve, a nerve that extends along the forearm and the hand and supplies various muscles and the skin of these parts.

median palatine suture, the line between the two portions of the bone that forms the back part of the hard palate inside of the mouth.

median plane, an imaginary line that divides the body into right and left halves. Also called **cardinal sagittal plane, midsagittal plane.** Compare **frontal plane.**

median rhomboid glossitis, a swelling of a diamond-shaped area on the back of the tongue. It is often caused by alcohol, hot drinks, or spicy foods. It may also be caused by a fungus infection (candidiasis).

median toxic dose (TD$_{50}$), the dose of a drug that causes side effects in one-half of the patients to whom it is given.

mediastinum /mē′dē-əstī′nəm/, a portion of the space in the middle of the chest, between the sacs containing the two lungs. It extends from the breastbone (sternum) to the spine. It contains all of the chest organs, except the lungs.

mediate, to cause a change to occur, as stimulation by a hormone.

Mediatric, a trademark for a food supplement with multivitamins, minerals, hormones, and a central nervous system stimulant (methamphetamine hydrochloride).

Medicaid, a federally paid, state operated program of medical assistance to patients with low incomes. It is authorized by Title XIX of the Social Security Act. Under broad federal guidelines, the individual states determine benefits, eligibility, rates of payment, and methods of distribution.

Medicaid mill, *informal.* a health program or service that solely or mostly serves patients eligible for Medicaid. Such services are found mainly in low-income areas where there are few other health services.

medical assistant, a person who, under the direction of a physician, does many routine administrative and nontechnical clinical tasks in a hospital, clinic, or similar facility.

medical care, services related to continuing health, preventing illness, and treating illness or injury.

medical center, 1. a health-care facility. **2.** a hospital, especially one staffed and set up to care for many patients and for a large number of diseases and disorders, using modern technology.

medical consultation, a procedure whereby, on request by one physician, another physician reviews a patient's medical history, examines the patient, and makes suggestions about care and treatment. The medical consultant often is a specialist with experience in a specific field of medicine.

medical history. See **health history.**

medical indigency /in′dijen′sē/, the lack of money to pay for medical care, especially a person or family barely able to manage other basic living expenses.

Medicare, federally paid national health insurance. It is for certain persons over 65 years of age. The program is divided into two parts. Part A protects against costs of medical, surgical, and mental hospital care. Part B is a voluntary medical insurance program paid in part from federal funds and in part from premiums paid by persons enrolled in the program. Medicare enrollment is offered to persons 65 years of age or older who can receive Social Security or railroad retirement benefits. Other persons over 65 years of age, as federal employees and aliens, may not be permitted to join. Medicare was set up by Title XVIII of the Social Security Act of 1965.

medicated enema, medication given by a solution directed through the anus into the lower portion of the large intestine (rectum). It is usually used before operations on patients scheduled for bowel surgery.

medicated tub bath, a bath in which a drug is put in water, usually to treat skin disorders, as psoriasis. The water temperature is usually between 96° F (35.6° C) and 100° F (37.8° C). The temperature may be as high as 103° F (39.4° C) in treating psoriasis vulgaris. Most medicated baths are half-hour treatments. A folded towel or waterproof pillow is placed behind the head. A towel is draped over the shoulders for comfort. In certain conditions, the patient may scrub the affected skin areas with a brush and washcloth. In others, the physician may advise that the skin should not be scrubbed at all. After the bath the skin is patted dry. Ointment, cream, or other skin medication is applied.

medication, a drug or other substance that is used as a drug or remedy for illness.

medicine, 1. a drug or a remedy for illness. 2. the art and science of the diagnosis, treatment, and prevention of disease and keeping good health. 3. the art of treating disease without surgery. Two major divisions of medicine are academic medicine and clinical medicine. Some branches of medicine are **environmental medicine, family medicine, forensic medicine, internal medicine, physical medicine. —medical,** *adj.*

Medihaler-Epi, a trademark for a stimulant (epinephrine bitartrate).

Medihaler-Ergotamine Aerosol, a trademark for a painkiller (ergotamine tartrate).

meditation, a state of consciousness in which the individual tries to stop awareness of the surroundings so the mind can focus on a single thing, as a sound, key word, or image. It leads to a state of rest and relief from stress. A wide variety of meditation therapies are used to clear the mind of stressful outside disturbances.

Mediterranean fever. See **brucellosis.**

medium, *pl.* **media,** a substance through which something moves or through which it acts. A **contrast medium** is a substance, as a dye, that has a different quality than body tissues. It causes contrasts of body structures when used with x-ray films. A **culture medium** is a substance that provides a food environment for the growth of microorganisms or cells.

medium-chain triglycerid (MCT), a sweet, clear, oily fluid (glycerin ester) combined with an acid and distinguished from other triglycerides by having eight to 10 carbon atoms. MCTs in foods are usually high in calories and easily digested.

Medrol, a trademark for an adrenal hormone drug (methylprednisolone disodium phosphate).

Medrol Acetate, a trademark for an adrenal hormone drug (methylprednisolone acetate).

medroxyprogesterone acetate, a female sex hormone, progestin. It is given to treat menstrual disorders caused by unbalanced hormones.

★CAUTION: Known or suspected pregnancy, blood clots, stroke, liver problems, cancer of the breast or genitals, abnormal vaginal bleeding, missed abortion, or known allergy to this drug prohibits its use.

★ADVERSE EFFECTS: Among the more serious side effects are blood clots, stroke, and liver disease (hepatitis).

medulla /mədul′ə/, *pl.* **medullas, medullae,** 1. the most inner part of a structure or organ, as the adrenal medulla, or inner part of the adrenal gland.

medulla oblongata, a vital part of the brain. It continues as the bulblike part of the spinal cord just above the opening into the skull (foramen magnum). It is one of three parts of the brain stem. It contains mostly white substance with some gray substance. The medulla contains the heart, blood vessel, and breathing centers of the brain. Thus, any injury or disease in this area is often fatal.

medullary carcinoma, a soft cancer of a thin layer of cells covering various body parts (epithelium) containing little or no fiberlike tissue. A small percentage of breast and thyroid tumors are medullary carcinomas. Also called **carcinoma medullare, carcinoma molle, encephaloid carcinoma.**

medullary cystic disease, a lifelong disease of the kidney. It is marked by the slow beginning of excess urea in the body (uremia). The disease appears in young children or adolescents, who pass large volumes of watered down urine with greater-than-normal amounts of salt (sodium). Kidney dialysis is the usual treatment for the disease as the uremia continues and becomes worse. See also **uremia.**

medullary fold. See **neural fold.**

medullary groove. See **neural groove.**

medullary plate. See **neural plate.**

medullary sponge kidney, a birth defect of the kidney. It leads to widening of the tubes that collect urine in the kidney. Patients with this defect often develop a kidney stone or an infection of the kidney because the urine flow is reduced or stopped. Treatment includes drugs to increase the acid in the urine. A diet low in calcium and high in fluids must be followed to reduce the danger of forming stones.

medullary tube. See **neural tube.**

medulla spinalis. See **spinal cord.**

medulloblastoma /mədul'ōblastō'mə/, a brain cancer that develops from leftover embryonic nerve cells. The tumor usually starts in the brain (cerebellum). It occurs most often between 5 and 9 years of age. It affects more boys than girls. Although medulloblastomas can be treated with radiation, they grow rapidly, and radiotherapy usually allows one to live for only 1 or 2 years longer.

mefenamic acid /mef'ənam'ik/, a drug given to treat mild to moderate pain.
★CAUTION: Stomach and intestinal ulcers or swelling, kidney problems, or known allergy to this drug prohibits its use. It is used carefully in patients with asthma.
★ADVERSE EFFECTS: Stomach upset and diarrhea are the most common side effects. Other stomach and intestinal symptoms, dizziness, drowsiness, or skin rash occasionally result. Serious blood disorders rarely occur.

Mefoxin, a trademark for an antibiotic (cefoxitin sodium).

mega-, megalo-, mego-, a combining form meaning 'great or huge.'

megabladder. See **megalocystis.**

megacaryocyte /meg'əker'ē·əsīts'/, a very large bone marrow cell. Megacaryocytes are needed to make platelets in the marrow. They are normally not in the blood circulation. Also spelled **megakaryocyte.** See also **platelet.** –**megacaryocytic,** *adj.*

megacaryocytic leukemia /meg'əker'ē·ōsit'ik/, a cancerous disease of blood-forming tissue in which megacaryocytes increase abnormally in the bone marrow and move in the blood in large numbers.

Megace, a trademark for a female sex hormone used as an anticancer drug (megestrol acetate).

megacolon /meg'əkō'lən/, massive, abnormal widening of the large intestine (colon) that may be inborn or may develop later in life. **Congenital megacolon** (Hirschsprung's disease) is caused by the lack of autonomic nerve centers in the smooth muscle wall of the colon. **Toxic megacolon** is a serious result of ulcerative colitis and may lead to a tear in the colon, blood poisoning, and death. Surgery is the usual treatment for toxic and inborn megacolon. **Acquired megacolon** is the result of a long-term inability to defecate. It usually occurs in children who are psychotic or mentally retarded. The colon is widened by being overfilled with feces. Laxatives, enemas, and psychiatric treatment are often necessary. See also **Hirschsprung's disease.**

megadose, a dose that is greatly in excess of the amount usually prescribed or recommended.

megaesophagus /meg'ə·isof'əgəs/, abnormal widening of the lower parts of the esophagus. It results from the failure of the muscle at the opening to the stomach to relax and allow food to pass from the esophagus into the stomach. See also **achalasia.**

megalencephaly /meg'əlensef'əlē/, a condition with an abnormal overgrowth of brain tissue. In some cases brain tissue overgrowth is linked to mental retardation or a central nervous system disorder, as epilepsy.

megaloblast /meg'əlōblast'/, an abnormally large, immature, red blood cell that does not function.

megaloblastic anemia, a blood disorder marked by making and spreading abnormal red blood cells (megaloblasts). These red blood cells are usually linked to very dangerous anemia in which there is a lack of vitamin B_{12} or folic acid. Effective treatment is to inject vitamin B_{12}. See also **nutritional anemia.**

megalocephaly. See **macrocephaly.**

megalocystis /meg'əlōsis'tis/, an abnormal condition occurring mostly in girls, marked by a large and thin-walled bladder. Reducing the size of the bladder or changing the flow of urine through the small intestine (ileum) may be done by surgery to correct this condition. Also called **megabladder.**

megalomania /meg'əlōmā'nē·ə/, an abnormal mental state with delusions of grandeur in which one believes oneself to be a person of great importance, power, fame, or wealth. See also **mania.**

megaloureter /meg'əlōyŏŏrē'tər/, an abnormal condition marked by great widening of one or both ureters leading from the kidney to the bladder. It results from failure of the smooth muscle in the ureters. Treatment may include surgery.

megavitamin therapy, a type of treatment that involves giving large doses of certain vitamins and minerals.

megestrol acetate /məjes'trōl/, a hormone anticancer drug. It is given to treat cancer of the uterus and, more commonly, to relieve symptoms of the late stages of uterine and breast cancer.
★CAUTION: Allergy to the drug or pregnancy prohibits its use.
★ADVERSE EFFECTS: Some patients have had hair loss and blood clots while using the drug.

megrim. See **migraine.**

meibomian gland /mēbō'mē·ən/, one of several oil glands that release a fatty material (sebum) from their ducts on the outer side of each eyelid. The glands are buried in the supporting tissues (tarsal plate) of each eyelid. Also called **tarsal gland, palpebral gland.**

Meigs' syndrome /megz/, a pooling of fluid in the chest linked to a tumor of the ovaries or other pelvic tumor.

meiosis /mī·ō'sis/, dividing a sex cell, as it matures, into two, then four ova or spermatozoa (gametes). The nucleus of each gamete receives one-half of the number of chromosomes in the body cells of the species. In humans, meiosis results in gametes each containing 23 chromosomes, including one sex chromosome. Also called **meiotic division.** Compare **mitosis.**

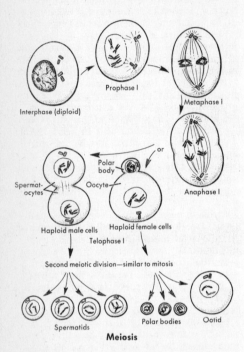

Interphase (diploid)

Prophase I

Metaphase I

Spermat-ocytes

Polar body

Oocyte

or

Anaphase I

Haploid male cells

Haploid female cells

Telophase I

Second meiotic division—similar to mitosis

Spermatids

Polar bodies

Ootid

Meiosis

Meissner's corpuscle. See **tactile corpuscle.**

melancholia /mel'angkō'lē·ə/, excess sadness; melancholy.

melanin /mel'ənin/, a black or dark brown color that occurs naturally in the hair, skin, and in the iris and choroid membrane of the eye. See also **melanocyte.**

melanocyte /mel'ənōsīt', məlen'ōsīt/, a body cell able to make the color of skin, hair, and eyes (melanin). Such cells are found throughout the bottom (basal) cell layer of the skin. They form melanin color from an amino acid (tyrosine). Melanin grains are then moved to nearby basal cells and to hair. A melanocyte stimulating hormone from the pituitary glands controls the amount of melanin made in a specific person.

melanocyte stimulating hormone (MSH), a hormone, released by the pituitary gland, that controls the amount and appearance of melanin color in skin cells.

melanoderma /mel'ənōdur'mə/, any abnormal darkening of the skin caused by large amounts of melanin or by chemical compounds of iron or silver.

melanoma /mel'ənō'mə/, any of a group of skin cancers that are made up of melanocytes. Most melanomas form flat, dark skin patches over several months or years. They occur most commonly in fair-skinned people having light-colored eyes. Any black or brown spot having an irregular border, color appearing to move beyond that border, a red, black, and blue color seen on close examination, or a nodelike surface may mean there is a melanoma. It is usually removed by surgery for laboratory examination. Outcome depends on the kind of melanoma, its size and depth, its location, and the age and condition of the patient. Kinds of melanoma are **amelanotic melanoma, benign juvenile melanoma, lentigo-maligna melanoma, nodular melanoma, primary cutaneous melanoma, superficial spreading melanoma.** Compare **blue nevus.** See also **Hutchinson's freckle.**

melanosis coli, an abnormal condition in which the mucous membrane of part of the large intestine (colon) is black or dark brown in color.

melanotrichia linguae. See **parasitic glossitis.**

melasma. See **chloasma.**

melatonin /mel'ətō'nin/, a hormone released into the bloodstream by the pineal gland in the brain. It follows a 24-hour rhythm with blood levels up to 10 times greater at night than during the day. The hormone seems to stop a number of endocrine gland functions, including the gonadotropic hormones. It also seems to decrease the color of the skin. When injected into a patient, melatonin causes drowsiness. Decreased release of melatonin occurs when calcium deposits or tumor formation destroys or damages the pineal gland. Decreases in melatonin can result in too-early puberty or in sex gland problems.

melena /məlē'nə/, abnormal, black, tarry stools containing digested blood. It usually results from bleeding in the stomach. It is often a sign of peptic ulcer or small bowel disease. See also **gastrointestinal bleeding.**

-melia, a combining form meaning "condition of the limbs," as in phocomelia or abnormally short or absent arms or legs.

melioidosis /mel'ē·oidō'sis/, an infection caused by the bacterium *Malleomyces pseudomallei.* **Severe melioidosis** involves pneumonia, pus in the chest, lung sores, blood poisoning, and liver or spleen problems. **Chronic melioidosis** is linked to bone swelling, multiple open sores of the internal organs, and the growth of abnormal body openings (fistulas) from the sores. The disease is most commonly seen in China and Southeast Asia. It is acquired by direct contact with infected animals. Human-to-human infection is unlikely. Treatment using antibiotics for several months is usually successful.

Mellaril, a trademark for a tranquilizer (thioridazine).

melphalan /mel'fələn/, an anticancer drug. It is given to treat cancer tumors, including multiple myeloma.

★CAUTION: Pregnancy, recent use of anticancer drugs or having radiation treatment, or known allergy to this drug prohibits its use.

★ADVERSE EFFECTS: Among the more serious side effects are bone marrow disorders, nausea, and vomiting.

membrana tectoria, the broad, strong ligament helping to connect the spinal column to the skull. Also called **occipitoaxial ligament.**

membrana tympani. See **tympanic membrane.**

membrane, a thin layer of tissue that covers a surface, lines a space, or divides a space, as the stomach membrane that lines the stomach wall. The main kinds of membranes are **mucous membrane, serous membrane, synovial membrane, cutaneous membrane.**

membranous labyrinth, a network of three fluid-filled, membrane-lined ducts hanging in the bony half-circle canals of the inner ear. They are linked to the sense of balance. The ducts contain a fluid called endolymph.

memory, the ability or power that enables one to remember and to recall, through unconscious means of association, previous sensations, impressions, ideas, concepts, and all information that has been consciously learned. Kinds of memory include **affect memory, anterograde memory, kinesthetic memory, long-term memory, screen memory, short-term memory, visual memory.** See also **amnesia, déjà vu.**

memory cell. See **lymphocyte.**

menadione /men'ədī'ōn/, a form of vitamin K_3. It is given to treat a lack of vitamin K and prothrombin, other than the type one is bornwith. Also called **menaphthone** /mənaf'thōn/ .

★CAUTION: It is not used in pregnancy, for overdose of drugs used to stop blood clotting, or to act against heparin. Known allergy to this drug prohibits its use.

★ADVERSE EFFECTS: Among the most serious side effects are a form of jaundice of the nervous system (kernicterus) in the newborn, and hemolytic anemia in certain patients. Stomach upset, rashes, and headaches also may occur.

menarche /menär'kē/, the first menstruation and the beginning of the menstrual cycle in females. It usually occurs between 9 and 17 years of age. See also **pubarche.**

Mendel's laws, basic laws of inheritance of physical traits. They are based on the breeding experiments of garden peas by the 19th-century Austrian monk Gregor Mendel. They are usually stated as two laws, called the law of segregation and the law of independent assortment. The law of segregation says that each characteristic of a species, or trait, as color, is represented in cells by a pair of units, now known as genes. The genes separate during a type of cell devision (meiosis) so that each egg cell or sperm (gamete) receives only one of the two genes for each trait. The second law says that the members of gene pairs on different chromosomes separate independently from other genes on the same chromosomes during meiosis. This means that the gametes may show all possible groups of traits. Actually, genes on the same chromosome tend to separate in groups. This discovery was made after Mendel. Also called **mendelian laws, mendelian genetics.** See also **chromosome, crossing over, dominant gene, linkage, meiosis, recessive gene.**

Mendelson's syndrome, a kind of chemical pneumonia resulting from breathing stomach acid into the lungs. It usually occurs when a person vomits while drunk, is drowsy from anesthesia, or unconscious. Also called **pulmonary acid aspiration syndrome.**

Menest, a trademark for a form of estrogen.

Meniere's disease /mānē·erz'/, a disease of the inner ear with periods of dizziness (vertigo), nerve deafness, and buzzing or ringing in the ear (tinnitus). The cause is not known. Occasionally the condition shows up after middle ear infection or a head injury. There also may be nausea, vomiting, and heavy sweating. Attacks last from a few minutes to several hours. Treatment includes a low-salt diet and antihistamines or other drugs. In very bad cases, surgery on the labyrinth or vestibular nerve linked to the sense of balance may be required. Because sudden movements often worsen the dizziness, a patient usually prefers to move at his or her own rate. The patient should have help while walking.

meninges /minin'jēz/, *sing.* **meninx** /mē'ningks, men'-/, any one of the three membranes that cover the brain and the spinal cord. They are the tough outer layer (dura mater), a thin inner layer (pia mater), and a spiderweblike middle layer (arachnoid). The pia mater and the arachnoid can become infected by a bacterial swelling. This may cause life-threatening problems. **–meningeal,** *adj.*

meningioma /minin'jē·ō'mə/, a tumor of the meningeal membranes covering the brain and spinal cord. Meningiomas often grow slowly. They usually contain blood vessels. The tumors may vary in shape and structure. They may invade the skull, causing weakening of the bones and pressure on the brain tissue. Meningiomas usually occur in adults. They follow in some cases after a head injury.

meningism /minin'jizəm/, an abnormal condition with irritation of the brain and the spinal cord. The symptoms look like those of meningitis. In meningism, however, there is no actual swelling of the meninges.

meningitis /min'inji'tis/, *pl.* **meningitides,** any infection or swelling of the membranes covering the brain and spinal cord. Usually pus-forming, it involves the fluid of the brain and spine in the space between the membranes that cover the brain. Symptoms are a bad headache, vomiting, and pain and stiffness in the neck. The most common causes are bacterial infection with *Streptococcus pneumoniae, Neisseria meningitidis,* or *Haemophilus influenzae*. Aseptic meningitis may be caused by other kinds of bacteria, by chemical irritation, tumor, or by viruses. Meningitis caused by coxsackievirus or echovirus is limited and disappears naturally. Others are worse, as those caused by herpes viruses or poliomyelitis viruses. Yeasts as *Candida* and fungi as *Cryptococcus* may cause a harsh, often fatal, meningitis. Tuberculous meningitis, almost always fatal if untreated, may result in many nervous system problems even with the best treatment. Bacterial meningitis should be treated right away with antibiotics. Except for adenine arabinoside, advised for herpes simplex meningitis, there is no specific treatment for viral infections of the meninges. Antifungus drugs given for several weeks may prevent death from fungal meningitis. Yet serious side effects may occur.

meningocele /mining'gōsēl'/, a saclike bump, or rupture, of either the brain or spinal membranes (meninges) through a defect in the skull or the spinal column. It forms a lump (hernial cyst) that is filled with fluid from the brain and the spine. It does not contain nerve tissue. The defect is called a cranial meningocele or spinal meningocele, depending on where it is. It can be easily repaired by surgery. See also **myelomeningocele, neural tube defect.**

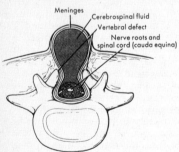

Meninges
Cerebrospinal fluid
Vertebral defect
Nerve roots and spinal cord (cauda equina)

Meningocele (cross-sectional view)

meningococcal polysaccharide vaccine, either of two active drugs used to fight meningococcal disease bacteria. It is used for vaccination against meningococcal meningitis.
★CAUTION: Reduction of the natural resistance to disease or sudden infection prohibits its use.
★ADVERSE EFFECT: The most serious side

effect is a dangerous allergic reaction.

meningococcemia /mining'gōkoksē'mē·ə/, a disease caused by *Neisseria meningitidis* bacteria in the bloodstream. The beginning of symptoms is sudden. Chills, pain in the muscles and joints, headache, pinhead-sized spots of bleeding under the skin, sore throat, and collapse will occur. Other symptoms are rapid heart beat and fast breathing and pulse rate. Body temperature may rise and fall. The best treatment is with antibiotics. However, the blood circulation may collapse.

meningococcus /mining'gōkok'əs/, a bacterium. It is often found in the nose and throat of persons who are carriers but not ill themselves. The organism may cause blood poisoning or spinal meningitis. Meningococcal infections are not easily spread. However, crowded conditions, as may be found in army camps, group the number of carriers together and reduce some people's ability to resist the disease. Skin tumors, with bleeding beneath the skin, are major clues to the diagnosis. Early treatment with antibiotics is needed for a cure. Several meningococcal vaccines are available. See also **meningitis. –meningococcal,** *adj.*

meningoencephalocele /mining'gōensef'əlōsēl'/, a saclike lump (cyst) that contains brain tissue, cerebrospinal fluid, and the brain's covering (meninges). It pushes through a defect in the skull. The condition is commonly linked to other defects in the brain. Also called **encephalomeningocele.** See also **neural tube defect.**

meningomyelocele. See **myelomeningocele.**

meniscectomy /men'isek'təmē/, surgical removal of one of the crescent-shaped cartilages of the knee joint. Long-term pain from a torn cartilage and unstable or locking of the joint are the usual reasons for surgery. After surgery, keeping the leg propped up reduces swelling. Exercises help to maintain muscle strength. Crutch walking usually begins about the fourth day. Normal walking begins after 2 weeks.

meniscus /minis'kəs/, a curved part of cartilage in the knees and other joints. See also **meniscectomy.**

Menke's kinky hair syndrome /men'kēz/, a disorder affecting the normal absorption of copper from the intestine. It is characterized by the growth of sparse, kinky hair. Infants with the syndrome have brain problems, slowed growth, and early death. Early diagnosis and injections of copper may stop brain damage.

meno-, a combining form meaning 'related to the menses,' as in menopause or menorrhea.

menometrorrhagia /men'ōmet'rōrā'jē·ə/, excess menstrual and uterine bleeding that is not caused by menstruation. It may be a sign of cancer, especially cancer of the cervix.

menopause /men'əpôz/, the end of menstruation. Commonly used to refer to the period ending the female reproductive phase of life (climacteric). Menses stop naturally with the decline of monthly hormonal cycles between 45 and 60 years of age. It may stop earlier in life as a result of illness or the surgical removal of the uterus or both ovaries. As the production of estrogen by the ovaries and pituitary gonad-stimulating hormones decreases, ovulation and menstruation happen less often and eventually stop. Variations in the circulating levels of the hormones occur as the levels decline. Hot flushes are the only general symptom of menopause that nearly every woman has. They can often be controlled with estrogen but are seldom so bad as to need therapy. Hot flushes will stop in time without hormonal treatment. Occasionally, heavy irregular bleeding occurs at this time, usually linked to fiberlike tumors or other uterine disorders. Estrogens given in large doses may be effective. However, a hysterectomy is sometimes required to control uterine bleeding.

menorrhagia /men′ərā′jē·ə/, abnormally heavy or long menstrual periods. Menorrhagia occurs sometimes during the reproductive years of most women's lives. If the condition becomes long-term, anemia from excessive blood loss may result. Abnormal bleeding after menopause always needs to be checked to rule out cancer. Menorrhagia is a fairly common result of fiberlike tumors of the uterus. It may be so bad as to require a hysterectomy. Also called **hypermenorrhea.**

menorrhea /men′ôrē′ə/, the normal release of blood and tissue from the uterus. See also **menorrhagia, menstruation.**

menostasis /minos′təsis/, an abnormal condition in which the products of menstruation cannot escape the uterus or vagina because of a blockage of the cervix (stenosis), or the opening of the vagina.

menotropins, a preparation of gonad-stimulating hormones from the urine of women who have gone through menopause. They are given with chorionic gonadotropin to cause ovulation in women and to make sperm (spermatogenesis) in men.

★CAUTION: High gonad-stimulating hormone levels in the urine, thyroid or adrenal gland problems, pituitary gland tumor, abnormal bleeding, ovarian lumps (cysts), pregnancy, or known allergy to this drug prohibits its use.

★ADVERSE EFFECTS: Among the more serious side effects are overstimulation of the ovaries, blood clots, multiple pregnancies, and possible birth defects.

menoxenia, any abnormality linked to menstruation.

Menrium, a trademark for a drug for menopause symptoms. It contains estrogens and a sedative (chlordiazepoxide).

menses /men′sēz/, the normal flow of blood and cast off uterine cells that occurs during menstruation. The first day of the flow of the menses is the first day of the menstrual cycle. Also called **catamenia.**

menstrual age, the age of an embryo or fetus as counted from the first day of the last menstrual period.

menstrual cycle, the repeating cycle of change in the membrane lining (endometrium) of the uterus. The temporary layer of the endometrium sheds during menstruation. It then regrows, thickens, is kept for several days through ovulation, and sheds again at the next menstruation. The average length of the cycle, from the first day of bleeding of one cycle to the first of another, is 28 days. However, the length and character vary greatly among individual women. Menstrual cycles begin at puberty. They end with the menopause. The three phases of the cycle are the **proliferative phase, secretory phase,** and **menstrual phase.** See also **oogenesis.**

menstrual phase, the last of the three phases of the menstrual cycle. It is the one in which menstruation occurs. The cast off mucosal lining of the endometrium is shed, leaving the permanent layer (stratum basale). Bleeding occurs. The average blood loss is 30 ml. The days of the menstrual cycle are counted from the first day of the menstrual phase. Compare **proliferative phase, secretory phase.**

menstrual sponge, a small natural sponge or a piece of artificial sponge to which a loop of string is attached. It is placed in the vagina to absorb the menstrual flow. It is removed by pulling the string. It may be washed, squeezed dry, and reused as necessary through menstruation. Menstrual sponges are not commonly used today. They are not easily available.

menstruation, the periodic discharge through the vagina from the nonpregnant uterus. It is made up of a bloody mass containing cast off tissue from the shedding of the membrane lining (endometrium). The average length of menstruation is 4 to 5 days. It recurs at about 4-week intervals throughout the reproductive life of nonpreganant women. Kinds of menstruation are **anovular menstruation, retrograde menstruation, vicarious menstruation.** See also **menstrual cycle.** −**menstruate,** v.

mental, of, relating to, or characteristic of, the mind (psyche).

mental deficiency. See **mental retardation.**

mental disorder, any disturbance of emotional balance, as shown in abnormal behavior or mental problems. It is caused by genetic, physical, chemical, biologic, mental, or social and cultural factors. Also called **emotional illness, mental illness, psychiatric disorder.**

mental handicap, any mental defect or characteristic resulting from a birth defect, serious injury, or disease that causes thinking problems and prevents a person from taking part in activities normal for a particular age group. See also **mental retardation.**

mental health, a state of mind in which a person who is healthy is able to cope with and adjust to the stresses of everyday living.

mental health consultation, any communication between two or more health-care professionals regarding a problem in treating mental and emotional disorders (psychotherapy).

mental health consultation nurse, a nurse with a master's degree and special training and experience in mental health care.

mental illness. See **mental disorder.**

mental retardation, a disorder marked by less-than-average general intellectual function with problems in the ability to learn and to act socially. The disorder is twice as common among men as among women. It may be named according to the intelligence quotient as: borderline, IQ 71 to 84; mild, IQ 50 to 70; moderate, IQ 35 to 49; severe, IQ 20 to 34; and profound, IQ below 20. Treatment is made up of educational programs and training according to the level of retardation. Emphasis is placed on prevention, as genetic counseling, checking the amniotic fluid for defects (amniocentesis), and general health care for pregnant women and for the baby after delivery. This is done especially for the poor and other high-risk groups. See also **amniocentesis, Down's syndrome, Hurler's syndrome, intelligence quotient, phenylketonuria, Tay-Sachs disease.**

menthol, an anti-itching drug with a cooling effect that relieves discomfort. It is part of many skin creams and ointments.

mentholated camphor, a mixture of equal parts of camphor and menthol. It is used in drugs and causes a skin swelling so as to relieve a swelling on a deeper level (counterirritant).

mentum /men′təm/, the chin, especially of the fetus.

mepenzolate bromide, a drug given to treat stomach and intestine problems, and peptic ulcer.
★CAUTION: Narrow-angle glaucoma, asthma, blockage of the urinary or stomach and intestinal tracts, dangerous ulcerative colitis, or known allergy to this drug prohibits its use.
★ADVERSE EFFECTS: Blurred vision, central nervous system effects, rapid heart beat, dry mouth, little sweating, or allergic reactions may occur.

Mepergan, a trademark for a central nervous system drug. It contains a narcotic (meperidine hydrochloride) and an antihistamine (promethazine hydrochloride).

meperidine hydrochloride, a narcotic painkiller. It is used to treat moderate to severe pain. It is also used before surgery to relieve pain and anxiety.
★CAUTION: Head injuries, asthma, kidney or liver problems, unstable heart condition, simultaneous use of a monoamine oxidase inhibitor, or known allergy to this drug prohibits its use.
★ADVERSE EFFECTS: Among the most serious side effects are drowsiness, dizziness, nausea, constipation, sweating, difficulty in breathing, slowed blood circulation, and drug addiction.

mephenytoin /mifen′ətō′in/, a drug to fight convulsions. It is given to control seizures in epilepsy when less dangerous drugs have not been effective.
★CAUTION: It is seldom used in pregnancy. Known allergy to this drug or to any hydantoin prohibits its use.
★ADVERSE EFFECTS: Among the most serious side effects are rash, fever, liver disorders, and various blood problems. The frequency of side effects limits the use of this drug.

mephobarbital /mef′ōbär′bital/, a sedative drug used to fight convulsions. It is given to treat anxiety, nervous tension, inability to sleep, and epilepsy.
★CAUTION: An inherited disorder (porphyria) or known allergy to this drug or to barbiturates prohibits its use.
★ADVERSE EFFECTS: Among the more serious side effects are drug addiction, lack of vitamin D, excitement, skin rash, and stomach upset.

Mephyton, a trademark for a vitamin K product (phytonadione).

meprobamate /miprō′bəmāt/, a sedative. It is given to treat anxiety and tension and as a muscle relaxer.

meralgia /miral′jə/, a pain in the thigh.

meralgia paresthetica /per′esthet′ikə/, a condition with pain, tingling, and numbness on the surface of the thigh. The cause is that a nerve is trapped in the inguinal ligament, which extends from the hipbone to the pubic bone.

mercaptopurine, an anticancer and immune suppressing drug. It is given to treat many cancers, including acute lymphocytic leukemia.

mercurial /mərkyŏŏr′ē·əl/, referring to mercury, especially a drug with the element mercury.

mercurial diuretic, any one of several drugs that have mercury. Mercurial diuretics prevent sodium and chloride from being reabsorbed and potassium from being released through the kidney. The main use for the drugs is to treat fluid pooling from heart disease, cirrhosis of the liver, or lack of urine in kidney disease. Flushing, hives, fever, and nausea and vomiting are common side effects. Blood disorders, mercury poisoning, and harsh allergic reactions are among the more serious side effects of the mercurial diuretics.

mercurialism. See **mercury poisoning.**

mercury (Hg), a metal element used in dental devices, thermometers, and blood pressure measuring instruments. It forms many poisonous compounds.

mercury poisoning, a serious condition caused by swallowing or breathing mercury or a mercury compound. A long-term form results from breathing the vapors or dust of mercury compounds or from repeated swallowing of very small amounts. It leads to irritability, excess saliva, loosened teeth, gum disorders, slurred speech, trembling, and staggering. Symptoms of sudden mercury poisoning appear in a few minutes. They include a metal taste in the mouth, thirst, nausea, vomiting, severe stomach pain, bloody diarrhea, and kidney failure that may result in death. Treatment may include flushing the stomach with milk and egg white or baking soda (sodium bicarbonate). Drugs may be given that hook onto mercury so it can be released from the body. Free mercury, as in thermometers, is not absorbed by the stomach or intestines. However, dangerous vapors may get through ordinary dust masks, causing poisoning by breathing the vapors. Mercury compounds are found in farming chemicals and in certain antiseptics and dyes. They are used heavily in industry. Industrial wastes containing mercury have been located in some areas. Seafood from contaminated waters has caused serious public health problems. Also called **hydrargyrism, mercurialism.** See also **Minamata disease.**

mercy killing. See **euthanasia.**

merisis /mer'isis/, an increase in size as a result of cell division and adding new material instead of the cell expanding. Also called **multiplicative growth.** See also **hyperplasia.**

meromelia /mer'əmēl'yə/, being born without any part of a limb, as in phocomelia.

Meruvax, a trademark for an active vaccinating drug (live rubella virus vaccine).

mesangial IgA nephropath. See **Berger's disease.**

mesangium /mesan'jē·əm/, a tuftlike network of blood vessels in the kidney that helps support the small blood vessels between the arteries and veins (capillaries). The mesangial cells help to fight infection and often contain large molecules or inflammatory agents that may aid in diagnosis of a kidney disorder when examined in a laboratory.

Mesantoin, a trademark for a drug to control convulsions (mephenytoin).

mescaline /mes'kəlēn, -lin/, a mind-altering, poisonous alkaline drug. It comes from the flowering heads of the cactus *Lophophora williamsii.* Closely related chemically to epinephrine, mescaline causes an irregular heart rate, sweating, widened eye pupils, and anxiety. The drug, taken in capsules or dissolved in a drink, causes hallucinations of sight, as color patterns and distortions of space. It does not usually cause confusion. North American Indians used mescaline in religious ceremonies to cause a heightened sense of well-being and a feeling of ecstasy. Also called **peyote.**

mesencephalon /mes'ensef'əlon/, one of the three parts of the brain stem. It is mostly made up of white matter with some gray matter. A red nucleus is in the mesencephalon. It contains the ends of nerve fibers from the other parts of the brain. Deep inside the mesencephalon are nuclei of several skull nerves. The mesencephalon also contains nerve nuclei for certain hearing and seeing reflexes. Also called **midbrain.** –**mesencephalic** /mes'ensifal'ik/, *adj.*

mesenteric node, a node in one of three groups of lymph glands serving parts of the intestine. The mesenteric nodes receive lymph from the small and large intestine and the appendix.

mesentery proper, a broad, fan-shaped fold of stomach wall membrane (peritoneum). It connects the membranes (jejunum and ileum) of the small intestine with the back wall of the abdomen. It holds the small intestine and various nerves and arteries of the abdomen.

mesiodens, a extra tooth that develops between two upper front teeth.

mesioversion, 1. a condition in which one or more teeth are closer than normal to the middle. **2.** a condition in which the upper or lower jaw is farther forward than normal.

mesoderm /mes'ōdurm/, the middle of the original three tissue cell layers of the growing embryo. It lies between the outer (ectoderm) and the inner (endoderm) layers. Bone, connective tissue, muscle, blood, blood vessel and lymph tissue, and the membranes of the heart and abdomen all come from the mesoderm.

mesomorph /mes'əmôrf'/, a person whose body shape is made up mainly of muscle, bone, and connective tissue, structures that develop from the middle (mesodermal) tissue cell layer of the embryo. Compare **ectomorph, endomorph.** See also **athletic habitus.**

mesonephric duct, a duct of the human embryo. It creates in the male the passageways of the reproductive system (ductus epididymidis, ductus deferens, seminal vesicle, ejaculatory duct). In the female, it becomes part of the ligament of the ovaries. Also called **wolffian duct.**

mesonephros, a type of excreting organ that develops in the embryo. It is made up of a series of twisting tubes that form urine filters (glomerulus) and connect with a duct (mesonephric duct). In humans the organ works only during early embryonic growth. However, the duct system is kept and placed in the male reproductive system. Also called **mesonephron, middle kidney, wolffian body.** See also **mesonephric duct.**

mesoridazine, a tranquilizer. It is given to treat psychotic disorders, behavior problems in mental diseases, and alcoholism.
★CAUTION: Parkinson's disease, use at the same time of central nervous system depressant drugs, liver or kidney problems, falling blood pressure, or known allergy to this drug

or similar drugs prohibits its use.

★ADVERSE EFFECTS: Among the more serious side effects are low blood pressure, liver problems, many nerve and brain reactions, blood disorders, and allergic reactions.

mesosalpinx /mes'ōsal'pingks/, a border of the broad ligament in which the fallopian tubes lie.

mesothelioma /mes'ōthē'lē-ō'mə/, *pl.* **mesotheliomas, mesotheliomata,** a cancer of the membranes of the lungs, heart, or stomach. It is linked to earlier contact with asbestos. The tumor may form thick sheets covering the internal organs. The outlook for recovery is poor. Also called **celothelioma.**

mesothelium /mes'ōthē'lē-əm/, a layer of cells that lines the body cavities of the embryo. It continues after birth as a covering on membranes, as the pleura of the chest and pericardium of the heart.

messenger RNA (mRNA), an RNA (ribonucleic acid) part that sends information from DNA (deoxyribonucleic acid) to the protein-making ribosomes of cells. See also **deoxyribonucleic acid, ribonucleic acid, ribosome.**

Mestinon, a trademark for a nerve and muscle-blocking drug (pyridostigmine). It is used as an aid to anesthesia and to treat myasthenia gravis.

mestranol /mes'trənōl/, an estrogen combined in some drugs with a progestin as a birth-control pill.

metabolic /met'əbol'ik/, referring to **metabolism.**

metabolic acidosis, acidosis in which excess acid is added to the body fluids or bicarbonate is lost from them. In starvation and in uncontrolled diabetes mellitus, sugar (glucose) is not present or is not available to burn for body fuel. The blood plasma bicarbonate of the body is used up in neutralizing substances (ketones) that result from the breakdown of body fat used for energy in the lack of glucose. Metabolic acidosis also occurs when carbohydrates are burned without enough oxygen, as in heart failure or shock. Excess blood potassium is often seen with the condition.

metabolic alkalosis, an abnormal condition marked by great loss of acid in the body or by increased levels of base bicarbonate. The acid loss may be caused by heavy vomiting, not enough replacement of minerals, or too-many adrenal hormones. The condition may also be caused by using too-much baking soda (bicarbonate of soda) and other antacids during the treatment of peptic ulcers. Signs and symptoms of metabolic alkalosis may include breathing difficulty, headache, drowsiness, irritability, nausea, vomiting, and rapid heart beat. Severe, untreated metabolic alkalosis can lead to coma and death.

metabolic disorder, any disorder that interferes with normal digestion and use of food in the body.

metabolic equivalent (MET), the amount of oxygen taken in per kilogram of body weight per minute when a person is at rest.

metabolic rate, the amount of energy released or used in a given unit of time. The metabolic rate is listed in calories as the amount of heat released during metabolism at the cell level. See also **basal metabolic rate.**

metabolism, the sum of all chemical processes that take place in the body as they relate to the movement of nutrients in the blood after digestion, resulting in growth, energy, release of wastes, and other body functions. Metabolism takes place in two steps. The first step is the constructive phase (anabolism), Smaller molecules (amino acids) are converted to larger molecules (proteins). The second step is the destructive phase, (catabolism). Larger molecules (as glycogen) are converted to smaller molecules (as glucose). Exercise, body temperature, hormone activity, and digestion can increase the rate of metabolism. See also **acid-base metabolism, anabolism, basal metabolism, catabolism. –metabolic,** *adj.*

metabolite /mitab'əlīt/, a substance made by metabolic action or one necessary for a metabolic process. An essential metabolite is one needed for an important metabolic process. For example, urea and ammonia are metabolites of proteins.

-metacin, a combining form for indomethacin-type substances used to reduce swelling or inflammation.

metacarpus /met'əkär'pəs/, the middle portion of the hand. It consists of five slender bones numbered from the thumb side, metacarpals I through V. **–metacarpal,** *adj., n.*

metagenesis /met'əjen'əsis/, the regular mixing of sexual with asexual methods of reproduction within the same species, as occurs in some organisms. **–metagenetic, metagenic,** *adj.*

Metahydrin, a trademark for a diuretic used in the treatment of high blood pressure (trichlormethiazide).

metal fume fever, a job-related disorder. It is caused by breathing fumes of metal compounds. Symptoms are similar to those of influenza. The condition occurs among workers in welding, casting, and other occupations dealing with metals. Access to fresh air and treatment of the symptoms usually relieve the condition. Also called **brassfounder's ague, zinc chill.** Compare **siderosis.**

metamodel, (in neurolinguistics) a theory that language represents experience, as in a map or a model, rather than being an experience itself.

metamorphopsia /met'əmôrfop'sē-ə/, a defect in seeing. Objects are seen as distorted in shape, resulting from a disease of the retina, as a fluid leak at the back of the eye.

Metandren, a trademark for an androgen (methyltestosterone).

metanephrine /met′ənef′rin/, a main byproduct (metabolite) of the nerve signal carriers, epinephrine and norepinephrine, found in the urine.

metaplasia /met′əplā′zhə/, the change of normal tissue cells into an abnormal form in response to chronic stress or injury.

metaphyseal dysostosis /mətaf′izē′əl, met′əfiz′-ē-əl/, an abnormal condition that affects the skeletal system. It is marked by a disturbance of mineral deposits in the growth area of growing bones. The result is dwarfism or bone deformities, as bowlegs. Cartilage-hair hypoplasia is one form of the disorder. It is marked by severe dwarfism and sparse, short, brittle hair. Mental retardation is not usually linked to metaphyseal dysostosis.

metaphyseal dysplasia, an abnormal condition marked by defective growth of the long bones. The ends of the affected bone become large and the middle becomes smaller. Metaphyseal dysplasia most often affects the femur or the tibia of the legs.

metaphysis /mətaf′əsis/, an area of bone in which the shaft (diaphysis) and ends (epiphysis) meet.

metaproterenol sulfate /met′əprōter′inôl/, a bronchial tube widening drug. It is given in the treatment of bronchial asthma.
★CAUTION: Irregular heart rhythms linked to rapid heart beat or known allergy to this drug prohibits its use.
★ADVERSE EFFECTS: Among the more serious side effects are rapid heart beat, high blood pressure, and heart attack.

metaraminol bitartrate, a drug used to restore blood pressure. It is given to treat very low blood pressure and shock that may occur after surgery.
★CAUTION: Known allergy to this drug prohibits its use. It is not used as the sole drug for falling blood pressure linked to low blood volume.
★ADVERSE EFFECTS: Among the more serious side effects are irregular heart rhythms, tissue damage at the injection site, high blood pressure, tremors, and nausea.

metaruricyte, a red blood cell with a nucleus. Such cells are not normally found in the blood of adults.

metastasis /mətas′təsis/, pl. **metastases** /-sēz/, **1.** the process by which tumor cells are spread to distant parts of the body. Because cancers have no enclosing capsule, their cells may escape and be transported by the lymph circulation or the bloodstream to hook onto lymph nodes and other organs far from the original tumor. **2.** a tumor that develops in this way. –**metastatic,** adj., **metastasize,** v.

metastatic calcification, the process whereby calcium salts gather in previously healthy tissues. It is caused by excess levels of blood calcium, as in abnormal activity of the parathyroid gland.

metatarsalgia /met′ətärsal′jə/, a painful condition around the foot bones. It is caused by new calcium formations or another abnormality of the foot. Also called **Morton's foot, Morton's neuroma, Morton's toe.**

metatarsal stress fracture, a break or rupture of a metatarsal bone of the foot. It is caused by lengthy running or walking. Also called **fatigue fracture, march fracture.**

metatarsus, a part of the foot, made up of five bones numbered I to V, from the large toe. Each bone has a long, slender body, and connects with the first row of toe bones (phalanges) at the outer end. –**metatarsal,** adj.

metatarsus valgus, a birth defect of the foot in which the front part points out away from the middle of the body and the heel remains straight. Also called **duck walk, toeing out.**

metatarsus varus, a birth defect of the foot in which the front part points in toward the middle of the body and the heel remains straight. Also called **intoe, metatarsus adductus, pigeon-toed, toeing in.**

Metatensin, a trademark for a heart drug. It contains a diuretic (trichlormethiazide) and a high blood pressure drug (reserpine).

Metchnikoff theory, a theory that living cells absorb disease organisms. It is proved in the process of engulfing (phagocytosis) and the digestion of harmful microbes by white blood cells (leukocytes).

meteorism, gathering of gas in the stomach or the intestine, usually with a bloated abdomen.

meteorotropism /mē′tē·ərətrō′pizəm/, a body reaction to influences of climate shown by biological occurrences, as sudden death, attacks of arthritis, and chest pain (angina) during weather changes. –**meteorotropic,** adj.

meter (m), a metric unit of length equal to 39.37 inches. Also spelled **metre.**

methacycline hydrochloride, an antibiotic given to treat many infections.
★CAUTION: Kidney or liver disease, pregnancy, early childhood, or known allergy to this drug or similar drugs prohibits its use.
★ADVERSE EFFECTS: Among the more common side effects are stomach and intestinal problems, sensitivity to light, potentially serious additional infections, and allergic reactions. Discoloration of teeth may occur in children exposed to the drug before 8 years of age.

methadone hydrochloride, a narcotic drug used for anesthesia or as a substitute for heroin. It allows withdrawal without severe reactions. Methadone does not cause a heightened sense of well-being, sleepiness, or stupor. It is not given to pregnant women or to patients with liver disease.

methanol, a clear, colorless, toxic, liquid distilled from wood. Drinking methanol paralyzes the eye nerve. It may cause death. Also called **wood alcohol.**

metharbital, drug used to treat epilepsy.
★CAUTION: Known allergy to barbiturates prohibits its use. It is used with care in pregnancy or liver disease.
★ADVERSE EFFECTS: Among the more common side effects are loss of voluntary muscle control, irritability in children, and confusion in elderly patients. Rashes and other allergic reactions also may occur.

methazolamide, a diuretic drug. It is given to treat glaucoma.

methdilazine /methdil′əzēn/, an antihistamine, it is given to relieve itching.
★CAUTION: Asthma, glaucoma, or known allergy to this drug or similar drugs prohibits its use. It is not given to newborn infants or nursing mothers.
★ADVERSE EFFECTS: Among the more serious side effects are bone marrow disorders and involuntary muscle movements. Dry mouth and drowsiness commonly occur.

methemoglobin /methē′məglō′bin, methem′-/, a form of hemoglobin in which the iron component is changed so it cannot carry oxygen and thus does not help the normal breathing of body tissues. See also **hemoglobin.**

methemoglobinemia, the presence of a form of hemoglobin that cannot carry oxygen (methemoglobin) in the blood, causing a bluish discoloring of the skin because the red blood cells are unable to release oxygen.

methenamine, an antibiotic given to treat urinary tract infections.
★CAUTION: Liver or kidney disease or known allergy to this drug or to similar drugs prohibits its use.
★ADVERSE EFFECTS: Among the most serious side effects are severe stomach and intestinal disturbances and rashes.

Methergine, a trademark for a drug that causes the uterus to contract, to control bleeding after childbirth (methylergonovine maleate).

methionine (Met), amino acid needed for proper growth in infants and for nitrogen balance in adults. It is also given in the treatment of liver diseases. See also **amino acid, protein.**

methocarbamol, a skeletal muscle-relaxing drug given to treat skeletal muscle spasm.
★CAUTION: Kidney disease, central nervous system defects, or known allergy to this drug prohibits its use.
★ADVERSE EFFECTS: Side effects may include low blood pressure and rapid heart beat. Drowsiness, dizziness, and nausea may occur.

method, a technique or procedure for creating a desired effect, as a surgical procedure, a laboratory test, or a diagnostic technique.

methotrexate, an anticancer drug given to treat severe skin inflammation (psoriasis) and many cancers.

methoxsalen, a drug applied to the skin to increase skin darkening (pigmentation). It is also given for repigmentation in loss of skin color (vitiligo).
★CAUTION: Liver disease, use (of any drug) at the same time that may cause light sensitivity reactions, or known allergy to this drug prohibits its use.
★ADVERSE EFFECTS: Among the most common side effects are central nervous system effects and skin burns. Stomach and intestinal discomfort and allergic reactions also may occur.

methscopolamine bromide, a nervous system-depressing drug. It is given to treat overactivity of the stomach and intestines and to treat peptic ulcer.
★CAUTION: Glaucoma, asthma, blockage of the tract or of the stomach or intestines, severe ulcerative colitis, or known allergy to this drug prohibits its use.
★ADVERSE EFFECTS: Blurred vision, central nervous system effects, rapid heart beat, dry mouth, little sweating, or allergic reactions may occur.

methsuximide /methsuk′simīd/, a drug used to treat convulsions in petit mal epilepsy.
★CAUTION: Known allergy to this drug or to any similar drug prohibits its use.
★ADVERSE EFFECTS: Among the more common side effects are blood disorders, liver and kidney damage, and a nervous system disease (systemic lupus erythematosus).

methyclothiazide /meth′əklōthī′əzīd/, a diuretic and high blood pressure drug. It is given to treat high blood pressure and pooling of fluid (edema).

methylbenzethonium chloride, an anti-infective skin medication. It is given for the prevention and treatment of diaper rash and other skin disorders.
★CAUTION: Known allergy to this drug prohibits its use.
★ADVERSE EFFECTS: There are no known serious side effects. Local skin irritation may occur.

methyldopa, a drug prescribed to reduce high blood pressure.

methylergonovine maleate, an artificial drug that causes contractions of the uterus. It is given to prevent or to treat failure of the uterus to return to normal size, bleeding, or other problems after childbirth.
★CAUTION: It is not given during pregnancy or given by injection into a vein, except in life-threatening situations. High blood pressure, general body poisoning, or known allergy to ergot alkaloid drugs prohibits its use.
★ADVERSE EFFECTS: Among the most serious

side effects are convulsions and death. High blood pressure, nausea, blurred sight, and headaches also may occur. Side effects are more common after giving the drug by intravenous (IV) injection.

methylphenidate hydrochloride, a central nervous system-stimulating drug. It is given to treat overactivity in children and to treat a sleep disorder (narcolepsy) in adults.
★CAUTION: Glaucoma, severe anxiety, tension, mental depression, or known allergy to this drug prohibits its use. It is not given to children under 6 years of age.
★ADVERSE EFFECTS: Among the more serious side effects are nervousness, inability to sleep, and loss of appetite. Allergic reactions and rapid heart beat may occur.

methylprednisolone, an adrenal hormone given to treat inflammatory conditions, including rheumatic fever and rheumatoid arthritis.

methyltestosterone /meth′iltəstos′tərōn/, a male sex hormone. It is given to treat a lack of testosterone, bone weakening (osteoporosis), female breast cancer. It is also given to stimulate growth, weight gain, and the making of red blood cells.
★CAUTION: Cancer of the male breast or prostate, heart, kidney, or liver disease, excess blood calcium, known or suspected pregnancy, breast feeding, or known allergy to this drug prohibits its use.
★ADVERSE EFFECTS: Among the more serious side effects are excess blood calcium, the pooling of fluids, irreversible male features in female patients, and liver disease (jaundice).

methyprylon /meth′əpri′lon/, a sedative and hypnotic drug. It is given to treat an inability to sleep (insomnia).
★CAUTION: Known allergy to this drug prohibits its use.
★ADVERSE EFFECTS: Among the more common side effects are occasional dizziness and excitability. Headache, rash, and stomach upset also may occur.

methysergide maleate /meth′isur′jīd/, a blood vessel relaxing drug. It is given to relieve migraine headache.
★CAUTION: Pregnancy, severe infection, liver or kidney disorders, heart, lung, or circulation system disease, or known allergy to this drug prohibits its use. It is not to be given to children.
★ADVERSE EFFECTS: Among the more common side effects are mild upset stomach and heartburn.

Meticorten, a trademark for an adrenal hormone (prednisone).

metoclopramide hydrochloride /met′əklō′prəmīd/, a stomach and intestinal-stimulating drug. It is given to stimulate stomach activity, to increase the strength of stomach contractions and to stop vomiting.

★CAUTION: Epilepsy, simultaneous use of drugs that cause nervous system reactions, adrenal gland disorders, stomach bleeding, blockage, or ulcer, or known allergy to this drug prohibits its use.
★ADVERSE EFFECTS: Among the more common side effects are central nervous system reactions, usually in children, and stomach and intestinal disturbances. Drowsiness and allergic reactions with a rash also may occur.

metolazone /mətō′ləzōn/, a diuretic and high blood pressure drug. It is given to treat fluid pooling (edema) and high blood pressure.

"me-too" drug, *informal.* a drug product that is similar, identical, or closely related to a drug for which a manufacturer has gotten a new drug application. The "me-too" drug is placed on the market by a company other than the holder of the new drug application. Because of its similarity to the approved drug, it is assumed that the new drug has been recognized as safe and effective. Further clinical tests are not required of the new supplier. However, information regarding the biological effectiveness and other data, and labeling of the product must meet Food and Drug Administration standards.

metopic /mətō′pik/, referring to the forehead.

metoprolol tartrate, a nerve signal blocker drug, given to treat high blood pressure.
★CAUTION: Slow heart rate, heart diseases, breathing disorders, or known allergy to this drug prohibits its use.
★ADVERSE EFFECTS: Among the more serious side effects are fatigue, abnormally slow heart rate, lung spasms, and stomach upset.

metralgia /mətral′jē·ə/, tenderness or pain in the uterus. Also called **metrodynia.**

metric equivalent, any value in metric units of measurement that equals the same value in English units, as 2.54 centimeters equal 1 inch or 1 liter equals 1.0567 quarts.

metric system, a decimal system of measurement based on the meter (39.37 inches) as the unit of length. The gram (15.432 grains) is the unit of weight or mass. The liter (0.908 US dry quart or 1.0567 US liquid quart) is the unit of volume.

metritis /mətrī′tis/, swelling of the walls of the uterus. Kinds of metritis are **endometritis, parametritis.** Also called **uteritis.** See also **puerperal metritis.**

metrodynia. See **metralgia.**

metronidazole, an antimicrobe drug. It is given to treat infections from amebas, certain bacteria, and *Trichomonas.*
★CAUTION: First three months of pregnancy, blood disorders, central nervous system disorders, or known allergy to this drug prohibits its use.
★ADVERSE EFFECTS: Among the more serious side effects are severe stomach and intestinal

distress, dizziness, blood disorders, and nervous system problems. A metal taste in the mouth is commonly noted.

-metropia, -metropy, a combining form meaning 'condition of the deflecting ability of the eye.'

metrorrhagia /met'rōrā'jē-ə/, uterine bleeding other than that caused by menstruation. It may be caused by tumors in the uterus or may be a sign of a cancer of the urinary and genital glands, especially cervical cancer.

Metubine, a trademark for a neuromuscular blocking drug (metocurine iodide). It is used to assist in anesthesia.

metyrapone, a diagnostic test drug. It is used to test hypothalamus and pituitary gland functions.

metyrosine /mətir'əsēn/, a high blood pressure drug, given to treat an adrenal gland disorder.
★CAUTION: Known allergy to this drug prohibits its use.
★ADVERSE EFFECTS: Among the more serious side effects are central nervous system reactions, including trembling and drooling. Drowsiness is common. Diarrhea and anxiety may occur.

Mexate, a trademark for a drug that controls or kills cancer cells (methotrexate).

Meynet's node /mānāz'/, any of the numerous nodes that may develop in the capsules surrounding joints and in tendons affected by rheumatic diseases, especially in children.

Mezlin, a trademark for a partly artificial penicillin antibiotic (mezlocillin sodium).

mezlocillin sodium, an antibiotic given for respiratory, abdominal, urinary tract, gynecological, and skin infections. It is also given for bacterial blood poisoning.
★CAUTION: Allergy to any of the penicillins prohibits its use.
★ADVERSE EFFECTS: The most serious side effects are excess sensitivity, convulsions, abdominal pain, blood disorders, and changes in liver and kidney functions.

M.F.D., abbreviation for *minimal fatal dose.*

mg, abbreviation for **milligram.**

MI, abbreviation for **myocardial infarction.**

micellar chromatography /mīsel'ər/, a method of monitoring very small quantities of drugs in blood serum, urine, or saliva. The technique eliminates the need to remove proteins that usually interfere with analysis of these body fluids. Micellar chromatography is used to monitor levels of prescribed drugs, as well as illicit drugs, such as LSD and THC.

-micin, a combining form for antibiotics produced by Micromonospora strains.

miconazole nitrate /mīkon'əzōl/, an antifungus drug used to treat certain fungus infections of the skin and vagina. It is also injected to treat systemic fungus infections.
★CAUTION: Known allergy to this drug prohibits its use.

★ADVERSE EFFECTS: Among the more common side effects of skin or vaginal use are irritation and burning. When used by injection, nausea, itching, vein swelling, and anemia may occur.

micrencephalon /mī'krənsef'əlon/, an abnormally small brain. See also **microcephaly.**

micro-, micr-, mikro-, a combining form meaning 'small.'

microaerophile, a microorganism that requires oxygen for growth. It needs it at a lower quantity than that in the atmosphere. Compare **aerobe, anaerobe. –microaerophilic,** *adj.*

microangiopathy, a disease of the small blood vessels, in which a membrane of capillaries thickens (diabetic microangiopathy), or in which clots form in the arterioles and the capillaries (thrombotic microangiopathy).

microbe, a microorganism. **–microbial,** *adj.*

microbiology, the branch of biology that studies microorganisms, including algae, bacteria, viruses, protozoa, fungi, and rickettsiae.

microcephaly /mī'krōsef'əlē/, a birth defect with an abnormally small head in relation to the rest of the body. It also leads to slowed growth of the brain. The result is some degree of mental retardation. The face is generally normal. The condition may be caused by heredity, an accident while an embryo or fetus, as exposure to irradiation, chemical agents, or mother's infection, or an injury, especially during the last 3 months of pregnancy. There is no treatment. Also called **microcephalia, microcephalism.** Compare **macrocephaly.**

microcheiria /mī'krōkī'rē-ə/, a birth defect with abnormally small hands. The condition is usually linked to other abnormal conditions or to bone and muscle disorders. Also spelled **microchiria.**

microcirculation, the flow of blood throughout the system of smaller vessels, particularly the capillaries, of the body.

microcyte /mī'krəsīt/, an abnormally small red blood cell. It often occurs in iron deficiency and other anemias.

microcytic anemia, a blood disorder marked by abnormally small red blood cells. It is usually linked to long-term blood loss or a disease of eating, as iron deficiency anemia. Compare **macrocytic anemia.**

microdactyly /mī'krōdak'təlē/, a birth defect with abnormally small fingers and toes. The condition is usually linked to bone and muscle disorders.

microdrepanocytic /mī'krōdrep'ənōsit'ik/, referring to a blood disorder in which both abnormally small red blood cells (microcytes) and sickle cells (drepanocytes) are present, as occurs in sickle cell-thalassemia.

microfilament, a small, threadlike structure found in most cells, it functions as a support system.

microfilaria /mī′krōfiler′ē·ə/, *pl.* **microfilariae,** the beginning form of any filarial worm, common in tropical areas. Certain bloodsucking insects take in these forms from an infected person or animal. They then develop in the body of the insect and become infective larvae. See also **filariasis.**

microgenitalia, a condition marked by abnormally small outer genitals.

microglia /mīkrog′lē·ə/, small cells that form part of the central nervous system. They collect waste products of the nerve tissues of the body.

micrognathia /mī′krōnā′thē·ə/, slowed growth of the jaw, especially the lower jaw. Compare **macrognathia. –micrognathic,** *adj.*

micromelic dwarf, a dwarf whose arms and legs are abnormally short.

Micronor, a trademark for a birth-control pill. It contains a progestin (norethindrone).

micronutrient, an organic compound, as a vitamin, or a chemical element, as zinc or iodine. Micronutrients are needed only in small amounts for the normal processes of the body. Also called **microelement, minor element, trace element.**

microorganism, a tiny animal or plant able to carry on living processes. It may or may not be a cause of disease. Kinds of microorganisms include **bacteria, fungi, protozoa, viruses.**

microphage /mī′krəfāj/, a white blood cell able to take in and digest small things, as bacteria. Compare **macrophage. –microphagic,** *adj.*

microphthalmos /mī′krəfthal′məs/, a birth defect marked by abnormal smallness of one or both eyes.

micropodia, a birth defect with abnormal smallness of the feet. The condition is often linked to other defects or to bone disorders.

micropsia /mīkrop′sē·ə/, an abnormal condition of seeing. A person sees objects as smaller than they really are. It often occurs during hallucinations. **–microptic,** *adj.*

microscopic, referring to very small objects, visible only when seen with a microscope. Compare **gross.**

microsomal enzymes, a group of enzymes that plays a role in the metabolism of many drugs.

microsomia, having an abnormally small and underdeveloped, yet otherwise perfectly formed, body with normal relationships of the various parts. See also **primordial dwarf.**

Microsporum, a type of fungus that causes ringworm epidemics in children.

microthermy, a treatment in which heat is given off by radio waves. It is used in physical therapy.

microtome /mī′krətōm/, a device, used in laboratory tests, that cuts samples of organ tissue into very thin slices for microscopic study in a hospital laboratory.

microvascular, referring to the portion of the body's circulatory system that is made up of the tiny blood vessels (capillaries) that link the arteries and veins.

microwave interstitial system, a microwave-generated system used to create a heat field in certain tumors that are no more than 2 inches beneath the skin. The microwaves produce a temperature of about 109°F to destroy the tumor cells. The treatment can be monitored on a video screen that shows the location of the tumor and the heat applicators.

micturition reflex, a normal reaction to a rise in fluid pressure within the urinary bladder. It causes the bladder wall to contract and a circular band of muscle (sphincter) to relax and open the urethra. This results in a flow of urine. Voluntary control of this reflex normally prevents undesired urination, as occurs in infancy.

Midamor, a trademark for a diuretic (amiloride hydrochloride).

midarm muscle circumference, a measure of muscle shrinking (wasting) in the upper arm calculated by subtracting the skin fold of the triceps muscle in the upper arm from the circumference of the midupper arm.

midbody, 1. the middle of the body, or the middle area of the trunk. 2. a mass of granules that appears in the middle of a cell during a phase (mitotic anaphase) of cell division.

middle cardiac vein, one of five blood veins of the heart muscle.

middle ear, the portion of the ear beyond the eardrum. It contains tiny bones (auditory ossicles) in a space inside the temporal bone. It is separated from the outer ear by the eardrum (tympanic membrane) and from the inner ear by the oval window on the cochlea. The auditory (eustachian) tube carries air from the back of the throat into the middle ear. Compare **external ear, internal ear.**

middle lobe syndrome, a local collapse of the middle lobe of the right lung. It is linked to a long-term infection, cough, wheezing, and inflammation of the lung. Blockage of the tube from the throat (bronchus) may occur. The condition is caused by the swelling of a cuff of lymph glands, resulting from tuberculosis or another swelling during childhood. The middle lobe bronchus is thus put under pressure, with collapse resulting in the blocked part of the lung. Treatment includes antituberculosis drugs, adrenal gland hormones, or surgical removal of the lobe.

middle mediastinum, the widest part of the space between the lungs (mediastinum), containing the heart, parts of the aorta, pulmonary arteries, a vein (superior vena cava), and nerves of the diaphragm.

midforceps, a childbirth operation in which forceps are placed on the head of the baby when the head has reached an easy-to-reach level of the mother's pelvis. In some cases, as severe fetal distress, midforceps may be the most rapid and the safest means of childbirth. Difficult midforceps delivery is likely to be more harmful to the baby and the mother than cesarean section.

midlife transition, a period between early adulthood and middle adulthood that occurs between 40 and 45 years of age.

midline, an imaginary line that divides the body into right and left halves.

Midrin, a trademark for a central nervous system drug. It contains a nerve impulse stimulant (isometheptene mucate), a tranquilizer (dichloralphenazone), and a painkiller (acetaminophen). It is used to treat migraine headaches.

midstream catch urine specimen, a urine specimen collected during the middle of a flow of urine. Some medical laboratories need the midstream catch urine for certain tests, rather than a urine sample containing the first or last part of the flow.

midupper arm circumference (MAC), an indication of upper arm muscle shrinking (wasting) based on the measurement of the circumference at the midpoint of the upper arm.

midwife, a person who assists women in childbirth. Among the responsibilities of the midwife are overseeing the woman's pregnancy, labor, delivery, and recovery after birth. The midwife may assist the birth alone, without the help of a physician. The midwife may get the help of a physician when necessary or handle emergency measures as required. The midwife may practice in a hospital, clinic, maternity home, or in a mother's own home. The midwife, whose practice may include well-child care, family planning, and some aspects of gynecology, is often an important source of health counseling in the community. Also called **obstetrix.**

migraine, a throbbing headache, usually occurring on only one side of the head. It is marked by severe pain, sensitivity to light, and other disturbances during the first phase. Attacks may last for hours or days. The disorder occurs more often in women than in men. The chances that a patient will have migraines may be inherited. The exact cause for the disorder is not known. The head pain is related to widening of blood vessels, which may be the result of chemical changes that cause spasms of the vessels. Allergic reactions, excess carbohydrates, iodine-rich foods, alcohol, bright lights, or loud noises can begin attacks. Migraine may begin with sensations called auras. These may be seeing disturbances, as flashing lights or wavy lines, or a strange taste or odor. Other disturbances are tingling, dizziness, ringing in the ears, or a feeling that part of the body is distorted in size or shape. The first phase may also include nausea, vomiting, chills, excess urination, sweating, swollen face, irritability, and extreme tiredness. After an attack the patient often has dull head and neck pains and a great need for sleep. Aspirin seldom helps during an attack. Drugs that narrow arteries of the head can usually stop the headache from developing if taken early enough. Also called **hemicrania, megrim.**

migrainous cranial neuralgia /mīgrā′nəs/, a variation of migraine, it is marked by very painful, throbbing headaches. It is often accompanied by a widening of blood vessels around the temples, sweating, tears, a runny nose, droopy eyelids, and swelling of the face. The headaches usually occur in groups within a few days or weeks. A long period without a headache may follow. A usual attack begins suddenly with a burning sensation in an eye or temple. The resulting pain may last 1 or 2 hours. The pain may be helped by antihistamines. Also called **cluster headache, histamine headache, Horton's headache.** See also **migraine.**

migratory polyarthritis, arthritis of a number of joints, one after another, and finally settling in one or several. It occurs in patients with gonorrhea. It develops a few days to a few weeks following the first signs of gonorrheal urethritis. The patient usually has a light fever and 1 to 5 days of pain in various joints, with signs of swelling. Large joints are most affected. After the swelling goes down, the skin over the joint may peel. Also called **migratory gonorrheal polyarthritis.**

migratory thrombophlebitis, an abnormal condition in which blood clots in both deep veins and those near the skin. It may be linked to cancer, especially cancer of the pancreas. The disorder often shows up several months before other signs of cancer. Also called **thrombophlebitis migrans.** See also **thrombophlebitis.**

Mikulicz's syndrome /mik′yŏŏlich′ēz/, an abnormal swelling of the saliva glands and tear glands. It is found in many diseases, including leukemia and tuberculosis. Also called **Mikulicz's disease.**

mild, referring to gentleness, subtlety, or low intensity, as a mild infection.

milia neonatorum, a skin condition marked by tiny lumps (cysts). They occur on the face and, occasionally, on the body of a newborn. The cysts disapppear by normal shedding of the skin within a few weeks following birth. They leave no scars.

miliaria /mil′ē·er′ē·ə/, tiny blisters and pimples, often red. They are caused by blockage of sweat ducts during periods of heat and high humidity. Backup pressure may cause sweat to escape under the skin, causing itching and prickling. Prevention and treatment include a cooling environment, air circulation, baths, and dusting powders. Also called **prickly heat.**

miliary /mil'ē·er'ē/, describing a condition with very small tumors, the size of millet seeds, as in miliary tuberculosis, which is marked by tiny tubercules throughout the body.

miliary carcinosis, a condition with many tiny cancer nodes.

miliary tuberculosis, a form of tuberculosis with spreading through the bloodstream of the germs (tubercle bacilli). In children it is linked to high fever, night sweats, and, often, swelling of the membranes covering the brain and spinal cord (meningitis). Other symptoms are fluid in the chest cavity and inflammation of the stomach and intestinal lining (peritonitis). A similar illness may occur in adults. Then there are weeks or months of mild symptoms, as weight loss, weakness, and light fever. Many small objects looking like millet seeds may show up on chest x-ray films. The liver, spleen, bone marrow, and membrane covering of the brain (meninges) are often affected.

milium, *pl.* **milia** /mil'ē·ə/, a very small, white lump (cyst) of the skin. It is caused by a blockage of hair follicles and sweat glands. One kind is seen in newborn infants. It disappears within a few weeks. Another type is found mainly on the faces of middle-aged women. Milia may be treated with a harsh cleanser or by cutting and draining. Also called **whitehead.**

milk, a liquid released by the mammary glands of animals that suckle their young. After breast feeding, people consume the milk of the cow and that of many other animals, including goats. It is a valuable nutrient for adults. It is nearly a complete food for infants, especially breast milk. Milk does not contain the necessary amount of iron. Its vitamin C content depends on the amount in the mother or the animal making the milk. Some individuals show an allergic reaction to milk because of a lack of the enzyme lactase. See also **breast milk.**

milk-alkali syndrome, a condition in which the pH level of the body fluids is higher than normal (alkalosis), caused by consuming too much milk, antacid medications containing calcium, or other sources of alkaline substances. The condition results in too much calcium in the blood (hypercalcemia), too little calcium excreted in the urine (hypocalciuria), and calcium deposits in the kidneys and other tissues. The patient may experience symptoms of nausea, headache, weakness, and kidney damage. Milk-alkali syndrome tends to occur most frequently in older adults with peptic ulcers.

milk baby, an infant with iron-deficiency anemia. It is caused by drinking excess amounts of milk and without adding iron-rich foods in the diet.

Milk babies are overweight and have pale skin and poor muscle growth. They are likely to get infections. See also **anemia.**

milk bath, a bath taken in milk for cosmetic reasons or for a skin disease.

milk-ejection reflex, a normal reflex in a nursing mother. It is caused by stimulation of the nipple, resulting in release of milk from the glands of the breast. Also called **let-down reflex.**

milker's nodule, a smooth, brownish-red tumor of the fingers or palm. The disease is gotten from tumors on the udder of a cow infected with cowpox virus. No treatment is needed because the infection acts as a vaccination.

milk fever, *nontechnical.* a fever that begins with the beginning of milk release (lactation) in the female breast. It used to be considered a normal reaction to lactation. Now it is known to mean an infection is present.

milking, a procedure used to release the contents of a duct or tube, to test for tenderness, or to get a specimen for study. The examiner presses the structure with a finger and moves the finger firmly along the duct or tube to its opening. Also called **stripping.**

milk leg. See **phlegmasia alba dolens.**

Milkman's syndrome, a form of bone softening characterized by multiple absorption stripes on both sides in a symmetrical pattern in long bones and the pelvis and shoulder that have lost calcium. The abnormalities appear on x-ray films. The syndrome is named for American radiologist Louis A. Milkman.

milk of magnesia, a laxative and antacid containing magnesium hydroxide. It is given to relieve constipation and acid indigestion.

★CAUTION: Kidney disease, symptoms of appendicitis, or known allergy to this drug prohibits its use.

★ADVERSE EFFECTS: Among the most serious side effects are diarrhea and excess blood magnesium, usually occuring in patients who have kidney disease.

milkpox. See **alastrim.**

milk sugar. See **lactose.**

milk therapy, a food treatment, used to treat Curling's ulcer in patients who have been severely burned. Cool, homogenized milk is given in doses of 1 to 2 ounces (30 ml to 60 ml) every hour through a nose tube. As the milk is better absorbed and tolerated, feedings are increased to 150 ml of milk per kilogram of body weight daily. An example is 9,000 ml or 9 quarts for a 60-kg, or 132-pound person.

milk tooth. See **deciduous tooth.**

milligram (mg), a metric unit of weight equal to one thousandth (10^{-3}) of a gram.

milliliter (ml), a metric unit of volume that is one thousandth (10^{-3}) of a liter.

millimeter (mm), a metric unit of length equal to one thousandth (10^{-3}) of a meter.

millipede /mil'ipēd'/, a many-legged, wormlike

insect. Certain species squirt irritating fluids that may cause a skin disease.

Milontin, a trademark for a drug used to treat convulsions (phensuximide).

Miltown, a trademark for a drug to help the patient sleep (meprobamate).

Milwaukee brace, a device that helps to keep the torso and the neck of a patient rigid. It is used to treat or correct spinal deformities and usually made of strong but light metal and fiberglass supports lined with rubber to protect against rubbing.

mimic spasm, undesired movements of a small group of muscles, as of the face. The spasm is usually psychological in origin. It may be made worse by stress or anxiety and is generally brought under control quickly. Multiple grimacing and blinking spasms occur in Gilles de la Tourette's syndrome. Also called **tic.**

Minamata disease /min'əmä'tə/, a severe, wasting, nerve disorder. It is caused by eating seed grain cooked with water containing mercury or of seafood taken from waters polluted with industrial mercury wastes. The term is taken from a tragedy involving Japanese who ate seafood from Minamata Bay. Mercury passes through the placenta in pregnant women, causing the inborn form of the disease. Symptoms may not appear for several weeks or months. They include numbness of the mouth, arms, and legs, and narrowed sight. Other symptoms are difficulties with speech, hearing, muscular abilities, and concentration, weakness, emotional problems, and stupor. Continuing to take in mercury causes serious damage to the kidneys, stomach, and intestines. Severe cases may result in coma and death. See also **mercury poisoning.**

mind, **1.** the part of the brain that is the seat of mental actions. It allows one to know, reason, understand, remember, think, feel, react, and adapt to all external and internal stimulations or surroundings. **2.** the combined conscious and unconscious processes of the individual that act on and direct mental and physical behavior. **3.** the condition of the intellect or understanding in contrast to emotion and will. See also **brain, intellect, psyche.**

mineral, **1.** an inorganic substance occurring naturally in the earth's crust. It has a certain chemical makeup and, usually, a crystallike structure. **2.** a nutrient that is eaten in food as a compound, as table salt (sodium chloride) rather than as a free element. Minerals are important in regulating many body functions.

mineral deficiency, the inability to use one or more of the mineral elements needed for human nutrition. Causes may be a birth defect, digestive disorder, or lack of that mineral in the diet. The symptoms vary, depending on the specific function or functions of the element in helping growth and keeping the body healthy.

Minerals are part of all the body tissues and fluids. They are important factors in keeping physiological processes going. They act in nerve responses, muscle contractions, and the changes of nutrients in foods. They regulate electrolyte balance and the making of hormones. They strengthen skeletal structures. All mineral deficiencies are treated by adding the specific element to the diet, either as a pill or in the right foods. See also specific minerals. See also **electrolyte.**

mineralization, adding any mineral to the body.

mineralocorticoid, a hormone, released by the adrenal glands, that keeps blood volume normal. It causes the kidney to retain sodium and water. It increases the release through urination of potassium and hydrogen ions. An excess of mineralocorticoid causes fluid to gather, high blood pressure, a lack of potassium, too much alkaline, and a slight increase in salt in the blood. A lack of the hormone results in low blood pressure, collapse of the circulation, excess potassium, and heavy salt loss. Without the hormone an adult may lose as much as 25 g of salt a day. Injury and stress increase mineralocorticoid release. See also **alkalosis.**

mineral oil, a laxative, stool softener, skin softener, and a solvent for dissolving substances for medicines. It is given to prevent and treat constipation, and is also given to prepare the bowel for surgery or examination.

★CAUTION: Symptoms of appendicitis, constipation, blockage or ulcer of the intestines, pregnancy, or known allergy to this drug prohibits its use.

★ADVERSE EFFECTS: Among the more serious side effects are laxative addiction, lack of vitamins, and stomach cramps.

miner's cramp. See **heat cramp.**

miner's elbow, a swelling of a membrane in the elbow joint. It is caused by resting the weight of the body on the elbow, as in some coal mining activities. The condition is sometimes seen in children and adults who lean on their elbows. See also **bursitis.**

miner's pneumoconiosis. See **anthracosis.**

Minerva cast /minur'və/, a body cast applied to the body and head, with spaces cut out for the face area and ears. The section around the body extends to the breastbone and lower rib border. The cast is used for keeping the head and part of the body rigid in the treatment of neck and chest injuries and spinal infections in the neck. Also called **Minerva jacket.**

minim (min), a measurement of volume in a drug measuring system. It is roughly equal to one drop of water. Sixty minims equal 1 fluid dram and 1 minim equals 0.06 milliliters.

minimal brain dysfunction. See **attention deficit disorder.**

minimal care unit, a unit for the treatment of patients in a hospital who are able to move about and meet many of their own daily living needs but need some nursing care.

Mini-Mental State Examination, a brief psychological test designed to differentiate between three types of mental disorders: dementia, in which mental functions deteriorate and break down; psychosis, a major disorder with a physical or emotional source; and affective disorders, characterized by severe and inappropriate emotional responses and mood and thought disturbances. It may include ability to count backward by 7s from 100, identify common objects such as a pencil and a watch, write a sentence, spell simple words backward, and show knowledge of surroundings by identifying the day, month, and year, as well as town and country.

minimization, (in psychology) thought disturbance in which the effects of one's behavior are minimized. See also **magnification.**

Minipress, a trademark for an anti-high blood pressure drug (prazosin hydrochloride).

Minocin, a trademark for an antibiotic (minocycline hydrochloride).

minocycline hydrochloride /min′əsī′klēn/, an antibiotic active against bacteria, rickettsia, and other organisms. It is given to treat many infections.

★CAUTION: Use carefully with kidney or liver disorders. Known allergy to this or similar antibiotics prohibits its use.

★ADVERSE EFFECTS: Among the more common side effects are stomach and intestinal disturbances, light sensitivity, loss of the sense of balance, and various allergic reactions. Use during pregnancy or in children under 8 years of age may result in discolored teeth.

minor element. See **micronutrient.**

minor surgery, any surgery procedure that does not need general anesthesia or breathing assistance.

minoxidil, a blood vessel widener. It is given to treat severe high blood pressure.

★CAUTION: Adrenal gland tumors or known allergy to this drug prohibits its use.

★ADVERSE EFFECTS: Among the most serious side effects are rapid heart beat and other heart disorders, salt and water storing, and excess hair growth. Stomach and intestinal disturbances also may occur.

Mintezol, a trademark for a drug used to treat worm problems (thiabendazole).

miosis /mī-ō′sis/, **1.** narrowing of the muscle of the iris, causing the pupil of the eye to become smaller. Certain drugs or an increase in light on the eye result in miosis. **2.** an abnormal condition in which excess narrowing of the iris results in very small, pinpoint pupils. Compare **mydriasis.** –**miotic,** *adj.*

miotic /mē-ot′ik/, any substance or drug, as pilocarpine, that causes narrowing of the pupil of the eye. Such drugs are used to treat glaucoma. –**miosis,** *n.*

mirage /miräzh′/, a seeing illusion caused by the bending of light waves through air layers of different temperatures, as sheets of water that seem to shimmer over stretches of hot pavement. Individuals under heavy stress are especially likely to interpret these images in wild, unrealistic ways.

mirror speech, abnormal speech in which the order of syllables in a word is reversed.

miscarriage. See **spontaneous abortion.**

missed abortion, a condition in which a dead, immature embryo or fetus is not released from the uterus for 2 or more months. The uterus becomes smaller and symptoms of pregnancy slow down. Infection and disorders of the clotting of the mother's blood may follow. The fetus and placenta may decay. Less commonly, the fetus becomes calcified calcium and the placenta is absorbed by the uterus.

missile fracture, a fracture caused by a fast-moving object, as a bullet or a piece of shrapnel.

mite, an insect with a flat, almost transparent body and four pairs of legs. Examples include tiny relatives of ticks and spiders, as chiggers and scabies mites. Some female mites burrow into the skin and lay eggs that hatch into larvae. The movements of the larvae cause heavy itching. See also **scabies.**

mite typhus. See **scrub typhus.**

Mithracin, a trademark for an anticancer drug (plicamycin).

mitleiden, physical symptoms resulting from emotional problems sometimes experienced by expectant fathers.

mitochondrion /mī′tōkon′drē·on/, *pl.* **mitochondria,** a small, threadlike organ within the cytoplasm of a cell that controls cell life and breathing. It occurs in varying numbers in most living cells. Exceptions are bacteria, viruses, and red blood cells. Mitochondria are the main source of cell energy. Also called **chondriosome.**

mitolactol /mī′təlak′tôl/, an anticancer drug used for many cancers, including Hodgkin's disease.

mitomycin, an antibiotic given to treat certain cancers.

★CAUTION: Lack of clotting or other blood disorders or known allergy to this drug prohibits its use.

★ADVERSE EFFECTS: The most serious side effect is bone marrow disease. Stomach and intestinal disturbances, hair loss, and skin reactions commonly occur.

mitosis /mītō′sis, mit-/, a type of cell division. It occurs in body cells and results in forming two identical cells, or daughter cells. Mitosis is the process by which the body makes new cells for both growth and repair of injured tissue. Kinds of mitosis are **heterotypic mitosis, homeotypic mitosis, multipolar mitosis, pathologic mitosis.** Also called **indirect division.** Compare **meiosis.**

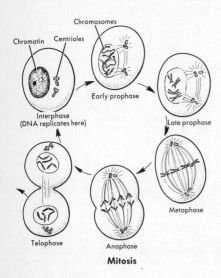

Chromosomes
Chromatin Centrioles
Early prophase
Interphase (DNA replicates here)
Late prophase
Metaphase
Telophase Anaphase
Mitosis

mitotane /mī'tətān/, an anticancer drug. It destroys normal and cancerous adrenal gland cells. It is given to treat cancer of the adrenal cortex.
★CAUTION: Known allergy to this drug prohibits its use.
★ADVERSE EFFECTS: Among the more serious side effects are stomach and intestinal symptoms, drowsiness, and hormone disorders.

mitral /mī'trəl/, referring to the mitral valve of the heart.

mitral regurgitation, a lesion of the mitral valve of the heart that causes the flow of blood back from the lower chamber (left ventricle) into the upper chamber (left atrium). The condition may result from a birth defect. Other causes are rheumatic fever, expansion of the left ventricle, and swelling of the heart muscle. Symptoms include breathing discomfort, fatigue, and irregular heart rate. Congestive heart failure may eventually occur. Treatment depends on the dangerousness of the condition. Surgery may be needed in cases of congestive heart failure. Also called **mitral insufficiency.** See also **valvular heart disease.**

mitral valve, one of the four valves of the heart. It is located between the upper chamber (left atrium) and the lower chamber (left ventricle). It is the only valve with two small flaps (cusps). The mitral valve allows blood to flow from the left atrium into the left ventricle. It normally stops blood from flowing back into the atrium. Narrowing of the ventricle forces the blood up against the valve. This closes the two cusps so the flow of blood is moved from the ventricle into the main artery of the body (aorta). Also called **bicuspid valve, left atrioventricular valve.**

mitral valve prolapse (MVP), sticking out of one or both small flaps (cusps) of the mitral valve back into the upper chamber of the heart (left atrium) during narrowing of the lower chamber (ventricle). This results in failure of the valve to close properly and a flow of blood back into the atrium. Most patients feel no symptoms. Some may have chest pain, an irregular heart rate, weakness, or breathing difficulty. The condition may lead to swelling of the left side of the heart. See also **valvular heart disease.**

mitral valve stenosis, a narrowing of the mitral valve of the heart. It is caused by the small flaps (cusps) of the valve sticking together (adhesions). The problem usually results from rheumatic heart disease. Excess growth of the heart's left atrium develops. This may be followed by right-sided heart failure and fluid gathering in the lungs. Reduced blood pumping causes weakness, breathing difficulty, and bluish skin color. Surgery on the valve may be necessary to remove the adhesions. The valve may be replaced by an artificial heart valve. See also **valvular heart disease, valvular stenosis.**

mittelschmerz /mit'əlshmerts/, lower abdominal pain in the area of an ovary during ovulation. It usually occurs in the middle of the menstrual cycle. For many women, mittelschmerz is useful in identifying ovulation. Thus they know the time when pregnancy is most likely to occur.

Mittendorf's dot, an eye anomaly characterized by presence of a small opaque floating spot at the back of the lens. It is a remnant of an artery that was present in the eye during embryonic development. The object usually does not affect vision.

mixed cell sarcoma, a tumor made up of two or more kinds of cells, not including fibrous tissue. Also called **malignant mesenchymoma.**

mixed connective tissue disease (MCTD), a disease marked by the combined symptoms of two or more white fiber tissue diseases, as synovitis, polymyositis, and systemic lupus erythematosus. This condition may cause joint pain, inflammation of the muscles, arthritis, swollen hands, and breathing difficulty.

mixed dentition, a phase of tooth growth when some of the teeth are permanent and some are baby teeth (deciduous).

mixed infection, an infection by several different microorganisms, as in some open sores, pneumonia, and infections of wounds. Many combinations of bacteria, viruses, and fungi may be involved.

mixed leukemia, a cancer disease of blood-forming tissues. It is marked by an excess of many different kinds of white blood cells, in contrast to a single type of white cell, as in lymphocytic or monocytic leukemia.

mixed tumor, a growth made up of more than one kind of tumor tissue.

mixed venous blood, blood that is composed of blood from the heart and from tissues of all body systems in proportion to the amount of each returned to the heart. Normally mixed venous blood is present in the artery leading from the heart to the lungs (pulmonary artery). Blood samples drawn from the right atrium or right ventricle may be incompletely mixed.

mixture, 1. a substance made up of parts that are not chemically combined. The parts may not occur in a fixed combination. 2. a liquid drug containing one or more drugs. Compare **compound, solution.**

ml, abbreviation for **milliliter.**

MLD, abbreviation for **minimum lethal dose.**

mm, abbreviation for **millimeter.**

MMR, abbreviation for **measles, mumps, and rubella virus vaccine live.**

Moban, a trademark for a tranquilizer (molindone).

Mobidin, a trademark for a painkiller (magnesium salicylate).

Mobitz I heart block, a second-degree heart block. Symptoms include weakness, dizziness, and, in some cases, fainting spells. It may happen after a mild heart attack and is usually a temporary condition needing no treatment. Also called **Wenchebach heart block.**

Mobitz II heart block, a second-degree heart block. Loss of conciousness (syncopal attacks), occurring without warning when the patient is upright or lying down, is common in Mobitz II block. It may be temporary or suddenly become a complete block. Long-term therapy means implanting a pacemaker.

Möbius' syndrome /mē′bē·əs/, a disorder of body growth. It is marked by paralysis on both sides of the face and is usually linked to seeing difficulties or other nervous system disorders, speech problems, and various defects of the arms and legs. The condition is caused by a defect involving the skull nerves that control the muscles. Also called **congenital facial diplegia, congenital oculofacial paralysis, nuclear agenesis.**

moderator band, a thick bundle of muscle in the middle of the right lower chamber (ventricle) of the heart. It is missing in some individuals and is of varying size in others. The band usually contains part of the fibers needed to conduct signals to contract the heart.

Moderil, a trademark for a high blood pressure drug (rescinnamine).

Modicon, a trademark for a birth-control pill. It contains an estrogen (ethinyl estradiol) and a progestin (norethindrone).

modified milk, cow's milk in which the protein content has been reduced and the fat content increased to make it similar to human breast milk. See also **formula, infant.**

modified radical mastectomy, surgery in which a breast is completely removed with some but not all underlying chest muscle and some of the nearby lymph nodes. The pectoralis major chest muscle is not removed. The operation treats early and easily spotted cancers of the breast. It is reported to be as successful as the more complicated radical mastectomy. Compare **radical mastectomy, simple mastectomy.** See also **mastectomy.**

Moeller's glossitis /mel′ərz/, a swelling of the tongue. It is marked by a sensation of burning or pain and a sensitivity to hot or spicy foods. Also called **glossodynia exfoliativa.** See also **glossitis.**

mohel /mō′əl, môhāl′/, an ordained Jewish circumciser.

moist gangrene. See **gangrene.**

molar, any of the 12 molar teeth, six in both the upper and lower dental arch. Each of the upper molars has three roots. The lower molars are larger than the uppers, and each has two roots.

molar pregnancy, pregnancy in which a cystlike mole (hydatid mole) instead of an embryo grows from the tissue of the early stage of the fertilized egg. The signs of pregnancy are all heightened. The uterus grows more rapidly than is normal. Morning sickness is often severe and constant. Blood pressure is likely to be high. Blood levels of female hormones are very high. The mole must be removed, because it may develop into a form of cancer. See also **hydatid mole.**

molar solution, a solution that contains 1 mole of solute per liter of solution.

mold, a fungus.

molding, the natural process by which a baby's head is shaped during labor as it is squeezed into and through the birth canal by the forces of labor. The head often becomes quite long. The bones of the skull may be caused to overlap slightly, without skull damage. Most of the changes caused by molding go back to normal during the first few days of life. See also **cephalhematoma.**

molecule, the smallest unit of a substance that has the properties of an element or compound. A molecule is made up of two or more atoms that are chemically combined. See also **atom, compound.**

molindone hydrochloride, a tranquilizer. It is given to treat schizophrenia.

★CAUTION: Severe central nervous system disease or known allergy to this drug prohibits its use.

★ADVERSE EFFECTS: Among the most serious side effects are central nervous system reactions, falling blood pressure, drowsiness, and other reactions characteristic of the phenothiazine tranquilizers.

molluscum /məlus′kəm/, any skin disease marked by soft, rounded masses or nodes.

molluscum contagiosum, a disease of the skin and mucous membranes, it is caused by a virus found worldwide and marked by scattered white pimples. Palms of the hands and soles of the feet are not affected. The disease occurs most often in children and in adults with a likelihood of getting an infection. It is carried from person to person by direct or indirect contact and lasts up to 3 years, although individual tumors last for only 6 to 8 weeks. Untreated, the tumors eventually disappear by themselves without scarring.

-monab, a combining form for identical antibodies that are formed from a single cell.

-monam, a combining form for monobactam (monocyclic beta-lactam) antibiotics.

Mönckeberg's arteriosclerosis, a form of hardening of the arteries in which many calcium deposits are found in the lining of the artery. There is little blockage of the open part. Also called **medial arteriosclerosis.**

Monday morning fever. See **byssinosis.**

Monge's disease. See **altitude sickness.**

Mongolian spot, a harmless, bluish-black spot, occurring over the sacrum between the hipbones or the buttocks of some newborns. It is especially common in blacks, Native Americans, Southern Europeans, and Orientals. The spot usually disappears during early childhood.

mongolism, mongoloid idiocy. See **Down's syndrome.**

moniliasis. See **candidiasis.**

Monistat, a trademark for an antifungus drug (miconazole nitrate).

monitrice, a childbirth coach who is specially trained in the Lamaze method of childbirth. The coach gives emotional support and leads the mother through labor and childbirth. The mother uses the specific techniques for breathing, concentration, and massage taught in the Lamaze classes to prepare for childbirth.

monoamine oxidase (MAO), an enzyme that makes nervous system hormones, as epinephrine, inactive. Also called **amino oxidase.** See also **monoamine oxidase inhibitor.**

monoamine oxidase (MAO) inhibitor, any of a group of drugs used mainly to treat depression. These drugs also help control anxiety and are especially useful for anxiety linked to abnormal fears (phobias). MAO inhibitors are sometimes used to treat migraine headache and high blood pressure. The effects of the drugs vary greatly from patient to patient. Among the most common side effects are drowsiness, dry mouth, blood pressure that falls as one stands up, and constipation. Overdose may cause trembling, a heightened sense of well-being, or psychotic behavior. MAO inhibitors interact with many drugs, one of which is ephedrine, which is in many common cold remedies. Certain foods are likely to cause severe high blood pressure linked to headache, irregular heart rate, and nausea. Patients taking MAO inhibitors are given a list of foods to avoid. Among these foods are cheeses, red wine, smoked or pickled herring, beer, and yogurt. See also **amine pump.**

monobenzone, a drug given to treat abnormal skin coloration (pigmentation), as disseminated vitiligo. It is not used for minor conditions, as freckles.

★CAUTION: Known allergy to this drug prohibits its use.

★ADVERSE EFFECTS: The most serious side effect is excess and irreversible skin bleaching. Common reactions are irritation and allergic reactions of the skin.

monoblast /mon′əblast/, a large, immature white blood cell. Some leukemias show by an excess amount of immature blood cells (monoblasts) in the marrow and an abnormal presence of these forms in blood circulation. Compare **megaloblast, myeloblast.** See also **bone marrow, leukocyte.**

monoblastic leukemia, a cancer of blood-forming organs. It is marked by the spread of immature white blood cells (monoblasts) and giant white blood cells (monocytes). Both children and adults get the disease. Also called **monocytic leukemia, Schilling's leukemia.**

Monocid, a trademark for a cephalosporin-type antibiotic (cefonicid sodium).

monoclonal /mon′əklō′nəl/, referring to a group of identical cells or organisms that are made from a single cell (cloned).

monoclonal gammopathy. See **gammopathy.**

monocyte /mon′əsīt/, the largest of the white blood cells. They have two to four times the diameter of a red blood cell.

monocytic leukemia /mon′əsit′ik/, a cancer of blood-forming tissues in which the major cells are giant white blood cells (monocytes). The disease is marked by discomfort, weakness, fever, loss of appetite, weight loss, a large spleen, bleeding gums, skin disorders, and anemia. There are two forms: **Schilling's leukemia,** and the more common **Naegeli's leukemia.** Also called **histiocytic leukemia.**

monocytosis /mon′ōsītō′sis/, a large amount of giant white blood cells (monocytes) in the circulation.

monofactorial inheritance, an inherited trait or condition that depends on a single specific gene. Compare **multifactorial inheritance.**

monomphalus /mənom'fələs/, twins that are joined at the navel. Also called omphalopagus.

mononeuritis multiplex. See multiple mononeuropathy.

mononeuropathy, any disease or disorder that affects a single nerve trunk. Some common causes of disorders involving single nerve trunks are electric shock, radiation, and broken bones that may press or cut nerve fibers. Casts and bandages that are too tight may also damage a nerve by pressure. Accidental injection of penicillin and other drugs into the sciatic nerve can seriously injure the nerve. The nerve trunks beyond the spinal cord are especially open to pressure and damage.

mononuclear cell, a white blood cell, including lymphocytes and monocytes, with a round or oval nucleus.

mononucleosis /mon'ōnōō'klē-ō'sis/, an abnormal increase in the number of mononuclear white blood cells in the circulation. See also infectious mononucleosis.

monopus /mon'əpəs/, a person who was born with a foot or leg missing.

monorchism /mon'ôrkiz'əm/, a condition in which only one testicle has come down into the male scrotum. Also called monorchidism. See also cryptorchidism. –monorchidic, adj.

monosaccharide, a carbohydrate made up of one basic sugar unit.

monosomy /mon'əsō'mē/, a birth defect characterized by the lack of one chromosome from the normal set of 23 pairs. In humans, the condition usually involves the lack of one of the sex chromosomes, as occurs in the XO condition in Turner's syndrome. Compare trisomy.

monotropy /mənot'rəpē/, a condition in which a mother appears to be able to bond with only one infant at a time. When one of a pair of twins is taken home from the hospital earlier than the other, the mother often reports that she does not feel that the baby brought home later is hers.

monovulatory /mənō'vyələtôr'ē/, a normal condition in which the ovaries release one ovum during each menstrual cycle. Compare diovulatory.

monozygotic (MZ), referring to offspring grown from one fertilized egg (zygote), as occurs in identical twins. Compare dizygotic.

monozygotic twins, two offspring born of the same pregnancy and grown from one fertilized egg that splits into equal halves. This results in separate fetuses. Such twins are always of the same sex. They have the same genes and have identical blood groups. They closely look like each other in all characteristics. Monozygotic twins may have single or separate placentas and membranes. This depends on the time when they divided. Monozygotic twinning is equally common to all races. It happens in about one-third of all twin births. Also called enzygotic twins, identical twins, true twins, uniovular twins. Compare dizygotic twins. See also Siamese twins.

monster, a fetus that is badly disfigured and usually will not live. Kinds of monsters include compound monster, double monster, single monster.

mons veneris, a pad of fatty tissue and rough skin that lies over the lower front bones of the female pelvis. After puberty, it is covered with pubic hair. Also called mons pubis.

Montgomery straps, bands of adhesive tape used to keep in place dressings that must be changed often. Also called Montgomery tapes.

Montgomery's tubercle, one of several oil glands on the areas (areolae) surrounding the nipples of the breasts. The glands normally get larger during pregnancy. The oily material released by the glands of each areola oils and protects the breast from infection and injury during breast feeding. Also called Montgomery's gland.

mood, a long-lasting emotional state that influences one's whole personality and life functioning. See also affect.

moon face, a condition in which a rounded, puffy face occurs in patients given large doses of steroid drugs, as those with rheumatoid arthritis or acute childhood leukemia. Features return to normal when the drug is stopped.

MOPP /mop/, an abbreviation for a drug combination used to treat cancer. It contains three antitumor drugs—Mustargen (mechlorethamine), Oncovin (vincristine sulfate), Matulane (procarbazine hydrochloride)—and prednisone, an adrenal gland hormone. MOPP is given to treat Hodgkin's disease.

morbidity, an illness or an abnormal condition or quality.

morbilli. See measles.

morbilliform /môrbil'ifôrm/, describing a skin condition that looks like the rash of measles.

Morgagni's globule /môrgan'yēz/, a substance that may form from fluid clotting between the eye lens and the saclike capsule in which it is held, especially in cataract.

morgue, a unit of a hospital for storing and doing autopsies on dead persons.

Morita therapy, an alternative therapy founded by Shomer Morita that focuses on the emotionally unstable (neurotic) symptoms of the patient. The goal of therapy is character building, which enables the patient to live responsibly and constructively, even if the symptoms continue.

morning-after pill, informal. A large dose of an estrogen given by mouth to a woman within 24 to 72 hours after sexual intercourse. The purpose is to stop conception, most commonly in an emergency, as rape or incest. The woman is warned that the drug, taken over a short period of time, may cause serious problems if contraception fails. These include clots, severe nausea and vomiting. Other problems are the risk of cancer-causing effects on the fetus or birth defects. See also **diethystilbestrol.**

morning dip, a significant decline in the functioning of the breathing system in some persons with asthma during early morning. A similar decrease can occur in normal persons after peaking in the afternoon. The asthmatic person tends to experience a morning dip and a high point in midafternoon.

morning sickness. See **nausea and vomiting of pregnancy.**

Moro reflex /môr′ō/, a normal reflex in a young infant caused by a sudden loud noise. It results in drawing up the legs, an embracing position of the arms, and usually a short cry. Also called **startle reflex.**

morphea /môr′fē·ə/, local hardening of the skin, with yellowish or ivory-colored, rigid, dry, smooth patches. It may lead to a hardness of tissue (sclerosis) elsewhere in the body. It is more common in women than men. Also called **Addison's keloid, circumscribed scleroderma, localized scleroderma.**

morphine sulfate, a narcotic given to reduce pain.
★CAUTION: Drug addiction or known allergy to this drug prohibits its use.
★ADVERSE EFFECTS: Among the more serious side effects are increased brain pressure, heart disturbances, breathing difficulties, and drug addiction.

morphology, the study of the physical shape and size of a specimen, plant, or animal.

Morquio's disease (MPS IV) /môrkē′ōz/, a disorder of carbohydrate use. It results in abnormal muscle and bone growth in childhood. Dwarfism, hunchback, and knock-knees may occur. The disease may first show as the child, learning to walk, uses an abnormal, waddling gait. See also **mucopolysaccharidosis.**

mortality, 1. the condition of being subject to death. 2. the death rate, noted as the number of deaths per unit of population for a specific region, age group, disease, or other grouping.

mortar, a cup-shaped dish in which materials are ground or crushed by a club-shaped device (pestle) in making drugs.

Morton's foot, Morton's neuroma. See **metatarsalgia.**

Morton's plantar neuralgia, a severe throbbing pain that affects a branch of the nerves of the sole (plantar) of the foot.

Morton's toe. See **metatarsalgia.**

morula /môr′ələ/, a solid, spheric mass of cells resulting from the cell divisions of the fertilized egg in the early stages of growth during pregnancy.

Morvan's disease, an opening of the spinal cord causing tissue changes in the arms and legs, as numbness and tingling of the forearms and hands, and continuous, painless skin lesions on the fingertips.

mosaicism /mōzā′isiz′əm/, a condition in which an individual, developed from a single fertilized egg (zygote), has two or more cell populations that are different. Most commonly seen in humans is a variation in the number of chromosomes in the body cells. Normally, all body cells would have the same number of chromosomes.

mosaic wart, a group of neighboring warts on the sole (plantar) of the foot.

mosquito bite, a bite of a bloodsucking insect of the subfamily Culicidae. It may result in a severe allergic reaction in an allergic person, an infection, or, most often, an itching sore. Mosquitoes are carriers of many infectious diseases. They are attracted by moisture, carbon dioxide, estrogens, sweat, or warmth.

-motine, a combining form for antiviral quinoline derivatives.

motion sickness, a condition caused by uneven or rhythmic motions in any combination of directions. Severe cases are characterized by nausea, vomiting, dizziness, and headache. Mild cases are characterized by headache and general discomfort. Antihistamines are used to stop the effect. Kinds of motion sickness are **air sickness, car sickness, seasickness.**

motor, 1. referring to motion, as the body involved in movement, or the brain functions that direct body movements. 2. referring to a muscle, nerve, or brain center that makes or takes part in motion.

motor aphasia, the inability to say remembered words because of a lesion in the brain. It involves brain tissue known as Broca's motor speech area in the left side of the brain in right-handed patients. The condition most commonly is caused by a stroke. The patient knows what to say but cannot make the mouth movements for the words. Also called **ataxic aphasia, expressive aphasia, frontocortical aphasia, verbal aphasia.**

motor apraxia, the inability to carry out certain planned movements or to handle small objects, although one knows the use of the object. It is caused by a lesion in a part of the brain on the opposite side of the arm that cannot move. Also called **cortical apraxia, innervation apraxia.** See also **apraxia.**

motor area, a portion of the brain (cerebral cortex) that includes the centers that cause the voluntary muscles to contract. Removing the motor area from one of the brain's sides (hemispheres) causes paralysis of voluntary muscles. This happens especially to the opposite side of the body. Various parts of the motor area are linked to different body structures, as the lower arm, face, and hand. The parts linked to more complicated movements are larger than those linked to general body movements.

motor coordination, the coordination of all body functions that involve movement.

motor dysfunction, any type of disorder that affects movement, it is found in children with learning disabilities. Also called **motor deficit, motor disorder.**

motor end plate, a broad band of fibers of the motor nerves that are attached to voluntary muscles. Motor nerves from the brain and spinal cord enter the coverings of voluntary muscle fibers and spread like the roots of a tree.

motor fiber, one of the fibers in the spinal nerves that carry movement signals to muscle fibers.

motor lag, an unusually long period between the time a stimulus for movement is received and the motor response.

motor neuron, one of various nerve cells that carry nerve signals from the brain or from the spinal cord to muscle or gland tissue. Also called **motoneuron.** Compare **sensory nerve.** See also **nervous system.**

motor neuron paralysis, an injury to the spinal cord that causes damage to motor neurons. It results in various degrees of loss of movement, depending on where the damage is.

motor planning, the ability to plan and execute skilled task that one does not usually perform. Also called **motor praxis.**

motor seizure, a temporary disturbance in brain function, it is caused by abnormal nerve signals that begin in a local motor nerve area of the brain. The effects depend on where the abnormal electric activity is, as chewing movements caused by excess signals in the motor area of the brain controlling the jaws. The disturbance may spread. It also may end in a group of reflex movements or lead to a general convulsion. Also called **focal motor seizure.** See also **epilepsy, focal seizure.**

motor unit, a working structure made up of a motor nerve cell and the muscle fibers to which it supplies nervous energy.

Motrin, a trademark for an anti-inflammatory drug (ibuprofen).

mountain fever, mountain tick fever. See **Colorado tick fever, Rocky Mountain spotted fever.**

mouse, a hand-controlled device that moves the cursor on a computer screen. Rolling the device on a flat surface causes the cursor to move in the same direction. See also **joystick, trackball.**

mouth, the open cavity at the upper end of the digestive tube. The opening, located in front of the teeth. It is surrounded externally by the lips and cheeks and internally by the gums and teeth. The mouth receives fluids from the salivary glands. The mouth cavity connects with the voicebox (pharynx) and is covered at the top by the hard and the soft palates. The tongue forms the large part of the floor of the cavity.

mouthstick, a device that can be manipulated with the mouth and used to type, push buttons,

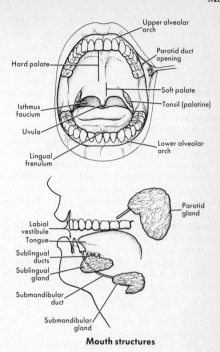

Mouth structures

turn pages, or operate power wheelchairs and other equipment for paralyzed patients.

mouth-to-mouth resuscitation, a procedure in artificial resuscitation done most often with chest compressions. The victim's nose is sealed by pinching the nostrils closed. The head is tilted back. Air is breathed by the rescuer through the victim's mouth and into the lungs. See also **cardiopulmonary resuscitation.**

mouth-to-nose resuscitation, a procedure in artificial resuscitation. The mouth of the victim is covered and held closed. Air is breathed through the victim's nose. See also **mouth-to-mouth resuscitation.**

movement decomposition, an abnormal change in voluntary movement in which the movement occurs in a sequence of separate, isolated steps, rather than a normal, smooth, flowing pattern.

moxibustion /mok'səbus'chən/, a method of relieving pain or changing the workings of a system of the body. Moxa, wormwood, or another slow-burning substance is lit and held as near to the point on the skin as possible without causing pain or burning. It is sometimes used with acupuncture.

MPD, abbreviation for *maximum permissible dose.*

MPL + PRED, an anticancer drug combination of melphalan and prednisone.

MS, abbreviation for **multiple sclerosis.**

MTX + MP + CTX, an anticancer drug combination of methotrexate, mercaptopurine, and cyclophosphamide.

mucin /myōo'sin/, a carbohydrate that is the main part of mucus. It is present in most glands that release mucus. Thus mucin is the oily material that protects body surfaces from rubbing or wearing down.

mucinoid, looking like mucin.

mucinous carcinoma, a tumor that is sticky because of the large amount of mucin released by its cells. Also called **colloid carcinoma, gelatiniform carcinoma, gelatinous carcinoma.**

mucocutaneous /myōo'kōkyōotā'nē·əs/, referring to the mucous membrane and the skin.

mucocutaneous leishmaniasis. See **American leishmaniasis.**

mucocutaneous lymph node syndrome (MLNS), a sudden illness with fever mainly of young children. Symptoms include inflamed membranes of the mouth, "strawberry tongue," and swollen lymph nodes in the neck. A rash on the body, redness and shedding of the skin on the arms and legs are other symptoms of this illness. Joint pain, diarrhea, ear disorders, pneumonia, and heart rhythm changes are additional symptoms. The cause is unknown. No clear-cut environmental, seasonal, or geographical factors have been discovered. Person-to-person contact has not been found to be a cause. Some people may inherit a condition that makes them unable to resist the disease. Treatment includes aspirin in large doses. It may be given over a long period of time. Also called **Kawasaki disease.**

mucoepidermoid carcinoma, a cancer of gland tissues, especially the ducts of the salivary glands.

mucoid /myōo'koid/, looking like mucus.

mucogingival junction, the tissue that separates the gums from the membranes lining the mouth.

mucolytic /myōo'kəlit'ik/, anything that dissolves or destroys the mucus.

mucomembranous /myōo'kəmem'brənəs/, referring to a mucous membrane, as the lining of the small intestine or the bladder.

mucopolysaccharidosis (MPS) /myōo'kōpol'ēsak'-əridō'sis/, pl. **mucopolysaccharidoses,** one of a group of inherited disorders of carbohydrate use. They are marked by greater-than-normal gatherings of substances making up sugars and mucins in the tissues. Symptoms include skeletal deformity, especially of the face, mental retardation and slowed growth. There is a lowered life expectancy. The disorders may be found before birth by testing fetal cells present in amniotic fluid. After birth, a diagnosis is made through urine testing, x-ray films, and a family history. There is no successful treatment. Kinds of mucopolysaccharidosis include **Hunter's syndrome (MPS II), Hurler's syndrome (MPS I), Morquio's disease (MPS IV).**

mucoprotein /myōo'kōprō'tēn, -tē·in/, a chemical compound present in all connective and supporting tissue that contains carbohydrates combined with protein.

mucopurulent /myōo'kōpyōor'yələnt/, referring to a combination of mucus and pus.

mucosa /myōokō'sə/, pl. **mucosae,** mucous membrane. –**mucosal,** adj.

mucositis, any inflammation of a mucous membrane, as the lining of the mouth and throat.

mucous /myōo'kəs/, referring to mucus or the release of mucus.

mucous colitis. See **irritable bowel syndrome.**

mucous membrane, any one of four major kinds of thin sheets of tissue cells that cover or line various parts of the body. Mucous membranes line openings or canals of the body that open to the outside. Examples include linings of the mouth, digestive tube, breathing passages, and the genital and urinary tracts. It releases mucus, and absorbs water, salts, and other substances. Compare **serous membrane, skin, synovial membrane.**

mucous plug, a collection of thick mucus in the cervix of the uterus. It is often released just before labor begins. The plug may be dry and firm. More often it is partly fluid and streaked with blood.

mucous shreds. See **shreds.**

mucus /myōo'kəs/, the sticky, slippery material released by mucous membranes and glands. It has mucin, white blood cells, water, and cast-off tissue cells. –**mucoid,** adj., **mucous,** adj.

mud bath, placing warm mud on the body to help the body become healthy.

Mudrane, a trademark for a lung drug. It contains a smooth muscle-relaxing drug (theophylline), a stimulating drug (ephedrine hydrochloride), a drug to free up sputum (potassium iodide), and a drug to help the patient sleep (phenobarbital).

mulibrey nanism, an inherited disorder, with dwarfism, heart disorders, poor muscle tone, and defects of the skull and face. Yellow dots inside the eyeball are typical. The name of the condition comes from the first two letters of the body sites of the main defects: muscle, liver, brain, and eyes.

müllerian duct, one of a pair of tubes in the human embryo that become the fallopian tubes, uterus, and vagina in females.

Müller's maneuver, an effort to inhale against a closed airway or opening between the vocal cords (glottic). The effort decreases pressure in the lungs and chest and expands gas in the lungs.

multidisciplinary health-care team, a group of health-care workers who are members of different disciplines, each one providing specific services to the patient.

multifactorial, referring to any condition or disease caused by two or more factors. Examples are diseases that involve inherited and environmental factors. Many disorders, as spina bifida, neural tube defects, and Hirschsprung's disease, are considered to be multifactorial.

multifactorial inheritance, the likelihood to develop a physical appearance, disease, or condition that represents many inherited and environmental factors, as body build and blood pressure. See also **polygene.**

multiform, an organ, tissue, or other object that may appear in more than one shape.

multigenerational model, a model of family therapy that focuses on equivalent role relationships over a period of time. The family is viewed as an emotional system where patterns of interacting and coping, as well as unsolved problems, can be passed from one generation to the next and can cause stress. The goal is to help the family members become more distinct as individuals.

multigenerational transmission process, the repetition of relationship patterns, including divorce, suicide, or alcoholism, associated with emotional problems that can be traced through several generations of the same family.

multigravida /mul'tigrav'idə/, a woman who has been pregnant more than once. Compare **multipara, primagravida.**

multiinfarct dementia, a form of brain disease with the rapid failure of mental functioning. It is caused by a blood vessel disease. Symptoms include emotional upsets and defects in memory, abstract thinking, and judgment. There also may be nervous system defects, as walking abnormalities, mild paralysis, and numbness in the arms and legs. The condition is more likely to affect men than women. It may be caused by a stroke. See also **dementia, senile psychosis.**

multipara /multip'ərə/, *pl.* **multiparae,** a woman who has given birth to more than one living child. Compare **multigravida, nullipara, primipara.**

multipenniform, a body structure having a featherlike shape. It occurs mainly in sheets of muscles that become narrow to join tendons. Compare **bipenniform, penniform.**

multiple family therapy, a method of treating emotional problems (psychotherapy) in which four or five families meet weekly to discuss problems or issues that they have in common.

multiple fracture, **1.** a fracture causing several fracture lines in one bone. **2.** the fracture of several bones at one time or from the same injury.

multiple idiopathic hemorrhagic sarcoma. See **Kaposi's sarcoma.**

multiple impact therapy, a method of treating emotional problems (psychotherapy) in which families come together for intensive work meetings over a 3-day weekend or weeklong encounter.

multiple lipomatosis, an inherited disorder with deposits of fat in the tissues of the body. This fat is not available for use by the body, even in starvation.

multiple mononeuropathy, an abnormal condition with failure of several nerve trunks. It may be caused by various diseases, as uremia, diabetes mellitus, and some inflammatory disorders.

multiple myeloma, a cancer of the bone marrow. The tumor is made up of blood cells. It destroys bone tissue, especially in flat bones, and causes pain, fractures, and bone deformities. A common effect is an abnormal curving of the spine. There also may be anemia, weight loss, breathing problems linked to rib fractures, and kidney failure. Also called **multiple plasmacytoma of bone, myelomatosis, plasma cell myeloma.**

multiple neuroma. See **neuromatosis.**

multiple peripheral neuritis, swelling or breakdown of nerves of the arms and legs. Symptoms include numbness, tingling in the arms and legs, hot and cold sensations, and slight fever. There also may be pain, weakness, loss of reflexes, and in some cases, paralysis. The disorder may be caused by poisoning. Poisons may include antimony, arsenic, carbon monoxide, copper, lead, mercury, and various drugs, as drugs for epilepsy, tuberculosis, and cancer. Multiple peripheral neuritis may occur in alcoholism, hardening of the arteries, beriberi, long-term stomach and intestine diseases, diabetes, leprosy, and rheumatoid arthritis. Therapy consists of removal of the poison or treatment of the disease, rest, and drugs for pain. Also called **peripheral polyneuritis, peripheral polyneuropathy.** See also **Guillain-Barré syndrome.**

multiple personality, an abnormal condition in which two or more well-developed personalities exist within the same individual. Awareness of the others among the various personalities may not occur. Each may take over at a particular time. Change from one to another is usually sudden and linked to stress. The condition is most often seen in young females. It may be treated with hypnosis, mind-altering drugs, or psychotherapy. Also called **split personality.**

multiple plasmacytoma of bone. See **multiple myeloma.**

multiple pregnancy, a pregnancy in which there is more than one fetus in the uterus.

multiple sclerosis (MS), a disease characterized by loss of the protective myelin covering of the nerve fibers of the brain and spinal cord. It begins slowly, usually in young adulthood, and continues throughout life. There are cycles in which symptoms worsen or become milder. The first signs are numbness, or abnormal sensations in the arms and legs or on one side of the face. Other early signs are muscle weakness, dizziness, and sight disturbances, as double vision and partial blindness. Later in the course of disease there may be extremes in emotions, loss of muscle control, abnormal reflexes, and difficulty in urinating. Because many other conditions cause similar symptoms, the diagnosis of MS is slow and difficult. As the disease continues, the periods of relief from symptoms grow shorter and disability becomes greater. There is no specific treatment for the disease. Drugs are used to treat the symptoms that occur with sudden episodes of symptoms. Physical therapy may help to delay or stop specific disabilities. The patient is told to live as normal and active a life as possible. Also called **disseminated multiple sclerosis.**

multisynaptic, referring to a system of nerve cells needing a series of connections (synapses) between nerve cells.

mummified fetus, a fetus that has died in the uterus and has dried up.

mumps, a viral disease characterized by a swelling of the salivary glands near the neck. It is most likely to affect children between 5 and 15 years of age. However, it may occur at any age. In adulthood the infection may be severe. Antibodies from the mother usually prevent this disease in children under 1 year of age. Mumps is most contagious during the late winter and early spring. The mumps virus lives in the saliva of the affected patient and is carried in droplets or by direct contact. The symptoms of mumps usually last for about 24 hours. They include loss of appetite, headache, discomfort, and light fever. These signs are followed by earache, saliva gland swelling, and a temperature of 101° to 104° F (38.3° to 40° C). The patient feels pain when drinking sour liquids or when chewing. The saliva glands may become swollen. The treatment of mumps includes keeping the patient isolated. Drugs are given to reduce pain and fever. The patient must drink enough fluids to avoid dehydration caused by fever and loss of appetite. Drinking fluids may be difficult for the patient who cannot swallow because of swollen saliva glands. Patients with mumps are also told to avoid spicy foods and must avoid foods that require much chewing. All cases of mumps are reported to health authorities. Vaccination within 24 hours of being exposed to the disease may halt the spread of the disease to others or may reduce its effects. The chance for recovery from mumps is good. However, the disease sometimes involves complications, as arthritis, and inflammation of the pancreas, heart muscle, ovary, and kidney. About one-half of the men with swelling of the testicles suffer some damage to the testicles. Sterility rarely results. Also called **epidemic parotitis, infectious parotitis.**

mumps live virus vaccine, an active drug given for vaccination against mumps.

★CAUTION: Halted immunity, use of steroid drugs, sudden infection, pregnancy, known allergy to chicken proteins, neomycin, or to this drug prohibits its use.

★ADVERSE EFFECTS: Among the most serious side effects are fever, inflamed saliva glands, and allergic reactions.

Mumpsvax, a trademark for a mumps live virus vaccine.

Munchausen's syndrome /mun'chousənz/, a condition in which a patient falsely claims to be sick or injured so as to receive medical treatment and hospitalization. The patient may imagine the symptoms and history of a real disease. The unreal symptoms will get better with treatment. However, the patient may then seek treatment later for another imaginary disease. Also called **pathomimicry.**

mural, something that is found on or against the wall of a cavity, as a mural blood clot (thrombus) on an inside wall of the heart.

Murchison fever. See **Pel-Ebstein fever.**

murine typhus, a sudden virus infection, it is caused by *Rickettsia typhi* and carried by the bite of an infected flea. The disease is characterized by headache, chills, fever, muscle pain, and rash. The fever lasts about 12 days. A dull-red rash, mainly on the body, appears about the fifth day. This lasts for 4 to 8 days. Recovery is usually rapid but death can occur in elderly or feeble patients. Antibiotics are given. Prevention involves getting rid of the rats that carry the fleas. Also called **endemic typhus, flea-borne typhus, new world typhus, rat typhus, urban typhus.** See also **Brill-Zinsser disease, epidemic typhus.**

murmur, a low-pitched fluttering or humming sound in the body, as a heart murmur.

Murocoll, a trademark for an eye medicine.

Murphy's sign, a test for gallbladder disease in which the patient is asked to inhale while the examiner's fingers are held at the border of the liver at the bottom of the rib cage. Inhaling causes the gallbladder to descend onto the fingers, producing pain if the gallbladder is inflammed. The test is used in the diagnosis of gallbladder cancer, as well as inflammation of the gallbladder (cholecystitis).

muscae volitantes. See **floater.**

muscle, a kind of tissue made up of fibers that are able to contract, causing and allowing movement of the parts and organs of the body. There are two basic kinds: striated muscle and smooth muscle. All skeletal muscles are striated, long, and voluntary. They respond quickly to stimulation but are paralyzed by any stopping of nerve supply. Smooth muscle, found in internal organs, is short and involuntary. It reacts slowly to stimulation but does not entirely lose its ability to contract if the nerves are damaged. The heart muscle (myocardium) is sometimes called a third (cardiac) kind of muscle. However, it is basically a striated muscle that does not contract as quickly as the skeletal muscles. Also, it is not completely paralyzed if it loses its nervous system stimulation. See also **cardiac muscle, smooth muscle, striated muscle.**

muscle bridge, a band of heart wall (myocardial) tissue over one or more of the large arteries supplying the heart. It may cause narrowing of the artery during the tightening (systole) of the heart.

muscle relaxant, a drug that reduces the ability of muscle fibers to contract. Such drugs are used to gain a lighter level of anesthesia during surgery and to control breathing of patients on ventilators other uses are to reduce muscle contractions in shock therapy and muscle spasms in convulsions. The drugs are also used in the treatment of leg cramps at night. Muscle-relaxant drugs act in several ways. Some lengthen the relaxation of muscle fibers. Others stop nerve impulses from causing muscle contractions.

muscle-setting exercise, a method of keeping muscle strength and tone. It is done by contracting and relaxing a skeletal muscle, or any group of muscles, without moving that part of the body. Such exercises can prevent breakdown of the muscles, if there are abnormal conditions involving the joints.

muscle tone, a normal state of balanced muscle tension.

muscular, referring to a muscle.

muscular dystrophy, a group of inherited diseases. They are characterized by weakness and wasting of skeletal muscles without the breakdown of nerve tissue. In all forms of muscular dystrophy there is a slow loss of strength with increasing disability and deformity. Each type of the disease differs in the muscles affected, the age at which it begins, and the rate of its progress. The basic cause is unknown. However, it appears to be an inherited disorder of body functioning. Diagnosis is based on examining a piece of muscle, muscle tests, and a family history. Treatment consists mainly of physical therapy and surgery to reduce deformity. See also **Becker's muscular dystrophy, distal muscular dystrophy, Duchenne's muscular dystrophy, limb-girdle muscular dystrophy, myotonic muscular dystrophy.**

muscular system, all of the muscles of the body, including the smooth, cardiac, and striated muscles, considered as one structural group. See also **Color Atlas of Human Anatomy.**

muscular tumor. See **myoma.**

musculature, the arrangement and condition of the muscles.

musculoskeletal /mus′kyo͞olo̅skel′ətəl/, referring to the muscles and the skeleton.

musculoskeletal system, all of the muscles, bones, joints, and related structures, as the tendons and connective tissue, that function in the movement of the parts and organs of the body. See also **Color Atlas of Human Anatomy,** skeleton.

musculoskeletal system assessment, an evaluation of the condition and functioning of the muscles, joints, and bones and of the body. The patient's general appearance, posture of the body, age, blood pressure, pulse, breathing, handgrip, skin conditions as bruises or rashes, and allergies are checked. Recent weight loss or gain are also checked. The physician asks about any pain or swelling in muscles, joints, and bones. The physician also asks about weakness in arms and legs; limitations in movements; unsteadiness on the feet; or need for assistance. Also noted are any previous problems, as spinal surgery, poliomyelitis, partial paralysis, cerebral palsy, parkinsonism, stroke, syphilis, bone diseases, tuberculosis, alcoholism, and defects of sight or hearing. The presence of muscle contractures, deformities, paralysis, footdrop, or wristdrop, the range of motion of arms and legs, and the use of crutches, cane, or walker is noted. Diseases or conditions checked include injury to the spinal cord, nerve damage, arthritis, bursitis, multiple sclerosis, muscular dystrophy, myasthenia gravis, fracture, and broken disk. Laboratory studies are important. Diagnosis may require x-ray films of bones, examining pieces of bone or muscle, draining joints, and electromyogram tests of muscles.

mushroom poisoning, a condition caused by eating certain mushrooms, particularly two species of the genus *Amanita.* Muscarine, a substance in *Amanita muscaria,* causes poisoning in a few minutes to 2 hours. Symptoms include tears, excess saliva, sweating, vomiting, difficult breathing, stomach cramps, diarrhea. In severe cases, convulsions, coma, and failure of the circulation may occur. Atropine is usually given in treatment. More deadly but slower-acting phalloidine, a substance in *A. phalloides* and *A. verna,* causes similar symptoms. It also causes liver damage, kidney failure, and death in 30% to 50% of the cases. Treatment includes emptying the stomach. This is followed by a saltwater enema. Intensive care and removing the poison from the blood by cleansing the blood (hemodialysis) may prevent death. In some patients, drinking alcohol complicates mushroom poisoning.

mushroom worker's lung, a type of allergy common among workers in the mushroom-growing industry. Symptoms of the sudden form of the disease include chills, cough, fever, breathing difficulty, loss of appetite, nausea, and vomiting. The long-term form of the disease is characterized by weakness, constant cough, weight loss, and breathlessness during exercise.

Mustargen Hydrochloride, a trademark for an anticancer drug (mechlorethamine hydrochloride).

-mustine, a combining form for drugs that control or kill cancer cells, particularly amine derivatives.

mutacism /myo͞o′təsiz′əm/, the incorrect use of /m/ sounds.

mutagen /myo͞o′təjən/, any chemical or physical agent that causes a gene change (mutation) or speeds up the rate of mutation. **–mutagenic,** *adj.,* **mutagenicity,** *n.*

mutagenesis /myo͞o′təjen′əsis/, the cause of a genetic change (mutation). See also **teratogenesis.**

Mutamycin, a trademark for an anticancer drug (mitomycin).

mutant, any individual or organism with genetic material that has had a change (mutation).

mutant gene, any gene on a chromosome that has had a change, as the loss, gain, or exchange of genetic material, which affects the normal inheritance of a trait.

mutation, an unusual change in a person's genes that occurs by itself with or without the influence of a mutagen, as x-rays. The alteration changes the physical trait carried by the gene. Genes are stable units, but a mutation often is passed on to future generations. **–mutate,** *v.,* **mutational,** *adj.*

mutism /myo͞o′tizəm/, the inability or refusal to speak. The condition often results from an emotional conflict. It is most commonly seen in patients who are psychotic, neurotic, apathetic, or depressed. A kind of mutism is **akinetic mutism.**

muton /myo͞o′ton/, the smallest part of a DNA molecule that can cause a change (mutation). See also **deoxyribonucleic acid (DNA).**

mutual support group, a type of group in which members organize to solve their own problems. They are led by the group members themselves who share a common goal and use their own strengths to gain control over their lives.

MX gene, a human gene that helps the body resist viral infections. Presence of the gene helps explain why some individuals are better able to resist certain viral infections, as the flu, than others.

myalgia /mī·al′jə/, a muscle pain. It may be linked to many infectious diseases, as influenza, measles, malaria, rheumatic fever, and poliomyelitis. Muscle pain occurs in many other disorders, as swelling of connective and muscle tissue, excess release of parathyroid hormones, low blood sugar, and muscle tumors. Many drugs also may cause myalgia. See also **epidemic myalgia. –myalgic,** *adj.*

myalgic asthenia, a general feeling of weakness and muscular pain. It is often caused by psychological stress.

Myambutol, a trademark for an antibiotic (ethambutol hydrochloride).

myasthenia /mī′əsthē′nē·ə/, abnormal weakness of a muscle or a group of muscles. It may be the result of a neuromuscular problem, as in myasthenia gravis. **–myasthenic,** *adj.*

myasthenia gravis, an abnormal condition of long-term tiredness and muscle weakness. It occurs especially in the face and throat and results from a defect in the movement of nerve signals between nerve fibers to muscles. Symptoms begin gradually. They start with drooping upper eyelids, double vision, and weakness of facial muscles. The weakness may then extend to other muscles, as the breathing muscles. Muscular use worsens the symptoms. The disease occurs most often in young women and in men over 60 years of age. Restricted physical activity and bed rest are ordered. Anticholinesterase drugs that stimulate nerve signals are usually given before meals. Myasthenic crisis may need emergency respiratory care. The patient's diet is changed if the ability to chew and swallow food is affected.

myasthenia gravis crisis, sudden increase in intensity of myasthenia gravis. Causes include infection, surgery, emotional stress, or a wrong size dose of a drug. Common symptoms include breathing difficulty, extreme tiredness, increased muscular weakness, swallowing and speaking difficulties, and fever. The patient may be anxious, restless, irritable, unable to move the jaws or to raise one or both eyelids. If the condition is caused by drugs, there may be loss of appetite, nausea, vomiting, and diarrhea. Excess saliva sweating, tears, blurred sight, dizziness, and muscle cramps and spasms may also occur. Emergency treatment includes getting oxygen into the lungs. Oxygen may have to be given with special equipment. An opening into the throat (tracheostomy) may be made. The patient's bed should be tilted so the head is 30 degrees higher than the foot. If an eyelid is affected, the eye may be covered with a patch. Soothing eyedrops may be given. Walking and other physical exercises are ordered. Range of motion exercises of arms and legs are done several times a day. Rest periods are kept to avoid tiredness and another episode.

mycelium /mīsē′lē·əm/, *pl.* **mycelia,** a mass of threadlike strands (filaments) found on most fungi. Also called **hypha.**

mycetismus /mī′sitiz′məs/, mushroom poisoning.

mycetoma /mī′sətō′mə/, a serious fungus infection involving skin, connective tissue, and bone. One kind of mycetoma is **Madura foot.**

-mycin, a combining form for antibiotics produced by Streptomyces strains.

Mycitracin, a trademark for a combination of drugs containing three antibiotics (polymyxin B sulfate, bacitracin, and neomycin sulfate).

myco-, myc-, myceto-, myko-, a combining form meaning 'related to fungus.'

mycobacteriosis /mī′kōbak′tirē·ō′sis/, a tuberculosislike disease caused by mycobacteria other than *Mycobacterium tuberculosis.*

Mycobacterium /mī'kōbaktir'ē·əm/, a kind of rod-shaped bacterium with two important species. *Mycobacterium leprae* causes leprosy. *M. tuberculosis* causes tuberculosis.

Mycolog, a trademark for a skin cream. It contains a hormone (triamcinolone acetonide), two antibiotics (neomycin sulfate and gramicidin), and an antifungus drug (nystatin).

mycology /mīkol'əjē/, the study of fungi and fungus diseases

mycomyringitis. See **myringomycosis.**

mycophenolic acid /mī'kōfinō'lik/, an antibiotic that also stops the growth of fungi.

Mycoplasma /mī'kōplaz'mə/, microscopic organisms without rigid cell walls. They are considered to be the smallest of all free-living organisms. One species is a cause of mycoplasma pneumonia, pharyngitis, and other infections.

mycoplasma pneumonia, a contagious disease of children and young adults. It is caused by *Mycoplasma pneumoniae.* The disease has a 9- to 12-day period with no symptoms. It is followed by a dry cough and fever. Symptoms include harsh or reduced breath sounds and fine bubbling or crackling noises on breathing in. There may be complications of swollen sinuses (sinusitis), chest pain (pleurisy), nerve inflammation, or heart muscle disorders. In untreated adults, long-term cough, weakness, and discomfort are common. Antibiotics, bed rest, a high-protein diet, and enough fluids help recovery. Infants and people in poor health must avoid contact with patients having mycoplasma pneumonia. Also called **Eaton-agent pneumonia, primary atypical pneumonia, walking pneumonia.**

mycosis /mīkō'sis/, any disease caused by a fungus. Some kinds of mycoses are **athlete's foot, candidiasis, diaper rash. –mycotic,** *adj.*

mycosis fungoides /fung·goi'dēz/, a skin cancer looking like eczema. Symptoms include a skin tumor, followed by small skin sores and tumors looking like those of Hodgkin's disease in lymph nodes and stomach and intestinal organs.

Mycostatin, a trademark for an antifungus drug (nystatin).

mycotic, referring to a disease caused by a fungus.

mycotic aneurysm, a widening in a blood vessel caused by the growth of a fungus. It usually occurs as a result of a heart disease (bacterial endocarditis). See also **bacterial aneurysm.**

mycotoxicosis /mī'kōtok'sīkō'sis/, poisoning that affects the whole body, it is caused by poisons produced by fungal organisms.

mydriasis /midrī'əsis/, widening of the pupil of the eye. It is caused by contraction of the widening (dilator) muscle of the iris, a covering of muscle fibers that moves out like the spokes of a wheel around the pupil. With a decrease in light or the action of certain drugs, the dilator pulls the iris outward. This makes the pupil larger.

mydriatic and cycloplegic agent, any one of several eye drugs that widen the pupil and paralyze the eye muscles. Such drugs are used in examination of the eye, and before and after many eye surgeries. They are also used in some tests for glaucoma. Blurred vision, thirst, flushing, fever, and rash may result from the drugs. In children and elderly patients, more serious side effects may occur.

myelacephalus, a fetal monster. It is usually a separate, genetically identical twin, whose form and parts are barely recognizable.

myelatelia /mī'ələtē'lē·ə/, any growth defect involving the spinal cord.

myelin /mī'əlin/, a fatty substance found in the coverings of various nerve fibers. The fat gives the normally gray fibers a white, creamy color. **–myelinic,** *adj.*

myelinated /mī'əlinā'tid/, referring to a nerve having a myelin sheath.

myelinic neuroma, a nerve tumor made up of myelinated nerve fibers.

myelinization /mī'əlin'īzā'shən/, growth of the myelin sheath around a nerve fiber.

myelinolysis /mī'əlinol'isis/, a disease that dissolves the myelin sheaths around certain nerve fibers. It occurs in some alcoholic and undernourished patients.

myelin sheath, a fatty layer of myelin that wraps the signal-moving fibers (axons) of many nerve cells in the body. The fat content gives these coverings a whitish look. Various diseases, as multiple sclerosis, can destroy the myelin wrappings.

myelitis /mī'əli'tis/, a swelling of the spinal cord with linked motor or sensory nerve dysfunction. Some kinds of myelitis are **acute transverse myelitis, leukomyelitis, poliomyelitis.**

myeloblast, a bone marrow cell from which a kind of white blood cell (granulocytic leukocyte) begins. In certain leukemias, a marked increase in myeloblasts is seen in the marrow and found in the circulating blood. **–myeloblastic,** *adj.*

myeloblastic leukemia, a cancer of blood-forming tissues. It is marked by many immature white blood cells (myeloblasts) in the circulating blood and tissues.

myelocele /mī'əlōsēl'/, a saclike bulge of the spinal cord through a break in the spinal column, which is seen at birth. See also **myelomeningocele, neural tube defect.**

myeloclast /mī'əlōclast'/, a cell that breaks down the myelin sheaths of nerves of the central nervous system.

myelocystocele /mī'əlōsis'təsēl'/, a lumpy (cystic) tumor of spinal cord substance that extends out through a break in the spinal column. See also **myelomeningocele, neural tube defect, spina bifida.**

myelocystomeningocele /mī′əlōsis′tōməning′gōsēl/, a lumpy (cystic) tumor. It contains both spinal cord substance and membrane (meninges) that extends out through a break in the spinal column. See also **myelomeningocele, neural tube defect, spina bifida.**

myelocyte /mī′əlōsīt/, an immature white blood cell, it is normally found in the bone marrow. These cells appear in the circulating blood only in certain forms of leukemia. **–myelocytic,** *adj.*

myelocythemia /mī′əlōsīthē′mē·ə/, an excess level of immature white blood cells (myelocytes) in the circulating blood, as in acute myelocytic leukemia.

myelocytic leukemia. See **acute myelocytic leukemia, chronic myelocytic leukemia.**

myelodiastasis /mī′əlōdī·as′təsis/, breakdown and decay of the spinal cord.

myelodysplasia, imperfect growth of any part of the spinal cord, especially of the lower part.

myelofibrosis. See **myeloid metaplasia.**

myelogenous leukemia. See **acute myelocytic leukemia, chronic myelocytic leukemia.**

myelogram /mī′əlōgram′/, **1.** an x-ray film of the spinal cord taken after the injection of a dye. It shows any distortions of the spinal cord, spinal nerve roots, and the surrounding space. **2.** a count of the different kinds of cells in a sample of bone marrow.

myeloid /mī′əloid/, **1.** referring to the bone marrow. **2.** referring to the spinal cord.

myeloid leukemia. See **acute myelocytic leukemia, chronic myelocytic leukemia.**

myeloid metaplasia, a disorder in which bone marrow tissue develops in abnormal sites. Anemia, a large spleen, immature blood cells in the circulation, and blood cell formation in the liver and spleen are signs of the disorder. Myeloid metaplasia may be linked to cancer, leukemia, excess red blood cells, or tuberculosis.

myeloidosis /mī′əloidō′sis/, a general overgrowth of red bone marrow. See also **Hodgkin's disease, multiple myeloma.**

myeloma /mī′əlō′mə/, a bone-destroying tumor. It may develop at the same time in many sites. Thus it causes large areas of patchy destruction of the bone. The tumor occurs most often in the ribs, vertebrae, pelvic bones, and flat bones of the skull. Intense pain and sudden fractures are common. Kinds of myeloma are **endothelial myeloma, extramedullary myeloma, giant cell myeloma, multiple myeloma, osteogenic myeloma.**

-myeloma, a combining form meaning a 'tumor made up of cells normally found in bone marrow.'

myelomalacia /mī′əlōmələ′shē·ə/, abnormal soft-

ening of the spinal cord. It is caused mainly by a poor blood supply.

myelomatosis. See **multiple myeloma.**

myelomeningocele /mī′əlōməning′gōsēl′/, a central nervous system hernia. A sac containing the spinal cord, its membrane covering (meninges), and cerebrospinal fluid extends out through a break in the vertebral column. The condition is caused mainly by the failure of the nerve (neural) tube to close during growth during pregnancy. It may also result from the reopening of the tube from an abnormal increase in cerebrospinal fluid pressure. The defect occurs in approximately 2 in every 1,000 live births and is obvious at birth. The hernia may be located at any point along the spinal column, but it usually occurs in the lower back. The saclike structure may be covered with a thin layer of skin. It may also be covered with a fine membrane that can be easily broken. This makes the risk of infection greater. Usually the condition is linked to varying degrees of paralysis of the legs and to defects as clubfoot and joint deformities. Loss of anal and bladder control are also common. Hydrocephalus is the most common defect linked to myelomeningocele. It occurs in almost 90% of the cases where the defect is located in the lower back. Hydrocephalus is usually obvious at birth. It may appear shortly afterward. Immediate surgery is necessary if the break is leaking fluid from the brain and spine. When surgery of the spinal break is done, other linked problems are addressed. These include shunt correction of hydrocephalus and antibiotic therapy to reduce the chance of meningitis. Urinary tract infections and pneumonia are also treated. Surgery is done for correction of hip, knee, and foot deformities. Prevention and treatment of urinary tract complications are also important. Improved surgical techniques and other treatments have increased the survival rate. However, they cannot change the physical disability and deformity, mental retardation, and long-

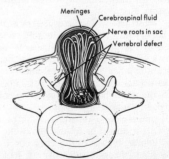

Meninges
Cerebrospinal fluid
Nerve roots in sac
Vertebral defect

Myelomeningocele (cross-sectional view)

term urinary tract and lung infections that the children may have. With proper and long-term 'meningomyelocele. Compare **menigocele.** See also **neural tube defect, spina bifida cystica.**

myelomere /mī′əlōmir′/, any of the embryonic parts of the brain or spinal cord during fetal growth during pregnancy.

myelopathic anemia. See **myelophthisic anemia.**

myelopathy /mī′əlop′əthē/, any disease of the spinal cord.

myelophthisic anemia /mī′əlofthiz′ik/, a defect of the red blood cell forming tissues of the bone marrow. It causes anemia. Also called **myelopathic anemia.**

myelopoiesis /mī′əlōpō·ē′sis/, the formation and growth of the bone marrow.

myeloradiculodysplasia /mī′əlōrədik′yəlōdisplā′-zhə/, any growth defect of the spinal cord and spinal nerve roots.

myelosuppression, the halting of blood cell and platelet production in bone marrow.

myesthesia /mī′esthē′zhə/, sense of any sensation in a muscle, as touch, direction of movement, contraction, relaxation, or stretching.

myiasis /mī′yəsis/, infection or infestation of the body by the larvae of flies. They usually enter through a wound or an ulcer. They rarely come through the intact skin.

myitis. See **myositis.**

Myleran, a trademark for an anticancer drug (busulfan).

Mylicon, a trademark for an intestinal gas drug (simethicone).

mylohyoideus /mī′lōhī·oi′dē·əs/, one of a pair of flat triangular muscles that form the floor of the mouth. It acts to raise the tongue. Also called **mylohyoid muscle.**

myocardial infarction (MI), a blockage of a heart artery. It is caused by a kind of hardening of the arteries (atherosclerosis) or a blood clot. This results in a dead tissue area in the heart muscle. Myocardial infarction often begins with a crushing, viselike chest pain that may move to the left arm, neck, or upper abdomen. It sometimes seems like indigestion or a gallbladder attack. The patient becomes ashen, clammy, short of breath, faint, anxious. The patient may feel that death is near. Typical signs are rapid heartbeat, a barely felt pulse, low blood pressure, above normal temperature, and heartbeat irregularities. Emergency treatment of MI may require cardiopulmonary resuscitation (CPR) before the patient is taken to an intensive cardiac care unit of a hospital. In sudden MI, oxygen, heart drugs, and anticoagulants are usually given. Sleeping pills and painkillers are also given. Iced drinks and cold foods are avoided. The patient is usually given a low-sodium, low-cholesterol diet. Stool softeners and laxatives may be used to prevent straining.

myocardiopathy /mī′ōkär′dē·op′əthē/, any dis-

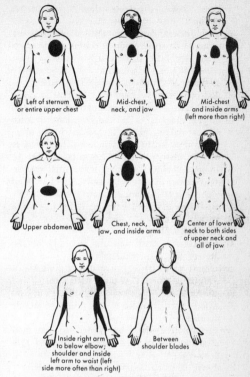

Left of sternum or entire upper chest

Mid-chest, neck, and jaw

Mid-chest and inside arms (left more than right)

Upper abdomen

Chest, neck, jaw, and inside arms

Center of lower neck to both sides of upper neck and all of jaw

Inside right arm to below elbow; shoulder and inside left arm to waist (left side more often than right)

Between shoulder blades

Locations of pain from heart attack

ease of the heart muscle. Also called **cardio-myopathy.**

myocarditis /mī′ōkärdī′tis/, an inflammation of the heart muscle. It may be caused by a viral, bacterial, or fungal infection. It may also be caused by rheumatic fever, a chemical agent, or result from a connective tissue disease. Myocarditis most often occurs as a sudden viral disease. It may lead to heart failure. Treatment includes painkillers, oxygen, anti-inflammatory drugs, and rest to prevent shock or heart failure.

myocardium /mī′ōkär′dē·əm/, a thick layer of muscle cells that forms most of the heart wall. The myocardium contains few other tissues, except for blood vessels. It is covered inside by a smooth membrane (endocardium). The tissue of the myocardium that causes it to contract is made up of fibers like skeletal muscle tissue. The fibers are about one-third as large in diameter as those of skeletal muscle. They branch often and are joined to form a network that is more or less continuous. Myocardial muscle contains less connective tissue than skeletal muscle. Specially changed fibers of myocardial muscle make up the contraction signal system of the heart. This includes the sinoatrial node, the atrioventricular node, the atrioventricular bundle, and the Purkinje fibers. Most of the myocardial fibers contract the heart. The heart uses free fatty acids as its main fuel, as well as important amounts of sugar and a small amount of amino acids. Oxygen, which affects the ability of muscle tissue to contract, is an important food for the myocardium. Without an oxygen supply, myocardial contractions decrease in a few minutes. The heart normally takes in about 70% of the oxygen reaching it by the coronary arteries. Myocardial oxygen use increases with an overactive thyroid (hyperthyroidism). It decreases with an underactive one (hypothyroidism). In anemia, the total use of myocardial oxygen may increase greatly because of increased blood supply demands resulting from the disorder. An enlarged heart may develop if the anemia is chronic. **–myocardial,** *adj.* Compare **epicardium.**

Myochrysine, a trademark for an antirheumatic drug (gold sodium thiomalate).

myoclonus /mī·ok'lənəs/, a spasm of a muscle or a group of muscles. **–myoclonic,** *adj.*

myodiastasis /mī'ōdī·as'təsis/, an abnormal condition in which there is separation of muscle bundles.

myofacial pain dysfunction syndrome. See **temporomandibular joint pain dysfunction syndrome.**

myofibril, a slender strand of muscle tissue.

myogelosis /mī'ōjəlō'sis/, a condition in which there are hardened areas or nodes within muscles, especially the gluteal muscles of the buttocks. There are no serious results of this condition. No treatment is necessary.

myogenic /mī'ōjen'ik/, referring to muscles, especially heart and smooth muscles that do not require nerve signals to begin and continue contractions.

myoglobin /mī'əglō'bin/, a form of hemoglobin found in muscle tissue. It is the cause of the red color of muscle and its ability to store oxygen.

myoglobinuria, myoglobin in the urine.

myokinase. See **adenylate kinase.**

myoma /mī·ō'mə/, *pl.* **myomas, myomata,** a common, noncancerous tumor on the uterus. It develops most often after 30 years of age in women, especially black women, who have never been pregnant. Heavy menstruation, backache, constipation, and pain with menstruation or intercourse are common symptoms. They develop in relation to the size, location, and rate of growth of the tumor. Blockage of a ureter may result if a large myoma puts pressure on it. A myoma may cause sterility if it blocks the fallopian tube. It also can interfere with fetal growth. It can cause difficult childbirth and bleeding if it is in or near the cervix. Also called *(informal)* **fibroid.**

myoma previum. See **leiomyoma uteri.**

myoma striocellulare. See **rhabdomyoma.**

myomectomy /mī'ōmek'təmē/, the surgical removal of muscle tissue.

myomere. See **myotome.**

myometritis /mī'ōmətrī'tis/, a swelling of the muscle wall (myometrium) of the uterus.

myometrium /mī'ōmē'trē·əm/, the muscular layer of the wall of the uterus.

myonecrosis /mī'ōnekrō'sis/, the death of muscle fibers. **Progressive** or **clostridial myonecrosis** is caused by a bacterium of *Clostridium* that cannot live in oxygen. It is seen in deep wound infections. Progressive myonecrosis is linked to pain, tenderness, a brown watery discharge, and a rapid gathering of gas in the tissue of the muscle. The affected muscle turns a blackish-green color. Treatment includes thorough wound cleaning, giving penicillin, and using oxygen under pressure to destroy the bacteria. Also called **gas gangrene.**

myoneural /mī'ōnōōr'əl/, referring to a muscle and its nearby nerve, especially to nerve endings in muscles.

myoneural junction. See **neuromuscular junction.**

myopathy /mī·op'əthē/, a disorder of skeletal muscle characterized by weakness, wasting, and changes within muscle cells. Examples include any of the muscular dystrophies. A myopathy is different from a muscle disorder caused by nerve dysfunction. See also **muscular dystrophy. –myopathic,** *adj.*

myope /mī'ōp/, an individual who is nearsighted or has myopia.

myopia /mī·ō'pē·ə/, a condition of nearsightedness. Causes include lengthening of the eyeball or an error in deflecting rays so that parallel rays of light are focused in front of instead of on the retina. Some kinds of myopia are **chromic myopia, curvature myopia, index myopia, pathologic myopia.** Also called **nearsightedness, short sight.**

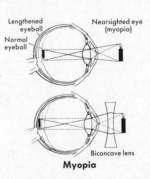

Lengthened eyeball · Normal eyeball · Nearsighted eye (myopia) · Biconcave lens

Myopia

myorrhexis /mī'ərek'sis/, a tearing or break in a muscle. **–myorrhectic,** *adj.*

myosarcoma /mī′ōsärkō′mə/, a cancer of muscle tissue.

myosin /mī′əsin/, a protein that makes up nearly one-half of the proteins in muscle tissue. An interaction between myosin and another protein, actin, makes muscle contraction possible.

myositis /mī′əsī′tis/, a swelling of muscle tissue, usually of the voluntary muscles. Causes of myositis include injury, infection, and invasion by parasites. Kinds of myositis include **epidemic myositis, interstitial myositis, parenchymatous myositis, polymyositis, traumatic myositis.** Also called **myitis.**

myositis fibrosa, a swelling of the muscles caused by an abnormal growth of connective tissue. Also called **interstitial myositis.** See also **myositis.**

myositis ossificans /əsif′əkanz/, an inherited disease in which muscle tissue is replaced by bone. It begins in childhood. Early symptoms are stiffness in the neck and back. It continues to rigidity of the spine, body, arms, and legs. Certain drugs may prevent the abnormal deposits of bone. There is no cure once it has occurred.

myositis purulenta, any bacterial infection of muscle tissue. It results in the formation of abscesses.

myositis trichinosa /trik′ənō′sə/, swelling of the muscles from infection by the parasite *Trichinella spiralis.* See also **trichinosis.**

myostroma /mī′əstrō′mə/, the framework of muscle tissue.

myotatic reflex. See **deep tendon reflex.**

myotenotomy, division of a tendon done by surgery.

myotome /mī′ətōm/, **1.** a group of muscles stimulated by a single spinal nerve segment. **2.** an instrument for cutting or dissecting a muscle.

myotomy /mī·ot′əmē/, the cutting of a muscle, done to get to tissues underneath. It is also used to relieve constriction in a circular band of muscles (sphincter), as in the esophagus or the pylorus of the stomach.

Myotonachol, a trademark for a nerve stimulating drug (bethanechol chloride).

myotonia /mī′ətō′nē·ə/, any condition in which muscles do not relax after contracting. **–myotonic,** *adj.*

myotonia atrophica. See **myotonic muscular dystrophy.**

myotonia congenita /konjen′itə/, a mild form of skeletal muscle wasting (myopathy) seen in infants. The only effects of the disorder are large and stiff muscles. Also called **Thomsen's disease.** See also **myopathy.**

myotonic muscular dystrophy, a severe form of muscular dystrophy, it is characterized by drooping eyelids, facial weakness, and speaking difficulties. Weakness occurs first in the hands and feet. It occurs later in the shoulders and hips. There is no specific treatment. How-

ever, exercises are used to relieve symptoms. Also called **myotonia atrophica, Steinert's disease.** See also **muscular dystrophy.**

myotonic myopathy, any of a group of disorders characterized by increased skeletal muscle contractions and decreased relaxation of muscles after contraction. Kinds of myotonic myopathy include **myotonia congenita, myotonic muscular dystrophy.**

myringectomy /mir′injek′təmē/, surgical removal of the eardrum (tympanic membrane).

myringitis /mir′injī′tis/, swelling or infection of the eardrum.

myringomycosis /miring′gōmīkō′sis/, a fungus infection of the eardrum. Also called **mycomyringitis.**

myringoplasty /miring′gōplas′tē/, surgical repair of breaks in the eardrum with a tissue graft. It is done to correct hearing loss. The openings in the eardrum are made larger. The grafting material is sewn over them, and antibiotics are put on the area. A packing of absorbable gelatin sponge is put on to hold the graft in place.

myringotomy /mir′ing·got′əmē/, surgical opening of the eardrum to relieve pressure or release pus from the middle ear. After the fluid is gently sucked out, ear drops may be used to improve drainage. If pain increases, it may have to be done again. Severe headache or confusion are possible side effects. Also called **tympanotomy.** See also **myringoplasty.**

Mysoline, a trademark for a drug used to control convulsions (primidone).

mysophobia /mē′sə-/, an anxiety disorder. It is characterized by an abnormal fear of dirt, contamination, or getting dirty. Also spelled **misophobia. –mysophobic, misophobic,** *adj.*

myxedema, the most severe form of decreased activity of the thryroid (hypothyroidism). Signs include swelling of the hands, face, feet, and tissues around the eye. The disease may lead to coma and death.

myxo-, a combining form meaning 'relating to mucus.'

myxofibroma /mik′sōfībrō′mə/, a fiberlike tumor that contains jellylike (myxomatous) tissue. Also called **myxoma fibrosum.**

myxoma /miksō′mə/, a tumor of connective tissue. These tumors may grow to huge size. They are usually pale gray, soft, and jellylike. They may occur under the skin. They are also found in bones and in the genitals and urinary tract. **–myxomatous,** *adj.*

myxoma fibrosum. See **myxofibroma.**

myxopoiesis /mik′sōpō·ē′sis/, making mucus.

myxosarcoma /mik′sōsärkō′mə/, a cancer that contains some jellylike (myxomatous) tissue. Also called **myxoma sarcomatosum.**

myxovirus /mik′sōvī′rəs/, any of a group of viruses usually carried by mucus. Some kinds of myxoviruses are the viruses that cause influenza, mumps, and croup.

N

N, **1.** abbreviation for **normal. 2.** symbol for **nitrogen.**

Na, chemical symbol for **sodium.**

Nabothian cyst /nabō′thē·ən/, a lump (cyst) formed in a nabothian gland of the uterine cervix, commonly found in routine pelvic examination of women of reproductive age, especially in women who have had children. The pearly white, firm cyst seldom causes side effects.

Nabothian gland, one of many small, mucus-releasing glands of the uterus.

nadir /nā′dər/, the lowest point, such as the blood count after it has been depressed by chemotherapy.

nadolol, a nerve blocking drug given for chest pain (angina pectoris) and high blood pressure.

★CAUTION: Asthma, certain heart disorders, or known allergy to this drug prohibit its use.

★ADVERSE EFFECTS: Among the more serious side effects are spasms of the bronchial tubes, slow or irregular heart beat, heart failure, weakness, and tiredness. Stomach and bowel problems, rashes, and other allergic reactions also may occur.

Naegeli's leukemia. See **monocytic leukemia.**

nafcillin sodium, an antibiotic, given to treat infections caused by penicillin-immune staphylococci.

★CAUTION: Known allergy to this drug or to other penicillins prohibits its use.

★ADVERSE EFFECTS: Among the more serious side effects are allergic reactions, nausea, and vomiting.

Nägele's obliquity. See **asynclitism.**

Nägele's rule /nā′gələz/, a method for estimating the date of childbirth. Three months are taken from the first day of the last menstrual period, and 1 year plus 7 days are added to that date. See also **estimated day of confinement.**

Nager's acrofacial dysostosis /nā′gərz/, a condition of defective bone growth. Defects include joining of the lower arm bones, imperfect tissue growth, or the lack of a long bone of the lower arm or of the thumbs. Also called **dysostosis mandibularis.**

Nahrungs Einheit Milch (nem) /nä′rŏōngz īn′hīt milsh, -mil*kh*/, a unit of feeding that is equal to 1 g of breast milk.

nail, **1.** a flat, structure with a horny surface at the end of a finger or toe. Each nail has a root, body, and edge. The root joins the nail to the finger or toe by fitting into a groove in the skin. The nail ground substance (matrix) has long ridges, which are seen through the body of the nail. The matrix joins the body of the nail to the connecting tissue under the finger or toe. The whitish moon shape (lunula) near the root is less firmly joined to the connective tissue, which gives it a pale color. The cuticle is joined to the nail just ahead of the root. The nails grow longer when cells at the root divide. They grow thicker during the making of the cells of the part under the lunula. **2.** any of many metal nails used in bone and joint surgery to join bones or pieces of bone.

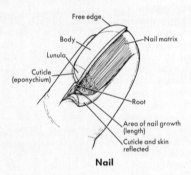

Nail

nal-, a combining form for narcotic agonists or antagonists related to normorphine.

Naldecon, a trademark for a drug with two stimulants (phenylpropanolamine hydrochloride and phenylephrine hydrochloride) and two antihistamines (chlorpheniramine maleate and phenyltoloxamine citrate).

Nalfon, a trademark for an anti-inflammatory drug used to relieve the pain of rheumatoid arthritis (fenoprofen calcium).

nalidixic acid, an antibiotic given to treat urinary tract infections.

★CAUTION: Kidney or liver disease, a history of seizures, or known allergy to this drug prohibits its use.

★ADVERSE EFFECTS: Among the more serious side effects are mild nervous system and stomach problems. Seizures and increased skull pressure may occur.

naloxone hydrochloride, a drug used to reverse narcotic depression or for sudden narcotic overdose.

★CAUTION: Known allergy to this drug prohibits its use.

★ADVERSE EFFECTS: Among the most serious side effects, when given to addicted patients, are those linked to narcotic withdrawal.

naltrexone hydrochloride, a drug, taken by mouth, used to block the effects of pain-relieving narcotic drugs (opioids) that contain opium, derivatives of opium, or synthetic drugs that act like opium. It is prescribed for patients recovering from addiction to drugs as heroin, morphine, and methadone.

★CAUTION: Acute hepatitis or liver failure prohibits use of the drug. Periodic liver function tests are recommended for all patients. Patients must be completely free of opioids before taking naltrexone to prevent severe withdrawal symptoms. Breathing may be depressed deeply for some time if a patient is given a large emergency dose of an opioid pain-reliever after taking naltrexone.

★ADVERSE EFFECTS: The most serious adverse reactions are stomach pain, cramps, nausea, vomiting, headache, sleep problems, and joint and muscle pain. Some adverse effects may actually be withdrawal symptoms rather than reactions to naltrexone.

NAMI, abbreviation for **National Alliance for the Mentally Ill.**

nandrolone decanoate /nan'drəlōn/, a male sex hormone given to treat a lack of testosterone, bone breakdown, female breast cancer, stimulation of growth, weight gain, and the making of red cells.

★CAUTION: Cancer of the male breast or prostate, liver disease, pregnancy or suspected pregnancy, or known allergy to this drug prohibits its use.

★ADVERSE EFFECTS: Among the most serious side effects are hormone disturbances, depending on the age of the patient. Excess hair growth, acne, liver disorders, and acid-base problems also occur.

nandrolone phenpropionate, a drug with male sex hormones given to treat bone breakdown, some anemias, and breast cancers of women.

★CAUTION: Cancer of the breast in males and some females, pregnancy, kidney disease, or known allergy to this drug prohibits its use.

★ADVERSE EFFECTS: Among the more serious side effects are excess hair growth, acne, various hormone effects depending on the age and sex of the patient, male features in females, liver disorders, excess blood calcium in women with breast cancer, and gathering fluid and salt.

nanism /nā'nizəm, nan'-/, an abnormal smallness or stunted growth; dwarfism. Kinds of nanism are **mulibrey nanism, Paltauf's nanism, pituitary nanism, renal nanism, senile nanism, symptomatic nanism.** Also called **nanosomia.** **–nanus,** *n.*

nano-, a combining form meaning 'small, or related to smallness or dwarfism.'

nanocephalic dwarf. See **bird-headed dwarf.**

nanocephaly /nā'nōsef'əlē, nan'-/, a growth defect characterized by a very small head. Also called **nanocephalia, nanocephalism. –nanocephalous,** *adj.,* **nanocephalus,** *n.*

nanocormia /nā'nōkôr'mē·ə/, an abnormal small-

ness of the body in relation to the head, arms, and legs. **–nanocormus,** *n.*

nanomelia /nā'nōmē'lē·ə, nan'-/, abnormally small arms and legs in relation to the head and body. **–nanomelous,** *adj.,* **nanomelus,** *n.*

nanophthalmos /nā'nofthal'məs, nan'-/, the condition when one or both eyes are abnormally small. The small size may not affect the person's sight. Also called **nanophthalmia.** See also **microphthalmos.**

nanosomus, a very short person; a dwarf.

nape, the back of the neck.

naphazoline hydrochloride /nəfaz'əlēn/, a drug which shrinks blood vessels, given to treat nasal congestion and some eye disorders.

★CAUTION: Glaucoma or known allergy to this drug or allergy to related drugs prohibits its use.

★ADVERSE EFFECTS: Among the most serious side effects are drowsiness and heart problems. Irritation to nasal mucous membranes and more congestion also may occur.

naphthalene poisoning, a toxic condition caused by swallowing naphthalene or paradichlorobenzene. They cause nausea, vomiting, headache, stomach pain, muscle spasm, and convulsions. Treatments include making the patient vomit, flushing the stomach with water, a salt-water laxative, and baking soda (sodium bicarbonate). Naphthalene and paradichlorobenzene are part of mothballs and moth crystals. Paradichlorobenzene is also used as an insecticide.

naphthol camphor, a blend of camphor and betanaphthol, used on the skin as an antiseptic.

napkin-ring tumor, a tumor that surrounds a tubelike structure of the body, as the intestine. It usually destroys the function of an organ and narrows its open area (lumen).

napping, periods of sleep, usually during the day. They may last from 15 to 60 minutes without reaching the level of deep sleep.

Naprosyn, a trademark for an anti-inflammatory, antifever, and pain-relieving drug (naproxen).

naproxen, a nonsteroid drug given for the relief of swelling symptoms of arthritis.

Naqua, a trademark for a diuretic and a high blood pressure drug (trichlormethiazide).

Naquival, a trademark for a blood pressure drug containing a diuretic (trichlormethiazide) and a high blood pressure drug (reserpine).

Narcan, a trademark for a drug reversing the effects of narcotics (naloxone hydrochloride).

narcissism /när'sisiz'əm/, an abnormal interest in oneself, especially in one's own body and sexual characteristics; self-love. Compare **egotism.** See also **narcissistic personality.**

narcissistic personality, a personality characterized by behavior and attitudes that show an abnormal love of the self. Such a person is self-centered and self-absorbed, is very unrealistic concerning abilities and goals, wavers between building up and tearing down others, and, in general, assumes that he or she has the right to more than is reasonable in relationships with others. Compare **narcissism.**

narco-, a combining form meaning 'related to stupor or a stuporous state,' as in narcolepsy, narcotic.

narcoanalysis, an interview conducted while the patient is in a state of drowsiness caused by drugs so that inhibitions are reduced and responses will be more truthful.

narcolepsy /när'kəlep'sē/, a disease characterized by sudden sleep attacks, sleep paralysis, and sight or hearing hallucinations at the onset of sleep. It begins in adolescence or young adulthood and lasts throughout life. Its cause is unknown, and no defects are found in the brain. Patients with narcolepsy have an uncontrollable urge to sleep many times in 1 day. Sleep periods may last from a few minutes to several hours. Temporary loss of muscle tone occurs during waking hours (cataplexy), or while the patient is asleep. Narcolepsy may be difficult to diagnose because not all patients with the disorder have all of the symptoms. Amphetamines and other stimulating drugs are used to stop the attacks. **–narcoleptic,** adj.

narcoleptic /när'kəlep'tik/, **1.** referring to a condition or substance that causes an uncontrollable desire for sleep. **2.** a patient with narcolepsy.

narcosis /närkō'sis/, a state of insensibility (stupor) caused by narcotic drugs. See also **narcotic.**

narcotic, 1. a substance that produces insensibility (stupor). **2.** a narcotic drug. Narcotic painkillers (analgesics), made from opium or made artifically, change one's sense of pain. They also cause a heightened sense of well-being, mood changes, mental confusion, and deep sleep. They may slow breathing and coughing, narrow the pupils, cause muscle spasms, vomiting, and nausea, and reduce contractions of the intestines. Repeated use of narcotics may result in physical and psychological addiction. Among the narcotic drugs given for relief of pain are butorphanol tartrate, hydromorphone hydrochloride, morphine sulfate, pentazocine lactate, and meperidine hydrochloride.

narcotic antagonist, a drug used mainly to work against the effects of narcotics. The narcotic antagonists nalorphine, levallorphan, and naloxone are usually given by injection.

narcotic antitussive. See **antitussive.**

Nardil, a trademark for an antidepressant drug (phenelzine sulfate).

nares /ner'ēz/, sing. **naris,** the openings in the nose that allow the passage of air to the throat (pharynx) and lungs during breathing. See also **anterior nares, posterior nares.**

narrow-angle glaucoma. See **glaucoma.**

nasal, referring to the nose and nasal cavity. **–nasally,** adv.

nasal airway, a flexible, curved piece of rubber or plastic, with one wide, trumpetlike end and one narrow end that can be inserted through the nose into the throat.

nasal cannula, a device for delivering oxygen by way of two small tubes that are inserted into the nostrils.

nasal cavity, one of 2 of openings (cavities) that open on the face through the nose and join the throat. Each passage is narrower at the top than at the bottom.

nasal decongestant, a drug that provides relief of symptoms in short- and long-term nasal problems and infected sinuses (sinusitis). Most are over-the-counter products made of a drug that shrinks blood vessels, as ephedrine or phenylephrine, and an antihistamine. A steroid drug may be added to reduce swelling. Long-term use or a dose greater than usual may cause more widening of blood vessels and severe clogging.

nasal drip, a method of giving liquid to a dehydrated infant by a tube placed through the nose and into the esophagus.

nasal fossa, one of the two chambers of the nasal opening (cavity). They are separated by the nasal wall, open externally through the nostrils, and internally into the throat. Each is divided into a smelling (olfactory) section and a breathing (respiratory) section. The olfactory section is located in the top of the fossa. It contains receiving cells and nerves for the sense of smell. The respiratory area is lined with mucous membrane, many glands, nerves, and a group of widened veins and blood spaces. This area is easily irritated, causing the membrane to swell, blocking the breathing passages and the openings of sinuses.

nasal glioma, a tumor made up of nerve tissue in the nasal opening (cavity).

nasal instillation of medication, putting (instilling) a drug into the nostrils by drops from a dropper or by a spray. Drops should be put in each nostril with the head tilted back. The mouth should remain open, and the head should stay in the tilted back position for several minutes to let the drug spread through the nasal passages. Nasal spray can be given to the patient in a sitting position. The patient should spit (expectorate) any solution that runs down into the throat.

nasalis /näzal'is/, one of the muscles of the nose.

nasal polyp, a round, long bit of overgrown mucous membrane that extends into the nasal cavity.

nasal septum, the wall dividing the nostrils. It is made up of bone and cartilage covered by mucous membrane.

nasal sinus, any one of the many openings (cavities) in various bones of the skull. A sinus is lined with mucous membrane which lines the nasal cavity and is very sensitive. When irritated, the membrane may swell and block the sinuses. The nasal sinuses are divided into frontal sinuses, ethmoidal air cells, sphenoidal sinuses, and maxillary sinus. Also called **air cells of the nose.**

nascent, just born; beginning to exist.

nasion /nā′zion/, a pushed in space where the top of the nose meets the forehead.

nasogastric feeding /nā′zōgas′trik/, putting liquid food directly into the stomach using a tube that is inserted through the nose into the stomach. Also called **gavage feeding.**

nasogastric intubation, placing a nasogastric tube through the nose into the stomach. It is used to remove gas or stomach contents; to give drugs, food, or fluids; or to get a specimen for laboratory tests. After surgery and in any condition in which the patient can digest food but not eat it, the tube may be put in and left in place for tube feeding until the patient can eat normally. The tube is put in the nostril, where it is pushed forward and downward. The patient must bend the neck forward, take shallow, rapid breaths, and help move the tube into the stomach by swallowing. For the patient's comfort, the tube is chosen to fit well and to be right for the purpose of the procedure. A tight fit is irritating, and a small tube might not allow the food to pass through. The tube is accepted most easily with the full help of the patient. Resistance, gagging, and wincing may be lessened by a slow steady progress, and by proper lubrication of the tube and placement of the patient. In many hospitals a physician inserts the tube the first time. If left in place, the tube is attached with tape to the nose and to the cheek or jaw.

nasogastric tube, any tube passed into the stomach through the nose. See **nasogastric intubation.**

nasojejunal tube /nā′zōjijōō′nəl/, a weighted tube inserted through the nose to allow natural movement caused by the wavelike, rhythmic contraction of smooth muscles from the tube-shaped part of the stomach (pylorus) into the top of the small intestine (jejeunum).

nasolabial reflex /nā′sōlā′bē·əl/, an infant's quick backward movement of the head, arching of the back, and stretching of the limbs in response to a light touch to the tip of the nose with an upward sweeping motion. The reflex disappears by about 5 months of age.

nasolacrimal /nā′zōlak′riməl/, referring to the nasal opening (cavity) and nearby tear (lacrimal) ducts.

nasolacrimal duct, a channel that carries tears from the tear (lacrimal) sac to the nasal opening (cavity).

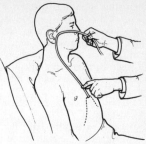

Measuring the length of tubing

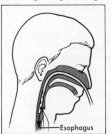

Nasogastric intubation

nasopharyngeal angiofibroma /nā′sōfərin′jē·əl/, a noncancerous tumor of the nose and throat. It is made of fiberlike connecting tissue with many blood vessel spaces. The tumor begins in puberty and is more common in boys than in girls. Typical signs are nose and eustachian tube blockage, muffled speech, and difficult swallowing. Also called **juvenile angiofibroma, nasopharyngeal fibroangioma.**

nasopharyngeal cancer, a cancer of the throat area behind the nose (nasopharynx). Depending on the site of the tumor, there may be nasal blockage, middle ear swelling (otitis media), hearing loss, sense or motor nerve damage, destruction of the skull bones, or disorders of the lymph nodes of the neck. Exposure to dusts of nickel, chromium, wood, and leather and to isopropyl oil increases the risk of nasopharyngeal cancer. High levels of Epstein-Barr virus antibodies are found in Chinese patients with the cancer, and there is evidence it is hereditary.

nasopharyngeal fibroangioma. See **nasopharyngeal angiofibroma.**

nasopharyngoscopy /nā′sōfer′ing·gos′kəpē/, a technique in physical examination in which the nose and throat are viewed using a laryngoscope, a fiberoptic device, a flashlight, and a dilator for the nostrils. **–nasopharyngoscopic,** *adj.*

nasopharynx /nā′sōfer′ingks/, one of the three parts of the throat, behind the nose and reaching from the back of the nasal opening to the soft palate. On the back wall of the nasopharynx are the pharyngeal tonsils. Swollen or large pharyngeal tonsils may completely block the passage of air from the nose into the throat. Compare **laryngopharynx, oropharynx.** See also **tonsil.** –**nasopharyngeal,** *adj.*

nasotracheal tube, a tube put into the windpipe (trachea) through the nose and throat. It is often used to give oxygen and in other breathing therapies.

natal, 1. referring to birth. **2.** referring to the buttocks (nates).

nates /nā'tēz/, *sing.* **natis,** the large fleshy knobs at the lower back of the body made up of fat and the gluteal muscles. Also called **buttocks.**

National Alliance for the Mentally Ill (NAMI), a national organization for family members of severely mentally ill (psychotic) patients.

National Eye Institute (NEI), a division of the National Institutes of Health, set up to support research in the normal workings of the human eye and seeing system. See also **eye, vision.**

national health insurance, a government-financed health insurance program providing complete benefits to most or all of the population. Compare **Medicaid, Medicare.**

National Health Service Corps (NHSC), a program of the United States Public Health Service (USPHS) in which health-care persons work in areas that are underserved. Nurses, physicians, and dentists serve in rural and urban areas, usually in local health-care agencies. The USPHS pays most of the salary of each member.

National Institute of Child Health and Human Development (N.I.C.H.H.D.), the part of the National Institutes of Health that is concerned with the growth, development, and health of the children of the United States.

National Institutes of Health (N.I.H.), an agency within the United States Public Health Service made up of several institutions and divisions, including the Bureau of Health Manpower Education, the National Library of Medicine, the National Cancer Institute, and several research institutes and divisions.

National Institute of Mental Health (NIMH), a branch of the (U.S.) National Institutes of Health within the Alcohol, Drug Abuse, and Mental Health Administration. It is responsible for federal research and education programs dealing with mental health.

National Organization of Victims Assistance, a private, nonprofit organization of victims and witness assistance practitioners, criminal justice professionals, researchers, former victims, and others committed to the recognition of victims' rights.

natriuresis /nātrēy·oŏorē'sis/, the release of more-than-normal amounts of salt (sodium) in the urine. It may be caused by diuretic drugs that help release sodium or from various disorders of chemical and physical processes that take place in the body. -**natriuretic,** *adj.*

natriuretic /nā'trēyoŏoret'ik/, referring to increased salt (sodium) filtering in the kidneys, allowing more sodium to be released with the urine.

natural childbirth, labor and childbirth (parturition) done with little or no medicine. Some experts think it is safest for the baby and most satisfying for the mother. It needs a normal pregnancy, a large-enough birth canal, strong interest by the mother, physical and emotional preparation, and constant, strong support of the mother during labor and birth. See also **Lamaze method.**

natural dentition, the entire set of natural teeth, made of original (deciduous) or permanent teeth or a mixture of the two. See also **tooth.**

natural family planning method, any method of family planning that does not require a drug or a device to avoid pregnancy. Some methods pinpoint the time of ovulation to increase the chance of the egg being fertilized. Natural family planning methods need knowledge, the help and desire of the parents, plus correctly noting and recording the menstrual cycle information. Kinds of natural family planning include **basal body temperature method of family planning, calendar method of family planning, ovulation method of family planning, symptothermal method of family planning.**

natural immunity, a usually inborn and permanent form of immunity to a specific disease. Kinds of natural immunity include **individual immunity, racial immunity, species immunity.** Also called **genetic immunity, innate immunity.** Compare **acquired immunity.**

naturalistic illness, an illness thought to be caused by impersonal factors, as an imbalance in the Oriental yin and yang or the Hispanic model of hot and cold forces.

naturally acquired immunity. See **acquired immunity.**

natural pacemaker, any heart-pacing site in the heart tissues, as the sinoatrial node.

natural radiation, radioactivity in the soil and rocks or that reaches the earth from space as radiation from the sun and particles from beyond the solar system.

natural selection, the natural processes by which animals and plants best suited to the environment survive and those that are unfit die out. Compare **artificial selection.**

Naturetin, a trademark for a diuretic and blood pressure drug (bendroflumethiazide).

nature versus nurture, a name given to a long-standing debate regarding the influence of nature versus the influence of the environment in the development of personality. Nature is represented by instincts and genetic factors and nurture by social influences.

naturopathy /nā'choŏorop'əthē, nach'-/, a system of disease treatment using natural foods, light, warmth, massage, fresh air, regular exercise, and the avoidance of drugs. Supporters believe that illness can be healed naturally by the body.

Nauheim bath /nou′hīm/, a bath taken in water through which carbon dioxide is bubbled. It is used with an exercise plan to treat heart conditions. Also called **Nauheim treatment.**

nausea /nô′zē-ə, nô′zhə/, a sensation leading to the urge to vomit. Common causes are motion sicknesses, early pregnancy, intense pain, emotional stress, gallbladder disease, food poisoning, and various infections. -**nauseate,** *v.*, **nauseous,** *adj.*

nausea and vomiting of pregnancy, a common condition of early pregnancy. There may be frequent and long-lasting nausea, often in the morning, with vomiting, weight and appetite loss, general weakness, and discomfort. The cause is not known. It usually does not begin before the sixth week after the last menstrual period and ends by the 12th to the 14th week of pregnancy. Relief is often gotten by eating frequent small, easily digested meals, and not allowing the stomach to be empty. Drugs may be given for severe cases. Nausea and vomiting after the 16th week is unusual and is called persistent nausea and vomiting of pregnancy. Severe vomiting of pregnancy means the patient must go to the hospital. Also called **morning sickness.**

Navane, a trademark for a tranquilizer (thiothixene).

navel, the point on the abdomen at which the umbilical cord joined the fetal abdomen. In most adults it is a pushed in space. In some it is a small lump of skin. It is located about halfway between the breastbone and the genital area. Also called **belly button, umbilicus.**

navicular /nəvik′yo͞olər/, having the shape of a boat, as the navicular bone in the wrist.

navicular bone. See **scaphoid bone.**

NBRC, abbreviation for *National Board for Respiratory Care.*

near drowning, a state in which a person has survived conditions that usually cause drowning. Cardiopulmonary resuscitation (CPR) is done at once, followed by hospitalization. The return of consciousness does not necessarily mean the patient will recover. Strong, close treatment may be needed for several days. Compare **drowning.** See also **hypothermia.**

nearsightedness. See **myopia.**

nebula, *pl.* **nebulae,** a slight eye (corneal) spot or scar that usually does not block sight and can be seen only by special lighting.

nebulization, a method of giving a drug by spraying it into the nose. The drug may be given with or without oxygen to help carry it into the lungs.

nebulize, to give a liquid in a fine spray.

nebulizer, a device for making a fine spray. Nasal sprays are given by a nebulizer. Also called **atomizer.**

Necator, a small worm (nematode) that is an intestinal parasite and causes hookworm disease.

necatoriosis, hookworm disease caused by *Necator americanus,* the most common North American hookworm. The larvae live in the soil and reach the human intestines through bad food and water or through the skin of the feet and legs. Symptoms include diarrhea, nausea, stomach pain, and anemia in the worst cases. Treatment consists of fixing the anemia if present, followed by worming drugs. Prevention includes getting rid of soil pollution and avoiding direct skin contact with the soil. See also **ancylostomiasis, hookworm.**

neck, a narrowed section, as the part of the body that connects the head with the body. Other examples are the neck of the upper arm bone (humerus) and the neck of the upper leg bone (femur).

neck dissection, surgical removal of the lymph nodes of the neck to stop the spread of cancers of the head and neck. The neck (cervical) system of lymph nodes and lymphatic ducts is removed entirely using a general anesthetic. Compare **radical neck dissection.**

neck righting reflex, an involuntary response in newborns. Turning the head to one side while the infant is lying face down (supine) causes the shoulders and body to turn in the same direction and allows the child to roll over from the supine to the back (prone) position. Lack of the reflex or its being present beyond about 10 months of age may mean there is central nervous system damage.

necorbiosis lipoidica, a skin disease recognized by thin, shiny, yellow to red spots (plaques) on the shins or forearms. These plaques may forms crusts or ulcers. Usually linked to diabetes mellitus, necrobiosis lipoidica occurs most often in women. Treatment includes control of the diabetes and sometimes the use of skin drugs.

necrolysis /nekrol′isis/, breakdown or shedding of dead tissue. Compare **necrosis.** −**necrolytic,** *adj.*

necrophilia, 1. a morbid liking for being with dead bodies. 2. a morbid desire to have sexual contact with a dead body, usually of a man to perform a sexual act with a dead woman. -**necrophile, necrophiliac,** *n.*

necropsy. See **autopsy.**

necrosis /nekrō′sis/, local tissue death that occurs in groups of cells because of disease or injury. In **coagulation necrosis,** blood clots block the flow of blood, keeping blood from nearby tissue. In **gangrenous necrosis,** lack of blood combined with bacterial decay causes rotting of tissue. See also **gangrene.**

necrotic /nekrot′ik/, referring to the death of tissue in response to disease or injury.

necrotizing enteritis, an acute inflammation of the small and large intestine by the bacterium *Clostridium perfringens.* Symptoms are strong stomach pain, bloody diarrhea, and vomiting. Some patients recover completely or survive with long-term bowel obstruction. A hole in the intestine, dehydration, poisoning of the intestinal area (peritonitis), or blood poisoning may cause death.

necrotizing enterocolitis (NEC), a sudden inflammatory bowel disorder that occurs mainly in premature or low birth-weight infants. Symptoms include destruction of the stomach and intestinal lining, which leads to a break in the bowel and poisoning of the intestinal area (peritonitis). Its cause is unknown. It may involve a lack of ability to fight normal intestinal bacteria rather than an infection from invading germs. Premature birth, low blood volume, respiratory distress syndrome, infection, a blood exchange transfusion, and feeding with special bottle formulas may lead to the condition. The disease causes blood to move away from the stomach and intestinal tract. This leads to convulsions narrowing the blood vessels to the intestines. The reduced blood supply in turn interferes with the normal making of mucus and with other bowel functions. The result is tissue death with bacterial invasion of the intestinal wall. Bottle-fed infants are more likely to get the disorder, maybe because formula lacks the substances found in breast milk that may protect the intestinal lining from damage and bacterial invasion. Symptoms usually develop several days after birth and include a below-normal temperature, drowsiness, poor feeding, vomiting of bile, a bloated abdomen, blood in the stools, and decreased or absent bowel sounds. Signs of worsening are difficult breathing, liver disease (jaundice), abnormally low amounts of urine, a tender abdomen, and redness and swelling of the abdomen wall. Untreated, eventual breathing failure leads to death. Treatment includes stopping feeding by mouth and giving food by vein (intravenously). Blood transfusions and antibiotics may be needed. Improvement usually occurs within 48 to 72 hours after treatment starts. Feedings by mouth usually are not begun for 10 days to 2 weeks. Total intravenous food is necessary during that time. Surgery for the damaged bowel segment may be needed.

necrotizing vasculitis, a swelling of blood vessels in which there is tissue death and overgrowth of the inner layer of the veseel wall. This may result in blocking the blood flow. Necrotizing vasculitis may occur in rheumatoid arthritis, systemic lupus erythematosus, small artery swelling, and a disease of blood vessels and connective tissue (progressive systemic sclerosis). It is usually treated with adrenal hormone drugs.

need-fear dilemma, a conflict in which the need to experience closeness is accompanied by fear of the experience.

needle bath, a shower in which fine jets of water are sprayed over the body.

needle biopsy, the removal of a part of living tissue for microscopic examination by putting a hollow needle through the skin or the surface of an organ or tumor and turning it within the cell layers. See also **aspiration therapy.**

needle filter, a device for filtering drugs that are drawn into a syringe before giving them.

needle holder, a surgical device (forceps) used to hold and pass a sewing needle through tissue. Also called **suture forceps.**

negative, 1. referring to a laboratory test result that a substance or a condition is not present. **2.** meaning that on physical examination a disease is not present; often meaning that there is no medical problem.

negative adaptation. See **habituation.**

negative anxiety, an emotional or psychological condition in which anxiety keeps a person from normal functioning and from doing usual daily activities.

negative feedback, a decrease in a body function in response to stimulation. For example, when the release of certain hormones reaches a certain level, a signal is given by another hormone to slow the release. Thus a constant level is kept.

negative identity, the taking on of an identity that conflicts with the accepted values and expectations of society.

negative pressure, less-than-standard atmospheric pressure, as in a vacuum or at an altitude above sea level. Some breathing assistance devices have a negative pressure that help a patient to breathe out. See also **IPPB.**

negative punishment, a form of behavior modification in which removing something after a certain behavior occurs decreases the probability that the behavior will occur again.

negative reinforcer, (in psychology) a stimulus that, when presented immediately following occurrence of a particular behavior, will decrease the rate of that behavior. See also **reinforcement.**

negativism, a behavior attitude marked by resistance or refusal to cooperate with reasonable request. The response may be passive, as the stiff postures seen in catatonic schizophrenia, or active, as in a contrary act, like sitting down when asked to stand.

NegGram, a trademark for an antibiotic (nalidixic acid).

neglect, a condition that occurs when a parent or guardian is unable to or fails to provide minimal physical and emotional care for a child or other dependent person.

Neisseria gonorrhoeae, a bacterium that causes the venereal disease gonorrhea. Also called **gonococcus.** See also **gonorrhea.**

Neisseria meningitidis. See **meningococcus.**

Nelson's syndrome, a hormone disorder that may follow removal of the adrenal gland, as in Cushing's disease. There is a large increase in the making of adrenocorticotropic hormone (ACTH) and melanocyte stimulating hormone (MSH) by the pituitary gland. Treatment includes radiation to slow pituitary function and, sometimes, surgical removal of the pituitary. See also **Cushing's disease.**

nematocides, chemicals used to kill nematode worms.

nematode /nem′ətōd/, a parasitic worm of the phylum Nematoda. All roundworms belong to the phylum, including *Ancylostoma duodenale, Ascaris lumbricoides, Enterobius vermicularis, Necator americanus, Strongyloides stercoralis,* and several other species.

Nembutal, a trademark for a barbiturate (pentobarbital) used as a sedative.

neo-, ne-, a combining form meaning 'new,' as in neonatal.

neobehaviorism, a school of psychology that stresses experimental research and laboratory tests to study behavior and information difficult to measure, as fantasies, love, and stress. See also **behaviorism.**

neoblastic, referring to a new tissue or new growth.

neoglottis, a vibrating structure that replaces the voice apparatus (glottis) to produce speech after the surgical removal of the voicebox (laryngectomy). Also called **pseudoglottis.**

neologism /nē·ol′əjiz′əm/, a word made up by a psychiatric patient that has meaning only to the patient.

neomycin sulfate, an antibiotic given to treat infections of the intestine, sudden liver disorders, and skin infections.

★CAUTION: Kidney dysfunction, intestinal blockage, or known allergy to this drug or to any related drug prohibits its use.

★ADVERSE EFFECTS: Among the more serious side effects are nausea, vomiting, diarrhea, and failure of the digestive system to absorb food. Long-term treatment in patients with kidney disease may result in side effects. Allergic reactions may occur with use of this drug on the skin.

neonatal, the period of time covering the first 28 days after birth.

Neonatal Behavior Assessment Scale, a scale for checking an infant's alertness, reactions, irritability, and interaction with people. It is used to test the nervous system condition and the behavior of a newborn infant. Some researchers believe that the quality of the parent-child relationship may be predicted from the scale.

neonatal breathing, breathing in newborn infants that begins when fluid in the lungs is forced out by pressure of the chest during delivery or reabsorbed from the lungs into the bloodstream and lymph system. Air enters the lungs after birth, but forceful breathing is needed to keep the lungs full. These forces come from temperature changes, touching sensations, blood gas tension, and certain reflexes. Newborns are highly sensitive to carbon dioxide during the first weeks, which helps control breathing. However, control of breathing rhythm is not fully developed at birth.

neonatal death, the death of a live-born infant during the first 28 days after birth. Early neonatal death is usually one that occurs during the first 7 days. Compare **infant death, perinatal death.**

neonatal developmental profile, the growth status of a newborn infant based on three examinations: a chronological-age inventory, a brain and nerve examination, and a Neonatal Behavior Assessment score.

neonatal hyperbilirubinemia. See **hyperbilirubinemia of the newborn.**

neonatal intensive care unit (NICU), a hospital unit with special equipment for the care of premature and seriously ill newborn infants. See also **intensive care unit.**

neonatal mortality, the rate of infant deaths during the first 28 days after live birth. It is noted as the number of such deaths per 1,000 live births in a specific geographical area or population in a given time period.

neonatal jaundice. See **hyperbilirubinemia of the newborn.**

neonatal period, the period from birth to 28 days of age. It is the time of the greatest risk to the infant. About 65% of all deaths that occur in the first year of life happen in this 4-week period.

neonatal pustular melanosis, a temporary skin condition of the newborn. Blisters that appear at birth fill with pus. The sores disappear within 72 hours, leaving dark spots that gradually fade by about 3 months of age.

neonatal thermoregulation, the protection of body temperature of a newborn infant, which may be affected by evaporation, conduction, radiation, and convection. To prevent the loss of body heat through evaporation, the infant is dried with a warm towel immediately after birth. Wrapping the baby in a warm blanket or covering the baby as he or she lies on the mother's skin and by warming all equipment used for the infant prevents loss of heat by conduction. Placing the baby under a heater, on a warmed, padded surface, skin-to-skin with the mother reduces loss of heat by radiation. Avoiding drafts, air-conditioning vents, and low temperatures prevents loss of heat by convection. Infant bassinettes have high sides to prevent cross drafts. Because the surface area of the head of a newborn is quite large compared to the body, heat loss from the head may be great; therefore, a cap or fold of blanket is placed around the head. The armpit (axillary) temperature of an infant is normally between 97.5° F (36.5° C) and 98.6° F (37° C), and the rectal temperature is normally 1° higher than the axillary temperature.

neonatal tyrosinemia. See **tyrosinemia.**

neonatal unit, a unit of a hospital that provides care and treatment for newborn infants through 28 days of age, and longer if necessary.

neoplasia /nē′ōplā′zhə/, the new and abnormal development of cells that may be harmless (benign) or cancerous (malignant). **-neoplastic,** *adj.*

neoplastic fracture, a fracture resulting from bone tissue weakened by a tumor. Also called **pathologic fracture.**

Neosporin, a trademark for a skin drug containing antibiotics (polymyxin B sulfate, neomycin sulfate, and bacitracin zinc).

neostigmine bromide /nē′ōstig′mēn/, a nerve-stimulating drug given to treat myasthenia gravis.

★CAUTION: Bowel obstruction, urinary infection, or known allergy to this drug or to other bromides prohibits its use.

★ADVERSE EFFECTS: Among the more serious side effects are severe breathing problems, excess saliva, and intestinal cramps.

Neo-Synephrine Hydrochloride, a trademark for a blood vessel constricting drug (phenylephrine hydrochloride).

nephrectomy, the surgical removal of a kidney. It is done to remove a tumor, drain a sore (abscess), or treat kidney bloating caused by urine pooling (hydronephrosis).

-nephric, a combining form referring to the kidneys.

nephritic gingivitis, a kind of mouth and gum swelling linked to kidney failure. Symptoms include pain, an odor of ammonia, and increased saliva. Also called **uremic gingivitis.**

nephritis /nefrī′tis/, any disease of the kidney marked by swelling and abnormal function. Kinds of nephritis include **acute nephritis, glomerulonephritis, hereditary nephritis, interstitial nephritis, parenchymatous nephritis, suppurative nephritis.**

nephro-, nephr-, a combining form referring to the kidneys.

nephroangiosclerosis /nef′rō·an′jē·ōsklerō′sis/, destruction of the small renal arteries, linked to high blood pressure. This condition is present in some patients with high blood pressure between 30 and 50 years of age. Early signs are headaches, blurred vision, and a diastolic blood pres-

sure greater than 120 mm Hg. Examination of the retina shows bleeding. The heart is usually large, especially the left chamber (ventricle). Proteins and red blood cells are found in the urine. Heart and kidney failure may occur if the disease is untreated. Treatment includes diet and high blood pressure drugs. Kidney dialysis is used when preventive measures fail. Also called **malignant hypertension.** See also **hypertension, renal failure.**

nephrocalcinosis /nef′rōkal′sinō′sis/, an abnormal condition of the kidneys in which deposits of calcium form in the filtering units. It usually occurs at the site of a previous swelling or breakdown.

nephrogenic /nef′rōjen′ik/, beginning in the kidney.

nephrogenic ascites, the presence of fluid in the abdominal (peritoneal) cavity of patients having kidney dialysis for kidney failure. Its cause is unknown. See also **ascites.**

nephrogenic diabetes insipidus, a condition in which the kidneys do not hold urine, resulting in increased urination, excess thirst, and very watered-down urine. The release of antidiuretic hormone (ADH) by the pituitary gland is normal, and all kidney function is normal, but there is no response to ADH. See also **diabetes insipidus.**

nephrolith, a stone formed in a kidney. **-neprolithic,** *adj.*

nephrolithiasis /nef′rōlithī′əsis/, the presence of stones in the kidney. See also **renal calculus.**

nephrolytic, referring to the breakdown of the structure and function of a kidney.

nephron /nef′ron/, a filtering unit of the kidney, resembling a tiny funnel with a long stem and two twisted tubes. Each kidney contains about 1.25 million nephrons. Each nephron is made up of a renal corpuscle containing a ball of blood vessels (glomerulus) surrounded by a Bowman's capsule and several long tubes. Urine is formed in the renal corpuscles and in the tubes by filtering, reabsorption, and release. The collecting tubes carry the urine to the kidney pelvis and the ureters. Also called **nephrone** /nef′rōn/. See also **kidney, renal corpuscle.**

nephropathy /nefrop′əthē/, any swelling or breakdown disorder of the kidney. See also **kidney disease.**

nephropexy /nef′rəpek′sē/, an operation to make stable a floating or drooping (ptotic) kidney.

nephroptosis /nef′roptō′sis/, a downward movement or dropping of a kidney.

nephroscope, an instrument used to break up and remove kidney stones. The nephroscope is inserted through the body wall, and the stones are found using x-rays. An ultrasonic probe giving off high-frequency sound waves breaks the stones into small pieces that are easily removed.

nephrostomy, a surgical technique in which a tube (catheter) is inserted into the kidney pelvis for drainage.

nephrotic syndrome, a kidney disease marked by protein in the urine, abnormally low blood protein (albumin), and fluid gathering in the tissues. It occurs in kidney glomerular disease, blood clotting in a kidney vein, and as a result of other diseases, as diabetes mellitus, systemic lupus erythematosus, and multiple myeloma. Treatment depends on the cause of disease. The nephrotic syndrome is usually successfully treated with adrenal gland hormones. Diuretics are used to control fluid pooling, but dialysis may be needed. Also called **nephrosis.**

nephrotomy, a surgical incision into the kidney.

nephrotoxic, anything poisonous or destructive to a kidney.

nephrotoxin, a poison specifically destructive to the kidneys.

nephrouterolithiasis /nef′rōyoo′tərōlithī′əsis/, stones in the kidneys and the tubes that carry urine from the kidney into the bladder (ureters).

Neptazane, a trademark for a diuretic (methazolamide).

nerve, one or more bundles of signal-carrying fibers that connect the brain and the spinal cord with other parts of the body. Nerves carry inward (afferent) signals from receiving organs toward the brain and spinal cord, and outward (efferent) signals to the various organs and tissues. Each nerve consists of an outer sheath enclosing a bundle of nerve fibers. The sheath is made up of joining tissue. Single nerve fibers are wrapped in a membrane (neurilemma) in which some nerve fibers are also enclosed in a fatty insulating substance (myelin). See also **axon, dendrite, neuroglia, neuron.**

nerve accommodation, the ability of nerve tissue to adjust to a constant source and strength of stimulation so that some change in either strength or length of stimulation is needed to get its attention.

nerve block anesthesia. See **conduction anesthesia.**

nerve compression, harmful pressure on one or more nerve branches, resulting in nerve damage and muscle weakness (atrophy). Any nerve that passes over a bony knob is at risk. The degree of damage depends on the amount and length of time of pressure. Activities in routine occupations may put unnecessary pressure on certain nerves. Crossing the legs while seated may put pressure on the femoral nerve. Compare **nerve entrapment.**

nerve entrapment, nerve damage and muscle weakness (atrophy) caused by entrapping a nerve. Nerves that pass over rigid knobs or through narrow bony and fiberlike tissue tunnels are particularly at risk of being trapped. Common signs of this disorder are pain or numbness and muscular weakness. Nerve damage occurs more often when joints are affected by swelling, as in rheumatoid arthritis. One of the most common types of entrapment is **carpal tunnel syndrome.** Compare **nerve compression.**

nerve fiber, a slender thread (filament) of a nerve cell (neuron), which usually carries signals away from the nerve cells. Some fibers are insulated (myelinated) by a fatty substance (myelin), and some fibers are uninsulated (unmyelinated). Some myelinated fibers carry signals of pressure, temperature, touch, and sharp pain. Others are linked to abdominal organs. Unmyelinated fibers carry signals of lengthy, burning sensations from the abdomen and outer body.

nerve growth factor (NGF), a protein looking like insulin with hormonelike action that affects the growth and care of nerve cells.

nerve impulse. See **impulse.**

nervous breakdown, *informal,* any mental condition that disrupts normal functioning.

nervous system, an intricate system of nerve cells that starts, oversees, and controls all of the functions of the body. It is divided into the central nervous system, made up of the brain and spinal cord, and the peripheral nervous system, which includes the cranial nerves and spinal nerves. These nerves combine and communicate to interact with all organs and tissues of the body with inward (afferent) and outward (efferent) nerve fibers. Afferent fibers carry sense signals, as pain and cold, to the central nervous system. Efferent fibers carry motor signals and movement commands from the central nervous system to the muscles and other organs. Somatic nerve fibers are linked to bones, muscles, and skin. Visceral nerve fibers are linked to the internal organs, blood vessels, and mucous membranes. The many functions of the nervous system are linked through a vast system of tiny structures, as neurons, axons, dendrites, and ganglia. Compare **parasympathetic nervous system, sympathetic nervous system, visceral nervous system.** See also the **Color Atlas of Human Anatomy.**

Nesacaine, a trademark for a local anesthetic (chloroprocaine).

Netromycin, a trademark for an antibiotic (netilmicin).

nettle rash, a fine, itching eruption resulting from skin contact with the stinging nettle. The common weed has leaves containing histamine. The stinging and itching lasts from a few minutes to several hours.

network therapy, a type of treatment for mental and emotional disorders that is conducted in the patient's home, in which all persons interested or involved in a particular problem or crisis participate.

Neufeld nail /noi′felt/, an orthopedic nail used

for repairing a break of the upper leg bone (femur).

neural /nŏŏr'əl/, referring to nerve cells and their fibers.

neural canal. See **neurocele.**

neuralgia /nŏŏral'jə/, a painful condition caused by a variety of disorders that affect the nervous system. The term is usally linked to an affected body area, as facial neuralgia. –**neuralgic,** *adj.*

neural impulse. See **impulse.**

neural tube, the tube of tissue that lies along the central axis of the early embryo. It gives rise to the brain, spinal cord, and other parts of the central nervous system. Failure of the tube to close causes a number of birth defects, as spina bifida. Also called **cerebromedullary tube, medullary tube.** See also **neural tube defect, neural tube formation.**

neural tube defect, any defect of the brain and spinal cord caused by failure of the neural tube to close during growth during pregnancy. The defect often results from an abnormal increase in spinal fluid pressure on the neural tube during the first 3 months of pregnancy. It may occur at any point along the spinal column. The amount of deformity and disability depends on how much of the neural tube is affected. The most severe defect is total lack of the skull and defective brain growth. Other serious defects, usually linked to severe mental and physical disorders, occur most often at the base of the skull. Most neural tube defects involve incomplete joining of one or more parts of the spinal column. Such defects include spina bifida cystica, meylomeningocele, and meningocele. In all of these conditions there is constant risk of a break in the saclike lump of nerve tissues and a danger of infection. Immediate surgery is often necessary. Many neural tube defects can be found during pregnancy by ultrasonic scanning of the fetus in the uterus. Such tests are done during the 14th to 16th weeks of pregnancy to allow abortion. See also **meningocele, myelomeningocele, spina bifida cystica.**

neurapraxia, the interruption of nerve conduction without loss of continuity of the long part of the nerve cell (axon).

neurasthenia /nŏŏr'əsthē'nē·ə/, **1.** a condition of nervous exhaustion and physical tiredness that often follows depression. **2.** a stage in the recovery from schizophrenia in which the patient is listless and apparently unable to cope with routine activities and relationships. –**neurasthenic,** *adj.*

neurilemma /nŏŏr'əlem'ə/, a layer of cells that surrounds the segments of myelin coverings (sheaths) of nerve fibers. Each myelinated nerve fiber has a covering (neurilemma) cell for each segment. The nerve fibers of the brain and the spinal cord are not surrounded by neu-

rilemma. Also called **Schwann's sheath.** See also **nerve, myelin sheath.**

neurilemoma. See **schwannoma.**

neurinoma /nŏŏr'inō'mə/, *pl.* **neurinomas, neurinomata,** a tumor of the nerve covering (sheath). It is usually harmless but may become a cancer. A kind of neurinoma is **acoustic neurinoma.** See also **schwannoma.**

neuritis /nŏŏrī'tis/, *pl.* **neuritides,** swelling of a nerve. Some of the signs are nerve pain (neuralgia), sensitivity of the skin, loss of feeling, paralysis, muscular weakness, and slowed reflexes.

neuro-, neur-, a combining form referring to nerves.

neuroblastoma /nŏŏr'ōblastō'mə/, *pl.* **neuroblastomas, neuroblastomata,** a cancer made up of primitive cells that come from the tissues of life in the womb. The tumor may begin in any part of the nervous system, but it is most common in the adrenal glands of young children. Neuroblastomas spread early and widely to lymph nodes, liver, lung, and bone. Symptoms may include an abdominal mass, breathing difficulty, and anemia. Active adrenal gland tumors may cause irritability, flushing, sweating, high blood pressure, and fast heart beat. Early treatment with surgery, radiation, and chemicals is often successful. A kind of neuroblastoma is **Pepper syndrome.**

neuro check, *nontechnical.* a brief nerve test, usually done on coming to an emergency service of a hospital. The level of consciousness is noted as alert and aware, drowsy, listless, or in a coma. The movements of the arms and legs are noted to be voluntary or involuntary. The pupils of the eyes are checked for equal widening, reaction to light, and ability to focus. See also **neurologic assessment.**

neurocirculatory asthenia, a psychological disorder of nervous and circulation irregularities, including breathlessness, irregular heart rate, dizziness, trembling, chest pain, and increased tiredness. The symptoms often result from or are linked to psychological stress.

neurocoele /nŏŏr'əsēl/, a system of openings (cavities) in the central nervous system. It consists of the openings (ventricles) of the brain and the central canal of the spinal cord, which begin from the neural tube during the early growth of pregnancy. Also called **neural canal.**

neurocytoma /nŏŏr'ōsītō'mə/, a tumor made up of nerve cells. Also called **neuroma.**

neurodermatitis, an itching skin disorder seen in anxious, nervous patients. Scratches and skin thickening are found on exposed areas of the body, as the forearms and forehead.

neurofibroma /nŏŏr'ōfibrō'mə/, *pl.* **neurofibromas, neurofibromata,** a fiberlike growth of nerve tissue. Many growths of this type in the nervous system are often linked to many defects in other tissues. See also **neurofibromatosis.**

neurofibromatosis /noōr'ōfi'brōmətō'sis/, an inherited condition marked by many fiberlike growths (neurofibromas) of the nerves and skin, and light brown (café au lait) spots on the skin. There may also be defects of the muscles, bones, and abdominal organs. Many large, stalklike soft tissue tumors may develop. An example is the famous case of the "Elephant Man," in 19th-century England. Bone changes may result in skeletal defects, especially curving of the spine. Neurofibromas may develop in the intestinal tract, bladder, endocrine glands, and skull nerves. The disorder occurs in 1 of 2,500 to 3,000 live births. Sometimes it is linked to meningocele, spina bifida, or epilepsy. Also called **multiple neuroma, neuromatosis, von Recklinghausen's disease.**

neurogen /noōr'əjən/, a substance within the early growing embryo that stimulates the making of the neural plate, which leads to the growth of the tissue of the nervous system.

neurogenic arthropathy, a condition of nerve damage, and the gradual and usually painless breakdown of a joint. A major cause of this condition is thought to be a minor injury that is not noticed by the patient due to numbness in the injured tissue. Inadequate rest and care worsen such injuries and prevent proper healing. See also **Charcot's joint.**

neurogenic bladder, a urinary bladder disorder that can be caused by a tumor of the nervous system. To prevent infection and keep kidney functions, treatment aims at emptying the bladder completely and regularly. Kinds of neurogenic bladder are **spastic bladder, reflex bladder, flaccid bladder,** Also called **neuropathic bladder.**

neurogenic fracture, a fracture linked to the destruction of the nerve supply to a bone.

neurogenic shock,, a form of shock due to blood vessels widening in the arms and legs as a result of damage in the nervous system.

neuroglia /noōrog'lē·ə/, the supporting or connective tissue cells of the central nervous system. Kinds of neuroglia include **astrocytes, oligodendroglia, microglia.** Compare **neuron.** **-neuroglial,** adj.

neurohormonal regulation, control of an organ or a gland by the combined effect of nervous system and hormone activity.

neurohumor, a chemical substance made and carried by a neuron. It is needed for the activity of nearby neurons or nearby organs or muscles. Kinds of neurohumoral substances are **acetylcholine, dopamine, epinephrine, norepinephrine, serotonin.** Also alled **neurotransmitter.**

neurohypophyseal hormone, a hormone released by the pituitary gland. Kinds of neurohypophyseal hormones are **oxytocin, vasopressin.** See also **pituitary gland.**

neurohypophysis, the back lobe of the pituitary gland, the source of antidiuretic hormone (ADH) and oxytocin. Nervous system stimulation controls the release of both substances into the blood. ADH hormone causes the cells in the kidney tubules to reabsorb more water, thereby reducing the amount of urine. The neurohypophysis releases oxytocin under proper stimulation from the hypothalamus of the brain. Oxytocin causes strong contractions of the pregnant uterus and causes milk to flow from breasts. Sucking the nipples of the breast by a nursing infant starts the release of this hormone. Also called **posterior pituitary gland.**

neurolemma. See **neurilemma.**

neurolepsis, an altered state of consciousness marked by reduced physical movement, anxiety, and by indifference to the surroundings. Sleep may occur, but usually the patient can be woken up and can respond to commands. Antipsychotic drugs usually cause neurolepsis.

neuroleptanalgesia, a form of pain relief achieved by giving a neuroleptic and a painkiller. Anxiety, physical movement, and sensitivity to pain are reduced. The patient is quiet and indifferent to the environment and surroundings. Sleep may or may not occur. The patient is conscious and can respond to commands.

neuroleptanesthesia, a form of anesthesia achieved by giving a neuroleptic agent, a narcotic analgesic, and nitrous oxide in oxygen. The anesthesia is given slowly, but consciousness returns quickly after the patient stops breathing nitrous oxide.

neuroleptic, 1. referring to neurolepsis. **2.** a drug that causes neurolepsis, as droperidol. Also called **neurolept.** See also **antipsychotic.**

neurolinguistic programing, a communication approach that involves both verbal and nonverbal messages, sensory experience and awareness or perception through patterns of behavior that can be observed and perceived.

neurologic assessment, an examination of a patient's nervous system. A careful neurological assessment is an important aid to the physician in making a diagnosis and choosing treatment. The physician will ask about weakness, numbness, headaches, pain, tremors, nervousness, irritability, or drowsiness. There will be questions about memory loss, periods of confusion, hallucinations, and loss of consciousness. The patient's general appearance, facial expression, attention span, responses to stimulation, emotional state, coordination, balance, and ability to follow commands are noted. Skin color and temperature; pupil size and reactions to light; breathing rate, rhythm, and quality; and chest movements and breath sounds are observed. The pulse is checked; ears and nose are examined for possible drainage. Strength of the handgrip and reflexes are tested. Speech is examined for slurring and ability to say certain words. The physician may ask about other diseases, as high blood pressure, cancer, and narrowing of the aorta; past illnesses linked to head injury; seizures, motor or sensory nerve, or emotional disturbances; and neurological, medical, or surgical procedures. There may be questions about sleep patterns, drugs, personality changes, relationships with family and friends, and any family history of seizures, stroke, mental illness, tumors, or sudden death. For a complete examination, spinal fluid analysis, complete blood count, x-ray films of the spinal cord (myelogram), ultrasound brain record (echoencephalogram), brain scan made with radioisotopes to locate possible tumors, computerized x-ray films of the brain (tomogram), and tests of sugar and mineral levels may be needed.

neuroma /nŏŏrō'mə/, *pl.* **neuromas, neuromata,** a noncancerous tumor made up mainly of nerve cells and nerve fibers. It may be soft or very hard and may vary in size up to 6 inches or more. Pain moves from the tumor to the ends of the affected nerve. It is not usually constant but may become continuous and severe. Kinds of neuromas include **acoustic neuroma, cystic neuroma, false neuroma, multiple neuroma, myelinic neuroma, neuroma cutis, nevoid neuroma, traumatic neuroma.**

neuroma cutis, a skin tumor that contains nerve tissue and may be very sensitive to pain.

neuroma telangiectodes. See **nevoid neuroma.**

neuromatosis /nŏŏr'ōmətō'sis/, a disease marked by numerous noncancerous tumors of nerve cells and fibers (neuromas). Also called **multiple neuroma.** See also **neurofibromatosis.**

neuromodulator, a substance that changes transmission of nerve impulses.

neuromuscular /nŏŏr'ōmus'kyŏŏlər/, referring to the nerves and the muscles.

neuromuscular blockade, the blocking of a muscle contraction caused by the nervous system, possibly causing muscle weakness or paralysis.

neuromuscular blocking agent, a drug that interferes with the sending or receiving of signals from motor nerves to skeletal muscles. Neuromuscular blocking agents are used to cause muscles to relax in anesthesia, to aid putting an airway tube into the throat, electroshock therapy, and in treating tetanus, encephalitis, and poliomyelitis. Neuromuscular blocking drugs can cause spasm of the bronchial tubes, very high body temperature, falling blood pressure, or breathing paralysis. They must be used carefully, especially in patients with myasthenia gravis or with kidney, liver, or lung disorders, and in elderly and weak patients. See also **muscle relaxant.**

neuromuscular junction, the place where the ends of a nerve fiber and a fiber of skeletal muscle contact. Also called **myoneural junction.** See also **motor end plate, myelin, nerve.**

neuromuscular spindle, a small bundle of delicate muscle fibers, surrounded by a capsule, in which sensory nerve fibers end. The spindles contain up to four nerve fibers that pierce the capsule and surround the muscle fibers.

neuromyal transmission, the passage of a nerve signal from a motor neuron to a muscle fiber at the place where nerves and muscles meet.

neuromyelitis /nŏŏr'ōmī'əlī'tis/, an abnormal condition marked by inflammation of the spinal cord and nearby nerves. See also **peripheral nervous system.**

neuron /nŏŏr'on/, the basic nerve cell of the nervous system. It contains a nucleus within a cell body with one or more fibers (axons or dendrites) extending from it. Neurons are named according to the direction in which they carry signals and to the number of fibers they extend. Sensory neurons carry nerve signals toward the spinal cord and brain. Motor neurons carry nerve signals from the brain and spinal cord to muscles and gland tissue. Usually multipolar neurons have one axon, to carry signals away from the cell body and several dendrites to carry signals toward the cell body. Most of the neurons in the brain and spinal cord are multipolar. Bipolar neurons, which are fewer than the other types, have only one axon and one dendrite. All neurons have at least one axon and one or more dendrites and are slightly gray in color when clustered, as in the brain and spinal cord. Also spelled **neurone.**

neuronitis /nŏŏr'ənī'tis/, an inflammation of a nerve or nerve cell, especially the cells and roots of spinal nerves.

neuropathic bladder. See **neurogenic bladder.**

neuropathic joint disease, a wasting disease of one or more joints marked by swelling, instability of the joint, bleeding, heat, and changes in bone tissue. Pain is usually less severe than would be expected for the damage to the joint. The disease results from an underlying disease, as syphilis, diabetes, leprosy, or a defect in pain sensation. Early recognition of the disease and guarding of the joint may prevent further damage. Surgery is seldom effective, and it may be necessary to cut off the limb. Also called **Charcot's joint.**

neuropathy /nŏŏrop'əthē/, any abnormal condition marked by swelling and wasting of the nerves, as that linked to lead poisoning. –**neuropathic,** *adj.*

neuroplegia /nŏŏr'ōplē'jē·ə/, nerve paralysis caused by disease, injury, or the effect of drugs given to achieve **neuroleptanalgesia** or **neuroleptanesthesia.** See also **lytic cocktail.**

neurosarcoma, a cancer made up of nerve tissue, connective tissue, and blood vessels. Also called **malignant neuroma.**

neurosis, 1. any faulty or inefficient way of handling worry or inner conflict. It usually involves using unconscious defense mechanisms that may finally lead to a neurotic disorder. An example is anorexia nervosa, which may begin as an unconscious defense against facing sexual maturity and leads to a life-threatening disorder requiring forced feeding and psychotherapy. 2. *informal.* an emotional disturbance other than psychosis. See also **neurotic disorder, neurotic process.**

neurosurgery, any surgery involving the brain, spinal cord, or nerves. Brain surgery is done to treat a wound, remove a growth or foreign body, relieve pressure on the brain caused by bleeding, cut out an infected sore, treat parkinsonism, or relieve pain. Kinds of brain surgery include craniotomy, lobotomy, hypophysectomy. Surgery of the spine is done to correct a defect, remove a growth, repair a ruptured disk, or relieve pain. Kinds of spinal surgery include fusion, laminectomy. Surgery on nerves is done to remove a growth, relieve pain, or join a cut nerve. One kind of nerve surgery is **sympathectomy.**

neurosyphilis, infection of the central nervous system by syphilis organisms. If the brain is affected, partial paralysis may result. If the spinal cord is infected, wasting of the spinal cord (tabes dorsalis) with severe pains in the arms and legs may result. See also **syphilis, tabes dorsalis. –neurosyphilitic,** *adj.*

neurotendinous spindle, a sheath of tendon and nerve fibers. Nerve fibers pierce the side of the capsule, subdivide, and end between the tendon fibers. The tendons with nerve endings respond more easily to stretching actions of muscle. Also called **organ of Golgi.**

neurotic, 1. referring to neurosis or to a neurotic disorder. 2. one who is afflicted with a neurosis. 3. *informal.* an emotionally unstable person.

neurotic disorder, any mental disorder marked by symptoms that are distressing, unacceptable, and foreign to one's personality. Examples include severe anxiety, obsessions, and compulsive acts. The ability to function may be affected, but behavior generally stays within acceptable norms and sense of reality is unchanged. There is no proof of a physical cause. The disorder is not simply a reaction to stress and may be long-lasting or return if untreated. Kinds of neurotic disorders include **anxiety neurosis, obsessive-compulsive neurosis, psychosexual disorder, somatoform disorder.** See also **neurosis, neurotic process.**

neurotic process, a process in which an unconscious conflict, as a struggle between an idealized self-image and the real self, leads to feelings of anxiety. Defense mechanisms are used to avoid these uncomfortable feelings. Personality change and the symptoms of neurosis result.

Neurotics Anonymous, a self-help group for persons with emotional problems, based on the format of Alcoholics Anonymous.

neurotmesis /noor'ōtmē'sis/, a nerve injury in which the nerve is completely cut by a wound or traction. It requires surgical repair, but recovery is unpredictable.

neurotoxic /noor'ōtok'sik/, anything having a poisonous effect on nerves and nerve cells, as the effect of lead on the brain and nerves.

neurotoxin /noor'ōtok'sin/, a poison that acts directly on the tissues of the central nervous system. It may move along the motor nerves to the brain, as the venom of certain snakes. Other examples are made by certain bacteria or by the cell breakdown of certain bacteria, as the botulism toxin or *Clostridium botulinum.*

neurotransmitter, any chemical that changes or results in the sending of nerve signals across spaces (synapses) separating nerve fibers. Neurotransmitter chemicals are released from knobs at the ends of axons into gaps between nerve fibers (synaptic clefts). Tiny sacks within these knobs each store thousands of neurotransmitter molecules. When a nerve signal reaches the knob, the neurotransmitter molecules squirt into the synaptic cleft and bind to receptors on the nearby nerve fiber. This flow lets the signal move across to the next nerve fiber. Kinds of neurotransmitters include **acetylcholine chloride, gamma-aminobutyric acid, norepinephrine.**

neutral, a state exactly between two opposing values, qualities, or properties, as when a substance is neither acid nor alkaline. See also **acid, base, pH.**

neutralization, the interaction between an acid and a base that makes a solution that is neither acidic nor basic. The usual products of neutralization are a salt and water.

neutral rotation, the placement of a leg or arm that is turned neither toward nor away from the body's middle. When lying on the back with the leg neutrally rotated, the toes should point straight up.

neutral thermal environment, an artificial environment that keeps the body temperature normal to save oxygen and body energy. An incubator or Isolette for a premature, sick, or low birth-weight infant creates such an environment. See also **incubator, Isolette.**

neutropenia /noo'trōpē'nē·ə/, an abnormal drop in the number of white blood cells (neutrophils) in the blood. Neutropenia is linked to leukemia, infections, rheumatoid arthritis, vitamin B_{12} deficiency, and a large spleen. Compare **leukopenia.** See also **neutrophil.**

neutrophil /noo'trəfil/, a grainlike white blood cell (leukocyte). Neutrophils are the circulating white blood cells necessary for removing or destroying bacteria, cell debris, and solid particles in the blood. An increase in neutrophils is the most common form of abnormally high levels of blood cells (leukocytosis) and may result from sudden infection, drunkenness, bleeding, and cancer.

neutrophilic leukemia. See **polymorphocytic leukemia.**

nevoid neuroma, a nerve tissue tumor that contains many small blood vessels. Also called **neuroma telangiectodes.**

nevus /nē′vəs/, a colored skin spot that is usually harmless but may become cancerous. Any change in color, size, or texture or any bleeding or itching of a nevus should be checked. Also called **birthmark, mole.** See also **blue nevus, junction nevus, nevus flammeus.**

nevus flammeus /flam′ē·əs/, a flat, blood vessel tumor that is present at birth and ranges in color from pale red to deep reddish purple. It is usually on the back of the head and rarely is a problem. On other parts of the body, it tends to be darker and, unlike the scalp tumor, does not resolve by itself. These tumors are most often on the face. The color varies with the skin depth of the blood vessels involved. On the face, the tumor stays and acquires a thick wartlike surface. Nevus flammeus is usually on only one side of the face and follows the nerve affecting the skin. Cosmetic creams can hide the tumor and special techniques, as cryotherapy, can improve the appearance of the rough skin. Laser therapy is an experimental treatment. Also called **port-wine stain.**

newborn, a recently born infant; neonate.

newborn intrapartal care, care of the newborn in the delivery area after birth and before the mother and infant move to the postbirth unit. During newborn intrapartal care, the throat and mouth of the infant are cleaned to remove excess mucus as the head is born. The baby is then put on the mother's stomach and covered with a warm, dry blanket or put by the nurse in an infant warmer. Apgar scores are given at 1 minute of age and at 5 minutes of age. Sometimes, another is given at 10 minutes of age. The baby is handled gently and quietly. Bright lights are often avoided, and contact with the mother is suggested. The nurse is usually the first person to examine the baby. Most newborns are healthy and do not need any medical care. If a baby has good color, is alert, can cry and suck, urinate, defecate, and respond to sound and light, the baby is almost always healthy and normal. If there are no problems, the nurse may put silver nitrate drops in the eyes, trim and clamp the umbilical cord, inject vitamin K, take footprints for identification, and diaper and wrap the baby. If abnormal function is seen, expert help may be called for as emergency measures are begun. Bleeding from the umbilical cord, hard breathing, and various other abnormal conditions may occur.

new drug, a drug for which the Food and Drug Administration needs proof of safety and effectiveness before its use is approved in the United States.

new growth, a tumor.

New World leishmaniasis. See **American leishmaniasis.**

New World typhus. See **murine typhus.**

Nezelof's syndrome /nez′əlofs/, an abnormal condition marked by a lack of immune responses and little or no specific making of antibodies. The cause of Nezelof's syndrome is not known. It affects both male and female brothers and sisters, pointing to a possible hereditary disorder. A theory is that it may be caused by lack of growth of the thymus gland, leading to a lack of thymus cells (T cells). Nezelof's syndrome causes increasingly severe, frequent, and finally fatal infections. Signs that often are seen in infants or in children up to 4 years of age include frequent pneumonia, middle ear infection, fungus infections, nose and throat infections, diarrhea, and a large spleen. The disease may make the lymph nodes and tonsils larger in some infants, but these structures may be totally lacking in others. Affected children may show a tendency to develop cancer. Infection is the usual cause of death. Initial treatment of Nezelof's syndrome may include monthly injections of gamma globulin or monthly infusions of fresh frozen blood plasma and the heavy use of antibiotics to fight infections. The plasma infusions are especially helpful if the patient cannot make certain immunoglobulins. Immune function linked to T cells can usually be temporarily restored within weeks by a fetal thymus transplant. Repeated transplants are needed to keep the immunity.

niacin /ni′əsin/, a white, crystal-like, vitamin of the B complex group that dissolves in water, usually found in various plant and animal tissues. It acts in the breakdown and use of all major foods. It is necessary for healthy skin, normal working of the stomach and intestinal tract, caring for the nervous system, and production of the sex hormones. It may also improve circulation and reduce high blood cholesterol levels. Rich sources of both niacin and its originator, tryptophan, are meats, poultry, fish, liver, kidney, eggs, nuts, peanut butter, brewer's yeast, and wheat germ. Symptoms of a lack include muscular weakness, general tiredness, loss of appetite, various skin spots, bad breath, swelling of the mouth, lack of sleep, irritability, nausea, vomiting, frequent headaches, tender gums, tension, and depression. A severe lack leads to a niacin deficiency syndrome (pellagra). The vitamin is not stored in the body and any excess in the diet is released. Also called **nicotinic acid.** See also **pellagra.**

niacinamide, a B complex vitamin. It is closely related to niacin but lacks blood vessel widening action. Also called **nicotinamide.**

nickel (Ni), a silvery-white metal element. Large numbers of people are allergic to nickel. Nickel causes more cases of allergic skin reaction (dermatitis) than all other metals combined.

nickel dermatitis, an allergic contact skin inflammation (dermatitis) caused by the metal, nickel. Exposure comes usually from jewelry, wristwatches, metal clasps, and coins. Sweating makes the rash worse. Treatment includes avoiding exposure to nickel and reducing sweating. See also **contact dermatitis.**

Niclocide, a trademark for a worming drug (niclosamide).

niclosamide /niklō'səmīd/, an antiworm (anthelmintic) drug given to treat beef tapeworm and fish tapeworm infestations.
★CAUTION: Known allergy to this drug prohibits its use. Its safety in pregnant or nursing mothers or small children has not been proven.
★ADVERSE EFFECTS: Among the most serious side effects are rectal bleeding, irregular heart rate, loss of hair, excess tissue fluid, nausea, and vomiting.

Nicobid, a trademark for two coenzymes (niacin and niacinamide) used as a vitamin supplement.

Nicorette, a trademark for a nicotine chewing gum used to help patients trying to quit cigarette smoking.

nicotinamide. See **niacinamide.**

nicotine, a colorless, quick-acting poison in tobacco that is one of the major reasons for the ill effects of smoking. It is used to fight insects in farming and to fight parasites in veterinary medicine. Swallowing large amounts of nicotine causes excess saliva, nausea, vomiting, diarrhea, headache, dizziness, slowing of the heart beat and, in severe cases, paralysis of breathing muscles. Treatment includes rinsing the stomach with a weak solution of potassium permanganate, followed by activated charcoal, and giving artificial respiration and oxygen, as needed. Pentobarbital is used to control seizures, ephedrine for low blood pressure, and nerve-blocking agents to control abdominal symptoms.

nicotine poisoning, poisoning from swallowing nicotine. In nicotine poisoning, excitement of the central and autonomic nervous systems is followed by depression of these systems. In fatal cases, death is from dysfunction of the breathing center.

nicotine polacrilex, a nicotine chewing gum used to help patients trying to quit cigarette smoking.
★CAUTION: Use by patients after a heart attack or those with severe or worsening chest pain (angina pectoris), or life-threatening changes in pattern of the heart beat (dys-

rhythmias) is prohibited. It should be used cautiously in patients with hyperactive thyroid, high blood pressure, insulin-dependent diabetes, or peptic ulcers. Drug dosages may have to be adjusted in patients taking other drugs whose effects may increase when the patient stops smoking. Patients should be monitored to ensure that they do not become dependent on the nicotine in the gum.
★ADVERSE EFFECTS: The most serious side effects include burning and soreness of the mouth, lightheadedness, headache, hiccups, nausea, vomiting, and excessive production of saliva.

nicotinic acid. See **niacin.**

nicotinyl alcohol /nik'ətē'nil/, an alcohol used as a blood-vessel widener to treat blood vessel disease, blood vessel spasm, varicose ulcers, bed sores, itching (chilblains), Ménière's syndrome, and dizziness.

nidation /nīdā'shən/, the process by which an embryo burrows into the membrane lining (endometrium) of the uterus. Also called **implantation.** See also **placenta, uterus.**

-nidazole, a combining form for substances used to treat diseases caused by protozoa (metronidazole-type).

NIDDM, abbreviation for **non-insulin-dependent diabetes mellitus.**

Niemann-Pick disease /nē'monpik'/, an inherited disorder of fat use in which a substance (sphingomyelin) collects in the bone marrow, spleen, and lymph nodes. The disease, which in North America is most common among Jewish people, begins in infancy or childhood. Effects include a large liver and spleen, anemia, swelling of lymph nodes, and slow mental and physical breakdown. There is no effective treatment, and children with the disease usually die within a few years of the beginning of symptoms. See also **sphingomyelin lipidosis.**

nifedipine, a coronary artery widening drug given to treat several types of chest pain (angina).
★CAUTION: Known allergy to this drug prohibits its use.
★ADVERSE EFFECTS: Among the more serious side effects are low blood pressure, irregular heart rate, difficult breathing, nausea, dizziness, flushing, and headache.

-nifur, a combining form for nitrofuran derivatives.

night blindness, poor vision at night or in dim light due to a lack of vitamin A, a birth defect, or other causes. Also called **day sight, nyctalopia.**

nightcare program, a medical service for patients who use hospital services regularly for some nighttime hours, although fulltime care in the hospital is not needed.

nightmare, a dream occurring during rapid eye movement (REM) sleep that brings out feelings of strong, inescapable fear, terror, distress, or extreme anxiety, usually awakening the sleeper. Compare **pavor nocturnus, sleep terror disorder.**

night vision, an ability to see dimly lit objects. It stems from a condition linked to the rod cells of the retina. The rods contain a highly light-sensitive chemical, rhodopsin, or visual purple, which is necessary for being able to see in dim light. Night vision is sharpest at the edge of the retina because of the grouping of rods there. Night vision may be reduced by a lack of vitamin A, an important part of rhodopsin.

nigrities linguae. See **parasitic glossitis.**

N.I.H., abbreviation for **National Institutes of Health.**

nikethamide /nīketh′əmīd/, a central nervous system-stimulating drug given to treat depression of the central nervous and respiratory systems.

★CAUTION: Known allergy to this drug prohibits its use.

★ADVERSE EFFECTS: Among the most serious side effects at high doses are rapid heart beat, high blood pressure, muscle spasms, and convulsions. General weakness and feeling of fear may also result.

Nikolsky's sign /nikol′skēz/, easy removal of the top layer (stratum corneum) of the skin from the bottom layer by rubbing apparently normal skin areas. It occurs in pemphigus and a few other blister-forming (bullous) diseases.

Nilstat, a trademark for an antifungus drug (nystatin).

NIMH, abbreviation for **National Institute of Mental Health.**

ninth cranial nerve. See **glossopharyngeal nerve.**

nipple, a small cylindric bump just below the center of each breast. The tip of the nipple has about 20 tiny openings to the milk (lactiferous) ducts, which carry milk from lobes where it is made. The skin of the nipple is surrounded by the skin of the areola. The color of the nipple and areola in women who have never been pregnant ranges from rosy pink to brown, depending on the skin color of the individual. In pregnancy, the skin of the nipple darkens but lightens again when nursing of the infant ends. Stimulation of the nipple in men, as well as women, causes it to become erect. In women the nipple becomes larger and more sensitive after puberty.

nipple cancer, a cancer of the nipple and areola that is usually linked to a cancer in another part of the breast. It usually starts in the nipple and spreads to the areola. Also called **Paget's disease of the nipple.**

nipple discharge, a sudden release of fluid from the nipple. It may be normal, as colostrum in pregnancy, or a sign of disease.

nipple shield, a device to guard the nipples of a nursing mother. It is usually made of soft rubber and has a tab on one side to hold it in place. The baby nurses from a nipple in the center of the shield. It is used to let sore or cracked nipples heal while milk is still being made. Also called **nipple protector.**

Nipride, a trademark for a blood vessel-widening drug (sodium nitroprusside).

niridazole /nirid′əzōl/, a drug used to treat a liver fluke (schistosomal) infection. In the United States it is available from the Centers for Disease Control.

nirvanic state /nirvä′nik, nirvan′ik/, (in Zen meditation) a state in which mental processes stop, often leading to a drastic change in personality.

Nissl body /nis′əl/, any of the large grainlike structures in the cytoplasm of nerve cells.

nit, the egg of a parasitic insect, as a louse. It may be found attached to human or animal hair or to clothing. See also **pediculosis.**

nitrazine paper, an absorbent strip of paper that turns specific colors when exposed to solutions of acid or base. Also called **pH paper.**

nitric acid /nī′trik/, a colorless, highly toxic acid that gives off suffocating brown fumes of nitrogen dioxide when exposed to air.

nitrite /nī′trīt/, a salt of nitrous acid used as a blood-vessel widener and to fight spasms. Among the nitrites used in medicine are amyl, ethyl, potassium, and sodium nitrite.

nitritoid reaction, a group of side effects, including low blood pressure, flushing, lightheadedness, and fainting, caused by medications containing arsenic or gold. It is similar to the effects of nitrites.

nitrobenzene poisoning, poisoning due to the absorption into the body of nitrobenzene, a pale yellow, oily liquid used in shoe dyes, soap, perfume, and artificial flavors. Exposure in industry is usually by breathing the fumes or absorbing it through the skin. Symptoms of sudden poisoning include headache, drowsiness, nausea, loss of muscle control, bluish skin color, and, in severe cases, breathing failure. Contaminated clothing is removed and the skin is washed with vinegar, followed by soap and water. Oxygen, blood transfusion, and, in severe cases, blood cleansing (hemodialysis) may be needed. Long-term exposure to nitrobenzene on the job may cause headache, weakness, loss of appetite, and anemia.

Nitrobid, a trademark for a coronary artery-widening drug (nitroglycerin), used to treat chest pain (angina pectoris) caused by heart problems.

nitrofuran, one of a group of antimicrobial drugs used to treat infections caused by protozoa or by certain bacteria. Nitrofurazone, one of the drugs, is used to treat skin wounds and infections, particularly burns. Furazolidone is used to treat bacterial and protozoal diarrhea and swelling of the intestines (enteritis). Nitrofurantoin is used to treat urinary tract infections. Use of nitrofuran drugs internally is linked to many side effects, the most common being nausea and diarrhea. Serious side effects include nerve disorders, allergic reactions, lung swelling, and blood abnormalities. Nitrofurans can cause anemia in some patients.

nitrofurantoin /nī′trōfyo͞oran′tō·in/, an antibiotic given to treat certain urinary tract infections. ★CAUTION: Kidney disorders or known allergy to this drug prohibits its use. It is not given to children under 1 year of age or to pregnant or nursing women. ★ADVERSE EFFECTS: Among the most serious side effects is lung inflammation that can lead to the making of fiberlike material (fibrosis), nervous system disorders, and anemia in certain patients. Stomach and intestinal disturbances and fever are common.

nitrofurazone, an antibiotic given to prevent and treat infection in second- and third-degree burns and to treat infections of the skin and mucous membranes. ★CAUTION: Known allergy to this drug prohibits its use. ★ADVERSE EFFECTS: Among the most serious side effects are severe allergic reactions and new infections.

nitrogen (N), an element that is a gas at normal temperatures. Nitrogen makes up about 78% of the atmosphere and is a part of all proteins and of most physical substances. Nitrogen follows a cycle from a gas in the atmosphere into certain bacteria and then into green plants. The plants are eaten by animals and humans, and by decay or waste the nitrogen goes back into the soil. In a 24-hour period the nitrogen released by a healthy person in the urine, feces, and sweat, together with nitrogen kept in skin and hair, equals the nitrogen taken in food and drink. The process of protein use explains this nitrogen balance. Nitrogen compounds, as nitroglycerin amyl nitrite, are blood vessel wideners (vasodilators) often used to relieve symptoms of chest pain (angina pectoris), but exactly how they work is not known.

nitrogen balance, the relationship between nitrogen taken into the body, usually as food, and nitrogen released from the body in urine and feces. Most of the body's nitrogen is blended into protein. Positive nitrogen balance occurs when the intake of nitrogen products for making tissue is greater than the nitrogen released. Negative nitrogen balance occurs when more nitrogen is released than is taken in, causing the waste or destruction of tissue.

nitroglycerin, a coronary artery-widening drug (vasodilator) given for the prevention or relief of chest pain (angina pectoris). ★CAUTION: Known allergy to this drug prohibits its use. ★ADVERSE EFFECTS: Among the most serious side effects are falling blood pressure, flushing, headache, and fainting.

nitrosamines, compounds that may cause cancer, produced by reactions of nitrates with certain substances normally present in the body. They are produced by bacteria in saliva and in the intestine from nitrates in vegetables and in nitrate-treated fish, poultry, and meats. More than 70% of nitrates consumed are from vegetables.

nitrosourea /nītrō′sōyo͞oorē′ə/, an anticancer drug used to treat brain tumors, bone tumors, Hodgkin's disease, gland cancers, liver tumors, long-term leukemias, and cancers of the breast and ovaries. They have been less successful in treating cancers of the lungs, head, neck, and stomach and intestinal tract. Like other anticancer drugs, they can have severe side effects, including bone marrow disorders. Nausea and vomiting are common side effects. Carmustine and lomustine are typical examples of this group of drugs. See also **alkylating agent.**

Nitrospan, a trademark for a coronary artery dilator (nitroglycerin).

Nitrostat, a trademark for a coronary artery-widening drug (vasodilator) (nitroglycerin).

nitrous oxide (N_2O), a gas used as an anesthetic in dentistry, surgery, and childbirth. It gives light anesthesia, delivered in various mixtures with oxygen. Nitrous oxide does not provide deep-enough anesthesia to be used alone for major surgery. It is not given to patients with a lack of oxygen in the blood, lung disease, or intestinal blockage.

Nizoral, a trademark for an antifungus drug (ketoconazole).

NMR, abbreviation for **nuclear magnetic resonance.**

NMR imaging, the use of nuclear magnetic resonance (NMR) techniques to make pictures of the internal structure and reactions of the body. It uses the nuclei of the hydrogen atom, the most common element in the body, and a part of all body tissues. Radio waves sent at the body make the hydrogen nuclei give off light particles (photons), which form an NMR signal. A computer uses the NMR signal to make an image of the internal body that is as good or better than x-ray films.

Nocardia /nōkär′dē·ə/, a genus of bacteria, some species of which cause disease, as *Nocardia asteroides*, which causes a fungal infection of the feet (madura foot). See also **nocardiosis.**

nocardiosis /nōkär′dē·ō′sis/, an infection marked by pneumonia and by abscesses in the brain and tissues under the skin. The organism enters the breathing tract and spreads by the bloodstream. Surgical drainage of sores and sulfonamide therapy for 12 to 18 months may be necessary. Without treatment the disease is usually fatal.

nociceptive /no'sēsep'tiv/, referring to a nerve that receives painful stimuli.

nociceptor, a free nerve ending that usually reacts to tissue injury, but may also be stimulated by chemical substances in the body.

no code, a note written in a patient record telling the staff members not to attempt to revive the patient in case of heart or lung failure. It is signed by a qualified, usually senior or attending, physician. This note is usually given only when a patient is so seriously ill that death is near and cannot be avoided. Also called **DNR.**

noctambulation. See **somnambulism.**

nocturia /noktŏŏr'ē·ə/, urination, especially excess urination at night. It may be a symptom of prostate or kidney disease, or it may occur in persons who drink excess amounts of fluids, especially alcohol or coffee, before bedtime. Also called **nycturia.** Compare **enuresis.**

nocturnal, 1. referring to or occurring at night. **2.** describing an individual or animal that is active at night and sleeps during the day.

nocturnal emission, involuntary release of semen during sleep, usually linked to an erotic dream. Also called **wet dream.**

nocturnal paroxysmal dyspnea, an abnormal condition of the breathing system in which sudden attacks of shortness of breath, heavy sweating, rapid heart beat, and wheezing awaken the patient from sleep. The attacks may be caused by nightmares, noises, or coughing. It is usually linked to heart failure or fluid in the lungs, and is relieved by getting up and opening a window. See also **dyspnea.**

nodal event, an event that may cause anxiety, as birth, death, divorce, marriage, or a child leaving home.

node, 1. a small, rounded mass. **2.** a lymph node.

nodular, a small, firm, knotty structure or mass. See also **node, nodule.**

nodular cutaneous angiitis, an inflammatory condition of small arteries, with tumors of the skin.

nodular melanoma, a skin tumor that is usually bluish-black and nodelike and sometimes surrounded by an area of pale, uncolored skin. The tumor is always raised and may be dome-shaped. Most often found in adults in middle age, it is one of the three major types of melanoma, occurring in 10% to 15% of melanoma patients. See also **lentigo-maligna melanoma, superficial spreading melanoma.**

nodule, a small node or nodelike structure.

noise pollution, in an environment, a noise level that is uncomfortable.

Noludar, a trademark for a sedative (methyprylon).

Nolvadex, a trademark for a breast cancer drug (tamoxifen).

noma /nō'mə/, a sudden ulcer disease of the mucous membranes of the mouth or genitals. The condition is most often seen in children with poor nutrition and cleanliness. There is rapid and painless breakdown of bone and soft tissue along with a bad odor. Bacteria may be involved. Healing eventually occurs but often with disfiguring defects. Also called **gangrenous stomatitis.**

non-A, non-B (NANB) hepatitis, viral hepatitis that is caused by a virus other than the types that cause hepatitis A or hepatitis B. It caused more than 90% of the cases of hepatitis in the United States, occurring in patients receiving multiple blood transfusions. NANB hepatitis is usually milder than types A or B but is otherwise similar, and treatment is the same as for other forms.

nonadhesive skin traction, a kind of skin traction in which foam-backed traction straps that do not stick to the skin are used to attack traction weights. They are usually used when only temporary traction is needed. The straps spread the traction pull over a wide area of the skin surface and decrease the risk of skin damage to the patient. Compare **adhesive skin traction.**

nonbacterial thrombic endocarditis, a type of heart muscle inflammation (endocarditis) with tissue growth that affects the heart valves. It may be the first step in the development of bacterial endocarditis. The valve growths may cause blood clots that result in death. This disease affects equal numbers of men and women of all ages. It causes heart murmurs in about 30% of the cases, and tends to affect the valves on the left side of the heart. There is no successful treatment of nonbacterial thrombic endocarditis. Blood-thinning (anticoagulant) drugs may reduce the risk of arterial blood clots. See also **Libman-Sacks endocarditis.**

noncompliance, the failure of a patient to follow a physician's medical advice. The patient may have a health belief, a cultural or spiritual value, an economic difficulty, or a personal problem with the physician, which results in missing appointments or not using drugs as ordered.

non compos mentis, a legal term applied to a person declared to be mentally incompetent.

nondirective therapy, a psychotherapeutic approach in which the psychotherapist does not give advice or interpret. Instead, the patient is helped to identify conflicts and to understand his or her own feelings and values. Compare **directive therapy.** See also **client-centered therapy.**

nondisjunction, failure of matching pairs of chromosomes to split properly during cell division (meiosis or mitosis). As a result, the daughter cells do not receive a matching set of complete chromosomes. One daughter cell usually receives an extra chromosome and the other daughter cell lacks a complete set. Nondisjunction causes many birth defects. Compare **disjunction**. See also **monosomy, trisomy**.

nonfat milk. See **skimmed milk**.

nongonococcal urethritis (NGU), an infection of the urethra marked by a mild urination problem and a small to moderate amount of discharge. The discharge may be white or clear, thin or mucuslike, with pus cells. The infection is often caused by a parasite, *Chlamydia trachomatis*. Untreated NGU may result in urethral narrowing, swelling of the prostate and epididymis, and long-term swelling of the urethra in males. Women may develop wasting of the cervix and pus-filled cervical mucus. An infant passing through the cervix and vagina of a mother infected with *C. trachomatis* may develop eye, nose, and throat infections in the first few days after birth and pneumonia at 3 to 4 months of age. Most cases of NGU are successfully treated with antibiotics. Sexual partners should be treated whether or not they have symptoms. Nearly 50% of all cases of an inflamed urethra are nongonococcal. See also **nonspecific urethritis**.

non-Hodgkin's lymphoma, any kind of cancer of the lymph tissues other than Hodgkin's disease. Also called **lymphosarcoma**.

non-insulin-dependent diabetes mellitus (NIDDM), a type of diabetes mellitus in which patients are not dependent on injections of insulin. They are not likely to develop ketosis although they may use insulin for correction of symptoms, as excess sugar in the blood (hyperglycemia). They also can develop ketosis during infection or stress. The disease usually begins after 40 years of age, but can occur at any age. About 60% to 90% of patients are overweight. In these patients, the condition is often improved by weight loss. There are probably several causes for the development of diabetes mellitus. One is that the patient is born with the likelihood of getting it. Environment and lifestyle along with this likelihood probably start the symptoms. Previously called adult onset diabetes, ketosis-resistant diabetes, maturity onset diabetes, maturity onset type diabetes, MOD, stable diabetes. Also called **Type II diabetes mellitus**. See also **diabetes mellitus, ketosis**.

noninvasive, referring to a test or treatment that does not require the skin to be broken or a cavity or organ of the body to be entered, as taking a blood pressure reading with a stethoscope and sphygmomanometer.

nonionizing radiation, radiation that does not make the tissue radioactive.

nonosteogenic fibroma /non'ostē-əjen'ik/, a common bone tumor, usually affecting the ends of the large long bones. It often does not cause symptoms and is only discovered during x-ray tests made for other reasons.

nonproductive cough, a cough caused by irritation or inflammation that does not clear the breathing tract. Certain cough drugs, as ammonium chloride, potassium iodide, and terpin hydrate, increase breathing tract sputum and may cause productive coughing. If one needs to stop the coughing, cough medicines (antitussives) that stop the cough reflex may be given, including codeine or dextromethorphan. Cleaning the throat may be necessary when sputum causes severe breathing difficulty and coughing is nonproductive. Compare **productive cough**.

nonprotein nitrogen (NPN), the nitrogen in the blood that is not a part of protein. Examples include the nitrogen linked to urea and uric acid. About 50% of the nonprotein nitrogen in the blood is linked to urea. Measurement of NPN is part of tests of kidney function.

nonrapid eye movement (NREM). See **sleep**.

nonreflex bladder. See **flaccid bladder**.

nonshivering thermogenesis, a natural method by which newborns can produce body heat by increasing the amount of energy used.

nonspecific urethritis (NSU), an inflammation of the urethra not known to be caused by a specific disease organism. The start of symptoms is often linked to sexual intercourse. The sudden phase is not often seen in women, but a long-term phase is a common urinary tract problem among them. The condition is marked by urethral discharge in men and by reddening of the urethral mucosa in women. Treatment with antibiotics is not always successful. See also **nongonoccal urethritis**.

nonstress test (NST), an evaluation of the response of the heart rate of the fetus to natural contractions or to an increase in fetal activity.

nonthrombocytopenic purpura, a disorder marked by purplish or reddish skin areas that does not involve a decrease in the number of platelets in the blood.

nontoxic, not poisonous. Also called **atoxic**.

nontropical sprue, a condition due to an inborn inability to digest foods that contain gluten. See also **celiac disease**.

nonulcerative blepharitis, a condition of greasy scales on the edges of the eyelids around the lashes, and increased blood (hyperemia) and thickening of the skin. Nonulcerative blepharitis is often linked to greasiness (seborrhea) of the scalp, eyebrows, and the skin behind the ears.

nonverbal communication, the sending of a message without the use of words. It may involve any or all of the five senses. See also **body language**.

Noonan's syndrome, a disorder occurring only in males, marked by short stature, low-set ears, webbing of the neck, and skeletal problems. Testicular function may be normal, but fertility is often decreased. The XY karyotype is normal. The cause is unknown. See also **Turner's syndrome.**

norepinephrine /nôr'epinef'rin/, a hormone that increases blood pressure by blood vessel narrowing but does not affect the heart's output. It is released by the adrenal glands and is available also as a drug, levarterenol, given to keep normal the blood pressure in severe cases of low blood pressure.

norepinephrine bitartrate, a blood vessel narrowing drug given to treat heart and circulation disorders.
★CAUTION: Low blood volume, blood clotting (coagulation) disorders, or known allergy to this drug prohibits its use.
★ADVERSE EFFECTS: Among the more serious side effects are local tissue death at the injection site, abnormally slow heart beat, headache, and high blood pressure.

norethindrone /nôreth'indrōn/, a hormone given to treat abnormal uterine bleeding and endometriosis. It is a part of birth-control pills.
★CAUTION: Blood clotting (coagulation) difficulties, liver disease, unusual vaginal bleeding, breast cancer, missed abortion, or known allergy to this drug prohibits its use. It should not be used during pregnancy.
★ADVERSE EFFECTS: Among the more serious side effects are breakthrough bleeding, lack of menstruation, stomach and intestinal problems, breast changes, and male features in a female fetus.

norethindrone acetate and ethinyl estradiol, a female sex hormone combination given for birth control, endometriosis, and excess menstrual bleeding.
★CAUTION: Blood clotting (coagulation) disorders, heart disease, breast or reproductive organ cancer, unusual vaginal bleeding, gallbladder disease, liver tumor, or known allergy to this drug prohibits its use. It is not given to women over 40 years of age or during breast feeding, pregnancy, or suspected pregnancy. It is given carefully to women who smoke.
★ADVERSE EFFECTS: Among the more serious side effects are blood clots, uterine tumors, porphyria disturbances (porphyria), liver disease (jaundice), and stroke.

Norflex, a trademark for a skeletal muscle relaxant and antihistamine (orphenadrine citrate).

Norgesic Forte /nôrjē'zik fôrt'/, a trademark for a drug containing a muscle relaxant (orphenadrine citrate) and APC (aspirin, phenacetin, and caffeine), used to relieve mild to moderate pain of short-term muscle and bone disorders.

norgestrel /nôrjes'trəl/, a hormone given alone or with estrogen as a birth-control drug.
★CAUTION: Blood clotting, liver dysfunction, unusual vaginal bleeding, breast cancer,

missed abortion, or known allergy to this drug prohibits its use.
★ADVERSE EFFECTS: Among the more serious side effects are lack of menstrual flow, abnormal uterine bleeding, breast changes, and male features in a female fetus.

Norinyl, a trade name for a birth control drug containing a progestin (norethindrone) and an estrogen (mestranol).

Norlestrin, a trade name for a birth-control drug containing an estrogen (ethinyl estradiol) and a progestin (norethindrone acetate).

Norlutin, a trade name for a progestin (norethindrone).

norma basalis, the base of the skull with the lower jaw removed.

normal, 1. describing a usual, regular, or typical example of a set of objects or values. **2.** referring to persons in a nondiseased population.

normal dental function, the correct and healthy action of opposing teeth during chewing.

normal diet. See **regular diet.**

normal dwarf. See **primordial dwarf.**

normal human serum albumin, a solution made from proteins taken from healthy donors used to treat low blood protein, low blood volume, or shock.

normoblast /nôr'məblast/, an immature red blood cell that still has a nucleus. After the nucleus is released, the young red blood cell (erythrocyte) becomes known as a reticulocyte. Compare **erythrocyte.** See also **reticulocyte.** **–normoblastic,** *adj.*

normochromic /nôr'məkrō'nik/, referring to a red blood cell of normal color, usually because it contains the right amount of hemoglobin. Compare **hypochromic.** See also **red cell indices.**

normocyte /nôr'məsīt/, an ordinary, normal, adult red blood cell of average size.

Normodyne, a trademark for a drug (labetalol hydrochloride) used to treat high blood pressure.

normoglycemic, referring to a normal blood glucose level.

normotensive, referring to normal blood pressure. **–normotension,** *n.*

Norpace, a trade name for a drug given to correct abnormal heart rates (disopyramide phosphate).

Norpramin, a trademark for an antidepressant (desipramine hydrochloride).

Nor-QD, a trademark for a birth-control drug containing a progestin (norethindrone) but no estrogen.

North American blastomycosis, an infection caused by breathing the fungus *Blastomyces dermatitidis.* It may resemble bacterial pneumonia. Painless, wartlike, or ulcerated skin tumors occur on the face and hands. The disease may involve bones and the brain; many abdominal organs can be infected. Treatment is with an antifungus drug, amphotericin B, or, in severe cases, a combination of amphotericin B and sulfonamides. Also called **Gilchrist's disease.** Compare **paracoccidioidomycosis.**

North Asian tick borne rickettsiosis, an infection caught in Asia from Armenia to Mongolia. Caused by *Rickettsia siberica,* it is carried by ticks, and is like Rocky Mountain spotted fever with a pimply rash on the palms and soles, fever, and large lymph nodes. Rarely fatal, it responds quickly to treatment with chloramphenicol. No vaccine is available. Also called **Siberian tick typhus.** See also **boutonneuse fever, relapsing fever.**

Northern blot test, a test for identifying the presence or absence of particular mRNA molecules and nucleic acid hybridization. See also **Southern blot test.**

nortriptyline hydrochloride, an antidepressant given to treat mental depression.
★CAUTION: Taking monoamine oxidase inhibitors at the same time, recent heart attack, or known allergy to this drug or to related drugs prohibits its use. It is used carefully in patients with a seizure disorder or a heart disease.
★ADVERSE EFFECTS: Among the more serious side effects are drowsiness and stomach and intestinal, heart, and nervous system reactions. This drug interacts with many other drugs.

nose, a structure on the front of the skull that is a passageway for air to and from the lungs. The nose filters the air, warming, moistening, and checking it for foreign bodies that might irritate the lining of the breathing tract. The nose is the organ of smell and aids in speaking. The external portion, which grows out of the face, is much smaller than the internal portion, which lies over the roof of the mouth. The hollow interior portion is divided by a wall (septum) into a right and a left cavity. Each cavity is subdivided into a top, middle, and bottom opening by bony ridges (nasal conchae). The external nose has two nostrils and the internal portion has two rear nostrils (posterior nares). Four pairs of sinuses drain into the nose. Mucous membrane with hairlike projections (cilia) lines the nose. The mucous membrane contains the smelling (olfactory) cells that connect with the nerves needed for the sense of smell.

nosebleed, abnormal bleeding from the nose. Emergency treatment includes seating the patient upright with the head held forward to prevent swallowing blood. Pressing both thumbs directly under the nostril and above the lips may block the blood supply to the nose. Pressure with both forefingers on each side of the nostril often slows bleeding by blocking the main arteries and their branches. If bleeding continues, insert cotton or other absorbent material into the nostril and press on the arteries to slow bleeding. Cold com-

presses on the nose, lips, and the back of the head often help control bleeding. Continued bleeding needs treatment by a physician. Also called **epistaxis.**

NOSIE, abbreviation for *nurses' observation scale for inpatient evaluation.*

nosocomial /nos′əkō′mē·əl/, referring to a hospital.

nosocomial infection, an infection aquired during hospitalization. Also called **hospital-acquired infection.**

nostrils. See **anterior nares.**

notch, a gap or a depression in a bone or other organ, as the sciatic notch, a groove in the hipbone.

notifiable, referring to conditions, diseases, and events that must, by law, be reported to a government agency. Examples include birth, death, smallpox, serious communicable diseases, and certain violations of public health regulations.

notomelus /nətom′ələs/, a birth defect in which one or more extra limbs are attached to the back.

nourish, to furnish or supply the necessary foods for maintaining life.

nourishment, any substance that nourishes and supports the life and growth of a person.

Novahistine, a trade name for a drug containing an antihistamine (chlorpheniramine maleate) and a decongestant (phenylpropanolamine).

Novocain, a trade name for a local anesthetic (procaine hydrochloride).

noxious /nok′shəs/, something that is harmful, causes injury, or endangers health.

NPH Iletin, a trademark for an insulin (isophane).

NPO, abbreviation for a Latin phrase *non per os* meaning "nothing through the mouth."

NREM, abbreviation for **nonrapid eye movement.** See also **sleep.**

Nubain, a trade name for an artificial painkiller (nalbuphine hydrochloride) used with an anesthetic.

nucha /nōō′kə/, *pl.* **nuchae,** the back of the neck (nape). **–nuchal,** *adj.*

nuchal cord, a condition in which the umbilical cord is wrapped around the neck of the fetus in the uterus or as it is being born. Usually the loop or loops of cord are gently slipped over the infant's head. The shoulders may come through a single loose loop. The condition occurs in more than 25% of births, more often with long cords than with short ones.

nuchal rigidity, a resistance to bending of the neck, seen in patients with meningitis.

nuclear family, a family unit made up of the biological parents and their children. Breakup of a marriage results in breakup of the nuclear family. The nuclear family is less efficient than an extended family in providing necessary services to family members, as in raising children and care of older family members. Compare **extended family, matrifocal family.**

nuclear family emotional system, the organization of interaction between family members and how much these patterns promote unity.

nuclear fission. See **fission.**

nuclear hyaloplasm. See **karyolymph.**

nuclear magnetic resonance (NMR), a situation in which the nuclei of certain atoms (phosphorous) in a strong magnetic field will absorb radio waves. The energy of the radio waves absorbed by the nucleus causes release of light particles that form an image of organs and processes inside the body. See also **NMR imaging.**

nuclear medicine, a branch of medicine that uses radioactive chemical elements (isotopes) in the diagnosis and treatment of disease.

nuclear problem, (in psychology) an underlying reason for a person's reaction to an event.

nuclear sap. See **karyolymph.**

nuclear scanning, a method of medical diagnosis. The size, shape, location, and function of various body parts is seen using radioactive material and a device that senses the radioactivity in the body. Also called **radionuclide organ imaging.**

nucleic acid /nōōklē'ik/, a chemical compound involved in making and storing energy, and carrying hereditary characteristics. Kinds of nucleic acid are **deoxyribonucleic acid, ribonucleic acid.** See also **nucleotide.**

nucleocapsid /nōō'klē·ōkap'sid/, a capsulelike protein coat that surrounds nucleic acid. Some viruses are made only of bare nucleocapsids.

nucleocytoplasmic /nōō'klē·ōsī'tōplas'mik/, relating to both the nucleus and cytoplasm of a cell.

nucleocytoplasmic ratio, the balance between the nucleus and the cytoplasm of a cell. This balance is usually steady for a certain cell type. An increase in the nucleus is a sign of cancer. Also called **karyoplasmic ratio, nucleoplasmic ratio.**

nucleolus /nōōklē'ələs/, pl. **nucleoli** /nōōklē'əli/, any of the small, dense structures made up mostly of ribonucleic acid and located in the cytoplasm of cells. Nucleoli are needed to make cell proteins.

nucleon, a term applied to protons and neutrons within the nucleus.

nucleophilic, referring to some molecules (nucleic acids and proteins) with electrons that can be shared and thus form bonds with alkylating agents.

nucleoplasm /nōō'klē·əplaz'əm/, the protoplasm of the nucleus, as opposed to the protoplasm of the cell outside of the nucleus. Also called **karyoplasm.** Compare **cytoplasm.** **–nucleoplasmic,** adj.

nucleotide /nōō'klē·ətīd/, any of the parts into

which nucleic acid is split by the action of the enzyme nuclease.

nucleus /nōō'klē·əs, nyōō'-/, **1.** the main controlling body in a living cell, usually surrounded by a membrane. It contains genetic codes for continuing life systems of the organism and for controlling growth and reproduction. **2.** a group of nerve cells of the central nervous system that have the same function, as supporting the sense of hearing or smell.

nucleus pulposus, the central part of each disk between the vertebrae. It consists of a rubbery substance that loses some ability to recover from strain with age. In elderly persons, the nucleus pulposus may be suddenly put under pressure by unusual exercise or by injury, and squeeze out through the cartilage, causing a protruding disk and extreme pain.

Nuhn's gland, a gland in tissues on the bottom and near the tip of the tongue.

null cell, a kind of white blood cell (lymphocyte) that grows in bone marrow. Stimulated by an antibody, these cells can apparently attack certain cells directly and are known as "killer," or K, cells. Compare **B cell, T cell.** See also **cytotoxin, immune gamma globulin.**

nulligravida /nul'igrav'ədə/, a woman who has never been pregnant.

nullipara /nəlip'ərə/, pl. **nulliparae,** a woman who has not given birth to a living infant. The term "para 0" means nulliparity. Compare **multipara, primapara.** **–nulliparity,** n., **nulliparous,** adj.

numbness, a partial or total lack of feeling in a part of the body, due to anything that interrupts the sending of signals from sensory nerve fibers. Numbness is often seen with tingling.

nummular dermatitis /num'yələr/, a skin disease marked by round blisters or eczemalike tumors on the forearms and front of the calves. The cause is unknown.

Numorphan Hydrochloride, a trademark for a narcotic painkiller (oxymorphone hydrochloride).

Nupercainal, a trademark for a local anesthetic (dibucaine hydrochloride).

Nuremberg tribunal, an international court created by the United Nations War Crimes Commission to find, catch, try, and punish persons accused of war crimes during World War II. It led to the writing of laws governing the use of human beings in medical research. The court found Nazi physicians guilty of crimes against humanity in doing experiments on human beings who were not volunteers and who did not consent. See also **Helsinki accords.**

nurse, a person educated and licensed in the practice of nursing. See also **nursing, registered nurse.**

nurse anesthetist, a registered nurse qualified by advanced training to manage the anesthetic care of a patient in some surgical situations.

nurse midwife, a registered nurse qualified by special training in childbirth and newborn infant care. The nurse midwife manages the care of women having a normal pregnancy, labor, and childbirth.

nursery diarrhea, diarrhea of the newborn. In nurseries, outbreaks of diarrhea due to certain bacteria or viruses can be life-threatening to an infant. The newborn may be infected at birth by the mother's stool or infected later by the hands of hospital workers. Care includes restoring fluid and mineral balance and giving antibiotics.

nurse's aide, a person who does basic nonmedical tasks in the care of a patient, as bathing and feeding, making beds, and moving patients.

nurses' observation scale for inpatient evaluation (NOSIE), a systematic, objective scale used by nurses to rate patient behavior.

nurses' station, an area in a clinic, unit, or hospital ward that is the administrative center for nursing care for a certain group of patients.

nursing, 1. acting as a nurse, giving care that encourages and promotes the health of the patient being served. **2.** breast feeding an infant.

nursing assessment, noting by a nurse of the needs, desires, and abilities of a patient. Assessment includes the symptoms and signs of the condition, the patient's spoken and nonspoken communication, medical history, and any other information available. Among the physical aspects noted are temperature and blood pressure, skin color and condition, physical and sensory nerve function, nutrition, rest, sleep, activity, urination and defecation, and level of consciousness. Assessment is important because it gives the scientific basis for a complete nursing care plan.

nursing-bottle caries, tooth decay that occurs in children between 18 months and 3 years of age who are given a bottle at bedtime. It results in excess exposure of the teeth to milk or juice. Cavities (caries) form because pools of milk or juice may become food for acid-making bacteria. The acid destroys tooth enamel. Preventive measures include stopping the bedtime feeding or giving water instead of milk or juice in the nighttime bottle. Also called **bottle-mouth syndrome.**

nursing health history, information collected by nurses about a patient's current health, changes-in-life patterns, social and cultural roles, and mental and emotional responses to illness.

nursing home. See **extended care facility.**

nursing observation, an objective note made by a nurse of the various aspects of a patient's condition.

nursing process, the process that is a basis for the practice of nursing. It includes all of the steps taken by the nurse in caring for a patient: information collection, diagnosis, planning, treatment, and evaluation.

nursing specialty, a nurse's particular professional field of practice, as surgical, pediatric, obstetric, or psychiatric nursing.

nursing theory, a framework of concepts and purposes designed to guide the practice of nursing.

Nursoy, a trademark for an allergy-free (hypoallergenic) food supplement for infants.

nurture, to feed, rear, foster, or care for, as in the nourishment, care, and training of growing children.

nutation, nodding, especially involuntary nodding due to some nervous system disorders.

nutcracker esophagus. See **symptomatic esophageal peristalsis.**

Nutramigen, a trademark for a milk substitute formula made from a soybean product and is milk sugar (lactose)-free. It is given to infants who are unable to absorb a substance in milk (galactosemia) and as a protein supplement for patients who cannot digest lactose. See also **Pro Sobee, Soyalac.**

nutrient, a substance that provides nourishment and aids in the growth and development of the body.

nutrient artery of the humerus, one of a pair of branches of the arteries near the middle of the arm.

nutrition, 1. nourishment. **2.** the sum of the steps involved in taking in nutrients and in their use by the body for proper functioning and health. The stages are ingestion, digestion, absorption, assimilation, and excretion. **3.** the study of food and drink as related to the growth and health of living organisms.

nutritional anemia, a disorder marked by inadequate making of red blood cells due to a lack of iron, folic acid, or vitamin B_{12}, or other food disorders. See also **iron deficiency anemia, megaloblastic anemia, pernicious anemia.**

nutritional care, the procedures involved in getting the proper foods, especially for the hospitalized patient. Depending on the patient's condition, food needs may be met by regular meals with menus selected from the ordered diet, by tube feeding, or by feeding through a vein (intravenous). Patients who are unable to feed themselves are assisted. Additional foods, when ordered by a physician, and fluids are offered between meals. Tooth cavities, loose teeth or dentures, gum problems, nausea, vomiting, diarrhea, or constipation may affect food care. If indicated, as may be with overweight patients or those with disorders needing a highly restricted diet, the intake of food is limited.

nutrition alteration: less than body requirements, a condition of poor nutrition due to an inability, based on psychological, biological, or other factors, to swallow or to digest food or to absorb nutrients in the right amount for normal health. The characteristics of the condition may include loss of weight, eating less food than is necessary, lack of interest in food, change in the taste of food, feelings of fullness right after eating small amounts, stomach pain for no other reason, sores in the mouth, diarrhea, pale skin, weakness, and loss of hair.

nutrition alteration: more than body requirements, a condition of poor nutrition due to an excess intake of food in relation to the needs of the body. The characteristics of the condition include excess weight, low activity level, and bad eating habits, as eating when not hungry. The main characteristics, one of which must be present for the diagnosis to be made, include weight gain of 20% greater than the ideal for the height and body build of the patient, and triceps skin fold measurements greater than 15 mm (¾ inch) in men and 25 mm (1 inch) in women.

nutrition alteration: potential for more than body requirements, an inherited or familial likelihood to become overweight. It may begin as an excess intake of calories during adolescence and other periods of rapid growth, frequent, closely spaced pregnancies, and faulty attitudes toward food and eating. The problem may include the use of solid foods as a major part of the diet before 5 months of age, using food as a reward, an increase in the beginning weight at the start of each pregnancy, or bad eating patterns, as eating in response to social situations or the time of day. The main characteristics include excess weight in one or both parents and rapidly increasing measurements of the infant's or child's weight as compared to others of the same age.

nutritionist, one who studies and puts into practice the rules and science of nutrition.

nyctalopia. See **night blindness.**

nycto-, a combining form referring to night or darkness.

nyctophobia /nik'tō-/, an obsessive, irrational fear of darkness.

nycturia. See **nocturia.**

nylidrin hydrochloride /nil'idrin/, a blood vessel-widening drug given to treat circulation problems of the skin and inner ear.

★CAUTION: Sudden heart disease, rapid heart beat, Graves' disease (thyrotoxicosis), chest pain (angina pectoris), or known allergy to this drug prohibits its use.

★ADVERSE EFFECTS: The most serious side effect is falling blood pressure with dizziness, rapid heart beat, nausea, and weakness.

nymphomania, a psychosexual disorder of women marked by an excessive desire for sexual satisfaction, often due to an unconscious conflict, as a desire to disprove lesbianism or frigidity. See also **psychosexual disorder.**

nystagmus /nīstag'məs/, involuntary, rhythmic movements of the eyes back and forth, up and down, around, or mixed. Jerking nystagmus, marked by faster movements in one direction than in the opposite direction, is the most common. Pendular nystagmus has eye movements that are about equal in both directions. Jerking nystagmus occurs normally when a person watches a moving object. It may be a sign of barbiturate overdose or of another disorder. A disorder of the inner ear may cause rolling eye movements and is usually seen with dizziness and nausea. Other causes are various diseases of the retina of the eye and multiple sclerosis. Miners, after many years of working in darkness, may have eye movements that are very quick, increase on upward gaze, and are often linked to dizziness, head trembling, and sensitivity to light.

nystatin /nis'tətin/, an antifungus antibiotic given to treat fungal infections of the stomach and intestinal tract, vagina, and skin.

★CAUTION: Known allergy to this drug prohibits its use.

★ADVERSE EFFECTS: There are no known serious side effects. Mild stomach distress and mild skin reactions may occur.

nystaxis. See **nystagmus.**

O

O, symbol for **oxygen atom.**

oat cell carcinoma, a cancer that usually begins in the surface layer cells of one of the breathing tubes leading to the lungs. Tumors caused by these cells do not form areas of tissue but usually spread along the lymph system. One third of all cancerous tumors of the lung are of this type. Usually surgery cannot be done, and chemotherapy and radiation do not work. Thus, the outlook is poor. Also called **small cell carcinoma.**

obesity, an abnormal increase in the amount of fat, mainly in the stomach and intestines, and in tissues beneath the skin.

Obetrol, a trademark for a drug that has central nervous system stimulants (dextroamphetamine and amphetamine).

OB-Gyn, *informal.* abbreviation for **obstetrics and gynecology.**

objective, referring to a condition, as a health change, that is seen by others and is not subjective. An objective finding is often a physical sign, something that can be measured, as compared to a symptom, which is a subjective finding, as pain or nausea that another person cannot see or feel.

objective data collection, gathering health information relating to a patient's problem by a doctor or nurse through direct physical examination. This includes looking at the patient (observation); examining with the hands, as feeling for tissue masses (palpation); listening for sounds in the body (auscultation); laboratory tests; x-ray tests; and other tests. Compare **subjective data collection.**

obligate aerobe, an organism that cannot grow without free oxygen. See also **aerobe.**

obligate anaerobe, a living thing that cannot grow in oxygen, as *Clostridium tetani* and *C. botulinum.* Some anaerobes can live in an area in which most, but not all, oxygen has been taken away. See also **anaerobe, anaerobic infection.**

oblique, a slanting angle or any change from an up and down (vertical) or a sideways (horizontal) line. Some muscles have an oblique pattern.

oblique bandage, a bandage put on using spiraling circles in slanting turns, usually to an arm or leg.

oblique fissure of the lung, the grooves marking the division of the lower and middle lobes in both the right and left lung.

oblique fracture, a break in a bone at a slanting (oblique) angle.

obliquus externus abdominis, one of a pair of muscles in the area of the stomach and intes-

tines. It helps to hold the contents of this area and helps in urination, defecation, vomiting, childbirth, and forced breathing out. Both sides acting together flex the vertebral column. Also called **descending oblique muscle, external oblique muscle.**

obliquus internus abdominis, one of a pair of muscles in the area of the stomach and intestines that functions to hold the contents of this area and assists in urination, defecation, vomiting, childbirth, and forced breathing out. Both sides acting together flex the vertebral column. Also called **ascending oblique muscle, internal oblique muscle.**

observation, **1.** the act of watching carefully and closely. **2.** a report of what is seen or noticed.

obsession, a thought or idea with which the mind is always concerned and that usually deals with something irrational. The thought is not easily removed just by thinking or talking it through. It usually leads to a compulsion, as an uncontrollable urge to clean a room that is not dirty. See also **compulsion, obsessive compulsive neurosis. −obsessive,** *adj.*

obsessional personality, a type of personality in which continuous, abnormal, uncontrollable, and unwanted thoughts lead to compulsive actions. The thoughts may be made up of single words, simple ideas or desires, or, more commonly, a group of ideas linked to past events or to events in the future. A patient with an obsessional personality is on time, orderly, neat, and can be depended on, but is filled with feelings of not being good enough, of being insecure, and of guilt. The patient also is open to threat, worry, and not being able to make decisions.

obsessive compulsive, marked by or relating to the high risk of performing acts or rituals over and over, usually as a way of lowering tension or getting rid of worries and fear.

obsessive compulsive neurosis, a neurotic condition marked by being unable to resist or stop continuous, abnormal, and uncontrollable urges, thoughts, or fears that are different from the patient's judgments. The problem usually appears after the early teen-age years resulting from fear, feelings of guilt, and worrying about punishment. Treatment may be made up of psychotherapy to find the basic fears and help the patient to tell the difference between real dangers and unreal dangers. Also called **psychasthenia.**

obsessive compulsive personality, a type of personality in which there is an uncontrollable need to do certain acts or rituals. This behavior may go from simple personal habits, as saying certain words over and over before doing something, to more serious and uncontrollable acts, as continous washing of hands or changing of clothes. A patient with this kind of personality is usually orderly and neat, is always on time, can be depended on. There is also a high risk of being rigid and stubborn and to act superior to others. When the acts or rituals become abnormal and more obvious, they can get in the way of everyday actions in society, becoming neurotic reactions.

obstetric anesthesia, any of various ways of giving a drug to put the patient to sleep (anesthetic) during childbirth. It includes local anesthesia for a cut made during surgery to widen the opening of the birth canal (episiotomy), or regional anesthesia for labor or childbirth, as by nerve block. Anesthesia for using surgery to make a cut to form a new opening for childbirth (cesarean section) may be done with a nerve block or by general anesthesia. Light breathing anesthesia with a mixture of nitrous oxide and oxygen is commonly given when forceps are needed or when a difficult vaginal birth is likely to happen.

obstetric forceps, forceps used to assist birth of the fetal head. They vary in length, shape, and way of action, but are all made up of a handle, a shank, and a curved blade.

obstetric position. See **lateral recumbent position.**

obstetrician, a physician who specializes in obstetrics.

obstetrics, the branch of medicine dealing with pregnancy and childbirth, including the workings of the female reproductive tract and care of the mother and fetus throughout pregnancy, childbirth, and the period right after childbirth. —**obstetric, obstetrical,** *adj.*

obstipation, a condition of serious and continuing constipation caused by a blockage in the intestines. See also **constipation.**

obstruction, **1.** something that blocks or clogs an opening or passageway. **2.** the condition of being blocked or clogged. —**obstruct,** *v.,* **obstructive,** *adj.*

obstructive airways disease, any blockage of the breathing tract that may be linked to symptoms of inflammation or unusual conditions in the bronchial tubes leading to the lungs, and a disorder caused by destructive changes in the tissues of these airways (emphysema). See also **acute bronchitis, bronchial asthma, chronic obstructive pulmonary disease (COPD), cystic fibrosis.**

obstructive anuria, a condition marked by being almost completely unable to urinate because of a blockage of the urinary tract. See also **obstructive uropathy.**

obstructive jaundice. See **cholestasis.**

obstructive uropathy, any disease that blocks the flow of urine. The condition may lead to kidney disorders and a higher risk of urinary infection.

obtund /obtund'/, **1.** to deaden pain. **2.** to make the patient deadened to unpleasant activities or pain by reducing the level of being awake, as by anesthesia or a strong narcotic painkiller.

obtundation, the use of a drug that reduces pain by blocking feelings at some level of the central nervous system, as in use of anesthesia before surgery, use of narcotics to control pain, and use of a tranquilizer as a calming drug.

obturator /ob'tərā'tər, ob'tyərā'tər/, a device used to block a passage or a canal or to fill in a space, as a rubberized device (prosthesis) placed in the mouth to bridge the gap in the roof of the mouth in a cleft palate.

obturator externus, the flat, triangle-shaped muscle covering the outer surface of the front wall of the pelvis. It rotates the thigh to the side.

obturator foramen, a large opening on each side of the lower part of the hipbone.

obturator internus, a muscle that covers a large area of the lower part of the pelvis, where it surrounds the obturator foramen. It rotates the thigh to the side and pushes out and raises the thigh when it is flexed.

obturator membrane, a tough fiberlike membrane that covers the obturator foramen of each side of the pelvis.

occipital artery, one of a pair of branched arteries from the external carotid arteries that supplies blood to parts of the head and scalp.

occipital bone, the cuplike bone at the back of the skull that has a large opening (the foramen magnum) that links with the spinal canal.

occipital lobe, one of the five lobes of each side (hemisphere) of the brain. It lies under the occipital bone of the skull.

occipitofrontalis /oksip'itōfrətal'is/, one of a pair of thin, broad muscles covering the top of the skull. The occipitofrontalis contains branches of the nerves for the face. It is the muscle that pulls the scalp and raises the eyebrows.

occiput /ok'sipət/, *pl.* **occiputs, occipita** /oksip'itə/, the back part of the head. Also called **occiput cranii.**

occlusal adjustment, grinding the surfaces of the teeth to make the fit better between different parts of the mouth, including teeth, the roots of teeth and the bone beneath the gum, muscles used in chewing, and the joints between the upper and lower jaws (temporomandibular joints).

occlusal conturing, changing tooth surfaces by grinding rough spots, as uneven high points or crooked teeth.

occlusal form, the shape of the facing (occluding) surfaces of a tooth, a row of teeth, or any dental structure.

occlusal radiograph, an x-ray film made inside the mouth with the film placed between the facing (occlusal) tooth surfaces.

occlusal recontouring, reshaping the biting surface of a natural or artificial tooth.

occlusal relationship, the fit between the lower teeth and the upper teeth when they are in contact.

occlusal trauma, an injury to a tooth and roots and bone beneath the gum caused by the pressure of crooked teeth resulting from accidents, problems at the corners of the jaws (temporomandibular joints), and teeth grinding.

occlusion, **1.** a blockage in a canal, artery or vein, or passage of the body. **2.** any contact between the biting or chewing surfaces of the upper and lower teeth. **–occlude,** *v.,* **occlusive,** *adj.*

occlusive /əcloo'siv/, referring to something that causes a blockage or closing, as a taped bandage.

occlusive dressing, a bandage that prevents air and germs from reaching a wound. It stores moisture, heat, body fluids, and drugs and may be made up of a sheet of thin plastic fastened with tape.

occult, hidden or hard to see directly, as occult blood.

occult blood, blood that comes from an unknown place, with unclear signs and symptoms. It may be found by using a chemical test or by using a microscope to look closer at the blood. Occult blood is usually in the stools of patients with stomach and intestinal diseases.

occult carcinoma, a small cancer that does not cause serious symptoms. It may stay in one place and be found only at an autopsy following death from another cause, or it may spread (metastasize) through blood or lymph and be found in the results of tests done to look at the patient's disease. Also called **latent carcinoma.**

occult fracture, a broken bone that cannot be seen at first by using x-ray tests but may show up on x-ray films weeks later. It has the usual signs of pain and injury and may cause soft tissue swelling.

occupational accident, an injury caused by an accident to an employee that happens in the workplace. Accidents account for more than 95% of workplace injuries. In most cases the injured worker is paid for the injury.

occupational asthma, an unusual condition of the breathing system caused by coming into contact with things that cause allergies and itching while in the workplace. The condition is most common among patients who work with soaps, Western red cedar, cotton, flax, hemp, grain, flour, and stone. See also **asthma, byssinosis, occupational lung disease.**

occupational disability, a condition in which a worker is unable to do a job properly because of an occupational disease or a workplace accident.

occupational disease, an illness that is caused by doing a certain job, usually from coming into contact with things that cause diseases, or from doing certain actions over and over again.

occupational health, the state of a worker being able to work well enough and hard enough to do his or her job well, not to miss work because of illness, to have few claims for disability payments, and to be able to work for a long time.

occupational history, a part of the health record in which questions are asked about the patient's job, source of income, effects of the work on health or the patient's health on the job, length of the job, and whether the patient is happy with the job. Certain side effects may be linked to a certain job or place of work. For example, a carpenter might be asked about muscle and bone problems or a taxi driver about problems of the urinary tract.

occupational lung disease, any of a group of unusual problems in the lungs caused by breathing dusts, fumes, gases, or vapors in a place where a patient works. See also **chronic obstructive pulmonary disease, metal fume fever, occupational asthma, silo fillers' disease.**

occupational medicine, a part of medicine that deals with preventing medical problems relating to work and especially to the health of workers in different kinds of workplaces and jobs.

occupational neurosis, a mental problem in which symptoms keep the worker from doing the necessary work for a job, as in writer's cramp. The symptoms are not caused by the job; rather, they may be a sign of a mental problem.

occupational therapist, a person who works with patients who need help in activities of daily living and who is licensed to do this therapy.

occupational therapy, the training of patients with physical injury or illness, mental disease, or learning problems to work and live by themselves despite any health problem that keeps the patient from living a normal life.

ochronosis /ō'krənō'sis/, a condition marked by deposits of brown-black color in connective tissue and cartilage. It is often caused by alkaptonuria or poisoning with phenol. Bluish spots may be seen on the whites of the eyes, fingers, ears, nose, genitals, mouth, and armpits. The urine may be dark-colored. See also **alkaptonuria.**

ocular /ok'yŏŏlər/, **1.** referring to the eye. **2.** an eyepiece or system of lenses, as in a microscope.

ocular hypertelorism, a birth defect marked by a very wide bridge of the nose and more distance between the eyes. The condition is often linked to other head and face problems and some mental retardation. Also called **orbital hypertelorism.**

ocular hypotelorism, a birth defect characterized by a narrowing of the bridge of the nose and an abnormally small distance between the eyes. It results in a form of cross eye (convergent strabismus). The condition is often linked to badly formed parts of the head and face, and some slow mental growth (mental retardation). Also called **orbital hypotelorism.**

ocular myopathy, a slow weakening of the muscles that move the eyeball. There may be less and less movement of the eye and drooping of the upper lid. The problem may affect one or both eyes and may be caused by damage to the third skull nerve necessary for eye movement, a brain tumor, or a disease that affects nerves and muscles.

ocular spot, an unusual loss of vision in the eye. A shower of red and black dots may be seen in the eye following bleeding in an eye vessel. Cloudiness in the lens is caused by cataracts. In one disease (asteroid hyalitis), often linked to diabetes, small white calcium deposits are found in the watery substance (vitreous humor) between the lens and retina.

oculocephalic reflex, a test of the condition of the brain stem. When the patient's head is quickly moved to one side and then to the other, the eyes will usually take a moment to catch up with the head movement and then slowly move to the middle position. Failure of the eyes to do either of these things properly means a brain stem tumor is on the opposite side of the head. Also called **doll's eye maneuver.**

oculogyric crisis /ok'yŏolōjī'rik/, condition in which the eyes are deviated and in a fixed position, usually up and sideways, for minutes or several hours. It happens in patients who have recovered from sleeping sickness (encephalitis) but have signs of another brain disease (parkinsonism). In some cases the eyes are held down or sideways and there may be a sudden muscle movement (spasm) or closing of the lids. Oculogyric crises may be set off by emotional stress. Patients with the problem often have symptoms of mental problems.

oculomotor nerve, either of a pair of cranial nerves that controls eye movements, supplying certain outside (extrinsic) and inside (intrinsic) eye muscles. Also called **nervus oculomotorius, third cranial nerve.**

Ocusert Pilo, a trademark for a nerve drug (pilocarpine).

odontectomy, the removal of a tooth.

odontiasis /ō'dontī'əsis/, the process of the teeth coming in.

-odontic, 1. a combining form referring to the size of teeth, as in macrodontic. **2.** a combining form referring to a type of dental treatment, as in orthodontic.

odontitis /ō'dontī'tis/, unusual growth of an immature (unerupted) tooth, usually caused by a swelling of the cells that make new teeth (odontoblasts) rather than of the mature (erupted) tooth. It may be caused by infection, tumor, or injury.

odontodysplasia, an unusual condition in the growth of the teeth, marked by bad forming of the outer layers of the teeth (enamel and dentin). Also called **ghost teeth.**

odontoid process, the lump on the upper surface of the second cervical backbone (axis) in the neck. It is the place around which the first cervical backbone (atlas) turns, allowing the head to turn. Also called **dens.**

odontogenic /ōdon'tōjen'ik/, referring to the growth of tissues that make teeth.

odontogenic fibroma, a tumor of the jaw that does not lead to cancer.

odontogenic fibrosarcoma, a cancer of the jaw.

odontogenic myxoma, a tumor of the jaw that does not lead to cancer.

odontoid ligament. See **alar ligament.**

odontoid vertebra. See **axis.**

odontology /ō'dontol'əjē/, the scientific study of the shape, form, and makeup of the teeth and of the other parts of the mouth.

odontoma, a toothlike growth that looks like a hard tumor. It is made up of tooth tissues, as cementum and enamel, that may be in the form of teeth. Also called **gestant anomaly.**

odor, a scent or smell. The sense of smell is set off when molecules in the air carry the odor (olfactory) to the first cranial nerve located inside the nose.

odynophagia /od'inōfā'jə/, a strong feeling of burning, squeezing pain while swallowing. It is caused by irritation of the mucous membranes or a muscle problem of the esophagus (gastroesophageal reflux), a germ or fungus infection, a tumor, or chemical irritation.

Oedipus complex, a sexually excited feeling by a child for the parent of the opposite sex, usually with strong negative feelings for the parent of the same sex. Experts disagree on the cause, as the parents' supporting it, or its commonness, because it is not found in all countries.

ofloxacin, a type of antibiotic (carboxygluoroquinolone type).

Ogen, a trademark for a female sex hormone (estropipate).

oil, any of a large number of fatty liquid substances that will not mix with water. Oil may stay the same for long periods of time or can be turned easily into a vapor and can be gotten from animal, vegetable, or mineral matter. An oil is sometimes different from a solid fat by being liquid at a temperature of 68° F (20° C).

ointment, a creamlike medicine used on the skin and having one or more drugs. Various ointments are used as local painkillers, anesthetics, anti-infectives, astringents, irritants, or decoloring (depigmenting) and skin softening (keratolytic) agents. Also called **salve, unction, unguent.**

Old Age, Survivors, Disability and Health Insurance Program, a national government program that provides health-insurance benefits for people over 65 years of age and for disabled people under 65 years of age. It is controlled by the Social Security Administration. This program is usually called Medicare. See also **Medicare.**

Old World leishmaniasis. See **oriental sore.**

olecranon /ōlek'rənon/, a bump on the lower arm bone (ulna) that forms the point of the elbow. It fits into the dent (olecranon fossa) of the upper arm bone (humerus) when the forearm is straightened out.

olecranon bursa, the bursa of the elbow. See also **bursa.**

olecranon fossa, the dent in the back surface of the upper arm bone (humerus) that receives the olecranon of the lower arm bone (ulna) when the forearm is straightened out. Compare **coronoid fossa.**

oleic acid /ōlē'ik/, a colorless, liquid fatty acid found in vegetable and animal fats. In store products, oleic acid is found in lotions, soaps, ointments, and food additives.

oleovitamin /ō'lē·ōvī'təmin/, a mixture of fish liver oil or vegetable oil that can be eaten and contains one or more of the vitamins that are dissolved by fat or similar substances.

oleovitamin A, an oily mixture, usually fish liver oil, which may be plain or watered down with a vegetable oil that can be eaten, containing the natural or artificial form of vitamin A. See also **vitamin A.**

oleovitamin D₂. See **calciferol.**

olfactory /olfak'tərē/, referring to the sense of smell. **–olfaction,** n.

olfactory anesthesia. See **anosmia.**

olfactory center, the part of the brain responsible for making sense of odors. It is made up of a complex group of nerve cells located in the brain.

olfactory foramen, one of several openings in the criblike plate of the bone in the roof of the chamber behind the nose (nasal cavity).

olfactory nerve, one of a pair of nerves linked to the sense of smell. The olfactory nerve is also called cranial nerve I and is made up of many thin threads that spread through the mucous membrane of the smell-sensing area in the chamber behind the nose (nasal cavity). The fibers form a grouping under the mucous membrane and rise in tiny holes in the criblike (ethmoid) bone of the nasal cavity. Passing into the skull, the fibers form links with the fibers of the cells in the olfactory bulb, a relay center between the nose and the brain. The olfactory bulb and the olfactory tract are parts of the portion of the brain linked to the sense of smell.

oligodactyly /ol'igōdak'tilē/, a birth defect that usually takes the form of the lack of one or more of the fingers or toes. Also called **oligodactylism, oligodactylia. –oligodactylic,** adj.

oligodendroglioma /ol'igōden'drōglī·ō'mə/, pl. **oligodendrogliomas, oligodendrogliomata,** a brain tumor made up of cells that usually are part of the tissue around nerve cells. The tumor may grow to a large size. It grows in a number of different places of the brain. Also called **oligodendroblastoma.**

oligohydramnios, an unusually small amount or lack of amniotic fluid.

oligodontia /ol'igōdon'shə/, a dental problem that usually takes the form of having fewer than the normal number of teeth.

oligogenic /ol'igōjen'ik/, referring to inborn traits brought about by only one or a very few genes.

oligomeganephronia /ol'igōmeg'ənefrō'nē·ə/, a type of inborn kidney problem that usually takes the form of a lack of filtering units and too many other kidney tissues. Also called **oligomeganephronic renal hypoplasia. –oligomeganephronic,** adj.

oligomenorrhea, unusually light menstruation or menstruation that does not occur as often as is normal. **–oligomenorrheic,** adj.

oligospermia /ol'igōspur'mē·ə/, lack of enough sperm in the semen. Compare **azoospermia.**

oliguria /ol'igyŏor'ē·ə/, a reduced ability to make and excrete urine, usually less than 500 ml (1 pint) a day. A result is that the waste products of the body's chemical processes (metabolism) cannot be released properly. It may be caused by body fluids and minerals that get out of balance, by kidney tumors, or by a urinary tract blockage. Also called **oliguresis.** Compare **anuria. –oliguric,** adj.

Ollier's disease. See **enchondromatosis.**

Ollier's dyschondroplasia /ol'ē·āz'/, a problem of bone growth in which the tissue necessary for bone growth spreads through the bones. It causes unusual and rough growth and, over time, badly formed bones. The long bones and the hip bone are the ones most often changed by this problem. Surgery to correct badly formed bones may be necessary and helpful, but the patient often becomes an invalid. A kind of dyschondroplasia is **hereditary multiple exostoses.** Also called **multiple enchondromatosis.**

-olol, a combining form for beta blockers.

-oma, a combining form meaning a 'tumor.'

omalgia, pain in the shoulder.

omarthritis, swelling of the shoulder joint.

ombudsman, a person who investigates and helps to solve patients' problems and complaints linked to a hospital's services. Also called **patient representative.**

omentum, *pl.* **omenta, omentums,** an extension of the abdominal lining (peritoneum) that surrounds one or more nearby organs in the stomach and bowel area (abdomen). See also **greater omentum, lesser omentum.** –**omental,** *adj.*

Omnipen, a trademark for an antigerm drug (ampicillin).

omo-, oma-, a combining form referring to the shoulder.

omphalitis, a disorder of the navel characterized by redness, swelling, and pus in severe cases.

omphalo-, omphal-, a combining form referring to the navel (umbilicus).

omphalocele /om'fəlōsēl'/, a hernia of intestinal organ material through a hole in the intestinal wall at the navel. The hole is usually closed surgically soon after birth. Compare **gastroschisis.**

Omsk hemorrhagic fever (OHF) /ômsk/, a serious infection, seen in regions of the USSR. It is caused by a virus carried by an infected tick or by handling infected muskrats. The disease is marked by fever, headache, nosebleeds, stomach and uterine bleeding, and bleeding in other body areas. Patients who are otherwise healthy usually recover.

onanism. See **masturbation.**

onchocerciasis /on'kōsərkī'əsis/, a condition where worms multiply rapidly in the patient's body (filariasis), common in Latin America and Africa. It is characterized by bumps (nodules) under the skin, an itching rash, and eye tumors. The disease is carried by the bites of black flies *Onchocera volvulus* that place their eggs under the skin. The insect eggs move under the skin and into the eyes, and fiberlike bumps grow around the growing adult worms. Allergic reactions to the dying larvae include extreme itching, a rash, skin thickening, loss of skin color, and possible increased growth of certain body parts (elephantiasis). Problems in and around the eye because of this condition may include corneal swelling, swelling of the iris, and, rarely, blindness. Doctors can tell the patient has this condition if they find worm larvae in the skin or in the patient's eye. Treatment includes drugs to kill the larvae and surgery to take out the nodules in order to remove adult worms. Protective clothing should be worn in black fly areas. Also called **river blindness.**

onco-, a combining form referring to a swelling or tumor.

oncofetal protein, a protein made by or linked to a tumor cell, particularly an embryological tumor. An example of an oncofetal protein is alpha-fetoprotein.

oncogene, a gene that may possibly cause cancer to grow. Normally, such genes play a role in the growth and spread of cells, but when changed in some way by a cancer-causing agent, as radiation, they may cause the cell to be changed to a cancer.

oncogenesis /ong'kōjen'əsis/, the process of the growth of a tumor through the action of biological, chemical, or physical agents. Compare **carcinogenesis, sarcomagenesis, tumorigenesis.** –**oncogenic** /ong'kōjen'ik/,*adj.*

oncogenic virus, a virus that is able to cause the growth of a cancer. More than 100 oncogenic viruses are known to exist. In the laboratory, oncogenic viruses have been injected into and grown in all major groups of animals, including primates. Many "slow viruses," which may remain nonactive for years, are thought to cause cancer in humans.

oncology /ongkol'əjē/, the branch of medicine that deals with the study of tumors.

Oncovin, a trademark for an anticancer drug (vincristine sulfate).

oncovirus /ong'kōvī'rəs/, a family of viruses linked to certain cancers (leukemia and sarcoma) in animals and, possibly, in humans.

Ondine's curse /ondēnz'/, an inability to breathe, caused by loss of automatic control of breathing. The term is taken from a fairy tale. A problem in the breathing center's reaction to the buildup of carbon dioxide leaves the patient with too much carbon dioxide and lack of oxygen in the blood. However, the patient is fully able to breathe on his or her own. This condition may cause the pickwickian syndrome or the sleep apnea syndrome, and it may be one cause of sudden infant death syndrome (SIDS). Ondine's curse may be caused by drug overdose, as with opiate narcotics; it may follow bulbar poliomyelitis or encephalitis; or it may set in after surgery that involves the brain stem or the higher parts of the spinal cord.

one-and-a-half spica cast, a bone cast used for keeping the body rigid from the nipple line, one leg as far as the toes, and the other leg as far as the knee. For keeping the patient still, a slanted crossbar joins the parts of the cast covering the legs. This type of cast is used during recovery of surgery to repair the hip or a broken upper leg and for repairing hips that are badly formed.

one-to-one care, a way to organize nursing services in a hospital by which one nurse controls all nursing care given one patient for the length of one shift.

-onide, a combining form for a type of steroids applied to the skin (derived from acetal).

-onium, a combining form for quaternary ammonium derivatives.

onlay, a part of a partial denture that can be taken out, extended to cover (onlay) the whole chewing surface of a tooth. Compare **inlay.**

ontogeny /ontoj'ənē/, the life history of one living thing from a single-celled egg to the time of birth, including all phases of cell division and growth. Compare **phylogeny.**

onychia /ōnik'ē·ə/, swelling of the area of the finger under the nail (nail bed). Compare **paronychia.**

onychogryphosis /on'ikōgrifō'sis/, a thickened, curved, clawlike overgrowth of fingernails or toenails.

onycholysis /on'ikol'isis/, the coming apart of a nail from its bed. It is linked to psoriasis, dermatitis of the hand, fungus infection, bacteria infection, and many other conditions.

onychomycosis /on'ikōmīkō'sis/, any fungus infection of the nails.

ooblast /ō'əblast/, the female germ cell from which the egg grows.

oocyesis /ō'əsī·ē'sis/, a pregnancy with an embryo growing within the ovary instead of the uterus where it normally grows.

oocyst /ō'əsist/, a malarial or similar parasite, which after it is fertilized grows a surrounding (cyst) wall around itself.

oocyte /ō''əsīt'/, a not-fully-developed egg.

oogenesis /ō'əjen'əsis/, the growth of female eggs (ova). Growth actually begins during life in the womb when the very first germ cells in the fetal ovary make cells called oogonia. By the time of birth, the oogonia have multiplied and grown into primary oocytes. Each one has a layer of cells around it that form the primitive ovarian follicle. The oocytes stay this way until they are sexually mature. Then every month, one, or sometimes two, of the primary oocytes break into a large secondary oocyte and a much smaller body that does not do anything. The second division begins at about the time of ovulation, resulting in one large mature egg, or ootid, and one or more smaller bodies that soon break apart. The mature egg has the haploid number of the mother's chromosomes that will join with the sperm during fertilization to form the zygote. If fertilization does not occur, the egg breaks apart and is released during menstruation. A female baby is born with all the primary oocytes that will be used during her reproductive life. Only a small amount of these live until puberty, and only a small number will be ovulated. Follicles that have primary oocytes are found in different stages of growth in the ovary of the sexually mature woman. Also called **ovogenesis.** Compare **spermatogenesis.** See also **gametogenesis, meiosis, menstrual cycle, ovulation. –oogenetic,** *adj.*

oogonium /ō'əgō'nē·əm/, *pl.* **oogonia,** a cell from which an oocyte grows in the fetus during life in the womb. Also called **ovogonium.** See also **oogenesis.**

oophorectomy /ō'əfərek'təmē/, surgery to remove one or both ovaries. It may be done to take out a lump (cyst), a tumor, or a sore, to treat endometriosis, or, in breast cancer, to take out the part of the body that makes the female sex hormone (estrogen), which helps to start some cancers. If both ovaries are removed, the patient will not be able to have children and menopause is started. In women who have not yet gone through menopause, one ovary or a part of one ovary may be left in place unless a cancer is present. The operation often is done with a removal of the uterus (hysterectomy). Unless a cancer is present, estrogen may be given to avoid the side effects of menopause. Also called **ovariectomy.**

oophoritis /ō'əferī'tis/, inflammation of one or both ovaries, usually occurring with inflammation of the fallopian tubes (salpingitis).

oophorosalpingectomy /ō'əfôr'əsal'pinjek'təmē/, surgery to remove one or both ovaries and the fallopian tubes. The purpose may be to take out a lump (cyst), tumor, or a sore, or to treat endometriosis. If both tubes are taken out, the patient can no longer have babies and menopause is started. Doctors will begin to give the patient estrogen, unless a cancer is present, to take away the unpleasant side effects when menopause begins.

ooplasm /ō'əplaz'əm/, the outer part (cytoplasm) of the egg cell (ovum). Also called **ovoplasm.**

oosperm /ō'əspurm/, a fertilized egg; the cell caused by the joining of the sperm and the egg after fertilization occurs; a zygote.

ootid /ō'ətid/, the mature eggs.

opacity, the condition of a thing that cannot be seen through (opaque or nontransparent), as a cataract opacity.

opaque, referring to a substance or surface that neither carries nor lets light come through.

open amputation, a kind of surgery to remove parts of the body (amputation) in which a straight cut is made without skin flaps. Open amputation is done if an infection is likely, is already happening, or has been coming back. The cut (cross section) is left open to drain away fluids, and the skin is pulled back to keep the section from closing. Drug treatment to keep an infection from starting is begun, and surgery is used to close the cut when the infection is gone. Compare **closed amputation.** See also **gangrene.**

open-angle glaucoma. See **glaucoma.**

open bite, an abnormal dental condition in which the lower front teeth do not touch the upper front teeth when the jaws are closed. Compare **closed bite.**

open charting, a way to keep medical records in which the patient can look at his or her own chart.

open drainage. See **drainage.**

open drop anesthesia, the oldest and most simple way to put the patient to sleep (anesthetize) during surgery or other medical procedures. A liquid anesthetic is dripped, one drop at a time, onto a loosely woven cloth or mask held over the patient's face. Chloroform and ether are the major general anesthetics used this way. Anesthetics are no longer used this way in modern countries.

open fracture, See **compound fracture.**

open operation, surgery that allows a full view of the parts of the body or organs being worked on.

operant conditioning, a way of learning used in treatment to change the way a patient thinks or does things (behavior therapy). The patient is rewarded for the right response and punished for the wrong response. Also called **instrumental conditioning.**

operating microscope, a small microscope that is worn like glasses in front of each eye and is used in surgery where the things being operated on are very small, especially surgery of the eye or ear. Also called **surgical microscope.**

operating room (O.R.), a room or area in a hospital where patients are made ready for surgery, have surgery, and recover from the effects of the anesthetic needed for the surgery.

operation, any surgery, as an appendectomy or a hysterectomy.

operative cholangiography, a way of using x-ray tests to outline the largest tubes that carry the liquid made by the liver (bile) from the liver. It is done during surgery by injecting a dye into the tubes. It is usually done to find gallstones in the bile tract. See also **cholangiography.**

operculum /ōpur′kyoŏləm/, *pl.* **opercula, operculums,** a covering, as the mucous plug, that blocks the tube or channel of a uterus that has a fertilized egg in it. **–opercular,** *adj.*

ophthalmia /ofthal′mē-ə/, serious swelling of the outer surface (conjunctiva) or of the deeper parts of the eye. Some kinds of ophthalmia are **ophthalmia neonatorum, sympathetic ophthalmia, trachoma.**

ophthalmia neonatorum /nē′ōnətôr′əm/, an irritation of the outer part of the eye that causes pus to form and also causes swelling of the outer part of the eye (cornea) in newborn babies. It is caused by the eyes coming into contact with chemicals, viruses, or germs. Irritation of the outer part of the eye caused by chemicals usually is the result of putting silver nitrate in the eyes of a newborn baby to keep a virus infection from starting. Also called **neonatal conjunctivitis.** See also **conjunctivitis.**

ophthalmic administration of medication, giving a drug by slowly pouring a cream or ointment or by slowly dripping drops of a liquid drug in the outer surface of the eye (conjunctiva). The patient should be placed comfortably, lying back on a bed or sitting up with the neck leaned backward. The loose tissue between the eyeball and the eyelid (conjunctival sac) is uncovered by a gentle pull on the tissue just below the lower eyelid. The drug is placed in the

sac as the patient looks away from the eyedropper. The eyedropper is not allowed to touch the eye, and the drug is not placed directly on the outer surface of the eye. The eyelid is slowly released, and the patient rolls the eye around a few times to spread the drug over the whole surface of the eye.

ophthalmology /of′thalmol′əjē/, the branch of medicine that deals with the working, makeup, structures, and diseases of the eye, and finding their causes and treatments for them. **–ophthalmologic, ophthalmological,** *adj.*

ophthalmoplegia /ofthal′məplē′jə/, the loss of movement of the motor nerves of the eye. Ophthalmoplegia of both eyes may come about quickly with serious myasthenia gravis, serious vitamin B$_1$ (thiamin) shortage, or botulism. In some patients with myopathic ophthalmoplegia, problems also may occur in arm and leg muscles.

ophthalmoscope /of′thalmol′əskōp/, a tool for looking at the inside of the eye. It includes a light, a mirror with a single hole through which the doctor may look, and a dial that has several lenses of different powers.

Ophthochlor, a trademark for an antibiotic (chloramphenicol) used to treat eye infections.

Ophthocort, a trademark for an eye drug that has an adrenal hormone (hydrocortisone acetate) and antibiotics (chloramphenicol and polymyxin B sulfate).

opiate, **1.** a narcotic drug that contains opium, drugs made from opium, or any of several partly artificial or artificial drugs that behave like opium. **2.** referring to chemicals that cause sleep or help ease pain. Morphine and other opiates like it may cause unwanted side effects, as nausea, vomiting, dizziness, and constipation. In some cases a patient treated with an opiate may become confused. Some patients may also become more sensitive to pain after the opiate has worn off. Allergic reactions to opiates, as itching (urticaria) and other skin rashes, may occur. Patients with low amounts of blood are more likely to have their blood pressure lowered because of morphine and other drugs like it. Opiates should be used very carefully in overweight patients and in those with head injuries, or any problems linked to breathing. In patients with a large prostate, morphine may cause a serious buildup of urine, making it necessary to use a tube in the urinary tract (catheter). Also called **opioid.**

opisthorchiasis /ō′pisthôrkī′əsis/, infection with a kind of *Opisthorchis* liver worms commonly found in Asia, the Pacific Islands, and parts of Europe. Cancer of the bile ducts may be a late result. The disease is best prevented by avoiding eating raw fish or freshwater fish that have not been cooked long enough.

opisthotonos /ō′pisthot′ənəs/, a continuous severe spasm of the muscles causing the back to arch back, the head to bend back on the neck, the heels to bend back on the legs, and the arms and hands to flex rigidly at the joints.

opium, a dried or partly dried milky sap from the unripe capsules of the opium poppy (*Papaver somniferum* and *Papaver album*) producing nearly 10% or more of morphine. It is a narcotic painkiller, a drug that brings on sleep or hypnosis, and a drug that reduces the flow of body liquids (astringent). Opium contains several alkaloids, including codeine, morphine, and papaverine. See also **codeine, morphine sulfate, opium tincture, papaverine hydrochloride, paregoric.**

opium alkaloid, any of several substances taken from the unripe seed pods of the opium poppy (*Papaver somniferum*), a kind of plant that grows only in the Near East. Three of the alkaloids—codeine, papaverine, and morphine—are used in medicine for pain relief, but their use risks physical or psychological addiction. Morphine is the basic, most common drug of its kind against which the painkiller effect of newer drugs for pain relief are tested. The opium alkaloids and the semiartificial drugs that are made from them, including heroin, act on the central nervous system, causing loss of pain, a change in mood, drowsiness, and mental slowness. The effects in a patient who has pain are usually pleasant; a higher sense of well-being and pain-free sleep are common, but nausea and vomiting sometimes occur. In usual doses, the relief from pain is achieved without loss of consciousness. Morphine and other opiates cause the level of actual pain to go down, and what is left is less uncomfortable to the patient. The opium alkaloids have several other effects on the different systems of the body: Coughing is halted; the brain waves look like those of sleep; the pupils get smaller; breathing is slowed; the workings of the stomach and intestines are slowed; and biliary and pancreatic fluids are reduced. Morphine was used to treat diarrhea for hundreds of years before it was used as a painkiller. It is still the best constipating drug available.

opium tincture, a painkiller and antidiarrhea drug given to treat too-much intestinal activity, cramping, and diarrhea.
★CAUTION: Drug addiction, the presence of poison in the bowel, or known allergy to this drug prohibits its use.
★ADVERSE EFFECTS: Among the more serious side effects are drug addiction, an enlarged colon, and central nervous system effects.

Oppenheim reflex /op′ənhīm/, a different type of Babinski's reflex. It is caused by firmly stroking downward on the front and inner surfaces of the lower leg, causing the great toe to straighten out and causing the fanning of other toes. It is a sign of central nervous system disease. Compare **Chaddock reflex, Gordon reflex.** See also **Babinski's reflex.**

Oppenheim's disease, an inborn disorder of infants, marked by flabby muscles, especially in the legs, and the lack of or very slow deep muscle reflexes. The infant seems unable to move during its first few months of life and almost a third of the patients do not survive for 1 year. Also called **amyotonia congenita.** See also **myotonia congenita.**

opportunistic infection, an infection caused by a virus or by germs that are usually not harmful to normal persons. The patient becomes infected because his or her ability to fight off diseases has been reduced by diseases, as diabetes mellitus or cancer; by surgery, as a cerebrospinal fluid shunt; or a tube in the heart or urinary tract. The result is an unusual infection with a common germ or virus.

opsonin /op′sənin/, a substance that clings to foreign material, a germ or virus, or other germ or virus fighter (antigen). It speeds the destruction of that material faster by white blood cells (leukocytes) and other cells able to digest germs and viruses. **–opsonize,** *v.*

optic, referring to the eyes or to sight. Also **optical.**

optic atrophy, wasting away of the optic disc in the innermost part of the eye (retina), caused by a breakdown of optic nerve fibers. In primary optic atrophy, the disc is white with sharp outer edges, and the central depression is large. In secondary atrophy the disc is gray, its outer edges are blurred, and the depression is filled in. Optic atrophy may be caused by a birth defect, swelling blockage of the central retinal artery or internal carotid artery, or by alcohol, arsenic, lead, nicotine, or other poisons. Breakdown of the disc may be seen with arteriosclerosis, diabetes, glaucoma, hydrocephalus, anemia, and different types of nervous system disorders.

optic disc, the small blind spot on the surface of the retina. It is the only part of the retina that is not sensitive to light. At its center is the entrance of the central artery of the retina. Also called (*informal*) **blind spot, discus nervi optici.**

optic glioma, a tumor made up of cells that grow slowly on the optic nerve or in the optic chiasm, a crossing over of fibers from the left and right eyes. It causes loss of sight in the patient, and he or she will often have uneven eyes (strabismus), bulging eyeballs (exophthalmos), and eyes that cannot be moved.

optician, a person who grinds and fits eyeglasses and contact lenses by prescription.

optic nerve, the second cranial nerve made up mainly of rough fibers that start in the retina, travel through the thalamus at the base of the brain, and join with the visual cortex at the back of the brain. At the optic chiasm the fibers from the inner half of the retina of each eye cross to the optic tract of the other side. The fibers left over from the outer half of each retina are uncrossed and pass to the visual cortex on the same side. The visual cortex works to sense light and shade and to sense objects by decoding nerve signals from the retina. The optic nerve is cranial nerve II and comes from a part of the front part of the brain. The optic nerve fibers therefore are matched with a tract of fibers within the brain rather than to the other skull nerves.

optics, a field of study that deals with sight and the way that the workings of the eye and the brain are linked in order to sense shapes, patterns, movements, distance, and color. **–optic, optical,** *adj.*

optic stalk, one of a pair of slim structures that become the optic nerve. In the embryo the optic stalk grows during the second week and attaches the optic vesicle to the wall of the brain. The stalk becomes complete during the seventh week of pregnancy.

optic system assessment, a testing of the eyes for current and past disorders or injuries that may result in problems in the patient's sight. The patient is tested to check if sight is blurred, double, reduced, or lacking in one or both eyes, or reduced in darkness or in bright light. The physician asks if halos or lights are seen and if when the patient runs into strange objects he or she is unable to see objects held too close or too far; if the eyes water, itch, feel tender, painful, or tired; and if an injury to the eye, face, or head has ever happened. Other observations include the way a patient looks overall, his or her temperature and blood pressure, the kind of eyeglasses or contact lenses worn, the amount of tears he or she has, the ability to blink, his or her being likely to rub the eyes, and the ability to focus. A report is made about outer eye itchiness (conjunctivitis), any discharge coming from the eye, bleeding in the eye, swelling or drooping of the eyelids, bulging eyes, eye unevenness, rolling of the eyes, swelling of the whites of the eyes, eyelid redness or swelling, cuts, bruises, or something (as dirt or sand) in the eye. Also noted are signs of aging, glaucoma, cataract, retinal detachment, or the presence of multiple sclerosis, diabetes mellitus, myasthenia gravis, gonorrhea, thyroid dysfunction, sinus problems, or brain injury or tumors. The patient's report of eye surgery or treatment earlier in his or her life, head or face injury, arteriosclerosis, kidney disease, retinal degeneration, being unconscious for long periods of time (coma), treatment with oxygen, and drug misuse are noted, as well as a family history of glaucoma or diabetes. Also looked at are the patient's job and hobbies to see if the patient is exposed to any possible dangers (and note is made of any safety steps taken), the patient's use of alcohol, and

use of drugs, especially antibiotics, eye drugs, and certain drugs that increase the passing of urine (diuretics). Testing may include a test of what the patient can see, x-ray film of the eyes and skull, an eye examination, a test for eyeball pressure (tonometry), brain scan, and using a microscope to look at scrapings from the outer surface of the eyeball.

optometry /optom′ətrē/, the practice of testing the eyes for the ability to focus and see, making corrective lenses, and suggesting eye exercises. See also **optician.**

OPV, abbreviation for **oral poliovirus vaccine.**

oral administration of medication, giving a tablet, a capsule, an elixir, or a solution or other liquid form of a drug by mouth. Enough water to oil the solid forms or to water down the liquid forms is given for swallowing with the drugs. Drugs with an unpleasant taste may be given with something with enough flavor to hide the taste. Drugs that are bad for the teeth should be given through a straw. Patients who have a hard time swallowing pills or capsules may find it easier to swallow the drug if they look up as they swallow. Ways of giving drugs by mouth are **buccal administration of medication, sublingual administration of medication.**

oral airway, a curved tubelike device of rubber, plastic, or metal put in the throat while the patient is unconscious because he or she has been given a drug (general anesthesia) to make the patient sleep during an operation or other procedure. This tube helps allow free passage of air and helps to keep the tongue from falling back over the windpipe. The artificial airway is not taken out until the patient begins to awaken and is once again able to cough and swallow correctly.

oral cancer, a cancer on the lip or in the mouth. It usually occurs in patients around 60 years of age and is eight times more common in men than in women. Causes for the disease are alcoholism, heavy use of tobacco, poor mouth care, poorly fitting dentures, syphilis, a low iron disease (Plummer-Vinson syndrome), and betel nut chewing. Lip cancer may result from overexposure to sun and wind and pipe smoking. Leathery plaques, painless red patches, or a painless sore in the mouth area may be the first sign of oral cancer. Local pain usually appears later, but lymph nodes may also quickly get the disease. Small primary tumors may be treated by surgical removal or radiation and more extensive mouth tumors by surgery, with the disease lymph nodes being taken out, and radiation treatment.

oral character, a type of behavior beginning in the oral stage of infancy. It may be marked by either feeling good about the future, feeling good about oneself, and carefree giving that shows the pleasurable aspects of infancy, or feeling bad about the future, feeling nothing is worthwhile, being nervous, and enjoying hurting others as ways to show problems and worries that the patient had when he or she was a baby. See also **oral stage, psychosexual development.**

oral contraceptive, an oral steroid drug for birth control. The two major steroids used are progestogen and a combination of progestogen and estrogen, both related to female sexuality. The steroids act by stopping the making of gonadotropin-releasing hormone by the hypothalamus. Therefore the pituitary gland does not release gonadotropins that usually cause the ovary to release an egg cell. This causes the endometrium lining of the uterus to become thin and the cervical mucus to become thick, thus stopping the sperm from getting through it. Before birth-control pills are given, the woman should have a complete physical examination. While on the drug, she should be examined after 3 months and then once a year. Combination steroids are given for 3 weeks with no drug in the fourth week to allow for withdrawal bleeding (menstruation). If heavy (breakthrough) bleeding occurs, the estrogen dose may need to be made higher. If there is an absence or very low level of bleeding (amenorrhea), the progestogen may need to be lowered. Conditions that usually keep the patient from using birth-control pills include pregnancy, diabetes mellitus, liver disease, high levels of blood fats, blood clotting problems, coronary heart disease, and sickle cell disease. Patients who are mentally depressed or who have migraine headaches and those who are heavy cigarette smokers usually need more frequent medical checkups. An increased risk of circulation disease occurs in women more than 35 years of age who have used birth-control pills for more than 5 years and who smoke cigarettes or who have other risk factors. Amenorrhea may occur in women who stop taking birth-control pills, particularly those who have a history of little or no menstrual flow. The risk of pregnancy when birth-control pills are used correctly is less than 0.2% a year. See also **contraception.**

oral dosage, referring to taking a drug by mouth.

oral hygiene, the practice of brushing the teeth to take away bits of food, germs, and plaque. It includes massaging the gums, using dental floss or a water tool to help circulation and take away bits of food, or cleaning dentures and making sure of their proper fit to keep the gums from getting swollen, red, or itchy.

oral mucous membranes, the tissues lining the mouth that may be changed by different types of diseases, injuries, and treatments. Conditions that can cause changes in tissues of the mouth cavity include radiation to the head or neck, chemical or mechanical injury, bad mouth care, infection, eating badly or not having enough to eat, the effect of certain drugs, loss of water in the body, and breathing through the mouth. The symptoms of damage to the mucous membranes include mouth pain or discomfort, a coated tongue, dry mouth, mouth tumors or ulcers, a lack of or decrease in saliva, bleeding gums, tooth cavities, and bad breath.

oral poliovirus vaccine (OPV), a drug of changed live poliovirus that makes a patient immune to poliomyelitis. It is often given for a vaccination against poliomyelitis. Also called **Sabin vaccine.**
★CAUTION: Problems with the body's natural ability to resist infection and disease, using steroids at the same time, cancer, or severe infection prohibits its use.
★ADVERSE EFFECTS: Side effects are uncommon. Cases of vaccine-caused disease that makes someone unable to move have occurred but are very rare.

oral sadism, a kind of hateful sexual excitement dealing with the mouth shown by behavior as biting, chewing, and other such actions linked to eating habits. Compare **anal sadism.**

oral stage, the first stage of psychosexual growth, occurring in the first 12 to 18 months of life when the feeding experience and other mouth-related activities are the main source of pleasure. To a great extent, experiences during this stage cause later feelings about food, love, being accepted and rejected, and other parts of the links between the patient and friends or family and the way people act.

orbicularis oculi, the muscular part of the eyelid made up of the palpebral, orbital, and lacrimal muscles. The palpebral muscle closes the eyelid gently; the orbital muscle closes it harder, as in winking. Also called **orbicularis palpebrarum.**

orbicularis oris, the muscle that goes around the mouth, made up partly of fibers taken from other face muscles, as the buccinator, that are placed into the lips, and partly of fibers that are in the lips. It closes and purses the lips.

orbit, one of a pair of bony, cup-shaped openings in the skull that contain the eyeballs and various eye muscles, nerves, and blood vessels that deal with the eyeballs.

orbital fat, a semifluid cushion of fat that lines the bony opening or cave in the skull (orbit) that houses the eye. Loss of the fat causes the eye to look sunken. The fat may be replaced by tumor or other abnormal tissue in certain diseases.

orbital pseudotumor, a swelling of the orbital tissues of the eye, marked by bulging eyes and swollen eyelids. The cause is not known.

orchidectomy /ôr′kidek′təmē/, using surgery to take out one or both testicles. It may be done for serious disease or injury to the testicles or to control cancer of the prostate by taking out a source of male sex (androgenic) hormones. Also called **orchiectomy.**

orchiopexy /ôr′kēpek′sē/, an operation to move an unlowered testicle into the sac that holds the testicles (scrotum), and attach it so that it will not move back into the intestinal area. Sometimes a threadlike stitch (suture) is attached to the lower scrotum and taped to the inner thigh.

orchitis /ôrkī′tis/, inflammation of one or both of the testicles, marked by pain. It is often caused by mumps, syphilis, or tuberculosis. Treatment includes supporting and raising the scrotum, cold packs, and painkillers. **–orchitic,** *adj.*

Oretic, a trademark for a drug to increase the passing of urine (diuretic) (hydrochlorothiazide).

Oreticyl, a trademark for a blood pressure drug containing a diuretic (hydrochlorothiazide) and a high blood pressure drug (deserpidine).

Oreton, a trademark for a male sex hormone (testosterone).

Oreton Methyl, a trademark for a male sex hormone (methyltestosterone).

orexigenic /ôrek′sijen′ik/, a substance that increases the desire to eat.

oreximania /ôrek′simā′nē-ə/, a condition of extreme appetite and of too-much eating. It often results from an unusual or unnatural fear of becoming thin when there is no great chance of that happening. Compare **anorexia nervosa.**

orf, a skin disease caused by viruses and gotten from sheep, in which painless blisters may become red, oozing bumps, finally crusting and healing. Treatment is not necessary. The condition is limited and heals by itself. After having the infection the patient is safe from the infection for the rest of his or her life (immunity).

organ, a structural part of a system of the body, made up of tissues and cells that allow it to do a certain job, as the liver, spleen, or heart. Each one of the organs that occur in pairs, as the lungs, can function by itself. The liver, pancreas, spleen, and brain may continue normal or near normal function with more than 30% of its tissue damaged, destroyed, or taken out by surgery. Also called **organon, organum. –organic,** *adj.*

organelle /ôrgənel′/, any of different bits of living substance found within most cells, as the mitochondria, the Golgi complex, and the centrioles.

organic, 1. referring to any chemical compound that has carbon in it. Compare **inorganic. 2.** referring to an organ.

organic brain syndrome. See **organic mental disorder.**

organic dust, dried bits or dust of plants, animals, fungi, or germs that are fine enough to be carried by the wind. Many kinds of this dust cause different types of breathing problems if they are breathed in. See also **asthma, bagassosis, byssinosis, hay fever.**

organic dust toxic syndrome (ODTS), any respiratory illness caused not by allergy or infection, but by inhaling organic dust from moldy hay or other agricultural products. Symptoms include shaking chills or sweats, cough or shortness of breath, headache, loss of appetite, and muscle pain. See also **farmer's lung, hypersensitivity pneumonitis.**

organic mental disorder, any mental or behavior problem linked to temporary or lifelong brain disorder caused by a physical problem of brain tissue. Causes may include cerebral arteriosclerosis, lead poisoning, or neurosyphilis. Also called **organic brain syndrome.**

organism, any individual living animal or plant able to live by using organs and bits of living substance found in most cells (organelles) in a way that each organ depends on the others.

organizer, any part of an embryo that causes structural growth in some other part. Kinds of organizers include **nucleolar organizer, primary organizer.**

organ of Corti, the true organ of hearing, a spiral within the inner ear containing hair cells that are stimulated by sound waves. The hair cells change the waves into nerve impulses that are sent by the auditory nerve to the brain. Also called **spiral organ of Corti.**

organ of Giraldès. See **paradidymis.**

organ of Golgi. See **neurotendinous spindle.**

organogenesis, the growth of organs and organ systems during life in the womb. The period goes from roughly the end of the second week through the eighth week of pregnancy. During this time the embryo grows and changes rapidly and is very likely to be damaged by infections, drugs, radiation, or other agents in the mother that can cause birth defects. Anything that alters the normal processes of organogenesis can stop the growth of a body part, resulting in one or more birth defects. Also called **organogeny.**

organoid, 1. looking like an organ. **2.** any structure that looks like an organ physically or by the way it works, especially an abnormal tumor mass.

organoid neoplasm, a tumor that looks like a body organ. Compare **histoid neoplasm.**

organotherapy, the treatment of disease by giving animal endocrine glands or the substance that comes from them. Whole glands are no longer put into patients, but substances taken from animal organs are widely used. Also called **Brown-Séquard's treatment.** **–organotherapeutic,** *adj.*

organotypic growth /ôr′ganōtip′ik/, the normal growth and multiplication of tissue cells, as occurs naturally as tissues and organs grow. Compare **histiotypic growth.**

orgasm, the sexual climax, a series of strong muscle tightenings of the genitals over which there is no control. It is experienced as very pleasurable and is set off by intense sexual excitement. **–orgasmic,** *adj.*

orgasmic platform, clogging of the lower vagina during sexual intercourse.

oriental sore, a skin disease caused by the parasitic one-celled organism *Leishmania tropica.* It is carried by the bite of the sand fly. This form of leishmaniasis, marked by skin ulcers, occurs mainly in Africa, Asia, and some Mediterranean countries. Oriental sore causes no general body symptoms, but the sores may cause other infections. Treatment may include infrared treatment and injection of ulcers with an antimony. Also called **Aleppo boil, cutaneous leishmaniasis, Delhi boil, Old World leishmaniasis, tropical sore.** See also **leishmaniasis.**

orientation, being aware of where one is with regard to time, place, and knowing who the people around you are. Disorientation is usually a symptom of physical brain disease and most mental diseases.

orifice /ôr′ifis/, the entrance or outlet of any opening in the body, as the vaginal orifice. Also called **ostium.** **–orificial,** *adj.*

origin, the fixed end of a muscle attachment. Compare **insertion.**

Orimune, a trademark for a live poliovirus vaccine taken by swallowing.

Orinase, a trademark for an antidiabetic drug (tolbutamide) taken by swallowing.

Ornade, a trademark for a drug that has a decongestant (phenylpropanolamine hydrochloride), an antihistamine (chlorpheniramine maleate), and a nerve signal blocker (isopropamide iodide), used for the relief of symptoms of upper breathing tract problems.

ornithine, an amino acid that is not a part of proteins, but is a substance made while food is being made into energy by the body.

ornithine carbamoyl transferase, an enzyme in the blood that increases in patients with liver disease and other diseases.

Ornithodoros /ôr′nithod′ərəs/, a type of tick, some kinds of which carry the spirochetes of relapsing fevers.

ornithosis. See **psittacosis.**

orphan drug, any drug that may be open to use by physicians and patients in countries other than the United States but that has not been taken on by a drug company in the United States. An orphan drug may not be for sale or use in the United States because there would not be enough of it sold to allow the company to spend large amounts of money to develop and make it. Also the drug may not have been approved by the Bureau of Drugs of the Food and Drug Administration, or the drug may be a natural substance. It is very hard legally to keep other companies from making other drugs like it if it is a natural substance. Many orphan drugs are drugs made in Europe or Asia that can be bought and used in the United States as experimental drugs. The U.S. Orphan Drug Act of 1983 offers federal money to companies and research groups to make and sell drugs that before now have not been available in the United States.

oropharynx /ôr′ōfer′ingks/, one of the three parts of the throat (pharynx). It goes from the soft palate in the back of the mouth to the level of the hyoid bone below the lower jaw. It contains the tonsils. Compare **laryngopharynx, nasopharynx.** **–oropharyngeal,** *adj.*

Oroya fever. See **bartonellosis.**

orphenadrine citrate, a drug that relaxes skeletal muscles given to treat serious muscle strain. ★CAUTION: Myasthenia gravis, allergic reactions to similar drugs, or known allergy to this drug prohibits its use.

★ADVERSE EFFECTS: Among the most serious side effects are dry mouth, rapid heart beat, and allergic reactions.

orphenadrine hydrochloride, a nerve signal blocker and antihistaminic drug given to treat parkinsonism.

★CAUTION: Myasthenia gravis or other condition that keeps doctors from using nerve signal-blocking drugs or a known allergy to this drug prohibits its use.

★ADVERSE EFFECTS: Among the most serious side effects are nerve signal-blocking side effects and allergic reactions.

orthodontia. See **orthodontics.**

orthodontic appliance, any device used to change tooth position. Kinds of devices are fixed, movable, active, retaining, within the mouth (intraoral), and outside the mouth (extraoral).

orthodontic band, a thin metal ring, usually made of stainless steel, fitted over a tooth for attaching orthodontic devices to a tooth.

orthodontics /ôr′thədon′tiks/, a branch of dentistry that deals with crooked teeth (malocclusion) and problems of badly aligned teeth.

orthogenesis /ôr′thəjen′əsis/, the theory that evolution is controlled by factors within the living thing (organism) and follows a set path of development rather than as a result of only the strongest and best-suited animals and plants surviving (natural selection) and other factors in the world around each living thing. **–orthogenetic,** *adj.*

orthogenic, referring to treating children and helping to make them normal when they have mental or emotional problems. See also **orthopsychiatry.**

orthomyxovirus /ôr'thōmik'sōvī'rəs/, a member of a family of viruses that includes several that cause the flu (human influenza).

Ortho-Novum, a trademark for a birth-control pill that has a female sex hormone (mestranol) and a progestin (norethindrone).

orthopantogram /ôr'thōpan'təgram/, an x-ray film showing a view of all of the teeth, jaw bones, and nearby structures on a single film.

orthopedics, the branch of medicine that deals with the skeleton, its joints, muscles, and other related structures.

orthopedic traction, a way to keep a patient very still in a device attached by ropes and pulleys to weights that pull on a body part. At the same time, a force in the opposite direction (countertraction) is continued. Traction is used mainly to change the position of bones and keep broken bones rigid. It also is used to overcome muscle spasm, to stretch taped bandages (adhesions), to correct certain badly formed bones, and to help correct permanent tightening of muscles (contractures) caused by arthritis. Traction may be used directly on the skin by attaching the rope-pulley-weight system to bands of adhesive, moleskin, or foam rubber or to a splint attached to a body part. Side arm traction is a kind of skin traction used to line up a broken upper arm bone after the bones have been set into new positions after surgical cutting (open reduction). Skeletal traction may be used directly on a bone in which a wire or pin is put in while the patient is unconscious (under anesthesia) during open reduction of a broken bone. The ends of the pin coming through the skin on both sides of the bone are covered with corks. The pins are attached to a slinglike device, which in turn is attached to the traction rope. Skin or skeletal traction used on a leg allows the patient to move more easily in bed because the leg is balanced with weights and any slack in the ropes attached to the weights caused by the patient's movements is taken up by the traction device. A girdle that fits over the pelvis is used to stop low back pain and a halter is used to stop neck pain. Neck traction may also be used when a broken neck bone is thought to have occurred. During the first stages of traction, the injured part of the body is checked often for pulse, color, warmth, motion, feeling, and swelling.

orthopnea /ôrthop'nē·ə/, an abnormal condition in which a patient must sit or stand to breathe deeply or comfortably. It occurs in many disorders of the heart and breathing systems, as asthma, emphysema, pneumonia, and chest pain (angina pectoris). See also **dyspnea.** –**orthopneic,** adj.

orthopsychiatry, the branch of psychiatry that studies mild mental and behavior disorders, especially in children, and tries to create new ways to help emotional growth.

orthoptic /ôrthop'tik/, referring to normal two-eyed (binocular) sight.

orthoptic examination, testing of the ability of the two eyes to work together correctly, resulting in a single image. If the patient has diplopia, two images are seen. If the patient has amblyopia only one picture may be seen by the working eye. Three-dimensional sight (stereoscopic) training may help two-eyed sight in some conditions.

orthoptist /ôrthop'tist/, a person who tests eye muscles and teaches exercise programs designed to correct problems of the eyes and eye muscles not working together smoothly.

orthosis /ôrthō'sis/, a system designed to control, correct, or make up for a badly shaped bone. Orthosis treatment often uses special braces. –**orthotic** /ôrthot'ik/,adj., n.

orthostatic hypotension, unusually low blood pressure that occurs when a patient stands after sitting or lying down. The falling blood pressure may cause the patient to faint. Also called **postural hypotension.**

orthostatic proteinuria, the presence of protein in the urine of some people who have been standing. It disappears when they lie back and is not medically important. It usually occurs in teen-agers. Also called **orthostatic albuminuria, postural albuminuria, postural proteinuria.**

orthotist /ôr'thətist/, a person who designs, builds, and fits braces or other bone devices.

orthotonos /ôrthot'ənəs/, a straight, rigid posture of the body caused by a muscle spasm. It may happen after being poisoned by strychnine or after a tetanus infection. The neck and all other parts of the body are in a straightened-out position but not as much as in opisthotonos. Compare **emprosthotonos.**

Ortolani's test /ôr'təlä'nēz/, a test of the stability of the hip joints in newborns and infants. The baby is placed on its back, with the hips and knees bent at right angles. The legs are pushed out until the outside of the knees touch the table. The examiner's fingers are stretched out along the outside of the thighs, with the thumbs holding the insides of the knees. The knees are turned to the inside and to the outside. A click or a popping feeling (Ortolani's sign) may be felt if the joint is not strong, because the end of the thigh bone (femur) moves out of the hip joint under pressure from the examiner's hands. See also **congenital dislocation of the hip.**

Orudis, a trademark for a nonsteroidal agent (ketoprofen) used to treat inflammation.

os /os/. See **bone.**

oscilloscope, an instrument with a TV-like screen that shows current electric changes made by heart pumpings or other workings of the body. As used in the study of the heart (cardiology), the oscilloscope can act as a nonstopping device to check different signs of the heart's workings (electrocardiogram).

Osgood-Schlatter disease /oz'goodshlat'ər/, swelling or partial coming apart of the point of attachment of the knee cap (patellar) ligament on the lower leg bone. It is caused by longterm irritation or from too much use of a thigh muscle (quadriceps). The condition is seen mainly in athletic adolescent boys and is marked by swelling and tenderness near the top of a lower leg bone (tibia). Swelling increases with exercise or any movement that straightens out the leg. Treatment may require keeping the knee completely rigid in a cast. If the leg does not heal, surgery may be necessary. Also called **Osgood's disease, Schlatter's disease, Schlatter-Osgood disease.**

Osler's nodes /ōs'lərz/, tender, reddish or purplish bumps of the soft tissue on the ends of fingers or toes. The condition is seen in an infection of the heart lining and valves (mild bacterial endocarditis), and usually lasts only 1 or 2 days.

Osler-Weber-Rendu syndrome /ōs'lərweb'əran-doo'/, an inherited circulation problem. It is marked by bleeding from widened surface blood vessels (capillaries) in the skin and mucous membranes. Small red-to-violet sores are found on the lips, mouth and nasal mucous membranes, tongue, and tips of fingers and toes. The thin, widened vessels may bleed on their own or as a result of only minor injury, becoming more and more severe. Bleeding from the small sores is often heavy and may result in serious blood shortage (anemia). Bleeding sores easily found on open surfaces may be treated with pressure. Blood replacement may be necessary for severe bleeding, and iron deficiency anemia may need continuous treatment. Also called **hereditary hemorrhagic telangiectasia, Rendu-Osler-Weber syndrome.**

osmethesia, the ability to sense and know the difference between odors; the sense of smell.

osmoceptors, receivers in the hypothalamus of the brain that respond to pressure caused by two different fluids being kept apart by a tissue (osmotic pressure), thereby regulating the making of the antidiuretic hormone.

osmosis /ozmō'sis, os-/, the movement of a fluid, as water, through a special tissue (semipermeable membrane) from a solution that has a lower amount of a dissolved substance to one that has a higher amount. The tissue allows the fluid to go through it, but does not allow the substance dissolved in the fluid to pass through. Movement through the tissue happens until the levels of dissolved material in the solutions become equal. See also **permeable, semipermeable membrane.**

osmotic diarrhea, a form of diarrhea that can develop when water is retained in the bowel because substances that do not absorb water have accumulated there. Consuming too much of certain sugar substitutes (hexitols, sorbitol, and mannitol) used in candies, chewing gum, and dietetic foods can lead to osmotic diarrhea. The severity of the condition relates directly to the amount of sugar substitutes consumed and improves when the quantity consumed is reduced. Also called **chewing gum diarrhea, dietetic food diarrhea.**

osmotic diuresis, urine release caused by certain substances in tubes of the kidney, as urea or glucose, that cannot be absorbed.

osmotic fragility, sensitivity to change in osmotic pressure of red blood cells. Exposed to a lower osmotic pressure (hypotonic concentration) of salt in a solution, red cells may absorb more and more water and swell until they burst. Exposed to a higher osmotic pressure (hypertonic concentration) of salt in a solution, red cells give off fluid, shrink, and break up.

osphresis, olfaction; the sense of smell.

osseous labyrinth, the bony part of the inside of the ear. It is made up of three openings: the vestibule, the semicircular canals, and the cochlea, carrying sound vibrations from the middle ear to the acoustic nerve. All three openings have a fluid called perilymph. Also called **labyrinthus osseus.**

ossicle /os'ikəl/, a small bone, as the hammer (malleus), the anvil (incus), or the stirrup (stapes), the ossicles of the inner ear. **–ossicular,** *adj.*

ossification /os'ifikā'shən/, the growth of bone. **Intramembranous ossification** is bone growth that has membrane growth go before it, as in the forming of the roof and the sides of the skull. **Intracartilaginous ossification** is bone growth that has the growth of rods of cartilage go before it, as that forming the bones of the arms and legs.

ossifying fibroma, a slow-growing, noncancerous tumor of bone, seen most often in the jaws, especially the lower jaw. The tumor is made up of bone that grows within fiberlike connective tissue.

ostealgia, any pain that is linked to an abnormal condition within a bone, as osteomyelitis. **–ostealgic,** *adj.*

osteitis /os'tē·ī'tis/, an inflammation of bone, caused by infection, wasting away of bone, or injury. Swelling, tenderness, dull, aching pain, and redness in the skin over the affected bone are signs of the condition. Some kinds of osteitis are **osteitis deformans, osteitis fibrosa cystica.** See also **osteomyelitis, Paget's disease.**

osteitis deformans. See **Paget's disease.**

osteitis fibrosa cystica, a condition in which normal bone is replaced by lumps (cysts) and fiberlike tissue. It is usually linked to excess production of thyroid hormone (hyperparathyroidism).

osteoanagenesis /os'tē·ō·an'əjen'əsis/, the forming or rebuilding of bone tissue by the body. Also called **osteanagenesis.**

osteoarthritis /os'tē·ō·ärthrī'tis/, a common form of arthritis in which one or more joints have tissue changes. Lumps (cysts) may form in bone tissue. Cartilage that normally cushions the joint becomes soft and breaks down. Small pieces of bone and cartilage may become loose and get caught inside the joint, causing pain or forming bony spikes (osteophytes) that point out into the joint. Swelling of the membrane lining the joint is common. Its cause is unknown but may include chemical, mechanical, inborn, metabolic, and endocrine factors. Emotional stress often worsens the condition. The condition usually begins with pain after exercise or use of the joint. Stiffness, tenderness to the touch, rubbing noises (crepitus), and a large joint develop. Badly formed bones or joints, and joints becoming out of place (subluxation) may occur over time. When the hip, knee, or the spine are involved, this causes more problems of movement and use of joints than osteoarthritis of other areas. Treatment includes rest of the joints that are affected, heat, and antiswelling drugs. Injections of adrenal hormone drugs into the joint may give relief. Surgery is sometimes necessary and may reduce pain and greatly improve the working of a joint. Replacing the hip and joining together the parts of the joint are some of the kinds of surgery that are used in treating serious cases of osteoarthritis. Also called **degenerative joint disease.** Compare **rheumatoid arthritis.**

osteoblast, a cell that begins in the embryo and, during the early growth of the skeleton, works in forming bone tissue. Osteoblasts bring together the substances that form the bone grouping and over time grow into osteocytes. Also called **osteoplast.** See also **ossification.** **–osteoblastic,** *adj.*

osteoblastoma /os'tē·ōblastō'mə/, *pl.* **osteoblastomas, osteoblastomata,** a small, noncancerous bone tumor. It occurs most often in the spine or bones of the legs or arms. Children and young adults most often get this condition. The tumor causes pain and loss of bone tissue. When possible, using surgery to take out the tumor is the best treatment. Also called **osteoid osteoma.**

osteochondroma /os'tē·ōkondrō'mə/, a noncancerous tumor made of bone and cartilage.

osteochondrosis /os'tē·ōkondrō'sis/, a disease that affects the bone-forming centers in chil-

dren. It begins by destroying and killing bone tissue, followed by regrowth of bone tissue. Kinds of osteochondrosis include **Legg-Calvé-Perthes disease, Osgood-Schlatter disease, Scheuermann's disease.**

osteoclasia /os'tē·ōklā'zhə/, **1.** a condition when bony tissue is destroyed and absorbed by large bone cells (osteoclasts). It may occur during growth or the healing of broken bones. **2.** the destruction of bone by disease. See also **osteolysis.**

osteoclasis /os'tē·ok'ləsis/, a process in which a surgeon purposely breaks a bone that is badly shaped and reshapes it in a normal condition. Also called **osteoclasty.** **–osteoclastic,** *adj.*

osteoclast, 1. also called **osteophage.** a large bone cell that works in periods of growth or repair. During healing of broken bones, or during certain diseases, osteoclasts carve paths through bone tissue around the break. Osteoclasts are set off by parathyroid hormone and also by a substance made by white blood cells (lymphocytes) in diseases, as multiple myeloma and lymphomas. See also **ossification. 2.** a tool used during surgery in the breaking or rebreaking of bones in order to repair a badly shaped bone.

osteoclastic, 1. referring to osteoclasts. **2.** destructive to bone.

osteoclastoma /os'tē·ōklastō'mə/, *pl.* **osteoclastomas, osteoclastomata,** a giant cell tumor of the bone that occurs most often at the end of a long bone. It often appears as a tissue mass that has a thin shell of new bone around it. The tumor may be harmless (benign) but is more often cancerous. It causes pain, loss of the ability of the bone to work correctly, and, in some cases, weakness followed by broken bones. Also called **giant cell myeloma, giant cell tumor of bone.**

osteocyte, a bone cell; a fully grown osteoblast that has become buried in the bone material (matrix). It is found in a small opening and sends out new shapes that connect (anastomose) with those of other osteoblasts to form a system of tiny canals within the bone grouping. **–osteocytic,** *adj.*

osteodystrophy, any basic problem in bone growth. It is usually linked to problems in calcium and phosphorus use by the body and kidney disease, as in kidney osteodystrophy. Also called **osteodystrophia.**

osteogenesis, the beginnings and growth of bone tissue. Also called **osteogeny.** See also **ossification. –osteogenetic, osteogenic,** *adj.*

ostegenesis imperfecta, an inborn problem that causes poor growth of connective tissue. It is marked by abnormally brittle and fragile bones that are easily broken by the slightest injury. In its worst form, the disease may be seen at birth, when it is known as osteogenesis imperfecta congenita. The newborn baby has multiple broken bones because of bones forming badly and bone turned to minerals. Most infants with this condition die shortly after birth, although a few survive as badly deformed dwarfs with normal mental growth if no head injury has happened. If the disease happens later, it is called osteogenesis imperfecta tarda and is usually less serious. Symptoms may appear when the child begins to walk, but they become less serious with age, and the high risk of having broken bones gets lower and often goes away after puberty. Other factors include bluish eyeballs, clear skin, ligaments that stretch too far, poor tooth growth, getting nosebleeds often, sweating too much, mild fever, deafness, and a high risk of bruising easily. There is no known cure for the disease. Extreme care must be taken in handling patients, especially infants who have a serious condition, to keep broken bones from happening. Giving the patient magnesium oxide may lower the broken bone rate and the sweating, fever, and constipation linked to the condition. Also called **brittle bones, fragilitas ossium, hypoplasia of the mesenchyme, osteopsathyrosis.**

osteogenic, made up of or starting from any tissue that the body uses in the growth or repair of bone. Also **osteogenous** /os′tē·oj′ənəs/.

osteogenic sarcoma. See **osteosarcoma.**

osteoid /os′tē·oid/, referring to or looking like bone.

osteolysis /os′tē·ol′isis/, the destruction of bone tissue, caused by disease, infection, or poor blood supply. The condition often affects bones of the hands and feet. It is seen in disorders that affect blood vessels, as in Raynaud's disease, scleroderma, and systemic lupus erythematosus. **–osteolytic,** adj.

osteoma /os′tē·ō′mə/, pl. **osteomas, osteomata,** a tumor of bone tissue.

osteomalacia /os′tē·ōmələā′shə/, an abnormal softening of the bone. There is a loss of calcium in the bone material (matrix), along with weakness, broken bones, pain, loss of desire to eat, and weight loss. The condition may be caused by not enough phosphorus and calcium in the blood to allow proper hardening of the bones. This lack of minerals may be caused by poor diet, a lack of vitamin D, or not getting enough sunlight, which the body needs to make use of vitamin D. Other causes are a disorder that disturbs the normal absorption of minerals and nutrients from the intestine. Osteomalacia causes and also makes worse many other diseases and conditions. Treatment usually includes giving the necessary vitamins and minerals. See also **adult rickets, hyperparathyroidism, Paget's disease, rickets.**

osteomyelitis /os′tē·ōmī·əlī′tis/, an infection of bone and bone marrow. It is most often caused by germs that enter the bone during an injury or surgery. The germs may also reach the bone directly from a nearby infection or through the bloodstream. Staphylococci germs are often part of the cause of this problem. The long bones in children and the spinal bones in adults are often places of infection caused by germs spreading through the bloodstream. Continuing and increasing bone pain, tenderness, local muscle spasm, and fever are symptoms of the disease. Treatment includes bed rest and anti-infection drugs by injection for several weeks. Surgery may be necessary to take out dead bone and tissue, to fill holes, and to use artificial devices to keep the diseased bones and joints from moving. Long-term osteomyelitis may go on for years with periods of many or fewer symptoms in spite of treatment.

osteon /os′tē·on/, the basic unit of compact bone. It is made up of the haversian canal and 4 to 20 layers of rounded plates of hard bone (lamellae).

osteonecrosis /os′tē·ōnəkrō′sis/, the destruction and death of bone tissue, as caused by not-enough blood (ischemia), infection, cancer, or injury. **–osteonecrotic,** adj.

osteopath /os′tē·ōpath′/, a physician who specializes in bone diseases (osteopathy). Also called **osteopathist.**

osteopathy /os′tē·op′əthē/, the practice of medicine that uses all of the usual techniques of drugs, surgery, and radiation, but looks more at the links between the organs and the muscle and skeletal system. Osteopathic physicians may correct structural problems by changing the position of bones in the treatment of health problems.

osteopenia, a condition where the bone has not gotten enough mineral, usually because more bone cells are dying in the body than new ones are being made by the body.

osteopetrosis, an overall increase in bone density. It is usually caused by faulty bone resorption resulting from a lack of large bone cells (osteoclasts). In its worst form, the bone marrow cavity is destroyed, causing severe low levels of blood (anemia), a badly shaped skull, and pressure on the skull nerves, which may cause deafness and blindness and lead to an early death. A milder form is marked by short height, fragile bones that break easily, and a likelihood to develop a bone disease (osteomyelitis). Both kinds are inborn diseases. Also called **Albers-Schönberg disease, ivory bones, marble bones, osteosclerosis fragilis.** See also **osteoclast. –osteopetrotic,** adj.

osteopoikilosis, an inborn condition of the bones, marked by many areas of dense calcium deposits all over the bone tissue. It causes a spotty look on x-ray film. Osteopoikilosis is usually harmless, most often without symptoms, and of unknown cause. Also called **osteosclerosis fragilis congenita. –osteopoikilotic,** adj.

osteoporosis, a loss of normal bone density, marked by thinning of bone tissue and the growth of small holes in the bone. It occurs most frequently in women who have gone through menopause, patients who are inactive or paralyzed, and in patients taking steroid hormones. The disorder may cause pain, especially in the lower back, frequent broken bones, loss of body height, and various badly formed parts of the body. Osteoporosis is sometimes linked to other disorders, as the effects of too much parathyroid hormone (hyperparathyroidism). Estrogen, a female sex hormone, is often used to prevent postmenopausal osteoporosis, but use of the hormone also has the risk of causing cancer of the uterus.

osteopsathyrosis. See **osteogenesis imperfecta.**

osteosarcoma /os'tē·ōsärkō'mə/, a type of cancer made up of bone cells. Also called **osteogenic sarcoma.**

osteosclerosis, an abnormal increase in the density of bone tissue. The condition occurs in different kinds of diseases and is often linked to poor blood ciruclation in the bone tissue, infection, and the forming of tumors. It may be caused by faulty bone resorption. See also **achondroplasia, osteopetrosis, osteopoikilosis.** **–osteosclerotic,** *adj.*

osteotomy, the sawing or cutting of a bone. Kinds of osteotomy include block osteotomy, in which a section of bone is removed; cuneiform osteotomy to remove a bone wedge; and displacement osteotomy, in which a bone is rebuilt using surgery to change bone alignment on the areas that carry most of the body's weight.

ostomy /os'təmē/, *informal.* using surgery to make an artificial opening in the body to allow the release of urine from the bladder or of feces from the bowel. A cut (stoma) in the wall of the abdomen is made using surgery. An ostomy may also be done to correct a physical problem or to treat a blockage, infection, or injury of the urinary or intestinal tract. Each procedure is named for the place of the ostomy in the body and its organs, as a colostomy, cecostomy, or cystostomy.

ostomy care, the care given to the person with a cut made during surgery in the bladder, ileum, or colon for the short-term or long-term passage of urine or feces. In most cases the opening is covered with a temporary disposable bag in the operating room. The bag is changed when needed and the way the substance looks, its color, and the amount that has drained are noted. Mucus usually begins to drain from the opening (stoma) within 48 hours after the operation, fecal drainage within 72 hours. A long-term device is attached to the stoma as soon after surgery as possible. Each time the short-term or long-term device is changed, the skin

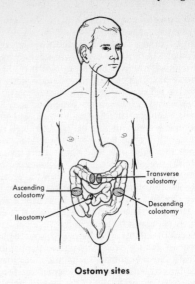

Transverse colostomy

Ascending colostomy

Descending colostomy

Ileostomy

Ostomy sites

around the stoma is washed with soap and water, rinsed carefully, and patted dry with a clean towel. If the skin is reddened or worn away, karaya powder, by itself or mixed with an ointment, is spread over the area before the device is put back in. A sticky substance may be used to keep a tight seal with the device, and deodorant drops or other odor controllers are added to the ostomy bag. The patient's diet must be planned according to the kind of ostomy. A patient with an ileostomy may need food high in sodium and potassium, as bananas, citrus juices, molasses, and cola. He or she should stay away from fried, highly seasoned, and rich foods; nuts; raisins; raw fruits other than bananas; and anything that causes gas or diarrhea. Gas-causing foods include cabbage, beans, broccoli, cauliflower, and corn. The patient should also stay away from foods that cause bad odors, as onions, eggs, and fish, and certain flavorings. A diet of foods that the body can easily digest and absorb is best for most ostomy patients. How much fluid the patient drinks should also be closely watched.

ostomy irrigation, a way to clean, start, and control the release of an opening in the body made during surgery to allow better discharge of feces or urine. Fluids used to clean out the opening are often tap water and salt (saline) or drugs dissolved in a liquid. Tools needed are irrigator tips, tubes (catheters), drainage bags that allow the tube to be put in, a container used during the cleaning of the device, and shields to keep leaking from occurring. Loop and double-barrel colostomies with two openings need to have their parts cleaned separately.

otalgia /ōtal′jē·ə/, pain in the ear. Also called **otodynia, otoneuralgia.**

OTC, abbreviation for *over the counter,* describing a drug that can be bought without a prescription.

Othello syndrome, a mental problem marked by the patient always thinking his or her spouse is unfaithful and by excess jealousy. This condition may be seen with rage and violence.

otic /ō′tik, ot′ik/, referring to the ear. Also **auricular.**

otics /ō′tiks, ot′iks/, drugs used to treat swelling of the outer ear canal or to take out excess ear wax (cerumen).

otitis /ōti′tis/, inflammation or infection of the ear. Kinds of otitis are **otitis externa, otitis interna, otitis media.**

otitis externa, swelling or infection of the outside canal of the ear or the larger part (auricle) outside the head. The main causes are allergy, germs, fungi, viruses, and injury. A patient may be allergic to nickel or chromium metal in earrings, to chemicals in hair sprays, cosmetics, hearing aids, and certain drugs. *Staphylococcus aureus, Pseudomonas aeruginosa,* and *Streptococcus pyogenes* are common germ causes. Herpes simplex and herpes zoster viruses are often other causes. Eczema, psoriasis, and seborrheic dermatitis also may affect the outer ear. Bruises of the ear canal may become infected, and swimming too much may wash out the ear wax that protects the ear and remove skin fats, leading to infection. Otitis externa is more common during hot, humid weather. Treatment includes aspirin or similar painkillers, careful cleaning, antibiotics to treat infection, or hormone creams to lower swelling.

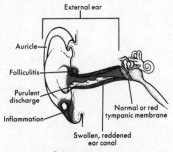

Otitis externa

otitis media, swelling or infection of the middle ear, a common disease of childhood. Acute otitis media is usually caused by *Haemophilus influenzae* or *Streptococcus pneumoniae.* Chronic otitis media is usually caused by germs as *Proteus, Klebsiella,* and *Pseudomonas.* Allergy, fungus, and several viruses also may be causes. An upper chest breathing infection often happens before the onset of otitis media. Germs and viruses get into the middle ear through the eustachian tube, which opens into the mouth and throat. Blockage of the eustachian tube and gathering of fluids may increase pressure within the middle ear, forcing infection into the porous mastoid bone (tympanic membrane). Symptoms of acute otitis media include a sense of fullness in the ear, with impaired hearing, pain, and fever. Usually only one ear gets this disorder. A tumorlike cyst (cholesteatoma) may grow in the middle ear. Deafness may occur if many infections cause a broken eardrum. Pneumococcal otitis media may also spread to the membranes of the brain and spinal cord.

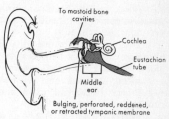

Otitis media

otocephaly /ōtōsef′əlē/, a birth defect marked by not having a lower jaw, a badly formed mouth, and joining of the ears on the neck. See also **agnathocephaly. –otocephalic, otocephalous,** *adj.*

otolaryngology a branch of medicine that deals with diseases and disorders of the ears, nose, and throat, and nearby parts of the head and neck.

otolith righting reflex /ō′təlith-/, a reflex that newborn babies cannot control in which tilting of the body when the infant is in an upright position causes the head to move back to the upright position. This uncontrollable movement allows the infant to raise the head and is important for the growth of later motor nerve workings. Not having this movement may mean there is something wrong with the baby's central nervous system.

otology /ōtol′əjē/, the study of the ear, including the diagnosis and treatment of its diseases and disorders.

otoplasty /ō′təoplas′tē/, using plastic surgery to rebuild the outer ear by taking out some of the cartilage in the ears in order to bring the outer ear closer to the head.

otorrhea /ō′tərē′ə/, any substance discharged from the external ear. Otorrhea may contain blood, pus, or cerebrospinal fluid. **–otorrheal, otorrheic, otorrhetic,** *adj.*

otosclerosis /ō′tōsklərō′sis/, an inborn problem of unknown cause in which abnormal bone formation in the canal labyrinth of the inner ear causes noises in the ear, then deafness. The deafness may come about any time between 11 and 30 years of age. Women get this condition twice as often as men. The condition may get worse during pregnancy. An operation to replace the stapes in the middle ear usually works to restore hearing for life. Also called **otospongiosis.**

otoscope /ō'təskōp'/, a tool used to look at the outer ear, the eardrum, and, looking through the eardrum, the tiny bones (ossicles) of the middle ear. It is made up of a light, a magnifying lens, and a device for blowing air into the ear (insufflation).

ototoxic /ō'tōtok'sik/, any substance having a bad effect on the eighth cranial (vestibulocochlear) nerve or the organs of hearing and balance. Common ototoxic drugs include certain antibiotics, aspirin, and quinine.

Otrivin, a trademark for a drug that makes blood vessels narrower (xylometazoline hydrochloride), used as a nasal decongestant.

ouabain /wəbā'in/, a heart tonic given to treat congestive heart failure and certain abnormal heart rhythms.

★CAUTION: Having a heart that beats with irregular patterns or a known allergy to this drug prohibits its use.

★ADVERSE EFFECTS: Among the more serious side effects are nausea, vomiting, sight problems, and abnormal heart beats.

ounce (oz), a unit of weight equal to ⅟₁₆ of 1 pound avoirdupois.

outbreeding, the making of offspring by the mating of individuals, plants, or other living things that are not related to each other. Compare **inbreeding.** See also **heterosis.**

outcome, the condition of a patient at the end of treatment or of a disease, including how well the patient is and the need for giving more care, drugs, support, or counseling.

outlet, an opening through which something can come out, as the pelvic outlet through which a baby comes during childbirth.

outlet contraction. See **contraction.**

outlet contracture, an abnormally small pelvic outlet. It is important in childbirth because it may not let the baby come through the birth canal.

outpatient, 1. a patient, not staying in a hospital, who is being treated in an office, clinic, or other walk-in ambulatory care facility. **2.** referring to a health-care facility for patients who do not need to be in a hospital. Compare **inpatient.**

ova and parasites test, a test using a microscope to look for parasites, as amebas or worms and their eggs (ova) in a patient's feces.

ovale malaria. See **tertian malaria.**

ovalocytosis. See **elliptocytosis.**

ovarian, referring to the ovary.

ovarian artery, a slim branch of the abdominal aorta that takes blood to an ovary. Compare **testicular artery.**

ovarian cancer, a cancer of the ovary. It occurs most often in women between 40 and 60 years of age and sometimes in adolescents. See also **ovarian carcinoma.**

ovarian carcinoma, a type of cancer of the ovaries that is not often found in the early stage. It occurs often in the fifth decade of life. The most common tumor of the reproductive system, ovarian carcinoma appears to be an increasingly common disease in the United States. Factors that increase the chance of getting the disease are not being able to have children (infertility), having few or no children, having children later than normal, repeated spontaneous abortion, endometriosis, Group A blood type, irradiation of pelvic organs, and exposure to chemicals that cause cancer, as asbestos and talc. After a beginning without symptoms, the tumor may have grown a great deal by the time it is found. In cases where the disease has grown for a long time the patient may have fluid pooling, swollen legs, and pain in the intestine area and backs of the legs. A pelvic examination each year after 40 years of age helps find the cancer at an early stage and helps the chances of recovery. As the disease grows, swelling and pain in the intestine area, abnormal vaginal bleeding, weight loss, and changes in urination and bowel movement patterns may be signs of the cancer in women who have gone through menopause. A pap smear may show cancer cells if the tumor is far along. A test using high-level sound waves (ultrasound examination) can show an ovarian tumor but does not show the difference between a harmless and cancerous tumor. A computed tomography (CT) scan may also help in finding an ovarian tumor. To be able to know for sure if the patient has a cancerous tumor, surgery on the intestine area is needed. The surgery that doctors suggest for ovarian cancer is to take out the uterus, ovaries, fallopian tubes, and the connecting membranes (omentum). About one-half of the tumors found to have cancer cannot be operated on. Postsurgery irradiation of the pelvis and pelvic lymph nodes should be done; radioisotopes are used in some cases.

ovarian cyst, a small globelike sac filled with fluid or semisolid material that grows in or on the ovary. It may only stay there for a short time and can be harmless or dangerous. Kinds of ovarian cysts include **chocolate cyst, corpus luteum cyst, dermoid cyst.**

ovarian pregnancy, a rare type of pregnancy in which the embryo grows in the ovary rather than in the womb.

ovarian varicocele, a varicose swelling of the veins of the broad ligament that helps support the ovaries. Also called **pelvic varicocele.**

ovarian vein, one of a pair of veins that come out from the broad ligament near the ovaries and the fallopian tubes. In some patients the ovarian veins have valves that get very large during pregnancy. Compare **testicular vein.**

ovariectomy. See **oophorectomy.**

ovary, one of the pair of female sexual reproduction organs (gonads) found on each side of the lower abdomen in a fold of the broad ligament, beside the uterus. At ovulation, an egg (ovum) is released from a small cavity (follicle) on the surface of the ovary. Ovulation is brought on by the gonadotrophic hormones, follicle stimulating hormone (FSH), and luteinizing hormone (LH). The fully grown ovarian follicle also releases the hormones estrogen and progesterone. Each ovary is normally firm, smooth, and looks like an almond in size and shape.

Ovcon, a trademark for a birth-control pill containing a female sex hormone (ethinyl estradiol) and a progestin (norethindrone acetate).

overbite, the up and down (vertical) overlapping of lower teeth by upper teeth. Compare **overclosure, overjet.**

overclosure, an abnormal condition in which the lower jaw rises too far.

overcompensation, an extreme attempt to overcome a real or unreal physical or mental problem. The patient may not be aware of his or her trying to solve the problem. See also **compensation.**

overdenture, a denture that can be totally or partly taken out and that is supported by the remaining tooth roots to give better support and make the denture more secure.

overinclusiveness, a type of mental problem seen in some schizophrenia patients. The patient is unable to think or speak well because of an inability to keep unimportant ideas and facts out of his or her mind.

overjet, a side to side (horizontal) pushing out of upper teeth beyond the lower teeth. Also called **horizontal overlap.** Compare **overbite, overclosure.**

overload, anything that pushes the body beyond its normal limits and may harm its health.

overoxygenation, an abnormal condition in which the amount of oxygen in the blood and other tissues of the body is greater than normal, and the amount of carbon dioxide is less than normal. The condition is marked by a fall in blood pressure, being less able to breathe, weakness, making errors in judgment, having numb hands and feet, not wanting to eat, nausea, and vomiting.

over the counter (OTC), referring to a drug that the consumer can buy without a prescription.

overweight, more-than-normal body weight after taking into account height, body build, and age.

oviduct. See **fallopian tube.**

oviferous /ōvif′ərəs/, bearing or able to make egg cells (ova).

ovoflavin /ō′vəflā′vin/, a riboflavin (vitamin B_2) taken from the yolk of eggs.

ovogenesis. See **oogenesis.**

ovoglobulin /ō′vəglob′yŏolin/, a protein (globulin) taken from the white of eggs.

ovogonium. See **oogonium.**

ovolacto vegetarian. See **lactoovo vegetarian.**

ovoid arch, a dental arch that curves smoothly from the molars on one side to those on the other side to form one-half of an oval.

ovomucoid /ō′vəmyŏo′koid/, referring to a glycoprotein, similar to mucin, taken from the white of eggs.

ovotestis /ō′vətes′tis/, a sexual reproductive organ (gonad) that has tissue like that of the ovary and testicles; a male and female (hermaphroditic) gonad. **–ovotesticular,** adj.

ovovitellin. See **vitellin.**

Ovral, a trademark for a birth-control pill that has a progestin (norgestrel) and a female sex hormone (ethinyl estradiol).

Ovrette, a trademark for a birth-control pill that has a progestin (norgestrel).

ovulation, releasing an egg (ovum) from the ovary after the breaking of a mature small cavity (follicle). It is caused by the new activity of cyclic ovarian and pituitary hormones. Ovulation usually occurs on the 14th day following the first day of the last menstrual period and often causes brief, sharp lower intestine area pain on the side of the ovulating ovary. See also **mittelschmerz, oogenesis. –ovulate,** v.

ovulation method of family planning, a natural method of family planning that depends on watching changes in the type and amount of cervical mucus as a means of telling the time of ovulation during the menstrual cycle. Because pregnancy occurs with fertilization of an egg (ovum) released from the ovary at ovulation, the method is used to increase or decrease the woman's chance of becoming pregnant. It allows the man and woman to cause or avoid insemination during the fertile period. The gonadotropic hormones, especially estrogen, cause changes in the amount and type of cervical mucus. In the first days after menstruation, a small amount of thick mucus is released by the cervix. These "dry days" are "safe days," with ovulation several days away. The amount of mucus then increases; it is pearly-white and sticky, and gets clearer and less sticky as ovulation gets nearer; these "wet days" are "unsafe days." During and just after ovulation the mucus is clear, slippery, and elastic; it looks like the uncooked white of an egg. The day on which this sign is most clear is the "peak day," probably the day before ovulation. The 4 days following the "peak day" are "unsafe"; fertilization might occur. By the end of the 4 days, the mucus becomes pearly-white and sticky again and decreases in amount until menstruation occurs, which begins a new cycle. During the first cycle, not having sexual intercourse may be necessary to allow watching the mucus without also having to watch semen or contraceptive foam, cream, or jelly. Looking closely at the mucus each day is needed even after several cycles because the length of the "safe" and "unsafe" periods and the time of ovulation are different from cycle to cycle, as they are from woman to woman. After childbirth, and during the time the mother has breast milk (lactation), the method is not safe until menstruation has become regular. The safeness of the method in knowing which are the most fertile days of the cycle is helped by using the basal body temperature method. This combined method is called the symptothermal method of planning. Supporters of the ovulation method say its strong points are that it is cheap and natural and works well. Opponents say that it is not being done by most people, that it requires a lot of teaching and self-motivation, and that it will only work well if the user can learn correctly how to watch the changes in the cervical mucus. Avoiding sexual intercourse may be necessary for up to 10 days by a woman whose menstrual cycles are long or are of irregular length. Also called **cervical mucus method of family planning.**

Ovulen, a trademark for a birth-control pill that has a female sex hormone (mestranol) and a progestin (ethynodiol diacetate).

Corona radiata

Polar body

Zona pellucida

Cytoplasm

Nucleus

Ovum

ovum, *pl.* **ova,** **1.** an egg. **2.** a female germ cell released from the ovary at ovulation.

oxacillin sodium, a penicillinase-immune penicillin antibiotic given to treat severe infections caused by penicillin-immune staphylococci.

★CAUTION: Known allergy to this drug or to any other penicillin prohibits its use.

★ADVERSE EFFECTS: Among the most serious side effects are severe allergic reactions, stomach and intestinal disturbances, and itching in the anal and genital areas.

oxandrolone, a male sex hormone given to treat lack of testosterone, osteoporosis, and female breast cancer, and to start or increase growth, weight gain, and red blood cell production.

★CAUTION: Cancer of the male breast or prostate, liver disease, pregnancy or suspected pregnancy, or known allergy to this drug prohibits its use.

★ADVERSE EFFECTS: Among the more serious side effects are excess hair growth (hirsutism), acne, liver disease, too many or too few minerals in the body, and different hormone effects in some patients.

oxazepam /oksā′zəpam/, a mild tranquilizer given to help lower tension and nervousness.

oxidation, **1.** any process in which the amount of oxygen of a chemical compound is increased. **2.** any reaction in which the positive charge of a chemical compound or a radical is increased because of a loss of electrons. **–oxidize,** *v.*

oxidative water, water made by the oxidation of molecules of food substances, as the changing of sugar to water and carbon dioxide in processes within a tissue cell.

oxidize, to combine or cause to combine with oxygen. **–oxidation,** *n.,* **oxidizing,** *adj.*

oxidizing agent, a chemical compound that easily gives up oxygen and attracts hydrogen from another compound.

Oxsoralen, a trademark for a skin-coloring drug (methoxsalen).

oxtriphylline /oks′trəfil′ēn/, a bronchial tube-widening drug given to treat bronchial asthma, bronchitis, and emphysema.

★CAUTION: Known allergy to this or a related drug prohibits its use. It is used carefully in patients with ulcers or with heart disease for whom making the heart beat faster might be harmful.

★ADVERSE EFFECTS: Among the more common side effects are stomach and intestinal distress, irregular heart beat, nervousness, and not being able to sleep (insomnia).

oxybutynin chloride, a nerve drug given to treat a bladder that is not working correctly (neurogenic).

★CAUTION: Glaucoma, problems of the stomach and intestinal or urinary tract, or known allergy to this drug or to other drugs like it prohibits its use.

★ADVERSE EFFECTS: Among the more serious side effects are reduced sweating, urinary bloating, blurred sight, rapid heart-beat, and severe allergic reactions.

oxycephaly /ok′sisef′əlē/, a birth defect of the skull in which premature closing of the joints or seams (sutures) of the skull results in increased upward growth of the head, giving it a long, narrow look with the top pointed or cone shaped. Also called **oxycephalia, acrocephaly,**

hypsicephaly, steeple head, tower head, tower skull, turricephaly. See also **craniostenosis.** –oxycephalus, *n.,* oxycephalous, *adj.*

oxycodone hydrochloride, a narcotic painkiller used to treat moderate to severe pain.
★CAUTION: It is used carefully in many conditions, including head injuries, asthma, kidney or liver disease, or unstable heart condition. Known allergy to this drug prohibits its use.
★ADVERSE EFFECTS: Among the most serious side effects are sleepiness, dizziness, nausea, constipation, breathing and circulation problems, and drug addiction.

oxygen (O), a tasteless, odorless, and colorless gas that is necessary for human life. In breathing therapy, oxygen is given to increase the amount of oxygen and thus to lower the amount of other gases in the blood. In anesthesia, oxygen is a carrier gas for the delivery of anesthetic drugs to the tissues of the body. An overdose of oxygen can cause poisoning that cannot be reversed in patients with lung problems, especially when things are made worse by long-term gathering in the body of carbon dioxide. Giving high levels of oxygen over a long time may cause damage to infants' eyes that cannot be reversed. Oxygen itself is not flammable or explosive, but because a room with high levels of oxygen will help cause fire and explosion, there must be no flames or electric sparks when oxygen is being given. See also **oxygen toxicity.**

oxygenation, the process of combining or treating with oxygen. –oxygenate, *v.*

oxygen consumption, the amount of oxygen in milliliters per minute necessary for normal body functions.

oxygen mask, a device used to give oxygen. It is shaped to fit snugly over the mouth and nose and may be held in place with a strap or with the hand. The mask has valves allowing oxygen to be breathed in or pumped into the lungs and carbon dioxide to be breathed out. Oxygen flows at a set rate through a tube to the mask, often through a bag that can be pumped by hand.

oxygen therapy, any procedure in which oxygen is given to a patient to relieve oxygen shortage (hypoxia). If hypoxia is the result of heart disease, a high level of oxygen may be given by a mask. Humidity and drugs in aerosol form may be given with oxygen. The giving of oxygen may help relieve low blood pressure, heart rhythm disorders, rapid heart beat, headache, confusion, nausea, and the nervousness that goes with hypoxia. It also allows the cells of the body to carry on normal functions once again.

oxygen toxicity, a condition of oxygen overdose that can cause dangerous tissue changes, as a form of blindness (retrolental fibroplasia) or a type of emphysema (bronchopulmonary dysplasia).

oxygen transport, the process by which oxygen is absorbed in the lungs by the hemoglobin in red blood cells and carried to tissue cells all over the body. This process is possible because hemoglobin is able to combine with large amounts of oxygen when it is at high levels, as in the lungs, and to release this oxygen when the oxygen level is low, as in the body tissues. See also **hemoglobin.**

oxyhemoglobin /ok′sēhē′məglō′bin, -hem′-/, the product of the combining of hemoglobin with oxygen. It is a loosely bound chemical complex that releases oxygen molecules easily in the tissue cells.

Oxylone, a trademark for a hormone cream (fluorometholone).

oxymetazoline hydrochloride /ok′sēmətaz′əlēn/, a decongestant given to treat nasal congestion.
★CAUTION: Hyperthyroidism, diabetes, use of a monoamine oxidase inhibitor within 14 days, or known allergy to this drug prohibits its use.
★ADVERSE EFFECTS: Among the more serious side effects are continued congestion, central nervous system activity, and, in children, a severe shocklike syndrome with coma, falling blood pressure, and slow heart beat.

oxymetholone, a male sex hormone given to treat a lack of testosterone, an abnormal bone disease (osteoporosis), and female breast cancer; and to increase the rate of growth, weight gain, and the making of red blood cells.
★CAUTION: Cancer of the male breast or prostate, liver disease, pregnancy or suspected pregnancy, or known allergy to this drug prohibits its use.
★ADVERSE EFFECTS: Among the more serious side effects are excess hair growth (hirsutism), acne, liver disease, having too much or too little minerals in the body, and, depending on the age of the patient, different hormone effects.

oxymorphone hydrochloride, a narcotic painkiller given to reduce moderate to severe pain, as a drug before surgery, and during anesthesia.
★CAUTION: Drug addiction or known allergy to this drug prohibits its use.
★ADVERSE EFFECTS: Among the more serious side effects are drug addiction, urinary bloating, and breathing or circulation problems.

oxyopia /ok′sē·ō′pē·ə/, unusually good sight. A patient with normal (20/20) vision when standing 20 feet from the standard Snellen eye chart can read the seventh line of letters, each of which is ⅛-inch high. A patient with oxyopia can read smaller letters at that distance. Also called **oxyopy** /ok′sē·ō′pē/.

oxytetracycline, an antibiotic given to treat germ and rickettsial infections.
★CAUTION: Pregnancy, early childhood, or known allergy to this or to other tetracyclines prohibits its use. The drug is used carefully in patients who have kidney or liver disease.

★ADVERSE EFFECTS: Among the more serious side effects are stomach and intestinal ailments, being sensitive to light, possible new and serious infections, and different kinds of allergic reactions. The teeth of children exposed to the drug in the uterus or before 8 years of age may become badly discolored.

oxytocic /ok′sitō′sik/, **1.** referring to a substance that is like the hormone oxytocin. **2.** any one of many drugs that start the smooth muscle of the uterus to pull in (contract). An oxytocic can cause and increase rhythmic contractions in the uterus at any time, but high doses are needed for such responses in early pregnancy. These drugs are often used to start labor at the end of pregnancy (term). They are also used to control bleeding after childbirth, to correct uterine muscle tone after childbirth, to cause uterine contractions after childbirth by surgical opening (cesarean section) or other uterine surgery, and to cause an abortion. The U.S. Food and Drug Administration has ruled that oxytocin is not to be used to end a pregnancy just because the patient desires to do so and should be used only in cases where continued pregnancy is seen as a greater risk to the mother or to the fetus than the risk of causing labor by drugs. These drugs are used very carefully in pregnant women with severe blood pressure problems, partial placenta previa, a fetus that may be larger than the pelvic opening, or more than one fetus. The risk of using these drugs is much higher in mothers who have just had uterine surgery or who have had a recent disease or injury. The most serious side effect is continued spasmodic contractions of the uterus that may cause death of the fetus or a break in the uterus.

oxytocin /ok′sitō′sin/, an oxytocic given to start uterine contractions in bringing on or increasing labor, and to contract the uterus to control bleeding following childbirth. See also **oxytocic.**

oxytocin challenge test, a test to see if the fetus is able to tolerate continuation of pregnancy or the likely stress of labor and childbirth. Other tests to check the well-being of the fetus may be done before physicians decide on an emergency childbirth by surgical opening (cesarean section) or causing labor.

ozena /ōzē′nə/, a condition of the nose marked by a decrease of the bony ridges and mucous membranes inside the nose. Symptoms include crusting of nasal fluids, discharge, and, especially, a very bad smell. Ozena may occur after long-term swelling of the nasal mucosa.

ozone shield, the layer of ozone, a form of oxygen, that hangs in the atmosphere from 20 to 40 miles above the surface of the earth and protects the earth from excess ultraviolet radiation.

ozone sickness, an abnormal condition caused by the breathing of ozone that may get into jet aircraft at altitudes over 40,000 feet. It is marked by headaches, chest pains, itchy eyes, and sleepiness. Exactly why and how ozone causes this condition is not known. It is more common early in the year and occurs most often in flights over the Pacific Ocean.

P

PA, abbreviation for **physician's assistant.**

PABA, abbreviation for **paraaminobenzoic acid.**

pabulum /pab′yələm/, any substance that is a food or nutrient.

pacemaker, 1. a group of special nervous tissue at the junction of a large vein (superior vena cava) and the right chamber (atrium) of the heart. It causes the heart to contract, and the right and left chambers (atria) carry the signal on to another area (atrioventricular node). The node then causes the lower chamber of the heart to contract. A misplaced (ectopic) natural pacemaker may cause abnormal heart contractions. 2. an artificial device for keeping a normal rhythm of heart contraction through electric signals to the heart muscle. A pacemaker may be permanent, sending the stimulus at a constant and fixed rate. It may also fire only on demand, as when the heart does not contract at a certain rate. Also called **cardiac pacemaker.**

pacemaker installation fluoroscopy, using x-ray techniques to watch during the placement of an artificial pacemaker to make sure it is done correctly.

pachometer. See **pachymeter.**

pachycephaly /pak′ēsef′əlē/, an abnormal thick skull, as in acromegaly. Also called **pachyceph-** alia. **–pachycephalic, pachycephalous,** *adj.*

pachydactyly /pak′ēdak′tilē/, abnormally thick fingers or toes. **–pachydactylic, pachydactylous,** *adj.*

pachyderma, thick skin.

pachymeter /pakim′ətər/, an instrument used to measure thickness, especially of thin structures, as a membrane or a tissue. Also called **pachometer.**

pachyonychia congenita /pak′ē·ōnik′ē·ə/, a birth defect with thick nails on the fingers and the toes, and with thick skin on the palms of the hands and soles of the feet. The surface of the tongue has a whitish coating.

pacifier, 1. something that soothes or comforts. 2. a nipple-shaped object used by infants and children for sucking. Pacifiers can be dangerous if they are too small or made poorly. The object can be swallowed or get stuck in the throat and block the air passage. The safest pacifiers are made in one piece, so that only the nipple fits into the mouth, with an easy-to-hold handle.

Pacini's corpuscles /päsē′nēz/, many special sense organs that look like tiny white bulbs (like a tiny onion), each joined to the end of one nerve fiber in the skin, and connective tissue of many parts of the body, especially the

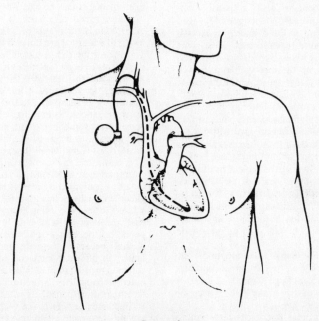

Pacemaker

575

palm of the hand, sole of the foot, genitals, and joints. They give in under pressure. Also called **pacinian corpuscles.** Compare **Golgi-Mazzoni corpuscles, Krause's corpuscles.**

pack, **1.** a treatment in which the body or a part of it is wrapped in hot or cold, wet or dry towels, or in ice for many reasons. Cold packs are used to bring down high temperatures and swellings or to cause lower body temperatures (hypothermia) during heart surgery or organ transplants. **2.** a tampon. **3.** a dressing to cover a wound or to fill the space left after removing a tooth.

package insert, a leaflet the FDA says must be placed inside the package of a prescription drug. The drug maker has to describe the drug, tell its generic name, tell when it should or should not be used, and give warnings, precautions, side effects, form, the correct dose, and how it should be taken.

packed cells, blood cells taken from the liquid portion (plasma) of the blood. It is often given in severe anemia to restore normal levels of hemoglobin and red cells without overloading the bloodstream with excess fluids. See also **bank blood, component therapy, pooled plasma.**

pad, **1.** a mass of soft material used to cushion shock, prevent wear, or soak up wetness. Abdominal pads are used to soak up fluids or to keep organs apart during surgery. **2.** a mass of fat that cushions many structures, as the fat pad of the knee cap.

Paget's disease of bone /paj'əts/, a disease of unknown cause, usually affecting middle-aged and elderly people. Bone tissue breakdown and changed bone repair occurs. Most cases are mild and without symptoms. However, bone pain may be the first symptom. Bowed lower leg bones (saber shins), forward curve of the spine (kyphosis), and many broken bones are caused by the soft, abnormal bone. The skull gets bigger and headaches and warmth over the places affected are caused by more blood flowing through them. Excess calcium is found in the urine. Other problems are broken bones, kidney stones if the patient has to stay in bed, heart failure, deafness or blindness, and bone cancer (osteosarcoma). No treatment is needed for mild cases. A high-protein, high-calcium diet may be ordered, unless the patient has to stay in bed. Also called **osteitis deformans.**

Paget's disease of the nipple. See **nipple cancer.**

pagophagia /pā'gōfā'jē·ə/, an abnormal condition with a craving to eat large amounts of ice. It is linked to a lack of iron in the diet. **–pagophagic, pagophagous,** *adj.*

PAHA sodium clearance test, a test for noting kidney damage or muscle diseases. The test uses a chemical (paraaminohippuric acid) for finding out the rate at which the kidneys remove this from the blood and urine.

pain, an unpleasant sense caused by signals from some sense nerve endings. It is a basic symptom of inflammation and is an important clue to the cause of many disorders. Pain may be mild or severe, chronic, acute, cutting, burning, dull, or sharp, exactly or poorly located, or referred. See also **referred pain.**

pain assessment, an examination of the things that make a patient's pain worse or better. It is used to diagnose and treat disease or injury. Reactions to pain vary widely among different people and depend on many different physical and mental factors. Specific diseases and injuries and the health, pain level, fear and anxiety, and ethnic background all affect reactions to pain. Patients also express their feelings of pain in different ways. A physician may ask a patient to describe the cause of the pain, if known, how strong it is, its location, and when it started. The patient should note anything that happened before the pain started, and how the pain is treated or handled. Severe pain causes pale skin, cold sweat, "goose bumps," wide pupils, and higher levels of the pulse, breathing rate, blood pressure, and muscle tension. When brief, strong pain starts to go away, the pulse may be slower and the blood pressure lower than before the pain began. If pain occurs often or is long term, the pulse rate and blood pressure may not go up much. If pain lasts for many days, the ability to fight infections may be lost. The patient's tone of voice, speed of speech, cries, groans, or other sounds, face and body movements, or trying to withdraw are noted by the physician. The size of the pain area, its tenderness, and the effects of body movement and pressure on the pain are also watched. The length of pain is noted in terms of hours, days, weeks, months, or years. Pain patterns are linked to many sensations, as burning, sticking, aching, or rhythmic throbbing. Some may give meanings to pain, as a test of one's worth, punishment, or as a sign of an illness getting worse. This may affect the strength of pain and mask its importance. It is hard to relieve strong or long-term pain, but a patient can learn to live almost normally even with some pain.

pain intervention, relieving pain caused by disease and injury. Useful pain intervention depends on the type of pain, the physical and mental sources of the pain, and the patterns linked to different kinds of pain. The most common method of pain intervention is to give narcotic painkillers, as morphine. Many believe that using painkillers without taking into account mental help is not useful. Nearly everyone has a mental and emotional, as well as physical, effect of pain. For that reason, pain intervention often uses methods that combine both mental and physical measures. Methods of pain intervention for short-term pain are different from those for long-term pain. Short-term pain in the first 24 to 48 hours after surgery is often hard to relieve, even with narcotics. Some believe that a patient who has had many surgeries becomes more sensitive to pain. The type of pain intervention also depends on how the patient describes the pain. Mild pain is sometimes relieved by having the patient watch television, have visitors, or read. Moderate pain may be relieved by a mixture of these actions and giving drugs. Intervention to relieve severe pain often includes giving narcotics, working with the patient and family or hospital workers. "Waking imagined analgesia," in which the patient thinks about past pleasant events, as relaxing on an ocean beach, is useful. In relieving all types of pain, removing anything that makes pain worse is a goal. Pain often gets worse in a cold room because the patient's muscles tend to contract. Putting on something cold, as with an ice pack, often relieves pain by bringing down swelling. Dealing with pain gets harder as the patient gets more tired. Tranquilizers may make pain worse, because they block otherwise useful ways of reducing pain. Overactivity may cause tiredness and fear, thus making the pain worse. Religious beliefs may help the patient to lessen pain or raise the ability to deal with it. Religious beliefs, however, may make pain worse if the patient sees the pain as punishment. Some drugs used to relieve pain are mild nonnarcotic painkillers and much more powerful and possibly addictive opiates, as morphine. Morphine given to relieve pain, cough, or diarrhea treats only the symptoms. It is used with care in patients with many diseases. Morphine can mask the symptoms or the course of the disease. Repeated daily use of any opiate drug will lessen the response to the drug, so the dose will have to be made larger over time. The risk of becoming mentally or physically dependent on any drug is always present. The narcotic painkillers act on the central nervous system, but the nonnarcotic drugs (as the salicylates) act on where the pain is. Some nonnarcotic drugs can bring down swelling and fever, as aspirin, indomethacin, or ibuprofen. In patients who are allergic to or are unable to take aspirin, acetaminophen may be used. Pain intervention in fatal illnesses uses many drugs that relieve pain and cause a sense of well-being and calm in patients who would otherwise suffer greatly. Painkilling mixtures of opiates and alcoholic mixtures may be given. Nerve block may be done by injecting alcohol. A nerve may also be cut to reduce pain. Other techniques include acupuncture and hypnosis. Behavior modification is another example, in which the treatment is to reduce drugs and exercise more over time, teach the patient to control body actions (biofeedback), and electric nerve actions that change pain signals to the brain. See also **pain assessment.**

pain mechanism, the group of nerves that carry unpleasant senses and feelings of pain through the body, most often linked to disease and injury with tissue damage. Because pain varies so much among people and because everyone responds differently to pain, medical science really does not understand the pain mechanism. Two ideas about it are the gate control theory and the pattern theory. The gate control theory says that pain signals in the nervous system excite a group of small nerve cells that form a "pain pool." These nerve cells become overactive until they reach a level where a supposed gate opens up and allows the pain signals to go to higher brain centers. The gates are thought to be in the spinal cord and the brain stem. The pattern theory says that the strength of a signal causes a pattern, which the brain senses as pain. This pain feeling is controlled by the strength and amount of activity of nervous system end organs. Some believe that two chemical substances made by the body (bradykinin and histamine) cause pain. Newly identified painkillers made by the body are the enkephalins and the endorphins. Some studies show that the enkephalins are 10 times as strong as morphine in lowering pain. The most recent pain theories include emotions as important in the pain mechanism. Past activity, fear, and causes for acting greatly affect everyone's feelings of pain. The fear of pain is second only to the fear of death for most people. It is known that fear and worry often make pain worse.

pain receptor, any of the many free nerve endings in the body that warn of possible harmful changes, as excess pressure or temperature. The free nerve endings making up most of the pain receptors are found mainly in the skin and in some mucous membranes. They also appear in the eye (cornea), in the root covers of hairs, and around sweat (sudoriferous) glands. Any kind of activity, if it is strong enough, can act on the pain receptors in the skin and the mucosa, but only major changes in pressure and some chemicals can act on the pain receptors in the inner organs. Referred pain results only from acting on the pain receptors in deep structures, as the organs in the abdomen, the joints, and the skeletal muscles, but never from pain receptors in the skin.

pain spot, any spot on the skin where something can cause pain.

paint, 1. to apply a drug solution to the skin. 2. a drug solution that is used in this way. Kinds of paint include **antiseptic, germicide, and sporicide drugs.**

pain threshold, the point at which a stimulus, usually one linked to pressure or temperature, starts pain receptors working and causes a feeling of pain. Patients with low pain thresholds have pain much sooner and faster than patients with high pain thresholds.

palatal, 1. referring to the palate. **2.** referring to the surface of an upper tooth facing the tongue.

palate, the roof of the mouth. It is divided into the hard palate and the soft palate. **–palatal, palatine,** *adj.*

palatine arch, the vault-shaped muscle forming the soft palate between the mouth and the throat. The uvula hangs from the back of the arch.

palatine bone, one of a pair of bones of the skull, forming the back part of the hard palate, and part of the nasal space.

palatine tonsil, one of a pair of almond-shaped masses of spongy (lymphoid) tissue on either side of the soft palate (palatine) arches. They are covered with mucous membrane and contain many lymph sacs (follicles) and many spaces.

palatitis, a swelling of the hard palate.

paleogenesis. See **palingenesis.**

paleogenetic, referring to a trait or structure of a living thing or species that began in an earlier generation.

palingenesis, 1. the regrowth of a lost part. **2.** the hereditary carrying of family traits, especially defects, from one generation to the next. Also called **paleogenesis.** Compare **cenogenesis. –palingenetic, palingenic,** *adj.*

palladium (Pd), a hard, silvery metal element used in high-grade surgery instruments and in dental devices.

palliate /pal'ē·āt/, to soothe or relieve. **–palliation,** *n.,* **palliative** /pal'i·ətiv/, *adj.*

palliative treatment, treatment to relieve or lessen pain or other uncomfortable symptoms but not to cause a cure. Some kinds of palliative treatment are the use of narcotics to relieve pain in late cancer, making a hole in the colon (colostomy) to bypass a tumor of the bowel that cannot be removed by surgery, and the removal of dead tissue in a patient with cancer. Compare **definitive treatment, expectant treatment.**

pallium. See **cerebral cortex.**

pallor, an abnormal paleness or lack of color in the skin.

palm, the lower side of the hand, between the wrist and bases of the fingers, when the hand is held stretched out with the thumb toward the body's middle. **–palmar,** *adj.*

palmar aponeurosis, connective tissue (fascia) that surrounds the muscles of the palm. Also called **palmar fascia.**

palmar crease, a groove across the palm of the hand.

palmar erythema, a swelling redness of the palms of the hands.

palmar fascia. See **palmar aponeurosis.**

palmaris longus, a long, slender muscle of the forearm. It flexes the hand.

palmar metacarpal artery, one of several arteries bringing blood to the fingers.

palmar reflex, a reflex that curls the fingers when the palm of the hand is tickled.

palmature, an abnormal condition in which the fingers are webbed.

palmomental reflex, an abnormal nerve effect caused in some people by scratching the palm of the hand at the base of the thumb. The muscles of the chin and corner of the mouth on the same side of the body as the scratching contract. It is sometimes seen in normal people but a strong reflex may occur in nervous system disease, heavy pressure on the brain, and a type of face paralysis. Also called **palm-chin reflex.**

palpate, the use of the hands or fingers to examine.

palpation, a technique used in physical examination in which the examiner feels the texture, size, feel, and location of parts of the body with the hands. **–palpable,** *adj.,* **palpate,** *v.*

palpatory percussion, a technique in physical examination in which body movements are looked at by using light pressure with the flat of the hand.

palpebra. See **eyelid.**

palpebral commissure. See **canthus.**

palpebral conjunctiva. See **conjunctiva.**

palpebral fissure, the opening between the upper and lower eyelids.

palpebral gland. See **meibomian gland.**

palpebra superior, *pl.* **palpebrae superiores,** the upper eyelid, larger and more movable than the lower eyelid.

palpebrate, 1. to wink or blink. **2.** having eyelids.

palpitate, to flutter or throb rapidly, as in the very fast beating of the heart under conditions of stress and in patients with heart problems.

palpitation, a pounding or racing of the heart. It is linked to normal emotion responses or with some heart disorders. Some people may complain of pounding hearts and show no sign of heart disease. Others, with serious heart disorders, may not detect these palpitations.

palsy /pôl'zē/, an abnormal condition with a loss of motor or sense nerve working, or a form of paralysis. Some kinds of palsy are **Bell's palsy, cerebral palsy, Erb's palsy.**

Paltauf's dwarf. See **pituitary dwarf.**

Paltauf's nanism, dwarfism linked to excess making or growth of lymph tissue.

Pamine, a trademark for a nerve drug (methscopolamine bromide).

panacea /pan'əsē'ə/, **1.** a remedy for everything. **2.** an ancient name for an herb or a potion with the ability to heal.

panacinar emphysema /panas′ənər/, a form of emphysema that affects all parts of the lung. It causes the air sacs (alveoli) to grow larger and slow down and destroys the blood vessel bed of the lung. Also called **panlobular emphysema.**

Panafil, a trademark for a skin drug with an enzyme (papain).

panarthritis, a swelling of many joints of the body. –**panarthritic,** *adj.*

pancake kidney, a birth defect in which the left and right kidneys are joined into a single mass in the pelvis. The fused kidney has two collecting systems and two tubes (ureters) but often becomes blocked because of its abnormal position.

pancarditis, a swelling of the whole heart.

Pancoast's syndrome, 1. a group of many signs linked to a tumor in the lung. The signs are pain in the arm, an x-ray shadow at the top of the lung, and weakening of the muscles of the arm and the hand. The signs are caused by the damaging effects of the tumor on the nerve in the neck (brachial plexus). **2.** an abnormal condition caused by bone destruction in a part of one or more ribs, and sometimes involving the backbones.

Pancoast's tumor. See **pulmonary sulcus tumor.**

pancolectomy, the removal of the whole colon. An opening must also be made in the small intestine (ileostomy).

pancreas /pan′krē·əs/, a fish-shaped, grayish-pink gland about 5 inches long that stretches across the back of the abdomen, behind the stomach. It releases insulin, glucagon, and some enzymes of digestion. With a lumpy surface, the pancreas is divided into a head, a body, and a tail. Small ducts from the releasing cells empty into the main duct that runs the length of the organ. The main duct empties into the intestine at the same spot as the exit of the common bile duct. About 1 million cell units (islands of Langerhans) are buried in the pancreas. Beta cells of the islands release insulin, which helps control the body's use of carbohydrate. Alpha cells of the islands release glucagon, which counters the action of insulin. Other units of the pancreas release enzymes that help digest fats and proteins.

pancreatectomy /pan′krē·ətek′təmē/, the removal of all or part of the pancreas. It is done to remove a cyst or tumor, treat swelling of the pancreas, or repair an injury. During the operation, the stomach and intestines are reattached. After surgery the patient is given a low-sugar, low-fat diet. If the whole pancreas is removed, a type of diabetes develops that needs strict control of both diet and insulin dose.

pancreatic cancer /pan′krē·at′ik/, a cancer of the pancreas. Symptoms are loss of appetite, gas in the intestines, weakness, a large weight loss, stomach or back pain, liver disease (jaundice), itching, and signs of diabetes. The patient may pass clay-colored stools. Insulin-releasing tumors cause low blood sugar (hypoglycemia), especially in the morning. Symptoms of peptic ulcer may be felt. In some cases, there may be diarrhea, low blood potassium, and a lack of stomach acid. Exploratory surgery is often needed to make a good diagnosis. Some cancers in the pancreas may be treated by removal of part of the gland, the common bile duct, the first part of the intestine (duodenum), and part of the stomach. Pancreatic cancer occurs three to four times more often in men than in women. It is on the rise in the industrial areas of the world. People who smoke more than 10 to 20 cigarettes a day, who have diabetes mellitus, or who have been exposed to a toxic chemical (polychlorinated biphenyl compounds) are most likely to get pancreatic cancer.

pancreatic dornase, an enzyme from beef pancreas that has been used to treat lung infections and cystic fibrosis.

pancreatic duct, the main releasing channel of the pancreas. Also called **duct of Wirsung.**

pancreatic enzyme, any one of the digestion enzymes released by the pancreas. See also **chymotrypsin, pancreatic juice.**

pancreatic hormone, any one of several hormones released by the pancreas. Major hormones are insulin and glucagon. They are released by cells in a special space (islands of Langerhans) of the pancreas. See also **glucagon, insulin.**

pancreatic insufficiency, any condition with not-enough release of pancreatic hormones or enzymes. A disease of pancreatic tissue is the usual cause. Loss of appetite, failure of the body to absorb food, stomach pain, discomfort, and heavy weight loss often occur. Alcohol-caused pancreatitis is the most common form. It is best to treat the cause of the condition.

pancreatic juice, the fluids released by the pancreas. They are made as a reaction to the arrival of food in the first part of the intestine (duodenum). Pancreatic juice contains water, protein, salts, and many enzymes. The juice is needed to break down proteins into amino acids, to turn fats in the diet to fatty acids, and to change starch to simple sugars.

pancreaticolienal node /pan′krē·at′ikōlī·ē′nəl/, a bump (node) in one of the groups of lymph glands in the organs of the abdomen and pelvis. Also called **splenic gland.** Compare **gastric node, hepatic node.**

pancreatin /pan′krē·ətin′/, pancreas enzymes from swine or cattle given to aid digestion to replace natural human pancreas enzymes in cystic fibrosis and surgery to remove the pancreas.

★CAUTION: Known allergy to this drug or to pork or beef protein prohibits its use.

★ADVERSE EFFECTS: There are no known serious side effects. Large doses may cause nausea or diarrhea.

pancreatitis /pan'krē·ətī'tis/, a swelling of the pancreas. **Acute pancreatitis** is often the result of damage to the gallbladder (biliary tract) by alcohol, injury, infection, or drugs. Symptoms are severe abdominal pain moving to the back, fever, loss of appetite, nausea, and vomiting. There may be yellowing of the skin (jaundice). Sores (pseudocysts) in pancreas tissue are a serious problem. Fluids are given through the veins and nonmorphine painkillers are also given. Acute pancreatitis is often fatal. The causes of **chronic pancreatitis** are like those of the acute form. When the cause is alcohol abuse, there may be calcium deposits and scars in the smaller ducts of the pancreas. There is stomach pain, nausea, and vomiting, as well as undigested fat and protein in the feces. Insulin levels may go down. Some patients get diabetes mellitus. Treatment includes removal of part of the pancreas when pain cannot be relieved by drugs. A pancreas extract is given to replace missing enzymes, and vitamin supplements are needed.

pancreatoduodenectomy /pan'krē·a'tōdoo'ōdə-nek'təmē/, surgery in which the head of the pancreas and the loop of intestine (duodenum) that surrounds it are removed. The operation is done in some forms of biliary tract cancer.

pancreatolith, a stone in the pancreas.

pancuronium bromide, a skeletal muscle-relaxing drug given to aid anesthesia and the use of mechanical breathing equipment.
★CAUTION: It is used with care in patients with a nerve disease (myasthenia gravis), kidney and liver disease, and in pregnancy. Known allergy to this drug or to related drugs prohibits its use.
★ADVERSE EFFECTS: The most serious side effect is difficult breathing.

pancytopenia /pan'sītəpē'nē·ə/, a marked reduction in the number of red and white blood cells and platelets. See also **anemia, aplasia.** –**pancytopenic,** adj.

pandemic, a disease that occurs throughout a population, as a large influenza epidemic.

panencephalitis /pan'əsef'əlī'tis/, swelling of the whole brain. The beginning may not be noticed (insidious), yet continue slowly with motor nerve and mental failure. It is often caused by a virus. See also **rubella panencephalitis, subacute sclerosing panencephalitis.**

panendoscope, an instrument that allows a wide view of the inside of the bladder. See also **cystoscope.**

panesthesia, the total of all feelings felt by a person at one time. Compare **cenesthesia.**

panhypopituitarism /panhī'pōpitoo'itəriz'əm/, general faulty working of the pituitary gland. **Postpubertal panhypopituitarism** may be caused by the death of pituitary gland tissue, caused by blockage of pituitary flow during or after giving birth. Signs of the disorder are failing to make breast milk (lactate), lack of menstruation (amenorrhea), weakness, an inability to stand cold temperatures, drowsiness, and loss of sex drive (libido) and of body hair. There may be heart and blood pressure disorders, early wrinkling of the skin and wasting of the thyroid and adrenal glands. Hormones are given to treat it. Also called **hypophyseal cachexia, pituitary cachexia, Simmonds' disease.** See also **prepubertal panhypopituitarism.**

panhysterectomy /pan'histərek'təmē/, the removal of the uterus and cervix. Compare **radical hysterectomy, total hysterectomy** under **hysterectomy.**

panic, a strong, sudden fear or feeling of worry that causes terror that may result in being unable to move or in senseless, uncontrolled behavior.

panivorous /paniv'ərəs/, referring to eating only bread. –**panivore,** n.

panlobular emphysema. See **panacinar emphysema.**

panniculus, pl. **panniculi,** a membrane made of many sheets of fiberlike tissue (fascia) covering a structure in the body.

pannus /pan'əs/, an abnormal condition of the eye (cornea) in which it becomes filled with blood vessels and grainy tissue just under the surface. Pannus may occur with many eye diseases.

panophthalmitis /pan'ofthalmī'tis/, a swelling of the whole eye, usually caused by a bacteria infection. Symptoms are pain, fever, headache, drowsiness, and swelling. As the infection continues, the iris appears muddy and gray. Treatment is giving strong antibiotics. In some cases, surgery may need to be done.

Pan Oxyl, a trademark for an acne drug (benzoyl peroxide).

panphobia, an irrational, vague fear of some unknown evil. Also called **panophobia, pantophobia.** –**panophobic,** adj.

panphobic melancholia, obsolete. a state of depression with an irrational fear of everything. See also **bipolar disorder, phobia.**

Panteric, a trademark for an enzyme (pancreatin).

pantomography, a technique for taking x-ray pictures of the dental arches and related structures of both the upper and lower jaws on a single film.

Pantopon, a trademark for a narcotic painkiller drug with opium alkaloids.

pantothenic acid /pan'təthen'ik/, a member of the vitamin B complex. An important element in food, it is widely found in plant and animal tissues.

Panwarfin, a trademark for a drug used to stop blood clotting (warfarin sodium).

papain /pəpā'ēn/, an enzyme from the fruit of the papaya used to clean wounds and help in healing.

Papanicolaou test, a simple method of examining tissue cells shed by a body organ. It is used most often to detect cancers of the cervix, but it may be used for tissue samples from any organ. A smear is usually taken by collecting a few loose cells in the vagina. The technique allows early diagnosis of cancer and has helped lower the death rate from cervical cancer. The findings are grouped into the following classes: Class I, only normal cells seen; Class II, cells linked to swelling; Class III, mild abnormal cells (dysplasia); Class IV, severe dysplasia, suspicious cells; Class V, cancer (carcinoma) cells seen. Also called *(informal)* **Pap test.** See also **Pap smear.**

papaverine hydrochloride, a smooth muscle-relaxing drug given to treat heart or abdomen organ spasms.

★CAUTION: Complete heart block or known allergy to this drug prohibits its use.

★ADVERSE EFFECTS: The most serious side effects are liver disease (jaundice), high blood pressure, and irregular heart rate.

paper doll fetus. See **fetus papyraceus.**

papilla /pəpil'ə/, *pl.* **papillae, 1.** a small pimple or nipple-shaped bump, as the cone-shaped (conoid) papillae on the surface of the tongue. **2.** the optic papilla, a tiny white disc in the retina of the eye, the entrance of the optic nerve. It is known as the "blind spot."

papillary /pap'əlerē/, referring to a papilla.

papillary adenocarcinoma, a cancer with small bumps (papillae) of connective tissue with blood vessels that reach into organ spaces (follicles), glands, or lumps (cysts). The tumor is most common in the ovaries and thyroid gland. Also called **polypoid adenocarcinoma.**

papillary adenocystoma lymphomatosum, a tumor with spongy (lymphoid) tissues that grows in the saliva glands. Also called **adenolymphoma, Warthin's tumor.**

papillary adenoma, a noncancer tumor in which the membrane lining of glands forms bumps that grow into or out of the surface of a space.

papillary carcinoma, a cancer with many fingerlike bumps. It is the most common type of thyroid tumor.

papillary duct, any of the thousands of urine collecting, small tubes that go through the center of the kidney and join with others to form the ducts that lead to the ureters. See also **kidney.**

papillary muscle, any of the muscles joined to the tendons (chordae tendineae) in the chambers (ventricles) of the heart. The papillary muscles help to open and close the heart valves.

papillary tumor. See **papilloma.**

papillate, marked by nipplelike (papillae) bumps.

papilledema, *pl.* **papilledemas, papilledemata,** swelling of the optic disc caused by high pressure in the skull. The coverings (sheaths) that surround the optic nerves are parallel to the membrane covering of the brain. Thus, high pressure is sent forward from the brain to the optic disc in the eye to cause the swelling.

papilliform, shaped like a papilla.

papillitis /pap'ili'tis/, an abnormal condition with swelling of a papilla, as the lacrimal papilla of the eyelid.

papilloma /pap'ilō'mə/, a noncancer tumor with a branching or stalk. Also called **papillary tumor.**

papillomatosis /pap'ilōmətō'sis/, a condition in which there is widespread growth of abnormal nipplelike bumps.

papillomatosis coronae penis. See **hirsutoid papilloma of the penis.**

papillomavirus /pap'ilōməvī'rəs/, the virus that causes warts in humans.

papovavirus /pap'əvəvī'rəs/, one of a group of small viruses that may cause cancer. The human wart is caused by a kind of papovavirus, but it rarely turns into cancer.

pappataci fever. See **phlebotomus fever.**

pappus, the first growth of beard with downy hairs.

Pap smear, *informal.* a sample of discarded tissue skin (epithelial) cells and cervical mucus collected during a pelvic examination for a cancer test using the Papanicolaou system. See also **Papanicolaou test.**

Pap test, *informal.* Papanicolaou test.

papular scaling disease, a skin disorder in which there are raised, dry, scalelike bumps. Some kinds of papular scaling diseases are **lichen planus, pityriasis rosea, psoriasis.** Also called **papulosquamous disease.**

papulation, the growth of papules.

papule /pap'yo͞ol/, a small, solid, raised pimplelike skin bump, as of acne. Compare **macule.** –**papular,** *adj.*

papulosquamous disease. See **papular scaling disease.**

papyraceous, being paperlike.

papyraceous fetus. See **fetus papyraceus.**

-para, a combining form meaning a 'woman who has given birth to children in a number of pregnancies.'

paraaminobenzoic acid (PABA) /per'ə·amē'-nōbenzō'ik/, a substance often linked to the vitamin B complex, found in cereals, eggs, milk, and meat. It is present in blood, urine, spinal fluid, and sweat. It is used as a sunscreen. It partially joins with the horny layer of the skin to fight removal by water and sweat. PABA may also be useful in treating some skin diseases.

paraaminosalicylic acid (PAS, PASA), a drug given to treat tuberculosis.

★CAUTION: Known allergy to the drug prohib-

its its use. It may interact with other drugs.
★ADVERSE EFFECTS: Among the most serious side effects are nausea, vomiting, diarrhea, and stomach pain.

parabiotic syndrome, a condition that can occur between identical twin fetuses so that one gets more placental blood than the other. One twin may become anemic and the other have an excess of blood.

paracentesis /per′əsentē′sis/, a procedure in which fluid is taken from a space of the body. A cut is made in the skin and a hollow tube is passed through into the space to allow the fluid to flow out into a collecting device.

paracervical block, a local anesthetic that is injected into a nerve network (plexus) on each side of the uterine cervix during labor. It is often a useful anesthesia for childbirth.

paracetamol. See **acetaminophen.**

paracoccidioidomycosis /per′əkoksid′ē·oi′dōmīkō′- sis/, a long-term, sometimes fatal fungus infection. It causes ulcers of the mouth, voicebox (larynx), and nose. Other effects include large, draining lymph nodes, cough, breathing difficulty, weight loss, and tumors of the skin, genitals, and intestines. The disease occurs in Mexico and Central and South America. It is caused by breathing in spores of the fungus. Treatment demands many years of antibacteria drugs (sulfonamides). Also called **paracoccidioidal granuloma, South American blastomycosis.** Compare **North American blastomycosis.**

Paradione, a trademark for a drug used to fight seizures (paramethadione).

paradoxic agitation, a period of unexpected excitement that sometimes follows the use of a sleeping pill or tranquilizer.

paradoxic breathing, a condition in which part of the lung empties when breathing in and fills when breathing out. The condition often is linked to an open chest wound or rib cage damage.

paradoxic intention, a treatment for phobias that has a patient do what he or she fears and if possible to overdo it to the point of humor.

paraffin bath, placing heat on a surface of the body using paraffin. The part is quickly sunk in heated liquid wax and then taken out so that the wax surrounds it. It is done several times, and then the whole surface is wrapped in a loose-fitting plastic bag or in paper towels. It is effective for heating injured or swollen areas, especially the hands, feet, and wrists. It is used for patients with arthritis and rheumatism or any joint problem. Also called **wax bath.**

Paraflex, a trademark for a skeletal muscle relaxing drug (chlorzoxazone).

Parafon Forte, a trademark for a drug with a painkiller (acetaminophen) and a skeletal muscle-relaxing drug (chlorzoxazone). It is used to relieve painful muscle and bone conditions.

paraganglion, *pl.* **paraganglia,** any of the small groups of special cells linked to the groups of nerve cells (ganglia) of the nervous system. The paraganglia release the hormones epinephrine and norepinephrine. Also called **chromaffin body.** See also **epinephrine, norepinephrine.**

paragonimiasis /per′əgon′imī′əsis/, a long-term infection with a lung fluke (*Paragonimus kellicotti*). It occurs most often in North American minks and can be carried to humans. The disease symptoms include bronchitis, bloody sputum, pain, diarrhea, brain damage with paralysis, eye disorders, and seizures. The disease may also be caused by eating fluke cysts in infected freshwater crabs or crayfish. Cooking shellfish long enough prevents the disease.

parainfluenza virus, a virus that causes lung infections in infants and young children, and, less commonly, in adults. There are four types of the virus. Types 1 and 2 parainfluenza viruses may cause a form of bronchitis or croup. Type 3 is a cause of croup, bronchitis, and bronchopneumonia in children. Types 1, 3, and 4 are linked to throat swelling and the common cold. Compare **influenza, rhinovirus.**

paraldehyde /peral′dəhīd/, a clear, colorless, strong-smelling liquid used as a lotion and may be given to cause hypnosis or sleep.

parallel play, a form of play among a group of children, mainly toddlers, in which each one engages in a separate activity that is close to but not affected by or shared with the others. Compare **cooperative play.** See also **associative play, solitary play.**

paralysis, *pl.* **paralyses,** the loss of muscle function or the loss of feeling, or both. It may be caused by many problems, ranging from injury to disease and poisoning. Paralyses may be named for the cause, the effects on muscle tone, their spread, or the part of the body affected. See also **flaccid paralysis, spastic paralysis.** –paralytic, *adj.*

paralysis agitans. See **Parkinson's disease.**

paralytic ileus, a lowering in or lack of intestine activity that may come after surgery, injury to the wall of the abdomen, or in severe kidney disease. It may also be linked to a broken backbone or broken ribs, heart attack, severe ulcers, heavy metal poisoning, or any severe disease. Paralytic ileus is the most common cause of blocked intestines. The symptoms are a tender and bloated abdomen, lack of bowel sounds, lack of gas, and by nausea and vomiting. There may be fever, too-little urine, mineral imbalance, too-little fluids, and breathing problems. The loss of fluids and minerals may be heavy. Unless they are replaced, the condition may lead to too-low blood volume of tightly packed blood cells. It can lead to kidney failure, shock, and death. The patient most often has to go to the hospital. Fluids are given through the veins, and drugs to make the digestive tract contract (peristalsis) are given. When the output goes up and the bowel sounds return, small amounts of warm tea or a carbonated drink may be given. Also called **adynamic ileus.**

paralytic shellfish poisoning. See **shellfish poisoning.**

paramedic, a person who is an assistant to a physician, especially a person in the military, trained in emergency medicine. **–paramedical,** *adj.*

paramedical personnel, health-care workers other than physicians, dentists, foot doctors, and nurses who have special training in health care. Kinds of paramedical personnel include **Emergency Medical Technician, audiologists, x-ray technologists.** Also called **allied health personnel.**

paramethadione /per′əmeth′ədī′ōn/, an antiseizure drug given to prevent seizures in petit mal epilepsy.

★CAUTION: Blood disorders, severe kidney or liver damage, or known allergy to this drug prohibits its use.

★ADVERSE EFFECTS: Among the more serious side effects are skin reactions, blood disorders, and liver disease (hepatitis). Drowsiness and day blindness may occur.

parametritis /per′əmetrī′tis/, an inflammation of the structures around the uterus. See also **pelvic inflammatory disease.**

parametrium /per′əmē′trē·əm/, *pl.* **parametria,** the tissue of the uterus that extends into the ligament, which helps support it. Compare **endometrium, myometrium.**

paramitome. See **hyaloplasm.**

paramnesia /per′amnē′zhə/, **1.** a memory defect in which one believes one remembers events that never happened. **2.** a condition in which words are remembered and used without knowing their meaning. Compare **déjà vu.**

paramyxovirus, a member of a family of viruses that includes the viruses that cause mumps and some lung infections.

paranasal, near or alongside the nose.

paranasal sinus, one of the spaces in many bones around the nose, as the frontal sinus in the forehead.

parangi. See **yaws.**

paranoia /per′ənoi′ə/, a mental disorder marked by a complex system of thinking. Delusions of persecution and grandeur usually center on one major theme, as a job situation or an unfaithful spouse. The delusions most often begin slowly, becoming complex, logical, and highly organized. The result is that they can be most convincing. The person may appear normal in actions, speech, thinking, and emotions, aside from the delusions. Symptoms include being wary of others, unwilling to change habits, being resentful, hostile, very angry, and de-

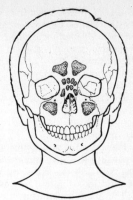

Paranasal sinuses

manding unrealistic things of others. Persons with the disorder often strongly resist treatment, although psychotherapy and behavior therapy may be useful in the early stages. Also called **paranoea** /per′ənē′ə/. Compare **paranoid schizophrenia.**

paranoiac /per′ənoi′ak/, a person with symptoms of paranoia.

paranoia hallucinatoria. See **acute hallucinatory paranoia.**

paranoia quaerula. See **querulous paranoia.**

paranoid /per′ənoid/, **1.** looking like paranoia. **2.** a person with a paranoid disorder. **3.** *informal.* a person who is too suspicious or who feels overly persecuted.

paranoid disorder, a large group of mental disorders marked by a damaged sense of reality and continuing delusions. Kinds of paranoid disorders include **acute paranoid disorder, paranoia, shared paranoid disorder.**

paranoid ideation, a too-strong belief or suspicion, most often without delusions, that one is being bothered or persecuted.

paranoid personality disorder, having extreme distrust of others. The person's own mistakes and failures are blamed on others.

parasitic glossitis, a fungus infection of the tongue, which develops a dark furry patch on the surface. The "fur" is easily broken. No discomfort is felt and a simple mouthwash may be used. The patch may go away and later come back. Also called **black hairy tongue, black tongue.**

parasitic thrombus, a group of bodies and spores of malaria parasites that may form a clot in the blood vessels of the brain in malaria.

parasympathetic, referring to a part of the nervous system. The actions of the parasympathetic part are started by the release of a chemical (acetylcholine), and affect body resources. Parasympathetic nerve fibers slow the heart and cause intestine activity (peristalsis).

They also help release fluids from tear, saliva, and digestion glands. They begin the release of bile and insulin, widen some blood vessels, and narrow the pupils, esophagus, and tubes in the lung (bronchioles). They also relax muscles during urination and defecation. Some parasympathetic nerve fibers also extend to the sex organs and cause blood vessels to widen in the clitoris and the penis.

parasympathetic nervous system. See **autonomic nervous system.**

parasympatholytic. See **anticholinergic.**

parasympathomimetic /per′əsim′pəthōmimet′ik/, referring to a substance causing effects like those caused by acting on a parasympathetic nerve. The parasympathomimetic drugs include those used to treat urine buildup and to counter the action of some muscle-relaxing drugs. Also called **cholinergic.**

parasympathomimetic drug. See **cholinergic.**

parataxic distortion /per′ətak′sik/, a mental defense action in which one's interactions with others are sensed and judged based on past experience. See also **transference.**

parathion poisoning /per′əthī′on/, a harmful condition caused by swallowing, breathing in, or taking in through the skin a chemical used to kill insects (parathion). Symptoms include nausea, vomiting, stomach and bowel cramps, confusion, headache, lack of muscle control, seizures, and breathing difficulty. Emergency treatment is needed.

parathyroid gland, one of many small structures, usually four, joined to the lobes of the thyroid gland. The parathyroid glands release a hormone that helps to keep the level of blood calcium normal. This action in turn keeps muscle tone, blood clotting, and cell membranes normal. Parathyroid failure most often causes excess muscle contractions (tetany) that can be treated by giving calcium salts or parathyroid extracts.

parathyroid hormone (PH), a hormone released by the parathyroid glands that acts to keep a constant level of calcium in body tissues. The hormone controls the movement of calcium in the body and controls its passing out of the body. Loss of the parathyroid glands results in low blood calcium, leading to muscle spasms, seizures, and death if the hormone is not replaced. See also **hypoparathyroidism.**

parathyroid injection, a cattle parathyroid hormone given to control blood levels of calcium, especially in treating hypoparathyroidism.
★CAUTION: Excess blood calcium, muscle overactivity not caused by hypoparathyroidism, excess calcium in the urine, or known allergy to this drug prohibits its use.
★ADVERSE EFFECTS: Among the most serious side effects are excess blood levels of calcium and allergic reactions.

paratrooper fracture, a break of the end of the lower leg bone and the ankle. It often occurs when a person jumps from a high platform and lands feet first on the ground, putting a high force on the ankles.

paratyphoid fever, a bacteria infection, caused by *Salmonella.* Symptoms look like typhoid fever, although milder. See also **rose spots, *Salmonella,* salmonellosis, typhoid fever.**

paraurethral duct. See **Skene's duct.**

Paredrine, a trademark for a nerve drug (hydroxyamphetamine hydrobromide).

paregoric, a mixture of opium, camphor, and other items given to treat diarrhea and as a painkiller.
★CAUTION: Known allergy to this or a similar drug prohibits its use. It should not be used when diarrhea is caused by a poison.
★ADVERSE EFFECTS: There are usually no side effects.

parenchyma /pəreng′kimə/, the working tissue of an organ as opposed to supporting or connective tissue.

parenchymal cell, any cell that is a working part of an organ.

parenchymatous neuritis /per′əngkim′ətəs/, a swelling affecting a nerve. Also called **axial neuritis, central neuritis.** See also **neuritis.**

parent, a mother or father; one who has offspring. **–parental,** *adj.*

parental grief, the behavior reactions that mark the grieving process and result in getting used to the death of a child. See also **death, grief reaction.**

parenteral /pəren′tərəl/, not in or through the digestion. An example is taking a drug by injection instead of by mouth. **–parenterally,** *adv.*

parenteral absorption, taking up substances in the body by structures other than the digestive tract.

parenteral dosage, referring to a drug given so that it bypasses the digestive tract, as by injection.

parenteral nutrition, food given other than by mouth, as by a vein. Fluids usually contain salt (saline) with glucose, amino acids, minerals (electrolytes), vitamins, and drugs. They are not a total diet but keep fluids and minerals balanced after surgery and in other conditions. See also **total parenteral nutrition.**

parent figure, 1. a parent or someone else who cares for a child. The parent figure gives physical, social, and emotional support needed for normal growth. **2.** a person who is an ideal parent with traits needed for forming the perfect parent-child bond.

parent image, a concept that a child forms concerning the roles and traits of the mother and father. See also **imago, primordial image.**

Parents Anonymous, a self-help group for parents who have abused their children or who feel that they are likely to abuse them. See also **child abuse.**

paresis /pərē'sis, per'isis/, **1.** less-than-total paralysis related in some cases to nerve swelling. **2.** a late sign of the third stage of syphilis (neurosyphilis) with paralysis, tremors, seizures, and mental decline, caused by damage to brain nerve cells. Paresis from untreated syphilis most often occurs in the third to fifth decades of life but may occur at an early age in patients with inborn syphilis. Also called **dementia paralytica, general paresis, paralytic dementia.** –paretic, *adj.*

paresthesia, any feeling others cannot sense, as numbness, tingling, or a "pins and needles" feeling. Some factors, as posture, activity, rest, swelling, congestion, or disease may change the feeling. When in the hands or feet, it is sometimes called **acroparesthesia.**

paretic dementia. See **general paresis.**

pargyline hydrochloride /per'jəlēn/, a monoamine oxidase (MAO) inhibitor used to treat moderate to severe high blood pressure.

paries /pā'ri·ēz/, *pl.* **parietes** /pərī'itēz/, the wall of an organ or space in the body. –parietal, *adj.*

parietal /pərī'ətəl/, **1.** referring to the outer wall of a space or organ. **2.** referring to the parietal bone of the skull, or the parietal lobe of the brain.

parietal bone, one of a pair of bones that form the sides of the skull.

parietal lobe, a part of each side of the brain that rests in the part of the skull (cranium) next to the bone on the side of the skull (parietal). Damage to the lobe causes disorders of speaking (aphasia) and sight. The parietal lobe also helps to tell the sizes, shapes, and textures of objects.

parietal lymph node, a small gland that filters the lymph passing through vessels in the chest, abdomen, and pelvis. See also **lymph, lymphatic system, lymph node.**

parietal pain, a sharp feeling of distress in the membrane lining the chest. The pain is made worse by breathing and chest movements. Causes include pneumonia, tuberculosis, cancer, or fluid building up from heart, liver, or kidney disease. Harmful actions do not cause pain in the membrane (pleura) covering the lungs. Pain coming from the chest wall membrane is felt over the affected area. However, pain from the central part of the diaphragm, separating the chest from the abdomen, is felt in back of the shoulder area.

parietal peritoneum, the part of the large membrane in the body that lines the wall of the abdomen. Also called **parietal pleura.** Compare **visceral peritoneum.** See also **peritoneal cavity.**

-parin, a combining form for heparin derivatives.

Parinaud's conjunctivitis /per'ənōz/, an eye membrane (conjunctiva) disorder that most often affects only one side and is followed by swollen and tender nearby lymph nodes. The condition may be linked to many infections, as rabbit fever (tularemia) and cat-scratch fever. Also called **Parinaud's oculogranular syndrome.**

parity, a system for labeling a woman by the number of live and dead children she has given birth to at more than 28 weeks of pregnancy. The total number of pregnancies is noted by the letter "P" or the word "para." A para 4 (P4) gravida 5 (G5) has had 4 births after 28 weeks out of 5 pregnancies and 1 abortion or miscarriage before 28 weeks. Another system uses the total number of pregnancies, followed by the number of on-time births, the number of premature infants, the number of abortions or miscarriages before 28 weeks of pregnancy, and the number of children currently living.

parkinsonism, a nerve system disorder with symptoms of tremor, rigid muscles, mild paralysis, slow shuffling gait, and difficulty in chewing, swallowing, and speaking. It is caused by damage to nerves in the motor system of the brain. Signs of parkinsonism look like those of Parkinson's disease and may be caused by brain swelling, syphilis, malaria, polio, or carbon monoxide poisoning. Parkinsonism often occurs in patients given tranquilizers. See also **Parkinson's disease.**

Parkinson's disease, a slowly growing disorder caused by damage to brain cells. Symptoms include tremors that occur while at rest, "pill rolling" movements of the fingers, and a masklike face. Other symptoms are a shuffling gait, a slightly bent posture, rigid muscles, and weakness. It is usually a disease of unknown cause (idiopathic) affecting persons over 60 years of age. However, it may occur in younger persons, especially following brain swelling (encephalitis) or poisoning by carbon monoxide, metals, or some drugs. Parkinson's disease patients may drool, have a heavy appetite, be unable to stand heat, have oily skin, be emotionally unstable, and have judgment problems. The symptoms are made worse by tiredness, excitement, and frustration. It rarely damages the ability to think and reason. Treatment of the disease is to correct the imbalance in some brain substances (dopamine, acetylcholine). A substance that is changed to dopamine in the body (levodopa) may be used. However, side effects, as nausea, vomiting, inability to sleep, blood pressure problems, and mental confusion may occur. A mixed drug (carbidopa-levodopa) causes fewer side effects. Patients with the disease are told to continue to work and stay active as long as possible. To prevent the spine from bending forward, they should lie on a firm mattress on the back and walk with the hands folded behind the back. Hand tremor while at rest is less noticed if the patient grasps the arms of the chair when seated. Some patients may be treated by cutting the nerve or injecting alcohol to destroy parts of the brain and to relieve rigid muscles or tremors. Also called **paralysis agitans.** /aj′itəns/.

Parlodel, a trademark for a parkinsonism drug (bromocriptine).

Parnate, a trademark for an antidepressant drug (tranylcypromine sulfate).

paronychia /per′ənik′ē·ə/, an infection of the fold of skin at the edge of a nail. Treatment is with hot compresses or soaks, antibiotics, and cutting open to drain.

paroophoritis /per′ō·of′ərī′tis/, swelling of the tissues around the ovary.

parosmia /pəroz′mē·ə/, any disorder of the sense of smell. See also **anosmia, cacosmia.**

parotid duct /pərot′id/, a tube that extends from the parotid saliva gland to the mouth. It opens on the cheek by the second upper molar tooth. Also called **Stensen's duct.** See also **parotid gland.**

parotid gland, one of the largest pair of saliva glands that lie inside the cheek just below and in front of the outer ear. Compare **sublingual gland, submandibular gland.** See also **salivary gland.**

parotitis /per′əti′tis/, swelling or infection of one or both saliva (parotid) glands. See also **mumps.**

-parous, a combining form referring to the number of offspring one has had.

paroxysm /per′əksiz′əm/, **1.** a marked rise in symptoms. **2.** a fit, seizure, or spasm. **–paroxysmal,** adj.

paroxysmal atrial tachycardia, a period of very rapid heart-beats that begins suddenly and ends suddenly.

paroxysmal cold hemoglobinuria (PCH), a disorder marked by red blood cell destruction and bloody urine, linked to exposure to cold.

paroxysmal hemoglobinuria, the sudden passage of hemoglobin in urine. It can occur following exposure to low temperatures. See also **Marchiafava-Micheli disease.**

paroxysmal labyrinthine vertigo. See **Ménière's disease.**

paroxysmal nocturnal dyspnea (PND), a disorder with sudden attacks of breathing problems, most often occurring after several hours of sleep lying down. It is most often caused by fluid in the lungs linked to a heart disease (congestive heart failure). There is also coughing, a feeling of being unable to breathe, cold sweat, and rapid heart beat. Sleeping with the head propped up on pillows may help breathing difficulty at night. The cause of the disease must be treated to prevent fluid buildup in the lungs.

paroxysmal nocturnal hemoglobinuria (PNH), a disorder in which red blood cells are destroyed, resulting in bloody urine, especially at night. A basic membrane defect in the red blood cells is involved. The cause is unknown, but it is linked to abnormal bone marrow. Occurring mainly in adults between 25 and 45 years of age, it has symptoms of stomach and bowel pain, back pain, and headache. Problems may be blood-clotting problems and a lack of iron. Treatment includes giving blood, iron, and drugs to halt bloot clotting.

paroxysmal supraventricular tachycardia, an abnormal heart rhythm more than 100 beats per minute and faster than 170 per minute.

parrot fever. See **psittacosis.**

pars /pärs/, a part. See also **part.**

Parsidol, a trademark for an antiparkinsonian drug (ethopropazine hydrochloride).

part, a portion of a larger area. Also called **pars.**

part-, a combining form meaning 'related to childbirth.'

parthenogenesis /pär′thənōjen′əsis/, a type of nonsexual reproduction in which a living thing grows from an unfertilized egg (ovum). Growth of the unfertilized ovum may be started by other than natural means. **–parthenogenetic, parthenogenic,** adj.

partial breech extraction. See **assisted breech.**

partial bypass, a system of blood flow in which a person's heart pumps and keeps a part of the blood flow while the rest of the flow depends on a pump.

partial crown, a dental device that replaces surfaces of a tooth.

partial hospitalization program, a health-care service that provides treatment to patients who use only day or night hospital services or adult day health services, rather than stay in the hospital 24 hours a day.

partially edentulous arch, a dental arch in which one or more, but not all, natural teeth are missing.

partial placenta previa, a condition of pregnancy in which the placenta partly covers the opening of the cervix. As the cervix widens in labor, the part of the placenta that lies over it breaks apart, causing bleeding. Depending on the amount of breakdown, the bleeding may result in bleeding that is possibly fatal to the mother and the baby. Treatment may be a cesarean birth. Partial placenta previa may be found before bleeding occurs by using ultrasound or feeling with the hands. See also **placenta previa.**

partial response, a condition in which a tumor becomes at least 50% but less than 100% smaller as a result of treatment.

parturition /pär′tyo͞orish′ən/, the process of giving birth.

parulis. See **gumboil.**

passive-aggressive personality, a behavior in which strong actions or opinions are given in an indirect, nonviolent manner, as pouting, being difficult or slow, stubborn, and forgetful.

passive-aggressive personality disorder, a behavior disorder with passive nonresponse to social demands. It results in long-term inability to act, lack of self-confidence, and poor personal interactions.

passive anaphylaxis. See **antiserum anaphylaxis.**

passive-dependent personality, a behavior marked by helplessness, inability to make a decision, and often clinging to and seeking support from others. Compare **aggressive personality, passive-aggressive personality.**

passive exercise, repeated movement of a part of the body as a result of force or willful effort of muscles directed by a physical therapist. Compare **active exercise.** See also **aerobic exercise, anaerobic exercise.**

passive immunity, a form of immunity from antibodies that are carried through the placenta to a fetus or through a breast substance (colostrum) from a mother to an infant. Passive immunity is also caused by injecting a drug (antiserum) for treatment or prevention. Passive immunity is not permanent and does not last as long as active immunity. See also **active immunity, immune response.**

passive lingual arch, a dental device that helps keep the tooth space and dental arch length normal when the baby teeth are lost too early.

passive play, play in which a person does not take part actively. For young children such activity may be to watch and listen to others, watch other children or animals, listen to stories, or look at pictures. For older children, passive play may be games and toys that need mental effort, as chess, reading, listening to music, or watching television. Compare **active play.**

passive smoking, the breathing in by nonsmokers of the smoke from other people's smoking. The amount of such smoke breathed in by a nonsmoker is small, but passive smoking can make lung diseases worse and can add to more serious diseases, as cancer, and can injure the health of nonsmoking spouses, infants, and unborn babies. Patients with long-term heart and lung diseases and allergies can be harmed.

passive transfer test. See **Prausnitz-Küstner test.**

passive transport, the movement of small molecules across the membrane of a cell by splitting. Passive transport is needed to absorb products of digestion by the cells lining the intestines. Compare **active transport, osmosis.**

passive tremor, an undesired trembling occurring when the patient is at rest, one of the signs of Parkinson's disease. Also called **resting tremor.**

Pasteurella /pas′tərel′ə/, a group of bacteria, including species that cause disease in humans. *Pasteurella* infections may be carried by animal bites.

pasteurization, the process of applying heat, most often to milk or cheese to kill or slow the growth of harmful bacteria. –**pasteurize,** *v.*

pasteurized milk, milk that has been treated by heat to destroy disease bacteria. By law, pasteurization needs a temperature of 145° F to 150° F for not less than 30 minutes. This is followed by a temperature of 161° F for 15 seconds and then rapid cooling.

past health, a patient's health history. It includes past injuries, allergies, operations, vaccinations, stays in the hospital, and any pregnancies or mental health history. The past health history is gotten from the patient or the patient's family by a physician and becomes part of the permanent record.

pastoral counseling department, the hospital chaplain service.

Patau's syndrome. See **trisomy 13.**

patch, a small, flat spot on skin that differs from the nearby area in color or texture. Also called **macule.**

patch test, a skin test for locating substances that cause allergies, especially those causing a skin condition (contact dermatitis). The substance, as food, pollen, or animal fur, is stuck to a patch that is placed on the patient's skin. Another patch, with nothing on it, is a control. After a time, usually 24 to 48 hours, both patches are removed. If the skin under the suspect patch is red and swollen and the control area is not, the test is said to be positive, and the person is likely allergic to that substance. Compare **Prausnitz-Küstner test, radioallergosorbent test.**

patella /pətel′ə/, a flat, triangle-shaped bone at the front of the knee joint. Also called **kneecap.**

patellar ligament, a part of a tendon of an upper leg muscle (quadriceps femoris). The ligament is a strong, flat band of tissue that stretches from the tendon above the knee across the kneecap (patella). It joins a bone of the lower leg (tibia).

patellar reflex, a tendon reflex caused by a sharp tap on the tendon just below the kneecap (patella). The normal response is a quick upward jerk of the leg at the knee. The reflex is stronger in disease of the nervous system. Also called **knee-jerk reflex, quadriceps reflex.** See also **deep tendon reflex.**

patent, the condition of being open and unblocked, as a patent airway.

patent ductus arteriosus (PDA), an abnormal opening between two arteries (pulmonary artery, aorta) caused by the fetal blood vessel (ductus arteriosus) failing to close after birth. The birth defect, seen mainly in premature infants, allows blood from the aorta to flow into the pulmonary artery. Blood must then flow through the lungs again before it is returned to the left chambers of the heart. This causes the heart to work harder. It is usually not corrected until the child is old enough to live through surgery. This also allows time for nature to close the defect. See also **congenital cardiac anomaly.**

Paterson-Kelly syndrome, a digestive system disorder linked to a lack of iron (iron deficiency anemia). Webs of tissue grow in the upper foodpipe (esophagus), making swallowing solids difficult. The webs are easily broken during examination or tube feeding and can cause bleeding. When the lack of iron is corrected, the webs disappear. Also called **Plummer-Vinson syndrome.**

-pathic, 1. a combining form referring to an illness or affected part of the body. **2.** a combining form referring to a form or system of treatment.

Pathilon, a trademark for a nerve signal blocker (tridihexethyl chloride).

pathogen /path'əjən/, any microorganism able to cause a disease. **–pathogenic,** *adj.*

pathogenicity, referring to the ability of a microorganism to cause a disease.

pathogenic occlusion, an abnormal closing of the teeth that may damage teeth, gums, and other parts of the mouth.

pathognomonic /pəthog'nəmon'ik/, a sign or symptom linked to a disease or condition, as Koplik's spots on the inside of the mouth, which are a sign of measles.

pathologic anatomy, the study of the structure and workings of the tissues and cells of the body as they relate to a disease.

pathologic fracture. See **neoplastic fracture.**

pathologic mitosis, any cell division that is not typical and results in an unequal number of chromosomes. It usually causes a defect, as occurs in cancer and genetic disorders.

pathologic myopia, a type of progressive near-sightedness with changes in the inside of the eyeball and bulging of the iris.

pathologic retraction ring, a ridge that may form around the uterus at the joining of the upper and lower parts during the second stage of a blocked labor. The lower part becomes bloated and thin, and the upper part becomes too thick. The ring, which may be felt through the wall of the abdomen, is a sign of a possible break in the uterus. Also called **Bandl's ring.** Compare **physiologic retraction ring, constriction ring.**

pathology, the study of the traits, causes, and effects of disease, as seen in the structure and workings of the body. **–pathologic,** *adj.*

pathomimicry. See **Munchausen's syndrome.**

pathway, 1. a group of nerve cells (neurons) that make a route for nerve signals from any part of the body to the spinal cord and the brain or from the nervous system to the muscles and organs. **2.** a chain of chemical reactions that makes many compounds one after the other.

-pathy, a combining form meaning a 'suffering or illness' of a certain kind.

patient, someone who receives health care.

patient advocate. See **ombudsman.**

patient compensation fund, a fund most often set up by state law and paid for by a charge on malpractice insurance premiums and used to pay malpractice claims.

patient dumping, the early discharge of Medicare or poor patients from hospitals for economic reasons. A 1986 federal rule requires hospitals to tell Medicare patients when they are admitted that they can challenge being discharged if they consider it too early. The rule was adopted after Medicare introduced a policy of paying hospitals according to a particular illness, regardless of the length of hospitalization, as an incentive for hospitals to reduce the length of time patients spend in the hospital.

patient interview, a step-by-step interview of a patient, to get information that can be used to develop a care plan. Also called **client interview.**

patient record, a group of papers that is a record of each time a patient had treatment and medical care. The record is private and is most often held by the hospital or other health-care service. Data in the record are given only to the patient, or with written permission. It has the patient's health history, laboratory test results, and other data. Also called *(informal)* **chart.**

patient representative. See **ombudsman.**

patient representative services, hospital services given by staff members dealing with patients' complaints and protecting patient's rights. See also **ombudsman.**

Patient's Bill of Rights, a list of patient's rights set up by the American Hospital Association. It offers some guides and protection to patients by stating the duties that a hospital and its staff have toward patients and their families during their stay in the hospital, but it will not hold up in court. (See chart on p. 589.)

pattern theory of pain. See **pain mechanism.**

patulous, referring to something that is open or spread apart.

Pauwel's fracture /pou'əlz/, a break of the neck of the upper leg bone (femur), near the socket of the hipbone.

Pavabid, a trademark for a smooth muscle-relaxing drug (papaverine hydrochloride).

A patient's bill of rights*

The American Hospital Association Board of Trustees' Committee on Health Care for the Disadvantaged, which has been a consistent advocate on behalf of consumers of health-care services, developed this bill of rights, which was approved by the AHA House of Delegates Feb. 6, 1973. The following rights are affirmed:

1. The patient has the right to considerate and respectful care.

2. The patient has the right to obtain from his physician complete current information concerning his diagnosis, treatment, and prognosis in terms the patient can be reasonably expected to understand. When it is not medically advisable to give such information to the patient, the information should be made available to an appropriate person in his behalf. He has the right to know, by name, the physician responsible for coordinating his care.

3. The patient has the right to receive from his physician information necessary to give informed consent prior to the start of any procedure and/or treatment. Except in emergencies, such information for informed consent should include but not necessarily be limited to the specific procedure and/or treatment, the medically significant risks involved, and the probable duration of incapacitation. Where medically significant alternatives for care or treatment exist, or when the patient requests information concerning medical alternatives, the patient has the right to such information. The patient also has the right to know the name of the person responsible for the procedures and/or treatment.

4. The patient has the right to refuse treatment to the extent permitted by law, and to be informed of the medical consequences of his action.

5. The patient has the right to every consideration of his privacy concerning his own medical care program. Case discussion, consultation, examination, and treatment are confidential and should be conducted discreetly. Those not directly involved in his care must have the permission of the patient to be present.

6. The patient has the right to expect that all communications and records pertaining to his care should be treated as confidential.

7. The patient has the right to expect that within its capacity a hospital must make reasonable response to the request of a patient for services. The hospital must provide evaluation, service, and/or referral as indicated by the urgency of the case. When medically permissible, a patient may be transferred to another facility only after he has received complete information and explanation concerning the needs for and alternatives to such a transfer. The institution to which the patient is to be transferred must first have accepted the patient for transfer.

8. The patient has the right to obtain information as to any relationship of his hospital to other health-care and educational institutions insofar as his care is concerned. The patient has the right to obtain information as to the existence of any professional relationships among individuals, by name, who are treating him.

9. The patient has the right to be advised if the hospital proposes to engage in or perform human experimentation affecting his care or treatment. The patient has the right to refuse to participate in such research projects.

10. The patient has the right to expect reasonable continuity of care. He has the right to know in advance what appointment times and physicians are available and where. The patient has the right to expect that the hospital will provide a mechanism whereby he is informed by his physician or a delegate of the physician of the patient's continuing health-care requirements following discharge.

11. The patient has the right to examine and receive an explanation of his bill regardless of source of payment.

12. The patient has the right to know what hospital rules and regulations apply to his conduct as a patient.

*Reprinted with the permission of the American Hospital Association, copyright 1975.

paraffin method, a method used to prepare a part of body tissue for a laboratory test. The tissue sample is treated with chemicals and buried in paraffin. The paraffin is then cut into very thin slices that can be studied under a microscope.

pavor /pā'vôr/, a reaction of excess terror to something frightening.

pavor diurnus /dī·ur'nəs/, a sleep terror disorder occurring in children during a daytime nap in which they cry out in fear and wake in fear and panic. See also **sleep terror disorder.**

pavor nocturnus /noktur'nəs/, a sleep terror disorder occurring in children during night sleep. See also **nightmare, sleep terror disorder.**

Pavulon, a trademark for a nerve and muscle drug (pancuronium bromide) used during anesthesia.

PCB, abbreviation for **polychlorinated biphenyls.**

PCP, abbreviation for **phencyclidine hydrochloride. 2.** abbreviation for *Pneumocystis carinii pneumonia.*

peak level, the highest amount, usually in the blood, that a substance reaches during a certain time, after which the amount gets smaller. An example is the highest blood glucose level reached during a glucose tolerance test.

peak method of dosing, giving a drug dose so that a certain maximum level is reached to cause a desired effect, as lowering the blood pressure.

peak mucus sign, a cloudy to clear white mucus that occurs in the vaginal area during times of high estrogen levels, as at the most fertile time. See also **spinnbarkeit.**

pearly penile papules. See **hirsutoid papillomas of the penis.**

pectin, a substance found in fruits and vegetables. It adds bulk to the diet, which is needed for the bowels to work correctly. See also **dietary fiber.**

pectineus /pektin'ē·əs/, one of the thigh (femoral) muscles. It moves the thigh and turns it toward the middle of the body.

pectoralis major, a large fan-shaped muscle of the upper chest wall. It flexes and rotates the arm in the shoulder joint, and pulls the shoulder in.

pectoralis minor, a thin, triangle-shaped muscle of the upper chest wall under the muscle of the upper chest wall (pectoralis major). It rotates the shoulder blade (scapula), draws it down and forward, and raises the upper ribs in forced breathing.

pectus excavatum. See **funnel chest.**

pederosis. See **pedophilia.**

pedia-, ped-, pedo-, a combining form referring to a child.

Pediaflor, a trademark for a dental drug (sodium fluoride). It is used to prevent cavities in children.

Pedialyte, a trademark for a balanced mixture of electrolytes.

Pediamycin, a trademark for an antibiotic (erythromycin ethylsuccinate).

pediatric dose, the correct amount, times of giving the dose, and total number of doses of a drug to be given to a child or infant. Such things as the age, weight, body surface area, and the action of the drug in the child must be kept in mind. Possible side effects also need to be considered. Many formulas have been made to figure the pediatric dosage from a standard adult dose. See also **Clark's rule, Cowling's rule, Young's rule.**

pediatric hospitalization, keeping a child or infant in a hospital for testing or treatment. No matter what the age or the degree of illness or injury, being in a hospital is a major crisis in a child's life, and may cause behavior reactions. Causes of stress include being separated from the parents and the home, breakdown of routines, loss of independence, and worry about injury or pain. Some hospitals tell parents to take part in the care of the child through rooming-in or visiting often. Being brought in because of an emergency makes the stress of being in the hospital worse.

pediatric nutrition, having a well-balanced diet. It should have the right foods and enough calories to help in growth and be correct for the many stages of a child's growth. Diet needs vary with age, activity level, and environment. They are also related to the rate of growth. In the prenatal period, growth is dependent on enough food in the mother's diet. During infancy the need for calories, especially protein, is important because of the rapid change in height and weight. Through the preschool and middle childhood years, growth is uneven and occurs in spurts, with a changing appetite and calorie use. In general, the average child uses 55% of energy on keeping the body working, 25% on activities, 12% on growth, and 8% on passing substances out of the body. The growth phase during adolescence needs more calories and vitamins, but food habits are often changed by emotional factors, peer pressure, and fad diets. A faulty diet, especially during important periods of growth, results in slowed growth or illness, as anemia from a lack of iron. A special problem is overfeeding in the early childhood years, which may lead to the child being overweight or an excess intake of vitamins. See also **dietary allowances,** and specific vitamins.

pediatrics /pē'dē·at'triks/, a branch of medicine concerned with the growth and care of children. Its special focus is on the diseases of children and their treatment and prevention. –**pediatric,** *adj.*

pediatric surgery, the special care of the child having surgery for injuries, defects, or diseases. In addition to the usual fears and emotional problems of illness and being in the hospital, the child is often worried about being put to sleep for the surgery. Younger children worry more about what will happen to them and how they will feel after waking up, whereas the older child fears the operation itself, possible death, the loss of control while asleep, and any change in the body or damage to body parts. See also **pediatric hospitalization.**

pediculicide /pədik'yōōlisīd'/, any drug that kills lice.

pediculosis /pədik'yōōlō'sis/, an infestation with bloodsucking lice. Lice cause severe itching, often resulting in infection from scratching the skin. Often only the eggs of the lice may be seen. Body lice lay eggs in the seams of clothing; crab and head lice attach their eggs to hairs. Lice are spread by direct contact with bedding, with people, or from borrowed combs, hats, and clothing. Body lice may carry some diseases. These include returning fevers, typhus, and trench fever. Treatment is to use shampoos, lotions, or creams with licekillers (pediculocides). After treatment, eggs are combed out of the hair with a fine-toothed comb. Lice and eggs on the eyelashes need a special ointment. Prevention is helped by careful washing, ironing, or dry cleaning any clothing or bedding that may have the lice in them. See also **crab louse, louse.**

Pediculus pubis. See **crab louse.**

pedigree, 1. line of descent. 2. a chart that shows the genetic makeup of a person's ancestors. It most often shows plain and shaded or partly shaded squares and circles to note normal males and females, those affected by the disease or trait, and those who are carriers of inherited diseases.

pedophilia /ped'əfil'ē·ə, -fēl'yə/, 1. an abnormal interest in children. 2. a disorder in which sexual activity with children is the desired way to get sexual pleasure. It may be heterosexual or homosexual. Also spelled **paedophilia. Also called pederosis.** See also **paraphilia.** –**pedophilic,** *adj.*

peds, *informal.* pediatrics.

peduncle /pədung'kəl/, a stalk or stemlike connecting part of a growth or tissue, as a peduncle graft. –**peduncular, pedunculate,** *adj.*

Peeping Tom. See **voyeur.**

Peganone, a trademark for an antiseizure drug (ethotoin).

Pel-Ebstein fever /pel'eb'stēn/, a fever that occurs in cycles of several days or weeks. Also called **Murchison fever.**

pell-, a combining form referring to the skin.

pellagra /pəlā′grə, pəlag′rə/, a disease resulting from a lack of a B complex vitamin (niacin) or an amino acid (tryptophan). Persons with diets made up of foods lacking in tryptophan, as cornmeal and porkfat, are at risk. Symptoms include scaly sores, especially on skin exposed to the sun, swelling of the mucous membranes of the mouth, diarrhea, and mental problems. These can range from depression and confusion to hallucinations. Treatment and prevention are to give niacin and tryptophan, usually with other vitamins, and a well-balanced diet with foods rich in these nutrients, as liver, eggs, milk, and meat. Compare **kwashiorkor.** –**pellagrous,** adj.

pellagra sine pellagra, a form of pellagra in which skin symptoms are absent. See **pellagra.**

pelvic, referring to the pelvis.

pelvic brim, the curved top of the bones of the hips. Below the brim is the pelvis.

pelvic cellulitis, a bacterial infection of the tissues (parametrium) around the cervix. It may occur after childbirth or an abortion. It may have spread from a first infection in the genitals. Symptoms include fever, chills, and sweats, stomach pain that spreads, or the uterus failing to return to its nonpregnant size. It is seen most often between the third and the ninth days after birth or abortion. If untreated, problems may be a large sore and infection of membranes in the abdomen (peritonitis). Treatment includes antibiotics, bed rest, and draining any sore that forms. Drugs may be given to reduce the size of the uterus.

pelvic classification, a system of measuring the lining up of the bones of the pelvis to find if they are suited for vaginal birth.

pelvic congestion syndrome, a condition marked by long-term low back pain, urinary difficulty, menstrual disorders, vague lower bowel pain, vaginal discharge, and discomfort during sexual intercourse. The cause of the symptoms is not understood. Women between 25 and 45 years of age are most often affected.

pelvic diaphragm, a group of pelvic muscles stretched like a hammock across the pelvic space. The muscles (levator ani, coccygeus) hold the contents of the abdomen, support the pelvic organs, and are pierced by the anal canal, urethra, and the vagina. Tissue and muscles linked to these structures hold up the pelvic diaphragm.

pelvic examination, a procedure in which the genitals are examined through looking, touching (palpation), tapping (percussion), and listening (auscultation). It should be done regularly during a woman's life. The woman empties her bladder, gets undressed, and puts on a special gown. She is made as comfortable as possible with her feet in stirrups and her buttocks at the very edge of the foot of the examining table, and is then draped. The breasts are examined, and the lower abdomen is felt. The space between the navel and the vagina is checked for any mass. The groin is checked for swollen lymph glands (lymphadenopathy) or hernias. If a mass is felt, the size is figured out. If there is a possible pregnancy, listening for fetal heart tones is done. The outer parts of the vagina are examined. Any swelling, discoloration, tumor, scar, lump (cyst), discharge, or bleeding is noted. Any fluids are examined and a sample is taken for tests. The pelvic muscles are checked. Hernia of the bladder (cytocele) or of the rectum (rectocele), or a falling (prolapse) of the uterus may be seen when the woman is asked to bear down. Because oils and jellies interfere with tests, examination with a device called a speculum is most often done without them. The speculum is coated with warm water, and placed slowly into the vagina. The woman may feel a stretching feeling. The speculum is gently opened and adjusted to show the cervix of the uterus. The color and condition of the vaginal lining are noted. Samples for tests are taken before the Pap test. For the Pap test, scrapings and fluids are taken. In the next part of the examination, the physician puts pressure to the outside of the lower abdomen in many places and directions to bring the uterus, fallopian tubes, and ovaries to where they may be felt. The size, shape, position, and other features of the organs and tissues are checked. Any discomfort is noted. Examination of the rectum is then done. The pelvic examination may discover any defect or disease and needs the help of the woman being examined. An inability to relax, being overweight, pelvic soreness, and heavy vaginal discharge can prevent a good examination. See also **female reproductive system assessment.**

pelvic exeneration, the removal of all reproductive organs and nearby tissues.

pelvic floor, the muscles and tissues surrounding the bottom of the pelvis.

pelvic inflammatory disease (PID), any inflammation of the female pelvic organs, especially one caused by bacteria. Symptoms include fever, foul-smelling vaginal discharge, pain in the lower abdomen, abnormal bleeding, and painful sexual intercourse. There may also be soreness or pain in the uterus, an ovary, or a fallopian tube. If an open sore has previously been seen, a soft, tender, fluid-filled mass may be found by the physician. A sample of mucus is taken for tests. Ultrasound may be used to locate the problem. Bed rest and antibiotics are usually ordered, but the open sore may need to be drained. Severe PID may need a hysterectomy to avoid fatal blood poisoning. If the cause is infection by a sexually carried disease, the woman's sexual partners are also treated with antibiotics. The full course of antibiotics should be taken by the woman. Failure to do so may result in a long-term form of PID. If there is already an open sore, the PID may become long-term. Severe PID is usually very painful. The woman may have to stay in bed and need narcotic painkillers. Repeated periods of a single severe attack of PID often results in scars, blocked fallopian tubes, and the inability to have children. See also **endometritis.**

pelvic inlet, the inlet to the true pelvis in a female. It is surrounded by the sacral and pubic bones. An infant must pass through the inlet to enter the true pelvis and be born through the vagina. The size of the inlet is an important measurement to be made in examining the pelvis in pregnancy.

pelvic minilaparotomy /min'ēlap'ərot'əmē/, an operation in which the lower abdomen is entered through a small cut. It is usually done to sterilize the tubes, but it is also done for diagnosis and to treat a pregnancy outside of the uterus, an ovarian lump (cyst), displaced tissue from the uterine lining (endometriosis), and an inability to have children. The cut (incision) is made in the middle fold of skin. Though small, it allows one to examine inside the abdomen. Each fallopian tube is brought up into the cut and the sterilization or other procedure is done. After each tube is replaced in its natural position, the cut is closed and a small, sterile dressing is placed over the cut. It is often done in the physician's office, although some women may need to stay in the hospital for a short time. Before leaving the hospital, patients are told how to look for danger signs of infection and how to take care of the cut at home. See also **bilateral tubal ligation, sterilization.**

pelvic outlet, the space surrounded by the bones at the bottom of the true pelvis, through which the fetus must pass during childbirth. It is bounded by the tip of the tailbone (coccyx), ligaments, and a joint of the pelvis (pubic symphysis). In men, the shape of the pelvic outlet is narrower than in women. In women, the shape and size of the pelvic outlet are not standard and are important in childbirth. The shapes are named by the length and width of the opening and by the thickness of the bones. See also **pelvic classification, pelvic inlet.**

pelvic pain, pain in the pelvic space, as occurs in appendicitis and a swollen ovary (oophoritis).

pelvic rotation, one of the major factors of walking patterns, with the movement of the pelvis to the right and the left. It is used to diagnose many diseases and abnormal conditions of bones and joints.

pelvic varicocele. See **ovarian varicocele.**

pelvifemoral, referring to the structures of the hip joint. Included are the muscles and the space around the bony pelvis and the head of the upper leg bone (femur).

pelvifemoral muscular dystrophy, a form of muscular dystrophy that begins in the hip. Also called **Leyden-Moebius muscular dystrophy.**

pelvimeter /pelvi ətər/, a device for measuring the pelvis.

pelvimetry /pelvim'ətrē/, measurement of the bony birth canal. Kinds of pelvimetry are **clinical pelvimetry, x-ray pelvimetry.**

pelvis /pel'viz/, pl. **pelves,** the lower part of the trunk of the body. It is made up of four bones: the two hip (innominate) bones on the front and sides, and the lower backbone (sacrum) and tailbone (coccyx) at the bottom of the spinal column. It divides into the greater (false) pelvis and the lesser (true) pelvis. The greater pelvis is the larger part of the space above a bony rim that divides the two parts. The lesser pelvis is below the rim. Its bony walls are more complete than those of the greater pelvis. The pelvis of a woman is usually wider and more circular than that of a man. **–pelvic,** *adj.* (See illustration on p. 593.)

pemoline /pem'əlēn/, a nervous system stimulant given to treat minimal brain defects and attention deficit disorders in children.
★CAUTION: Known allergy to this drug prohibits its use.
★ADVERSE EFFECTS: Some of the more serious side effects are inability to sleep, seizures, and hallucinations.

pemphigoid /pem'figoid/, a skin disease marked by blisters (bullae) and red patches or an itching rash. The skin effects may be linked to an inner cancer. Hormone drugs are used to treat it. Compare **pemphigus.**

pemphigus /pem'figəs, pemfi'gəs/, a disease of the skin and mucous membranes. It is marked by thin-walled blisters (bullae) on the skin or the mucous membrane. The bullae break open easily. The patient loses weight, becomes weak, and is at risk for infections. Treatment with hormones and other drugs has changed this disease from an often fatal one to one that can be controlled. The cause is unknown. Compare **pemphigoid.**

pendular nystagmus, unwillful rhythmic movements of the eyeballs in which both eyes move together in the same way at the same speed.

penicillamine (D-penicillamine), a drug given to bind with and remove metals from the blood. It is used to treat lead poisoning and also given to relieve symptoms of rheumatoid arthritis when other drugs have failed.
★CAUTION: Known allergy to this drug or a form of anemia prohibits its use. It is not given during pregnancy or to patients with kidney disorders.
★ADVERSE EFFECTS: Among the more serious

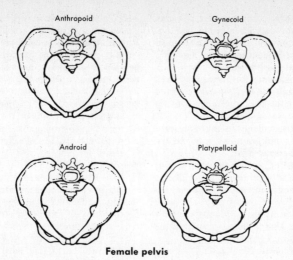

Anthropoid Gynecoid

Android Platypelloid

Female pelvis

side effects are fever, rashes, and blood disorders. Severe bone marrow disease is linked to long-term use of this drug.

penicillin /pen'isil'in/, any of a group of antibiotics taken from cultures of the fungus *Penicillium* or made in a laboratory. Many penicillins are given by mouth or injection to treat bacteria infections. Allergic reactions are common in patients who get penicillin. Side effects may appear even when the drug has not been used before. The reason for this may be an unnoticed use of a food or other substance with traces of the antibiotic. The most common allergic reactions to penicillin are rash and fever. Some patients have a severe skin swelling (erythema multiforme). The most common cause of allergic shock (anaphylaxis) is an injection of penicillin. See also **penicillinase-resistant penicillin, penicillin G, penicillin V.**

penicillinase /pen'əsil'ənās/, an enzyme made by some bacteria, including staphylococci, that stops the action of penicillin. This causes resistance to the antibiotic. It is used to treat the side effects of penicillin. Also called **beta-lactamase.**

penicillinase-resistant penicillin, one of the partly laboratory-made penicillins. They are not stopped from acting by the enzyme penicillinase. These antibiotics are used to treat infections caused by living things that make the enzyme.

penicillin G, an antibiotic given to treat many infections.

★CAUTION: Known allergy to this drug or any penicillin prohibits its use.

★ADVERSE EFFECTS: Among the more serious side effects are allergic reactions. Nausea and diarrhea sometimes occur.

penicillin G benzathine, a long-acting form of penicillin used to treat some streptococcal and other infections. It is given by slow, deep injection over 12 hours to several days.

★CAUTION: Allergy to this drug or to other penicillins prohibits its use.

★ADVERSE EFFECTS: The most serious side effect is allergic shock (anaphylaxis).

penicillin V, an antibiotic given to treat infections.

★CAUTION: Known allergy to this drug or to any penicillin prohibits its use.

★ADVERSE EFFECTS: Among the more serious side effects is allergic shock (anaphylaxis).

penicilliosis /pen'isil'ē-ō'sis/, a lung infection caused by a fungus, *Penicillium.*

penile cancer /pē'nīl/, a cancer of the penis that occurs mainly in men whose foreskin has not been removed. It is linked to genital herpesvirus infection and poor personal washing. Material (smegma) that gathers under the foreskin may be a factor, but the actual cancer-causing substance is unknown. Cancer of the penis often appears as a growth of tissue or a bleeding ulcer and spreads early in its growth. Treatment involves part or total removal of the penis and removal of lymph nodes in the groin and nearby tissue when needed. Radiation is often used. Anticancer drugs may also be given, especially in cancer that is spreading.

penis, the outer reproductive organ of a man. The penis is made up of three circular masses of spongy tissue covered with skin. Two of them (corpora cavernosa) partly surround a third one (corpus spongiosum). The corpus spongiosum contains the tube (urethra) that drains the bladder. The connective tissue (fascia) of the penis is parallel to the scrotum, which contains the testicles.

penniform /pen'ifôrm/, referring to the shape of a feather, especially in muscle fibers. Compare **bipenniform, multipenniform.**

pent-, penta, a combining form meaning 'five.'

pentaerythritol tetranitrate /pen'tə·erith'rətol/, a heart blood vessel-widening drug given to relieve chest pain (angina pectoris).
★CAUTION: Known allergy to this drug prohibits its use. It is not given in severe anemia, brain bleeding, or head injury.
★ADVERSE EFFECTS: Among the most serious side effects are low blood pressure and allergic reactions. Headaches and flushing also may occur.

pentamidine, an antiprotozoa drug that can only be gotten in the United States only from the Centers for Disease Control.

pentazocine hydrochloride /pentă'zəsēn/, a painkiller given to relieve moderate to severe pain.
★CAUTION: Known allergy to this drug prohibits its use. It should not be given to patients with head injury or those with a history of drug abuse and addiction.
★ADVERSE EFFECTS: Nausea and dizziness commonly occur. High doses may cause breathing and blood-flow problems. This drug can cause withdrawal symptoms in drug addicts.

pentazocine lactate. See **pentazocine hydrochloride.**

Pentids, a trademark for an antibiotic (penicillin G potassium).

pentobarbital, a tranquilizer and sedative given before surgery, to treat an inability to sleep, and to control seizures.

pentose, a sugar made by the body and also found in some fruits, as plums and cherries. Blood levels of pentose are higher after eating such fruits and in some diseases.

pentosuria /pen'təsŏŏr'ē·ə/, a condition in which a sugar (pentose) is in the urine. Pentosuria may be caused by an inherited defect.

Pentothal sodium, a trademark for a barbiturate drug (thiopental sodium), used as an anesthetic and to aid anesthesia.

pentoxifylline, an oral blood thinner used for the treatment of leg cramps that occur with exercise in patients with hardening of the arteries.
★CAUTION: Patients with disorders of the heart and blood vessels should be closely watched and their high blood pressure dosage reduced if needed. Patients taking more than one drug also should be closely watched.
★ADVERSE EFFECTS: Among the most serious side reactions are nausea, discomfort under the breastbone after eating (dyspepsia), dizziness, cramping chest pain (angina), abnormal heart beat (dysrhythmias), and low blood pressure.

Pen-Vee K, a trademark for an antibiotic (penicillin V potassium).

Pepper syndrome, a cancer of the adrenal glands that spreads to the liver.

pep pills, *slang.* amphetamines.

peps-, pept-, a combining form referring to digestion.

pepsin /pep'sin/, an enzyme released in the stomach that speeds up the breakdown of protein. Pepsin from pork and beef stomachs is sometimes used to aid digestion. See also **enzyme.**

pepsinogen /pəpsin'əjən/, a substance released by cells in the stomach and changed to the enzyme pepsin when stomach acid is present.

-peptic, a combining form referring to digestion.

peptic ulcer, a spot of breakdown or loss of mucous membrane of the stomach or any other part of the digestive system coming into contact with juices that have stomach acid and pepsin. Acute ulcers are almost always shallow and occur in groups. They may be without symptoms and heal without scars. Chronic ulcers are true ulcers. They are deep, single, and cause symptoms. The muscle coat of the wall of the tract is permanently damaged. A scar forms, and the mucous membrane may heal, but not the muscle under it. Peptic ulcers are caused by many uncertain factors. They include an excess amount of stomach acid, loss of covering of the mucous membrane, stress, inherited defects, and using some drugs. Chronic ulcers cause a gnawing pain in the upper stomach. The pain is not affected by a change in body position. Antacids and many, small bland meals may help. The cause is treated if known. A type of antihistamine (cimetidine) reduces the amount of acids, but may cause side effects. Other drugs can slow the action of stomach acid and help the pain. If there is bleeding, surgery may have to be done. The careful diagnosis of peptic ulcers is important because the early signs of cancer of the stomach and the small intestine are like those of peptic ulcers. In most cases, ulcers heal completely and pain may be controlled simply, often with the correct use of antacids and other drugs. The patient should eat many small meals made up of nonirritating foods. For many but not all patients, fatty, highly spiced, heavy, or high-fiber foods are likely to cause pain.

peptide /pep'tīd/, a molecule chain of two or more amino acids. See also **amino acid, polypeptide, protein.**

percent systole, an amount of time of each heartbeat that is used in removing blood from the lower heart chambers.

percephalus, *pl.* **percephali,** a fetus or person with a deformed head.

percept /pur'sept/, the mental sense of an object

that is perceived through the use of the sight, touch, or other senses.

perception, noting and sensing nerve signals from the sense organs. It often concerns the unconscious, as memory, that is the basis for understanding. See also **depth perception, extrasensory perception, facial perception, stereognostic perception. –perceptive, perceptual,** *adj.*

perceptual defect, any of a broad group of disorders of the nervous system that slow down the conscious sensing of nerve signals. Such conditions are caused by nerve cell damage in some parts of the brain. The cell damage can result from any illness or injury affecting the brain at any age or stage of growth. Mental damage can appear, as psychoses, delirium, dementia, or attention deficit disorder. They may result in some brain problems, as loss of language ability (aphasia) loss of ability to control muscles (apraxia), fits (epilepsy), or loss of memory.

perceptual deprivation, the lack of or reduced important signals. It may result from constant background noise or constant poor lighting.

perceptual monotony, a mental state caused by a lack of variety in the normal pattern of everyday signals.

Percodan, a trademark for a nervous system drug with two narcotic painkillers (oxycodone hydrochloride and oxycodone terephthalate).

Percogesic, a trademark for a lung drug with an antihistamine (phenyltoloxamine citrate) and a painkiller (acetaminophen).

percolation, the act of filtering any liquid through something liquids can pass through.

Percorten Acetate, a trademark for an adrenal gland hormone drug (desoxycorticosterone acetate).

percussion, a tapping in medical tests used to guess the size, borders, and texture of some chest organs and organs in the abdomen. It is also used to detect the presence and amount of fluid in a body space. **Immediate** or **direct percussion** refers to tapping (percussion) done by striking the fingers on the surface of the chest or abdomen. **Indirect, mediate,** or **finger percussion** is striking a finger of one hand on a finger of the other hand as it is placed over an organ. See also **cupping and vibrating, percussor, pleximeter. –percuss,** *v.,* **percussable,** *adj.*

percutaneous /pur′kyo͞otā′nē·əs/, a medical procedure done through the skin, as a biopsy. It also refers to fluid being taken out from below the skin using a needle, tube, or syringe, or a fluid put into a space by the same means.

percutaneous catheter placement, placing a tube (catheter) into a blood vessel (artery) through the skin, and moving it to a tissue or an organ to be studied. The skin where the tube goes in is deadened by medication. A special needle is put into the artery, and a long, flexible spring guide is passed through it. The needle is then removed, the catheter is moved to the desired place, and the guide is taken out.

percutaneous nephroscope, a thin fiberoptic device that can be inserted into the kidney through a skin incision. Light transmitted along the fibers enables the examiner to see the inside of the kidney. The device includes a tool for removing small stones.

percutaneous transluminal coronary angioplasty (PTCA), a technique to treat heart disease and chest pain (angina pectoris). Fatty material (plaques) in the blood vessels (arteries) of the heart are flattened against the vessel walls. It makes the blood flow better. A tube (catheter) is put into the vessel through the skin. A small balloon at the tip of the catheter is filled up and emptied many times to flatten the plaques. PTCA is done with x-ray or ultrasound machines so the catheter can be seen in the artery. When PTCA succeeds, the plaques stay flat and the symptoms of heart disease, including the pain of angina, are reduced.

Perez reflex /pərez′, per′ez/, the normal response of an infant. This includes crying, moving the arms and legs, and holding up the head and hips when on its back with a finger pressed along the spine from the lower back (sacrum) to the neck. If the reflex still occurs after 6 months of age, it may mean there is brain damage.

perfloxacin, an antibiotic of the carboxyfluoroquinolinone type.

perfluorocarbons, a group of chemicals that act somewhat like red blood cells by carrying oxygen through the blood vessels. They can sometimes be used to substitute for blood, regardless of the patient's blood type. They can be stored at room temperature and are free of infection-causing organisms. Also called **artificial blood.**

perforate, to make a hole. **–perforation,** *n.*

perforating fracture, an open broken bone caused by an object, as a bullet, making a small surface wound.

perforation of the uterus, an accidental break in the uterus, as may occur during an abortion or by a birth-control device (IUD).

perfusion, **1.** fluid passing through an organ or a part of the body. **2.** a method for giving a drug meant for a remote part of the body by sending it through the blood.

perfusion lung scan, an x-ray test of the lungs made after injecting a dye into the veins. It is used to diagnose a blood clot in the lungs.

Pergonal, a trademark for a hormone drug used to treat an inability to have children.

peri-, a combining form meaning 'around.'

Periactin, a trademark for an antihistamine used to relieve itching (cyproheptadine hydrochloride).

perianal abscess /per′ē·ā′nəl/, a pus-making infection beneath the skin around the anus.

Treatment includes hot soaks, antibiotics, and possibly cutting and draining it. If an abnormal channel (rectal fistula) is the cause of repeated perianal abscesses, surgery is often done.

periapical /per′ē·ap′ikəl, per′ē·ā′pikəl/, referring to the tissues around the root of a tooth, including the gums and bones.

periapical abscess, an infection around the root of a tooth, usually spread from tooth cavities. The abscess may go into nearby bone or, more often, to soft tissues. The infection may spread into the mouth or a sinus. There may be fever and nausea. Treatment includes drilling into the pulp of the tooth to drain it and relieve pain, followed by antibiotics, root canal treatment, or removing the tooth.

periapical fibroma, a mass of harmless connective tissue that may form at the root of a tooth with normal pulp.

periarteritis /per′ē·är′tərī′tis/, an inflammation of the outer coat of a blood vessel (artery) and the tissue around the vessel.

periarteritis gummosa. See **syphilitic periarteritis.**

periarteritis nodosa, a disease of the connective tissue with many large bumps (nodules) in groups along parts of middle-sized blood vessels (arteries). This causes blockage of the blood vessel, resulting in some places lacking blood (ischemia), bleeding, tissue death, and pain. The early signs of the disease are rapid heart beat, fever, weight loss, and stomach pain. The kidneys, lungs, and intestines may be affected. Other systems and organs of the body may also be affected. Treatment is giving a hormone drug. About 50% of patients live 4 years after the disease is found.

pericarditis /per′ikärdī′tis/, an inflammation of the membrane (pericardium) covering the heart. It is linked to injury, cancer, heart attack, and other diseases. The first stage is marked by fever, chest pain that moves to the shoulder or neck, breathing difficulty, and a dry cough. The physician may hear a rubbing sound around the heart. The patient becomes more anxious, tired, and unable to breathe unless standing or sitting. During the second stage, fluid gathers in the heart membrane, slowing down heart movement. Heart sounds become soft, weak, and distant. A bulge is seen on the chest over the heart. If the fluid has pus in it, a high fever, sweat, chills, and physical collapse also occur. Treatment includes bed rest with the head of the bed raised 45 degrees to make breathing easier. Drugs include antibiotics or antifungus drugs and painkillers. Surgery may be needed to remove fluid or to find the cause of the disease.

pericardium /per′ikär′dē·əm/, *pl.* **pericardia,** a double-layered sac of membranes around the heart. The inner part (serous pericardium) divides into a membrane that sticks to the heart's surface. The other lines the inside of the outer part (fibrous pericardium) of the sac. The most outer pericardium has tough, white, fiberlike tissue. It fits loosely around the heart and is fairly rigid. Between the two layers is the pericardial space. It contains fluid that oils tissue surfaces, allowing the heart to move easily while contracting. Injury or disease may cause fluid to fill the space. This divides the heart and the outer part of the sac. The fiberlike pericardium cannot stretch, causing the heart to constrict. See illustration on p. 596. **–pericardial,** *adj.*

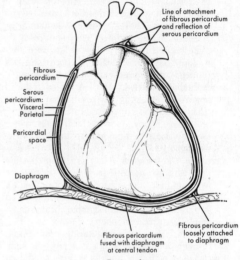

Line of attachment of fibrous pericardium and reflection of serous pericardium

Fibrous pericardium

Serous pericardium:
Visceral
Parietal

Pericardial space

Diaphragm

Fibrous pericardium fused with diaphragm at central tendon

Fibrous pericardium loosely attached to diaphragm

Pericardium

pericholangitis /per′əkōlanji′tis/, a swelling of the tissues around bile ducts in the liver. It is a problem caused by a disease of the intestines (ulcerative colitis) and is marked by fever, chills, and yellow skin (jaundice). See also **ulcerative colitis.**

perifolliculitis /per′ēfolik′yo͞oli′tis/, swelling of the tissue around a hair sac (follicle). Compare **folliculitis.**

perilymph /per′ilimf/, a clear fluid in the inner ear. Compare **endolymph.**

perimetrium /per′imē′trē·əm/, a membrane around the uterus.

perinatal /per′inā′təl/, referring to the time and process of giving birth or being born.

perinatal AIDS, AIDS transmitted to infants and children by their mothers during pregnancy, during delivery, or through infected breast milk.

perinatal death, 1. the death of a fetus weighing more than 1,000 g at 28 or more weeks of pregnancy. 2. the death of an infant between birth and 28 days after birth.

perinatal period, a period from 28 weeks of pregnancy to 28 days after birth.

perinatology, a branch of medicine that studies the anatomy and physiology of the mother and her infant. It also concerns the diagnosis and treatment of disorders during pregnancy, childbirth, and the 28 days after birth. **–perinatologic, perinatological,** *adj.*

perineal care, a method for cleaning the area around the anus and sex organs (perineum). Perineal care may be given by washing from front to back. A washcloth is used and changed after each stroke. The draped patient is helped into position on her back with a bedpan or on a pad that is later thrown away. A cleaning fluid is poured over the vulva. Then wet washcloths are used to clean more thoroughly. The patient is dried using sterile cloths, and the bedpan is removed. The patient then lies on her side for cleaning and drying the back. With perineal wound care, washcloths that are thrown away, soap, and a basin or a squeeze bottle of warm water are used. A fresh cloth is used for each stroke, again from front to back, in washing, removing soap, and drying. The back and front are cleaned and dried in the same way. Perineal wound care is done to take out fluids or dried blood from a wound and to avoid infecting the uterus and vagina with feces or urine. See also **postpartum perineal care.**

perineorrhaphy /per′inē·ôr′əfē/, a procedure in which a cut, tear, or defect in the space between the thighs (perineum) is repaired with stitches.

perineum /per′inē′əm/, the part of the body between the inner thighs on either side, with the buttocks to the rear and the sex organs at the front. The perineum holds up and surrounds the lower parts of the urinary and digestive tracts. **–perineal,** *adj.*

period, *nontechnical.* menses.

periodic, happening again and again. **–periodicity,** *n.*

periodic apnea of the newborn, a normal condition in the full-term newborn. Rapid breathing is followed by a brief period in which breathing stops (apnea). It usually occurs with rapid eye movement (REM) sleep. Apnea in the newborn not linked to REM sleep or with periodic breathing may be a sign of brain bleeding, seizures, or other disorders. See also **sleep, sudden infant death syndrome.**

periodic breathing. See **Cheyne-Stokes respiration.**

periodic hyperinflation, a normal unconscious sigh or deep breath that tends to occur when a person is not physically active. Because of the natural need for periodic deep breaths, an artificial sigh is often programmed into the pattern of mechanical devices that help patients to breathe (ventilators). See also **periodic deep inspiration.**

periodontal /per′ē·ōdon′təl/, referring to the space around a tooth.

periodontal cyst, a fluid-filled sac that occurs most often at the bottom of a tooth root. Cysts that occur at the side of a tooth root are less common.

periodontal disease, disease of the tissues around a tooth, as swelling of the periodontal ligament.

periodontal ligament (PDL), the fiberlike tissue that joins the teeth to the sockets (alveoli). It is made up of many bundles of connective tissue in groups and linked up with blood vessels, lymph vessels, and nerves. The periodontal ligament holds and supports the teeth.

periodontitis /per′ē·ōdontī′tis/, inflammation of the tissue that joins the teeth and sockets (periodontal ligament), the gums, and the jaw bone (periodontium). See also **periodontal, periodontal disease, periodontics.**

periodontoclasia, the loosening of permanent teeth.

periodontosis, a rare disease that affects young people, especially women, in which tooth (periodontal) tissues are destroyed. The cause is unknown.

periosteum /per′ē·os′tē·əm/, a fiberlike covering of the bones, except at their ends. It has an outer layer of connective tissue with some fat cells and an inner layer of fine stretchy fibers. Periosteum has the nerves and blood vessels that supply the bones. It is thick and rich in blood vessels over young bones but thinner and with fewer blood vessels in later life. Bones that lose periosteum through injury or disease often waste or die.

periostitis, inflammation of the fiberlike coverings of bones (periosteum). Infection or injury of them causes tenderness and swelling around the bone, pain, fever, and chills. In severe cases blood or a watery substance forms under them.

peripheral, referring to the outside surface or surrounding area of an organ or other structure.

peripheral acrocyanosis of the newborn, a normal, temporary condition of the newborn. It is marked by pale bluish skin on the hands and feet, especially the fingers and toes. The blueness fades as the baby begins to breathe easily but returns if the baby becomes chilled.

peripheral arteriovenography, an x-ray test of the blood vessels in the outer parts of the body, as the arms and legs. A special dye is injected into these vessels.

peripheral nervous system, the motor and sense nerves outside of the brain and spinal cord. The system has 12 pairs of skull nerves, 31 pairs of spinal nerves, and their many branches in body organs. Sense nerves carry signals to the brain and spinal cord (central nervous system). Motor nerves carry signals from the brain to other parts of the body. The sense and motor nerves travel together but divide at the spinal cord level. Some nerves (somatic) act on the body wall; others (visceral) supply internal organs. The autonomic nervous system is a part of the peripheral system. See also **autonomic nervous system.**

peripheral neuropathy, any disorder of the motor and sense nerves outside of the brain and spinal cord (peripheral nervous system). An example is numbness or tingling feelings (paresthesia).

peripheral odontogenic fibroma, a fiberlike connective tissue tumor involving the gums. It often has hard tissues caused by excess calcium.

peripheral plasma cell myeloma. See **plasmacytoma.**

peripheral polyneuritis, peripheral polyneuropathy. See **multiple peripheral neuritis.**

peripheral resistance, a resistance to the flow of blood. It is measured by the muscle tone and diameter of blood vessels.

peripheral vascular disease, any abnormal condition that affects the blood vessels outside of the heart and the major vessels. Different kinds and degrees of the disease have many signs and symptoms. These include numbness, pain, paleness, high blood pressure, and damaged pulses. Causes include being overweight, cigarette smoking, stress, and lack of activity. When linked to an infection of the heart (bacterial endocarditis), blood clots may form in tiny blood vessels (arterioles) causing tissue death (gangrene) in many parts of the body, as the tip of the nose, fingers, or toes. Treatment of severe cases may mean removing damaged body parts. Lesser problems may be treated with drugs. Some kinds of peripheral vascular disease are **arteriosclerosis, atherosclerosis.**

peripheral vision, an ability to see objects that are to the side of the body, rather than straight ahead.

peristalsis /per'istôl'sis, -stal'sis/, the wavelike, rhythmic contraction of smooth muscle. It forces food through the digestive tract, bile through the bile duct, and urine through the ureters.

peritoneal cavity /per'itōnē'əl/, a space between the outer (parietal) and the inner (visceral) layers of the membrane lining the abdomen (peritoneum). Normally, the two layers are in contact. The space is divided into a greater sac (peritoneal cavity) and a lesser sac (omental bursa). The omental bursa is in back of the stomach.

peritoneal dialysis, blood filtering (dialysis) process done to correct too-much or too-little fluid or electrolytes in the blood. It is also done to remove poisons, drugs, or other wastes the kidney normally gets rid of. The membrane of the abdomen (peritoneum) is used as a dialysis membrane. This form of dialysis may be done nightly for very ill children while they sleep and may also be done at home. A tube (cath-

eter) is put in place and connected to tubing that allows flow in and out. The amount and kind of fluid (dialysate) and the length of time for each cycle changes with the age, size, and condition of the patient. The fluid is first warmed to body temperature, and drugs used to stop blood clotting, antibiotics, or other additives may be given. Drugs may be given for pain. There are three phases in each cycle. During the first phase (inflow), the dialysate is sent into the peritoneal space. During the second phase (equilibration), the dialysate stays in the space. The needed substances pass to the blood. Waste products pass from the blood vessels through the peritoneum into the dialysate. During the third phase (outflow), the dialysate drains from the peritoneal space by gravity. Problems may occur, including puncturing (perforation) the bowel, infections, and bruises. Bruises often develop because the tissues are irritated by the catheter. See also **adhesions.**

peritoneal-dialysis solution, a fluid with many substances that is put into the membrane of the abdomen (peritoneum) to remove poisons from the body.

peritoneoscope. See **laparoscope.**

peritoneum /per'itənē'əm/, a large oiled membrane that covers the entire wall of the abdomen and is folded over the inner organs (viscera). It is divided into an outer (parietal) membrane and an inner (visceral) one. In men, the peritoneum is a closed sac. In women, it is passed through by the free ends of the fallopian tubes. The free surface of the peritoneum is oiled by fluid that permits the organs to glide against the wall and against one another. A part (mesentery) of the peritoneum fans out from the main membrane to hold the small intestine. See also **greater omentum, lesser omentum, transverse mesocolon.** –**peritoneal,** adj.

peritonitis /per'itənī'tis/, a swelling of the membrane that covers the wall of the abdomen (peritoneum). It is caused by bacteria or substances in the space in the abdomen by a wound or an abnormal hole (perforation) in an organ. Peritonitis is caused most often by a break in the appendix, but it also follows holes in other organs, as the spleen, liver, or fallopian tubes. Signs and symptoms of peritonitis include swelling, pain, nausea, vomiting, rapid heart beat, chills and fever, and rapid breathing. Shock and heart failure may follow. The patient should be placed in bed in a position halfway sitting up with the knees pulled up to make breathing easier and to make pus flow toward the lower abdomen. Oxygen, fluids given through the veins, large doses of antibiotics, and drugs to cause vomiting (emetics) are used. Pain is controlled with painkillers. Repair of the hole that caused the infection is often not done until the patient's condition is better. See also **appendectomy, appendicitis.**

peritonsillar abscess, an infection of tissue between the tonsil and throat, most often after an attack of tonsillitis. The symptoms include swallowing difficulty (dysphagia), pain moving to the ear, and fever. The tonsil and soft palate are red and swollen. Treatment includes penicillin, warm salt-water gargles, surgery, and drainage if needed. Also called **quinsy.** Compare **parapharyngeal abscess, retropharyngeal abscess.** See also **tonsillitis.**

Peritrate, a trademark for a blood vessel-widening drug (pentaerythritol tetranitrate).

periungual /per'ē·ung'gwəl/, referring to the space around the fingernails or the toenails.

permanent dentition, the coming in of the 32 permanent teeth, beginning with the first permanent molars at about 6 years of age. The process is complete by 12 or 13 years of age except for the four wisdom teeth. They may not come in until 18 to 25 years of age, or later. Also called **secondary dentition.** Compare **deciduous dentition.** See also **tooth.**

permanent tooth, one of the set of 32 teeth that appear during and after childhood and last until old age. In each jaw they include four incisors, two canines, four premolars, and six molars. The permanent teeth replace the 20 teeth (deciduous) of infancy, and also include 12 molars, three on each side of the upper and lower jaws, which come in later. The permanent teeth start to develop in the ninth week of pregnancy. They develop from the early dental tissue. As the permanent teeth grow in the fetus, they move back into the gum behind the deciduous teeth. The permanent teeth start to harden soon after birth. The teeth in the lower jaw grow somewhat faster than those in the upper jaw. They also come in first in the lower jaw. The first molars come in about 6 years of age. The two central incisors come in about 7 years of age. The two lateral incisors come in about 8 years of age. The first premolars come in about 9 years of age. The second premolars come in about 10 years of age. The canines come in between 11 and 12 years of age. The second molars come in between 12 and 13 years of age. The third molars come in after 17 and 25 years of age. The coming in of each tooth in the upper jaw lags only slightly behind that of the same tooth in the lower jaw. The third molars (wisdom teeth) in many people are badly placed or so deeply buried in bone that they must be removed. In some, one or all four of the third molars may not grow correctly. Compare **deciduous tooth.** See also **tooth.**

permeable, allowing fluids and other substances to pass through, as a permeable membrane. See also **osmosis.**

permissible dose, the amount of radiation that may be received by a person in a set period of time with no harmful results.

Permitil, a trademark for a tranquilizer (fluphenazine hydrochloride).

pernicious anemia /pərnish'əs/, a form of anemia, affecting mainly older patients. It results from a lack of a substance (intrinsic factor) that is needed to process the vitamin B_{12} (cyanocobalamin) needed for red blood cells. The making of red blood cells in bone marrow is stopped. The white blood cell count is lowered, and some white blood cells become abnormal. Extreme weakness, numbness and tingling in the arms and legs, fever, paleness, and loss of appetite and weight may occur. The condition is most often treated with injections of vitamin B_{12}, iron, and folic acid. See also **atrophic gastritis, intrinsic factor, nutritional anemia.**

pernio. See **chilblain.**

perochirus /pē'rōkī'rəs/, a person with deformed hands.

perodactyly /pē'rōdak'tilē/, a birth defect in which one or more of the fingers or toes are lacking. Also called **perodactylia.**

peromelia /per'əmē'lē·ə/, a birth defect in which one or more of the limbs are deformed. Also called **peromely** /pərom'əlē/. **–peromelus,** *n.*

peroneal /per'ənēəl/, referring to the outer part of the leg.

peroneal muscular atrophy, an abnormal inherited condition. It involves weakening or wasting of the foot and ankle muscles, and hammertoes. Affected people often have high arches and an awkward walk, caused by weak ankle muscles. Such people may be helped by surgery and leg braces that keep weak ankle joints rigid.

peronia /pərō'nē·ə/, a deformation.

perphenazine, an antipsychotic drug given to treat psychotic disorders and to control severe nausea and vomiting in adults.

PERRLA /pur'lə/, abbreviation for *pupils equal, round, react to light, accommodation.* It notes the condition of the eyes, the size and shape of the pupils, their reaction to light, and their ability to focus as normal. It is used to note results of an eye test.

Persa-Gel, a trademark for an acne drug (benzoyl peroxide).

Persantine, a trademark for a heart vessel-widening drug (dipyridamole).

persistent cloaca, a birth defect in which the intestinal, urinary, and reproductive ducts open into a common space. Also called **congenital cloaca.**

Persistin, a trademark for a nervous system drug with painkillers (aspirin and salicylsalicylic acid).

persona /pərsō'nə/, *pl.* **personae** /-nē/, the role that a person takes and presents to the world to satisfy the demands of society or as part of some mental conflict. The persona masks the person's inner being or unconscious self. Compare **anima**. See also **archetype**.

personal and social history, a person's story used in a health record, of the personal and social details of that person's life. It identifies the individual. Place of birth, religion, race, marriage status, number of children, military status, job history, and where one lives are usual in this part of the history. It may also include other data, as education, current living situation, and smoking, alcohol, and drug habits.

personal care services, the services done by health-care workers to help patients in meeting the demands of daily living.

personality, the pattern of behavior each person develops as a means of dealing with the surroundings and their cultural, ethnic, and other standards.

personality disorder, any of a large group of mental disorders with rigid and wrong behavior patterns. They damage a person's ability to act in society by severely limiting the ability to deal with the world.

perspiration, 1. the act or process of sweating; the release of fluid by the sweat glands through pores in the skin. 2. the fluid released by the sweat glands. It is made up of water with salt (sodium chloride), phosphate, urea, ammonia, and other waste products. Perspiration not only removes body wastes, but also helps control body temperature. Abnormal amounts of perspiration most often result from physical causes but may also come from severe emotional stress. Kinds of perspiration are **insensible perspiration, sensible perspiration.** See also **diaphoresis, sweat.**

Perthes' disease /per′täs/, abnormal changes in the growth of the bone substance in the head of the upper leg bone (femur) in children. It may begin with death and the breakdown of bone-forming tissues, followed by regrowth or rehardening of the bone. Also called **coxa plana, Legg-Calve-Perthes disease, pseudocoxalgia,Waldenström's disease.**

Pertofrane, a trademark for an antidepressant (desipramine hydrochloride).

pertussis. See **whooping cough.**

pertussis immune globulin, a passive vaccinating drug used against whooping cough.

★CAUTION: Known allergy to this drug prohibits its use.

★ADVERSE EFFECTS: Among the more serious side effects is allergic shock.

pertussis vaccine, an active vaccinating drug given to fight whooping cough (pertussis) when combined diphtheria, pertussis, and tetanus vaccine cannot be used.

★CAUTION: A lack of blood platelets (thrombocytopenia) or known allergy to the vaccine prohibits its use.

★ADVERSE EFFECTS: Among the most serious

side effects are severe allergic reactions, pain at the injection site, and fever.

perversion, 1. any varying from what is considered normal or natural behavior. 2. the act of causing a change from what is normal or natural. 3. *informal.* any of a number of sexual acts that vary from what is considered normal adult behavior. See also **paraphilia.**

pervert /pur′vərt/, 1. *informal.* a person who gets sexual pleasure from acts generally thought to be abnormal, especially when it is a substitute for normal sexual acts. 2. one whose sexual behavior varies from what is usually acceptable in a group but is not a disease.

pes /pēz/, the foot or a footlike structure.

pes cavus, a defect of the foot with a very high arch and very long toes. The condition may be present at birth or appear later because the muscles of the foot contract or become unbalanced, as in nerve or muscle diseases. Surgery is needed in severe cases, especially in children. In milder forms the pain can be relieved by special shoes. Also called **clawfoot, gampsodactyly, griffe des orteils** /grif′dezōrtä′ē/, **talipes cavus.**

pes planus, a flat arch of the foot. Also called **flatfoot.**

pessary /pes′ərē/, a device placed in the vagina to treat a failing uterus (prolapse), or other problems of the vaginal space. It is used to treat women whose older age or poor general condition prevents surgery. A vaginal cream with estrogen is usually given to cause the lining of the vagina to become thick and become better able to tolerate the pessary. Pessaries are also used in younger women in checking for a backward bending of the uterus (retroversion). Retroversion is the cause of pain if the pain is relieved by bending the uterus forward with the pessary in place and if it returns after the pessary is removed. The pessary is sometimes used in pregnancy to hold the uterus in a forward position. Pressure causes less stress on the neck of the womb. A pessary must be removed, usually daily, for cleaning. The woman may do this herself, or it may be done by someone else if she is unable to do it. Left in place, the pessary is likely to cause severe irritation, leading to an infection. One type of pessary is a rubber- or vinyl-covered wire rectangle that fits between the pubic bone and the back of the vagina, holding up the uterus and holding the cervix in place. Another kind of pessary is a rigid device made of plastic in the form of a large collar button. It has a canal through the stem that allows vaginal fluids to drain out. The large end of the pessary is placed deep in the vagina. The small end of the stem sticks out of the vagina (introitus). A **doughnut pessary** is a flexible rubber doughnut that is placed to support the uterus by blocking the canal of the vagina. An **inflatable pessary**

is a rubber doughnut that can be broken down and is fixed to a flexible stem with a valve. The pessary is put in when unfilled, filled with a squeeze bulb, and emptied for removal. A **Bee-cell pessary** is a soft rubber cube. In each face of the cube, a curved space acts as a suction cup when the pessary is in the vagina. A **diaphragm pessary** is a birth-control device also used to hold up the uterus and vagina.

pesticide poisoning, a condition caused by swallowing or breathing a substance used for pest control. See also **insecticide poisoning, malathion poisoning, parathion poisoning, rodenticide poisoning.**

petechiae /pētē′kē·ē/, *sing.* **petechia** /-ə/, tiny purple or red spots that appear on the skin because of small spots of bleeding under the skin. Petechiae range from pinpoint to pinhead size and are even with the skin surface. Compare **ecchymosis. –petechial,** *adj.*

petechial fever /pitē′kē·əl/, any illness with fever that has small spots (petechiae) on the skin, as in the late stage of typhoid fever.

petit mal seizure /pət′tē mal′, ptē′ mäl′/, a type of epileptic seizure. It is marked by a sudden, short-term loss of consciousness. Muscles may contract in the neck or arms, the face may twitch, or muscles may lose their tone. The seizures most often occur many times a day and are most common in children and adolescents. They are very common at the age of puberty. Someone having a typical seizure has a blank look and stops all willful movements. When consciousness returns, the person may start speaking again without knowing what had happened. Antiseizure drugs are used to prevent petit mal attacks. See also **epilepsy.**

P.E.T.N.S.R., a trademark for a blood vessel widener (pentaerythritol tetranitrate).

petrissage /pā′trisäzh′/, a type massage in which the skin is gently lifted and squeezed. Petrissage makes the blood flow easier and relaxes the muscles. Compare **effleurage, rolling effleurage.**

petrolatum gauze /pet′rəlā′təm/, gauze covered with white petroleum.

petroleum distillate poisoning, a harmful condition caused by swallowing or breathing in a petroleum producer, as fuel oil, model airplane cement, or other products. Nausea, vomiting, chest pain, dizziness, and severe depression of the nervous system are symptoms. Severe or fatal lung problems may occur. Vomiting should be avoided. Flushing the stomach (lavage) with water and oxygen, if needed, is useful. See also **gasoline poisoning, kerosene poisoning.**

Peutz-Jeghers syndrome, an inherited disorder with many growths in the intestines (polyps), and abnormal skin color over the lips and inside the cheeks. If blockage or bleeding occurs, the polyps may need to be removed.

Peyer's patches /pī′ərz/, groups of lymph nodes in the end of the small intestine (terminal ileum) near where it joins with the large intestine (colon). In some infections, as typhoid fever, they become open sores and can get swollen.

peyote /pā·ō′tē/, **1.** a cactus from which a hallucinogenic drug, mescaline, is made. **2.** mescaline.

Peyronie's disease /pārōnēz′/, a disease with a growth of fiberlike tissue on the erection tissue (corpora cavernosa) of the penis. The main symptom of Peyronie's disease is a painful erection. Treatment includes x-rays and adrenal hormone drugs. There is no known cure.

Pfizerpen-AS, a trademark for an antibiotic (penicillin G procaine).

PG, abbreviation for **prostaglandin.**

pH, a scale showing the levels of acid or alkaline in a solution. A value of 7.0 is neutral. Below 7.0 is acid. Above 7.0 is alkaline. See also **acid, acid-base balance.**

phacomalacia /fak′ōmələ′shə/, an abnormal condition of the eye in which the lens of the eye becomes soft, because of a soft milky covering (cataract).

phage. See **bacteriophage.**

-phage, -phag, a combining form meaning 'something that eats' a certain matter.

phagocyte /fag′əsīt/, a cell that is able to surround, eat, and digest small living things and cell wastes. **Fixed phagocytes** do not move in the blood. They include fixed cells and some connective tissue cells. **Free phagocytes** move in the blood and include white blood cells (leukocytes) and free cells. See also **macrophage. –phagocytic,** *adj.*

phagocytosis /fag′əsītō′sis/, the process by which some cells of the body, as cells that help the body fight bacteria, eat and get rid of small living things and cell wastes.

phakomatosis /fak′ōmətō′sis/, *pl.* **phakomatoses,** a group of inherited diseases marked by noncancerous tumorlike bumps (nodules) of the eye, skin, and brain. See also **cerebroretinal angiomatosis, encephalotrigeminal angiomatosis, neurofibromatosis, tuberous sclerosis.**

phalanx /fā′langks, *pl.* **phalanges** /fəlan′jēz/, any one of the narrowing bones making up the fingers of each hand and the toes of each foot. Each hand or foot had 14 phalanges. The fingers each have three phalanges. The thumb has two. The toes each have three phalanges. The great toe has two.

phallic stage, the period in mental and sexual growth between 3 and 6 years of age when awareness and playing with the genitals is the main source of pleasure. Not going beyond this stage may lead to very violent behavior in adulthood, or to other mental and sexual disorders. See also **psychosexual development.**

phallo-, phall-, a combining form meaning 'of or related to the penis.'

phalloidine /faloi′din/, a poison in the mushroom *Amanita phalloides*. Swallowing it results in bloody diarrhea, vomiting, severe stomach pain, kidney failure, and liver damage. About 50% of phalloidine poisonings are fatal. Also spelled **phalloidin.**

phantom, a mass of material like human tissue used to test the effects of radiation on human beings. Phantom materials can range from water to complex chemical mixtures.

phantom limb syndrome, a sense nerve feeling common after the removal of a limb. The patient has feeling in the missing limb. Some patients feel high levels of pain. See also **pseudesthesia.**

phantom tumor, an inflammation looking like a tumor, most often caused by muscles that contract or gas in the intestines.

pharmaceutic, referring to pharmacy or medical drugs.

pharmaco-, a combining form meaning 'of or related to drugs or medicine.'

pharmacokinetics /fär′məkōkinet′iks/, the study of the action of drugs in the body. It includes how the drug is used and gotten rid of, when it begins to act, and how long it acts. It also studies how the drug is changed into other things and what happens to its wastes.

pharmacology, the study of the making, ingredients, uses, and actions of drugs.

pharmacy, a place for making and giving out drugs.

pharyngeal reflex. See **gag reflex.**

pharyngeal tonsil, one of two masses of spongy lymph tissue on the back wall of the throat, behind the nasal space. During childhood these masses often swell with infected material and block air passing from the nose to the throat, preventing the child from breathing through the nose. Also called **adenoid.**

pharyngitis /fer′inji′tis/, a swelling or infection of the throat (pharynx), usually causing symptoms of a sore throat. Treatment depends on the cause, as in finding out whether the cause of the infection is a virus or a bacterium. Symptoms may be relieved by painkillers, drinking warm or cold liquids, or salt-water gargles. See also **strep throat.**

pharyngo-, pharyng-, a combining form meaning 'of or related to the throat (pharynx).'

pharyngoconjunctival fever /fəring′gōkon′-jungktī′vəl/, a virus infection with symptoms of fever, sore throat, and red eyes (conjunctivitis). The disease spreads quickly in warm weather. Infected water in lakes and swimming pools is a common cause of the infection. Also called **swimming pool conjunctivitis.** See also **adenovirus.**

pharynx /fer′inks/, the throat, a tubelike structure that extends from the base of the skull to the gullet (esophagus). It is just in front of the bones of the neck. It is a passage for both the breathing and digestive tracts. It also works in speech as it changes shape to allow one to form vowel sounds. The pharynx is made of muscle and is lined with mucous membrane. It is divided into three regions (nasopharynx, oropharynx, laryngopharynx). It contains the openings of the hearing (eustachian) tubes, nasal space (posterior nares), voice box (larynx), gullet (esophagus), and the tightening (fauces) between the mouth and the throat. It also contains the tonsils (palatine, pharyngeal, lingual). Also called **throat.** See also **laryngopharynx, larynx, nasopharynx, oropharynx.**

phase of maximum slope, the time during childbirth of rapid opening of the cervix and rapid lowering of the fetus. It occurs in the active phase of labor. See also **Friedman curve.**

-phasia, a combining form meaning a 'speech disorder.'

phenacemide /fənas′amīd/, an antiseizure drug given to treat severe epilepsy. It is used for mixed seizures that do not respond to other drugs.
★CAUTION: Pregnancy, behavior problems, or known allergy to this drug prohibits its use.
★ADVERSE EFFECTS: Among the more serious side effects are anemia, mental problems, and kidney and liver swelling.

phenacetin /fənas′itin/, a painkiller given to relieve pain and to lower fever.
★CAUTION: Known allergy to this drug prohibits its use. Repeated use should be avoided in anemia, heart, lung, liver, or kidney disease.
★ADVERSE EFFECTS: Among the more serious side effects are liver disease, fever, and skin rash.

Phenaphen, a trademark for a painkiller, antifever drug (acetaminophen).

phenazopyridine hydrochloride, a urinary tract painkiller given to relieve the pain of bladder swelling (cystitis) or other urinary tract infections.
★CAUTION: Kidney problems or known allergy to this drug prohibits its use.
★ADVERSE EFFECTS: Among the more serious side effects are headache and stomach and bowel problems.

phencyclidine hydrochloride (PCP) /fensī′klidēn/, a drug injected into a vein to put a patient to sleep for surgery. Because it can cause harmful hallucinations and other side effects, it is not used much in the United States.

phendimetrazine tartrate /fen′dīmet′rəsēn/, a drug given to lower the appetite in treating problems of being overweight caused by eating too much.
★CAUTION: Heart disease, high blood pressure, an overactive thyroid, sight problems (glaucoma), a history of drug abuse, use of nervous system-stimulating drugs, or monoamine oxidase inhibitors, or known allergy to this drug prohibits its use.

★ADVERSE EFFECTS: Among the more serious side effects are nervous system excitement, high blood pressure, an inability to sleep, dry mouth and addiction.

phenelzine sulfate, a monoamine oxidase (MAO) inhibitor given to treat depression.

pheniramine maleate /fənir'əmēn, -min/, an antihistamine given to treat many allergic reactions, including runny nose and skin rash.
★CAUTION: Asthma or known allergy to this drug prohibits its use. It is not given to newborn infants or nursing mothers.
★ADVERSE EFFECTS: Among the more serious side effects are drowsiness, skin rash, and allergic reactions. Dry mouth and rapid heart beat commonly occur.

phenmetrazine hydrochloride, a drug given to lower the appetite. It is used to treat an overweight condition caused by eating too much.
★CAUTION: Heart disease, high blood pressure, an overactive thyroid, sight problems (glaucoma), history of drug abuse, use of a nervous system-stimulating drug, or a monoamine oxidase (MAO) inhibitor, or known allergy to this or other drugs like it prohibits its use. It is not used for children under 12 years of age.
★ADVERSE EFFECTS: Among the most serious side effects are nervous system excitement, high blood pressure, an inability to sleep, and dry mouth.

phenobarbital, a barbiturate, antiseizure, and tranquilizing drug given to treat many seizure disorders and as a long-acting sleeping pill.

phenobarbital/phenytoin serum levels, the buildup of barbiturate (phenobarbital) and antiseizure drugs (phenytoin) in the blood. The levels are noted in patients who are likely to have seizures to keep the blood levels at a place where seizures will not occur, but not high enough to cause side effects. The effects of too-high a level of these drugs may include uncontrolled eye movements (nystagmus), loss of muscle control (ataxia), and tiredness.

phenocopy /fē'nōkop'ē/, a physical trait or condition caused by outside factors, but looks like a trait that is inherited. Conditions as deafness, mental retardation, and eye clouding (cataracts) can be inherited. They can also result from many other causes (for example, the rubella virus may cause inborn cataracts). Phenocopies may cause problems in helping people find out if they are likely to have children with birth defects. All such factors must be ruled out before any trait or defect found at birth can be labeled as inherited.

phenol /fē'nol/, a highly poisonous, harsh chemical taken from coal or plant tar or made in a laboratory. It has a strong odor and, as a fluid, is a strong cleaning fluid (carbolic acid).

phenol camphor, an oily mixture of camphor and phenol, used to sterilize things and to relieve toothache.

phenol coefficient, a measure of the cleaning action of a chemical as compared to carbolic acid. It is listed as the amount of the chemical that kills bacteria in 10 minutes, but not in 5 minutes, compared to a watering down of 1 part in 90 of carbolic acid that kills in the same time.

phenolphthalein /fē'nolthal'ē·in, -tha'lēn/, a laxative that acts by starting the motor nerve action of the lower intestines.

phenolphthalein laxative, a laxative that acts on the wall of the bowel. It is given to treat long-term constipation and to prevent straining. It is given to patients recovering from surgery and those with heart disease or high blood pressure.
★CAUTION: Symptoms of appendicitis, other stomach or bowel conditions that need surgery, or known allergy to this drug prohibits its use.
★ADVERSE EFFECTS: Among the most serious side effects are stomach and bowel pain, allergic reaction, dehydration, and laxative addiction.

phenol poisoning, harsh poisoning caused by swallowing compounds with phenol, as carbolic acid, creosote, and naphthol. Phenol poisoning causes burns of the mouth, seizures, and failure of all major systems. The skin around the mouth and nose should be washed, as well as any burns on the skin. The mouth, throat, gullet (esophagus), and stomach are flushed with water and charcoal. Oxygen, fluids given in the vein and painkillers may be needed. Narrowing (stricture) of the esophagus can happen because of a high level of tissue damage.

phenolsulfonphthalein, a dye to test the working of the kidneys. The test is done by measuring urine levels at regular periods after injecting a small amount of the dye.

phenomenon, a sign that is often linked to an illness or condition and is important in diagnosing something.

phenothiazine tranquilizers, any of a group of drugs used to treat mental problems, as an antihistamine to control vomiting and to put a patient to sleep before surgery. The most widely used drugs are chlorpromazine and prochlorperazine. These drugs have changed the way the mentally ill are treated, because they act on many organ systems of the body at once. All phenothiazine tranquilizers are not given to patients with severe nervous system problems or epilepsy. They are given with caution to those with liver disease. These drugs are not used in pregnancy. See also specific drugs.

phenotype, **1.** the traits of an individual or group one can see. They are caused by the interactions of family history and the outside world. **2.** a group of organisms that look like each other. Compare **genotype.** –**phenotypic,** *adj.*

phenoxybenzamine hydrochloride, a blood pressure drug given to control high blood pressure and sweating when a patient has adrenal tumors (pheochromocytoma).
★CAUTION: Low blood pressure or known allergy to this drug prohibits its use.
★ADVERSE EFFECTS: Among the more serious side effects are very low blood pressure and rapid heart beats.

phenprocoumon /fen'prōkoōmən/, a drug used to fight and prevent blood clotting and other blood problems.

phensuximide, an antiseizure drug given to prevent and treat seizures in petit mal epilepsy.
★CAUTION: Known allergy to this or a related drug prohibits its use.
★ADVERSE EFFECTS: Among the most serious side effects are blood disorders and kidney damage with blood in the urine.

phentermine hydrochloride /fen'tərmēn/, a drug given to lower the appetite to treat an overweight condition caused by eating too much.
★CAUTION: Hardening of the arteries, heart disease, high blood pressure, sight problems (glaucoma), overactive thyroid, or known allergy to this or other drugs like it prohibits its use.
★ADVERSE EFFECTS: Among the more serious side effects are an inability to sleep, rapid heart beat, and high blood pressure.

Phenurone, a trademark for an antiseizure drug (phenacemide).

phenylalanine (Phe) /fen'ilal'ənēn/, an amino acid needed for the normal growth of infants and children. It is also needed for normal protein use all through life. It is found in large amounts in milk, eggs, and other common foods. See also **amino acid, phenylketonuria, protein.**

phenylalaninemia /fen'ilaləninē'mē·ə/, the phenylalanine in the blood. See also **hyperphenylalaninemia.**

phenylbutazone, a nonsteroid anti-inflammatory drug given to treat severe symptoms of arthritis, bursitis, and other swelling conditions.

phenylephrine hydrochloride, a nervous system drug given to keep the blood pressure at a set level. It is also used in the nose and eyes to narrow blood vessels.
★CAUTION: Sight problems (narrow-angle glaucoma), use of monoamine oxidase inhibitors, or known allergy to this drug prohibits its use.
★ADVERSE EFFECTS: Among the more serious side effects are heart problems and a high rise in blood pressure. Allergic reactions may also occur.

phenylethyl alcohol, a colorless, pleasant smelling liquid with a burning taste. It is used to fight bacteria and to preserve drugs. Also called **benzyl carbonol.**

phenylketonuria (PKU) /fen'əlkē'tōnyoŏr'ē·ə, fē'nəl-/, a birth defect in which an enzyme needed to change an amino acid (phenylalanine) in the body into another substance (tyrosine) is lacking. Buildup of phenylalanine is poisonous to brain tissue. Signs include skin rashes (eczema), a mousy odor of the urine and skin, and mental retardation. Treatment is a diet free of phenylalanine. Phenylketonuria occurs about once in 16,000 births in the United States. Most states demand a screening test for all newborns. See also **Guthrie test, phenylpyruvic acid, tyrosine. –phenylketonuric,** *adj.*

phenylpropanolamine hydrochloride /fen'əlprō'pənol'əmēn/, a blood vessel-narrowing drug given to relieve a stuffy nose and other cold symptoms.
★CAUTION: High blood pressure, heart artery disease, simultaneous use of monoamine oxidase inhibitors, or known allergy to this drug prohibits its use.
★ADVERSE EFFECTS: Among the more serious side effects are nervousness, an inability to sleep, loss of appetite, and high blood pressure.

phenylpyruvic acid /fen'ilpīroō'vik/, a product of the breakdown of an amino acid (phenylalanine). Its presence in the urine is a sign of phenylketonuria.

phenyltoloxamine citrate /fen'iltəlok'səmēn, fē'nil-/, an antihistamine most often used in a drug with a painkiller.

phenytoin /fen'ətō'in/, an antiseizure drug given to treat grand mal and motor seizures and to control the heart rhythm.
★CAUTION: Known allergy to this drug or to related drugs prohibits its use. It is used with caution in patients with liver or blood problems and some heart disorders.
★ADVERSE EFFECTS: Among the more serious side effects are loss of muscle control, uncontrolled eye movements, and allergic reactions. This drug interacts with many other drugs.

pheochromocytoma /fē'ōkrō'mōsītō'mə/, *pl.* **pheochromocytomas, pheochromocytomata,** a tumor of the adrenal gland that causes too-much release of two hormones (epinephrine and norepinephrine). Signs include high blood pressure, headache, sweating, excess blood sugar, nausea, vomiting, and fainting spells. There may be weight loss and many heart problems. The tumor occurs most often in young people. Only a small number of the tumors are cancerous. Removal is the best treatment. Patients may also be treated with a drug that lowers levels of norepinephrine.

pheromone /fer'əmōn'/, a hormone substance released by a living thing that gets a response from another, most often of the opposite sex. Most pheromones have a strong odor.

-phily, a combining form meaning a 'fondness or a desire for something.'

phimosis /fimō'sis/, tightness of the foreskin (prepuce) of the penis that will not allow the foreskin to be pulled back. It may be the result of infection. Removing the foreskin (circumcision) is the usual treatment. Compare **paraphimosis.**

phimosis vaginalis /vaj'inā'lis/, an inherited narrowness or closing of the opening of the vagina.

phi phenomenon, a feeling of motion that is caused by lights that flash on and off at a certain rate. Also called **stroboscopic illusion.**

pHisoHex, a trademark for a cleanser with an anti-infective drug (hexachlorophene) used mainly before surgery. It should not be used for bathing infants.

phlebitis. See **thrombophlebitis.**

phlebo-, phleb-, a combining form meaning 'of or related to a vein or veins.'

phlebograph /fleb'əgraf'/, a device for making an x-ray or other graph record of the pulse.

phlebothrombosis /fleb'ōthrombō'sis/, an abnormal blood problem in which a clot forms in a vein. It is most often caused by poor blood flow, a blocked vein, or blood that clots faster than normal. In contrast to thrombophlebitis, the wall of the vein is not swollen. See also **thrombophlebitis.**

phlebotomus fever, a mild infection, caused by a virus carried to humans by the bite of an infected sandfly. Symptoms include fever, headache, eye pain, swelling, muscle pain, and a rash. Swollen spinal membranes (meningitis) may also occur. The disease is widespread in hot, dry areas where sandflies are common, as in Latin America. Bed rest, fluids, and aspirin are ordered. A second attack may occur a few weeks after the first. Also called **pappataci, sandfly fever, three-day fever.**

phlebotomy /fləbot'əmē/, entry into a vein to release blood, as in getting blood from a donor. It is done to treat an excess of red blood cells (polycythemia vera) and may be done every 6 months, or more often if needed. It is sometimes used to treat excess fluid in the lungs (pulmonary edema). Also called **venesection.**

phlegm /flem/, thick mucus released by the tissues lining the breathing passages.

phlegmasia alba dolens, a disorder of the vein of the upper leg (femoral), resulting in swelling and pain. It may occur after a severe fever illness or childbirth.

phlegmasia cerulea dolens, a severe form of blood clotting in a deep vein, most often the vein of the upper leg (femoral). It is sudden, strong, and has along with it swelling and loss of normal color in the leg beyond the blockage.

phlegmonous gastritis, a severe form of stomach inflammation (gastritis). It involves tissue of the stomach wall. It occurs as a result of an infection, peptic ulcer, cancer, surgery, or severe stress. It is an emergency. Treatment includes surgery, antibiotics, and painkillers.

phlyctenular keratoconjunctivitis, an inflammation of the cornea in the eye. Tiny bumpy sores occur from allergic material in bacteria or parasites. It is seen most often in children. A lack of vitamins may be a factor. The condition is treated with hormone drugs, but scars may remain on the eye. Also called **phlyctenulosis, scrofulous keratitis.** See also **eczematous conjunctivitis.**

-phobe, -phobiac, -phobist, a combining form meaning 'one who fears' something specific.

phobia /fō'bē·ə/, an anxiety problem with an overwhelming and irrational fear of a specific object. Examples include animals, an activity (as leaving home), or a physical situation (as heights). The patient may faint, have a racing heart rate, sweat, have nausea, and feelings of panic. The fear, which is not realistic, often results from something unpleasant in the past. The strong need to avoid the feared object or situation can alter regular behavior, which can result in changes in life patterns and interactions with others. Although the cause may be known, the patient feels unable to overcome the fear. Treatment is behavior treatment to reduce the anxiety. Some kinds of phobias are **agoraphobia, claustrophobia, photophobia.** Also called **phobic disorder, phobic neurosis, phobic reaction.** Compare **compulsion.** See also **simple phobia, social phobia.** –**phobiac,** *n.,* **phobic,** *adj.*

phobiac /fō'bē·ak'/, a person who has a phobia.

phocomelia /fō'kəmē'lē·ə/, a birth defect in which the upper part of one or more of the arms or legs is missing. The feet or hands or both are joined to the body by short, distorted stumps. it is seen as a side effect of a drug (thalidomide) taken during early pregnancy. Also called **seal limbs.** Compare **amelia.** –**phocomelic,** *adj.*

phocomelic dwarf, a dwarf in whom the long bones of any or all of the arms and legs are very short.

phonation, the production of speech sounds through vibration of the vocal folds.

-phone, a combining form meaning a 'device for hearing sounds.'

phonic, referring to voice, sounds, or speech.

phonocardiograph, a device that makes heart sound recordings. It is used to diagnose heart disorders. Two microphones are placed on the chest, one near the base of the heart, and the other over the top of the heart. The microphone placed over the base of the heart records the second heart sound (a short, sharp "dup") and the loudest murmurs. The microphone placed over the top of the heart records the sounds that may mean heart failure (atrial and ventricular gallops), as well as valve defect sounds. See also **gallop.** **–phonocardiographic,** *adj.*

phonology /fōnol'əjē/, the study of speech sounds, especially rules governing the way speech sounds are used in a given language.

phonophoresis /fō'nōfərē'sis/, a technique in which ultrasound waves are used to force medicines beneath the skin. Use for up to 10 minutes can drive a drug applied to the skin surface about 5 cm into muscle tissue. Drugs given by this method include hydrocortisone, aspirin, and lidocaine. Because the patient may be allergic to the medication, the technique is used with caution.

phosphatase /fos'fətāz/, an enzyme that starts chemical reactions with phosphorus. See also **catalyst, enzyme, phosphorus.**

phosphate, a salt of phosphoric acid. Phosphates are very important in living cells in storing and using energy. They also help carry genetic data within a cell and from one cell to another. See also **adenosine diphosphate, adenosine triphosphate, phosphoric acid.**

Phospholine Iodide, a trademark for an eye drug (echothiophate iodide).

phospholipid /fos'fōlip'id/, one of a class of chemical compounds, widely found in living cells. It contains phosphoric acid, fatty acids, and nitrogen. Two kinds of phospholipids are **lecithin, sphingomyelin.**

phosphoric acid, a clear, odorless liquid that is irritating to the skin and eyes and somewhat poisonous if swallowed. It is used in fertilizers, soaps, animal feeds, and some drugs.

phosphorus (P), a nonmetal chemical element. It is needed to digest protein, calcium compounds, and glucose. The body uses phosphorus in forms that are taken from milk, cheese, meat, egg yolk, whole grains, peas, and nuts. A lack of phosphorus can cause weight loss, anemia, and abnormal growth. Phosphorus is needed to make ATP (adenosine triphosphate), a major source of body energy, and for the breakdowns of sugar (glycolysis).

phosphorus poisoning, a condition caused by swallowing white or yellow phosphorus, sometimes found in rat poisons, fertilizers, and fireworks. Symptoms include nausea, throat and stomach pain, vomiting, diarrhea, and an odor of garlic on the breath. After a few days of seeming recovery, symptoms return with kidney and liver problems. Treatment includes flushing water through the stomach and giving mineral oil, vitamin K, fluids through the veins, and drugs to fight shock. One should not come into contact with the vomit and feces of the patient.

photo-, phot-, a combining form referring to light.

photoallergic, showing a delayed allergic reaction after being exposed to light. See also **photosensitive, phototoxic.**

photoallergic contact dermatitis, a skin reaction that occurs 24 to 48 hours after being exposed to light in a person who is put at risk by drugs or chemicals. The substance (photosensitizer) builds up in the skin and is changed to active allergic material by light. Avoiding both the substance and sunlight at the same time prevents the reaction. Treatment is the same as that for any other swelling of the skin. See also **photosensitizer.**

photochemotherapy, a kind of chemical treatment in which the effect of a drug is made stronger by exposing the patient to light. See also **chemotherapy.**

photophobia /fō'tō-/, **1.** abnormal reaction to light, as by the eyes. It occurs in albinos and many diseases that affect the eye membrane (conjunctiva) and cornea, as measles. **2.** an anxiety disorder marked by an unreal fear of light with a need to avoid light places. It is seen more often in women than in men and is most often caused by a conflict that has been ignored. Treatment is mental treatment to uncover the cause of the light phobia, followed by behavior treatment. **–photophobic,** *adj.*

photoscan, an x-ray picture that shows the spread of a radioactive drug in the body.

photosensitive, referring to a strong reaction of skin to sunlight often caused by certain drugs. A brief exposure to sunlight or to an ultraviolet lamp may cause swelling, pimples, hives, or acute burns in patients who are photosensitive. Treatment is to avoid sunlight or the drug causing the reaction. See also **photoallergic, photosensitizer, phototoxic.**

photosensitizer, anything that may cause an allergic reaction, as in the skin, when combined with light. Common photosensitizers are antibiotics (sulfanilamide), antiseptics (hexachlorophene), some birth-control pills, tranquilizers (phenothiazene), and a substance (psoralen) found in many plants, as carrots and mustard.

photosynthesis /fōtōsin'thəsis/, a process by which plants with green coloring (chlorophyll) make chemicals, mainly carbohydrates, from carbon dioxide and water. They use light for energy and to release oxygen.

phototherapy, to treat disorders by using light, as ultraviolet light. Ultraviolet light may be used to treat acne, bed sores, and other skin disorders. See also **photochemotherapy. –phototherapeutic,** *adj.*

phototherapy in the newborn, a treatment for a bile coloring disorder (hyperbilirubinemia) that causes yellowing (jaundice) in the skin of the newborn. The infant's bare skin, with eyes and sex organs covered, is exposed to a strong fluorescent light. The bluish light speeds up the release of the bile coloring (bilirubin) in the skin. The baby is turned often. The body temperature, heart, lungs, and blood pressure are closely checked. A side effect of phototherapy is fluid loss. An infant may need 25% more fluid during treatment. Excess bilirubin and skin yellowing (jaundice) that result from a blood cell disease or infection may be controlled with phototherapy. The real cause of the disease is treated separately. Recovery is usually complete.

phototoxic, showing a quickly growing reaction of the skin when it is exposed to a substance that causes the reaction (photosensitizer) and light. See also **photoallergic, photosensitive, photosensitizer.**

phototoxic contact dermatitis, sunburnlike response of skin that has been exposed to the sun after contact with something that puts the skin at risk. The skin may turn dark after the first reaction. Treatment is skin creams and lotions. See also **photosensitizer.**

-phrasia, a combining form meaning an 'abnormal condition of speech.'

-phrenia, a combining form meaning a 'disordered condition of mental action.'

phrenic /fren'ik/, **1.** referring to the diaphragm. **2.** referring to the mind.

phrenic nerve, one of a pair of branches of the fourth neck (cervical) nerve. It is known as the motor nerve to the diaphragm that helps to move it in breathing. Also called **internal respiratory nerve of Bell.** Compare **accessory phrenic nerve.**

Phthirus /thī'rəs/, a group of lice that suck blood, as the pubic or crab louse.

phycomycosis /fī'kōmīkō'sis/, a fungus infection. The fungi that cause the illness are common in the soil and are not often harmful. Severe infection in the lungs sometimes occurs with late diabetes mellitus that is untreated or out of control. See also **mucormycosis, zygomycosis.**

phylloquinone. See **vitamin K.**

phylogeny /filoj'ənē/, the growth of the structure of a race or species as it changed from simpler forms of life. Compare **ontogeny.** See also **comparative anatomy.**

physiatrist /fizē·at'rist/ a physician who works in physical medicine, treating conditions that require rehabilitation, as amputated limbs.

-physical, a combining form meaning 'natural.'

physical abuse, one or more times of forceful behavior that result in physical injury. It may cause damage to inner organs, sense organs, the nervous system, or the muscle and skeleton system of another person.

physical allergy, an allergic response to physical things, as cold, heat, light, or injury. Foreign material (antibodies) are commonly found in patients with physical allergies. Symptoms are itching, hives, and swelling beneath the skin (angioedema). The cause may be some cosmetics or drugs. Attempting to remove the cause may prevent the reaction. Treatment is antihistamines or other drugs. Compare **contact dermatitis.** See also **atopic.**

physical examination, a test of the body to find out its state of health, using any or all of the means of testing. The physical examination, medical history, and first laboratory tests are the basis on which a diagnosis is made and on which treatment is decided.

physical fitness, the ability to carry out daily tasks normally, without becoming too tired, and with enough energy left to meet emergencies or to enjoy leisure activities.

physical medicine, using physical therapy to return diseased or injured patients to a useful life. See also **rehabilitation.**

physical therapist, a person who is licensed to assist in testing and treating physically disabled patients. The physical therapist uses special exercise, applies heat or cold, uses sound waves, and other means.

physical therapy, the treatment of disorders with physical agents and methods. Some types are massage, moving muscles and bones, exercises, cold, heat, and light. They are done to assist in treating patients and in bringing back normal function after an illness or injury. Also called **physiotherapy.**

physician, 1. a health-care worker who has earned a degree of Doctor of Medicine (M.D.) after an approved course of study at an approved medical school. An M.D. most often enters a hospital internship program for 1 year of training after getting the degree before beginning practice or further training in a specialty. To practice medicine, an M.D. has to get a license from the state in which the services will be done. **2.** a health-care worker who has earned a degree of Doctor of Osteopathy (D.O.) by completing a course of study at an approved college of osteopathy. Osteopathic physicians and medical physicians follow nearly the same courses of training and practice. Osteopathic medicine places special stress on the physical defects of tissues as a cause of illness and on treatment that is moving body structures.

physician extender, a health-care worker who is not a physician but who does certain medical actions also done by a physician.

physician's assistant (PA), a person trained to assist a physician. A physician directs and oversees the physician's assistant. Some physician's assistants practice specific kinds of medicine, as helping during surgery, blood filtering (dialysis), or x-ray tests. Also called **physician's associate.**

physics, the study of the laws and effects of matter and energy, as related to motion and force.

physiologic contracture, a short-term condition in which muscles may contract and shorten.

Drugs, very high or low temperature, and buildup of lactic acid in the muscle are causes. Compare **functional contracture.**

physiologic dwarf. See **primordial dwarf.**

physiologic hypertrophy, an increase in the size of an organ or tissue because of a short-term change in normal body functions, as occurs in the walls of the uterus and in the breasts during pregnancy.

physiologic motivation, a body need, as food or water, that makes a person want to satisfy it. Also called **organic motivation.** Compare **achievement motivation, social motivation.**

physiologic occlusion, a closing of the teeth that allows a person to chew food more normally.

physiologic retraction ring, a ridge around the inside of the uterus that forms during the second stage of normal labor. It results from the lengthening of the muscle fibers of the lower part of the uterus and shortening of the muscle fibers of the upper part. The ridge grows between the two parts. Compare **constriction ring, pathologic retraction ring.**

physiologic third heart sound, a low-pitched extra heart sound heard early in heart muscle relaxation (diastole) in a healthy child or young adult. It is not important and most often goes away with age. The same sound, heard in an older person with heart disease, is abnormal and called a ventricular gallop. See also **gallop.**

physiology, 1. the study of the processes and workings of the human body. **2.** the study of the physical and chemical processes used in the working of living things and the parts that make them up. Compare **anatomy.**

physiotherapy. See **physical therapy.**

physostigmine salicylate, a drug given to treat nervous system side effects caused by drugs able to block normal nerve signals.
★CAUTION: Asthma, gangrene, diabetes, heart and blood vessel disease, or blocked intestines or urinary tract prohibits its use. It is not given to patients taking some nerve muscle-blocking drugs.
★ADVERSE EFFECTS: Among the most serious side effects are excess saliva, slow heart beat, seizures, and high blood pressure.

phytanic acid storage disease. See **Refsum's syndrome.**

phyto-, a combining form referring to plants.

phytohemagglutinin (PHA), a substance taken from a plant that causes red blood cells to clump together. An example is lectin from the red kidney bean. Also called **phytolectin.**

phytohemagglutinin test, a test to find persons who are carriers of cystic fibrosis. It is done by exposing white blood cells to a plant antibody (phytohemagglutinin). A normal reaction makes more cell protein. See also **cystic fibrosis.**

phytonadione. See **vitamin K₁.**

P.I., abbreviation in medical records for *present illness.*

pia mater /pē'ə mā'tər/, the most inner of the three membranes (meninges) covering the brain and the spinal cord. It carries a rich supply of blood vessels, which serve the nervous tissue. The cranial pia mater covers the surface of the brain dipping deeply into the many grooves. The spinal pia mater is thicker, firmer, and carries fewer blood vessels. Compare **arachnoid, dura mater.**

pian. See **yaws.**

pica /pī'kə/, a craving to eat things that are not foods, as dirt, clay, chalk, glue, ice, starch, or hair. It may occur with poor diet, with pregnancy, and in some forms of mental illness.

Pick's disease, a mental disorder that occurs in middle age. Affecting mainly the front part of the brain, it causes neurotic behavior, slow changes in personality, emotions, and abilities, as reasoning and judgment. See also **dementia.**

pickwickian syndrome, an abnormal condition with being overweight, breathing difficulty, tiredness, and excess red blood cells.

picornavirus /pīkôr'nəvī'rəs/, one of a group of small viruses (RNA) that cause polio, throat infections, brain swelling (meningitis), and other diseases. See also **virus.**

picrotoxin /pik'rōtok'sin/, a powerful nervous system-stimulating drug taken from the seeds of a Southeast Asian fruit, (*Anamirta cocculus*). It was used in the past to treat breathing problems caused by an overdose of barbiturate drugs.

PID, abbreviation for **pelvic inflammatory disease.**

P.I.E., abbreviation for *pulmonary infiltrate with eosinophilia,* an allergic reaction. Signs are invasion of the air sacs (alveoli) of the lungs with white blood cells and fluid, leading to lung swelling. It may be caused by parasite infections and by some drugs, as sulfonamides. One form of the illness, with fever, night sweats, cough, breathing difficulty, and weight loss, occurs in some drug allergies and bacteria, fungus, and parasite infections. A tropical form of the disease, with strong asthma attacks at night, is linked to a worm infection. See also **Löffler's syndrome.**

piebald /pī'bôld/, having patches of white hair or skin because of a lack of color-forming of pigment cells (melanocytes) in those areas. It is inherited. Compare **albinism, vitiligo.**

Pierre Robin's syndrome, a group of birth defects occurring together that includes a small lower jaw, cleft lip and cleft palate, and defects of the eyes and ears. Intelligence is most often normal. Plastic surgery may repair the defects, but speech or dental treatments and counseling are often needed.

pigeon breast, a birth defect with a breastbone that pushes out. It may cause heart and lung problems that sometimes need surgery. **–pigeon-breasted,** *adj.*

pigeon breeder's lung, a breathing disorder caused by allergic material in bird droppings. Also called **bird breeder's lung, hen worker's lung.**

pigment, 1. any organic coloring material made by the body tissues, as melanin. 2. any paintlike drug applied to skin surfaces. **–pigmentary, pigmented,** *adj.,* **pigmentation,** *n.*

pigmy. See **pygmy.**

pilar cyst. See **wen.**

piles. See **hemorrhoids.**

pill, a rounded or oval-shaped drug to be swallowed whole.

pilo-, a combining form meaning 'looking like or related to hair.'

pilomotor reflex /pī′lōmō′tər/, erection of the hairs of the skin in response to cold, emotion, or irritation of the skin. This normal reaction is lost below the level of some spinal cord injuries and may be too strong on the affected side in a patient with one-sided paralysis (hemiplegia). Also called **gooseflesh, horripilation, piloerection.**

pilonidal cyst /pī′lənī′dəl/, a hairy lump (cyst) that often grows in the skin of the lower back. The cysts may be noted at birth by a pushed-in space, sometimes a hairy dimple, in the middle of the back. These cysts most often do not cause any problems, but sometimes a space or tubelike hole (fistula) grows with an opening to the skin surface. This causes an infection. A fistula may also grow in the spinal tract from a cyst. If a cyst becomes infected, it is removed, and the space is closed after the infection has been treated.

pilonidal fistula, an abnormal channel with a tuft of hair, over or close to the tip of the tailbone (coccyx), but also occurring in other parts of the body. Also called **pilonidal sinus.**

pilosebaceous /pī′lōsibā′shəs/, referring to a hair sac (follicle) and its oil gland.

pilus /pē′ləs/, *pl.* **pili,** a hair or hairlike structure. Pili are used by some bacteria to join to human tissues while starting an infection.

Pima, a trademark for a cough syrup (potassium iodide).

pimaricin. See **natamycin.**

pimple, a small swelling of the skin, often an infection of a pore. See also **acne, furuncle, papule, pustule.**

pin, 1. to secure and hold fragments of bone with a nail in surgery. 2. a small metal rod or peg, used by dentists as a support in rebuilding a tooth.

pin-and-tube fixed orthodontic appliance, a dental device for correcting crooked teeth (malocclusion). It has a wire arch with posts that go into tubes joined to bands on the teeth.

pineal gland, a cone-shaped structure in the brain. No one knows exactly what it does. It may release a hormone (melatonin), which appears to stop the release of another (luteinizing) hormone. Also called **epiphysis cerebri, pineal body.** See also **luteinizing hormone.**

pineal hyperplasia syndrome, an abnormal condition caused by overgrowth of the pineal gland. It is marked by lack of response to insulin, dry skin, thick nails, hairiness, early tooth development, and premature sexual development. Although the teeth develop early, they are abnormally formed. External sex organs may reach adult size by the age of 4 years. Excessive amounts of acid and ketones in the blood (ketoacidosis) may develop even if the body produces high levels of insulin. Similar problems occur with some pineal tumors.

pinealoma /pin′ē-əlō′mə/, *pl.* **pinealomas, pinealomata,** a tumor of the pineal gland in the brain. It may result in fluid buildup in the brain (hydrocephalus), and disorders in walking. Early puberty occurs in some cases. Also called **pinealocytoma.**

pindolol, a drug given alone or with a fluid-releasing (diuretic) drug to treat high blood pressure.
★CAUTION: Asthma or heart disorders prohibits its use. It must be used with caution in patients with diabetes.
★ADVERSE EFFECTS: Among the most serious side effects are slow or rapid heart beat, low blood pressure, fainting, and stomach and bowel problems.

pine tar, a common part of creams, soaps, and lotions used to treat long-term skin conditions, as eczema or psoriasis.

ping-ponging, *slang.* an illegal practice in which a patient is passed from one physician to another so that a health program or service can charge someone else for many unneeded tests.

pinhole test, a simple eye test done in testing a person who has failing eyesight to find a lens defect (refractive error) caused by a disease. A refractive error may be corrected with glasses and is not dangerous. Loss of good vision from a disease is serious. It may mean a nervous system disease and blindness that could have been avoided. For the test, many pinholes are punched in a card, and the patient selects one and looks through it with one eye at a time, without wearing glasses. If sight is better, the defect is refractive; if not, it is physical. The pinhole effect results from blocking light waves from the side, those most distorted by refractive error.

Pinkus' disease. See **lichen nitidus.**

pinna. See **auricle.**

pinocytosis /pī′nōsītō′sis/, the process by which fluid is taken into a cell. The cell membrane develops a pouchlike space, fills with fluid from outside the cell, then closes around it, forming a tiny pond of fluid in the cell.

pinta, an infection of the skin in Latin America carried by flies or other insects. The bacterium enters the body through a break in the skin. A first tumor and the nearby lymph nodes slowly swell, followed in 1 to 12 months by a general red to slate-blue rash. Over time these tumors lose their color. The disease often results in a long-term discoloration of the skin. Treatment with penicillin G is useful. Also called **azula, carate, mal del pinto.** Compare **yaws.**

pin track infection, a condition in which treatment with traction is made more difficult by an infection of soft tissues or of bone (osteomyelitis). The infections may develop at traction pin sites. Signs of pin track infection are redness at the pin sites, pus draining and odor, pins slipping, high body temperature, and pain. A minor infection at the pin site is treated with antibiotics. Deeper infection at the pin sites more often means the pins need to be removed, and antibiotics given.

pinworm. See *Enterobius vermicularis.*

pions /pī'onz/, a kind of particle that can be made in nuclear reactions and used in some types of treatment. In treating brain tumors, pions can be made to go into the skull, save normal tissue, and give most of their energy to the tumor.

Pipracel, a trademark for an antibiotic (piperacillin).

piriformis /pir'ifôr'mis/, a flat, pyramid-shaped muscle lying partly in the pelvis and partly at the back of the hip joint. The piriformis moves the thigh and helps to extend it.

Pirquet test /pirkā'/, a skin test for tuberculosis infection. It is done by scratching the tuberculin material onto the skin. Also called **von Pirquet test.** See also **tuberculin test.**

pit and fissure cavity, a space that starts in tiny faults in tooth enamel, most often on the facing surfaces of molars and premolars.

Pitocin, a trademark for a uterus stimulating drug (oxytocin).

Pitressin, a trademark for a fluid gathering hormone drug (vasopressin).

pitting, 1. small, puncturelike dents in fingernails or toenails, often a result of a skin disorder (psoriasis). 2. a pushed-in space that remains for a short time after pressing fluid-swollen skin with a finger. 3. small, pushed-in scars in the skin or other organ of the body. 4. the removal by the spleen of material from within red blood cells without damage to the cells.

pituicyte, a cell of the pituitary gland.

pituitary adamantinoma. See **craniopharyngioma.**

pituitary cachexia. See **postpubertal panhypopituitarism.**

pituitary dwarf /pitoo'iter'ē/, a dwarf whose slowed growth is caused by a lack of growth hormone. It results from a defect of part of the pituitary gland, but in most cases the exact cause is unknown. The defect is mostly limited to a lack of the growth hormone (somatotropin), although other hormones may also be lacking. The body is normally shaped, with no face or skeleton defects, and there is normal mental and sexual growth. It is usually found in childhood. Also called **hypophyseal dwarf, Lévi-Lorain dwarf, Paltauf's dwarf.**

pituitary gland, the small gland joined to a gland (hypothalamus) at the base of the brain. It supplies many hormones that control many needed processes of the body. The pituitary is divided into a front lobe (adenohypophysis) and a smaller back lobe (neurohypophysis). The pituitary gland is larger in a woman than in a man and becomes larger during pregnancy. Also called **hypophysis cerebri.** See also **adenohypophysis, neurohypophysis.**

pituitary nanism, a type of dwarfism linked to another form of dwarfism (pituitary infantilism). See also **pituitary dwarf.**

pituitary stalk, a structure that connects the pituitary gland with another gland (hypothalamus) at the base of the brain.

pit viper, any one of a family of poisonous snakes found in the Western Hemisphere and Asia. Except for coral snakes, all poisonous snakes naturally found in the United States are pit vipers. See also **copperhead, cottonmouth, rattlesnake.**

pityriasis alba /pitərī'əsis/, a common skin disease mark by round or oval, finely scaling patches without skin color (pigment), usually on the cheeks. The itching sores are easy to spot and occur mostly in children and adolescents. Clearing of the sores is the usual outcome, but the condition may return. Treatment includes special creams.

pityriasis rosea, a skin disease in which a slightly scaling, pink rash spreads over unexposed parts of the body. The **herald patch,** a large, more scaly sore appears before the pink rash by several days. The smaller sores tend to follow the normal crease lines of the skin. Mild itching is the only symptom. The disease lasts 4 to 8 weeks and rarely returns.

pivot joint, a joint in which movement is limited by the joint to moving back and forth. The joint is formed by a pivotlike structure that may turn within a ring made partly of bone and of ligament. The elbow is a pivot joint. Also called **trochoid joint.** See also **synovial joint.**

PKU, abbreviation for **phenylketonuria.**

placebo /pləsē'bō/, an inactive substance given as if it were a real dose of a needed drug. The substance may be a salt-water solution, distilled water, or sugar, or a less-than-effective dose of a harmless substance, as a vitamin that dissolves in water. Placebos are used in drug studies to compare the effects of the inactive substance with those of an experimental drug. They are also given for patients who cannot be given a drug they may want or who do not need that drug. Placebo treatment is useful in some cases, and side effects often occur as they would from the actual drug. The benefit to the patient of a placebo may sometimes outweigh the ethical, moral, and legal problems raised by giving it.

placebo effect, a physical or emotional change occurring after a substance is taken that is not the result of any special effect of the substance. The change may be for the better, meeting the results the patient expects.

placement path, the direction of placing and removing a denture on its supporting structures.

placenta, a blood-rich structure through which the fetus takes in oxygen, food, and other substances and gets rid of carbon dioxide and other wastes. The placenta begins to form on about the eighth day of pregnancy when the first cells of the forming embryo (blastocyst) invades the wall of the uterus and becomes joined to it. The ball of cells is able to take in cells of the lining of the uterus, causing a small breakdown on the wall of the uterus in which an embryo buries itself. Because of high amounts of a hormone (progesterone) released by the ovary, the embryo and the placenta continue to grow. The embryo cell layer continues to invade the mother's tissues with fingerlike bumps (chorionic villi). Separating the villi are lakes of blood in the wasted wall of the uterus. The mother's blood flows into the lakes surrounding the villi, allowing food, gases, and other substances to pass into the fetal blood flow. The placenta is able to release large amounts of progesterone by the third month of pregnancy, enough to relieve the corpus luteum of that duty. At the end of pregnancy, the normal placenta weighs one-seventh to one-fifth of the weight of the infant. The mother's surface has a dark red, rough, liverlike look. The fetal surface is smooth and shiny. Large blood vessels fan out under the membranes from the umbilical cord. The time between the birth of the infant and the release of the placenta is the third and last stage of labor.

-placenta, a combining form meaning an 'organ shaped like a flat cake.'

placenta accreta, a placenta that invades the uterine muscle, making separation from the muscle difficult.

placenta battledore, a condition in which the umbilical cord is in the margin or edge of the placenta, instead of the normal central place.

placental dystocia, a prolonged or otherwise difficult delivery of the afterbirth (placenta). See also **dystocia.**

placental infarct, a bloodless, hard area on the fetus' or mother's side of the placenta.

placental hormone, one of the several hormones made by the placenta. See also **chorionic gonadotropin, estrogen, human placental lactogen, progesterone.**

placental insufficiency, an abnormal condition of pregnancy, marked by slowed growth of the fetus and uterus. Among defects that can result in placental insufficiency are defects of the placental membranes or of the umbilical cord, abnormal joining (implantation) of the placenta, and multiple pregnancy. Breaks in the placental membrane that cause fetal bleeding into the mother's blood flow may also occur. Also called **placental dysfunction.** See also **intrauterine growth retardation, postmature infant.**

placenta previa, a condition in which the placenta is buried abnormally in the uterus so that it partly or completely covers the opening of the cervix. It is the most common cause of painless bleeding in the third 3 months of pregnancy. Its cause is unknown. The possibility of the condition increases with each pregnancy from about 1 in 1,500 first pregnancies to about 1 in 20 after many pregnancies. Even slight widening (dilation) of the cervix can cause enough separation of an abnormally placed placenta to result in bleeding. If severe bleeding occurs, immediate cesarean section is

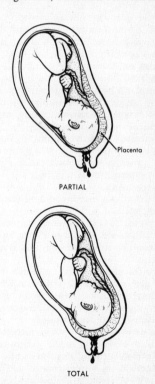

Placenta

PARTIAL

TOTAL

Placenta previa

usually needed to stop the bleeding and save the mother's life, regardless of the stage of the fetus' growth. Placenta previa may be diagnosed by ultrasound and treated with complete bed rest under close watching. Even at rest, bleeding can occur without warning. Most often the vagina is not examined if placenta previa is present or suspected. Feeling with the hands can cause and bring on bleeding. Cautious feeling may be done to find out the exact evidence of previa. Before this test, keeping the woman's body fluids stable is needed, and plans for blood transfer and cesarean section are made. If the placenta is next to or near, rather than touching or covering, the opening of the cervix, labor and birth through the vagina may be attempted. Also called *(informal)* **previa.**

placenta succenturiata, an extra, smaller placenta.

Placidyl, a trademark for a tranquilizer (ethchlorvynol).

plagiocephaly /plā′jē·ōsef′əlē/, a defect of the skull in which early or irregular closing of the borders of the skull results in the unequal growth of the head, making it look unbalanced. Also called **plagiocephalism.** See also **craniostenosis. –plagiocephalic, plagiocephalous,** *adj.*

plague, an infectious disease carried by the bite of a flea from a rodent infected with the bacillus *Yersinia pestis.* Plague is mainly an infectious disease of rats. The rat fleas feed on humans only when their normal hosts, most often rats, have been killed by the plague. Widespread human diseases occur after rat plague epidemics. Kinds of plague include **bubonic plague, pneumonic plague, septicemic plague.** See also *Yersinia pestis.*

plague vaccine, an active vaccinating drug made with killed plague bacilli. It is given to vaccinate against plague after a possible exposure or to protect travelers in high risk areas, as Southeast Asia.
★CAUTION: An inability to fight infections or strong infection prohibits its use.
★ADVERSE EFFECTS: Among the most serious side effects are allergic reactions, swelling at the injection site, headache, and general discomfort.

planar xanthoma, a yellow or orange flat patch or slightly raised pimple with foam. They occur in clusters in small areas, as the eyelids, or widely spread over the body. Also called **plane xanthoma, xanthoma planum.**

planned parenthood, a term applied to the use of birth-control methods, counseling, and family-planning programs and clinics. Planned parenthood supporters believe that it is the right of each woman to decide when to conceive and bear children and that care and in-

formation should be given to her to help her to become or to avoid becoming pregnant. See also **contraceptive.**

plantago seed /plantă′gō/, a bulk-forming laxative taken from *Plantago psyllium* seeds. It is given to treat constipation and diarrhea.
★CAUTION: Symptoms of appendicitis, blocked intestines, or ulcers prohibit its use.
★ADVERSE EFFECTS: Among the more serious side effects are blocked intestines and allergic reactions.

plantar /plan′tər/, referring to the sole of the foot. Also called **volar.**

plantar aponeurosis, the tough connective tissue (fascia) around the muscles of the soles of the feet. Also called **plantar fascia.**

plantaris /plantă′ris/, one of the muscles at the back of the leg. It flexes the foot and the leg. Compare **gastrocnemius, soleus.**

plantar neuroma, a tumor of the sole of the foot.

plantar reflex, the normal response of flexing the toes when the outer surface of the sole is firmly stroked from the heel to the toes. Compare **Babinski's reflex.**

plantar wart, a painful growth in the skin on the sole of the foot. Caused by the common wart virus, it occurs most often at points of pressure, as on the heel. There is a soft core surrounded by a firm, calluslike ring. Many tiny, black spots on the surface are bits of clotted blood in the wart. Treatment includes burning off (electrosurgery), freezing (cryotherapy), or using many drugs. See also **mosaic wart, wart.**

plantigrade /plan′tigrād′/, referring to the human walk. Walking on the sole of the foot with the heel touching the ground.

plaque /plak/, **1.** a flat, often raised patch on the skin or any other organ of the body. **2.** a patch of fatty buildup (atherosclerosis) on the lining of a blood vessel (artery). **3.** dental plaque, a thin film on the teeth made up of material found in saliva and often filled with bacteria.

Plaquenil Sulfate, a trademark for an antimalaria, antiarthritis, and lupus-suppressing drug (hydroxychloroquine sulfate).

-plasm, -plasma, a combining form meaning 'cell or tissue substance.'

plasma, the watery, colorless fluid in lymph and blood in which the white and red blood cells and platelets are hung. It has no cells and is made up of water, electrolytes, proteins, sugar (glucose), fats, bile coloring (bilirubin), and gases. Plasma is needed to carry the many parts of the blood through the bloodstream. It carries foods and wastes from the tissues, and keeps the acid-base balance of the body. Plasma and the fluid around body cells are much alike in their content of proteins. Plasma is important in keeping fluid pressure equal on either side of cell membranes, and also in exchanging fluids and other substances. Compare **serum.**

plasma-, a combining form meaning 'the liquid part of the blood.'

plasma cell, a cell found in the bone marrow, connective tissue, and, sometimes, in the blood. Plasma cells are used in the body's fight against disease and are formed in large numbers in bone marrow cancer (multiple myeloma). See also **B cell, multiple myeloma.**

plasma cell leukemia, an abnormal tumor of blood-forming tissues in which most of the cells in the blood are plasma cells. The disease may be caused by bone marrow cancer (multiple myeloma). In most cases plasma cell leukemia is fatal, but some patients respond to treatment with anticancer and hormone drugs.

plasma cell myeloma. See **multiple myeloma.**

plasmacytoma /plaz′məsītō′mə/, *pl.* **plasmacytomas, plasmacytomata,** a tumor with plasma cells. It may grow in the bone marrow, as in multiple myeloma, or outside of the bone marrow, as in some tumors of the inner organs and the membrane lining (mucosa) of the nose, mouth, and throat. Also called **peripheral plasma cell myeloma, plasma cell tumor.**

plasma membrane. See **cell membrane.**

plasmapheresis /plaz′məfərē′sis/, removing plasma from blood taken from a patient. It is also a mixture made from the cell parts of the plasma, and putting this mixture back into the patient. It is used to treat some diseases. Compare **leukapheresis, plateletpharesis.**

plasma protein, any of many proteins, which make up about 6% to 7% of the blood plasma in the body. These substances (as albumin, fibrinogen, prothrombin, and the gamma globulins) help to keep water balance and blood pressure normal. Fibrinogen and prothrombin are needed for blood clotting. The gamma globulins are important in keeping the body free of disease (immunoregulation). All of the plasma proteins except the gamma globulins are made in the liver. See also **antibody, serum.**

plasma-renin activity, the action of the enzyme renin, as measured in blood plasma. This aids in the diagnosis of adrenal gland disease linked to high blood pressure.

plasma volume, the total amount of plasma in the body. It rises in diseases of the liver and spleen and in a lack of vitamin C. It lowers in an adrenal gland disorder (Addison's disease), loss of fluids, and shock.

plasmid, any type of object inside a cell that has a genetic impact, as a molecule of DNA separate from the chromosome. Plasmids help bacteria to fight antibiotic drugs.

plasmidotrophoblast. See **syncytiotrophoblast.**

plasmin. See **fibrinolysin.**

Plasmodium /plazmō′dē·əm/, a type of protozoa that causes malaria. It is carried to humans by the bite of an infected Anopheles mosquito. *Plasmodium falciparum* causes the most severe form of malaria; *P. malariae* causes quartan malaria; *P. ovale* causes mild tertian malaria with oval red blood cells; and *P. vivax* causes common tertian malaria. See also *Anopheles,* **blackwater fever, malaria.**

plaster, **1.** any material made of a liquid and a powder that hardens when it dries. It can be used in shaping a cast to keep a broken bone aligned, as plaster of Paris. **2.** a home treatment made of a semisolid mixture placed on a part of the body, as a mustard plaster.

plastic surgery, the change, replacement, or rebuilding of the outer parts of the body. It is done to correct a structural or cosmetic defect. In corrective plastic surgery, the surgeon may use tissue from the patient or from another person or artificial material. The artificial tissue must not be irritating. It must have a texture that is right for the body part. It must also be able to hold its shape and form for a long time. Implants are often used in making breasts larger (mammoplasty). Skin grafts are common in plastic surgery. Simpler techniques (Z-plasty, Y-plasty) are often done instead of a graft in parts of the body covered by loose, stretchy skin, as the neck and throat. A coloring may be added to the skin of a graft to change the color of the graft to make it look like the surrounding skin. Scouring (dermabrasion) is used to remove pockmarks, scars from acne, or other signs of skin damage. Chemical peeling is used to remove small wrinkles on the face. Reconstructive plastic surgery corrects birth defects, repairs structures destroyed by injury, and replaces tissue removed in other surgeries. Cleft lip and cleft palate repair and other jaw and face (maxillofacial) surgeries, including those for the nose (rhinoplasty), ear (otoplasty), and wrinkles (rhytidoplasty), are also done. Correcting obvious defects may be very helpful for the patient in dealing with others and keeping a high sense of self-worth. See also specific procedures.

plate, a flat structure or layer, as a thin layer of bone.

platelet, the smallest of the cells in the blood. Platelets are disk-shaped and have no hemoglobin. They are needed for blood clotting. Compare **erythrocyte, leucocyte.** See also **hemoglobin.**

plateletpheresis, the removal of platelets from blood. The rest of the blood is put back into the patient. Also called **thrombapheresis, thrombotapheresis.** Compare **leukapheresis, plasmapheresis.**

platinized gold foil, a thin sheet of platinum stuck between two sheets of gold. It is used in dental techniques that need harder materials than those gotten from other materials.

Platinol, a trademark for an anticancer drug (cisplatin).

platinum (Pt), a silvery-white, soft metallic element. It is used in dentistry and to make chemicals that must be able to stand high temperatures.

platinum foil, a thin sheet of pure platinum used in dental devices and dentures. It is also used as the inside part of porcelain dental devices.

Platyhelminthes, a group of parasitic flatworms that includes tapeworms and flukes harmful to humans.

platypelloid pelvis /plat'əpel'oid/, a type of female pelvis in which the inlet is round, but the back section is made shorter by its flat and heavy border. Vaginal birth is not often possible in women who have platypelloid pelves. About 3%of women have this type of pelvis.

platysma /plətiz'mə/, one of a pair of wide muscles at the side of the neck. The platysma draws down the lower lip and the corner of the mouth. When the platysma fully pulls back, the skin over the collarbone is drawn toward the lower jaw, making the neck larger.

play, any action that is fun, entertaining, amusing, or diverting. It is important in childhood for normal personality growth and as a means for growing physically, mentally, and socially. Kinds of play include **active play, associative play, cooperative play, dramatic play, parallel play, passive play, skill play, solitary play.** See also **play therapy.**

play therapy, a form of mental treatment in which a child plays in a safe and guided place with games and toys set up by a health-care worker. This person watches by the behavior, affect, and speech of the child to gain data into the child's thoughts, feelings, and daydreams.

pleasure principle, the immediate need to satisfy instinctive drives. Compare **reality principle.**

pledget /plej'ət/, a small, flat compress made of cotton gauze, a piece of cotton, or material like it. It is used to wipe the skin, soak up fluids, or clean a small surface.

-plegia, a combining form meaning 'a paralysis' in a certain area.

Plegine, a trademark for a drug used to lower the appetite (phendimetrazine tartrate).

pleiotropy /plī·ot'rəpē/, the making by a single genc of a group of unrelated effects in a certain disorder.

plethora, a term given to the beefy red color of a newborn. The "boiled lobster" color of the infant's skin is caused by a very high level of red blood cells for the amount of blood. **–plethoric,** adj.

plethysmograph /pləthiz'məgraf'/, an instrument for listing changes in the size of hands, feet, and organs by measuring changes in the amount of blood. **–plethysmographic,** adj., **plethysmography,** n.

pleura /ploŏr'ə/, pl. **pleurae,** a frail, oily (serous) membrane surrounding the lung. The pleura is in two parts. The visceral pleura covers the surface of the lung, dipping into spaces between the lobes. The parietal pleura lines the chest wall, covers the diaphragm, and folds back over other structures in the chest space. The two parts of the pleura are separated from each other by a small amount of fluid that oils the space as the lungs fill and empty. See also **pleural cavity, pleural space. –pleural,** adj.

pleural cavity, the space within the chest (thorax) that holds the lungs. Between the ribs and the lungs are the chest linings (visceral and parietal pleurae).

pleural effusion, an abnormal buildup of fluid in the lungs. Symptoms are fever, chest pain, breathing difficulty, and a dry cough. The fluid comes from swollen lung surfaces caused by many things, as a blood clot in the lung, an injury, a tumor, or an infection. The cause is treated, and the fluid may be removed by suction or drained. Other treatment may include giving drugs to get rid of fluids and other drugs, giving oxygen, and using mechanical breathing.

pleural space, the small amount of space between the layers of the chest linings (pleurae).

pleurisy /ploŏr'əsē/, swelling of the linings (parietal pleurae) of the lungs. Symptoms include breathlessness and stabbing pain. It stops normal breathing with spasms on the affected side of the chest. A friction rub may be heard by the physician using a stethoscope. Pleurisy without fluid buildup is called dry (fibrinous). Causes include lung cancer, lung or chest wall sores, pneumonia, a blood clot in the lung, and tuberculosis. Permanent scars may result between the pleura and nearby surfaces. Treatment is pain relief and treatment for the disease causing the pleurisy. See also **pleural effusion, pleurodynia, pulmonary edema.**

pleurodynia /ploŏr'ōdin'ē·ə/, swelling of the muscles (intercostal) between the ribs and those that attach the diaphragm to the chest wall. Symptoms are sudden severe pain and tenderness, fever, headache, and loss of appetite. The pain is made worse by movement and breathing. The lungs are not affected. See also **epidemic pleurodynia.**

pleuropericardial rub, an abnormal coarse friction sound heard by the physician with a stethoscope. It is caused by the surfaces of the lung linings rubbing against each other. The sound is not affected by coughing. A pleural rub is a sign of swelling, tumor, or pleural disease. See also **breath sound, Kussmaul breathing, rale, rhonchi, wheeze.**

pleuroperitoneal cavity. See **splanchnocoele.**

pleuropneumonia, a combination of long lining swelling (pleurisy) and pneumonia.

pleurothotonos /ploŏr'əthot'ənəs/, an uncontrolled, severe, long-term contraction of the muscles of one side of the body. It results in a twisting of the body to that side and is usually linked to tetanus infection or strychnine poisoning. **–pleurothotonic,** *adj.*

plexiform neuroma, a tumor made of twisted bundles of nerve fibers. Also called **Verneuil's neuroma.**

plexor. See **percussor.**

plexus, *pl.* **plexuses,** a group of joined nerves, blood vessels, or lymph vessels. The body has many plexuses, as the cardiac plexus and the solar plexus.

plica /plī'kə/, *pl.* **plicae** /plī'sē/, a fold of tissue in the body, as the circular folds (plicae circulares) of the small intestine. **–plical,** *adj.*

plicae transversales recti, the crosswise (transverse) folds in the rectum that hold the weight of feces. Also called **Houston's valves.** See also **rectum.**

plicamycin, an anticancer drug given to treat cancer of the testicles, and excess blood calcium linked to cancer.
★CAUTION: Blood disorders, kidney or liver disease, bone marrow defect, or known allergy to this drug prohibits its use.
★ADVERSE EFFECTS: Among the more serious side effects are blood defects. Nausea and mouth swelling are common.

Plimmer's bodies, small, round objects found in cancer cells. They were once thought to be parasites that caused cancer. Also called **Behla's bodies.**

-ploid, a combining form meaning 'having a (specific) number of chromosome sets.'

plug, a mass of tissue cells, mucus, or other matter that blocks a normal opening or passage of the body, as a cervical plug.

Plummer's disease, a thyroid growth (goiter) with a harmful condition from an overactive thyroid or tumor. Also called **toxic nodular goiter.**

Plummer-Vinson syndrome /plum'ərvin'sən/, a disorder with severe and long-term iron deficiency anemia and swallowing difficulty caused by webs of tissue in the gullet (esophagus). Also called **sideropenic dysphagia.** Compare **Paterson-Kelly syndrome.**

plunging goiter. See **diving goiter.**

plutonium (Pu), an artificial, radioactive element. It is a very harmful waste product of nuclear power plants.

P.M.D., abbreviation for *private medical doctor.*

PMT, abbreviation for **premenstrual tension.**

PND, abbreviation for **postnasal drip.**

-pnea, -pnoea, a combining form meaning 'breath or breathing.'

pneumatic heart driver, a device that controls air under pressure brought to an artificial heart. It controls the heart rate and other heart functions.

pneumococcal /nōō'mōkok'əl/, referring to bacteria of the *Pneumococcus* group.

pneumococcal vaccine, an active vaccination drug with foreign bodies (antigens) of the 14

types of *Pneumococcus* linked to 80% of the cases of pneumococcal pneumonia. It is given to patients over 2 years of age who are at high risk of getting severe pneumococcal pneumonia.
★CAUTION: Pregnancy, early childhood (under 2 years of age), or known allergy to the vaccine prohibits its use.
★ADVERSE EFFECTS: Among the more serious side effects are swelling at the site of injection, fever, and allergic reactions.

pneumococcus /nōō'mōkok'əs/, *pl.* **pneumococci** /nōō'mōkok'sī/, a bacterium (*Diplococcus pneumoniae*), the most common cause of bacterial pneumonia. More than 85 subtypes are known. See also **lobar pneumonia, pneumonia.**

pneumoconiosis /nōō'mōkōnē·ō'sis/, any disease of the lung caused by the long-term breathing of dust, most often mineral dusts. See also **anthracosis, asbestosis, silicosis.**

pneumocystosis /nōō'mōsistō'sis/, a lung infection from a parasite (*Pneumocystis carinii*). commonly seen in infants or patients who are weak or at high risk. Symptoms are fever, cough, rapid breathing, and bluish skin (cyanosis). The death rate is near 100% in untreated patients. Also called **interstitial plasma cell pneumonia.**

pneumoderma. See **subcutaneous emphysema.**

pneumoencephalography /nōō'mō·ensef'əlog'rəfē/, a way of making x-ray pictures of the brain spaces. Air, helium, or oxygen is injected into the spinal cord to outline the spaces. See also **encephalography, ventriculography. –pneumoencephalographic,** *adj.*

pneumogastric nerve. See **vagus nerve.**

pneumomediastinum /nōō'mōmē'dē·əstī'nəm/, the presence of air or gas in the space between the lung lining (pleural) sacs of the chest. In infants, it may lead to a collapsed lung or air around the heart membrane (pericardium), as in those with breathing difficulty or lung swelling. In older children, it may result from bronchitis, asthma, whooping cough (pertussis), cystic fibrosis, or injury.

pneumonectomy, the removal of all or part of a lung.

pneumonia /nōōmō'nē·ə/, a swelling of the lungs, commonly caused by breathed-in bacteria (*Diplococcus pneumoniae*). Parts of the lungs become plugged with a fiberlike fluid. Pneumonia may also be caused by viruses, rickettsiae, and fungi. Symptoms of pneumonia are severe chills, a high fever (which may reach 105° F), headache, cough, and chest pain. An involved lower lobe of the right lung may cause a pain that is like appendicitis. Red blood cells leaking into the air sacs of the lungs causes a rust-colored sputum that may be a sure sign of pneumococcal infection. As the disease continues, sputum may become thicker and have pus. The patient may have painful attacks of coughing. Breathing often becomes painful, shallow, and rapid. The pulse rate goes up, often more than 120 beats a minute. Other signs may be heavy sweating and bluish skin. Stomach and bowel disorders and an outbreak of shingles (herpes simplex) on the face may also occur. Children with pneumonia may have seizures. The affected area of a lobe becomes filled with fluids and firm. A distinct breathing sound is heard by the physician. X-ray films are taken of the lungs. Laboratory tests of sputum and blood help in finding the cause. Treatment of pneumonia is bed rest, fluids, antibiotics, painkillers, and, if needed, oxygen. Ice packs or cold, wet compresses may be needed to lower the fever. Fever, loss of fluids, and breathing through the mouth result in a need for special care of the mouth and nose. Mild pneumonia is often treated at home. See also **aspiration pneumonia, bronchopneumonia, eosinophilic pneumonia, interstitial pneumonia, lobar pneumonia, mycoplasma pneumonia, viral pneumonia.**

pneumonic plague, a rapidly fatal form of plague with pneumonia. There are two forms: **primary pneumonic plague** is caused by the lungs being infected during bubonic plague; **secondary pneumonic plague** is caused by breathing infected bits of sputum from a patient with pneumonic plague. Compare **bubonic plague, septicemic plague.** See also **plague,** *Yersinia pestis.*

pneumonitis /nōo'mənī'tis/, *pl.* **pneumonitides,** an inflammation of the lung. It may be caused by a virus or be a reaction to chemicals or organic dusts, as bird droppings or molds. Dry cough is a common symptom. Treatment includes removing the things that caused it and giving hormone drugs to decrease the swelling. A kind of pneumonitis is **humidifier lung.** Compare **pneumonia.**

pneumothorax /nōo'mōthôr'aks/, a collection of air or gas in the chest (pleural space) causing the lung to collapse. It may be the result of an open chest wound that permits air to enter, the break of an air-filled blister (vesicle) on the lung's surface, or a severe bout of coughing. Pneumothorax may begin with a sudden, sharp chest pain. It is followed by difficult, rapid breathing, and normal chest movements stopped on the affected side. There may be rapid heart beat, a weak pulse, low blood pressure, sweating, fever, pale skin, and dizziness. The patient should stay quiet in bed, in a halfway upright position. Oxygen may be given. The air should be taken from the chest space at once. To remove the air, a tube is put in, and not removed until the air is no longer coming out through a water-seal draining system. Pain may be controlled with painkillers, but drugs that can cause slowed breathing are not used. Mechanical breathing may be given. The patient must learn how to turn, cough,

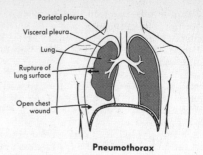

Pneumothorax

breathe deeply, and do passive exercises without making the condition worse. For example, stretching, reaching, or sudden movements must be not be done.

podalic, referring to the feet.

podalic version, the shifting of the position of a fetus to bring the feet to the outlet during labor.

podiatry /pədi'ətrē/, the diagnosis and treatment of diseases and other disorders of the feet.

podophyllotoxin, a substance taken from the roots of a common plant known as mayapple, or American mandrake. A drug (podyphillin) made from podophyllotoxin is given for some types of warts.

-poiesis, -poesis, a combining form meaning 'the making of.'

poikilo-, pecilo-, poecil-, a combining form meaning 'varied or irregular.'

poikilocytosis /poi'kilōsītō'sis/, an abnormal shape of red blood cells.

poikiloderma atrophicans vasculare, an abnormal skin condition with too-much skin coloring, tiny places of bleeding, and wasting of the outer layers. It may be even or patchy, in small areas or widespread. It is often long-term.

poikiloderma of Civatte, a common skin swelling with red patches on the face and neck that become dry and scaly. Skin coloring is found around hairs down the sides of the neck. The patient often has skin reactions to sunlight. Also called **reticulated pigmented poikiloderma.** See also **photosensitive.**

poikilothermic. See **cold-blooded.**

poison, any substance that damages health or destroys life when swallowed, breathed in or soaked up by the body in small amounts. Most doctors agree that, depending on the size of the dose, any substance can be harmful. Poisons are often divided into those that respond to treatments or antidotes and those for which there is no treatment. There are few workable antidotes. Treatment for poisoning is based mainly on getting the poison out the body before it can be absorbed. Making sure that the patient can breathe and has a good blood flow are important. Some substances that may be poisonous are the saps of some plants, bacteria poisons, animal poisons, chemicals, some metals, most gases, and many drugs. The harmful effects of poisons may or may not be able to be treated. The ability of body tissue to recover from poison is a measure of how strong the effect will be. Poisons that injure the nervous system often cause permanent damage because parts of the brain cannot regrow. The harmful effects of chemicals may be divided into local and system effects. Local effects, as those from swallowing harmful substances, involve the site of the first contact between the body and the poison. System effects depend on the soaking up and spread of the poison. System poisoning most often affects the nervous system but may also affect the blood flow, blood and blood-forming tissues, skin, and liver, kidneys, and lungs. Muscles and bones are less often affected. About 150,000 cases are reported to the National Clearinghouse for Poison Control Centers each year. Experts guess that the real number of cases is at least 10 times the number of reported cases. The total number of cases goes up each year. However, the rate of poisoning in children under 5 years of age has gone down, most likely because of safer packing of household drugs and products. About 60% of all poisoning involves children 1 to 2 years of age who have swallowed chemicals other than drugs. About 75% of the cases of poisoning in those over 15 years of age are drug-related. About 4,000 persons die each year in the United States from poisoning by liquid or solid substances. Another 7,000 persons are bitten by poisonous snakes, as the pit viper and coral snake. The saps or juices of plants, as poison ivy, poison sumac, and poison oak, may cause severe reactions through skin contact or by swallowing. Prompt treatment of poisoning from harmful chemicals and liquids is important. Some common treatments are vomiting and flushing the stomach with water. Most harmful effects of drugs occur shortly after taking them, but cancer-causing effects of chemicals may take 15 to 45 years to develop. See also **poisoning treatment.** **–poisonous,** *adj.*

poison control center, one of a nearly worldwide group of services that offer data about all aspects of poisoning, keep records of their rate and refer patients to treatment centers.

poisoning, 1. the act of taking or giving a poisonous substance. 2. the condition caused by swallowing, injecting, breathing in, or exposing someone to a poisonous substance. Finding what the poison is, and including labels on jars and bottles, is important for a quick diagnosis and treatment. See also specific types of poisoning.

poisoning treatment, the care given a patient who has been exposed to or who has taken a harmful drug or chemical. In the case of poisoning by mouth, the first thing to do is to remove the poison quickly. If vomiting does not occur, it should be started after first finding out what the poison is; if possible. However, if the poison is a part of gasoline, as kerosene, or a harsh or burning substance, vomiting should *not* be started. Before attempting to start vomiting, the victim, if conscious, should be given one or two glasses of milk or water. A carbonated beverage should never be given for poisoning by mouth. Because of the danger of high levels of salt (sodium) in the blood, the victim, especially a child, should not be given water with salt or mustard. Syrup of ipecac can be given, if handy, to start vomiting, and the dose can be repeated one time. But if the ipecac does not cause vomiting, working on the victim's gag reflex at the back of the throat may help. Ipecac should not remain in the stomach or be given with milk or charcoal, both of which can affect its action. In some cases, an antidote may be given to make the poison ineffective or to prevent its being taken in by the body, as by giving a mild mixture of vinegar or citrus juice to break down an alkali. As in other emergencies, a physician should be called to take charge of the case. If one is not available, the nearest Poison Control Center should be called for help.

Actions in selected situations with a conscious victim who has ingested poison*

Corrosive or caustic substances
Do not attempt to neutralize the substance.
Do not induce vomiting.
Offer the victim a glass of milk or water.

Noncorrosive substances
The decision on whether to induce vomiting is dependent on the substance ingested, the amount ingested, and the physical condition of the victim. In general, when pure petroleum distillates are ingested, vomiting is *not* indicated.
For other materials, vomiting may be induced. The Regional Poison Center can help in this evaluation.

Methods of inducing vomiting
1. Give 1 tbsp (15 ml) syrup of Ipecac followed by 1 glass of water. (Dose can be repeated once only if vomiting does not occur within 15 to 20 minutes.) Do not allow emetic to remain in stomach.
2. Physician's order: Apomorphine hydrochloride 0.03 mg/lb subcutaneously. (Contraindicated if respiratory depression is present or patient is comatose.) Apomorphine is rarely used. Can be reversed by the administration of naloxene.

*Information supplied by the American Association of Poison Control Centers, University of California Medical Center, San Diego.

poison ivy, any of several species of climbing vine (*Rhus*), with shiny, three-pointed leaves. Common in North America, it causes severe allergic reactions in many people. Blisters with itching and burning result that may be treated with lotions, cold compresses, or hormone lotions or creams. People who are extremely allergic to poison ivy may be given preventive treatment with a *Rhus* antigen after contact, before symptoms begin. Careful washing of the exposed skin after suspected contact may prevent the reaction. See also **rhus dermatitis, urushiol.**

poison oak, any of several species of shrub (*Rhus*), common in North America. Skin contact results in allergic skin swellings in many people. Symptoms and treatment are like those for poison ivy. See also **rhus dermatitis, urushiol.**

poison sumac /sŏŏ'mak/, a shrub (*Rhus*), common in North America. Skin contact results in allergic reactions in many people. Symptoms and treatment are similar to those for poison ivy. See also **rhus dermatitis, urushiol.**

poker spine. See **bamboo spine.**

Polaramine, a trademark for an antihistamine (dexchlorpheniramine maleate).

polar body, one of the small cells made during the division of female eggs (ova). It is not able to be fertilized. See also **oogenesis.**

polarity /pōler'itē/, **1.** the existence or display of opposing qualities, or emotions, as pleasure and pain, love and hate, or strength and weakness. It is important for mental treatment.

polarity therapy, a type of massage based on the idea that the body has positive and negative energy patterns that must be balanced to keep the body healthy.

polio, *informal.* poliomyelitis.

polioencephalitis /pō'lē·ō·ensef'əlī'tis/, a swelling of the gray matter of the brain caused by a virus (poliovirus).

polioencephalomyelitis /pō'lē·ō·ensef'əlōmī'əlī'tis/, swelling of the gray matter of the brain and the spinal cord, caused by a virus (poliovirus).

poliomyelitis /pō'lē·ōmī·əlī'tis/, a disease caused by a virus. There are mild forms of the disease and others that keep the body parts from moving at all (paralytic). One form without symptoms keeps the patient from ever having it again (immunity). The disease is carried from person to person. Stress increases the chance of getting the virus. Older people are more likely to get it in its serious form. More boys than girls are affected. More pregnant than nonpregnant women get the paralytic form. The mildest form lasts only a few hours with fever, headache, nausea, and vomiting. A longer-lasting form also includes irritation of brain membranes (meninges) with pain and stiffness in the back. Paralytic poliomyelitis begins with mild symptoms, which then go away. For several days the person seems well. The symptoms return, and pain, weakness, and paralysis start. The highest level of paralysis happens within the first week. In spinal poliomyelitis, viruses reproduce in the spinal cord, causing swelling and destroying nerve cells. The large muscles of the arms and legs are most often affected. Bulbar poliomyelitis is caused by viruses reproducing in the brain stem. The paralytic forms often happen at the same time. Treatment of the mild forms of the disease is usually bed rest, eating well, and not getting physically worn out. Treatment of the paralytic form includes a hospital stay where the patient is given hot packs, baths, exercise, and help in breathing when needed. As soon as the serious stage is over, work begins with the patient to rebuild his or her strength and muscle actions. The more quickly muscle function returns, the better the outcome. Because there is pain and muscle spasm during the serious period, the patient usually does not want to move. But this increases the chance for badly formed muscles to occur. The patient should exercise and work hard during the period that muscle strength is being rebuilt. Poliomyelitis can be prevented by getting vaccine shots. Families should get the whole series, especially before traveling in countries where the disease is still common. Poliomyelitis was seen mostly in the summer. Now, the few cases still seen happen at any time of the year. Also called (*informal*) **polio.** See also **poliovirus.**

poliomyelitis vaccine. See **poliovirus vaccine.**

poliosis /pō'lē·ō'sis/, loss of hair coloring. It may be an inborn problem and can occur over the whole body. It may also be gotten and be seen only in patches.

poliovirus, the virus that causes poliomyelitis. There are three different types of this very small virus. Getting infected by or vaccinated with one type does not keep the patient from getting the others.

poliovirus vaccine, a vaccine made from poliovirus to keep a person from getting the disease. TOPV (trivalent live oral vaccine), or Sabin vaccine, should be given to children under 18 years of age. IPV (inactivated poliovirus vaccine), or Salk vaccine, should be given to infants and children who have not formed a defense against the disease and for adults who have not been vaccinated. IPV is given by shot. Paralysis occurs rarely after giving TOPV.

pollakiuria /pol'əkēyŏŏr'ē·ə/, an abnormal condition with a need to pass urine often.

pollen coryza, swelling and reddening of the nose caused by coming into contact with pollens. Also called **hay fever.** See also **coryza.**

pollutant, an unwanted substance in the environment, usually with unhealthy effects. Pollutants can be in the atmosphere as gases or dust that irritates lungs, eyes, and skin, and as substances in drinking water, foods or beverages.

polyarteritis /pol'ē·är'tərī'tis/, a swelling of several arteries.

polyarteritis nodosa, a serious blood vessel disease in which small and medium-sized arteries become swollen and damaged. This causes the death of the tissues they supply with blood. Any organ or organ system may be affected. The disease attacks men and women between 20 and 50 years of age. Doctors do not know its cause. The disease may be sudden and cause death, or long-term and cause the patient to get worse and worse slowly. Symptoms are high temperatures, pain in the stomach and intestinal area, weight loss, and nerve damage. If the kidneys are affected, high blood pressure, fluid gain (edema), and a urine substance (urea) in the blood result. The disease may look like intestinal or heart disorders. The death rate is high, especially if the kidneys are involved. Treatment includes large doses of hormones. Physical therapy helps to keep muscles in good shape and slow being laid up.

polychlorinated biphenyls (PCB), a group of more than 30 chemical compounds used to make plastics, insulation, and chemicals to show the spread of flames. All can be poisonous and cancer-causing. Mild contact with these chemicals may cause a skin disorder (chloracne); serious contact may cause liver damage.

Polycillin, a trademark for an antibiotic (ampicillin).

polyclonal /pol'ēklō'nəl/, referring to a group of cells or living things that are exactly alike and come from several cells that are exactly alike.

Polycose, a trademark for a food supplement that has carbohydrates taken from cornstarch.

polycystic kidney disease (PKD), an abnormal condition of kidneys that have become too big and have many lumps (cysts). There are three forms of the disease. **Childhood polycystic disease (CPD)** does not occur often. Death usually occurs within a few years because the liver and kidney stop working. **Adult polycystic disease (APD)** may be gotten, or be present at birth, and may affect one kidney or both. There is pain in the outer side of the hip, thigh and buttock (flank) and high blood pressure. The kidneys stop working, causing urea in the blood (uremia) and death. **Congenital polycystic disease (CPD)** is a birth defect that affects all or only a small part of one or both kidneys. Kidney tissue that does not grow normally in the fetus causes death shortly after birth.

polycystic ovary syndrome, a disorder marked by a failure to ovulate or menstruate in a woman, an abnormal growth of body hair (hirsutism), and not being able to become pregnant. It is caused by the endocrine gland getting out of balance with higher levels of some hormones (testosterone, estrogen, and luteinizing) and lower giving off of FSH (follicle-stimulating hormone). Lower levels of FSH causes the ovarian follicles to grow only partly, which then do not release eggs (ova). Many lumps (cysts) may grow in the ovary. The affected ovary often gets to be twice in size and is covered by a smooth, pearly-white capsule. The higher level of a female sex hormone (estrogen) that is the result makes cancers of the breast and the uterus more likely. Treatment includes using female hormones or removal using surgery.

polycythemia /pol'ēsīthē'mē·ə/, an abnormal increase in the number of red blood cells. It may occur with lung or heart disease, or with being in high altitudes for a long time. Also called **Osler's disease, polycythemia vera.** See also **altitude sickness, erythrocytosis.**

polydactyly, a birth defect with more than the normal number of fingers or toes. Usually inborn, the defect can often be corrected by surgery shortly after birth. Also called **polydactylia, polydactylism, hyperdactyly.**

polydipsia /pol'ēdip'sē·ə/, having too much thirst. Several other conditions increase urination, which leads to low blood volume and thirst. These include diabetes and some kidney disorders. See also **diabetes insipidus, diabetes mellitus.**

polyesthesia, a disorder involving the sense of touch in which something that causes feeling in one area of the skin is felt at other sites as well as the area that has the true feeling.

polyestradiol phosphate, an anticancer drug given for cancer of the prostate and breast cancer.

★CAUTION: Male breast cancer, a blood clotting disorder (thrombophlebitis), or known allergy to this drug prohibits its use.

★ADVERSE EFFECTS: Among the more serious side effects are loss of sex drive, not being able to have sex, and growth of breasts in males.

polygene /pol'ējēn'/, any of a group of genes that alone have a small effect but work together to form a trait. Examples include genes that affect size, weight, or intelligence. Also called **cumulative gene, multiple factor, multiple gene.** See also **multifactorial inheritance.** –polygenic, adj.

polyhydramnios. See hydramnios.

polyleptic /pol'ēlep'tik/, any disease or condition that has many phases of high and low levels of seriousness of symptoms.

polyleptic fever, a fever that occurs in sudden attacks, as smallpox and relapsing fever.

polymer, a chemical compound formed by linking a number of small molecules (monomers). A polymer may be made up of different monomers or from many units of the same one.

polymicrogyria. See microgyria.

polymorphonuclear /pol'ēmôr'fōnōō'klē·ər/, a cell that has a nucleus with a number of segments (lobules) connected by a fine thread.

polymorphonuclear leukocyte, a white blood cell that has a segmented (lobular) nucleus; an eosinophil, basophil, or neutrophil. See also **basophil, epsonophil, granulocyte, neutrophil.**

polymorphous /pol'ēmôr'fəs/, referring to things that exist in many different forms, possibly changing in structure at different stages.

polymorphous light eruption, a common reaction to sunlight or ultraviolet light in patients who are sensitive to sunlight. Within 1 to 4 days after being in the light, small, red pimples and blisters appear on otherwise normal skin, then disappear within 2 weeks. Allergic reactions that do not appear right away may be the cause. Tanning lowers the seriousness of the reaction.

Polymox, a trademark for an antibiotic (amoxicillin).

polymyalgia arteritica. See **polymyalgia rheumatica.**

polymyalgia rheumatica, a long-term disease that swells the large arteries that may appear in people over 60 years of age. Two disorders are thought to be involved in the same disease with slightly different symptoms. One form (polymyalgia rheumatica) affects the muscles, with pain and stiffness of the back, shoulder, or neck, usually becoming more severe when the patient gets up in the morning. There may also be a headache. The other disorder (cranial arteritis) affects the arteries at the side and back of the head, causing a severe, throbbing headache. Serious problems that result from this disorder include not enough blood flow, heart attack, stroke, or blindness. Both forms of the disease will go away by themselves. Hormones are good for lowering swelling and in speeding recovery. Also called **polymyalgia arteritica.** See also **temporal arteritis.**

polymyositis /pol'ēmī'ōsī'tis/, inflammation of many muscles, usually with badly shaped muscles, swelling, not being able to sleep, pain, sweating, and tension. Some forms of polymyositis are linked to cancer. See also **dermatomyositis.**

polymyxin, an antibiotic used to treat some bacterial infections.
★CAUTION: Allergies to this drug prohibit its use. It is used very carefully in patients with kidney problems.
★ADVERSE EFFECTS: Among the more serious side effects are kidney damage and different nerve disorders. Pain or blood vessel irritation at the place of shots also may occur. Allergic reactions of the skin or mucous membranes are sometimes seen.

polymyxin B sulfate, an antibiotic given for infections, including urinary tract, blood, and eye infections.
★CAUTION: Known allergy to this drug prohibits its use. Extreme care is necessary when

it is given to people with kidney problems.
★ADVERSE EFFECTS: Among the more serious side effects are kidney and nervous system disorders, and drug fever. When used on the skin, allergies are the most common problem.

polyopia, a sight problem in which something is seen as many images; multiple vision. The condition can occur in one or both eyes. See also **diplopia.**

polyp, a small tumorlike growth that comes out from a mucous membrane surface.

polypeptide /pol'ēpep'tīd/, a chain of amino acids. A polypeptide is usually larger than a peptide but smaller than a protein. They are formed by partial breakdown of proteins or by connecting amino acids into chains. See also **amino acid, peptide.**

polyphagia /pol'ēfā'jē-ə/, eating to the point of being focused only on eating (gluttony). See also **bulimia.**

polypharmacy, the use of a number of different drugs by a patient who may have one or several health problems.

polyploidy /pol'əploi'dē/, the state or condition of having more than two complete sets of chromosomes.

polyposis, an abnormal condition with many tumors or growths (polyps) on an organ or tissue. See also **familial polyposis.**

polyradiculitis /pol'ērədik'yōōli'tis/, swelling and reddening of many nerve roots. See also **Guillain-Barré syndrome.**

polysaccharide, a carbohydrate that contains three or more molecules of simple carbohydrates. Examples include dextrins, starches, and gums.

polysomy /pol'əsō'mē/, having a chromosome that may be remade three times (trisomy), four times (tetrasomy), or more times. Among females with three, four, or five X chromosomes, instead of the normal two, mental retardation may occur more often. See also **Klinefelter's syndrome.**

Polysporin, a trademark for an eye and skin drug that has antibiotics (polymyxin B sulfate and bacitracin).

polythiazide, a drug given to treat high blood pressure and edema.

polyunsaturated fatty acid. See **fatty acid that can be dissolved further (unsaturated).**

polyuria /pol'ēyōōr'ē-ə/, the release of abnormally large amounts of urine. Some causes are diabetes (insipidus or mellitus), use of drugs that increase the passage of urine (diuretics), and too-much fluid intake.

Poly-Vi-Flor, a trademark for a children's drug given by mouth, it has several vitamins and sodium fluoride.

polyvinyl chloride (PVC), a common artificial material that releases hydrochloric acid when burned. This may be a cancer-causing substance that pollutes the environment.

POMP, an acronym for a drug combination, used in the treatment of cancer, that has three anticancer drugs, Purinethol (mercaptopurine), Oncovin (vincristine sulfate), methotrexate, and adrenal hormone (prednisone).

Pompe's disease, a form of muscle disease in which there is a buildup of glycogen. It results from a shortage of an enzyme (acid maltase). It usually causes death to infants. Children with Pompe's disease appear mentally retarded and lack normal muscle tone, seldom living beyond 20 years of age. In adults muscle weakness happens slowly, but the disease does not cause death. Also called **glycogen storage disease, type II.** See also **glycogen storage disease.**

pompholyx. See **dyshidrosis.**

Pondimin, a trademark for a drug to reduce appetite (fenfluramine hydrochloride).

ponos. See **kala-azar.**

pons /ponz/, *pl.* **pontes** /pon'tēz/, **1.** any bridge of tissue that connects two parts of a structure or an organ of the body. **2.** a mass of nerve cells on the surface of the brainstem. It has nuclei of various nerves, including the facial and the trigeminal nerves. Also called **bridge of varolius.**

Ponstel, a trademark for an anti-inflammatory and painkilling drug (mefenamic acid).

pontic, a part of a nonmoving partial denture, as an artificial tooth, usually placed in the space that had earlier had the natural tooth crown.

Pontocaine Hydrochloride, a trademark for a local anesthetic (tetracaine hydrochloride).

pooled plasma, a thin, colorless, or slightly yellow liquid part of whole blood for use when whole blood cannot be gotten. It does not break down in freeze-dried form, making it useful in surgery and other conditions. It is gotten from blood banks or made directly from donors. Of the total volume of normal blood, 55% to 65% is plasma. See also **bank blood, component therapy, packed cells.**

popliteal artery /pop'litē'əl/, a part of the femoral artery of the upper leg that continues below the knee. It splits into eight branches, and brings blood to different muscles of the thigh, leg, and foot.

popliteal node, a lymph node in one of the groups of lymph glands in the leg. About seven small popliteal nodes are found in the fat at the back of the knee.

popliteal pulse, the pulse of the popliteal artery, which can be felt behind the knee.

population, any group that is marked by a certain trait or situation.

population at risk, a group of people who share a trait that causes each member to be at risk to an event, as children who have not been given their shots (immunized) and are exposed to poliovirus or cigarette smokers who work with asbestos.

porcine graft, a short-term skin graft for humans made from the skin of a pig.

-pore, a combining form meaning 'passageway.'

pork tapeworm. See *Taenia solium.*

pork tapeworm infection, an infection of the intestine or the tissues, caused by the pork tapeworm (*Taenia solium*). This tapeworm can use humans as both a place for its young to grow and for the adult worm. Humans are usually infected with the adult worm after eating undercooked pork that has tapeworms in it. Infection is rare in the United States but relatively common in South America, Asia, and Russia. See also **cysticercosis, tapeworm infection.**

porphyria /pôrfir'ē·ə/, a group of inborn disorders in which there is an abnormal increase in biological colorings (pigments) (porphyrins). There are two major kinds of porphyria. **Erythropoietic porphyria,** in which large amounts of porphyrins are made in bone marrow, and **hepatic porphyria,** in which large amounts are made in the liver. Signs common to both are being sensitive to light, pain in the stomach and intestinal area, and nerve damage.

portacaval shunt, an artificial passage made using surgery to increase the flow of blood between the liver and digestive tract.

Portagen, a trademark for a substance added to food that has protein, carbohydrate, and fat.

portal hypertension, an increased blood pressure in the portal system caused by blockage in the liver's blood supply. It results in the spleen getting larger, high blood pressure, and varicose veins of the esophagus. Portal hypertension is often linked to alcoholic cirrhosis. Also called **renovascular hypertension.**

portal system, the network of veins that drains the blood from the stomach and intestinal portion of the digestive tract, spleen, pancreas, and gallbladder and carries blood from these organs to the liver.

portal vein, a short vein that carries blood from the stomach and intestinal organs to the liver.

portoenterostomy, surgery to open the bile duct. A part of the intestine is sewed to an opening in the liver. This lets bile flow directly into the intestine. The operation is successful in most cases. Without it, cirrhosis develops and causes an early death. Also called **Kasai operation.**

port-wine stain. See **nevus flammeus.**

position, **1.** any one of many postures of the body, as the anatomical position, prone, or supine position. See specific positions. **2.** the link between where a part of the fetus is in the womb, as the back of the head, chin, or shoulder blade (scapula) and where it is with respect to its location in the mother's pelvis.

positive, **1.** referring to a laboratory test showing that a substance or a reaction is present. **2.**

referring to physical examination showing that a sign is present, often meaning that there is disease change.

positive feedback, an increase in the working of an organ or system of organs in response to a signal, as urination increases once the flow of urine has started or as the uterus contracts more often and with greater strength once it has begun to contract in labor.

positive identification, the unknowing patterning of one's personality on that of another for whom one has much respect. See also **identification.**

positive signs of pregnancy, three unmistakable signs of pregnancy: heart tones of the fetus, heard through a stethoscope; fetal skeleton, seen on x-ray film or with other methods (ultrasound); and parts of the fetus, felt by pressing gently on the abdomen (palpation).

positron-emission tomography (PET), a computerized x-ray technique that uses radioactive substances to look at the body's processes. The patient either inhales or is injected with a radioactive substance that is mostly harmless. The computers of the PET device find gamma rays and change them into pictures that show the processes in the tissues being studied. See also **gamma ray.**

post-, a combining form meaning 'after or behind.'

postcommissurotomy syndrome, a condition that often follows heart valve surgery. Pain and fever may set in once in a while, lasting weeks or months, and then suddenly stop.

postconcussional syndrome, a condition that follows a head injury. Symptoms are dizziness, not being able to focus one's thoughts, headache, being sensitive to noise and other signals, and nervousness. It usually stops by itself without treatment. Also called **posttraumatic syndrome.**

posterior, referring to or placed in the back part of a structure. Compare **anterior.**

posterior Achilles bursitis, a painful heel condition caused by inflammation of the joint sac (bursa) between the Achilles tendon and the heel bone. It is commonly associated with Haglund's deformity.

posterior atlantoaxial ligament, one of five ligaments that link the first backbone (vertebra) below the skull (atlas) to the second backbone (vertebra) (axis). It helps movements that require turning of the head. Compare **anterior atlantoaxial ligament.**

posterior auricular artery, one of a pair of small branches of arteries from the outer carotid arteries that supply blood to parts of the ear, scalp, and other parts in the head.

posterior common ligament. See **posterior longitudinal ligament.**

posterior costotransverse ligament, one of the five ligaments of each joint in the spine, made

up of fibrous tissue linking each rib to the backbone above it. Compare **superior costotransverse ligament.**

posterior fontanel, a small triangular area where the bones meet at the back of a baby's skull. See also **fontanel.**

posterior longitudinal ligament, a thick, strong ligament attached to the back of each backbone and running from the base of the skull to the tailbone (coccyx). Also called **posterior common ligament.** Compare **anterior longitudinal ligament.**

posterior mediastinum, one of the several areas of the chest cavity. It contains the trachea, two bronchi, esophagus, thoracic lymph duct and many large lymph nodes, and different blood vessels, including a part of the aorta. Compare **anterior mediastinum, middle mediastinum, superior mediastinum.**

posterior nares, a pair of openings in the back of the nasal cavity. They connect the nasal cavity with the upper throat and allow the flow of air. Also called **choana.** Compare **anterior nares.**

posterior palatal-seal area, the area of soft tissues between the hard and soft palates. It is use by dentists to locate the proper place for a denture.

posterior pituitary, posterior pituitary gland. See **neurohypophysis.**

posterior tibial artery, one of the parts of the popliteal artery of the leg. It divides into eight branches, which supply blood to different muscles of the lower leg, foot, and toes. Compare **anterior tibial artery.**

posterior tibialis pulse, the pulse of the posterior tibialis artery felt on the ankle, just behind to the bulge of the ankle bone (talus).

posterior tooth, any of the upper and lower premolars and molars of the adult, or permanent teeth.

posterior vein of left ventricle, one of the five veins that drain blood from the heart muscle (myocardium).

posthepatic cirrhosis. See **cirrhosis.**

postictal /pōst'iktəl/, referring to the period of time following a serious muscle contractions that the patient cannot control (convulsion). –**postictus,** *n.*

postinfectious, occurring after an infection.

postinfectious encephalitis. See **encephalitis.**

postinfectious glomerulonephritis, the serious form of inflamed kidneys (glomerulonephritis). It may follow 1 to 6 weeks after a streptococcal infection, most often in childhood. Symptoms of the disease are bloody urine or shortage of urine, edema, and protein in the urine. There may be small problems with kidneys in adults, but most patients recover fully in 1 to 3 months. There is no specific treatment. Protein in meals should be limited and drugs to increase passage of urine (diuretics) may be needed until the kidney is working correctly again. See also **chronic glomerulonephritis, subacute glomerulonephritis.**

postmastectomy exercises, exercises that help keep muscles from tightening up and freezing of the joints following breast removal (mastectomy). The patient should flex and straighten out the fingers of the arm on the side where the breast was removed as well as the forearm as soon as she returns to her room after recovery from anesthesia and surgery. On the first day after surgery she squeezes a rubber ball in her hand. Brushing the teeth and hair are useful exercises. Other exercises include four that are called climbing the wall, arm swinging, rope pulling, and elbow spreading. They are done as follows:

★Climbing the wall: The patient stands facing a wall, toes close to the wall. The elbows are bent and the palms of the hands are placed on the wall at shoulder height. The hands are moved up the wall together until the patient feels pain or pulling on the place where the cut was made in surgery, returned to the starting position.

★Arm swinging: While standing, the patient bends forward from the waist, letting both arms relax and hang normally. The arms are swung together from the shoulders from left to right and then in circles straight out over the floor, swinging clockwise and counterclockwise. She straightens up slowly.

★Rope pulling: A rope is looped over a shower rod or a hook. Each end of the rope is held and the patient pulls one end of the rope then the other, raising one arm after the other to the height at which pain is felt at the surgical cut or pulling can be felt. The rope is shortened until the arm on the side where the breast was removed is raised almost directly overhead.

★Elbow spreading: The hands are clasped behind the neck and the elbows are slowly raised to chin level while holding the head straight. Slowly, the elbows are spread apart to the point at which pain or pulling is felt. With proper exercise, full range of motion returns, both arms can be extended fully and equally high over the head. The patient gains by having something active to do to help herself during the hard time of learning how to cope after mastectomy. Many activities of daily life give the patient good exercise, as reaching for things on high shelves, and gardening.

postmature, overly developed or matured. See also **dysmaturity. postmaturity,** *n.*

postmature infant, an infant born after the end of the forty-second week of pregnancy, usually with signs of the placenta becoming weak. The baby may have dry, peeling skin, long fingernails and toenails, and folds of skin on the thighs and, sometimes, on the arms and buttocks. Low blood sugar and potassium are common. Postmature infants often look as if they have lost weight in the uterus. It is necessary to keep the baby from having seizures and nerve system damage. To avoid the problem, labor may be brought on before the term of pregnancy reaches 42 weeks. To lower the risk of problems, the fetus and the mother may be closely watched with electronic devices through labor.

postmenopausal, referring to the period of life following menopause.

postmortem, examination after death. Also called **autopsy, necropsy, postmortem examination.**

postmyocardial infarction syndrome, a condition that may occur days or weeks after a serious heart attack. Symptoms are fever, inflamed heart with a friction rub, pleurisy, fluid buildup, and joint pain. It tends to happen again and again and often causes serious nervousness, sadness, and fear of another heart attack. Treatment includes aspirin and steroid hormones.

postnasal drip (PND), a drop-by-drop release of nasal mucus into the back of the throat, often with a bad taste, and bad breath. Causes are the nose being irritated, sinusitis, or too-much fluid being released by the nasal mucosa. Treatment includes nose drops or sprays, drugs to shrink blood vessels, cleaning of the sinuses to help drainage, and antibiotics. Treatment for allergies may be needed, and surgery may be necessary if the nasal passages are blocked by growths or a nose defect (deviated septum).

postnecrotic cirrhosis, a form of cirrhosis that may follow a swollen liver (hepatitis) or a problem like it. Also called **posthepatic cirrhosis.** See also **cirrhosis.**

postoperative, referring to the period of time following surgery. It begins with getting over the effects of anesthesia and goes through the time needed for the effects of the anesthetic or surgery to end.

postoperative atelectasis, the lung tissue falling in on itself, caused by the slowing of breathing caused by anesthetic drugs. Deep breathing and coughing should be done often after surgery to keep this condition from happening.

postoperative bed, a bed designed for a patient who is weak or unconscious when recovering from anesthesia. The bed is in the flat position and is made in a way that makes moving a patient from a stretcher into the bed easy.

postoperative cholangiography, a way to outline the major bile ducts. A special dye is injected into the common bile duct using a tube put in during surgery. It is usually done after an operation to remove the gallbladder (cholecystectomy) in order to show any gall stones that might still be in the body. See also **cholangiography.**

postpartal care, care of the mother and her newborn baby during the first few days after childbirth (puerperium). Changes that may have occurred while the baby was in the uterus are watched. The uterus pulls in after childbirth, and causes bleeding to slow. The liquids released from the uterus (lochia) change color during the first few days. A red liquid is released for up to a week, then turns yellow, and finally, becomes clear and sticky. The muscles around the stomach and intestinal area are soft, but muscle tone comes back with time and exercise. On the third day, the milk usually begins to fill the breasts. The bond between the mother and baby may become closer by contact between the mother and baby. Breast feeding, bottle feeding, nutrition, care of the navel and diaper areas, baby baths, safety, and exercises are taught to new mothers. Blood poisoning (toxemia), bleeding, and infection are the main medical problems after childbirth, but they are not common and can usually be avoided. Being tired, enlarged breasts, sadness, and minor blood clots (thrombophlebitis) are more common, but not usual.

postpartum /pōstpär′təm/, after childbirth.

postpartum depression, an abnormal condition that may follow childbirth. Symptoms range from mild "blues" to a severe, suicidal mental state where the patient loses touch with reality (psychosis). Severe depression occurs about once in every 2,000 to 3,000 pregnancies. The cause is not known. About one-third of patients have some degree of similar problems before pregnancy. The disorder happens again in later pregnancies in 25% of cases. Women at risk are those who did not prepare for the expected baby, who had plans for work or travel after the baby's birth that could not possibly come true, or who refuse to accept the fact of being a mother. If the disorder is severe, drugs or a hospital stay may be needed.

postperfusion syndrome, an infection that occurs between 2 and 4 weeks after the replacement of old blood with new blood (transfusion) that has a virus (cytomegalovirus). Symptoms are fever, liver disease (hepatitis), rash, and a higher level of white blood cells. No certain treatment is now ready for use.

postpericardiotomy syndrome, a condition that sometimes occurs days or weeks after surgery on the heart membrane (pericardium). Symptoms include pain and the patient finding it hard to breathe, often with no fever. It can be caused by damaged cells of the heart muscle and membrane. See also **pericarditis.**

postpill amenorrhea, failure of normal menstrual cycles to start again within 3 months

after birth-control pills have stopped being used. The disorder rarely lasts forever. See also **amenorrhea.**

postpolycythemic myeloid metaplasia, a common problem with an abnormal increase in red blood cells (polycythemia vera). A main symptom is low red blood cells (anemia) caused by damage to bone marrow. Red blood cells are made only in nonbone tissue, as the liver and spleen. This condition is often made worse by a bone disease (leukemia), especially if the patient has been treated with radiation. See also **myeloid metaplasia, polycythemia.**

postprandial, after a meal.

postpubertal panhypopituitarism, a lack of pituitary hormones, especially sex hormones, following pregnancy. Blood clots in the pituitary gland during or after childbirth cause pituitary tissue death (necrosis). Symptoms are weakness, not being able to make breast milk, loss of menstrual flow and body hair, and loss of sex drive. Other effects include slow heart beat, and wasting away (atrophy) of the thyroid and adrenal glands. Treatment includes giving thyroid, adrenal, and sex hormones. Also called **Simmonds' disease, hypophyseal cachexia, pituitary cachexia.**

postpuberty, a period of about 1 to 2 years following the time when the individual is able to have reproductive activity (puberty). Bone growth slows and the reproductive functions start working normally. Also called **postpubescence. —postpuberal, postpubertal, postpubescent,** *adj.*

postrenal anuria, a lack of urine-making caused by a block in the ureters.

postsynaptic, 1. located after a gap between nerves (synapse). **2.** occurring after a synapse has been crossed by a nerve signal (impulse). See also **synapse.**

posttraumatic stress disorder, a form of nervousness with a serious traction to a tragic event. Causes may be a natural disaster, an airplane crash, or physical torture. Symptoms include going over memories or nightmares again and again; having no interest in daily life; having bad, restless sleep; and headaches. Treatment is often the use of drugs to make the patient calm (sedation) and treatment to help the patient's mental state (psychotherapy). Also called **stress reaction, stress response syndrome.** See also **combat fatigue, shell shock.**

postural albuminuria. See **orthostatic proteinuria.**

postural drainage, the use of body position to drain fluids released from the breathing tubes (bronchi) and lungs into the throat. Coughing usually gets rid of these fluids from the throat. Positions are chosen that help drainage. Pillows and other devices are used to support or raise parts of the body. The patient begins with the body straight out and level, and the head is slowly lowered. Breathing in through the nose and breathing out through the mouth is best. Tapping and shaking the body over the affected area of the lungs helps to loosen the fluids. The patient is then helped to a position to cough and breathe deeply. Outcome of this method depends on using positions that allow drainage by gravity, and breathing well and deeply. See also **cupping and vibrating.**

postural hypotension. See **orthostatic hypotension.**

postural proteinuria. See **orthostatic proteinuria.**

postural vertigo. See **cupulolithiasis.**

posture, the position of the body with respect to the space around it. A posture is made by the muscles that move the limbs, by feeling in muscles and joints (proprioception), and by the sense of balance.

potassium (K), an alkali-metal element needed by all plants and animals to live. Potassium in the body helps to control the nerves and muscles. Foods that have potassium are whole grains, meat, beans (legumes), fruit, and vegetables. Most of it is taken in through the stomach and intestines. The amount of potassium released in the urine is about equal to the amount of potassium in the food and drink taken in. The kidneys play an important role in controlling the amount that is released or taken into the system. Potassium is most often lost from the body through increased release by the kidneys, the stomach and intestines, or the skin. Increased kidney release may be caused by chemicals or drugs that increase passage of urine (diuretics), other drugs, or by kidney disorders. Loss of potassium can also occur through vomiting, diarrhea, surgical drainage, or the long-term use of laxatives. Loss through the skin is rare but can result from sweating during too-much exercise when hot.

potassium chloride (KCl), a drug to treat low blood potassium and digitalis intoxication.

★CAUTION: Too-much blood potassium, use of certain drugs (spironolactone or triamterene), or known allergy to this drug prohibits its use.

★ADVERSE EFFECTS: Among the most serious side effects are high blood levels of potassium, and open sores (ulcers) in the small bowel.

potassium iodide, a drug to treat inflammation of the breathing tubes (bronchitis), asthma, and other disorders.

★CAUTION: Serious bronchitis, pregnancy, or known allergy to this or similar drugs prohibits its use.

★ADVERSE EFFECTS: Among the more serious side effects are allergy, goiter, low levels of thyroid (myxedema), bowel problems, and skin sores.

potassium penicillin V. See **penicillin V.**

-potent, a combining form meaning 'able to do' something.

potential diabetes. See **possibility of the body's not being able to process glucose.**

potential difference, the difference in electric charge between two points.

potential trauma, a change in mouth tissue that may occur because of teeth that are improperly aligned (malocclusion).

potentiate /pōten'shē·āt/, to increase the strength or amount of activity of something.

potentiation /pōten'shē·ā'shən/, a condition in which the effect of two drugs given together is greater than the effect of the drugs given each by themselves.

potentiometer /pōten'shē·om'ətər/, a device to measure the level of electric pressure (voltage).

Pott's disease. See **tuberculosis spondylitis.**

Pott's fracture, a break of the lower leg bone (fibula) near the ankle. It often occurs with tearing of a ligament. Also called **Dupuytren's fracture.**

potty-chair, a small chair that has an open seat over a pot that can be removed, used for the toilet training of young children.

poultice /pōl'tis/, a soft, moist, substance spread between layers of gauze or cloth and placed hot onto a body surface. It may help blood flow and reduce pain. A kind of poultice is a **mustard poultice.**

povidone-iodine /pō'vidōnī'ədīn/, an antigerm chemical used to disinfect wounds. It is also used to treat infections and burns.

★CAUTION: Known allergy to this drug or to iodine prohibits its use.

★ADVERSE EFFECTS: Among the more serious side effects are itching of the skin, redness, and swelling.

Powassan virus infection, a form of brain inflammation (encephalitis) caused by a virus carried by ticks found in eastern Canada and the northern United States.

powder bed, a treatment in which large areas of the body are kept in contact with a powdered drug. It is usually repeated three times a day. An already-made bed is made ready by placing a full-sized sheet the long way over the linen. The powder is spread on the sheet from a shaker. The patient lies on the powdered sheet. Folds of skin are pushed apart with gauze, and powder is shaken over the body. The powdered sheet is then wrapped around the body in order to keep the powder touching the body.

powdered gold, a finely powdered gold, used by dentists to fill tooth cavities.

powerlessness, a feeling of a lack of control over a health problem. The patient knows that any action taken by him or her will not change the outcome of the problem. The patient may show no interest in the kind of medical care, irritability, or giving in totally to the problem; and resentment, anger, guilt, or not believing the way the problem may turn out.

pox, 1. any of several skin disorders marked by a rash of pimples, small blisters, or pus-filled sores. 2. the pitlike scars of smallpox.

poxvirus, one of a group of like (family) viruses that includes the living things that cause smallpox and vaccinia.

PPLO, abbreviation for **pleuropneumonia-like organism.** See also *Mycoplasma.*

ppm, abbreviation for *parts per million.*

practitioner, a person with the training and skills to practice in a special medical field, as a physician or nurse.

Prader-Willi syndrome, a condition marked by an inborn lack of muscle tone, too-much appetite, being overweight, and mental slowness (retardation). When diabetes mellitus occurs with these other symptoms, the condition is called Royer's syndrome. The cause may be a lack of pituitary gland hormones.

Pragmatar, a trademark for a skin balm that has a drug to control eczema (cetyl alcohol-coal tar distillate), a skin-loosening chemical (salicylic acid), and a drug to control the scabies mite (precipitates sulfur).

pralidoxime chloride /pral′ədok′sēm/, a drug used to reverse the effect (antidote) of poisoning from insect and rodent poisons and to treat drug overdosage in myasthenia gravis.
★CAUTION: Known allergy to this drug prohibits its use. It should not be used in poisoning by carbamate insect poisons.
★ADVERSE EFFECTS: Among the most serious side-effect reactions are becoming dizzy, fast heart beat, fast breathing, and weak muscles.

Pramosone, a trademark for a skin balm that has a hormone (hydrocortisone acetate) and a local anesthetic (pramoxine hydrochloride).

pramoxine hydrochloride, a local anesthetic to take away pain and itching in skin disorders, anogenital itching, hemorrhoids, and fissure, and minor burns.

prandial /pran′dē·əl/, referring to a meal; it is used in relation to timing, as after eating (postprandial) or before eating (preprandial). **prandiality,** *n.*

Prausnitz-Küstner (PK) test /prous′nitskist′nər/, a skin test in which an allergic reaction in one person is given over to a person that does not have that allergy. It is done to help find out what substance (allergen) is causing the allergy. After closely looking at an allergic patient for different diseases, a small amount of the patient's blood serum is injected beneath the skin at several places on a person who is not allergic, who is usually a relative of the allergic patient. After 24 to 48 hours, substances that are thought to cause allergies (allergens) are put on these places on the nonal-

lergic person. An allergic reaction on the skin shows that the allergen is indeed the cause of an allergy in the patient. The test is only done when skin testing cannot be done directly on the allergic person. Also called **passive transfer test, PK test.** Compare **patch test, radioallergosorbent test.** See also **anaphylaxis.**

prazepam, a calming drug (tranquilizer) used to treat abnormal worry about the future (anxiety) disorders or symptoms of anxiety.

prazosin hydrochloride /prā′zəsin/, a drug used to treat high blood pressure and congestive heart disease.
★CAUTION: Known allergy to this drug prohibits its use. Use of this drug with beta blocker drugs causes loss of consciousness.
★ADVERSE EFFECTS: Among the more serious side effects are fast heart beat, fainting, drowsiness, chest pain (angina), and a sudden drop in blood pressure.

preadmission certification, a system in which physicians must have approval in advance to admit Medicare patients to hospitals except in emergency cases. The system is intended to determine whether the patient can be treated outside the hospital to lower the cost. Emergency admissions require approval after admission.

preagonal ascites, a quick buildup of fluid in the peritoneal cavity. It happens with the passage of blood serum from veins and arteries through the membranes around them. Preagonal ascites happens before death in some cases. See also **ascites.**

preaortic node /prē′ā·ôr′tik/, one of a series of lymph nodes that serves different organs in the stomach and intestinal area.

precancerous dermatitis. See **intraepidermal carcinoma.**

Precef, a trademark for a cephalosporin-type antibiotic (ceforanide).

precipitate /prəsip′itāt, -it/, 1. to cause a substance to separate or to settle out of a liquid in which it is dissolved. 2. a substance that has separated from or settled out of a liquid in which it is dissolved. 3. an event that occurs quickly or without being expected.

precipitate delivery, childbirth that occurs with such speed or in a place where the usual preparations cannot be made. See also **emergency childbirth.**

precision rest, a stiff denture support. It is made up of two tightly fitting parts. One part rests firmly against the gums.

precocious, referring to the early, often premature, coming on of physical or mental traits.

precocious dentition, the abnormally early coming out of the baby or permanent teeth. Compare **retarded dentition.**

preconscious, 1. coming before the development of being aware of the self (self-consciousness). 2. the mental process in which thoughts, ideas, feelings, or memories can be brought into awareness. The material is thus able to be recalled, although it may not be present in the conscious mind.

precordial /prēkôr′dē·əl/, referring to the precordium, which is the part of the chest over the heart.

precordial movement, any motion of the front wall of the chest in the area over the heart.

precordial thump, a cardiopulmonary resuscitation (CPR) technique in which the fist is used to give a sharp blow to the chest when the heart has stopped beating (cardiac arrest) and a defibrillator is not available to convert the irregular electrical impulses and contractions (ventricular fibrillation) of the heart to normal impulses. It may also slow down rapid contractions (more than 100 per minute), but can cause severe problems with heart rhythms. Repeated thumps, or "fist pacing," may be successful in some patients with slowed heart beat (brady-asystolic arrest) as a temporary measure.

precursor, a part of a person's health condition that is linked to a higher or lower risk of death than the average. An example is cigarette smoking, a precursor of lung cancer.

predeciduous dentition, the structure found in the mouth of the infant before the coming out of the baby teeth. See also **deciduous dentition, teething.**

prediabetes. See **previous abnormality of glucose tolerance.**

prednisolone /prednis′əlōn/, a hormone (glucocortocoid) used to treat swelling and reddening of the skin, eyes, and for stopping the body from having an immune response (immunosuppression) to an allergic substance.

prednisone /pred′nisōn/, a hormone (glucocorticoid) used to treat severe swelling and stopping the body from having an immune response (immunosuppression) to an allergic substance.

preeclampsia /prē′iklamp′sē·ə/, an abnormal pregnancy marked by very high blood pressure after the sixth month of pregnancy. Other symptoms of preeclampsia are protein in the urine and swollen ankles (edema). It occurs in 5% to 7% of pregnancies, and most often in the first pregnancy. It is more common in some areas of the world than others, and is found most often in the southeastern United States. The risk gets higher the more the patient weighs, hydatidiform mole, or having too much amniotic fluid (hydramnios). A type of kidney injury (glomeruloendotheliosis) is a common sign pf preeclampsia. After the pregnancy, the signs and symptoms of the disease go away and the kidney disorder heals. Preeclampsia is usually typed as mild or severe. A disorder is typed mild preeclampsia if one or more of the following signs come about after the sixth month of pregnancy: blood pressure of 140/90 mm Hg, or more; protein in the urine; or swelling from fluid buildup. A disorder is typed severe preeclampsia if one or more of the following is present: blood pressure of 160/110 mm Hg or more; protein in the urine; low levels of urine; eye or brain disorders; a bluish skin color; or fluid in the lungs. Preeclampsia causes the level of nitrogen to get out of balance, the patient becomes irritable, the reflexes react too strongly, there are kidney disorders, and the body's mineral is get out of balance. Further problems include placenta coming away from the uterus, blood cell destruction, bleeding in the brain, eye damage, fluid in the lungs, and lower birth weight of the fetus. The most serious problem is a condition of coma or seizures (eclampsia), which can result in the death of the mother and fetus. Healthy living conditions, including a diet high in protein, calories and other necessary parts of a good diet, and rest may help prevent the disorder. Treatment includes rest, use of a calming drug, magnesium sulfate and high blood pressure drugs. If eclampsia is about to occur, forced childbirth or childbirth by surgical opening (cesarean section) may be necessary. See also **eclampsia.** Also called **toxemia of pregnancy.**

preexcitation, early contraction of part of the heart muscle. See also **accessory pathway.**

preferential anosmia, being unable to smell certain odors. It is often caused by mental factors linked to a certain smell or the place in which the smell occurs.

preformation, an old theory that a complete person exists in a tiny form within a sperm or egg and after fertilization grows to normal baby size. Compare **epigenesis.**

preformed water, the water found in foods.

prefrontal lobotomy, surgery in which fibers linking the front part of the frontal lobe of the brain (prefrontal lobes) and the rest of the brain are cut. The technique is rarely used today but in the past was a common way to treat certain mental patients.

Pregestimil, a trademark for a food supplement for infants.

pregnancy, the process of growth and development within a woman's reproductive organs of a new individual. It goes from the time of conception through the phases where the embryo grows and the baby develops as the fetus to birth. Pregnancy lasts about 266 days (38 weeks) from the day the egg is fertilized by the sperm, but it may last 280 days (40 weeks; 10 lunar months; 9⅓ calendar months) from the first day of the last menstrual period (LMP). The date of childbirth, or estimated date of confinement (EDC) is based on the LMP even if a woman's periods are not regular. If a woman is certain that sexual intercourse occurred only once during the month of conception and if she knows the date on which sexual intercourse occurred, the EDC may be figured as 266 days from that date. Pregnancy begins after sexual intercourse at or near the time of the egg being released (ovulation). This is usually about 14 days before a woman's next expected menstrual period. Of the millions of sperm cells in the vagina during sexual intercourse, thousands may reach the female egg (ovum) in the outer end of the fallopian tube. But only one is able to enter the egg for union of the male and female germ cells, which causes conception. The fertilized egg (zygote) is a new cell with genes that are unique. This is the original body cell of the new individual. Its cells begin to divide as it moves to the uterus where it implants itself in the wall. Parts of the woman's body and the embryo combine to form the start of the placenta, which grows into the wall of the uterus. The job of the placenta is to provide the fetus with nutrients from the woman's body and remove waste made by the fetus. However, the blood of the fetus and the woman's body do not normally mix. The embryo (conceptus) is, in some ways, like a foreign tissue skin replacement (grafts) or an animal that lives off another animal (parasite) within the mother. Though the mother normally does not have an allergic reaction, all of her tissues and organs go through change, some of which will remain for the rest of her life.

★PSYCHOLOGICAL CHANGES: The effects of pregnancy on the woman's feelings are normal and healthy, but are very different processes than before pregnancy. A pregnant woman becomes very aware of the fast and unavoidable changes her body is going through. She finds new interest in herself. Her concern for the perfection of her baby, her looking ahead to labor, and her thoughts about the new or bigger role of motherhood all serve to increase her emotions.

★CARDIOVASCULAR CHANGES: The heart must pump 30% to 50% more blood during pregnancy. The increase begins at about the sixth week, reaches a peak about the 16th week, and begins to go down after the 30th week. It returns to normal, prepregnancy level about the sixth week following childbirth (postpartum). The pulse rate rises during pregnancy to about 80 to 90 beats per minute. Blood pressure may drop slightly after the 12th week of pregnancy and return to its usual level after the 26th week. The circulation of blood to the uterus near the end of pregnancy (term) is about one liter per minute, using about 20% of the total heart output. Total blood volume also increases in pregnancy.

★PULMONARY CHANGES: Though the breathing level (vital capacity) remains the same in pregnancy, the breathing rate and other factors increase. Lung reserves get smaller.

★KIDNEY CHANGES: The rate of blood being filtered by the kidneys increases from between 30% to 50% during pregnancy. The pattern of change is a lot like that of heart function. The urinary tract expands greatly (hydronephrosis of pregnancy). It is caused by pressure on the ureters from the uterus getting bigger. The way the body is positioned has greater effects on the way the kidney works because the uterus pushes on major blood vessels. The kidney works better when the woman is lying down than when she is standing and is better when lying on the side than when on the back.

★GASTROINTESTINAL CHANGES: Hormone effects that increase during pregnancy cause some smooth muscles to relax in the stomach and intestines. Heartburn may result. Lower bowel activity and pressure on the bowel from the uterus getting bigger may result in constipation. Nausea and vomiting may occur, usually early in pregnancy, probably caused by the effect of a hormone (human chorionic gonadotropin). The chance of getting gallbladder disease is slightly higher.

★ENDOCRINE CHANGES: The way the thyroid gland works changes in a way that looks like a disorder of too-much thyroid secretion. Adrenal gland hormone levels get higher and may be the cause of streaks on the skin in the intestinal area. Sugar processing by the body is changed and the need for insulin is increased. The placenta makes four hormones. One (human chorionic gonadotropin) keeps the corpus luteum living longer early in pregnancy. A second (progesterone) supplies the lining (decidua) of the uterus, and starts the growth of the breast milk sacs (acini). A third (estrogen) starts uterine and breast growth. The fourth (human placental lactogen) starts the growth of breast tissue to get ready for the breasts making milk (lactation).

★BREAST CHANGES: The breasts become firm and more painful early in pregnancy. This tenderness is a symptom of pregnancy. As the breasts get larger and softer, the tenderness disappears. The circular area (areola) around the nipple becomes more deeply colored, and its glands become larger. As the tubules and milk sacs of the breasts grow, a clear or whitish watery substance (colostrum) begins to come out from the nipple.

★SKIN CHANGES: Sweating increases. Redness of the skin can be easily seen. Hair growth may be started. Pinpoint bleeding in the skin is very common. Streaks (stria) over the intestinal area, breasts, and buttocks appear in some women. More skin pigment (melanin) cause freckles to get darker. The dark line (linea nigra) in the midline of the lower intestinal area becomes darker and longer. The skin over the nose and above the eyebrows may get darker. This is called chloasma, or the "mask of pregnancy."

★WEIGHT CHANGES: Normal weight gain is different for each woman, within wide limits. Average weight gain is 20 to 25 pounds, but greater increases are common without problems.

★NUTRITIONAL CHANGES: The body's need for iron, protein, and calcium increase more than the body's needed overall increase in intake of calories and other nutrients.

pregnancy gingivitis, an enlargement or overgrowth of the gum tissue caused by imbalanced hormones during pregnancy.

pregnancy luteoma. See **luteoma.**

pregnanediol /pregnăn′dē·ol/, a substance found in the urine of women during pregnancy or the phase of the menstrual cycle that has fluids being released. It is formed in the body tissues from a hormone (progesterone).

preload, the first stretch of heart muscle (myocardia) fiber as blood begins to flow into the lower heart chambers (ventricles). The amount of stretch affects the force and rate of movement (velocity) of the heart muscles pulling in after the chambers become filled with blood.

Preludin, a trademark for a drug to lower the desire for eating (phenmetrazine hydrochloride).

premalignant fibroepithelioma, a raised flesh-colored tumor formed out of ribbons of tissue on a stalk. The tumor occurs most often on the lower trunk of older people. It may have a basal cell cancer.

Premarin, a trademark for sex hormone drug (estrogen).

Premarin with Methyltestosterone, a trademark for a hormone drug that has Premarin and a male sex hormone (androgen) (methyltestosterone).

premarket approval (P.M.A.), the OK given by the federal government to medical equipment companies to sell their devices to doctors and hospitals.

premature, 1. not fully grown or mature. **2.** occurring before the usual time. **–prematurity,** *n.*

premature atrial contraction, a heart disorder in which a heart chamber (atrium) contracts earlier than it should. It may be caused by stress, caffeine, or nicotine. Premature atrial beats that occur once in a while usually are not dangerous, but premature atrial contractions that occur often may cause heart flutter as well as lower the amount of blood being pumped by the heart. Also called **premature atrial beat.**

premature contraction, any contraction of the heart chambers that occurs too soon with respect to the normal heart rhythm.

premature ejaculation, an uncontrolled, untimely spurting (ejaculation) of semen. It is often caused by worry during sexual intercourse. New ways can be learned by the man and his partner to make the length of time between erection of the penis and ejaculation longer. See also **ejaculation, erection.**

premature infant, any infant, no matter what birth weight, born before 37 weeks of pregnancy. Since exact age of the fetus is often hard to know, low birth weight is an easy way to tell if the infant is premature. Prematurity may be caused by blood disorders, long-term disease, serious infection, or multiple births. Especially in countries without free healthcare systems and payments to help poor people, it is most likely to occur among women from poor backgrounds with poor nutrition

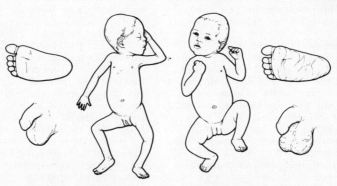

PREMATURE INFANT		TERM INFANT	
•Little subcutaneous fat	•Girls—labia majora	•More subcutaneous fat	•Girls—labia majora cover
•Poor muscle tone	separated, clitoris	•Good muscle tone	labia minora and clitoris
•Poorly developed	prominent	•Well-developed ear	•Boys—scrotum full, more
ear cartilage	•Boys—small scrotum,	cartilage	rugae
•Few creases on soles	few rugae	•Creases cover soles	
and palms		and palms	

Comparison of premature and term infants

and lack of prebirth medical care. The premature infant may appear small and scrawny, with a large head in relation to body size, and a weight of less than 2,500 grams (5.5 pounds). The skin is bright pink, smooth, shiny, and the blood vessels can be seen easily. The arms and legs are straight, not flexed, as in babies born full-term. There is little skin fat, little hair, few creases on the soles of the feet and palms, and poorly developed ear cartilage. Problems of premature babies include chilling, breathing problems, poor sucking and swallowing reflexes, and small stomachs. Other problems may include kidney, liver, and intestinal breakdown. The number of new problems and the number of premature infants that will survive is linked to the full growth of the organ systems at the time of birth. With treatment in a care unit for young babies, survival rates get better each year. Many very small babies now grow normally, and those who do not have seizures or breathing problems in the first few days after birth will not have serious damage. Also called **preterm infant.** Compare **postmature infant.**

premature labor, labor that occurs earlier in pregnancy than normal, either before the fetus has reached a weight of 2,000 to 2,500 grams (5 to 5.5 pounds) or before the 37th week of pregnancy. No one way to measure the fetus' weight or age is used to tell whether a birth is premature. If premature labor itself threatens to fetus, the outcome of pregnancy may be helped if labor can be put off. Guessing age and condition of the fetus wrongly can cause labor that is premature. Premature babies whose births have been brought about by a wrong diagnosis account for 15%of newborns in intensive care units. Also called **preterm labor.** See also **small for gestational age infant.**

premature rupture of membranes, the breaking open of the amniotic sac before the start of labor.

premature thelarche. See **thelarche.**

premature ventricular contraction (PVC), a contraction of a heart ventricle before it would normally occur. PVCs may occur once in a while, in a regular pattern, or as several in a row. They may be caused by stress, acidosis, minerals in the body getting out of balance, lack of oxygen, or a reaction to drugs. PVC often means the heart muscle is unsteady and may lead to ventricular flutter (fibrillation) and poor heart function. Also called **premature ventricular beat.**

premedication, any calming drug or other drug given before anesthesia or a test.

premenopausal, referring to the time of life before the menopause.

premenstrual tension (PMT), nervous tension, irritability, weight gain, fluid buildup, headache, and sore breasts that occur each month in the days just before the start of menstruation. There are several ideas on the cause for the condition. They include poor eating, stress, and hormones getting out of balance.

premolar /prēmō′lər/, one of eight teeth, four in the upper jaw and four in the lower jaw, found on the side and behind the canine teeth. The premolars appear during childhood and normally stay until old age. They are smaller and shorter than the canine teeth. The upper premolars are larger than the lower premolars. Also called **bicuspid.** Compare **canine tooth, incisor, molar.**

premonitory, an early symptom or sign of a disease. The term is often used to refer to minor symptoms that may come before a major health problem.

prenatal, occurring before birth. The term may refer both to the care of the woman and the growth and development of the fetus. Also called **antenatal.** See also **antepartal care.**

prenatal development, the entire process of growth that occurs between conception and birth. When an egg (ovum) is fertilized, it begins right then the process of fetal growth and birth. During the first 14 days the first cell formed by the union of sperm and egg (zygote) divides several times. It becomes a ball of cells that is ready to be attached to the wall of the uterus. From the start of the third to the end of the seventh week, this process deepens and then is finished. A very simple placenta appears, and the cell mass becomes a three-layered disk. Next, the basic structures of the body begin to form. A nerve tube grows as the first stage of a central nervous system. Simple blood vessels and blood cells, a heart tube, and umbilical cord vessels form and begin to work. Arm and leg buds may be seen, and the gut, lungs, and kidneys start to form. By the fifth week, the brain has begun to grow quickly, the heart tube splits into chambers, the roof (palate) of the mouth and the upper lip are formed, and the urinary and genital system develops. By the end of the seventh week, all basic body systems are present. The period of time from the eighth week to birth is called the fetal stage. From the eighth to the 10th week the fetus continues to grow and develop quickly. The head is almost one-half of its total length. The fetus floats in the amniotic fluid of the amniotic sac inside the uterus. The umbilical blood vessels in the cord are linked to a quickly growing placenta. By the 12th week the basic parts of the face are formed and the eyelids are present but not yet closed, as they have not split into upper and lower eyelids. There is a neck between the large head and the body, and tooth buds and nail beds have begun to form. The outer sex organs can be seen for the first time. From the 13th to the 16th weeks, the arms, legs, and trunk grow quickly, and the fetus moves a lot. Hair on the head appears. The skeleton of the fetus can be seen on an x-ray film. Breathing movements may sometimes be seen. Between the 17th and the 20th weeks of pregnancy, the mother often first feels the baby move. The fetus looks like a very small baby at this time. It has eyebrows and tiny nipples. The fetus has been seen at this age sucking its thumb and holding its own umbilical cord. At the 24th week, the outer ears are smooth and soft and the skin is wrinkled. The body is covered with downy hair (lanugo) and a fatty film (vernix) and weighs a little more than a pound. At 28 weeks, fat begins to develop under the skin, fingernails and toenails are present, the eyelids have split and the eyes may open, and the scalp hair has grown a lot. In a modern young baby (neonatal) intensive care unit, more than 80% of the babies born at 28 weeks will live. By the 32nd week, the fetus weighs between 3 and 4 pounds. The hair is fine and woolly, the fingernails and toenails have grown to the tips of the fingers and toes and there are one or two creases on the soles of the feet. The colored circles of the nipples (areolae) on the breasts can be seen. In females, the clitoris is large and the sexual lips (labia) are small and divided. At 36 weeks, the body and the arms and legs are fuller and more rounded. As the fetus reaches term, between 38 and 42 weeks, the fatty coating on the body starts to go away. In males, the testes are in the scrotum; in females, the labia majora meet in the midline and cover the labia minora and the clitoris. At 40 weeks, the average fetus weighs 7¼ pounds and is between 19 and 22 inches long. Prenatal growth may be affected by several things. Between 2 and 14 weeks of pregnancy, x-rays or other radiation and some drugs may have serious effects on body structures and workings. Various viruses, poor eating, injury, or disease in the mother may also affect a quickly growing structure or organ. After 14 weeks when all the organs, systems, and parts of the body have formed, harmful things may effect the workings of the fetus, but serious damage to the structures of the fetus is not likely to occur. See chart on pp. 632-633.

prenatal diagnosis, examining the developing fetus to find any inborn disorder or other problem. X-ray examination and tests using sound waves (ultrasound scanning) can show growth of the fetus and find certain defects. Through using a needle placed into the amniotic sac to withdraw fluids (amniocentesis), fetal cells may be obtained from the amniotic fluid to find inborn disorders and other inborn problems. Use of a device to see into the fetus (fetoscopy) allows fetal blood to be taken out from a blood vessel of the placenta and looked at for disorders, as thalassemia, sickle cell ane-

mia, and Duchenne's muscular dystrophy. Also called **antenatal diagnosis.** See also **amniocentesis, fetoscopy, genetic counseling, genetic screening.**

preoperational thought phase, a phase of child growth, during the age period of 2 to 7, when the child focuses on the use of spoken words as a tool to meet his needs.

preoperative, referring to the period of time before surgery. The preoperative period begins at the time when the surgery is decided on. Twelve hours before surgery, fluids and food by mouth are not allowed. It ends with the start of anesthesia in the operating room.

preoperative care, the care given a patient before surgery. The person's nutritional and health condition, medical and surgical history, allergies, physical handicaps, signs of infection, drugs being used, and waste elimination habits are noted and recorded. The signed informed-consent statement, the physician's orders for care before surgery, and the patient's I.D. bands are checked by a nurse. The nurse also checks to see if the patient is to receive blood, and that he or she understands how to use the call bell and knows the purpose of the bed's side rails. Blood pressure, temperature, pulse, and breathing are taken down, and any abnormal signs are reported to the physician. The physician is also told if the ECG (electrocardiogram), chest x-ray, or laboratory tests show any problems. Before bedtime, the patient showers, using an antigerm soap; nothing is given by mouth after midnight unless ordered by a physician. After preoperative drugs are given, the side rails of the bed are raised. Before leaving for the operating room, the patient urinates, and any dentures, contact lenses, and valuables are removed for safekeeping.

prepared cavity, a tooth cavity that has been made ready to be filled (restoration).

prepared childbirth. See **natural childbirth.**

prepayment, the paying before getting healthcare services, by holders of a health-insurance plan, as Blue Cross/Blue Shield.

preprandial, before a meal.

prepubertal panhypopituitarism, a lack of pituitary hormones, caused by damage to the pituitary gland. The condition occurs with a brain growth (cyst) or tumor in childhood. It causes the body to stay very small (dwarfism) with normal body shape below normal sexual development, low levels of hormone functions, and yellow, wrinkled skin. Diabetes insipidus may be present and there may be sight problems or even total blindness, but the patient's thinking is most often normal. The condition is treated with various needed hormones.

prepuberty, the period just before puberty, lasting about 2 years. During the period there are important body changes, such as quick growth

TIMETABLE OF HUMAN PRENATAL DEVELOPMENT
1 to 6 weeks

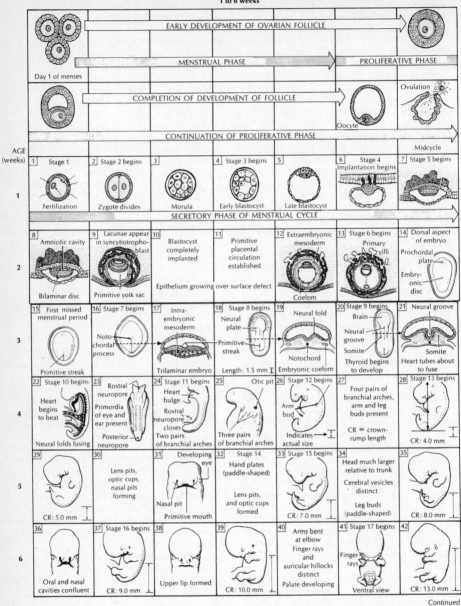

Continued.

and the first signs of pubic hair and other physical traits that come before sexual maturity. **–prepuberal, prepubertal.** *adj.*

prepuce /prē′pyo͞os/, a fold of skin that forms a cover that folds back, as the foreskin of the penis. **–prepucial, preputial,** *adj.*

prerenal anuria, a lack of urine being made caused by low blood pressure in the kidney. A certain level of blood pressure is needed to keep the kidney filtering correctly.

presbycardia /prez′bikär′dē·ə/, an abnormal heart condition, that affects mainly old persons. It is marked by the heart muscle losing its stretchiness and changes in the fibers of the

TIMETABLE OF HUMAN PRENATAL DEVELOPMENT
7 to 38 weeks

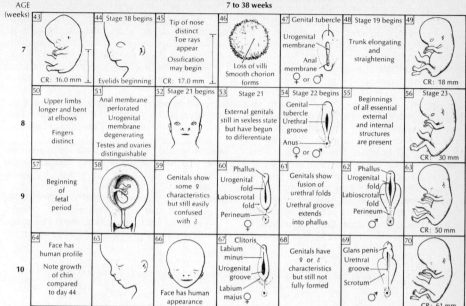

AGE (weeks)						
7	43 CR: 16.0 mm	44 Stage 18 begins / Eyelids beginning	45 Tip of nose distinct / Toe rays appear / Ossification may begin / CR: 17.0 mm	46 Loss of villi / Smooth chorion forms	47 Genital tubercle / Urogenital membrane / Anal membrane / ♀ or ♂	48 Stage 19 begins / Trunk elongating and straightening	49 CR: 18 mm
8	50 Upper limbs longer and bent at elbows / Fingers distinct	51 Anal membrane perforated / Urogenital membrane degenerating / Testes and ovaries distinguishable	52 Stage 21 begins	53 Stage 21 / External genitals still in sexless state but have begun to differentiate	54 Stage 22 begins / Genital tubercle / Urethral groove / Anus / ♀ or ♂	55 Beginnings of all essential external and internal structures are present	56 Stage 23 / CR: 30 mm
9	57 Beginning of fetal period	58	59 Genitals show some ♀ characteristics but still easily confused with ♂	60 Phallus / Urogenital fold / Labioscrotal fold / Perineum ♀	61 Genitals show fusion of urethral folds / Urethral groove extends into phallus	62 Phallus / Urogenital fold / Labioscrotal fold / Perineum ♂	63 CR: 50 mm
10	64 Face has human profile / Note growth of chin compared to day 44	65	66 Face has human appearance	67 Clitoris / Labium minus / Urogenital groove / Labium majus ♀	68 Genitals have ♀ or ♂ characteristics but still not fully formed	69 Glans penis / Urethral groove / Scrotum ♂	70 CR: 61 mm

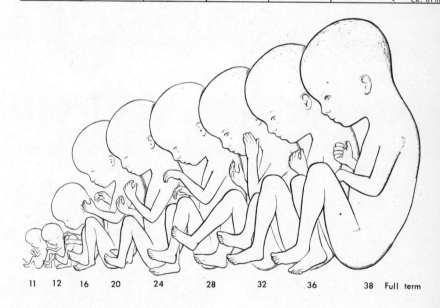

11 12 16 20 24 28 32 36 38 Full term

heart valves. It does not cause heart failure but makes older persons more subject to heart failure from other causes.

presbycusis, the normal loss of good hearing that goes with aging.

presbyopia /prez′bi·ō′pē·ə/, farsightedness caused by a loss of stretching of the lens of the eye. The condition often occurs with old age.

Compare **visual accommodation.** –**presbyopic,** *adj.*

preschizophrenic state, a period before an actual serious mental disorder (psychosis) appears when a person's behavior changes from normal although it but does not show the usual symptoms of a mental disorder, such as not being able to tell what is real (delusions), seeing things that do not exist (hallucinations), or a condition of unconsciousness (stupor).

prescreen, *informal.* a quick physical examination of a person who does not seem to be seriously ill. It may include taking a medical history of the patient.

prescribe, 1. to write an order for a drug, treatment, or process. **2.** to suggest or encourage a certain way to treat a patient for a disorder.

prescription, an order for drugs, treatment, or a device given by someone who has authority to do so, usually a doctor. The order is given to a person, such as a pharmacist, who has the power to fill the order. The prescription is usually in written form and has the name and address of the patient, the date, the ℞ symbol (superscription), the drug prescribed (inscription), directions to the pharmacist or other person who will fill the order (subscription), directions to the patient that must appear on the label, the prescriber's signature, and, usually, a code number that is needed to refill the original prescription.

prescription drug, a drug that can be given to the public only with a doctor's prescription. Only the Food and Drug Administration (a federal branch of government) can classify a drug as a prescription drug. See also **ethical drug.**

presenile dementia. See **Alzheimer's disease.**

presenting part, the part of the fetus that is closest to the opening of the cervix, just before or during labor.

present health, the health condition of a patient at that time, with any recent changes, as the symptoms that made the person get health care.

preservation, the uncontrolled repeating of the same words or a repeated muscle movement, no matter what caused it to start. The condi-

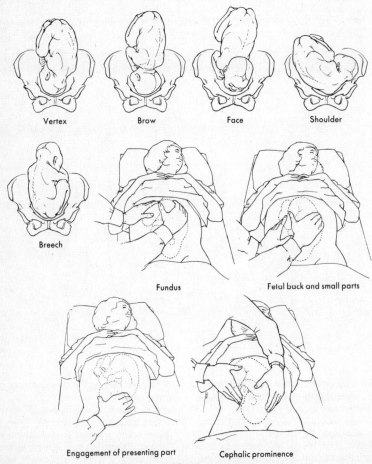

Vertex   Brow   Face   Shoulder

Breech

Fundus   Fetal back and small parts

Engagement of presenting part   Cephalic prominence

Palpation of fetal presentation

tion occurs in patients with brain damage or physical mental disorders. It may also appear in patients with schizophrenia.

pressor /pres'ər/, a substance that often causes blood pressure to go up.

pressure, a force, or stress, put against a surface by a fluid or an object.

pressure acupuncture, one kind of acupuncture in which pressure, as from the tip of a finger, is put on certain points of the body. See also **acupuncture.**

pressure area, an area of the mouth that is likely to get damage to the soft tissue by a denture or other dental device.

pressure bandage, a bandage put on to stop bleeding, stop swelling, or give support for varicose veins.

pressure dressing, a dressing put on firmly to put pressure on something, most often on a wound, to stop loss of blood.

pressure edema, 1. swelling of the legs caused by a pregnant uterus pushing against the large veins of the lower abdomen. **2.** a swelling of the scalp of the fetus after of the head has come out of the mother's body.

pressure point, 1. a point over an artery where the pulse may be felt. Pressure on the point often helps to stop the flow of blood from a wound past that point. **2.** a place that is very sensitive to pressure, as the phrenic pressure point, along the phrenic nerve on the right shoulder. Pressure at this place may be a sign of gallbladder disease.

presumptive signs, signs of a pregnancy that may not mean the woman is pregnant. Presumptive signs may include missing a menstrual period and morning sickness. See also **Chadwick's sign.**

presymptomatic disease, an early phase of disease when changes in the body have begun although no signs or symptoms are felt or seen.

presynaptic, 1. located near or before a nerve gap (synapse). **2.** something that occurs in a nerve before a synapse is crossed.

presynaptic element, any nerve cell structure, as a neuron, located before a synapse.

presystolic, referring to the period before systole or contraction of the heart muscle.

preterm infant. See **premature infant.**

preterm labor. See **premature labor.**

pretibial /prētib'ē-əl/, referring to the area in front of the lower leg bone (tibia).

pretibial fever, an infection in which one of the signs is a rash on the front of the legs. Other symptoms are headache, chills, fever, and muscle pain. Also called **Fort Bragg fever.**

prevalence /prev'ələns/, the number of all new and old cases of a disease during a certain period of time.

prevention, any action taken to prevent illness and help make for good health.

preventive, referring to things that slow, stop, or break up the path of an illness or to lower the risk of a disease.

preventive care, medical care that focuses on preventing disease and on keeping people in good health. It includes early finding of disease, finding those people at risk of getting certain diseases or health problems, counseling, and other ways to help patients avoid a health problem. Screening tests, health education, and getting vaccine shots (immunization) are common examples of preventive care.

preventive treatment, any procedure designed to keep a disease from occurring or a mild disorder from getting more severe. Various diseases are prevented by shots with vaccines, antiinfection measures, regular exercise, diet, enough rest, and screening programs to detect diseases. Also called **prophylactic treatment.**

previa /prē'vē-ə/, *informal.* placenta previa. Also spelled **praevia.**

previous abnormality of glucose tolerance, the condition of patients who before had had diabetic excess blood sugar (hyperglycemia) or a problem in the body's glucose tolerance but whose blood glucose levels have gone back to normal. Included are persons who had gestational diabetes and overweight persons whose blood glucose levels returned to normal. Previously called latent diabetes, prediabetes. See also **diabetes mellitus.**

previtamin. See **provitamin.**

priapism /prī'əpiz'əm/, a problem with the penis remaining erect too long. This is often painful and is not often linked to being sexually excited. It may be caused by urinary stone (calculi) or a sore inside the penis or the central nervous system. It sometimes occurs in men who have sickle cell anemia or severe leukemia. Treatment may include surgery.

priapitis /prī'əpī'tis/, swelling and redness of the penis.

prickle cell layer. See **stratum spinosum.**

prickly heat. See **miliaria.**

prilocaine hydrochloride /pril'ōkān/, a local anesthetic used to block the nerves and for regional anesthesia.

primaquine phosphate /prī'məkwin/, a drug used to treat malaria and keep it from coming back during recovery from the disease.

★CAUTION: Arthritis, use of bone marrow depressants or related drugs, or known allergy to this drug prohibits its use.

★ADVERSE EFFECTS: Among the more serious side effects are blood disorders, and pain in the stomach and intestines.

primary, 1. first in order of time, place, development, or importance. **2.** not gotten or taken from any other source or cause, as the original condition or set of symptoms in disease processes.

primary afferent fiber, a sensory nerve fiber that carries signals from the fibers of the muscle spindle to the central nervous system when the muscles contract. See also **gamma efferent fiber.**

primary amenorrhea. See **amenorrhea.**

primary amputation, removal of a body part using surgery (amputation) done after severe injury, when the patient has gotten over shock, and before infection has set in. Compare **secondary amputation.**

primary amyloidosis. See **amyloidosis.**

primary apnea, a total lack of breathing. It may come after a blow to the head and is common right after birth in the newborn baby who may not breathe until the carbon dioxide in the blood reaches a certain level. Reflexes are present and the heart is beating, but the skin color may be pale or blue. No treatment is needed, but keeping the body temperature steady, and clearing of the breathing passageways are usually done. Within seconds the baby usually begins breathing, becomes pinker, moves the arms and legs, and cries. Compare **periodic apnea of the newborn, secondary apnea.**

primary atelectasis, failure of the lungs to expand fully at birth. It is most often seen in babies born before full term or those drugged by anesthetics given to the mother. The infant is usually cared for in an incubator in which the temperature and humidity may be closely watched. Changing the position often of the infant is needed to help breathing, along with using a vacuum machine to suck out liquids released into the breathing tubes. Very slow feedings are given to avoid stomach bloating.

primary atypical pneumonia. See **mycoplasma pneumonia.**

primary biliary cirrhosis, a swelling of the liver. Symptoms are general itching, the liver getting larger, weight loss, and diarrhea with pale, bulky stools. Pinpoint bleeding in the skin, nose bleeds, or bleeding caused by blood coagulation defects may also occur. Broken bones and collapsed back bones may occur because of the body not absorbing vitamin D and calcium from the stomach and intestines. Doctors do not know the cause of the disease. The condition most often affects women 40 to 60 years of age. Treatment often includes taking vitamins A, D, E, and K to prevent and stop shortages caused by the body not absorbing enough nutrients from the intestines (malabsorption). When treatment is begun in the early stages of the condition, the outcome is excellent. The life expectancy is about 5 years for patients after the onset of liver disease (jaundice). Compare **secondary biliary cirrhosis.**

primary bronchus, one of the two main air passages that branch from the windpipe (trachea) and take air to the lungs. The bronchi, like the trachea, are made up of rings of cartilage, tissue made up of fibers, mucous membrane, and glands. A hook-shaped ridge (carina) at the bottom of the trachea separates the two primary bronchi. It is located to the left of the middle line so that the right primary bronchus is a more direct continuation of the trachea than the left. As a result, foreign objects that come into the trachea usually drop into the right bronchus rather than the left.

primary carcinoma, the first area where a cancer appears, the place where it started.

primary care, the first contact with a doctor for treatment of illness, that leads to a decision on a way to treat a health problem.

primary degenerative dementia. See **senile psychosis.**

primary dental caries, dental decay that occurs in the enamel of a tooth that was free of disease before.

primary dentition. See **deciduous dentition.**

primary gain, a benefit, such as getting over an emotional conflict and freedom from worry, which the patient is able to do by using a thought or action to block the bad thoughts (defense mechanism) or other mental process. Compare **secondary gain.**

primary host. See **definitive host.**

primary physician, the physician who usually takes care of a person; the physician who first sees a patient for the care of a health problem.

primary relationships, personal relationships with sexual partners, close friends, and family.

primary sensation, a feeling or sense that comes directly from something that causes the sensation (stimulus).

primary sequestrum, a piece of dead bone that totally comes away from healthy, nonbroken bone during the process of tissue death. Compare **secondary sequestrum.**

primary shock, a state of physical collapse much like fainting. It may be caused by slight pain or by fright. Primary shock is often mild, and will go away by itself in a short time. Severe injury may make the shock last longer and merge primary shock with secondary shock. Compare **hemorrhagic shock.**

primary tuberculosis, the childhood form of tuberculosis. It often occurs in the lungs, the back of the throat, or the skin. Infants are prone to infection. They also are especially open to quick and bodywide spread of the infection through their bodies. In childhood, the disease is often quickly over, with lymph gland disorders. The tuberculin test will show signs of having tuberculosis for the rest of one's life. See also **tuberculosis.**

prime mover, a muscle that acts directly to bring about a movement. Most movements of the body need the combined action of many muscles. Compare **antagonist, fixation muscle, synergist.**

primidone /prī′mədōn/, a drug to control muscle spasms (anticonvulsant) used to treat seizure disorders, including grand mal, psychomotor, and focal epilepsy-like seizures.

★CAUTION: Porphyria or known allergy to this or similar drugs prohibits its use.

★ADVERSE EFFECTS: The most serious side effect is shortage of red blood cells in the blood (anemia). Drowsiness, loss of control of those muscles we can control by will (ataxia), and dizziness are common.

primigravida /prim′igrav′idə/, a woman pregnant for the first time, shown by the term "gravida I" on the woman's medical records. Also called gravida. Compare multigravida, primapara. –primigravid, adj.

primipara /primip′ərə/, pl. primiparae, a woman who has given birth to one healthy infant, shown by the term "para 1" on the woman's medical records. Compare multipara, nullipara, primagravida.

primitive, formed early in the course of growing; existing in an early or simple form. Compare definitive.

primitive reflex, any unthinking action (reflex) normal in an infant or fetus. Having this in an adult usually means serious nerve disease. Some kinds of primitive reflexes are grasp reflex, Moro reflex, sucking reflex.

primordial /prīmôr′dē·əl/, 1. the most undeveloped or simple form of those cells or tissues that begin to grow in the early stages of the life of the embryo. 2. first or original; primitive.

primordial cyst, a fluid-filled sac that grows in the jaw from dental tissue in the embryo.

primordial dwarf, a person who is very short but is otherwise normal. The person has normally shaped body parts and normal mental and sexual development. The condition may be inborn, with some problem in the body being able to use growth hormones, or the disorder may occur with no real pattern within the population. Also called hypoplastic dwarf, normal dwarf, physiologic dwarf, pure dwarf, true dwarf. See also pituitary dwarf, pygmy.

primordial germ cell, any large round cells formed in the embryo that will be future eggs (ova) or sperm. They are formed outside the gonads and move later to the ovaries and testes. See also oogenesis, spermatogenesis.

primordium /prīmôr′dē·əm/, pl. primordia, the first phase in the embryo body when groups of cells that will develop in various organs, tissues, or structures, can be seen. Also called anlage, rudiment.

principal cell. See chief cell.

Principen, a trademark for an antibiotic (ampicillin).

principle, 1. a truth or rule of action. 2. a main beginning point or element from which anything continues. 3. a law on which others are based or from which others are taken.

Prinzmetal's angina, an unusual form of chest pain (angina) that occurs at rest rather than with activity. It can happen with blockage or spasms of the coronary arteries. Also called Prinzmetal's variant angina.

priority, actions planned in order of importance or urgency to the health of the patient, or other person at a given time.

Priscoline Hydrochloride, a trademark for a drug that enlarges blood vessels located away from the center of the body (tolazoline hydrochloride).

privileges, rights given to a physician or dentist by a hospital governing board to give care to the hospital's patients. Clinical privileges are limited to the doctor's license, experience, and skill. Emergency privileges may be given by a hospital in an emergency without regard to the physician or dentist's normal standing. Temporary privileges may be given to a physician or dentist to give health care to patients for a limited period or to a certain patient.

Privine Hydrochloride, a trademark for a drug that increases the activity of nerves (naphazoline hydrochloride).

p.r.n., (in prescriptions) abbreviation for a Latin phrase (pro re nata) meaning "as needed."

proaccelerin. See factor V.

probable signs, medical signs of a strong chance of pregnancy. Examples include enlargement of the abdomen, softening of the cervix (Goodell's sign), muscle contractions in the uterus (Braxton Hick's sign) and hormone test results that show pregnancy is likely. Compare presumptive signs.

Pro-Banthine, a trademark for an ulcer drug (propantheline bromide).

probenecid /prōben′əsid/, a uric acid and antibiotic drug used to treat an inborn form of arthritis (gout). It is also used to prolong the action of other drugs used to treat some infections, as gonorrhea.

★CAUTION: Kidney stones, blood disorders, or known allergy to this drug prohibits its use. It is not started during serious attack of gout. It is not given to children under 2 years of age. Use of drugs, as aspirin, lowers the effect of probenecid.

★ADVERSE EFFECTS: Among the most serious side effects are low levels of red blood cells in the blood (anemia), headache, frequent urination, and minor allergic reactions. It reacts with many other drugs.

problem, any health-care condition that needs testing and treatment.

probucol, a drug used to treat high cholesterol levels in patients who have not reacted well to diet, weight control, or other treatments.

★CAUTION: Known allergy to this drug prohibits its use.

★ADVERSE EFFECTS: Among the most serious

side effects are heart disorders, fainting, dizziness, and numbness.

procainamide hydrochloride /prōkān'əmīd/, a drug used to treat various heart disorders.
★CAUTION: Myasthenia gravis, heart block, or known allergy to this or drugs like it prohibits its use.
★ADVERSE EFFECTS: Among the more serious side effects are stomach and intestinal problems, allergic reactions, and white blood cell disorders.

procarbazine hydrochloride, an anticancer drug used to treat various cancers, including Hodgkin's disease and lymphomas.

Procardia, a trademark for a calcium channel blocker (nifedipine).

procaryon. See **prokaryon.**

procaryosis. See **prokaryosis.**

Procaryotae /prōker'ē·ō'tē/, a group of plants that includes bacteria.

procaryote. See **prokaryote.**

procerus /prəsir'əs/, one of three muscles of the nose. It pulls down the eyebrows and wrinkles the nose. Compare **depressor septi, nasalis.**

process, 1. a series of linked events that follow one after another from a given state or condition. **2.** a natural growth that comes out from a bone or other body part.

process schizophrenia, a form of mental disorder (schizophrenia) caused by tissue changes in the brain rather than by outside causes. The start of the disease is usually slow and moves slowly or rapidly to a mental state that cannot be reversed. Compare **reactive schizophrenia.** See also **schizophrenia.**

processus vaginalis peritonei, a pocket of the membrane in the embryo that goes through the stomach and intestinal wall (inguinal canal). In males it goes down into the scrotum to form a membrane around the testicles; in females it fails to grow further. Also called **Nuck's canal, Nuck's diverticulum.**

prochlorperazine, a drug used to combat mental disorders (antipsychotic) and control vomiting and nausea (antiemetic).

prochromosome. See **karyosome.**

procidentia, the falling or dropping down of an organ, such as the uterus.

procoagulant, an agent that promotes blood clotting. Examples include fibrinogen and prothrombin.

proconvertin. See **factor VII.**

procreation, the entire process of producing offspring. **–procreate,** v.

proctitis /proktī'tis/, swelling and reddening of the rectum and anus caused by infection, injury, drugs, allergy, or radiation injury. Serial or long-term symptoms are minor pain and the urge to defecate without being able to do so. Pus, blood, or mucus may be present in the stools, and straining (tenesmus) may be present. Also called **rectitis.**

procto-, proct-, a combining form referring to the rectum.

proctocele. See **rectocele.**

proctocolectomy /prok'tōkələk'təmē/, a surgical procedure in which the anus, rectum, and colon are removed. An artificial passage is created for the removal of feces. It is a common treatment for severe, uncontrollable ulcerative colitis. See also **ileoanal anastomosis.**

Proctocort, a trademark for an adrenal hormone (hydrocortisone).

proctology /proktol'əjē/, the branch of medicine that deals with treating disorders of the colon, rectum, and anus.

proctoscope, an instrument used to look at the rectum and the lower end of the colon. It consists of a light mounted on a tube. Compare **sigmoidoscope.**

proctoscopy, a checking of the rectum with a device designed to look at the inside of the intestine (proctoscope).

prodromal labor, the early period in childbirth before contractions of the uterus become strong and frequent enough to cause the enlargement of the uterine cervix.

prodrome, 1. an early sign of a health disorder or disease. **2.** an early stage of a disorder or disease. **–prodromal,** adj.

productive cough, a sudden, noisy movement of air from the lungs. It usually forces sputum from the breathing tract, clearing the air passages and allowing oxygen to reach the air sacs (alveoli). Coughing is brought on by irritation of the breathing tract. Inhaling deeply and then contracting the diaphragm and muscles between the ribs and exhaling with force helps patients with breathing tract infections bring on productive coughing. Drugs that turn mucus into liquid (mucolytic agents) in the breathing tract help bring it up so it can be forced out more easily. Other drugs, as atropine, reduce the amount of mucus. See also **nonproductive cough.**

Professional Standards Review Organization (PSRO), an organization formed under the Social Security Act Amendments of 1972 to look at the services given under Medicare, Medicaid, and Maternal Child Health programs. Physicians review the programs to decide if they are needed and to ensure they follow certain standards in proper settings.

progenitive, capable of creating offspring.

progenitor, 1. a parent or ancestor. **2.** anything or anyone that starts or goes before; a precursor.

progeny /proj'ənē/, **1.** offspring; an individual or living thing that comes from a mating. **2.** the descendants of a known or common ancestor.

progeria /prōjē'rē·ə/, an abnormal condition marked by early aging. It commonly begins with the appearance in childhood of gray hair, wrinkled skin, and small size. There may be the posture and body build of an aged person and a lack of pubic and facial hair. Death usually occurs before 20 years of age. Compare **infantilism.**

progestagen. See **progestogen.**

Progestasert, a trademark for a female sex hormone (progesterone).

progestational /prō'jestā'shənəl/, referring to a drug with effects like those of progesterone, the female sex hormone. Natural and synthetic kinds of progesterone are used to treat a disorder in which a woman who has menstruated normally stops menstruation (secondary amenorrhea) and has abnormal bleeding of the uterus. Progestational compounds are used in birth-control pills.

progesterone /prəjes'tərōn/, a natural progestational hormone used to treat various menstrual disorders and inability to become pregnant. ★CAUTION: Blood clotting, liver problems, breast cancer, missed abortion, or allergy to this drug prohibits its use. ★ADVERSE EFFECTS: Among the more serious side effects are pain at the place of injection, and problems in the body's chemical processes.

progestin 1. progesterone. **2.** any of a group of hormones, natural or synthetic, released by the corpus luteum, placenta, or adrenal cortex. They have progesteronelike effects on the uterus.

progestogen, any natural or synthetic female sex (progestational) hormone. Also spelled **progestagen.** Also called **progestin.**

prognathism /prog'nəthiz'əm/, condition in which the face looks abnormal because one or both jaws project forward. One form, called real prognathism, is present when both the lower and upper jaws grow longer or when the lower jaw is normal and the upper jaw grows longer than is normal. Another form (imaginary prognathism) is present when the lower jaw is shorter than normal and the upper jaw length is normal. **–prognathic,** *adj.*

prognosis, predicting the likely outcome of a disease based on the condition of the patient and the usual action of the disease.

progressive, referring to the process of the signs and symptoms of a disease or condition becoming more obvious and severe as it develops.

progressive myonecrosis. See **myonecrosis.**

progressive patient care, a system of care in which patients are placed in units on the basis of their needs for care. The needs are based on the degree of illness. The usual levels of progressive patient care are intensive care, intermediate care, and minimal care.

progressive relaxation, a way to combat tension and worry by tensing and relaxing groups of muscles in sequence.

progressive resistance exercise, a way to increase the strength of a weak or injured muscle by slowly increasing the force against which the muscle works. An example is the use of heavier and heavier weights over a period of time. Also called **graduated resistance exercise.** See also **active resistance exercise.**

progressive spinal muscular atrophy of infants. See **Werdnig-Hoffmann disease.**

progressive systemic sclerosis (PSS), the most common form of hardening of the skin (scleroderma).

projection, 1. anything that thrusts or juts outward, as from a bone. **2.** a subconscious way to defend oneself by attributing traits, ideas, or actions that one cannot accept in oneself on another person.

projectile vomiting, vomiting that is very forceful.

projective test, a mental test that uses inkblots, a series of pictures, or unfinished sentences to bring out responses that show the patient's true personality. See also **Rorschach test.**

prokaryocyte /prōker'ē·əsīt'/, a cell without a true nucleus. It may have nuclear material scattered throughout the cytoplasm. Bacteria, viruses, and other disease organisms are prokaryocytes. Also spelled **procaryocyte.** Compare **eukaryocyte.**

prokaryon /prōker'ē·on/, cell nucleus parts that are not bound by a membrane but are spread throughout the protoplasm of a cell outside the nucleus (cytoplasm). Compare **eukaryon.**

prolactin (PRL) /prōlak'tin/, a hormone that is made and released into the bloodstream by the pituitary gland. Prolactin, acting with other hormones, starts the growth of the mammary glands. After childbirth, it helps to start and maintain the making of breast milk. This occurs in response to suckling by the infant. When suckling stops, prolactin slows and the breasts stop making milk. Also called **lactogenic hormone, luteotropin.**

prolapse /prō'laps, prōlaps'/, the falling, sinking, or sliding of an organ from its normal position or place in the body, as a prolapsed uterus.

prolapsed cord, an umbilical cord that comes out of the mother beside or before the first part of the fetus to appear during childbirth.

proliferation, the rapid spread of like forms of tissues. The term often refers to increases of cells or lumps (cysts).

proliferative phase, the phase of the menstrual cycle following menstruation. Under the effect of FSH (follicle stimulating hormone) from the pituitary gland, the ovary makes more estrogen. This causes the lining of the uterus to become thick and rich in blood supply. The phase ends with releasing of the egg (ovulation). Compare **menstrual phase, secretory phase.**

proline (Pro), an unimportant amino acid found in many proteins of the body, especially collagen. See also **amino acid, protein.**

Proloid, a trademark for a thyroid hormone drug (thyroglobulin).

prolonged release, the trait or quality of a drug that is released over a long period of time. The most common form is a drug in a soft capsule that dissolves and has tiny pellets of the drug for release at different rates in the intestine. Special resins that cling to drugs and liquids that have slow-release drug granules mixed with them are also used to extend drug action.

Proloprim, a trademark for an antibiotic (trimethoprim).

promethazine hydrochloride, an antihistamine and calming drug used to treat motion sickness, nausea, irritation of the mucus in the nose (rhinitis), itching, and skin rash.

prompt insulin zinc suspension, a fast-acting insulin used to treat diabetes mellitus when a fast, intense response is needed. Its action is only slightly slower than a shot of insulin. See also **fast-acting insulin.**

promyelocyte /prōmī'ələsīt/, a large, simple white blood cell form not normally present in the circulation. It is a sign of leukemia.

pronation /prōnā'shən/, **1.** a lying-flat position, in which the body faces downward. **2.** the turning of the forearm so that the palm of the hand faces downward and backward. **3.** the lowering of the inner edge of the foot by turning it outward. **–pronate,** *v.,* **prone,** *adj.*

pronator teres, a muscle of the forearm. It turns the hand downward or backward (pronates).

prone, referring to the position of the body when lying face downward. Compare **supine.**

Pronemia, a trademark for a body-building drug containing iron, vitamin B_{12}, a chemical to allow vitamin B_{12} to be absorbed (intrinsic factor concentrate), vitamin C, and folic acid.

proneness profile, a process that predicts growth problems in the early years of a child's life. Screening may begin during prenatal care and continue after childbirth. Growth problems are predicted based on the health of the mother and infant at the time of childbirth, problems during pregnancy, childbirth, and the period right after childbirth. The infant is screened for alertness, activity, and response patterns.

Pronestyl, a trademark for a drug that slows the heart rate (procainamide hydrochloride).

pronucleus, *pl.* **pronuclei,** the nucleus of the egg or the sperm after fertilization but before the two sets of chromosomes have united to form the nucleus of the original cell of the embryo (zygote). Also called **germ nucleus, germinal nucleus.** See also **oogenesis, spermatogenesis.**

propantheline bromide, a drug used to treat peptic ulcer.

proparacaine hydrochloride /prōper'əkān/, a fast-acting, local anesthetic used for various eye (ophthalmological) procedures, including removing foreign objects from the eye. One drop gives 15 minutes of eye anesthesia. Also called **proxymetacaine.**

prophase /prō'fāz/, the first phase of nuclear division of tissue cells (mitosis) and of germ cells (meiosis). See also **anaphase, interphase, meiosis, metaphase, mitosis, telophase.**

prophylactic /prō'filak'tik/, **1.** keeping a disease from spreading. **2.** a drug that stops the spread of disease. See also **condom. –prophylactically,** *adv.*

prophylactic odontomy, a kind of dental surgery to take out harmful pits and crevices in the molars.

prophylactic treatment. See **preventive treatment.**

prophylaxis /prō'filak'sis/, prevention of or protection against disease. It may mean using a biological, chemical substance, or mechanical device to destroy germs or viruses or keep them from entering the body.

Propionibacterium, a kind of bacteria found on the skin of humans, in the gut of humans and animals, and in dairy products. One species (*P. acne*) is common in acne blisters.

propionicacidemia /prō'pē·on'ikas'idē'mē·ə/, an inborn defect in which the body is not able to use certain amino acids (threonine, isoleucine, and methionone). It causes mental and physical retardation. Acidosis is also caused by a buildup of substances that come from acid. A diet low in certain amino acids is the only treatment. **–propionicacidemic,** *adj.*

Proplex, a trademark for human clotting factor IX.

propositus /prōpoz'itəs/, a patient whose ancestry is traced to find the way a disease or a physical trait is passed on to members of the family.

propoxyphene /prōpok'səfēn/, a mild narcotic painkiller used to relieve mild to moderate pain.
★CAUTION: Use of calming or antidepressant drugs, current alcohol or drug abuse, or known allergy to aspirin prohibits use of this drug. It should be not used by people who may want to kill themselves, those who may tend toward alcohol or drug addiction, or pregnant women.
★ADVERSE EFFECTS: Among the more serious side effects are liver problems and severe slowing of the central nervous system from a drug overdose or reaction with another drug. Some patients may have nausea, dizziness, sleepiness, or vomiting when given the drug.

propoxyphene hydrochloride, a painkiller used to relieve mild to moderate pain.
★CAUTION: Known allergy to this drug or known narcotic addiction prohibits its use.
★ADVERSE EFFECTS: Among the more serious side effects are slowed or shallow breathing, excitement, and muscle spasms.

propranolol hydrochloride, a nerve-blocking agent used to treat chest pain (angina pectoris), irregular heart rhythm, and high blood pressure.

★CAUTION: Asthma, irregular heart rhythms, heart failure, use of monamine oxidase (MAO) inhibitors, or known allergy to this drug prohibits its use.

★ADVERSE EFFECTS: Among the more serious side effects are heart failure, heart block, breathing difficulty, stomach and intestine problems, and allergic reactions. Withdrawal symptoms may occur in some patients.

proprietary, referring to an institution or a product, as a drug or device, run or made for profit.

proprietary hospital, a hospital run as a profit-making organization. Many such hospitals are owned by physicians who run the hospital mainly for their own patients but also accept patients from other physicians.

proprietary medicine, any drug that is protected from competition from other drug makers because the chemicals it is made out of or the way it is made are secret or protected by trademark or copyright.

proprioception /prō′prē·əsep′shən/, feeling linked to cues from within the body. The cues help one to know the positions of body parts and the motions of the muscles and joints.

proprioceptor /prō′prē·əsep′tər/, any sensory nerve ending that responds to cues from within the body regarding movement and position of body parts. They are located in the middle ear, muscles, joints, and tendons. Compare **exteroceptor, interoceptor.** See also **mechanoreceptor.**

proptosis /proptō′sis/, bulging, pushing out or out of place of a body organ or area.

proscribe, to forbid. **–proscriptive,** *adj.*

prosencephalon /pros′ensef′əlon/, the part of the brain that has the thalamus and hypothalamus. It controls important body functions and affects thinking, appetite, and feelings. Also called **forebrain.** Compare **mesencephalon.** **–prosencephalic,** *adj.*

Pro Sobee, a trademark for a milk-substitute formula made from soybeans and has no milk in it. It is given to infants with a milk processing disorder (galactosemia) and patients who cannot drink milk without a harmful reaction. See also **galactosemia, lactose intolerance.**

prosopalgia. See **trigeminal neuralgia.**

prosopopilary virilism /pros′əpōpī′lərē/, a heavy growth of facial hair.

prospective study, a study to find a link between a health condition and a factor shared by some members of a group. The group selected is healthy at the beginning of the study. Some but not all of the members of the group share a certain health factor, as smoking. The study follows the group over a period of years, noting the rate at which a condition, as lung cancer, occurs in the smokers and in the nonsmokers. Compare **retrospective study.**

prostacyclin **(PGI₂),** a prostaglandin, it is formed mainly in human blood vessel walls and slows blood platelet clumping.

prostaglandin (PG) /pros′təglan′din/, one of several strong hormonelike fatty acids that act in small amounts on certain organs. They are made in tiny amounts and have many different effects. Prostaglandins given by nasal spray, in tablets, or dissolved in liquids cause changes in smooth muscle tone, hormone functions, and in the autonomic and central nervous systems. Prostaglandins are used to end pregnancy and to treat asthma and too-much stomach acid.

Prostaphlin, a trademark for an antibiotic (oxacillin sodium).

prostate /pros′tāt/, a gland in men that surrounds the neck of the bladder and the urethra. It releases a substance that makes semen into a liquid. It is a firm structure about the size of a chestnut, and is made up of muscular and glandular tissue. It is located in front of the rectum, through which it can be felt, especially when enlarged. The ducts that control ejaculation pass on an angle through the back part of the gland. The substance released by the prostate gland is made up of alkaline phosphatase, citric acid, and various proteolytic enzymes. **–prostatic,** *adj.*

prostatectomy /pros′tətek′təmē/, surgical removal of part of the prostate gland. It may be done for an enlarged prostate (benign prostatic hypertrophy). If the gland is cancerous, total removal may be necessary. The most common way (transurethral) uses an instrument put in through the urethra. Shavings of tissue from the prostate gland are cut off at the bladder opening. An opening between the scrotum and anus is used to remove tissue for examination when early cancer is suspected or when stones (calculi) are removed. Another opening is made above the penis and a large tube is placed in the bladder through an opening in the intestinal wall. After surgery, bloody urine is likely for several days. Problems that may occur after the operation include blocking of urine flow, inability to control urination, and sexual failure.

prostatic /prostat′ik/, referring to the prostate gland.

prostatic catheter, a tube that is about 16 inches long. It is used in men when an enlarged prostate gland blocks the urethra. The tube is used to drain the bladder, which is beyond the prostate.

prostatic ductule /duk′tyo͞ol/, any one of 12 to 20 tiny tubes that carry substances released by the prostate gland to the urethra.

prostatitis /pros′tətī′tis/, a swelling of the prostate gland, usually caused by infection. The patient feels urgent needs to urinate frequently and has a burning sensation during urination. It is treated with antibiotics, sitz baths, bed rest, and fluids. Compare **benign prostatic hypertrophy.**

prostatomegaly, enlargement of the prostate gland.

prosthesis /prosthē'sis/, *pl.* **prostheses, 1.** a device designed to replace a missing part of the body. **2.** a device designed and applied to make a part of the body work better, as a hearing aid or denture. See also **artificial limb, maxillofacial prosthesis, Starr-Edwards prosthesis.**

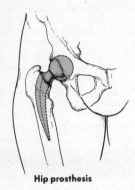

Hip prosthesis

prosthodontics /pros'thədon'tiks/, a branch of dentistry that deals with making artificial devices that take the place of missing teeth.

Prostin VR Pediatric, a trademark for a form of prostaglandin (alprostadil).

prostration, a condition of being severely worn out and unable to exert oneself further, as from heat or stress.

protamine sulfate /prō'təmēn/, a drug produced from fish sperm used to lower or reverse the effect of an overdose from a drug used to block blood clotting (heparin).

★CAUTION: Pregnancy, allergy to fish, or known allergy to this drug prohibits its use.

★ADVERSE EFFECTS: Among the more serious side effects are low blood pressure, troubled breathing, and slow heart beat.

protamine zinc insulin suspension, a long-acting insulin that is absorbed slowly at a steady rate. Some patients can be treated with only one injection daily.

protanopia. See **daltonism.**

protease /prō'tē·ās/, an enzyme that helps the breakdown of protein. See also **proteolytic.**

protein /prō'tē·in, prō'tēn/, any of a large group of complex, organic nitrogen compounds. Each is made up of linked amino acids that have the elements carbon, hydrogen, nitrogen, and oxygen. Some proteins also have sulfur, phosphorus, iron, iodine, or other necessary elements of living cells. Twenty-two amino acids have

been identified as necessary for body growth, development, and health. The body can make 14 of these amino acids, called nonessential, while the other eight must be obtained from food. Protein is the main building material for muscles, blood, skin, hair, nails, and the inside organs. It is needed to form hormones, enzymes, and antibodies and can be a source of heat and energy. It is necessary for proper release of body wastes. Foods high in protein are meat, poultry, fish, eggs, milk, and cheese. Complete proteins have the eight essential amino acids. Nuts and legumes, including navy beans, chick peas, soybeans, and split peas, are incomplete proteins, since they do not have all the essential amino acids. Protein shortage causes abnormal growth and certain diseases in children (kwashiorkor, marasmus). In adults it causes lack of long-term strength, weakness, depression, decreased ability to resist infection, poor healing of wounds, and slow recovery from disease. Too-much protein may cause fluids in the body to get out of balance.

protein-bound iodine (PBI), iodine that is attached (bound) to protein in blood serum. The measurement of PBI shows the level of a thyroid gland hormone (thyroxine) in the blood. Low PBI is a sign of too-low a thyroid level. A PBI of more than the normal values shows too-much thyroid.

protein-calorie malnutrition. See **energy-protein malnutrition.**

protein-hydrolysate injection, a fluid and nutrient restorer used to correct a low nitrogen balance and in other medical conditions where nutrients must be given by putting fluid directly in the vein.

★CAUTION: Kidney failure, lack of urine, severe liver disease, or known allergy to one or more of the amino acids prohibits the use of this drug.

★ADVERSE EFFECTS: Among the more serious side effects are low blood pressure, pain in the stomach and intestinal area, muscle spasms, and blood clotting.

protein metabolism, the ways by which protein in foods is used by the body for energy and to make other proteins. Food proteins are first broken down into amino acids, then absorbed into the bloodstream and used in body cells to form new proteins. Excess amino acids may be changed by liver enzymes for use as sources of energy. They may also be changed into glucose or fat to be stored. Urea, a waste from the body's use of protein, is released in urine and sweat. Growth and sex hormones start the forming of protein, while adrenal gland hormones often cause breakdown of body proteins. See also **homocystinuria, maple sugar urine disease, phenylketonuria.**

proteinuria /prō'tēnyoŏr'ē·ə/, having large amounts of protein in the urine, as albumin.

Proteinuria is often a sign of kidney disease or kidney problems brought on by another disease. However, proteinuria can also be caused by heavy exercise or fever. Also called **albuminuria.**

proteolipid /prō'tē-ōlip'id/, a compound of protein and fat (lipid) in which lipid forms more than half of the molecule. It occurs mainly in the brain.

proteolysis /prō'tē-ol'isis/, a process in which water added to the bonds that link protein units causes the protein molecule to break down. Many enzymes may cause this effect. The action of mineral acids and heat may also cause proteolysis.

proteolytic /prō'tē-əlit'ik/, referring to any substance that helps the breakdown of protein.

Proteus /prō'tē-əs/, a type of bacteria often linked to hospital (nosocomial) infections. It is normally found in feces, water, and soil. *Proteus* may cause urinary tract infections, wound infections, diarrhea, bacteria in the blood, and shock. Most kinds of this bacterium are controlled by antibiotics.

Proteus morgani, the kind of bacteria that causes diarrhea in infants.

Proteus vulgaris, a kind of bacteria that is often the cause of urinary tract infections. The bacterium is found in feces, water, and soil.

prothrombin /prōthrom'bin/, a blood plasma protein that forms thrombin, the first step in blood clotting. It is made in the liver if the body has enough vitamin K. Also called **factor II.** See also **blood coagulation.**

prothrombin time (PT), a test for blood clotting defects. A clotting substance (thromboplastin) and calcium are added to a sample of the patient's blood plasma and, at the same time, to a sample of normal blood plasma. The length of time needed to clot in both samples is compared. See also **blood clotting.**

proton, a positively charged electric particle that is in the nucleus of all atoms. The number of protons in the nucleus of an atom equals the atomic number of the element. Compare **electron, neutron.**

Protopam Chloride, a trademark for a drug used to combat nerve poisons (pralidoxine chloride).

protoplasm, the living substance of a cell, usually made up of water, minerals, and animal and vegetable compounds.

protoplast /prō'təplast/, the living substance (protoplasm) of a cell without the membrane that holds it in.

protoporphyria /prō'tōpôrfir'ē-ə/, higher levels of protoporphyrin in the blood and feces.

protoporphyrin /prō'tōpôr'firin/, a kind of coloring (porphyrin) that mixes with iron and protein to make many important body chemicals, as hemoglobin and myoglobin. See also **heme.**

protozoa /prō'təzō'ə/, *sing.* **protozoon,** single-celled, tiny living things that are the lowest form of animal life. Protozoa are more complex than bacteria, which are a form of plant life. About 30 kinds of protozoa cause diseases in humans. **–protozoal, protozoan,** *adj.*

protozoal infection, any disease caused by protozoa. Some kinds of protozoal infections are **amebic dysentery, malaria, trichomonas vaginitis.**

protracted dose, a low amount of radiation treatment given over a long period of time.

protrusio bulbi. See **exophthalmia.**

proud flesh, an overgrowth of granulation tissue. See also **pyogenic granuloma.**

Proventil, trademark for a drug to expand the breathing tubes (albuterol).

Provera, trademark for a hormone (medroxyprogesterone acetate).

provider, a hospital, clinic, or health-care professional, or group of health-care professionals who give a service to patients.

provirus, a stage in viral reproduction in which the viral genetic information has been mixed with the genes of the host cell. It may occur spontaneously or be caused by a specific stimulus to progress to a complete virus.

provitamin /prōvī'təmin/, a substance, found in certain foods, that the body may convert into a vitamin. Also called **previtamin.**

provocative diagnosis, a way of diagnosis in which the cause of a disorder is found by causing an attack of the disorder. For example, a substance that causes allergies (allergen) may be found by using various substances to bring on an allergic reaction.

proximal /prok'siməl/, a body part that is nearer to a point, as the trunk of the body, than other parts of the body.

proximal radioulnar articulation, the pivot joint of the elbow. The joint lets the lower arm move in circles. Also called **superior radioulnar joint.** Compare **distal radioulnar articulation.**

proximity principle, a rule that when two or more objects are close to each other they may be seen as a single unit.

prurigo /proŏrī'gō/, a swelling of the skin. It is marked by severe itching and many small pimples capped by tiny blisters. Later, because of repeated scratching, crusting and skin thickening may occur. Some causes of prurigo are allergies, drugs, and parasites. Treatment depends on the cause.

pruritus /proŏrī'təs/, the symptom of itching, a feeling that makes someone want to scratch. Scratching often causes secondary infection. Some causes are allergy, infection, liver disease (jaundice), or a tumor. Treatment is geared to the cause. Some relief may come from using antihistamines, starch baths, hormone creams, or cool water. **–pruritic,** *adj.*

pruritus ani, an itching of the skin around the anus. Some causes are contact dermatitis, hemorrhoids, pinworms, psoriasis, and fungus. Treatment is geared to the cause. Some relief may come from careful cleaning, soothing creams or lotions, hormone creams, and antihistamines.

pruritus vulvae, itching of the outer genitals of a female. The condition may become long-term and cause thickening and hardening of the skin, wasting away (atrophy), and cancer. Some causes of pruritus vulvae are skin disorders (dermatitis) and fungus (candidiasis). Treatment of the condition depends on the cause.

psammoma /samō'mə/, *pl.* **psammomas, psammomata,** a tumor that has small hard grains (psammoma bodies). It occurs in the brain tissue, pineal body, and ovaries. Also called **sand tumor.**

psammoma body, a round, layered mass of sand-like material found in some tumors and in some swollen tissue.

pseudesthesia /sōō'desthē'zhə/, a sensation felt without an outside cue or that is not felt with the cue, as phantom limb pain.

pseudo-, pseud-, a combining form meaning 'false.'

pseudoanorexia, a condition in which a person eats secretly while claiming to have no appetite and no ability to eat. Also called **false anorexia.**

pseudochylous ascites /sōō'dōkī'ləs/, the abnormal buildup in the peritoneal cavity of a milky fluid that is like chyle. It is a sign of a tumor or infection in the intestinal area. See also **ascites, chyle.**

pseudocoxalgia. See **Perthes' disease.**

pseudocyesis /sōō'dōsī·ē'sis/, a condition in which a woman thinks she is pregnant when she is not. Some signs and symptoms look like pregnancy, as failure to menstruate, although no egg has been fertilized. The condition may have a mental source or be caused by a tumor or hormone problem. Also called **false pregnancy, pseudopregnancy, spurious pregnancy.**

pseudocyst, a space or opening without a lining that has gas or liquid. Pseudocysts may occur in the pancreas when juices that help process food break through the normal ducts and collect in spaces or on surfaces of other organs. Draining by surgery is the usual treatment. See also **pancreatitis.**

pseudoephedrine hydrochloride, a drug that affects the nervous system, used to reduce congestion in the nose and the eustachian tube. ★CAUTION: Known allergy to self-controlling (autonomic) nervous system drugs prohibits its use. It may interact with drugs to control mental depression (MAO inhibitors) or high blood pressure. It is given with caution to patients who have high blood pressure, glaucoma, heart disease, diabetes, or urinary problems. ★ADVERSE EFFECTS: Among the more serious

side effects are an increase in the activity of the central nervous system, headache, and rapid heart beat.

pseudoephedrine sulfate. See **pseudoephedrine hydrochloride.**

pseudoglottis. See **neoglottis.**

pseudogout. See **chondrocalcinosis.**

pseudohermaphroditism, a condition in which a person has the body traits of both sexes though having either male testicles or female ovaries. Also spelled **pseudohermaphrodism.** See also **feminization, hermaphroditism.**

pseudojaundice, a yellow skin color caused by eating too-much carotene-rich food, as carrots. It is not caused by too-much bile pigment in the blood.

pseudomembranous enterocolitis. See **necrotizing enterocolitis.**

pseudomembranous stomatitis, a severe swelling of the mouth with a fluid release. It may result from bacteria or chemicals and may cause problems in swallowing, pain, fever, and swelling of the lymph glands.

Pseudomonas /sōōdom'ənas/, a kind of bacteria often found in wounds, burns, and infections of the urinary tract. They have light reflecting colors and are not controlled by antibiotics.

pseudopregnancy. See **pseudocyesis.**

pseudopsychopathic schizophrenia. See **latent schizophrenia.**

pseudosclerema. See **adiponecrosis subcutanea neonatorum.**

pseudotumor, a false tumor.

pseudotumor cerebri, a condition of headache, vomiting, swelling of the optic nerve, and a mild paralysis of the cranial nerves. Also called **benign intracranial hypertension, meningeal hydrops.**

pseudoxanthoma elasticum. See **Grönblad-Strandberg syndrome.**

psilocybin /sī'lōsī'bin, -sib'in/, a psychedelic drug that produces mood changes and may cause people to see things that are not there. An active ingredient of various Mexican mushrooms that causes people to hallucinate. It has no formal medical use in the United States. Psilocybin is controlled under Schedule 1 of the Comprehensive Drug Abuse Prevention and Control Act of 1970, which bans the prescription of psilocybin and many other drugs.

psittacosis /sit'əkō'sis/, a pneumonialike illness caused by a bacterium (*Chlamydia psittaci*). It is given to humans by infected birds, especially parrots. The symptoms include fever, cough, and severe headache. Antibiotics are usually used to treat it. Also called **ornithosis, parrot fever.** See also *Chlamydia*.

psoas major /sō'əs/, a long muscle in the lower (lumbar) area of the back. It moves the thigh in circles and bends the spine.

psoas minor, a long, slim muscle of the pelvis. It flexes the spine.

psoralen-type photosynthesizer, a chemical compound that contains psoralen, a substance that makes things sensitive to light. After being exposed to ultraviolet light, psoralens react to increase the coloring (melanin) in the skin. Natural psoralens are found in buttercups, carrot greens, celery, clover, dill, figs, limes, and parsley. Some psoralen-type chemicals are used in drugs to help skin tanning. They are also used to treat skin diseases, as psoriasis and vitiligo. Such drugs should be applied carefully to keep the skin from becoming too sensitive to light. Psoralens are also used in some perfumes, colognes, and hair creams. They can cause skin reactions.

psoriasis /sərī'əsis/, an inborn skin disorder in which there are red patches with thick, dry, silvery scales. It is caused by the body making too-many skin cells. Sores may be anywhere on the body but are more common on the arms, scalp, ears, and the pubic area. A swelling of small joints may go along with the skin disease. Treatment includes hormone creams, ultraviolet light, tar soap baths, creams and shampoos.

psoriatic arthritis, a form of rheumatoid arthritis linked to psoriasis of the skin and nails. It often occurs in joints of the fingers and toes.

PSRO, abbreviation for **Professional Standards Review Organization.**

psychasthenia. See **obsessive-compulsive neurosis.**

psyche /sī'kē/, the basic mental or spiritual being of the individual as opposed to the body or soma. Compare **soma.**

psychedelic /sī'kədel'ik/, **1.** describing a mental state of altered senses in which a person may see things that are not there (hallucinate). The person may feel very happy or fearful. It is caused by the use of drugs or other substances that affect the brain. **2.** describing any drug or substance that causes this state, as mescaline or psilocybin.

psychiatric disorder. See **mental disorder.**

psychiatric emergency service, a hospital service that treats patients with severe mental problems on a 24-hour-a-day basis.

psychiatric foster care, a service for mental patients who have been released from a hospital. They get care in an approved foster home.

psychiatric home care, a service for mental patients who have been released and get care in their home.

psychiatric inpatient unit, a hospital ward or like area used for the treatment of persons admitted to a hospital (inpatients) who need mental care around the clock.

psychiatry, the branch of medical science that deals with the causes, treatment, and prevention of mental, emotion, and behavior disorders. **–psychiatric,** *adj.*

psychic infection /sī'kik/, the spread of unreal fears (neurotic influences) to others. It may occur on a small scale, as in folie à deux, or on a large scale, as in the witch manias of the Middle Ages or the spread of panic in a crowd. Also called **psychic contagion.** See also **sympathy.**

psychic suicide, the ending of one's own life without the use of physical means or agents. An older person, widowed after many years of marriage, may lose "the will to live."

psychic trauma, an emotional shock or injury that leaves lasting effect on the subconscious mind. Common causes of psychic trauma are abuse or neglect in childhood, rape, and loss of a loved one.

psycho-, psych-, a combining form meaning 'of or related to the mind.'

psychoanalysis, a branch of psychiatry, founded by Sigmund Freud, that deals with the study of the mental aspects of human development and behavior. It is a system of mental treatment that uses the power of the unconscious mind. The theory uses such techniques as having patients rapidly say what a word or idea makes them think of (free association), and analyzing dreams and psychological defenses. Treatment is meant to help the patient become aware of his or her repressed mental conflicts and find their source, so the patient's abnormal behavior can be changed. See also **psychosexual development.**

psychoanalyst, a physician who works with mental treatment, usually a psychiatrist, who has had special training in analyzing the mind (psychoanalysis) and who uses psychoanalytic techniques.

psychobiology, the study of behavior in terms of the way the body and the mind work together. Also called **biopsychology.**

psychocatharsis. See **catharsis.**

psychodrama, a form of group therapy in which people act out their emotional problems in order to find new solutions (role playing). Also called **role-playing therapy.**

psychogenesis /sī'kōjen'əsis/, **1.** the development of the mind or a mental function. **2.** the development of a physical symptom or disease from mental rather than physical causes. Compare **somatogenesis.**

psychogenic /sīkōjen'ik/, starting in the mind. Compare **somatogenic.** See also **psychosomatic.**

psychogenic pain disorder, a disorder of continuing and severe pain for which there seems to be no physical cause. There also may be numbness or muscle spasm. The cause may be one or many emotional needs or conflicts. It may be treated by psychotherapy.

psychologic test, any of a group of standard tests designed to measure traits as intelligence; the desire or lack of desire to undertake activities; values; worries and fears.

psychologist, a person who specializes in the study of the structure and function of the brain and related mental processes of animals and humans. A clinical psychologist is one who is qualified by education and training to test and counsel patients with mental and emotional disorders.

psychology, the study of behavior and the functions and processes of the mind. See also **analytic psychology, animal psychology, behaviorism, clinical psychology, cognitive psychology, experimental psychology, humanistic psychology, social psychology.** –**psychologic, psychological,** *adj.,* **psychologically,** *adv.*

psychomotor, referring to self-controlled muscle movements often linked with nervous system activity.

psychomotor development, the skills developed by a child that use both the mind and muscles. These include being able to turn over, sit or crawl at will in infancy; and later to walk, talk, control urination and defecation, and begin to solve problems. They occur at these ages:

12 weeks	looks at own hand.
20 weeks	able to grasp objects voluntarily.
24 weeks	able to roll from back to front at will.
44 weeks	creeps with abdomen off the floor and imitates speech sounds.
15 months	able to walk without help.
24 months	has a vocabulary of 300 or more words and uses pronouns.
30 months	able to jump with both feet.
3 years	able to ride a tricycle and to feed self well.
4 years	able to hop and skip on one foot, catch and throw a ball; is independent, boasts, tattles, and shows off.
5 years	able to tie shoelaces, cut with scissors, tries to please, interested in facts about world, gets along more easily with parents.

psychomotor seizure, a brief loss of consciousness. It is part of a brain (temporal lobe) disorder with loss of judgment, uncontrolled behavior, and abnormal acts. No muscle spasms that can be seen occur, but there may be loss of consciousness or loss of memory for the whole event. During the seizure the individual may appear drowsy, intoxicated, or violent. Crimes or acts that go against normal social ways may be committed but normal activities, as driving a car, typing, or eating, may go on normally. The patient may see things that are not there (hallucinate), have a sense of unreality and distorted sense of time. Physical symptoms may include chest pain, shortness of breath, rapid heart beat, and abnormal sensations of smell and taste. Also called **psychomotor epilepsy.**

psychopath /sī'kōpath/, a person with a personality disorder whose behavior goes against normal social ways (antisocial). Also called **sociopath.**

psychopathia. See **psychopathy.**

psychopathic /sī'kōpath'ik/, referring to behavior that goes against normal social ways (antisocial). Also called **sociopathic.**

psychopathic personality. See **antisocial personality.**

psychopathy /sīkop'əthē/, any disease of the mind, inborn or one that develops. It may or may not involve lower than normal intelligence. Also called **psychopathia.**

psychopharmacology, the study of the effects of drugs on behavior and normal and abnormal mental functions.

psychophylaxis. See **mental hygiene.**

psychophysical preparation for childbirth, a program that prepares women for childbirth. They learn about the childbirth process, ways to exercise and improve muscle tone and strength, and ways to breathe and relax for comfort during labor. Different methods may be taught, as the Bradley, Lamaze or Read methods. The methods share several goals: to reduce the mother's fear and pain, to reduce the use of painkillers and anesthetic drugs in childbirth, and to increase the mother's participation. As a result, the patient will not need as much help from physicians during childbirth.

psychophysiologic disorder, any of a large group of mental disorders that involve an organ or organ system controlled by the autonomic nervous system. For example, a peptic ulcer may be caused or made worse by feelings. The disorders are named for the organ system involved, as heart and blood (cardiovascular), breathing (respiratory) or stomach and intestines (gastrointestinal). Also called **psychosomatic illness, psychosomatic reaction.**

psychophysiology, the study of the functions and processes of a living thing (physiology) as it relates to behavior. See also **psychophysiologic disorder.**

psychosexual, referring to the mental and emotional aspects of sex. See also **psychosexual development, psychosexual disorder.** –**psychosexuality,** *n.*

psychosexual development, the growth of the personality through a series of stages from infancy to adulthood. Each stage is usually a certain period of childhood and is linked to a way of getting pleasure from various bodily urges. Solving the conflicts of each of the stages should lead to normal development. Failure to solve these conflicts causes personality problems. The stages of development are oral, anal, phallic, latency, and genital. Also called **libidinal development.**

psychosexual disorder, any condition of abnormal sexual feelings, desires, or activities with mental causes. See also **gender identity disorder, paraphilia, psychosexual dysfunction.**

psychosexual dysfunction, any problem of sexual adjusting or disorder, as sexual failure (impotence) or lack of sexual excitement (frigidity), caused by a mental problem.

psychosis /sīkō′sis/, *pl.* **psychoses,** any major mental disorder with a physical or emotional source. The personality may not be able to function smoothly. Often there is also severe depression, excitement, and mistaken beliefs (illusions). There may be those with the disorder who may hold false beliefs (delusions) and see things that are not there (hallucinate). These disturbances may prevent the patient from functioning normally. Care in a hospital is often needed. See also **alcoholic psychosis, bipolar disorder, Korsakoff's psychosis, major affective disorder, organic mental disorder, paranoia, schizophrenia, senile psychosis.**

psychosocial assessment, a review of a patient's mental health, social position, and ability to function with other people. The patient's physical status, appearance, and behavior are reviewed for factors that may show emotional problems or mental illness. Posture, facial expressions, manner of dress, speech and thought patterns, and level of alertness are noted. The patient is asked about his or her patterns of daily living, including work schedule and recreation. Background data include a history of past mental problems, the patient's ways of coping with stress, and relationships with others. Major life changes, as serious illnesses, unemployment, marriage, divorce, or death of a loved one are also noted.

psychosomatic /sī′kōsəmat′ik/, the display of an emotional problem through physical disorders. See also **psychogenic, psychophysiologic disorder.**

psychosomatic illness. See **psychophysiologic disorder.**

psychosomatic medicine, the branch of medicine that deals with the links between mental and emotional reactions and the processes of the body. It is based on the idea that the body and mind cannot be divided and that both physical and mental methods should be used in the study and treatment of illness. Also called **psychosomatics.**

psychosomatic reaction. See **psychophysiologic disorder.**

psychosomatogenic, referring to factors that cause or lead to psychosomatic methods of dealing with problems.

psychosurgery, surgery that cuts certain nerve pathways in the brain. It is done to treat some cases of long-term anxiety, over-excitement (agitation), or disorders in which the patient is uncontrollably absorbed by a certain idea or action (obsessional neuroses). The surgery is performed only when the condition is severe and other treatments do not work. A limited section of the front lobe of the brain may be removed (prefrontal lobotomy), and connecting fibers in the frontal lobe cut. A marked change in personality is a result. Various ways that the patient thinks, judges, and feels are also affected by the surgery, depending on how much of the nerve tissue was destroyed, and the age, sex, and condition of the patient. Modern drugs are used instead of psychosurgery in many cases.

psychotherapeutics, the treatment of personality disorders by means of counseling (psychotherapy).

psychotherapist, one who practices psychotherapy. Various types of education and training are required to become a psychotherapist in different places. The ways psychotherapy is defined and licenses awarded also differ from state to state. Compare **psychoanalyst.**

psychotherapy, any of a number of ways to treat mental and emotional disorders by mental techniques instead of physical means. See also **behavior therapy, group therapy, humanistic existential therapy, interpersonal therapy, psychoanalysis.**

psychotic /sīkot′ik/, **1.** referring to psychosis. **2.** a patient who shows the symptoms of a psychosis.

psychotic insight, a stage in the development of a psychosis. It comes after a period of confusion, and fear of the future. At this point, the patient develops an idea that justifies a system of false beliefs. With the new insight, the factors that were confusing before become a part of the pattern of the delusion. While the pattern may seem incorrect to a normal person, it is seen by the mental patient as especially clear thinking.

psychotropic, having an effect on the mind.

psychotropic drugs, drugs that affect the mental functions or behavior of a person using them.

psychro-, a combining form referring to cold.

psyllium seed. See **plantago seed.**

PT, abbreviation for **physical therapist.**

pteroylglutamic acid. See **folic acid.**

pterygoideus lateralis, one of the jaw muscles used to chew food. The muscle opens the jaws and moves the lower jaw from side to side. Compare **masseter, temporalis.**

pterygoid plexus /tur′igoid/, a network of veins of the face and upper jaw.

ptomaine /tō′mān/, a group of nitrogen compounds found in decaying proteins. Because injection of the substances causes side effects, the compounds were at one time viewed as poisonous. Later studies showed that ptomaines were made by the normal digestion of proteins in the human intestine without ill effects.

ptosis /tō′sis/, the drooping of one or both upper eyelids. It is caused by weakness of the muscle that raises the eyelid, or failure of a nerve that controls the muscle. It can be treated by surgery to shorten the muscle.

-ptosis, a combining form meaning a 'prolapse of an organ,' or the dropping down of an organ.

ptotic kidney /tō′tik/, a kidney that is abnormally located in the pelvis. A ptotic kidney may be inborn or caused by an injury. It may not cause symptoms, but pregnancy may cause the blocking of the flow of urine from the kidney.

ptyalin /tī′əlin/, an enzyme in saliva that helps to digest starch. Also called **amylase.**

ptyalism /tī′əliz′əm/, too-much saliva, as sometimes occurs in the early months of pregnancy. It is also a sign of mercury poisoning. Also called **hyperptyalism.** See also **sialorrhea.**

pubarche /pyōōbär′kē, pyōōbärkē/, the start of sexual maturity (puberty). It is marked by the first signs of adult sexual traits.

puberty, the period of life at which both males and females are first able to make a pregnancy.

-pubic, a combining form relating to the front part of the pelvis.

pubic bone. See **pubis.**

pubic region, the lowest part of the intestinal area and below the navel. Also called **hypogastric region, hypogastrium.** See also **abdominal regions.**

pubic symphysis, the slightly movable joint of the front of the pelvis. It is formed by the left and right pubic bones. They are kept apart by a disk of cartilage and linked by two ligaments. Also called **symphysis pubis.**

pubis /pyōō′bis/, *pl.* **pubes,** one of the bones that helps form the hip. The left and right pubic bones join at the pubic symphysis. Compare **ilium, ischium.**

public health, a field of medicine that deals with the general health of the community. It is active in such areas as water supply, waste disposal, air pollution, and food safety.

public health nursing, a field of nursing that deals with the health needs of the community as a whole.

pubococcygeus exercises. See **Kegel exercises.**

pudendal block, a form of regional anesthetic given to reduce the pain of the second stage of labor. Pudendal block anesthetizes the female genital region (perineum, vulva, clitoris, labia majora, and perirectal area) without affecting the contractions of the muscles of the uterus.

pudendal canal. See **Alcock's canal.**

pudendal nerve, one of the branches of a nerve network that arises from the second, third, and fourth spinal nerves of the lower part of the spine (sacrum). The pudendal nerve branches carry nerve signals to the rectum and genital areas, and the penis or clitoris. See also **pudendal plexus.**

pudendal plexus, a network of nerves formed by the branches of the second, third, and fourth sacral nerves. Compare **lumbar plexus, sacral plexus.**

pudendum /pyōōden′dəm/, *pl.* **pudenda,** the outer genitals, especially of women. In a woman it includes the sexual lips (labia), the opening of the vagina, and the various glands. In a man it includes the penis, testicle sac (scrotum), and testicles. **–pudendal,** *adj.*

puer-, a combining form meaning 'child.'

puericulture /pyōō′ərikul′chər/, the bringing up and training of children. **–puericulturist,** *n.*

puerperal /pyōō·ur′pərəl/, **1.** referring to the time right after childbirth. **2.** referring to a woman who has just given birth.

puerperal fever, a bacterial infection and blood poisoning that sometimes follows childbirth. It may be caused by using pregnancy and childbirth methods that are not germ-free. The symptoms include fever, fast heart beat, swollen uterus, and bloody discharge (lochia). If not treated, kidney failure, shock, and death may occur. The germ causing the disease is most often one of the bacteria (streptococci) known to destroy blood. Puerperal fever was rare before hospital childbirth became common, early in the 19th century. Then it became a common problem that caused the deaths of thousands of mothers and infants. Death rates of 20% and higher were not uncommon for new mothers who gave birth in hospitals. An Austrian doctor, Ignaz Philipp Semmelweis, found that women attended by midwives were much less likely to get puerperal fever than those attended by physicians and medical students. Midwives did not examine the vaginas of women as often during labor and did not examine dead bodies. Semmelweis found that the disease was being carried by doctors and students from the infected bodies in postdeath examination (autopsy) rooms to women in labor. By requiring that hands and instruments used in childbirth be cleaned of bacteria, the death rate of mothers dropped. The rule of clean hands was not followed by most doctors for almost half a century because physicians would not believe that they were spreading the disease. Not until World War II did puerperal fever cease to be the leading cause of death in young mothers. Also called **childbed fever, puerperal sepsis.**

puerperal mania, a severe mental disorder that sometimes occurs in women after childbirth. It is a severe reaction of depression and then excitement (mania). See also **mania.**

puerperal sepsis, an infection acquired during childbirth.

puerperium /pyōō′ərpir′ē·əm/, the period of 6

weeks following childbirth. During this time the body changes brought about by pregnancy stop, and a woman gets used to the role of motherhood and a nonpregnant life.

Pulex /pyo͞o'leks/, a type of flea that carries certain infections, as plague and epidemic typhus.

pulmonary /po͞ol'məner'ē/, referring to the lungs or the breathing system. Also **pulmonic** /po͞olmon'ik/.

pulmonary acid aspiration syndrome. See **Mendelson's syndrome.**

pulmonary alveolus, one of the tiny air sacs in the lungs in which oxygen and carbon monoxide are exchanged.

pulmonary anthrax. See **woolsorter's disease.**

pulmonary atrium, any of the spaces at the end of an air cell (alveolar) duct into which air cells in the lungs (alveoli) open.

pulmonary compliance, a measure of the stretchiness of the lung tissue.

pulmonary disease, a disorder with cough, chest pain, shortness of breath, bloody sputum, abnormal breathing noises, and wheezing. Less common symptoms may be arm and shoulder pain, slight pain in the calf of the leg, swelling of the face, headache, hoarseness, pain in the joints, and drowsiness. Pulmonary diseases are of either a blocking (obstructive) or tightening (restrictive) nature. Obstructive breathing diseases are caused by an obstacle in the airway. It blocks the flow of air. Such blockages may be swelling of the mucus that lines the breathing tube (bronchial mucosa), or thick substances released by the breathing tubes. Severe obstructive breathing diseases include asthma and irritation of the breathing tube (bronchitis). Long-term cases may be combinations of emphysema and bronchitis. Such diseases lower lung expansion and make the work of breathing harder.

pulmonary edema, fluid in lung tissues. It is often caused by congestive heart failure but also occurs as a side effect of drugs, infections, inflammation of the pancreas, or kidney failure. Pulmonary edema also may follow a stroke, skull fracture, near drowning, the breathing in of poisonous gases, the rapid flow of whole blood, or fluids in the veins. In congestive heart disease, fluid from the blood is pushed through walls of tiny blood vessels (capillaries) in the lungs into open spaces of the lungs. The patient with pulmonary edema breathes quickly, shallowly, and with difficulty. The patient may be restless and hoarse and have pale or bluish skin. He or she may cough up frothy, pink sputum. The veins of the neck, arms, and legs are usually swollen. Severe pulmonary edema is an emergency. It is treated by placing the person in bed in a sitting position and giving narcotic painkillers to relieve pain, slow breathing, and anxiety. A heart tonic, a drug that acts quickly to increase the passing of urine (diuretic), and a drug to enlarge the breathing tubes may be given. Mechanical breathing help may be ordered by the doctor. Tourniquets may be placed on one arm or leg at a time and then moved to a different arm or leg after a short time. This is done to pool blood in the arms and legs, thereby reducing the load on the heart. The patient should exercise moderately, rest often, report any symptoms, avoid smoking, and follow the prescribed routines for drugs, diet, and return checkups.

pulmonary embolism (PE), the blockage of a lung (pulmonary) artery by foreign matter, as fat, air, tumor tissue, or a blood clot. It may be caused by damage to blood vessel walls; total slowing of blood flow, especially when linked with childbirth; congestive heart failure; or surgery. Symptoms are like those of a heart attack or a lung disorder (pneumonia). There may be breathing difficulty, sudden chest pain, shock, and bluish skin coloring. Death of lung tissue (pulmonary infarction) often occurs within 6 to 24 hours after the forming of a blood clot in the lungs. It is marked by bloody sputum, fever, abnormal heart rhythms, and enlarged neck veins. Two-thirds of patients with a massive pulmonary embolus die within 2 hours.

pulmonary emphysema, a disease of the lungs, marked by overly large air sacs (alveoli).

pulmonary function test (PFT), a test of the ability of the lungs to exchange oxygen and carbon dioxide during normal breathing. There are two general kinds of breathing function tests. One measures the ability of the bellows action of the chest and lungs to move gas in and out of air sacs (alveoli). The other kind measures the movement of gas molecules across the tissues of the alveoli.

pulmonary hypertension, a condition of abnormally high pressure within the arteries and veins of the lungs.

pulmonary stenosis, an abnormal heart condition, marked by enlargement of the right lower heart chamber (ventricle) with little increase in the amount of blood being pumped between contractions. Pulmonary stenosis is most often a birth defect, but it may also occur after birth. Severe pulmonary stenosis may cause heart failure and death, but mild to moderate forms of this disorder may cause very little harm to some people. Also called **pulmonic stenosis.** See also **congenital cardiac anomaly, valvular heart disease, valvular stenosis.**

pulmonary sulcus tumor, a destructive tumor that grows at the top of the lung and spreads through the ribs, backbones, and other nearby tissue. Also called **Pancoast's tumor.**

pulmonary trunk, a short, wide blood vessel that carries blood of the veins from the right lower heart chamber (ventricle) to the lungs.

pulmonary valve, a heart structure made up of three flaps (cusps) that grow from the lining of the pulmonary artery. The cusps close during each heart beat to keep blood from flowing back into the right lower heart chamber (ventricle). The cusps resemble tiny buckets when they are closed and filled with blood. When open, the valve allows blood to flow through the pulmonary artery and on to the lungs. Compare **aortic valve, mitral valve, tricuspid valve.**

pulmonary vein, one of a pair of large blood vessels that return blood from the left and right lungs to the left upper heart chamber (atrium). Compare **pulmonary trunk.**

pulmonary Wegener's granulomatosis, a fatal disease of young or middle-aged men. It is marked by grainy sores of the breathing tract, swollen arteries, and swelling of body organs.

pulmonic. See **pulmonary.**

pulp, any soft, spongy tissue, as that in the spleen, or the pulp chamber of a tooth. – **pulpy,** *adj.*

pulp canal, the space that has the pulp in the root of the tooth. Also called **root canal.**

pulp cavity, the space in a tooth that has the dental pulp. It is divided into the pulp chamber and the pulp or root canal.

pulpitis /pulpī'tis/, a swelling of the dental pulp. See also **caries.**

pulpless tooth, a tooth in which the dental pulp is dead or has been taken out. Also called **devital tooth.**

pulsatile, referring to a rhythmic pulsing.

pulse, 1. a rhythmic beating or vibrating movement. 2. the regular opening and contraction of an artery caused by the movement of blood from the heart as it contracts. The effect is easily found on arteries, as the wrist (radial) and under the chin (carotid) arteries. The pulse matches each beat of the heart. The normal number of pulse beats per minute in the average adult is from 60 to 100. Differences may be caused by exercise, injury, illness, and emotions. The average pulse rate for a newborn baby is 120 beats per minute. It slows throughout childhood and adolescence. Girls, beginning about 12 years of age, and women have higher rates than boys and men.

pulse deficit, a condition in which the pulse rate at the wrist is less than the rate of heart contractions.

pulseless disease. See **Takayasu's arteritis.**

pulse point, any one of the places on the surface of the body where the pulse can be easily felt. The most commonly used pulse point is over the radial artery at the wrist. Other pulse points are over the temporal artery in front of the ear and over the common carotid artery under the chin at the throat.

pulse pressure, the difference between the blood pressure while the heart is in contraction (sys-

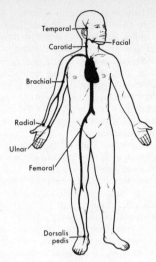

Pulse points

tolic) and the blood pressure while the heart is expanding and filling with blood (diastolic), normally 30 to 40 mm Hg.

pulsus alternans /pul'səs ôl'tərnanz/, a pulse that alternates between weak and strong beats. Also called **alternating pulse.**

pulvule, a gelatin capsule that has a dose of a drug in powder form.

pump, 1. a device used to move liquids or gases by suction or pressure, as a stomach pump. 2. a process by which a substance is moved, usually by chemical activity across a cell membrane, as a sodium pump.

pump lung. See **congestive atelectasis.**

punch biopsy, the removal of a sample of living tissue (usually bone marrow) to test, by means of an instrument with punch action.

punctum lacrimale /pungk'təm/, *pl.* **puncta lacrimalia,** a tiny opening in the edge of each eyelid that is linked to the tear (lacrimal) duct. It releases tears that travel from the lacrimal glands through the lacrimal ducts to the mucous membrane that lines the eyelids (conjunctiva) of the eye.

puncture wound, an injury caused by a cut of the skin by a narrow object, as a knife, nail, glass, or other material. In such an injury to the eye, a lung, or other organ, the object should not be taken out until the person has been taken to a medical facility. Minor puncture wounds are treated with thorough cleansing. If a puncture wound is allowed to close at the skin before deeper healing has occurred, pus will often form. A tetanus booster shot is usually given for such wounds.

pupil, an opening in the form of a circle in the iris of the eye. The pupil lies behind the cornea and in front of the lens. The pupil is the window of the eye through which light passes to the lens and the retina. Its size changes with contraction and relaxation of the fibers of the iris as the eye responds to changes in light, emotions, and other signals. See also **dilatator pupillae, sphincter pupillae. –pupillary,** *adj.*

pupillary reflex. See **accommodation reflex, light reflex.**

pupillary skin reflex. See **ciliospinal reflex.**

pure dwarf. See **primordial dwarf.**

pure vegetarian. See **strict vegetarian.**

purgative, a strong drug usually given by mouth, to bring about one or more bowel movements.

purge, 1. to empty the bowels, as with a laxative or drug given to cause vomiting (cathartic). **2.** a cathartic. **3.** to make free of an unwanted substance or an emotional problem. **–purgation,** *n.,* **purgative,** *n., adj.*

purine /pyŏŏr'ēn, -in/, any one of a large group of nitrogen compounds. They may be end products of digestion of proteins in the diet. Some purines are made in the body. Purines are in many drugs and other substances, including caffeine. Too-much blood uric acid may occur in people who are not able to use up and release purines. A low-purine diet or a purine-free diet may be necessary. Foods that are high in purines include anchovies and sardines, liver, kidneys, and other organ meats, legumes, and poultry. The foods with the lowest purine levels include vegetables other than legumes, eggs, fruit, cheese, nuts, sugar, and gelatin.

Purinethol, a trademark for an anticancer drug (mercaptopurine).

Purkinje fibers /pərkin'jə/, heart muscle fibers that help carry the electric signals that control heart contractions.

Purkinje's network /pərkin'jēz, pur'kinjēz, -jāz/, a network of muscle fibers that are spread through the heart. They carry the signals that contract the left and right lower heart chambers (ventricles) at almost the same time. The fibers that link to the Purkinje fibers start in the AV (atrioventricular) node in the right upper heart chamber (atrium) of the heart.

purpura /pur'pyŏŏrə/, a disorder with bleeding beneath the skin or mucous membranes. It causes black and blue spots (ecchymoses) or pinpoint bleeding.

purulent /pyŏŏr'ŏŏlənt/, making or having pus.

pus, a creamy, thick, pale yellow or yellow-green fluid that comes from dead tissue. Its main substance is white blood cells. Its most common cause is infection by bacteria. The color, makeup, quantity, or odor of pus indicate the cause of the infection.

pustular psoriasis, a form of a skin disorder (psoriasis) in which bright red patches and uninfected blisters show up all over the body. Groups of sores occur every few days in cycles that repeat for weeks or months. Hospital treatment may be needed to replace fluids in the body, and provide drugs and sedation. Compare **guttate psoriasis.** See also **psoriasis.**

pustule /pus'chŏŏl/, a small blister that usually has pus. **–pustular,** *adj.*

putrefaction, the decay of animal or plant tissue, especially proteins. It makes foul-smelling compounds, as ammonia. **–putrefactive,** *adj.*

putrefy, to decay, producing foul-smelling substances.

putrescine, a foul-smelling, poisonous substance made by an amino acid (ornithine) during the decay of animal tissues.

putromaine, any poisonous substance made by the decay of food within a living body.

PVB. See **VBP.**

PVC, abbreviation for **polyvinyl chloride.**

P.V. Carpine, a trademark for a drug to increase the activity of nerves (pilocarpine nitrate).

pyelogram /pī'əlōgram'/, an x-ray picture of the kidneys and tubes that carry urine from the kidneys to the bladder (ureters) taken after a dye has been injected. It shows the size and place of the kidneys, ureters and bladder, and any lumps or tumors within the kidneys. Also called **urogram.**

pyelolithotomy, surgery in which kidney stones are taken out of the top of the tube that carries urine from the kidney to the bladder (ureter).

pyelonephritis /pī'əlōnəfrī'tis/, a pus-forming infection of the kidney. **Acute pyelonephritis** is usually caused by an infection that moves upward from the lower urinary tract to the kidney. In females, it is often caused by bacteria in the opening of the urethra (meatus). Infection may spread to the kidney from other places in the body. The disorder comes on fast, with fever, chills, pain, nausea, and a frequent need to urinate. Testing of the urine (urinalysis) will show many bacteria and white blood cells. Antibiotics are given for 10 days to 2 weeks. **Chronic pyelonephritis** develops slowly after an infection of the kidney caused by bacteria. It may get worse and lead to kidney failure. Most cases are linked to some form of blockage, as a stone in the ureter. Treatment includes removing the blockage and long-term use of antibiotics.

pygmalianism /pigmā'lē·əniz'əm/, a mental problem in which the patient has sexual fantasies about an object that he or she has created.

pygmy, a very small person with normal body shape; an undeveloped dwarf. Also spelled **pigmy.**

pygo-, a combining form referring to the buttocks.

pygodidymus /pī'gōdid'əməs/, a badly formed fetus that has a double pelvis and hips.

pyknic /pik'nik/, describing a stocky body structure with short, round limbs; a full face; a short neck; and a tendency to become fat. See also **endomorph.**

pyloric orifice /pīlôr′ik/, the opening of the stomach into the duodenum.

pyloric sphincter, a thick muscular ring in the pylorus, separating the stomach from the first part of the small intestine (duodenum). Also called **pyloric valve.**

pyloric stenosis, a narrowing of the pyloric sphincter at the outlet of the stomach. It can block the flow of partly digested food into the small intestine. The condition occurs as a birth defect in one of 200 newborns. It also may develop in adults because of an ulcer. Forceful vomiting is a sign of the disorder in infants. Surgery is needed. The muscle fibers of the outlet are cut to widen the opening; the mucous membranes are left intact. See also **pyloromyotomy.**

pyloric ulcer. See **peptic ulcer.**

pyloromyotomy, Using surgery to separate the muscles of the pylorus. Also called **Fredet-Ramstedt's operation.** See also **pyloric stenosis.**

pyloroplasty /pīlôr′əplas′tē/, surgery done to relieve pyloric stenosis. In the treatment of an ulcer of the first part of the small intestine (duodenal), the operation allows the alkaline substances released by the duodenum to flow back into the stomach. Branches of the nerve that lead to the acid-releasing part of the stomach may be cut, lowering the acid levels of the stomach contents.

pylorospasm /pīlôr′əspaz′əm/, a spasm of the pyloric sphincter of the stomach.

pylorus /pīlôr′əs/, *pl.* **pylori, pyloruses,** a tube-shaped part of the stomach that angles from the main part of the stomach toward the first segment of the intestine (duodenum).

Pyocidin Otic, a trademark for a drug, used to treat ear infections (otic), that has a hormone (hydrocortisone) and an antibiotic (polymyxin B sulfate).

pyoderma /pī′ōdur′mə/, any pus-forming skin disease, as impetigo.

pyogenic /pī′əjen′ik/, pus-making.

pyogenic granuloma, a small, noncancerous mass of tissue, often found at the place of an injury. It may be a dull red color, with many tiny blood vessels that bleed easily. See also **granuloma.**

pyorrhea /pī′ərē′ə/, **1.** a releasing of pus. **2.** a pus-forming swelling of the gums. **–pyorrheal,** *adj.*

pyosalpinx /pī′ōsal′pingks/, a buildup of pus in a fallopian tube. See also **salpingitis.**

pyramidalis /piram′idā′lis/, one of the muscles of the intestinal area.

pyramidal tract, a nervous system pathway made up of nerve fibers in the white matter of the spinal cord. They carry motor nerve signals from the brain. These fibers, with nerve cell bodies in the brain, direct the activity of the muscles that can be controlled at will.

pyrantel pamoate, a drug used to treat a condition of having roundworms or pinworms.

★CAUTION: Known allergy to this drug prohibits its use. Caution should be used in patients with low levels of red blood cells (anemia) or severe malnutrition.

★ADVERSE EFFECTS: Among the more serious side effects are nausea, cramps in the stomach and intestines, diarrhea, dizziness, and skin rash.

-pyrexia, a combining form meaning any condition marked by fever.

Pyridium, a trademark for a painkiller (phenazopyridine hydrochloride).

pyridostigmine bromide /pir′idōstig′mēn/, a drug that increases the activity of the nerves used to treat myasthenia gravis.

★CAUTION: Blockage of the intestines or urinary tract, slow heart beat, low blood pressure, or known allergy to this or like drugs prohibits its use.

★ADVERSE EFFECTS: Among the more serious side effects are nausea, diarrhea, cramps in the stomach and intestines, muscle cramps, and weakness.

pyridoxine /pir′idok′sēn/, a vitamin that is part of the B complex group of vitamins. It helps to build and break down amino acids. The vitamin is needed to break down glycogen to glucose, make antibodies, and form heme in hemoglobin. Foods high in pyridoxine are meats, especially organ meats, whole-grain cereals, soybeans, peanuts, wheat germ, and brewer's yeast. Milk and green vegetables supply smaller amounts. Common symptoms of shortage are an acnelike skin disorder about the eyes, nose, mouth and behind the ears; cracked lips; nervousness; sadness; nerve irritation; and blood disorders. Several drugs prevent the use of pyridoxine, so extra amounts of the vitamin are needed with their use. Need for more pyridoxine occurs during pregnancy, infant nursing, heart failure, aging, and use of birth-control pills. Also called **vitamin B₆.**

pyridoxine hydrochloride. See **pyridoxine.**

pyrilamine maleate, an antihistamine used to treat different reactions, as swelling of the nose and skin rash.

★CAUTION: Asthma or known allergy to this drug prohibits its use. It is not given to newborn infants or nursing mothers.

★ADVERSE EFFECTS: Drowsiness, skin rash, dry mouth, and fast heart beat often occur.

pyrimethamine /pir′əmeth′əmēn/, a drug used to treat malaria and toxoplasmosis.

★CAUTION: Avoid use in some forms of malaria that do not respond to this drug. Care is needed in its use to treat toxoplasmosis because the doses needed may be poisonous.

★ADVERSE EFFECTS: Among the more serious side effects, mainly with large doses, are low levels of red blood cells (anemia), severe tongue swelling, low white blood cell levels, and muscle spasms.

pyrimidine /pərim′ədēn/, a nitrogen compound found in nucleic acids and in many drugs, including drugs that fight viruses.

pyro-, a combining form meaning 'related to fire or heat.'

pyrogen /pī′rəjen/, any drug or substance that causes a rise in body temperature, as some bacterial poisons. See also **fever. –pyrogenic,** *adj.*

pyrolagnia /pī′rōlag′nē·ə/, sexual pleasure from watching or setting fires.

pyromania /pī′rōmā′nē·ə/, an uncontrollable urge to set fires. The condition is found mainly in men. Those with the condition feel great tension before setting the fire and much pleasure while watching it burn.

pyromaniac /pī′rōmā′nē·ak/, a person who likes to set fires. **–pyromaniacal,** *adj.*

pyrosis. See **heartburn.**

Pyrroxate, a trademark for a drug that has a substance to stop muscle spasms (methoxyphenamine hydrochloride), an antihistamine (chlorpheniramine maleate), two painkillers (aspirin and phenacetin), and a stimulant (caffeine).

pyruvic acid /pīrōō′vik/, a compound formed by processing glucose where there is oxygen.

pyuria /pīyōōr′ē·ə/, white blood cells in the urine. It is a sign of infection of the urinary tract. Pyuria occurs in inflammation of the bladder, kidney, or urethra, and tuberculosis of the kidney. Pyuria conditions that have no bacteria may be caused by an infection from viruses of the bladder and urethra. Miliary pyuria causes blood, pus, and tissue cells, as well as bacteria, in the urine. See also **bacteriuria.**

Q

q.d., in prescriptions, abbreviation for *quaque die,* a Latin phrase meaning "every day." Also called **quotid.**

Q fever, a sudden feverish illness, usually involving the respiratory system, caused by the rickettsia *Coxiella burnetii (Rickettsia burnetii).* The disease is spread through contact with infected animals. This happens by breathing in the rickettsiae from their hides or other tissues, drinking infected raw milk, or contact with animal wastes containing the organism. The beginning is sudden. A high fever may persist for 3 weeks or more. The illness is especially common among those who work with sheep, goats, and cattle. Treatment with antibiotics usually works within 36 to 48 hours. People who are regularly exposed to domestic animals should be vaccinated against Q fever. Also called **Australian Q fever.** Compare **scrub typhus.**

q.h., in prescriptions, abbreviation for *quaque hora,* a Latin phrase meaning "every hour."

q.2h., in prescriptions, abbreviation for *quaque secunda hora,* a Latin phrase meaning "every 2 hours."

q.3h., in prescriptions, abbreviation for *quaque tertia hora,* a Latin phrase meaning "every 3 hours."

q.4h., in prescriptions, abbreviation for *quaque quarta hora,* a Latin phrase meaning "every 4 hours."

q.6h., in prescriptions, abbreviation for *quaque sex hora,* a Latin phrase meaning "every 6 hours."

q.8h., in prescriptions, abbreviation for *quaque octa hora,* a Latin phrase meaning "every 8 hours."

q.i.d., in prescriptions, abbreviation for *quater in die,* a Latin phrase meaning "4 times a day."

q.s., in prescriptions, abbreviation for *quantum sufficit,* a Latin phrase meaning "quantity required."

quack. See **charlatan.**

quadratus labii superioris. See **zygomaticus minor.**

quadriceps femoris, a group of four muscles of the thigh that functions to extend the leg.

quadriceps reflex. See **patellar reflex.**

quadrigeminal /kwod′rijem′inəl/, **1.** in four parts. **2.** a fourfold increase in size or frequency.

quadrigeminal pulse, a pulse in which a pause occurs after every fourth beat.

Quadrinal, a trademark for a respiratory drug. It contains a smooth muscle relaxant (theophylline calcium salicylate), a nerve stimulant (ephedrine hydrochloride), an expectorant (potassium iodide), and a sedative-hypnotic (phenobarbital).

quadriplegia /kwod′rəplē′jə/, paralysis of the arms, the legs, and the body below the level of an injury to the spinal cord. This disorder is often the result of a spinal cord injury in the area of the fifth to the seventh vertebrae. Automobile accidents and sporting mishaps are common causes. This condition affects about 150,000 Americans. Most of them are men between 20 and 40 years of age. The signs and symptoms of quadriplegia commonly include limpness of the arms and legs, and loss of muscle power and sensation below the level of the injury. Heart problems may also develop from any injury that damages the spinal cord above the fifth vertebra. At that level of the spinal cord, the injury may block signals from the sympathetic nervous system serving the heart muscle. A major cause of death from such an injury is breathing failure. Other symptoms may include low body temperature and abnormally slow heart beat. Impaired digestive system contractions and loss of normal reflexes may also occur. Diagnosis is based on a complete physical examination that includes the nervous system. X-ray pictures of the head, chest, and abdomen are taken to rule out other injuries. Spinal x-ray films show any fractures and spinal cord blockages. Emergency treatment starts at the accident scene. The neck and the spine of the patient are kept in line without movement (immobilized). Additional means to keep the neck and spine immobilized at the hospital may include using special traction equipment, inserting a urinary tube into the bladder (catheter), and therapy to ensure breathing function. Diuretics to reduce spinal cord swelling may be given. Surgery is commonly done to join unstable spinal sections and remove any bone fragments. Compare **hemiplegia, paraplegia.**

quadruplet /kwod′roopplit, kwodroo′plit/, any one of four offspring born at the same time during a single pregnancy. See also **Hellin's law.**

qualified, referring to a health professional or health facility that is recognized by an appropriate agency or organization as meeting good standards of performance. The standards relate to the professional ability of an individual or the eligibility of an institution to offer an approved health-care program.

qualitative, referring to the quality, value, or nature of something.

qualitative melanin test, a test for detecting a dark pigment (melanin) in the urine of patients with cancerous pigment cell tumors (melanomas).

qualitative test, a test that shows the presence or lack of a substance.

quality, referring to the penetrating power of a beam of x-rays. Greater penetrating power of an x-ray beam may be described as being "harder." Less energy in a beam is described as being "softer."

quality assessment measures, formal, organized evaluation of overall patterns or programs of care, including clinical, consumer, and systems evaluation.

quality factor, referring to the biological damage that radiation can produce. The same doses of different types of radiation can cause differing levels of damage.

quantitative test, a test that determines the amount of a substance per unit volume or unit weight.

quantum theory, a theory dealing with the interaction of matter and electromagnetic radiation. It applies particularly at the atomic and subatomic levels where radiation energy is made up of small units of energy called quanta. Also called **quantum mechanics.**

quarantine, 1. the isolation of patients with a communicable disease or of those exposed to a communicable disease during the contagious period. The purpose is to prevent spread of the illness. 2. the practice of holding travelers or ships, trucks, or airplanes coming from places of epidemic disease for the purpose of inspection or disinfection.

quartan /kwôr'tən/, happening again on the fourth day, or at about 72-hour intervals. See also **quartan malaria.**

quartan malaria, a form of malaria, caused by the protozoon *Plasmodium malariae.* It is characterized by fever attacks that occur every 72 hours. Also called **quartan fever.** Compare **falciparum malaria, tertian malaria.** See also **malaria.**

quartz silicosis. See **silicosis.**

Queckenstedt's test /kwek'ənstets/, a test for a blockage in the spinal canal in which the jugular veins on each side of the neck are under pressure, one at a time. The pressure of the spinal fluid is measured by an instrument connected to a lumbar puncture needle (catheter). Normally, pressure on the veins of the neck causes an immediate rise in spinal fluid pressure. If the spinal canal is blocked, no rise occurs. The test is not done if increased skull pressure is suspected. See also **spinal canal.**

Queensland tick typhus, an infection caused by *Rickettsia australis,* occurring in Australia, and carried by ticks. It looks like mild Rocky Mountain spotted fever. Treatment includes giving antibiotics. Prevention depends on avoiding tick bites and on removing attached ticks right away. Compare **boutonneuse fever, North Asian tickborne rickettsiosis, Rocky Mountain spotted fever.**

Quelidrine, a trademark for a respiratory drug. It contains two nerve stimulants (phenylephrine hydrochloride and ephedrine hydrochloride), an antihistamine (chlorpheniramine maleate), a cough drug (dextromethorphan hydrobromide), and a drug that releases sputum (ammonium chloride).

Quengle cast /kwen'gəl/, a two-section, hinged plaster cast. It keeps rigid the lower leg from the foot or ankle to below the knee and upper thigh to just above the knee. The two parts of the cast are connected by special hinges at knee level. The Quengle cast is used for the gradual correction of broken knees.

quercetin /kwur'sitin/, a yellow dye. It is found in oak bark, the juice of lemons, asparagus, and other plants. It is used to reduce abnormal small blood vessel (capillary) weakness.

querulous paranoia /kwer'yŏŏləs/, a form of paranoia. It is marked by very strong discontent and habitual complaining, usually about imagined slights by others. Also called **paranoia querulans.**

Questran, a trademark for a cholesterol control drug (cholestyramine resin).

Quibron, a trademark for a respiratory drug. It contains a smooth muscle relaxant (theophylline) and a drug that releases sputum (guaifenesin).

quick connect, a plastic or similar connecting device that is attached to or implanted in a patient who will be joined to an electromechanical apparatus, as an artificial heart.

quickening, the first feeling by a pregnant woman of movement of the baby in her uterus. It usually occurs between 16 and 20 weeks of pregnancy.

Quick's test, 1. a test for jaundice in which the patient is given a dose of sodium benzoate by mouth. It is broken down in the liver to form hippuric acid. The amount of hippuric acid present in the urine is measured. A large amount indicates little liver damage, and vice versa. 2. a test for hemophilia in which a solution of thromboplastin is added to oxalated blood plasma and calcium chloride. The faster a firm clot forms, the more prothrombin there is in the plasma, and vice versa.

quinacrine hydrochloride, an antiworm (anthelmintic) and an antimalarial drug. It is given to treat protozoa (giardiasis) and tapeworm (cestodiasis) infestations. It is also given to treat and suppress malaria.

★CAUTION: Pregnancy, use of primaquine at the same time, or known allergy to this drug prohibits its use. It is used carefully in patients having a history of psychosis and in patients over 60 years of age.

★ADVERSE EFFECTS: Among the more serious side effects are severe psoriasis, anemia, severe liver destruction, nausea, vomiting, and liver disease (jaundice).

Quinaglute, a trademark for a heart rhythm-control drug (quinidine gluconate).

Quincke's pulse /kwing'kēz/, an abnormal alternate paleness and reddening of the skin. It may be seen in several ways, as by pressing the front edge of the fingernail and watching the blood in the nail bed disappear and return. This pulsation is commonly seen in major blood vessel (aortic) problems and other abnormal conditions. It may also occur in otherwise normal individuals. It is caused by pulsation of groupings (plexuses) of small arteries and veins. Also called **capillary pulse.**

quinethazone /kwəneth'əzōn/, a diuretic and high blood pressure drug. It is given to treat high blood pressure (hypertension) and fluid pooling (edema).

Quinidex, a trademark for a heart rhythm-control drug (quinidine sulfate).

quinidine /kwin'ədēn, -din/, an antiarrhythmic drug given to treat heart rhythm irregularities. ★CAUTION: Known allergy to this drug prohibits its use. It should not be used in patients with heart block. ★ADVERSE EFFECTS: Among the most serious side effects are heart rhythm irregularities, high blood pressure, and cinchona alkaloid overdose (cinchonism). Rare, but possibly fatal, allergic reactions may occur. Diarrhea, nausea, and vomiting are common.

quinidine gluconate. See **quinidine.**

quinine /kwī'nīn/, a white, bitter, crystal-like alkaloid. It is made from cinchona bark and used in antimalaria drugs.

quinine sulfate, an antimalaria drug with anti-fever, pain relief, and muscle relaxant activity. It is given to treat malaria, particularly malaria caused by *Plasmodium falciparum,* and to treat night leg cramps. ★CAUTION: An inherited disorder (glucose 6-phosphate dehydrogenase deficiency) or certain heart disorders prohibits its use. ★ADVERSE EFFECTS: Among the more serious side effects are symptoms of cinchona drug overdose (cinchonism) or allergy to this drug, including ringing in the ears (tinnitus), headache, and visual, hearing, and stomach and bowel problems. Blood disorders and various allergic reactions also may occur.

Quinora, a trademark for a heart rhythm drug (quinidine sulfate).

quinsy. See **peritonsillar abscess.**

quint-, a combining form meaning 'fifth, or five-fold.'

quintan /kwin'tən/, happening again on the fifth day, or at about 96-hour intervals.

quintana fever. See **trench fever.**

quintuplet /kwin'tŏoplit, kwintŏo'plit/, any one of five offspring born at the same time during a single pregnancy. See also **Hellin's law.**

quotid. See **q.d.**

R

rabbit fever. See **tularemia.**

rabies /rā'bēz/,   a commonly fatal virus disease of the nervous system of mammals. It is carried from animals to humans by infected blood tissue, or saliva. The virus is found mainly in wild animals, as skunks, bats, foxes, and raccoons. Contact with an infected animal carries the virus to an unvaccinated dog or cat. Humans most often get the virus from a bite or exposure of a mucous membrane or break in the skin to the saliva of an infected animal. Infections also have resulted from breathing in the virus in an infected place. The virus moves along nerve pathways to the brain, and then to other organs. A dormant period ranges from 10 days to 1 year. The first symptoms are fever, headache, numbness, and muscle ache. After many days, severe brain swelling, confusion, very painful muscle spasms, seizures, paralysis, coma, and death result. There have been few nonfatal cases. Survival in those cases has been the result of extreme medical care. There is no treatment once the virus has reached the nervous system tissue. Immediate treatment of bites from rabid animals may prevent the disease. The wound should be cleaned with soap, water, and a disinfectant. A deep wound may be burned out and a vaccination drug (rabies immune globulin) injected directly into the base of the wound. For active vaccination, a series of injections into muscles with another vaccine (human diploid cell rabies vaccine) or duck embryo vaccine is begun. If the first is used, injections are given on the day of exposure and on days 3, 7, 14, 28, and 90. Great effort is made to find and examine the animal that is supposed rabid. It is first isolated and carefully watched. If the animal is well in 10 days, there is little danger of rabies being caused from the bite. Also called (obsolete) hydrophobia.   **–rabid** /rab'id/, adj.

rabies immune globulin (RIG),   a mixture of a vaccine (antirabies immune globulin) used with rabies duck embryo vaccine for possible treatment in patients who may have been exposed to rabies.

★CAUTION: Prior use of this drug or known allergy to it, to gamma globulin, or to thimerosal (Merthiolate) prohibits its use.

★ADVERSE EFFECTS: Among the more serious side effects are soreness at the site of injection, fever, and allergic reactions.

rabies vaccine (DEV),   a sterile mixture of killed rabies virus made from duck embryo. It is used to vaccinate and prevent rabies after exposure.

★CAUTION: A history of allergic reaction to chicken or duck eggs or to protein prohibits its use.

★ADVERSE EFFECTS: Among the most serious side effects are severe allergic reactions and pain and swelling at the site of injection.

race,   a vague, unscientific term for a group of genetically related people who share some physical traits.

racemose /ras'əmōs/,   describing a structure in which many branches end in nodelike forms like a bunch of grapes, as the air sacs (alveoli) of the lungs.

rachiopagus /rā'kē·op'əgəs/,   Siamese twins that are united back to back along the spinal column. Also called **rachipagus.**

rachischisis /rəkis'kəsis/,   a groove or cleft in one or more backbones at birth. See also **neural tube defect, spina bifida.**

rachitic /rəkit'ik/,   **1.** referring to rickets. **2.** looking like the condition of someone with rickets.

rachitic dwarf,   a person whose slowed growth is caused by rickets. See also **Fanconi's syndrome.**

rachitis /rəkī'tis/,   **1.** rickets. **2.** an inflammatory disease of the spine.

racial immunity,   a form of natural immunity shared by most members of a genetically related group. Compare **individual immunity, species immunity.**

racial unconscious.   See **collective unconscious.**

rackets,   (in psychology) feelings or behaviors used to cover other feelings.

rad /rad/,   abbreviation for radiation absorbed dose; the basic unit of a taken-in dose of ionizing radiation. See also **absorbed dose, rem.**

radarkymography,   a radar method for showing the size and outline of the heart. Using a radar tracking device, it shows images made by electric signals passed over the chest surface on a screen.

radial artery,   a blood vessel (artery) in the forearm. It divides into 12 branches to the forearm, wrist, and hand. (See illustration on p. 658.)

radial keratotomy,   an operation in which a series of tiny shallow cuts are made on the cornea of the eye. The small cuts cause the cornea to bulge slightly. This most often corrects the eye for mild to moderate nearsightedness (myopia). The operation is done using local anesthesia and lasts only 30 minutes. The patient does not need to go to the hospital.

radial nerve,   the largest branch of a group of nerves (brachial plexus) that supplies the skin of the arm and some of the muscles. Also called **musculospiral nerve.**

radial nerve palsy,   a condition in which the radial nerve is compressed against the arm bone

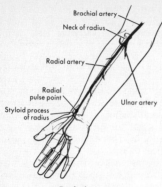

Brachial artery
Neck of radius
Radial artery
Radial pulse point
Ulnar artery
Styloid process of radius

Radial artery

(humerus), usually during deep sleep, resulting in symptoms of muscle weakness and loss of feeling.

radial pulse, the pulse of the blood vessel in the forearm (radial artery) felt on the thumb side of the wrist, over the end of the radius. The radial pulse is the one most often taken.

radial recurrent artery, a branch of the blood vessel of the forearm (radial artery), coming out just beyond the elbow. It supplies many muscles of the arm and the elbow.

radial reflex, a normal reflex in which flexing of the forearm is caused by tapping at the wrist. Flexing of the fingers may also occur if the reflex is very active.

radiant energy, the energy given off by radiation, as radio waves, visible light, and x-rays.

radiate, to move or spread from a common point. **–radiation,** n.

radiate ligament, a ligament that connects a rib with a backbone and a linked disk.

radiation, 1. the giving off of energy, rays, or waves. 2. the use of radioactive substance to diagnose or treat a disease. **–radiate,** adj., v.

radiation caries, tooth decay (caries) caused by radiation. This form of caries is often a side effect of radiation treatment for cancer of the mouth and jaw. See also **dental caries.**

radiation detector, a device for changing radiant energy to a form that can be seen. It is used to detect the presence and amount of radiation, which cannot be seen, felt, or otherwise noted by the human senses. A Geiger counter (Geiger-Müller detector) is an example of a radiation detector.

Radiation Effects Research Foundation (RERF), an organization that studies the long-term effects on survivors of atomic bombings of Hiroshima and Nagasaki during World War II. The studies have focused on the incidence of leukemia, which reached a plateau around 1950, then began declining, and the effects related to the different types of radiation produced by the two bombs, one fueled with ura-

nium and the other with plutonium. The RERF is successor to the Atomic Bomb Casualty Commission.

radiation hygiene, the art and science of protecting human beings from injury by radiation damage. Measures to lessen exposure to outside radiation include using protective barriers of radiation-absorbing material. Others are to ensure safe distances between people and radiation sources, lower exposure times, or use mixtures of all these.

radiation oncology, to treat cancer by using radiation.

radiation sickness, a condition resulting from exposure of the body to radiation. The seriousness of the condition depends on the amount of radiation, length of time of exposure, and the part of the body affected. Moderate exposure may cause headache, nausea, vomiting, loss of appetite, and diarrhea. Long-term exposure may cause an inability to have children (sterility), damage to the fetus in pregnant women, leukemia or other forms of cancer, loss of hair, and eye clouding (cataracts).

radiation therapy technologist, a health-care professional who assists and takes direction from radiation oncologists in the use of radiation in the treatment of disease.

radical, 1. drastic therapy, as to remove an organ, limb, or other part of the body. 2. a group of atoms that acts together as a part of a chemical compound. The group remains bound together when a chemical reaction moves it from one compound to another. A radical does not exist freely in nature.

radical dissection, the removal of tissue in a large area surrounding a surgery site. Most often it is done to find and remove all possible cancer tissue to lower the chance of the cancer returning.

radical mastectomy, removal of an entire breast, with the chest (pectoral) muscles, armpit (axillary) lymph nodes, all fat, and other nearby tissues. It is done to treat cancer of the breast. The woman often is very afraid and grieves in thinking she will not be feminine anymore. The period after surgery is physically and emotionally painful. Swelling of the arm on the affected side is the rule, because the armpit structures that drain the lymph from the arm are removed during surgery. Lung collapse may develop if deep breathing and coughing are not regularly done. A pressure dressing is most often applied to the cut and left in place until bleeding and draining have stopped. A drain is often left in the wound for many days. The woman may be fearful, depressed, angry, or withdrawn. Later in the time after surgery, the woman is helped in exercises for the arms and legs. She is also taught to do arm and shoulder exercises that get more complex over time. In discussion and in giving health care, the loss of the breast is dealt with openly. It is not good to avoid talking about it. On leaving the hospital, she is told to shower daily, to apply a lotion, as cocoa butter, to the cut, and to examine the remaining breast monthly. A volunteer service, Reach to Recovery, may help to counsel and support the woman before and after surgery. Chemical and radiation treatments may continue after surgery. The woman is told never to allow blood to be drawn from the affected arm. The use of injecting fluids or foods into the veins is also to be avoided in that arm, which will lack lymph nodes. Blood pressure measurement, vaccination, and other injections should be done on the other arm. Compare **modified radical mastectomy, simple mastectomy.** See also **mastectomy, Reach to Recovery.**

radical neck dissection, the removal of all lymph nodes and certain tissues under the skin of the neck. It is done to prevent the spread of cancer of the head and neck. The tumor, nearby tissues, and lymph nodes on the affected side are removed in one mass from the angle of the jaw to the shoulder, forward to the middle, and back again to the angle of the jaw. A total removal of the voicebox (laryngectomy) may be done as part of the surgery. Compare **neck dissection.**

radical therapy, 1. a treatment meant to cure, not only relieve symptoms. **2.** an extreme treatment; not conservative, as radical mastectomy rather than simple or partial mastectomy.

radical vulvectomy. See **vulvectomy.**

radicular cyst, a sac (cyst) that is joined to the tip of the root of a tooth.

radicular retainer, a type of dental device that lies in the body of a tooth, most often in the root.

radicular retention, dental treatment with metal projections placed into the root canals of pulpless teeth.

radioactive, giving off radiation as the result of the decay of the nucleus of an atom.

radioactive contamination, the unwanted buildup of radioactive material in the body or the area around the body, as clothing or tools. Any article found to be contaminated by a radioactive source in treating a patient must be gotten rid of following hospital or federal standards for removing radioactive waste.

radioactive decay, the breaking apart (disintegration) of the nucleus of an atom with the release of charged particles, photons, or both.

radioactive element, a chemical element subject to its nucleus with the release of alpha or beta particles or gamma rays. All elements with atomic numbers greater than 83 are radioactive. Many radioactive elements not found in nature have been made in laboratories. Some kinds of radioactive elements are radium and uranium.

radioactive iodine (RAI), a radioactive isotope of iodine. It is used as a tracer in medicine.

radioactive iodine excretion test, a method of checking thyroid gland action by measuring the amount of radioactive iodine in the urine. The patient is given an oral tracer dose of radioactive iodine (^{131}I). Normally, 5% to 35% of the dose is taken up by the thyroid. Absorption is higher in an overactive gland (hyperthyroidism) and lower in an underactive gland (hypothyroidism). Diarrhea can result in low values of radioactive iodine in the urine. A diseased kidney can cause high readings by lowering the amount that is gotten rid of.

radioactivity, the release of radiation (particles or waves) as a result of nuclear decay. Natural radioactivity is part of all chemical elements with an atomic number greater than 83.

radiobiology, the branch of science dealing with the effects of radiation on body systems. **–radiobiologic, radiobiological,** *adj.*

radiocarpal articulation. See **wrist joint.**

radiocurable, referring to the degree to which tumor cells can be destroyed by radiation.

radiograph, an x-ray picture.

radiography /rā′dē·ŏg′rəfē/, the use of radiation, as x-rays, to make shadow images on photographic film.

radioimmunoassay (RIA) /rā′dē·ō·imyōō′nōas′ā/, a method used to find the amount of a protein in the blood. A radioactive substance known to react in a certain way with the suspected protein is injected, and any allergic reaction is noted.

radioiodine /rā′dē·ō·ī′ədīn/, a radioactive isotope of iodine. It is used to treat some thyroid conditions. It is also used in many methods of diagnosis.

radioisotope /rā′dē·ō·ī′sətōp/, a radioactive isotope of an element.

radioisotope scan, an image of the gamma rays released by a radioactive isotope, showing its level in a body site, as the thyroid gland, brain, or kidney. Radioactive isotopes used in scanning may be given by mouth or injected in a vein.

radiologist, a physician who studies and practices radiology.

radiology, the branch of medicine that deals with radioactive substances, as in diagnosing and treating a disease.

radionecrosis, tissue death caused by radiation.

radionuclide /-nōō′klīd/, **1.** an isotope (nuclide) that has radioactive decay. **2.** any of the radioactive isotopes of cobalt, iodine, and other elements, used in nuclear medicine to treat tumors and cancers. They are also used for nuclear images of inner parts of the body. See also **nuclear scanning.**

radiopaque /-pāk′/, referring to anything that stops the passage of x-rays or other radiant energy. Bones are mostly radiopaque. They show as white areas on an x-ray film. Lead is very radiopaque. It is widely used to shield x-ray equipment and atomic power sources. See also **radioactive element, radioactivity, radiopaque dye. –radiopacity,** *n*.

radiopaque dye, a chemical that blocks the passage of x-rays. Radiopaque iodine mixtures are used to outline the inside of hollow organs, as heart chambers, blood vessels, and the bile ducts in an x-ray film. Compare **radiolucency.**

radiopharmaceutic, a drug that has a breakdown of unstable nuclei with the release of nuclear parts or photons.

radioresistance, the ability of cells, tissues, or organs to resist the effects of radiation. Compare **radiosensitivity. –radioresistant,** *adj*.

radiosensitivity, able to be changed by or reacting to radioactivity. Compare **radioresistant.** See also **radioactivity.**

radiosensitivity, the lack of ability of cells, tissues, or organs to resist the effects of radiation. Cells of the intestine are the most radiosensitive of the body. Cells that divide regularly but mature between divisions, as sperm are next. Long-lived cells that most often do not divide (mitosis) unless there is a good starting agent include the liver, kidney, and thyroid cells. Least sensitive are cells that have lost the ability to divide, as nerve cells.

radiosensitizers, drugs that raise the killing effect of radiation on cells.

radiotherapy, to treat cancer by using x-rays or gamma rays. It prevents the spread of cancer cells by lowering the rate of division (mitosis) or slowing the DNA making of the cells. It is painless, but the possible side effects include redness or darkening of the skin, shedding of skin cells, itching or skin pain, and hair loss. There is also possible fluid buildup, nausea, vomiting, headache, loss of ability to fight infection, and other problems. The patient lies on a table from which it is possible to talk to the radiotherapist in a nearby booth. After a dose of radiation, the patient is placed in a noninfecting room or, if needed, in isolation. Anyone, as friends, family, and staff members with an infection, especially one affecting the nose and throat, is not allowed to visit. Skin care is given after irradiation. The ink marks placed by the radiologist on the skin to set apart the treatment site are not removed. The treated place is not washed with water. Sterile mineral oil or another substance may be used. The patient wears loose garments and rests on an air mattress, foam pad, or sheepskin. A footboard or bed cradle is used to raise the top sheet and blanket. Cosmetics are not used, and underarm deodorants cannot be used if the armpit area is irradiated. If hair loss occurs, the patient may wear a wig or other head covering. High-protein foods, soothing jellies, and

ice cream are given. Other food is served when desired by the patient. Six small, bland feedings may be given rather than regular meals. Quiet periods are kept before and after meals. Antivomiting drugs and vitamins are given as needed. Feedings through the veins may be needed if the person's appetite declines. Before leaving the hospital, the patient learns to follow hospital practices for skin care, tooth brushing and mouthwashes, fluid intake and a high-protein, decent diet. Eating just before and after irradiation should not be done. The patient must avoid tight clothing, high or low temperatures, exposure to sunlight, tub baths or showers until allowed by a doctor. Patients with infections must also be avoided. Any problems, as signs of infection, an inability to eat, severe diarrhea, headache, or pain at the site of the therapy must be reported. Radiotherapy can control or stop many forms of cancers from growing and can relieve some tumors that cannot be operated on. Keeping a good diet and special care of the skin may allow the patient to avoid the most serious and unpleasant side effects of radiotherapy.

radium (Ra), a radioactive metal element of the alkaline earth group. Radium salts have been used as radiation sources to treat cancer but are now being replaced by cobalt and cesium.

radium insertion, putting the metal radium (Ra) into the body as the uterus, to treat cancer.

radius, *pl*. **radii,** one of the bones of the forearm. Its upper end is small and forms a part of the elbow joint. The lower end is large and forms a part of the wrist joint.

radix. See **root.**

radon (Rn), a radioactive, gaseous element. Radon is a decay product of radium and is used in radiation cancer therapy.

radon daughters, electrically charged ions that are produced when radon gas decays. They are regarded as a potential health hazard by the Environmental Protection Agency (EPA) because they tend to stick to surfaces, as the air sacs of the lungs, where they can cause radiation damage. Radon is released by rocks, soil, and groundwater and is a common source of background radiation, with levels that vary in different geographical areas.

radon seed, a small sealed tube of glass or gold with a decay product of radium (radon) put into body tissues to treat cancers.

rale, an abnormal breath sound. It is a bubbling noise heard in the chest while breathing in. Fine rales have a crackling sound caused by air entering the lower air sacs (alveoli) of the lungs that have a buildup of fluids. It is heard in congestive heart failure, pneumonia, or early tuberculosis. Coarse rales start in the larger bronchial tubes or windpipe (trachea) and have a lower pitch.

Ramsay Hunt's syndrome, a nerve disease caused by invasion of the face and hearing nerves by a virus (varicella zoster virus). It results in severe ear pain, facial nerve paralysis, dizziness, hearing loss, and often, mild brain inflammation (encephalitis). The dizzy feeling may last days or weeks but often goes away by itself. The paralysis of the face may be permanent. The hearing loss, which is most often short-term, may be partial or total. Treatment is to give steroid hormone drugs. Also called **herpes zoster oticus.**

ramus /rā′məs/, *pl.* **rami,** a small, branchlike structure extending from a larger one, as a branch of a nerve or blood vessel (artery). **–ramification,** *n.* **ramify,** *v.*

random genetic drift. See **genetic drift.**

random selection, a method of choosing subjects for a research study in which all members of a particular group have an equal chance of being selected.

random voided specimen, a sample of urine that has been passed from the body at any point during a 24-hour period.

range of motion exercise, any body action involving the muscles, joints, and movements in natural directions of arms and legs. Such exercises are used to treat bone and joint defects, to diagnose injuries, and to improve physical health. See also **abduction, extension, flexion, pronation, rotation.**

ranitidine, a histamine H_2 that slows stomach acid release used to treat small intestine (duodenal) and stomach ulcers and excess stomach acid conditions.

★CAUTION: Known allergy to this drug prohibits its use. The drug should be used in pregnancy only if clearly needed.

★ADVERSE EFFECTS: Among the most serious side effects are headaches and rashes.

Rankine scale, an absolute temperature scale calculated in degrees Fahrenheit. Absolute zero on the Rankine scale is −460° F, equivalent to −273° C. See also **Kelvin scale.**

ranula /ran′yoolə/, *pl.* **ranulae,** a large saclike (cystic) swelling in the floor of the mouth, most often caused by a blockage of the ducts of the saliva glands.

Ranvier's nodes /ränvē·āz′, räN-/, narrowings or gaps in the covering of a nerve fiber at more or less regular times.

rape, a sexual attack, homosexual or heterosexual. The legal definitions vary from state to state. Rape is a crime of violence or one done under the threat of violence. Its victims are treated for medical and mental injury. The victim is often frightened and feels at risk, degraded, and abused. General physical tests may reveal cuts, bruises, and other injuries. Pelvic or sex organ examinations may show injury to the inner or outer sex organs or anus. A careful physical examination is done and a detailed medical record is drawn up. Samples are gotten for laboratory tests and evidence. Ideally, emotional counseling is easy to have access to and offered right away to all victims of rape. In the case of a woman who has been raped by a man, a pregnancy test is done and injuries are treated. If the test is positive, birth-control pills may be given. Antibiotics are often given to prevent a venereal disease. A trained, concerned person of the same sex is told to stay with the victim. Privacy for the medical record and examination and police interview is given. The victim may or may not choose to talk to the police, but the police must be informed in every case. The victim must sign a special form to allow samples to be released to a law enforcement agency. In general, it is the role of medical staff members to examine, treat, and collect samples as needed, not to decide that rape has occurred. Before the victim leaves the hospital, it should be made certain that someone can be with the victim, because depression, anger, guilt, and fear are common following rape. See also **statutory rape.**

Rape preventive measures

Prevention of attack

Set house lights to go on and off by timer
Keep light on at all entrances
Place safety locks on windows and doors
Have key ready before reaching door of house or car
Look in car before entering
Insist on identification before letting a stranger in house; check identification with agency if suspicious
Do not list first name on mailbox or in telephone directory
Make arrangements with neighbor for needed assistance
Be alert when walking in street; walk in lighted areas
Walk down center of street if possible
Avoid lonely or enclosed areas

If attacked

Run toward a lighted house; yell "Fire"
Spit in rapist's face; act bizarre; vomit
Rip off rapist's glasses
Step hard on his foot (instep)
Aim at eyes—try to gouge eyes, scrape face
Hit throat at Adam's apple (larynx)
Use fighting and screaming with caution; this may scare some rapists, encourage others
Try talking to avoid rape
If powerless, make close observations about rapist, car, location

rape counseling, counseling by a trained person given to a victim of rape. Rape counseling ideally begins at the time the crime is first reported, as in an emergency room. The counselor offers support for the victim by accepting the person in a noncritical way. The victim's response to the assault is asked for, and three basic statements are made by the counselor: The counselor is sorry that the rape happened, is glad that the injuries are not worse, and does not think that the victim was wrong or did anything wrong. Counseling workers may support and be a link between the victim and medical, legal, and law-enforcement workers. This involves staying with the victim during medical tests, police or district attorney's questioning, and throughout the criminal justice process.

rape trauma syndrome, a phase of mental and emotional confusion and a longer phase of regrouping in the victim's life. The cause of the syndrome is the shock of the rape. The signs of rape shock are emotional and physical reactions. These are feelings of anger, guilt, embarrassment, fear of violence and death, humiliation, and a wish for revenge. There are many physical problems, as digestive problems, discomfort in the sex organs and urinary system, tension, and disturbed patterns of sleep, activity, and rest. The long-term phase of rape shock is marked by changes in the usual patterns of daily life, nightmares and irrational fears (phobias), and a need for support from friends and family. There may be alcohol or drug addiction, or the return of prior disorders, as mental illness. A silent reaction sometimes occurs in place of the rape trauma syndrome. Signs are a rise in fear during the interview about the rape, denying the rape happened, or refusing to discuss it, a sudden change in the victim's usual sexual relations, a marked change in sexual behavior, an increase in nightmares, and the sudden appearance of phobic reactions.

raphe /rā′fē/, a line that marks the joining of the halves of many similar parts of the body, as the raphe penis, which appears as a narrow, dark streak on the bottom of the penis. Also spelled **rhaphe.**

rapid-acting insulin. See **short-acting insulin.**

rapid eye movement (REM). See **sleep.**

rapport /rapôr′/, a sense of understanding, harmony, accord, confidence, and respect in a relation between two persons, as rapport between a therapist and patient in mental therapy.

raptus /rap′təs/, **1.** a state of intense emotional or strong excitement, often with uncontrollable actions; excess joy. **2.** any sudden or violent seizure or attack.

raptus haemorrhagicus /hem′ôrā′jikəs/, a sudden, heavy bleeding.

raptus maniacus /manī′əkəs/, a sudden, violent attack of mania. See also **mania.**

raptus melancholicus /mel′ənkō′likəs/, an attack of very high excitement or frenzy that occurs during the course of depression.

raptus nervorum /nervôr′əm/, a sudden, violent attack of nervousness that may be marked by cramps.

rash, a skin swelling. Kinds of rashes are **butterfly rash, diaper rash, drug rash, heat rash.**

Rashkind procedure /rash′kind/, making larger an opening in the heart wall (cardiac septum) between the right and left chambers (atria). It is done to relieve congestive heart failure in newborns by allowing better mixing between oxygenated blood from the lungs and blood from the rest of the body. It helps keep the infant alive until it is 2 to 3 years of age and a passage (shunt) can be created between the blood flow and the lungs. An emptied balloon is passed through a vein to an opening (foramen ovale) into the left chamber of the heart. The balloon is then filled and pulled through the opening, making it larger. Also called **balloon septostomy.**

Rasmussen's aneurysm /ras′myo͞osənz/, a breakdown of the wall of a blood vessel. It causes bleeding when it breaks.

ratbite fever, either of two infections carried to humans by the bite of a rat or mouse. It is marked by fever, headache, nausea, vomiting, and a rash. In the United States, the disease is more commonly caused by a *Streptobacillus moniliformis* bacterium. Its signs are a rash on palms and soles, painful joints, and prompt healing of the wound. It lasts an average of 2 weeks. In the Far East, ratbite fever is most often caused by a *Spirillum minus* bacterium. There is a rash on the arms and legs, no joint symptoms, fever, swelling at the site of the wound, and swollen lymph glands. It lasts from 4 to 8 weeks. It is common for the disease to return. Penicillin is used to treat either form of the disease. American ratbite fever is also called **Haverhill fever;** Asiatic ratbite fever is also called **sodoku.**

rate-pressure product, a measure of the amount of oxygen needed by the heart.

Rathke's pouch /rät′kēz/, a depressed area that forms in the roof of the mouth of an embryo around the fourth week of development. It later becomes the front section of the pituitary gland.

ratio, the relation of one quantity to one or more other quantities shown as a ratio of one to the others, and written either as a fraction (8/3) or linearly (8:3).

rational, 1. referring to a treatment based on an understanding of the cause and processes of a specific disease and the possible effects of the drugs or methods used in treating the disorder. **2.** sane; able to reason or act normally.

rationale /rash′ənal′/, a system of reasoning or a statement of the reasons used in explaining data or happenings.

rationalization, a way of making believable reasons to explain a behavior.

ratio solution, the relationship of a substance (solute) dissolved in a solution to the liquid (solvent) in which it is dissolved, written as a proportion, as 1:1000, or parts per thousand.

rattle, an abnormal sound heard in the lungs in some forms of lung disease. It is a coarse vibration caused by the movement of moisture and the division of the walls of small air passages during breathing.

rattlesnake bite, the bite of a poisonous pit viper with a series of hard parts at the tail end that make a rattlelike noise when shaken. More than 25 species of rattlesnakes are found in the Americas, including many parts of the United States. They have a blood poison in their venom and are the causes of most of the poisonous snake bites in the United States. See also **snakebite.**

rat typhus. See **murine typhus.**

Raudixin, a trademark for a blood pressure drug (purified *Rauwolfia serpentina*).

Rauwiloid, a trademark for a blood pressure drug (alseroxylon).

rauwolfia alkaloid, any one of more than 20 alkaloids taken from the root of a climbing shrub, *Rauwolfia serpentina,* which is native to India. Formerly used as a mental drug, it is today used to the treat high blood pressure. The main part of it is reserpine.

rauwolfia serpentina, the dried root from *Rauwolfia serpentina,* used as the source of a drug given to treat high blood pressure.

★CAUTION: Mental depression, peptic ulcer, ulcerative colitis, electroshock, or known allergy to this drug prohibits its use. It can interact adversely with MAO inhibitors.

★ADVERSE EFFECTS: Among the more serious side effects are symptoms looking like parkinsonism, sight problems (glaucoma), heart rhythm irregularities, and stomach and bowel bleeding.

Rauzide, a trademark for a heart drug with a fluid-releasing action (bendroflumethiazide) and a blood pressure drug (*Rauwolfia serpentina*).

ray, a beam of radiation, as heat or light, moving away from a source.

Raynaud's phenomenon /rānōz'/, sporadic attacks of blood flow interruptions (ischemia) of the fingers, toes, ears, and nose. The effect is caused by exposure to cold or by emotional stimulations. Symptoms are severe paling of the affected area, followed by bluish skin, then redness. There is also numbness, tingling, burning, and often pain. Normal color and feeling are replaced by heat. The attacks are often linked to other health conditions, as rheumatoid arthritis, shoulder girdle nerve compression, drug poisoning, some protein defects, high lung vessel pressure, and injury. It is called **Raynaud's disease** if the symptoms have occurred for at least 2 years and there is no evidence of another cause. Treatment depends on finding and treating any other disease.

Raynaud's phenomenon without a known cause occurs most often in young women 18 to 30 years of age, and may be controlled by protecting the body from the cold and by the use of mild tranquilizers and blood vessel-widening drugs.

Raynaud's sign. See **acrocyanosis.**

RBC, abbreviation for *red blood cell.* See **erythrocyte.**

RD, abbreviation for **registered dietitian.**

RDA, abbreviation for **recommended daily allowance.**

reabsorption, the process of something being absorbed again, as the removal of calcium from the bone back into the blood.

Reach to Recovery, a national volunteer service that offers counseling and support to women who have breast cancer and to their families. Many of the members have had their breasts removed themselves.

reaction, a response to a substance, treatment, or other stimulation, as an antigen –antibody reaction in immunology, or an allergic reaction.

reaction formation, a mental defense mechanism in which a patient avoids anxiety through behavior and attitudes that are the opposite of ignored impulses and drives. The false behavior conceals these feelings.

reactive depression, an emotional disorder marked by feelings of despair, sadness, and depression. The symptoms vary in strength and length. It is caused by an unrealistic reaction to some situation or conflict. The disorder is relieved when the situation is changed or the conflict is understood and solved.

reactive schizophrenia, a form of mental disease (schizophrenia) caused by outside factors rather than by physical changes in the brain. The beginning of the disease is most often rapid. Symptoms last a short time, and the patient appears well both before and following the episode.

reactor, 1. (in psychology) a family therapist who lets a family in therapy take the lead and then follows in that direction. 2. (in radiology) a cubicle in which radioisotopes are artificially produced.

Read method, a method preparing "natural childbirth" set up by Dr. Grantly Dick-Read. Read held that childbirth is a normal, physical process and that the pain of labor and birth is mental—the fear-tension pain syndrome. To lower tension, he suggested a group of breathing exercises for use during the many stages of labor. To help the mother relax and to function well in labor and recovery after birth, he set up a group of exercises to be done often in classes. They could also be done at home. The woman is helped to control labor and birth using the Read method in the following way. During the early and midfirst stage of labor, contractions are 2 to 5 minutes apart and last for 30 to 40 seconds. The mother lies on her back with her knees bent. Stomach breathing is used during contractions. Her hands are placed over her lower stomach, fingers touching. She breathes deeply and slowly—in through her nose and out through her mouth. The stomach wall rises with each breath in, which she can feel with her hands. The rate of breathing is no more than six breaths in 30 seconds, or 12 to 18 in one contraction. During the late part of the first stage of labor, contractions are 1½ to 2 minutes apart and last for 40 to 60 seconds. Rib cage (costal) breathing is used during contractions. Her hands are placed on her sides, over the ribs. She breathes in less deeply, feeling her ribs move sideways against her hands. Each breath is drawn in through her nose and breathed out through her mouth. The stomach wall does not rise and fall with this kind of breathing. The rate of breathing is no more than six breaths in 30 seconds, or 12 to 18 in one contraction. At the end of the first stage of labor, near full widening, contractions may be very strong, occurring every 1½ to 2 minutes and lasting 60 to 90 seconds. The mother lies on her back with her knees bent. Panting breaths are then used during the contractions. The mother holds one of her hands on her breastbone (sternum). It rises and falls as she pants lightly and rapidly through her mouth. Panting continues through the end of the first stage to full widening as the urge to push grows. Panting helps the woman not to push. During the second (expulsive) stage of labor after full widening of the cervix, the contractions occur every 1½ to 2 minutes, last 60 to 90 seconds. The woman has an urge to bear down and push. The woman lies back, head and shoulders held in a partly sitting position. She is helped to draw her legs up, holding them with her hands behind the lower thighs, thighs on her stomach and spread apart. As each contraction begins, she raises her head, takes a deep breath, tucks her chin on her chest, blocks the flow of air from her lungs, and bears down. During each contraction she may need to blow the air out, refill her lungs and push again two or three times. Throughout labor she is helped to understand what is occurring and to help with and accept the birth before it occurs. Many who support using some parts of the Read method strongly say that a woman in labor should not lie on her back. Falling blood pressure may result in this position, because the uterus can fall back onto the body's main blood vein (vena cava). This lowers the volume of blood returned to and leaving the heart. Low blood pressure (hypotension) for the mother follows. This results in a lack of oxygen for the fetus. Today, the woman using the Read method spends most of labor lying on her side or in a partly sitting position with her knees, back, and head supported. Compare **Bradley method, Lamaze method.**

reagent /rē·a′jənt/, a chemical substance known to react in a specific way. A reagent is used to find or make another substance in a chemical reaction.

reagin /rē′ājin/, a foreign body (antibody) linked to human Type I allergic disorders (atopy), such as asthma and hay fever. The antibody makes the skin and other tissues allergic. It starts the release of histamine and other substances that cause symptoms.

reagin-mediated disorder, an allergic reaction, as hay fever or an allergic response to an insect sting. It is caused by reaginic foreign bodies (antibodies) causing the release of histamine, serotonin, and other substances that cause allergy symptoms. Reactions range from a simple rash (wheal and flare) on the skin to near fatal allergic shock. The amount of mast cells (which hold the antibodies) in the skin, nose, and lungs makes those areas at risk to reagin-mediated reactions. Allergens that commonly cause these reactions are plant spores, pollens, animal danders, stings, blood proteins, foods, and some drugs. See also **allergy, generalized anaphylaxis, hay fever.**

reality orientation, an action that helps confused or deluded persons toward a sense of reality, as by repeating the hour, day, month, and weather.

reapproximate /rē′əprok′simāt/, to rejoin tissues divided by surgery or an accident. It is done to restore their proper places. **–reapproximation,** *n.*

reasonable care, the degree of skill and knowledge used by an able health-care worker in treating and caring for the sick and injured.

reasonably prudent person doctrine, a concept that a person with common sense will use standard care and skill in meeting the health-care needs of a patient.

rebase, a process of refitting a denture by replacing its base material without changing its relation with the other teeth.

rebirthing, a form of treatment for mental or emotional problems that focus on breathing. It is based on the theory that cutting the umbilical cord too soon forces the newborn to suddenly learn to breathe through fluid-filled lungs, resulting in terror and panic with every breath. The goal of treatment is to overcome this trauma so the person can use breathing as a supportive and creative part of life.

rebound, 1. recovery from illness. 2. a sudden muscle cramp after a time of relaxing. It is often seen in conditions in which some reflexes are lost.

rebound congestion, swelling and congestion of the mucous membranes of the nasal passages that follows the effects of decongestant medications.

rebound tenderness, a sign of swelling of the lining of the stomach and intestine wall (peritoneum) in which pain is caused by the sudden release of a hand that had been pressing on the stomach space. See also **appendicitis, peritonitis.**

rebreathing, breathing into a closed system, as a bag. Exhaled gas mixes with the gas in the system, and some of this mixture is then reinhaled. Rebreathing, which may result in progressively decreasing concentrations of oxygen and progressively increasing concentrations of carbon dioxide, can occur in poorly ventilated environments or during use of SCUBA or similar diving equipment.

rebreathing bag, a flexible bag joined to a face mask. The rebreathing bag may store gases used for anesthesia during surgery or for oxygen while trying to revive a nonbreathing patient. It may be squeezed to pump the gas or air into the lungs.

recannulate, to make a new opening through an organ or tissue, as opening a passage through a blocked blood vessel.

recapitulation theory, the notion that a human or other animal during the course of growth in the womb passes through stages that are like the structures of many species from which it may have grown from. Also called **biogenetic law, Haeckel's law.**

reception deprivation, an inability to receive stimuli properly because of damage to nerve endings, resulting in partial or total loss of feeling.

receptive aphasia, a sensory defect (aphasia) marked by a patient not being able to understand language. The patient may see or hear words but does not understand what they mean.

receptor, a sense nerve ending that responds to specific kinds of action.

receptor theory of drug action, the idea that certain drugs produce their effects by acting at some specific point on a cell, on a molecule within the cell, or on the cell membrane.

recessive gene, a gene that carries a trait that is masked or hidden if there is a ruling (dominant) gene at the same place on a matching chromosome. If genes on both chromosomes are nonruling (recessive) and cause the same trait, that trait is seen in the individual. Compare **dominant gene.**

reciprocal gene. See **complementary gene.**

reciprocal inhibition, a notion in behavior treatment that if a thing that causes worry (anxiety) occurs at the same time as a response that lowers anxiety, it may cause less anxiety. An example is the use of deep chest or stomach breathing; relaxing the deep muscles seems to lower anxiety and pain in birth. See also **systemic desensitization.**

Recklinghausen's canal /rek′linghou′sənz/, the small lymph spaces in the connective tissues of the body.

Recklinghausen's disease. See **neurofibromatosis.**

Recklinghausen's tumor, a noncancerous smooth muscle tumor with connective tissue and other elements. It occurs in the wall of the fallopian tube or uterus. Also called **adenomyosis of the uterus.**

reclining, leaning backward. **–recline,** v.

recombinant /rēkom′binənt/, referring to a cell or organism that results from the rejoining (recombination) of genes in the DNA molecule, whether because of natural or artificial causes. See also **recombinant DNA.**

recombinant DNA, a DNA molecule that has been broken into pieces that are then put back together in a new form. Parts of DNA material from another organism of the same or a different species may also be placed into the molecule. See also **genetic engineering.**

recommended daily allowances, the amount of foods, as vitamins, suggested as the needed part of one's daily food intake to stay healthy.

recon /rē′kon/, the smallest part of a gene that is able to be rejoined.

reconstitution, the repair of tissue damage.

reconstruction time, (in computed tomography) the period between the end of a scan and the appearance of an image.

record, a written form of communication that permanently reports information concerning the care of a patient.

Recovery, a self-help group that provides support for persons discharged from inpatient psychiatric hospitals.

recovery room (RR, R.R.), an area next to the operating room to which surgery patients are taken while still asleep, before being returned to their rooms. Life signs, as breathing, are carefully watched as the patient wakes up. The recovery room has machines and a specially trained nursing staff. See also **postoperative care.**

recreational therapy, a form of mental treatment in which games or other group actions are used as a means of changing unwanted behavior, making the patient have social interests, or making speaking to others easier in depressed, withdrawn patients.

recrudescence, a return of symptoms of a disease during a time of getting better.

recrudescent hepatitis, a form of viral hepatitis marked by a return of the disease during a time of getting better.

rectal anesthesia, general anesthesia done by putting the drug into the rectum. This is seldom done because the body does not always take up the drug.

rectal instillation of medication, putting (instilling) a drug pill, cream, or gel into the rectum. Some conditions treated by it are constipation and swelling (hemorrhoids). The pill may be self-oiled, or it may need to be oiled. The pill is gently placed past the anal muscle (sphincter). Sometimes a drug may be given in an enema. See also **enema.**

rectal reflex, the normal response (defecation) to feces in the rectum. Also called **defecation reflex.**

rectifier, an electrical device that converts alternating current (AC) to direct current (DC). Rectifiers are used to power x-ray tubes, which require a DC electrical source.

rectilinear scanner, a device that produces an image of a body organ by measuring radioactivity within the organ and recording it on film.

rectitis. See **proctitis.**

rectocele /rek′təsēl′/, a sticking out of the rectum and the back wall of the vagina into the vagina. The condition occurs after the muscles of the vagina and pelvic floor have been weakened by childbirth, old age, or surgery. It may mean an inborn weakness in the wall and may, if severe, cause painful sexual intercourse and difficulty in emptying the bowel. Surgery to rebuild the wall is often helpful and is joined with any other needed pelvic or vaginal repair. Also called **proctocele.** Compare **cystocele.**

rectosigmoid, a part of the body that includes the lower part of the large intestine (sigmoid colon) and the upper part of the rectum.

rectouterine excavation. See **cul-de-sac of Douglas.**

rectovaginal ligament, one of the four main ligaments that support the uterus and hold it in position. Also called **posterior ligament.**

rectum /rek′təm/, pl. **rectums, recta,** the part of the large intestine, about 12 cm long, that is parallel to the lower part of the large intestine (descending sigmoid colon), just before the anal canal. It follows the curve of the end of the backbone.

rectus abdominis, one of a pair of muscles of the stomach and intestines, reaching the whole length of the front of the stomach and intestines. The pair is divided by a tendon (linea alba). It flexes the spinal column, tenses the stomach and intestine walls, and helps to press the contents of the stomach and intestines.

rectus femoris, a muscle of the thigh and one of the four parts of another leg muscle (quadriceps femoris muscle). It flexes the leg. See also **quadriceps femoris.**

rectus muscle, any of many muscles of the body with a somewhat straight form. Some rectus muscles are **rectus abdominis, rectus capitis anterior,** and **rectus capitis lateralis.**

recumbent /rikum′bənt/, lying down or leaning backward. See also **reclining. –recumbency,** n.

recurrent bandage, a bandage that is wrapped many times around itself. It is most often used for the head or the end of a limb that has been cut off.

recurrent fever. See **relapsing fever.**

recurvatum /rē′kərvā′təm/, backward bending, as of the knee when caused by weakness of a leg muscle or a joint disorder.

red blindness, See **protanopia.**

red blood cell count (RBC), a measurement of the red blood cells (erythrocytes) in a sample of whole blood, commonly made with an electronic counting device.

red blood cell, red cell. See **erythrocyte.**

red cell indices, a series of signs that make a red blood cell sample. They are noted in terms of size, hemoglobin content, and hemoglobin amount. Red cell indices are useful in making diagnoses of many kinds of anemia.

red corpuscle. See **erythrocyte.**

Red Cross. See **American Red Cross, International Red Cross Society.**

red hepatization. See **hepatization.**

red infarct, a disorder that occurs in brain tissue that has become oxygen starved (ischemic) by lack of blood. With slowed blood flow, red blood cells leak into the working tissue of the brain. A well-formed pool of blood (hematoma) does not occur; only a buildup of red blood cells (erythrocytes).

red marrow, the red substance made up of connective tissue and blood vessels with early blood cells, cells that fight infection (macrophages), bone marrow cells (megakaryocytes), and fat cells found in the spaces of many bones. It occurs in the flat and the short bones, the bodies of the backbones, the breastbone, the ribs, and the joint ends of the long bones. Red marrow makes and releases white cells and red cells into the blood. Compare **yellow marrow.**

red tide. See **shellfish poisoning.**

reduce, 1. to restore a body part to its usual place after it has been moved. To reduce a broken bone, the ends or pieces are brought back into line. A rupture (hernia) may be reduced by returning the bowel to its normal place. If done by outside movement alone, it is said to be closed. If surgery is needed, it is said to be open. **2.** to decrease the amount, size, extent, or number of something, as of body weight.

reduction, 1. adding hydrogen to a substance. Also called **hydrogenation. 2.** removing oxygen from a substance.

reduction diet, a diet that is low in calories, used to lose weight. The diet should have fewer calories than the body uses each day while also having all foods needed to stay healthy. A diet of this type may allow 1,200 calories per day from the basic food groups. Meats are most often broiled, roasted, stewed, or lightly fried. Vegetables are steamed or eaten raw. Starches and fats are limited, and fresh fruits are eaten instead of desserts. Foods not to be eaten are sugar-sweetened soft drinks, fried foods, pastries, and most snack foods. A lack of vitamins and minerals may result if such a diet is not carefully planned. Also called **low-caloric diet, reducing diet.**

Reed-Sternberg cell, one of a number of large, abnormal cells in the lymph system in a cancer (Hodgkin's disease). The number and size of Reed-Sternberg cells found are the reason for the diagnosis of the specific type of Hodgkin's disease.

reefer. See **cannabis.**

reentry, the beginning of heart muscle contraction more than one time by the same electric signal. Reentry is one of the most common causes of heart rhythm problems.

referential index deletions, a neurolinguistical programming term that refers to leaving out the specific person being discussed.

referral, a process in which a patient or the patient's family is given more medical help. For example, a doctor may help a patient find a community health nurse after the patient leaves a hospital.

referred pain, pain felt at a place different from that of an injured or diseased organ or part of the body. The pain of heart vessel disease (angina) may be felt in the left shoulder, arm, or jaw. In disease of the gallbladder, pain may be felt in the right shoulder or chest.

referred sensation, a feeling or sensation felt at a place other than where the action occurs. Also called **reflex sensation.** See also **sensation.**

reflecting, a communication technique in which the listener picks up the feeling tone of the patient's message and repeats it back to the patient. It encourages the patient to continue with comments that provide further explanation.

reflex action, the unwilled working or movement of any organ or part of the body in response to a specific action. The reflex action occurs at once, without using the will or conscious thinking. See also **reflex arc.**

reflex apnea, an unwilled stopping of breathing caused by irritating, harmful vapors or gases.

reflex bladder. See **spastic bladder.**

reflex dyspepsia, faulty digestion that is linked to a disease or a change in an organ other than an organ of digestion. See also **dyspepsia.**

reflexology, a system of treating some disorders by massaging the soles of the feet, using methods like those of acupuncture.

reflux /rē'fluks/, an abnormal backward or return flow of a fluid, as when stomach contents go back into the gullet (esophagus) to cause heartburn. See also **gastroesophageal reflux, hepatojugular reflux, vesicoureteral reflux.**

reflux esophagitis, irritation and inflammation of the canal extending from below the tongue to the stomach (esophagus) that results when the stomach contents go back into the esophagus.

refractive error, an inability of the lens of the eye to focus, as occurs in nearsightedness and farsightedness.

refractory medium. See **medium.**

refraction, 1. a test to find and to correct light-focusing errors of the eye. 2. the change of direction of energy as it passes from one place to another of a different makeup.

refractometer, a device for finding what kinds of lenses may be needed to correct a sight defect in a patient's eyes.

refractory, referring to a disorder that resists treatment.

refractory period, the time after the excitement of a nerve cell or the pulling in of a muscle during which the cell membrane recharges. It is divided into two phases. During the first phase (absolute refractory period), the cell is not able to respond to any action, no matter how strong it is, because the electric charge is gone. During the second phase (relative refractory period), as the cell recharges, an action above a certain level (threshold) may start a response even though the normal electric level of the cell has not been reached.

reframing, looking at a situation from a perspective that differs from the actual experience, yet fits the "facts" equally well, thereby changing its entire meaning.

Refsum's syndrome /ref'sŏōmz/, a birth defect of fat processing in which a substance (phytanic acid) cannot be broken down. Symptoms are unsteadiness, defects of the bones and skin, nerve swelling, and an eye disorder (retinitis pigmentosa). Foods with animal fat and milk products should not be eaten. Also called **phytanic acid storage disease.**

regimen, a strictly controlled treatment, as a diet or exercise schedule.

regional, referring to a geographical area, as a regional medical service. It can also refer to a part of the body, as regional anesthesia.

regional anatomy, the study of the structures in the organs and the parts of the body. Kinds of regional anatomy are **surface anatomy** and **cross sectional anatomy.**

regional anesthesia, anesthesia of a part of the body by giving a numbing medication to block a group of sensory nerve fibers. Compare **general anesthesia, local anesthesia, topical anesthesia.** See also **anesthesia.**

regional control, the control of cancer in body parts that are the first stages of spread of the disease from the first site.

register, (in computed tomography) a device in the central processing unit (CPU) that stores information for future use.

registered nurse (RN), **1.** *U.S.* a professional nurse who has completed a course of study at a state-approved school of nursing and passed the State Board Test Pool Examination. A registered nurse may use the initials RN after the signature. RNs are licensed to practice by the states. **2.** *Canada.* a professional nurse who has completed a course of study at an approved school of nursing and who has taken and passed an examination given by the Canadian Nurses Association Testing Service. See also **nurse, nursing.**

registered respiratory therapist (RRT), a respiratory-care practioner who has successfully completed the registry examination of the National Board for Respiratory Care (NBRC). Usually a 2-year or 4-year college affiliation leading to an associate or bachelor's degree is required.

Registered Technologist (R.T.), a title given by the American Registry of Radiologic Technologists stating that a person can act as an x-ray technologist. See also **radiologic technologist.**

Regitine Hydrochloride, a trademark for a nerve-blocking drug (phentolamine hydrochloride).

regression, **1.** a backward movement (retreat) in conditions, signs, or symptoms. **2.** a return to an early form of behavior. **3.** a likelihood in growth to become more like the general population than of the parents, as when a child's adult height is closer to the average than that of tall or short parents. **–regress,** *v.*

Regroton, a trademark for a heart and blood vessel drug with a fluid-releasing drug (chlorthalidone) and a high blood pressure drug (reserpine).

regular diet, a full, well-balanced diet with all of the foods needed for growth, repair of tissues, and normal working of the organs. It contains foods with proteins, carbohydrates, fats, minerals, and vitamins in amounts that meet the specific caloric needs of the person. Also called **full diet, normal diet.**

regular insulin. See **insulin injection.**

regulative cleavage. See **indeterminate cleavage.**

regurgitation, **1.** the return of swallowed food into the mouth. **2.** the backward flow of blood through a defect in a heart valve, named for the affected valve. See also **reflux.**

rehabilitation, restoring a patient or a body part to normal or near normal after a disease or injury.

rehabilitation center, a center giving treatment and training for returning to normal (rehabilitation). The center may offer job training, physical treatment, and special training, as speech therapy. See also **rehabilitation.**

Reifenstein's syndrome /rī'fənstīnz/, an inherited form of male sexual dysfunction. It is marked by not being able to make sperm, testicles that have not lowered into the scrotum, femalelike breasts, and a lack of the male sex hormone (testosterone).

reimbursement, referring to a method of payment, commonly by a third-party payer. It could be a health-insurance agency paying for medical treatment or hospital costs.

reinforcement, a mental process in which a response is made stronger by the fear of punishment or the hope of reward.

reinforcement-extinction, a process of teaching socially acceptable behavior in which one learns to act in certain ways (reinforcement) or to avoid acting in certain ways (extinction). The goal is that the reinforced behaviors become normal and natural and those to be avoided disappear.

reinforcer, (in psychology) a consequence that makes it more likely that an act will be repeated.

Reiter's syndrome /rī'tərz/, an arthritic disorder of adult males. It is thought to result from a virus or fungus infection. It most often affects the ankles, feet, and lower back joints. It is commonly linked to an eye membrane disease (conjunctivitis) and swelling of the bladder tube (urethra). It may begin with unexplained diarrhea and a mild fever. Then there may be conjunctivitis 2 to 4 weeks later. Sores that later become ulcers may form on the palms and the soles. Arthritis often lasts after the first problems go away. Treatment is giving antibiotics to treat the infection and drugs to relieve the pain and swelling in the joint. The patient often recovers, but arthritic symptoms may continue off and on for many years.

rejection, **1.** an immune system response to bodies or substances that the body tissues see as foreign, as grafts or transplants. **2.** the act of keeping out or denying affection to another person.

Rela, a trademark for a skeletal muscle-relaxing drug (carisoprodol).

relapse, **1.** the reappearance of the symptoms of a disease from which a patient seems to have recovered. **2.** the return of a disease after the patient seems to have recovered. **–relapsing,** *adj.*

relapsing fever, any of many infections marked by times of fever and caused by many strains of *Borrelia* bacteria. The disease is carried by both lice and ticks and is often seen during wars and famines. It has occurred in the western United States but is more common in South America, Asia, and Africa. The first symptom commonly starts with a sudden high fever (104° to 105° F), with chills, headache, muscle pains, and nausea. A rash may appear over the trunk, arms, and legs. Yellow skin (jaundice) is common during the later stages.

Each attack lasts 2 or 3 days and peaks with high fever, heavy sweating, and a rise in heart and breathing rate. A quick drop in temperature is next, with a return to normal blood pressure. Victims often relapse after 7 to 10 days of normal temperature and recover over time. In a disease caused by lice, there is commonly only one relapse. In disease caused by ticks, many milder relapses may occur. For good diagnosis to be made, the bacterium must be seen on a blood smear taken during an attack. Treatment is with antibiotics, but they can cause a side effect, so treatment may be stopped during a high fever. Bed rest, sponge baths, and aspirin ease the symptoms. Clothing and bedding must be cleaned to destroy any lice or ticks. Also called **African tick fever, famine fever, recurrent fever, spirillum fever, tick fever.**

relapsing polychondritis, an inflammation and breakdown of cartilage. It is replaced by fiber-like tissue. Most commonly the ears and noses of middle-aged persons are affected. There are times of tender swelling, often with fever, joint pain (arthralgia), and an eye disorder (episcleritis). The disease results in floppy ears, a collapsed nose, hearing loss, or hoarseness and airway blockage because of damage in the voice box (larynx) and windpipe (trachea). Steroid hormone drugs make the disease less harsh.

relative biologic effectiveness (RBE), a measure of the ability of a specific radiation to kill cells, as for cancers. It is compared with a specific level of x-rays.

relative humidity, the amount of moisture in the air compared with the maximum the air could contain at the same temperature.

relative risk, the chance that a disease or side effect will occur given certain conditions or factors. It is compared with what would be expected. An example is the relative risk of lung cancer in someone who smokes cigarettes as compared with the risk in someone who does not smoke.

relaxation, 1. a lowering of tension, as when a muscle relaxes between contractions. **2.** a lowering of pain.

relaxation response, a mechanism that protects a person from stress by decreasing heart rate, lowering metabolism, and slowing breathing. It is the opposite of the "fight or flight," or stress, response.

relaxation therapy, treatment in which patients are taught to do breathing and relaxing exercises and to think about something good when a harmful action is done. The Lamaze method of childbirth uses relaxation therapy. Many yoga exercises and mental (biofeedback) methods may be used to suggest actions that would start relaxation. Some patients learn through relaxation therapy to relax stiff muscles at will,

to stop migraine attacks, or to lower their blood pressure. See also **Lamaze method.**

release therapy, a type of therapy used to treat children with stress and anxiety related to a specific, recent event.

releasing hormone (RH), one of many substances made by a part of the brain (hypothalamus) and released right into the pituitary gland through a connecting blood vein. Each of the releasing hormones acts on the pituitary to release a certain hormone. For example, the releasing hormone for growth hormone is a "message" sent to the pituitary to release growth hormone. Also called **releasing factor.**

releasing stimulus, (in psychology) an action or behavior by one individual that triggers a response in others. An example is yawning by one person that results in yawning by others in the group.

relief area, the part of tissue surface under a dental device on which pressures are lowered or removed.

relieving factor, an agent that relieves a symptom.

religiosity, a mental symptom in which excess or affected religious behavior is shown.

reline, to cover the tissue side of a denture with new material.

rem /rem, är′ē′em′/, abbreviation for *roentgen equivalent man.* A dose of radiation that causes in humans the same effect as one unit (roentgen) of x-rays or gamma rays. See also **sievert.**

REM /rem, är′ē′em′/, abbreviation for **rapid eye movement.** See also **sleep.**

remission, the partial or complete lack of symptoms of a long-term disease. Remission may be natural or the result of treatment. If the remission lasts for many years, the disease is said to be cured. Compare **cure.**

remittent fever, daily changes of a fever with increases and lack of symptoms (remissions) but never a return to normal.

remote afterloading, a radiation therapy method in which a device is placed in or on the patient and then loaded from a remote safe source with a strong radioisotope. Remote afterloading is used to treat head, neck, vaginal, and cervical tumors.

remotivation group, a group of mental patients that is set up to raise the interest, awareness, and speech among others of the withdrawn and inpatient members of the group.

removable orthodontic appliance, a dental device placed inside the mouth to correct crooked teeth (malocclusion). It can be removed or replaced by the patient.

REM rebound, the occurrence of greater-than-normal rapid eye movement (REM) activity (the portion of sleep when dreaming takes place) after a patient stops taking a drug that reduces REM time.

ren-, a combining form referring to the kidney.

renal /rē′nəl/, referring to the kidney.

renal angiography, an x-ray test of the kidney blood vessel (renal artery) and other blood vessels, after a dye is injected into the vessels.

renal anuria, a stop in urine making caused by a kidney disease.

renal artery, one of a pair of large branches of the stomach blood vessel (abdominal aorta) serving the kidneys, adrenal glands, and ureters. The left renal artery is somewhat higher than the right. Before reaching the kidney, each artery divides into four branches.

renal biopsy, the removal of a sample of kidney tissue (biopsy) for a microscope test. It is done to find the cause of a kidney disorder, to help find the stage of the disease, and to find the right treatment. An open biopsy which is a cut through the wall, offers a better view of the kidney and carries a lower risk of bleeding. A closed or through-the-skin (percutaneous) biopsy is done by drawing a piece of tissue through a hollow needle. The patient recovers more quickly and is likely to get an infection. An open biopsy is done in the operating room, but the closed one may be done in the patient's room. The kidney's location is marked on the patient's skin in ink for a needle biopsy. The patient is then placed face downward over a sandbag and soft pillow with the body bent at the level of the bottom of the rib cage. The shoulders are on the bed and the spine is in a straight line. An anesthetic is injected, and the doctor places the biopsy needle in the lower end of the kidney, because this area has the smallest number of large blood vessels. The needle is quickly taken out, and a pressure bandage is put on. The patient is kept in bed for at least 24 hours and is told not to lift any heavy objects for 10 days.

renal calculus, a stone (concretion) in the kidney. If the stone is large enough to block the tube (ureter) and stop the flow of urine from the kidney, it must be removed by surgery or other methods. Also called **kidney stone, nephritic calculus.** See also **nephroscope.**

renal calyx, the first unit in the system of funnel-like tubes (ducts) in the kidney. Each unit divides into two parts. The smallest duct (**minor calyx**), with many others, drains into a larger duct (**major calyx**). It then joins others to form the opening (renal pelvis) to the outside of the kidney. Urine is then emptied through the ureters.

renal cell carcinoma, a cancer of the kidney. The tumor may grow in any part of the kidney. It becomes a large mass that may grow into the branches of the kidney vein. Blood in the urine and pain are commonly present. Spread of the cancer, as to the lungs and bones, may occur early in the disease. Treatment is surgery and radiation. Also called **adenocarcinoma of the kidney, clear cell carcinoma of the kidney.** See also **Wilms' tumor.**

renal colic, sharp, strong pain in the lower back over the kidney that may also be felt in the groin. Renal colic is most often caused by a sudden widening of a bladder tube (ureter) with a spasm as a kidney stone sticks or passes through it. See also **urinary calculus.**

renal corpuscle. See **malpighian corpuscle.**

renal cortex, the soft, grainy, outer layer of the kidney. It has about 1.25 million tiny tubes. They remove body wastes from the blood in the form of urine.

renal diet, a diet given for long-term kidney failure. It is to control the intake of protein, potassium, sodium, phosphorus, and fluids. Carbohydrates and fats are the main sources of energy. Protein is limited and is often gotten from milk, eggs, and meat. Cereals, bread, rice, and pasta are the main sources of calories. Some vegetables and fruits may be eaten. Special flours and breads have been made that have no protein and are low in potassium and sodium. The low potassium level of the diet also makes it useful in conditions of excess blood potassium. Since this diet is not complete, vitamins and some minerals are needed. See also **Giordano-Giovannetti diet.**

renal dwarf, a dwarf whose slowed growth is caused by kidney failure.

renal failure, the inability of the kidneys to work. The condition may be short-term (acute) or long-term (chronic). **Acute kidney failure** is marked by very low amounts of urine and a rapid buildup of nitrogen wastes in the blood. It is caused by bleeding, injury, burns, poisoning, acute infection, or a blocked urinary tract. Many forms of acute renal failure are cured after the cause has been found. Treatment is to restrict the amount of fluids and substances that the kidney has to get rid of. Antibiotics and fluid-releasing drugs (diuretics) are also used. **Chronic renal failure** may result from many diseases. The early signs are fatigue and mental dullness. Later, a lack of urine, seizures, bleeding in the digestive tract, poor diet, and many nerve disorders may occur. The skin may turn yellow-brown and become covered with a crystal-like substance (uremic frost). Congestive heart failure and high blood pressure are problems that may occur. There is a constant amount of urine no matter how much water the patient drinks. Anemia often occurs. Treatment is to restrict the amount of water and protein taken in and the use of diuretics. When medical measures no longer work, long-term kidney filtering (dialysis) is often begun, and a kidney transplant is considered.

renal hypertension, high blood pressure resulting from kidney disease, as kidney cancer and kidney stones. Excess use of painkillers and some drug side effects may also result in renal hypertension. Treatment depends on the cause and may be antibiotics, fluid-releasing drugs (diuretics), or surgery. If untreated, the disorder is likely to result in kidney damage and heart disease.

renal nanism, dwarfism with bones failing to grow because of kidney disease.

renal osteodystrophy, uneven bone growth and loss of minerals caused by long-term kidney failure. See also **renal nanism, renal rickets.**

renal rickets, changes in the skeleton caused by long-term kidney swelling. See also **renal osteodystrophy.**

renal scan, an outline, or scan, of the kidneys made to find their size, shape, and exact place. It is used to help diagnose a tumor or other defects. The scan is done after injecting a radioactive substance, which causes the image.

renal tubular acidosis (RTA), a disorder caused by the kidneys being unable to use a salt (bicarbonate) properly and to put acid in the urine. Long-term disease can cause excess blood calcium and kidney stones. Depending on the treatment and the amount of kidney damage, the outlook for recovery is often good. Some common signs and symptoms, especially in children, may be loss of appetite, vomiting, constipation, slowed growth, having to urinate often, and rickets. In children and adults it can also cause urinary tract infections. Treatment is supposed to put back lost substances, as bicarbonate, and may be giving baking soda (sodium bicarbonate) tablets, potassium, vitamin D, and antibiotics. Surgery may be needed to remove kidney stones.

Rendu-Osler-Weber syndrome. See **Osler-Weber-Rendu syndrome.**

Renese, a trademark for a fluid-releasing drug (diuretic) and a high blood pressure drug (polythiazide).

renin /rē′nin/, an enzyme, made by and stored in a kidney area (juxtaglomerular apparatus) that surrounds each blood vessel as it enters a filter (glomerulus). The enzyme affects the blood pressure. Compare **rennin.**

rennin /ren′in/, a milk-curdling enzyme that occurs in the stomach juices of infants and is also in the substance (rennet) made in the stomach of cattle. It has been used to curdle by cheese makers, but now an artificial rennet is often used. Compare **renin.**

renogram, an x-ray image of the kidneys after injection of a radioactive drug. It evaluates kidney function by measuring levels of radioactivity over time.

renovascular hypertension. See **portal hypertension.**

reovirus /rē′ōvī′rəs/, a type of virus found in the breathing and digestive tracts in relatively healthy people. Some disorders, as upper breathing tract disease, may be caused by this virus.

replacement, the substitution of a missing part or substance with a like part or substance, as to replace lost blood with donor blood.

replication, 1. a means of reproducing, or copying; a folding back of a part to form a double. 2. the process by which chromosome material is doubled in the cell.

replicator, the part of the DNA molecule that starts and controls the doubling of the chromosome strands.

repolarization, the process by which the cell is brought back to its starting electric charge.

repression, 1. the act of holding back or down. 2. a mental defense mechanism in which unwanted thoughts, feelings, desires, or memories are pushed from the conscious into the unconscious mind. Because of the painful feeling of guilt or unpleasant content, the thoughts may remain hidden in the mind. They may, however, continue to affect behavior. Such repressed conflicts are a source of worry (anxiety) that may lead to other disorders. Compare **suppression.** –**repress,** v, **repressive,** adj.

repressive-inspirational approach, a way to discourage the breaking down of defense mechanisms in groups for treating mental or emotional problems. Members are encouraged to focus on positive feelings and group strengths. This approach is commonly used in groups of patients with chronic mental illness.

reproduction, 1. the process by which animals and plants make offspring. In humans, the germ cells, the male sperm and the female egg, join during fertilization to form the new person. 2. creating a like structure, situation, or factor. 3. remembering an early thought, sense, or lesson. See also **asexual reproduction, cytogenic reproduction, fertilization.**

reproductive endocrinology, the study of the maternal female hormone system, including the activities of the hypothalamus, pituitary, and ovaries from puberty through menopause.

reproductive system, the male and female sex glands, nearby ducts and glands, and the outer sex organs. They create offspring. In women these include the ovaries, fallopian tubes, uterus, vagina, clitoris, and vulva. In men these include the testicles, epididymis, vas deferens, seminal vesicles, ejaculatory duct, prostate, and penis. Also called **genital tract.**

repulsion, a force that divides two bodies or things.

required arch length, the total of the widths of all of the natural teeth in a dental arch.

RES, abbreviation for **reticuloendothelial system.**

rescinnamine /risin′əmin/, a drug used to treat mild high blood pressure that affects the heart, nervous system, or both.

★CAUTION: Mental depression, use of electroshock, or known allergy to this drug prohibits its use.

★ADVERSE EFFECTS: Among the more serious side effects are digestive, heart, and central nervous system problems.

research radiopharmaceutical, a drug in which a small amount of a radioactive element is put to study its spread in the body. It may later be used without a radioactive element.

resect, to remove tissue or an organ from the body by surgery. Resection of an organ may be part or complete.

reserpine /res'ərpēn/, a drug used to treat high blood pressure and some nerve disorders.

reserve, a possible ability of the body to keep life processes normal by changing to meet a need, as heart (cardiac) reserve or lung (pulmonary) reserve. See also **homeostasis.**

reservoir, a chamber or receptacle for holding or storing a fluid.

reservoir host, a nonhuman animal or other creature in which disease-causing things grow, as bacteria. They are a possible cause of human infection. Wild monkeys are reservoir hosts for the yellow fever virus, which can spread from the jungle to infect humans.

reservoir of infection, a constant source of infectious disease. People, animals, and plants may be reservoirs of infection.

resident, a doctor in training after an internship. The length of residency varies according to the doctor's specialty. See also **PGY.**

resident bacteria, bacteria living in a certain area of the body.

residential care facility, a health-care center, as a nursing home. It gives nonmedical care to patients who, because of physical, mental, or emotional disorders, are not able to live by themselves.

residual, referring to the part of a substance that stays after much of it has been removed. An example is residual urine that stays in the bladder after urination.

residual cyst, a lump (cyst) that stays in the jaw after the removal of a tooth.

residual dental caries, any decayed material left in a fixed tooth cavity.

residual volume, the air that stays in the lungs after breathing out as much as possible.

residue schizophrenia, a form of schizophrenia in which the patient has had at least one past psychotic episode, often with delusions and hallucinations. Signs of the illness, as withdrawal, strange behavior, and fuzzy thinking, may last. However, they are weaker than those in patients who are psychotic. See also **schizophrenia.**

resistance, fighting a force, as the body fighting infection.

resistance form, a shape given to a fixed tooth cavity to make sure it is strong and stable.

resocialization, the return of a patient to normal family and community life after a serious illness or a long-term hospital stay.

resonance, an echo or other sound made in the body by tapping (percussion) the skin over a body organ or space during a physical test. **–resonant,** *adj.*

resorcinated camphor /rizôr'sinā'tid/, a mixture of a mild irritant (camphor) and an antiseptic (resorcinol), used to treat lice infestations and itching.

resorcinol /rizôr'sinol/, an antiseptic used as a skin-peeling drug in skin diseases. It is also used in dyes and other products.

resorcinol test. See **Boas' test.**

resorption, the loss of tissue, as bone, by the breakdown of the tissue, which is soaked up by the blood. An example is the reduced size of the dental ridge of a jaw after a tooth has been taken out.

Respid, a trademark for a smooth muscle-relaxing drug (theophylline).

respiration, the give and take of oxygen and carbon dioxide in the body's tissues, from the lungs to the level of the cells. The rate changes with the age and condition of the person.

respirator, a machine used to aid or act as the breathing stimulant of patients with respiratory failure. See also **nebulizer, IPPB unit.**

respiratory /res'pərətôrē, rispīr'ətôr'ē/, referring to breathing (respiration).

respiratory acidosis, an abnormal condition with high blood levels of carbon dioxide. A lowered breathing rate slows the release of carbon dioxide, which then joins with water and makes large amounts of an acid (carbonic acid). This causes more acid in the blood. Many disorders can cause it, as a block in an airway, a muscle disease, chest injuries, pneumonia, and fluid in the lungs. It may also be caused by narcotics, sleeping pills, tranquilizers, or anesthetics, which hold down breathing reflexes. Some common signs and symptoms are headache, breathing difficulty, fine tremors, rapid heart beat, high blood pressure, and widened blood vessels. Failed treatment can lead to coma and death. Any block in an airway must be taken out at once. Treatment may be giving oxygen and lung drugs (bronchodilators) and baking soda (sodium bicarbonate). Compare **metabolic acidosis.** See also **metabolic alkalosis, respiratory alkalosis.**

respiratory alkalosis, an abnormal condition with low blood levels of carbon dioxide and large amounts of alkaline in the blood. The cause may or may not be a lung problem. Some lung causes are asthma and pneumonia. Other causes are aspirin poisoning, anxiety, fever, blood poisoning, and liver failure. The excess breathing linked to this disease commonly stems from excess anxiety. Deep and rapid breathing at rates as high as 40 breaths per minute is a major sign. Other symptoms are lightheadedness, dizziness, numbness or spasms of the hands and the feet, muscle weakness, and an irregular heart beat. Removing the cause of the condition is important in treatment. Severe cases, as those caused by excess anxiety, may be treated by having the patient breathe into a paper bag and breathe in exhaled carbon dioxide to make up for the loss being caused by rapid breathing (hyperventilation). Sedatives may also be given to slow the breathing rate. Compare **metabolic alkalosis.** See also **metabolic acidosis, respiratory acidosis.**

respiratory assessment, an evaluation of a patient's breathing system. The patient is asked about coughs, wheezes, shortness of breath, becoming tired easily, having chest or stomach pain, chills, fever, heavy sweating, dizziness, or swelling of the feet and hands. Signs of confusion, worry, restlessness, wide nostrils, bluish lips, gums, earlobes, or nails, swelling (clubbing) of the fingers, fever, loss of appetite, and sitting upright are noted. The patient's breathing is closely watched for slow, rapid, irregular, shallow, or waxing and waning (Cheyne-Stokes) breathing. The patient is also watched for long breathing-out phases, or times without breathing. Rapid, slow, or abnormal heart beats, or signs of congestive heart failure, as abnormal breathing sounds, fluid buildup, swollen spleen and liver, bloated stomach, or pain are recorded. The chest is checked for backbone defects. Tapping the chest (percussion) is done to check for drumlike sounds (tympany), dull or flat sounds, wheezing, friction rubs, or the carrying of spoken words through the chest wall. Also checked are lowered or absent breath sounds. Data important for the test may be allergies, recent exposure to infection, vaccinations, exposure to irritants, prior breathing disorders and operations, long-term conditions, current drugs, smoking habits, and the family history of breathing disorders. Tests are chest x-ray films, complete blood count, a heart rate test (electrocardiogram), and lung tests.

respiratory burn, tissue damage to the breathing system caused by breathing a hot gas or burning particles, as may occur in a fire or explosion. The patient often must have oxygen treatment and go to the hospital at once. Compare **smoke inhalation.**

respiratory center, a group of nerve cells in the brain that control the rhythm of breathing in response to changes in levels of oxygen and carbon dioxide in the blood and spinal fluid. Change in the amount of oxygen and carbon dioxide or hydrogen ion levels in the blood and spinal fluid starts nerve cells that send signals to the respiratory center, raising or lowering the breathing rate. This is needed for normal breathing. In patients with a carbon dioxide buildup, as in bronchitis or emphysema, the respiratory center does not respond to carbon dioxide, and the main reason for transfer is a lack of oxygen. If such patients breathe in a large amount of oxygen content, their breathing becomes lowered, leading to a further rise of blood carbon dioxide. The respiratory center is also harmed by barbiturates, anesthetics, tranquilizers and morphine.

respiratory cycle, breathing in followed by breathing out.

respiratory distress syndrome of the newborn (RDS), a lung disease of the newborn. It is marked by airless air sacs (alveoli), rigid lungs, more than 60 breaths a minute, a widened nose, cramps of rib cage muscles, grunting on breathing out, and fluid buildup in the arms and legs. The condition occurs most often in premature babies and in babies of mothers with diabetes. Causes include overfilled air sacs and, at times, a growth of a fiberlike (hyaline) bleeding in the lungs, lowered heart output, and very low blood oxygen. The disease resolves itself. The infant dies in 3 to 5 days or completely recovers with no aftereffects. Treatment is to correct shock, too much (acid), and lack of oxygen and to use constant positive airway pressure made just for infants to prevent collapse of the alveoli. Also called **hyaline membrane disease.**

respiratory exchange ratio (R), the amount of carbon dioxide breathed out compared to the amount of oxygen breathed in.

respiratory failure, the inability of the heart and lung systems to keep enough of a transfer of oxygen and carbon dioxide in the lungs. Respiratory failure may be caused by lack of oxygen (hypoxemic failure) or a transfer of gases problem (ventilatory failure). A sign of hypoxemic failure is excess breathing (hyperventilation). This occurs in diseases that affect the air sacs (alveoli) or supporting tissues of the lobes of the lungs, as alveolar edema, emphysema, fungus infections, leukemia, pneumonia, lung cancer, or tuberculosis. Ventilatory failure occurs in conditions in which kept lung fluids cause more airway resistance and lowered lung use, as in bronchitis and emphysema. Ventilation may also be lowered by a slowing of the breathing center by barbiturates or opiates. Other factors slowing breathing are oxygen problems, brain diseases, injury, or tumors of the nerve and muscle system or the chest. Respiratory failure in long-term lung diseases may be caused by added stress, as heart failure, surgery, anesthesia, or upper breathing tract infections. Treatment of respiratory failure includes clearing the airways by suction, giving lung drugs (bronchodilators), or making an airway (tracheostomy). Drugs given are antibiotics for infections, drugs that stop blood clotting for blood clots in the lungs, and electrolyte replacements for fluid imbalance. Oxygen may be given in some cases.

respiratory muscles, the muscles that expand and contract the chest during breathing.

respiratory rate, the normal rate of breathing at rest, about 12 to 16 breaths per minute. The rate may be more rapid in fever, lung infection, gas gangrene, left-sided heart failure, and other disorders. Slower breathing rates may result from head injury, coma, or narcotic overdose. See also **bradypnea, hyperpnea, hypopnea.**

respiratory rhythm, a regular cycle of breathing in and out, controlled by nerve signals carried between the muscles of breathing in the chest and the breathing centers in the brain. The normal breathing pattern may be changed by a long breathing phase in blocking diseases of the airway, as asthma, bronchitis, and emphysema, or by Cheyne-Stokes breathing in patients with raised brain pressure or heart failure.

respiratory syncytial (RS) virus (RSV), a member of a subgroup of viruses (myxoviruses) that cause epidemics of bronchitis, pneumonia, and the common cold in young children. It causes bronchitis and mild upper breathing tract infections in adults. Symptoms of infection with this virus include fever, cough, and severe tiredness. Some infants die. Treatment is rest and giving aspirin and nasal drugs. Compare **rhinovirus.** See also **bronchiolitis, bronchitis, bronchopneumonia, cold.**

respiratory system. See **respiratory tract.**

respiratory therapist, a person who, under the guidance of a doctor, gives oxygen and does chest exercises to help patients with breathing difficulties.

respiratory therapy (RT), any treatment that maintains or improves the function of the respiratory tract.

respiratory tract, the complex of organs and structures that transfers oxygen and carbon dioxide between the air outside and the blood flowing through the lungs. It also warms the air passing into the body. The speech function is helped by giving air for the throat (larynx) and the vocal cords. Every 24 hours about 500 cubic feet of air passes through the breathing tract of the average adult, who breathes in and out between 12 and 18 times a minute. The breathing tract is divided into the upper and the lower breathing tracts. Also called **respiratory system.**

respiratory tract infection, any infectious disease of the upper or lower breathing tract.

respiratory zone, the end air sacs in the lungs where gas actually enters and leaves the blood.

respite care, 1. health services provided for a brief period to a dependent older adult, either at home or in a health-care facility. 2. temporary care for a patient who requires specialized or intensive care or supervision normally provided by his or her family at home. Respite care provides the family with relief from demands of the patient's care.

responder, a tumor that shrinks by at least 50% as a result of chemotherapy, radiation, or other treatment.

response, (in psychology) a category of punishment in which reinforcement is either taken away or not given after an undesired response.

response time, 1. the period between the entering of information into a computer and the response. 2. the period between the application of a stimulus and the response of a cell or cells.

rest, a part of a dental device that supports a dental fixture, as a part denture.

rest area, a surface made on a tooth into which a dental device (rest) fits, supporting removable part denture.

resting tremor. See **passive tremor.**

restitution, the natural turning of the baby's head to the right or left after it has moved through the vulva.

rest jaw relation, the relation of the lower jaw to the upper jaw when the patient is resting comfortably in the upright position.

rest joint position, the position of a joint in which the joint surfaces are not pushed together and the support structures are relaxed. The position is used when moving a patient without the patient's effort.

restless legs syndrome, an irritating feeling of uneasiness, tiredness, and itching deep in the muscles of the leg. This occurs often in the lower part of the leg. There may also be twitching and sometimes pain. The only relief is walking or moving the legs. The condition may be linked to many nervous system disorders. Also called **anxietas tibiarum, Ekbom syndrome, Wittmaack-Ekbom syndrome.**

restoration, any tooth filling, inlay, crown, denture, or other dental device that restores or replaces lost tooth structure, teeth, or mouth tissues. Also called **prosthetic restoration.**

restoration contour, the shape of the surfaces of teeth that have been restored.

Restoril, a trademark for a sedative (temazepam).

restraint, any one of many devices used to hold and prevent the movement of patients to protect them from injury or to prevent them from pulling on any tubes or devices, as children in traction. Some kinds of restraints are specially made slings, jackets, or diapers. Restraints often cause emotional trauma for the patient and should be carefully used. Restraints that are too tight may cause skin irritation. Any that fit too loosely do not serve their purpose. Restraints are most often removed every 4 hours to check the skin condition and to give skin care.

restriction fragment, a fragment of viral or cel-lular nucleic acid produced by separation of the DNA molecule by certain enzymes (endo-nucleases).

restriction fragment length polymorphism (RFLP), a marker for a DNA segment of a chromosome that is linked with a hereditary disease. RFLPs have been used to find genes linked with several inherited disorders, includ-ing Huntington's disease.

restrictive disease, a breathing disorder charac-terized by decreased ability to expand the lungs or chest wall, resulting in lower lung vol-umes and capacities.

resuscitation, the process of keeping a patient in lung or heart failure alive. Resuscitation uses methods of artificial breathing and chest com-pression and treats the cause of the failure. See also **cardiopulmonary resuscitation. –re-suscitate,** v.

resuscitator /risus′itā′tər/, a device for pumping air into the lungs. It is made of a mask that fits snugly over the mouth and nose, a storage place for air, and a pump. Often oxygen may be added to the air.

retail dentistry, the practice of fee-for-service dentistry in a retail outlet, as a shopping center or a department store.

retained placenta, a condition in which all or part of the placenta remains in the uterus after birth.

retainer, the part of a dental device that con-nects a fixed (abutment) tooth with the hung part of a bridge. It may be an inlay, a part crown, or a complete crown. The word also means any clasp, attachment, or device for fix-ing or keeping rigid a dental fixture.

retaining orthodontic appliance, a device for holding the teeth in place, after tooth move-ment, until the desired place is made stable.

retarded, very slow. **–retard,** v., **retardation,** n.

retarded dentition, an abnormal delay of the coming in of the teeth caused by poor diet, placement of the teeth, a disorder, as a lack of thyroid, or other factors. Also called **delayed dentition.** Compare **precocious dentition.**

retarded ejaculation, the inability of a male to ejaculate after having achieved an erection. This often happens as men age.

retch, a strong attempt to vomit without bringing up anything. Compare **eructation, vomit.**

rete /rē′tē/, a grouping, as of blood vessels (arter-ies, veins). **–retial,** adj.

retention, **1.** to resist movement or being moved. **2.** the ability of the digestive system to hold food and fluid. **3.** the inability to urinate or defecate. **4.** the ability of the mind to remem-ber data. **5.** the ability of a dental device or filling to keep in place without moving under stress.

retention of urine, a high buildup of urine in the bladder. Causes include a loss of muscle tone

in the bladder, nerve damage to the bladder, a blocked tube (urethra), or the use of a narcotic painkiller, as morphine.

retention procedure, a method set up by state laws or mental-health codes for putting a pa-tient in a mental hospital. Most states name four types of retention: emergency, informal, involuntary, and voluntary.

reticular /ritik′yələr/, referring to a tissue or sur-face having a netlike pattern or structure of veins.

reticular activating system (RAS), a working sys-tem in the brain needed for the level of con-sciousness, from sleep to full attention. A group of nerve fibers in many parts of the brain (thalamus, hypothalamus, brain stem, and ce-rebral cortex) are part of the system.

reticular formation, a small, thick cluster of nerve cells in the brain stem. It controls breathing, heart beat, blood pressure, and other important workings of the body. The state of the body is constantly checked through joinings with the sense and motor nerve tracts. Certain nerve cells control the flow of hydro-chloric acid in the stomach. Other cells control movements of the face, eyes, and tongue.

reticulin, a substance found in the connective fibers of nerve cell (reticular) tissue.

reticulocyte /ritik′yələsīt/, an immature red blood cell with a meshlike pattern of threads and particles at the former site of the nucleus. These cells mainly make up less than 1% of the flowing red blood cells. A greater amount shows a higher rate of red cell making. Com-pare **erythrocyte.** See also **normoblast.**

reticulocytopenia /ritik′yəlōsī′təpē′nē·ə/, a de-crease below normal in the number of young red blood cells (reticulocytes) in a blood sample.

reticulocytosis, increase in the number of young red blood cells (reticulocytes) in the circulating blood. It may be a normal activity of the blood-forming tissues of the bone marrow in re-sponse to blood loss, an adjustment to living at a higher altitude, or therapy for anemia.

reticuloendothelial cells, cells lining blood and lymph vessels able to surround and kill (phago-cytose) bacteria, viruses, and gluelike (colloi-dal) particles or to form immune bodies against foreign bodies.

reticuloendothelial system (RES), a working sys-tem of the body mainly used to defend against infection and to dispose of the products of the breakdown of cells. It is made up of large cells (macrophages), the cells of the liver (Kuppfer cells), and the cells (reticulum) of the lungs, bone marrow, spleen, and lymph nodes.

reticuloendotheliosis /ritik′yəlō·en′dōthē′lē·ō′sis/, an increased growth and spread of the cells of a defense system of the body (reticuloendothe-lial system). See **reticuloendothelial system.**

reticulogranular, referring to a cloudy appearance of the lungs on a chest x-ray of a patient with respiratory distress syndrome.

reticulosarcoma. See **undifferentiated malignant lymphoma.**

reticulum cell sarcoma. See **histiocytic malignant lymphoma.**

-retin, a combining form for vitamin A_1 derivatives.

retina /ret'inə/, a 10-layered, frail nervous tissue membrane of the eye, parallel with the optic nerve. It receives images of outer objects and carries sight signals through the optic nerve to the brain. The retina is soft, semitransparent, and contains visual purple (rhodopsin), which gives it a purple tint. The retina becomes clouded if exposed to direct sunlight. The outer surface of the retina is in contact with the coating of the eye (choroid), the inner surface with the watery part of the eye (vitreous body). The retina is thinner in front, where it reaches nearly as far as the eyelids (ciliary body), and thicker toward the back, except for a thin spot in the exact center of the back surface where focus is best. See also **Jacob's membrane, macula, optic disc.**

Retin-A, a trademark for an acne drug (tretinoin).

retinaculum /ret'inak'yələm/, *pl.* **retinacula,** a structure that holds an organ or tissue in place.

retinaculum extensorum manus, the thick band of fiberlike sheets (antebrachial fascia) of the forearm that wraps tendons of the flexing (extensor) muscles of the forearm at the far ends of the forearm bones (radius, ulna). Also called **dorsal carpal ligament, extensor retinaculum of the hand.**

retinaculum flexorum manus, the thick, fiberlike band of sheets (fascia) that wrap the canal surrounding the tendons of the flexing muscles of the forearm at the wrist. Also called **flexor retinaculum of the hand, volar ligament.**

retinal /ret'inəl, retinal'/, **1.** the active form of vitamin A needed for night, day, and color vision. See also **retinene, vitamin A. 2.** referring to the retina of the eye.

retinal detachment, a division of the retina of the eye from the covering (choroid) in the back of the eye, most often resulting from a hole in the retina that allows the watery substance (vitreous humor) to leak between the choroid and the retina. Severe injury to the eye, as a bruise or penetrating wound, may be the cause, but in most cases retinal detachment is the result of internal changes in the vitreous chamber linked to aging or, less often, to swelling of the inner eye. In most cases retinal detachment develops slowly. The first symptom is often the sudden appearance of many spots floating loosely, hung in front of the affected eye. The patient may not seek help, because the number of spots tends to decrease during the days and weeks after the detachment. The patient may also notice a curious feeling of flashing lights as the eye is moved. Because the retina does not contain sense nerves that relay feelings of pain, the condition is painless. Detachment often begins at the thin outer edge of the retina and reaches gradually under the thicker, more central areas. The patient senses a shadow that begins at the side and grows in size, slowly edging in on central sight. As long as the center of the retina is unaffected, the sight, when the patient is looking straight ahead, is normal. When the center becomes affected, the eyesight is distorted, wavy, and unfocused. If the detachment is not halted, total blindness of the eye will result. The condition does not resolve itself. Surgery is often needed to repair the hole and prevent the

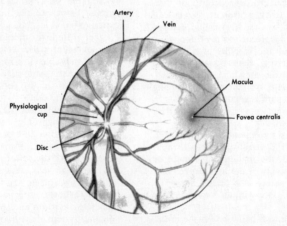

Retina

leakage of vitreous humor that divides the retina from its source of food, the choroid. If the condition is found early, when the hole is small and the amount of vitreous humor lost is not large, the retinal hole may be closed by causing a scar to form on the choroid and to join to the retina around the hole. The scar may be caused by heat, electric current, or cold. The degree of restored sight depends on the degree and length of division. Maximum sight is gained within 3 months after surgery. Unless replaced, a detached retina slowly dies after several years of detachment. Blindness resulting from retinal detachment cannot be treated.

retinene /ret'inin/, either of the two yellow colorings (carotenoid pigments) found in the rods of the retina that are sources of vitamin A and are set into motion by light. See also **retinal, retinol.**

retinoblastoma /ret'inōplastō'mə/, pl. **retinoblastomas, retinoblastomata,** an inherited cancer growing from eye (retinal) germ cells. Signs are lessened sight, unfocused eyes, a detached retina, and an abnormal pupil reflex. The rapidly growing tumor may invade the brain and spread to distant sites. Treatment includes removal of the eye and as much of the optic nerve as possible, followed by radiation and chemical treatments. It occurs in both eyes in about 30% of cases; the more affected eye is removed, and the other eye is treated with radiation, antibiotics, freezing (cryotherapy), or condensing protein (photocoagulation), singly or together. Because nearly 20% of the cases are carried as a ruling (dominant) trait with incomplete penetration, genetic counseling is urged.

retinocerebral angiomatosis. See **cerebroretinal angiomatosis.**

retinodialysis /ret'inōdī·al'isis/, a separation or tear in front of the retina where the support tissue (ciliary body) of the iris begins.

retinol /ret'inôl/, a form of vitamin A. It is found in the retinas of the eyes of mammals. Also called **vitamin A₁.**

retinopathy /ret'inop'əthē/, a nonswelling eye disorder resulting from changes in the eye (retinal) blood vessels.

retraction, 1. the moving of tissues to expose a part or structure of the body. 2. a backward movement of the teeth.

retraction of the chest, the visible sinking-in of the soft tissues of the chest between the ribs, as occurs with increased breathing effort. In infants, breastbone retraction also occurs with only a slight increase in breathing effort.

retractor, a surgery device for holding back the edges of tissues and organs to keep organs and tissues exposed.

retroaortic node /re'trō·ā·ôr'tik/, a node in one of the sets of lymph nodes behind the aorta that serve many structures in the stomach, intestines, and the pelvis.

retroclusion, a method of controlling bleeding from an artery by compressing it between tissues on either side. A needle is inserted through the tissues above the bleeding vessel, then turned around and down so it also passes through the tissues beneath the artery.

retroflexion, an abnormal placement of an organ in which the organ is tilted back and folded over on itself.

retroflexion of the uterus, a condition in which the body of the uterus is bent backward at an angle with the cervix, which usually does not move.

retrograde, 1. moving backward; moving in the opposite direction to that which is thought to be normal. 2. breaking down; going back to an earlier state or worse condition.

retrograde amnesia, the loss of memory for events occurring before a set time in a patient's life, often before the event that caused the amnesia. The condition may result from disease, brain injury or damage, or an emotional injury. Compare **anterograde amnesia.**

retrograde cystoscopy, a method in radiology for testing the bladder in which a tube (catheter) is put through the bladder tube (urethra) into the bladder, allowing the urine in the bladder to pass through the catheter. A radiopaque medium is introduced, filling the bladder, and the shape of the bladder is looked at, using many x-ray films or fluoroscopy, as the contrast medium is gotten rid of. See also **cystogram, retrograde pyelography.**

retrograde filling, a filling placed in the top part of a tooth root to seal the top part of the root canal. Also called **postresection filling.**

retrograde infantilism. See **acromegalic eunuchoidism.**

retrograde infection, an infection that spreads along a tube or duct against the flow of fluids or wastes, as in the urinary and lymph systems.

retrograde menstruation, a backflow of menstrual fluids through the uterine space and the fallopian tubes into the abdomen space. Pieces of matter from the uterus may become joined to the ovaries or other organs, causing endometriosis. Also called **regurgitant menstruation.**

retrograde pyelography, a method in radiology for testing the structures of the collecting system of the kidneys. It is very useful in finding a blockage in the urinary tract. A radiopaque dye is injected through a urinary tube (catheter) into the tubes of the kidneys.

retrogression, a return to a less complex state, condition, or behavior; breakdown. See also **regression.**

retrolental fibroplasia, a making of fiberlike tissue behind the lens of the eye, resulting in blindness. The disorder is caused by giving excess amounts of oxygen to premature infants.

retroperitoneal, referring to organs closely attached to the stomach and intestine walls and partly covered by the lining (peritoneum), rather than held up by that lining.

retroperitoneal fibrosis, a long-term swelling in which fiberlike tissue surrounds the large blood vessels in the lower back space. It often causes a narrowing of the middle of the bladder tubes (ureters), which may lead to urine bloating (hydronephrosis) and too much urea in the blood (azotemia). Sometimes it spreads up to involve the small intestine (duodenum), bile ducts, and the large blood vessel of the abdomen (superior vena cava). Symptoms include low back and stomach pain, weakness, weight loss, fever, and, with urinary tract involvement, excess urination, and other urinary problems. Methysergide, a drug taken to prevent migraine headaches, is one known cause of this condition. Treatment includes stopping the use of methysergide and beginning to release the ureters from the fibrosis through surgery.

retroperitoneal lymph node dissection, removal of lymph nodes behind the linings of the abdomen (peritoneum), most often done in an attempt to get rid of sites of lymph gland cancer or the spread of cancers that start in pelvic organs or the sex organs.

retropharyngeal abscess, a buildup of pus in the tissues behind the throat (pharynx) causing difficulty in swallowing, fever, and pain. Sometimes the airway becomes blocked. Treatment includes giving antibiotics and draining. It may be best to create an airway (tracheostomy). Compare **parapharyngeal abscess, peritonsillar abscess.**

retroplacental, behind the placenta.

retrospective study, a study in which a search is made for a relation between one (usually current) factor or condition and another that occurred in the past, as a study of the family histories of young women diagnosed as having clear cell tumors of the vagina, which showed a relation between giving a drug (diethylstilbestrol) to the mothers of the women during their pregnancies.

retrouterine /re′trō·yo͞o′tərin/, behind the uterus.

retroversion, 1. a common condition in which an organ is tipped backward, often without flexion or other distortion. The uterus may be retroverted in as many as 25% of normal women. Uterine retroversion is measured as first, second, or third degree, depending on the angle of tilt with respect to the vagina. No treatment is needed. **2.** an abnormal condition in which the teeth or other jaw structures are behind their normal places. Also called **retrusion.** –**retrovert,** v.

revascularization, restoring through surgery the blood flow to an organ or a tissue being replaced, as in bypass surgery.

reverse anaphylaxis. See **inverse anaphylaxis.**

reversed bandage, a roller bandage that is turned on itself with a half twist so that it lies smoothly, conforming to the contour of the arm or leg. See also **roller bandage.**

reverse isolation, isolation methods to protect a patient from infectious organisms that might be carried by the staff, other patients, or visitors or on droplets in the air or on equipment or materials.

reverse transcriptase (RT), an enzyme that is present in an RNA virus (retrovirus). It occurs in leukoviruses and some RNA tumor viruses. Also called **RNA-dependent DNA polymerase.** See also **retrovirus.**

reverse Trendelenburg, a position in which the legs are lower than the body and head, which are raised on a slanted, flat surface.

reversible brain syndrome, any of a group of severe brain disorders marked by an interruption of mental abilities, as in delirium. The disorder has a variety of biological causes, and recovery is possible.

review of systems (ROS), a system-by-system review of the person's health history of the body. It is begun during the first interview with the patient and completed during the physical examination, as physical findings prompt further questions. One outline of the systems and some of the signs and symptoms that might be noted or reported are as follows.

★SKIN: bruising, discoloration, itching, birthmarks, moles, ulcers, and changes in the hair or nails.

★BLOOD: abrupt or heavy bleeding, fatigue, swollen or tender lymph nodes, paleness, and a history of anemia.

★HEAD AND FACE: pain, injury, and difficulty seeing.

★EARS: ringing in the ears, change in hearing, discharge from the ears, deafness, and dizziness.

★EYES: change in sight, pain, swelling, infections, double vision, sight defects, blurring, and tearing.

★MOUTH AND THROAT: dental problems, hoarseness, difficulty in swallowing, bleeding gums, sore throat, ulcers, or sores in the mouth.

★NOSE AND SINUSES: discharge, nosebleed, sinus pain, or blockage.

★BREASTS: pain, change in shape or skin color, lumps, discharge from the nipple.

★BREATHING TRACT: cough, sputum, change in sputum, night sweats, shortness of breath, and wheezing.

★HEART SYSTEM: chest pain, difficulty in breathing, rapid heart beat, weakness, intolerance of exercise, varicose veins, swelling of tissues, known heart murmur, high blood pressure, or heart attack.

★DIGESTIVE SYSTEM: nausea, vomiting, diarrhea, constipation, quality of appetite, change in appetite, difficulty in swallowing, gas, heartburn, change in bowel habits, the use of laxatives, or other drugs to alter the function of the digestive tract.

★URINARY TRACT: lack of urine, change in color of urine, change in times of urination, pain with a desire to urinate, not being able to urinate, and fluid buildup.

★GENITAL TRACT: (female) menstrual history, use of birth-control pills and devices, discharge, pain or discomfort, itching, and a history of venereal disease.

★GENITAL TRACT: (male) penis discharge, pain or discomfort, itching, sores, blood in the urine, and a history of venereal disease.

★SKELETAL SYSTEM: heat, redness, swelling, limited movement, deformity, pain in a joint or a limb, the neck, or back, especially with movement.

★NERVOUS SYSTEM: dizziness, tremor, irregular muscle movements, difficulty in speaking, change in speech, paralysis, loss of sensation, seizures, and fainting.

★ENDOCRINE SYSTEM: tremor, rapid heartbeat, intolerance of heat or cold, too much urine, an excess thirst, excess speech, seizures, and goiter.

★MENTAL STATUS: nervousness, instability, depression, unreal fears, sexual problems, criminal behavior, lack of sleep, night terrors, mania, memory loss, and confusion.

Reye's syndrome /rāz'/, a combination of brain disease and fatty invasion of the inner organs that may come after a virus infection. It has been linked to influenza B, chicken pox (varicella), the enteroviruses, and the Epstein-Barr virus. It often affects patients under 18 years of age, causing a rash, vomiting, and confusion about 1 week after the beginning of the illness. In the late stage, there may be extreme confusion followed by coma, seizures, and stopped breathing. A liver test shows fatty breakdown and confirms the diagnosis. The death rate ranges from 20% to 80%, depending on the severity of symptoms. The cause of Reye's syndrome is unknown. There is no specific treatment. Insulin, antibiotics, and mannitol may be given. Prompt correction of any imbalance in vital functions is very important for the outcome of this disease.

RF (rheumatoid factor) test. See **latex fixation test.**

rhabdo-, rhabdi-, a combining form meaning 'rod-shaped', or referring to a rod.

rhabdomyoma /rab'dōmī·ō'mə/, pl. **rhabdomyomas, rhabdomyomata,** a tumor of striated muscle that may occur in the uterus, vagina, throat, or tongue, and may or may not be a cancer. A related disorder (congenital tumor nodules) occurs in the heart. Also called **myoma striocellulare.**

rhabdomyosarcoma, pl. **rhabdomyosarcomas, rhabdomyosarcomata,** a cancerous growth that occurs most often in the head and neck. It is also found in the sex organs and urinary tract, legs and arms, body wall, and abdomen. In some cases, the disease comes after an injury. The first symptoms depend on the site of the tumor. They are related to tissue or organ damage, as swallowing difficulty, vaginal bleeding, bloody urine, or a block in the flow of urine. The tumors occur in the head, neck, or body of young children. A different form is seen in the arms and legs of adolescents. One type of the adolescent form is most common in the legs of adults. Removal is rarely possible, because the tumor has nothing to stop it and tends to spread. Removing an affected leg or arm may help. Radiation and chemical treatments with anticancer drugs may lengthen the life of the patient.

rhabdovirus, a member of a family of viruses that includes the one that causes rabies.

rhagades /rag'ədēz/, cracks or breaks in the skin that has lost its stretching ability. It is very common around the mouth. See also **cheilosis.**

rhaphe. See **raphe.**

Rh$_o$(D) immune globulin, a vaccinating drug used to prevent Rh allergy after abortion, miscarriage, childbirth, or pregnancy outside of the uterus (ectopic).

★CAUTION: It is not given to those already vaccinated.

★ADVERSE EFFECTS: The most serious side effect is allergic shock.

Rheomacrodex, a trademark for a blood plasma expander (dextran 40).

-rheumatic, a combining form meaning 'relating to or showing traits of rheumatism.'

rheumatic aortitis, an inflammatory condition of the major blood vessel (aorta) in the body. It occurs in rheumatic fever and results in damage to the aorta wall that may develop into patches of scarlike tissue (fibrosis).

rheumatic arteritis, a problem linked to rheumatic fever in which there is swelling of blood vessels (arteries and arterioles). A blood clotting substance (fibrin) mixes with cell waste. This gets into, thickens, and stiffens the vessel wall. The vessel may be surrounded by bleeding.

rheumatic chorea. See **Sydenham's chorea.**

rheumatic fever, a disease that may develop within 1 to 5 weeks after recovery from a sore (strep) throat or from scarlet fever. It most often occurs in young children and may affect the brain, heart, joints, and skin. It is often sudden. Early symptoms are fever, joint pains, nose bleeds, stomach pain, and vomiting. The major effects of this disease are a form of arthritis in many joints. It also causes heart problems, as chest pain, and, in severe cases, symptoms of heart failure. Another disorder (Sydenham's chorea) may develop and is commonly the only, late sign of rheumatic fever. This may at first appear as an increased awkwardness and a habit of dropping objects. Irregular body movements may worsen, and sometimes the tongue and the face muscles are affected. Other problems may be skin disorders, as nodes beneath the skin or red patches with circular sores, a rise in the number of white blood cells, anemia, and protein in the urine. There is no specific diagnostic test for rheumatic fever. Returns of rheumatic fever are common. Except for heart inflammation, all effects of this disease often go away without any permanent problems. Mild cases may last 3 to 4 weeks. Severe cases with arthritis and heart swelling may last 2 to 3 months. Treatment of this disease is bed rest and keeping the patient from doing normal actions. Penicillin is often given, even if there is no sign of bacteria infection. Steroid drugs or aspirin may be used. Large amounts of fluids are given and joint pains are lessened by putting the patient in a comfortable position. See also **rheumatic heart disease.**

rheumatic heart disease, damage to heart muscle and heart valves caused by attacks of rheumatic fever. The heart damage may be found during the disease, or it may be discovered long after the disease has gone away. Heart murmurs result from narrowing or poor working of the valves. This causes changes in the size of the chambers of the heart and the thickness of their walls. Abnormal pulse rate and rhythm, heart block, and congestive heart failure are also common. Deaths are often caused by heart failure or infection in the heart. Long-term rheumatic heart disease may require no treatment except for close watching. If signs of poor heart action occur, heart drugs, fluid-releasing drugs (diuretics), and a low-sodium diet are often given. It may be necessary to correct or replace the valves. Patients with a history of rheumatic fever or signs of rheumatic heart disease may get daily doses of penicillin by mouth or monthly injections to protect against streptococcal infections. The antibiotics are given during childhood and adolescence. Patients with signs of deformed heart valves need preventive doses of antibiotics before surgery and dental work to prevent other infections. See also **aortic stenosis, mitral stenosis, rheumatic fever.**

rheumatism, *nontechnical.* any of many swelling conditions of the bursae, joints, ligaments, or muscles. Symptoms are pain, limited movement, and tissue damage. **–rheumatic, rheumatoid,** *adj.*

rheumatoid arthritis, a long-term, destructive connective tissue disease that results from the body rejecting its own tissue cells (autoimmune reaction). There is inflammation of the membranes (synovial) lining the joints and in-

creased release of synovial fluid. This leads to thickening of the synovial membrane and swelling of the joint. Rheumatoid arthritis first appears in early middle age, between 36 and 50 years of age. It occurs most commonly in women. The course of the disease varies. There are times when it goes away (remission), and times when it gets worse (exacerbations). The diagnosis is done by x-ray studies and blood tests. Rheumatoid arthritis is divided into four stages. Stage I, early effects, is based on x-ray films showing the first bone changes. Stage II, moderate rheumatoid arthritis, shows signs of some muscle wasting and loss of movement, in addition to x-ray findings. Stage III, severe rheumatoid arthritis, shows joint defects, much muscle wasting, soft tissue tumors, and bone and cartilage destruction. Stage IV, the terminal category, has all of the Stage III signs plus fiberlike or bony joining (ankylosis). Rheumatoid arthritis cases may also be named for functional capacity. Class I is patients with no loss of function. Class II is minor damage of functional capacity with some pain and stiffness. Class III is capacity limited to a few tasks. Class IV is the patient confined to a bed or a wheelchair.

Rheumatoid arthritis may first begin with general symptoms, as fatigue, weakness, and poor appetite. Other early signs are mild fever, anemia, and red blood cells changes. The symptoms listed by the American Rheumatism Association are morning stiffness, joint pain or tenderness, swelling of at least two joints; arthritic nodes found at pressure points (as the elbows), changes in the joint seen on x-ray films, a positive rheumatoid factor blood test, and changes in the content of synovial fluid. Rheumatoid factor (RF) is in blood and synovial fluid of most patients with rheumatoid arthritis. Higher amounts are found in the more severe forms of the disease. The basic treatment is rest, exercise to help joint function, drugs for pain relief and lowering the swelling, surgery to prevent or correct defects, and a good diet—with weight loss, if needed. Aspirin-type drugs are given. If the patient does not get better, other antiswelling drugs may be used. Steroids are given with caution because of side effects. These are peptic ulcer, slowed adrenal glands, and bone weakening (osteoporosis). Other treatments, as diathermy, ultrasound, warm paraffin applications, and exercise under water are sometimes used. Rheumatoid arthritis is not always progressive or deforming. Thus, early treatment may help the patient to recover and perhaps to avoid future attacks. Also called **arthritis deformans, atrophic arthritis.** Compare **ankylosing spondylitis.** (See chart on p. 681.)

rheumatoid coronary arteritis, a thickening of the lining of the heart blood vessels, which may result in lowered blood flow to the heart. The disease affects the connective tissue by swelling and fiber damage. It is commonly treated with corticoid hormone drugs. See also **glucocorticoid.**

rheumatoid factor (RF), a type of antibody often found in the blood of patients with rheumatoid arthritis. Rheumatoid factors are present in about 70% of such cases. They may also be found in other diseases, as tuberculosis, parasitic infections, and leukemia.

rheumatology, the study of disorders in which connective tissue and related body structures become swollen and break down. These disorders are sometimes referred to as rheumatism.

Rh factor, a substance (antigen) in the red blood cells of most people. A person with the factor is Rh+ (Rh positive). A person lacking the factor is Rh− (Rh negative). If an Rh− person receives Rh+ blood, red blood cells are destroyed and anemia occurs. An Rh+ fetus may be exposed to antibodies to the factor made in the Rh− mother's blood. Red cell destruction occurs and, if untreated, a fatal condition (erythroblastosis fetalis) results. Transfusion, blood typing, and cross-matching depend on Rh+ and ABO blood group labeling. The Rh factor was first found in the blood of a species of the rhesus (Rh) monkey. It is in the red cells of 85% of people. See also **erythroblastosis fetalis, Rh₀ (D) immune globulin.**

Rh incompatibility, a conflict between two groups of blood cells that are different because one group is RH+ and the other is RH−. See also **Rh factor.**

rhinencephalon /rī′nensef′əlon/, *pl.* **rhinencephala,** a part of each brain side (cerebral hemisphere) that contains the limbic system, which is linked to the emotions. See also **limbic system.** –**rhinencephalic,** *adj.*

rhinitis /rīnī′tis/, inflammation of the mucous membranes of the nose, with a nasal discharge. It may be seen with a sinus infection.

rhino-, rhin-, a combining form referring to the nose or to a noselike structure.

rhinopathy /rīnop′əthē/, any disease or defect of the nose.

rhinophycomycosis /rī′nōfī′kōmīkō′sis/, an infection of the sinuses around the nose caused by the fungus (phycomycete) *Entomophthora coronata.* The infection often spreads to surrounding tissues, including the eye and brain.

rhinophyma /rī′nōfī′mə/, a form of acne (rosacea). There is overgrowth of tissue, redness, prominent blood vessels, swelling, and defects of the skin of the nose. Treatment is scouring or surgery. See also **rosacea.**

rhinoplasty /rī′nəplas′tē/, a method in plastic surgery in which the structure of the nose is changed. Bone or cartilage may be removed, tissue taken from another part of the body, or artificial material planted to change the shape. Under local anesthesia cuts are made in the nose, and the nose is reshaped. After surgery, any breathing difficulty is reported at once and the patient is kept with the head and knees raised (mid-Fowler's position). Mouth care is given and ice compresses are applied to reduce the pain and fluid buildup (edema) that occur. Edema and discoloration around the eyes is

---

Rheumatoid arthritis

Clinical stages	Functional classification
Stage 1, early 1. X-ray films show no evidence of destructive changes. 2. X-ray films may show evidence of osteoporosis.	*Class I* No loss of functional capacity.
Stage II, moderate 1. X-ray films show evidence of osteoporosis, possibly with slight destruction of cartilage of subchondral bone. 2. Joints are not deformed, but mobility may be limited. 3. Adjacent muscles are atrophied. 4. Extraarticular soft-tissue lesions (as nodules and tenovaginitis) may be present.	*Class II* Functional capacity impaired but sufficient normal activities despite joint pain or limited mobility.
Stage III, severe 1. X-ray films show cartilage and bone destruction, as well as osteoporosis. 2. Joint deformity (as subluxation, ulnar deviation, or hyperextension) exists but not fibrous or bony ankylosis. 3. Muscle atrophy is extensive. 4. Extraarticular soft-tissue lesions (as nodules and tenovaginitis) are often present.	*Class III* Functional capacity adequate to perform few if any occupational or self-care tasks. *Class IV* Patient confined to bed or wheelchair and capable of little or no self-care.
Stage IV, terminal 1. Fibrous or bony ankylosis exists in addition to all criteria listed for stage III.	

expected to last for several days. It is most often done for cosmetic reasons.

rhinorrhea /rī'nôrē'ə/, **1.** the free release of mucus from the nose. **2.** the flow of spinal fluid from the nose following an injury to the head.

rhinoscopy /rīnos'kəpē/, the examination of the nasal passages to inspect the mucosa and detect swelling, defects, or a crooked nose. The nasal passages may be looked at from the front, by putting a device in the nostrils. They can also be looked at from behind, by putting a device in through the back of the throat. –**rhinoscopic,** *adj.*

rhinosporidiosis /rī'nōspərid'ē·ō'sis/, an infection caused by the fungus *Rhinosporidium seeberi.* It is marked by fleshy red growths (polyps) on the mucous membranes of the nose, the lining of the eye (conjunctiva), the back of the throat (nasopharynx), and the soft palate. The disease may be gotten by swimming or bathing in infected water. The most effective treatment is to burn off the growths (electrocautery).

rhinotomy /rīnot'əmē/, a surgery in which a cut is made along one side of the nose. It is done to drain pus from a sore or a sinus infection. Using local anesthesia the flap of skin and lining of the nose are turned back to offer a full view of the nasal passages for major sinus surgery.

rhinovirus /rī'nōvī'rəs/, any of about 100 distinct, small RNA viruses that cause about 40% of breathing illnesses. The infection is marked by a dry, scratchy throat; stuffy nose; tiredness; and headache. There is little fever. The fluids from the nose last 2 or 3 days. Children may also get a cough. The treatment is general and may be rest, painkillers, antihistamines, and decongestants. Complete recovery often occurs. See also **cold.**

rhitidosis /rit'idō'sis/, a wrinkling, as of the cornea of the eye. Also spelled **rhytidosis.**

rhizomelic /rī'zəmel'ik/, referring to the hip and shoulder joints.

rhizotomy /rīzot'əmē/, the cutting of the root of a spinal nerve to relieve pain.

Rh negative. See **Rh factor.**

Rhodesian trypanosomiasis, a form of African trypanosomiasis, caused by the parasite *Trypanosoma brucei rhodesiense.* The disease may take off rapidly, causing sleeping sickness (encephalitis), coma, and death in only a few weeks. Also called **kaodzera.** See also **African trypanosomiasis.**

rhodopsin /rōdop'sin/, the purple-colored part in the rods of the retina of the eye. They are formed by a protein (opsin) and a part of vitamin A (retinal). Rhodopsin gives the outer parts of the rods a purple color and adapts the eye to low density light. It breaks down when struck by light. It starts the sending of nerve signals. Short times of darkness allow the opsin and the retinal to remake the rhodopsin. This accounts for the short delay a person has in focusing in sudden or drastic changes in lighting, as when moving out of bright sunlight into a darkened room or from darkness into bright light. Closing the eyes is a natural reflex that allows the remaking of rhodopsin. Compare **iodopsin.**

RhoGAM, a trademark for a vaccinating drug (Rh₀ [D] immune globulin).

rhomboideus major /romboi'dē·əs/, a muscle of the upper back. It draws the shoulder blade toward the backbone while holding it up and drawing it slightly upward.

rhomboideus minor, a muscle of the upper back, above and parallel to another muscle of the upper back (rhomboideus major). It draws the shoulder blade toward the backbone while holding it up and drawing it slightly upward.

rhomboid glossitis. See **median rhomboid glossitis.**

rhonchi /rong'kī/, *sing.* **rhonchus,** abnormal sounds heard in an airway blocked by thick fluids, muscle spasms, tumors, or outside pressure. The constant rumbling sounds are lower when the patient breathes out, and they clear on coughing. Rhonchi may be sibilant or sonorous. Sibilant rhonchi are high pitched and are heard in the small tubes (bronchi), as in asthma. Sonorous rhonchi are lower pitched and are heard in the large bronchi, as in tracheobronchitis. Dry rales are called rhonchi. Compare **rale, wheeze.**

rhotacism /rō'təsiz'əm/, a speech disorder marked by a defective pronunciation of words with the sound /r/, by the excess use of the sound /r/, or by using another sound for /r/. Compare **lallation, lambdacism.**

Rh positive. See **Rh factor.**

rhus dermatitis, a skin rash resulting from contact with a plant of the genus *Rhus,* as poison ivy, poison oak, or poison sumac. See also **contact dermatitis.**

rhythm, the relation of one signal to nearby signals as measured in time, movement, or regular action.

rhythm method. See **natural family planning method.**

rhytid-, rhitid-, a combining form meaning 'wrinkle, or wrinkled.'

rhytidoplasty /ritid'ōplas'tē/, a method in plastic surgery in which the skin of the face is tightened, wrinkles are removed, and the skin is made to appear firm and smooth. A cut is made at the hairline, and excess skin is separated from the supporting tissue and taken away. The edges of the remaining skin are pulled up and back and stitched to the hairline. A pressure dressing is applied and left in place for 24 to 48 hours. Drugs are given after surgery for pain. The stitches are removed many days after surgery in a clinic or office. Also spelled **rhitidoplasty.**

rhytidosis. See **rhitidosis.**

rib, one of the 12 pairs of elastic arches of bone forming a large part of the chest (thoracic) skeleton. The first seven ribs on each side are called **true ribs** because they join to the breastbone (sternum) and the backbones (vertebrae). The other five ribs are called **false ribs.** The first three join the ribs above. The last two are free at their ends and are called **floating ribs.**

rib fracture, a break in a bone of the chest caused by a blow or crushing injury or by violent coughing or sneezing. The ribs most commonly broken are the fourth to eighth. If the bone is shattered or the break is displaced, sharp pieces may pierce the lung. The patient has pain, especially on taking a deep breath, and often breathes quickly and shallowly. The site of the break may be very tender to the touch. The crackling of bone pieces rubbing together may be heard. Breath sounds may be absent or show other signs of damage (rales and rhonchi). The location and nature of the break are found by chest x-ray films. The patient is watched for signs of blood or air in the chest, collapsed lung, pneumonia, and other problems. Broken ribs may be splinted with an elastic belt, an Ace bandage, or adhesive tape. To prevent irritation, the chest may be shaved and painted with benzoin before the adhesive tape is put on. If the patient needs to stay in the hospital, the patient is made to lie down and is helped in turning. The patient must learn how to breathe deeply, cough, and do exercises while wrapped in tape. If taping and painkilling drugs fail to relieve pain, the physician may do a regional nerve block by injecting the rib spaces above and below the break with 1% procaine.

riboflavin /rib′ōflā′vin/, a yellow crystal-like, heat-stable part of the B vitamin complex. It is a coenzyme in the breakdown of carbohydrates, fats, and proteins. It is also important in preventing some sight disorders, as cataracts. Small amounts of riboflavin are found in the liver and kidneys. It is not stored in any large amount in the body and must be gotten from the diet. Common sources are organ meats, milk, cheese, eggs, green leafy vegetables, meat, whole grains, and peas. A lack of riboflavin causes skin tumors, sensitivity to light and other eye disorders, trembling, sluggishness, dizziness, fluid buildup, inability to urinate, and vaginal itching. Also called **vitamin B₂.** See also **ariboflavinosis.**

ribonucleic acid (RNA) /rī′bōnoōklē′ik/, a nucleic acid, found in both the nucleus and cytoplasm of cells. It carries gene data from the nucleus to the cytoplasm. In the cytoplasm, RNA puts together proteins. See also **deoxyribonucleic acid.**

ribosome /rī′bəsōm/, a tiny organ (organelle) in the cytoplasm of cells. It is made of ribonucleic acid and protein that make protein. Ribosomes act with messenger RNA and transfer RNA to join together amino acid units into a larger protein molecule according to a series of reactions by a genetic code. See also **translation.**

rib shaking, a procedure in physical therapy in which constant downward pressure is applied with periodic shaking motions with the hands on the rib cage over an area being drained. It is done with the flat part of the palm of the hand over the lung segment being drained during 4 to 12 extended breaths by the patient through puckered lips.

rib vibration, a procedure in physical therapy, similar to rib shaking, done with downward vibrating pressure with the flat part of the palm during breaths.

rice diet, a diet made up only of rice, fruit, fruit juices, and sugar. Vitamins and iron are given. Salt is not used. It is sometimes given to treat high blood pressure, long-term kidney disease, and overweight. The diet is somewhat changed after the blood pressure is lowered and other symptoms are eased. It should not be followed for any length of time, because it may lead to diet problems, or imbalance. Also called **Duke diet, Kempner rice-fruit diet.**

rickets, a condition caused by the lack of vitamin D, calcium, and phosphorus. It is seen most often in infancy and childhood. It is marked by abnormal bone growth. Symptoms include soft bones causing defects, as bowlegs and knock-knees, swellings on the ends and sides of the bones, muscle pain, a swollen skull, chest defects, a curved spine, swollen liver and spleen, heavy sweating, and general tenderness of the body when touched. Prevention and treatment are a diet rich in calcium, phosphorus, and vitamin D and enough exposure to sunlight. Kinds of rickets include **adult rickets, celiac rickets, renal rickets, vitamin D resistant rickets.** See also **osteodystrophy, osteomalacia, vitamin D.**

rickettsia /riket′sē·ə/, any organism of the genus *Rickettsia.* Rickettsiae are small, round, or rod-shaped special bacteria. They live as viruslike parasites inside the cells of lice, fleas, ticks, and mites. They are carried to humans by bites from these insects. Rickettsial diseases have caused many of history's worst epidemics. The many species are told apart on the basis of the diseases they cause. The spotted fever group is Rocky Mountain spotted fever, rickettsialpox, and others. The typhus group is epidemic typhus, scrub typhus, murine typhus. Another group is Q fever and trench fever. Rickettsial diseases are uncommon in parts of the world where insect and rodent populations are well controlled. Antibiotics are often given to treat rickettsial diseases. **–rickettsial,** *adj.*

rickettsialpox /riket′sē·əlpoks′/, a mild infectious disease caused by *Rickettsia akari.* It is carried from mice to humans by mites. It is marked by a crusted sore, chills, fever, headache, tiredness, muscle pain, and a rash that looks like chickenpox. About 1 week after the symptoms begin, small pimples appear on any part of the body, but rarely on palms or soles. These become dry and form scabs. The scabs fall off, leaving no scars. Antibiotics help recovery. Prevention is getting rid of house mice. Also called **Kew Gardens spotted fever.** Compare Rocky Mountain spotted fever. See also **Rickettsia.**

rickettsiosis /riket′sē·ō′sis/, *pl.* **rickettsioses,** any of a group of infectious diseases caused by *Rickettsia* organisms.

rider's bone, a bony deposit that sometimes grows in horseback riders on the inner side of the lower end of the tendon of a thigh muscle. Also called **cavalry bone.**

ridge lap, the part of an artificial tooth that is next to or laps the bony ridge that remains around the socket of tooth that has been taken out.

Ridura, a trademark for a drug (auronofin) given by mouth to relieve arthritis.

Riedel's struma, Riedel's thyroiditis. See **fibrous thyroiditis.**

Rieder cell leukemia /rē′dər/, a cancer of blood-making tissues. It is marked by large numbers of early white blood cells in the blood.

-rifa, a combining form for antibiotics derived from rifamycin.

Rifadin, a trademark for an antibiotic (rifampin).

rifampin, an antibiotic used to treat or prevent tuberculosis, meningitis, and leprosy.

★CAUTION: Liver disorders or known allergy to this or like drugs prohibits its use.

★ADVERSE EFFECTS: Among the more serious side effects are liver disorders and symptoms looking like the flu. Stomach upset, aches and cramps, discolored urine, saliva, and sweat commonly occur. This drug interacts with many other drugs.

Rift Valley fever, an arbovirus infection of Egypt and East Africa spread by mosquitoes or by handling infected sheep and cattle. It is marked by abrupt fever, chills, headache, and general aching. It is followed by stomach pain, loss of appetite, loss of taste, and sensitivity to light. It lasts only a short time, and recovery is often complete. There is no specific treatment. A killed virus vaccine that protects for 2 years is available for those at risk, as laboratory workers and animal doctors.

Riga-Fede disease, a tumor of the tongue (lingual frenum) in some infants. It is caused by early teeth rubbing on it. Also called **Fede's disease.**

right atrial catheter, a small tube inserted directly into or close to the vein returning blood from the upper half of the body (superior vena cava), and threaded through the vein into the right atrium of the heart. The catheter may be left in place for an extended period.

right atrioventricular valve. See **tricuspid valve.**

right bundle branch block, a heart condition in which electric signals that normally travel along fibers on the right side of the heart fail to reach the right lower chamber (ventricle). This may be caused by a growth in the right bundle branch of fibers. A right bundle branch block is often linked to an enlarged right ventricle of the heart, especially in patients under 40 years of age. In older patients, a right bundle branch block is commonly caused by heart blood vessel (coronary artery) disease.

right coronary artery, one of a pair of branches of a part of the main artery (ascending aorta) of the body. It passes along the right side of the heart and divides into branches that supply both lower chambers (ventricles) and the right upper chamber (atrium). Compare **left coronary artery.**

right coronary vein. See **small cardiac vein.**

right-handedness, a natural favoring of the use of the right hand. Also called **dextrality.** See also **cerebral dominance, handedness.**

right-hand rule, a principle in physics in which the direction of electrical flow in a wire is related to the position of the imaginary lines of force of the magnetic field around the wire. Thus, if the fingers of the right hand are bent to represent the magnetic field and the thumb is then straightened, the thumb points in the direction of the electrical flow.

right hepatic duct, the duct that drains bile from the right lobe of the liver into the common bile duct.

right lymphatic duct, a vessel that carries lymph from the right upper area of the body into the blood. The duct joins two veins (right internal jugular and right subclavian) in the neck. At its opening are two valves that prevent blood from flowing back into the lymph system. Compare **thoracic duct.** See also **lymphatic system.**

right pulmonary artery, the longer, slightly larger of the two blood vessels (arteries) carrying blood from the heart to the lungs. It begins at the right lower heart chamber (ventricle) from a short blood vessel (pulmonary trunk), bends to the right, and divides into two branches at the root of the right lung. Compare **left pulmonary artery.**

right-sided heart failure, damage of the right side of the heart with clogging and high blood pressure in the veins and small vessels. It often relates to left-sided heart failure because both sides of the heart are part of the same circuit. What affects one side will affect the other over time. Thus, the most common cause of right-sided heart failure is left-sided heart failure. In failure linked to either side, the pumping action of the heart may be normal, lowered, or raised. Compare **left-sided heart failure.**

right subclavian artery, a large blood vessel (artery) with many important branches. It carries blood to the right side of the upper body.

right ventricle, the thin-walled lower chamber of the heart. It pumps blood received from the right upper chamber (atrium) into the lung (pulmonary) arteries to the lungs for oxygen. The right ventricle is shorter and rounder than the long, conic left ventricle. See also **heart.**

rigidity, a condition of hardness or stiffness. –**rigid,** *adj.*

rigor, 1. a rigid condition of the tissues of the body, as in rigor mortis. **2.** a violent attack of shivering that may come with chills and fever.

rigor mortis, the rigid stiffening of the muscles shortly after death.

Rimactane, a trademark for an antibiotic (rifampin).

rima glottidis. See **glottis.**

ringworm, a group of fungus skin diseases with itching, scaling, and, sometimes, painful tumors. Ringworm (tinea) is a general term that refers to infections of many causes on many body sites. The specific type is often named by a modifying term, as tinea capitis. Also called **tinea** /tin′ē-ə/.

Rinne tuning fork test /rin′ē/, a method of testing the ability to hear sounds of some frequencies. The test is done with tuning forks that cause sounds of 256, 512, and 1024 cycles per second. While each ear is tested, the other is covered. The stem of a vibrating fork is placed first 0.5 inches from the outside of the ear, then on the bone behind the ear. It is held until the sound is no longer heard at each of these positions. The person with normal hearing senses the sound for a longer time when conduction is by air outside of the ear, instead of by bone. In conductive hearing loss, the sound is heard for a longer time when conducted by bone than by air. In hearing loss from a sensory nerve disorder, the sound is heard longer when conducted by air, but hearing by both air and bone conduction is lowered.

-rinone, a combining form for an amrinone-type (cardiotonic) agent that increases the efficiency of heart contractions.

Rio Grande fever. See **abortus fever.**

Riopan, a trademark for an antacid (magaldrate).

risk factor, a factor that causes a person or a group of people to be at risk to an unwanted or unhealthful event, as cigarette smoking, which raises the chances of getting lung or heart disease.

risorius /risôr′ē-əs/, one of the 12 muscles of the mouth. It retracts the angles of the mouth, as in a smile.

Risser cast /ris′ər/, a fiberglass or plaster cast that surrounds the body and reaches over the neck as far as the chin. In rare cases it reaches over the hips to the knees. The cast prevents movement of the body. It is used to treat a spine disorder (scoliosis). Compare **body jacket, turnbuckle cast.**

risus sardonicus /rē′səs särdon′ikəs/, a wry, masklike grin caused by spasm of the face muscles, as seen in tetanus.

Ritalin Hydrochloride, a trademark for a nervous system-stimulating drug (methylphenidate hydrochloride).

Ritgen maneuver, a procedure used during birth to control delivery of the head. Upward pressure is applied from the base of the spinal column to extend the head during actual delivery, thereby protecting the muscles around the birth canal (perineum).

ritodrine hydrochloride, a nerve drug used in pregnancy to stop the uterus from contracting in labor that begins too soon.

★CAUTION: It is not given before the 20th week of pregnancy. Known allergy to this drug prohibits its use.

★ADVERSE EFFECTS: Among the more serious side effects are rapid heart beat, headache, nausea, and changes in blood pressure.

Ritter's disease, a bacterial infection of newborns that begins with red spots about the mouth and chin. The rash spreads over the entire body. General shedding of skin follows. Blisters and yellow crusts may also be present. Ritter's disease is often fatal unless treated with antibiotics. Also called **dermatitis exfoliativa neonatorum.** Compare **toxic epidermal necrolysis.**

river blindness. See **onchocerciasis.**

Rivinus' notch /rēvē′nəs/, an abnormality in the groove of the eardrum (tympanic membrane) where the soft upper part of the membrane attaches to the ear canal and to the first small bone (malleus or "hammer") in the middle ear.

RN, abbreviation for **registered nurse.**

RNA, abbreviation for **ribonucleic acid.**

Robaxin, a trademark for a skeletal muscle-relaxing drug (methocarbamol).

Robinul, a trademark for a peptic ulcer drug (glycopyrrolate).

Robitussin, a trademark for a cough syrup (guaifenesin). It is used in many cough drugs, and with an antihistamine it is used to stop coughing or to ease breathing.

Rocaltrol, a trademark for a calcium-controlling drug (calcitriol).

rocker knife, a knife that cuts with a rocking motion, designed for patients who have the use of only one hand.

rock fever. See **brucellosis.**

Rocky Mountain spotted fever (RMSF), an infectious disease carried by ticks in the warm zones of North America and South America. It is caused by bacteria *(Rickettsia).* Symptoms are chills, fever, severe headache, muscle pain, mental confusion, and rash. Red patches first appear on wrists and ankles. They spread quickly over the arms, legs, trunk, face, and on the hands and feet. Bleeding sores, constipation, and upset stomach are common. Early treatment with antibiotics is important. More than 20% of untreated patients die from shock and kidney failure. A diet high in protein is also important. Vaccination comes after recovery. Prevention includes the using of insect repellents and wearing protective clothing. Inspecting the body for ticks and careful removal of any found is needed. Care must be taken not to crush ticks, because infection may be gotten through breaks in the skin. Vaccination with killed vaccine is suggested for those often exposed to ticks. Also called **mountain fever, mountain tick fever, spotted fever.** Compare **murine typhus, rickettsialpox.** See also **boutonneuse fever, scrub typhus, typhus.**

rod, one of the tiny nerve cells shaped like a cylinder on the surface of the retina of the eye. Rods have a chemical (rhodopsin) that allows the eye to detect dim light. Compare **cone.** See also **rhodopsin.**

rodenticide poisoning, a harmful condition caused by swallowing a substance used to kill rats, mice, or other rodents. See also **phosphorus poisoning, poison, thallium poisoning, warfarin poisoning.**

rodent ulcer, a slowly growing form of skin cancer. See also **basal cell carcinoma.**

roentgen (R) /rent′gən, ren′jən/, the amount of x-rays or gamma rays that creates 1 electrostatic unit of ions in 1 ml of air. In radiology, the roentgen is the unit of the emitted dose. See also **gray, rad, rem.**

roentgenology, the study of the diagnostic and treatment uses of x-rays. See also **radiology, roentgen, x-ray.**

roentgen ray. See **x-ray.**

Roferon-A, a trademark for an anticancer drug (interferon-alpha-2a).

Rokitansky's disease. See **Budd-Chiari syndrome.**

role, a socially expected behavior pattern linked with an individual's function in various social groups. Roles provide a means for social participation and a way for significant others to test the meanings given to verbal and nonverbal behaviors.

role change, a situation in which status is retained while role expectations change, as when a nurse moves from the role of primary-care giver to administrator.

role clarification, gaining the knowledge, information, and cues needed to perform a role.

role induction interview, a technique that provides information to the patient in advance about the ways patients are expected to behave.

role playing, a method in which a person acts out a real or imagined situation as a means of understanding mental conflicts.

role-playing therapy. See **psychodrama.**

role reversal act, the act of taking on the role of another person to appreciate how that person feels, perceives, and behaves in relation to himself or herself as well as to others.

role strain, stress linked with expected roles or positions, felt as frustration. **Role ambiguity** is a type of role strain that occurs when the guidelines for an expected role are not given completely or clearly enough for the individual to tell what is desired and how to do it. **Role incongruence** is role stress that occurs when an individual makes a change in role requiring a significant change in attitudes and values. **Role overqualification** is a type of role stress that occurs when a role does not require full use of a person's resources

Rolfing. See **structural integration.**

roller bandage, a long, tightly wound strip of fabric that may vary in width. It is used as a circular bandage.

roller clamp, a device that can be moved to raise and lower the flow of a fluid through a tube into a vein during treatment.

rolling effleurage, a circular rubbing stroke used in massage. It relaxes muscles and helps the blood flow, especially on the shoulder and buttocks. It is done with the hand flat, the palm and fingers acting as a unit. Compare **effleurage, pétrissage.**

Romberg sign /rom′bərg/, a sign of loss of the sense of position in which the patient loses balance when standing erect, feet together, and eyes closed. Also called **Romberg test.**

Rondec-DM, a trademark for a drug with an antihistamine (carbinoxamine maleate), an antitussive (dextromethorphan hydrobromide), and a nasal and lung drug (pseudoephedrine hydrochloride).

Rondomycin, a trademark for an antibiotic (methacycline hydrochloride).

R-on-T phenomenon, a heart rhythm problem in which the ventricle contracts too soon.

rooming-in, a practice that allows mothers and new babies to remain together in the hospital as they would at home rather than being separated.

root, the part of an organ or a structure that is firmly joined to something, as the root of the tooth. Also called **radix.**

root canal. See **pulp canal.**

root canal file, a small metal device used for cleaning and shaping a root canal.

root canal filling, a material placed in the root canal system of a tooth to seal the space that used to hold the dental pulp.

root curettage, the scraping of the root surface of a tooth to remove plaque and help healthy gum tissues grow.

rooting reflex, a normal response in newborns when the cheek is touched or stroked along the side of the mouth. The infant turns the head toward the touched side and begins to suck. The reflex goes away by 3 to 4 months of age but it may last until 12 months of age.

root retention, a method to remove the crown of a root canal treated tooth and keep enough of the root and gums to hold a removable dental device (prosthesis).

Rorschach test /rôr'shäk/, a mental test set up by the Swiss psychiatrist Hermann Rorschach. It is made up of 10 pictures of inkblots. Five are in black and white, three are in black and red, and two are multicolored. The person studies the cards and responds by telling what images and emotions each design suggests. Replies are judged according to whether the response is to the entire image or only a part of it, and whether color, shading, shape, or location of certain picture parts are important. Other factors are whether movement is seen, and the complexity of each response. See also **Holtzman inkblot technique.**

rosacea /rōzā'shē·ə/, a long-term form of acne seen in adults. It is linked to widened blood vessels of the nose, forehead, and cheeks. Also called **acne rosacea.** See also **rhinophyma.**

rose fever, *informal.* a seasonal allergic nasal swelling caused by pollen, as of grasses. It is carried in the air at the time roses are in bloom. However, roses are not the cause of the common spring and summer allergic reactions.

Rosenthal's syndrome. See **hemophilia C.**

roseola /rōzē'ələ/, any rose-colored rash.

roseola infantum, an illness of infants and young children. There is an abrupt, high fever, mildly sore throat, and swollen lymph nodes. Seizures may occur. After 4 or 5 days the fever drops to normal and a faint, pink, pimplelike rash appears on the neck, body, and thighs. The rash may last a few hours to 2 days. There is no specific treatment or vaccine. Aspirin or acetaminophen are often used to try to control fever. Antiseizure drugs may be needed. Also called **exanthem subitum, sixth disease, Zahorsky's disease.**

rose spots, small reddish patches that occur on the upper stomach and chest lasting 2 or 3 days. They occur in typhoid and paratyphoid fevers.

rotating tourniquet, three tourniquets used in a rotating order to pool blood in the arms and legs. It is used to relieve fluid buildup in the lungs. Tourniquets are applied to the upper parts of three of the four arms and legs at one time. Every 15 minutes, in a clockwise pattern, a tourniquet is placed on the arm or leg not being wrapped, and one tourniquet is removed. As a result of this rotation, the blood vessels of each of the four limbs are narrowed for 45 minutes of each hour. A rotating tourniquet machine may be used in which blood pressure cuffs are automatically filled and emptied. Signs of blood clotting are watched

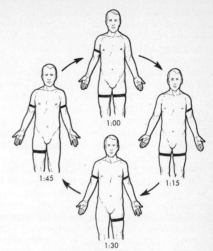

Rotating tourniquets

for. If the color of an arm or leg does not return to normal on release of a tourniquet, the physician is called. At the end of the treatment, one tourniquet is removed every 15 minutes in rotation.

rotation, 1. a turning around an axis. **2.** one of the basic kinds of motion allowed by many joints, as the rotation of the head on its central axis, the bones of the neck. **3.** the turning of a baby's head to go through the pelvis.

rotavirus, a double-stranded RNA molecule that appears as a tiny wheel, with a clearly defined outer layer, or rim, and an inner layer of spokes. The organism reproduces itself in the cells lining the intestine and is a cause of severe inflammation of the stomach and intestines (acute gastroenteritis) with diarrhea, especially in infants. Various types also infect domestic and wild animals. Human infections tend to peak during the winter months. See also **adult rotavirus (ADVR).**

Rotokinetic treatment table, a special bed that keeps patients completely immobilized and has an automatic turning device to turn from 90 to 270 degrees around a horizontal axis.

Rotor syndrome /rō'tər/, an inherited condition of the liver, with a mild yellowing of the skin (jaundice) but without other symptoms. The gallbladder works normally. See also **Dubin-Johnson syndrome, hyperbilirubinemia of the newborn.**

rotula. See **troche.**

roughage. See **dietary fiber.**

rouleaux /rōōlō'/, *sing.* **rouleau,** a clump of red cells in what looks like a stack of coins. It may sometimes be caused by abnormal proteins, but it is most often the result of red cells sticking to each other. Compare **hemagglutination.** See also **erythrocyte sedimentation rate.**

round ligament, 1. a curved fiberlike band of tissue that is joined at one end to the head of the upper leg bone (femur) and at the other to the ligament (transverse) of the hollow in the hipbone (acetabulum). **2.** a fiberlike cord reaching from inside the navel to the front part of the liver. It is the leftover part of a vein of the umbilical cord. **3.** in the female, a fiberlike band of tissue that reaches from the front surface of the uterus through a canal (inguinal) to the borders of the vaginal opening. It grows from the same tissue that becomes the sperm cord in the male.

roundworm, any worm of the class Nematoda, which includes the hookworm (*Ancylostoma duodenale*) and the pinworm (*Enterobius vermicularis*).

route of administration, any one of the ways in which a drug may be given. Examples are into a muscle (intramuscularly), in the nose (intranasally), into a vein (intravenously), in the mouth (orally), in the rectum (rectally), under the skin (subcutaneously), under the tongue (sublingually), on the skin surface (topically), or in the vagina (vaginally). Some drugs can be given only by one route. Taking the medication by the prescribed route allows for peak effectiveness. Taking the medication by another route may be damaging.

RR, R.R., abbreviation for **recovery room.**

-(r)rhage, a combining form meaning a break, or an excess release of fluid.

-(r)rhaphy, -(r)rhaphia, a combining form meaning a stitching in place.

-(r)rhea, -(r)rhoea, -(r)rhoeica, a combining form meaning 'release of fluid, flow.'

-(r)rhythmia, a combining form meaning a condition of the heart beat or the pulse.

RRT, abbreviation for **registered respiratory therapist.**

RSV, RS virus, abbreviation for **respiratory syncytial virus.**

R.T., abbreviation for **Registered Technologist.**

rubber, *informal.* a **condom.**

rubber dam, a thin sheet of latex rubber for separating one or more teeth during dental work.

rubbing alcohol, a disinfectant for skin and devices. It has 70% ethyl alcohol by volume. The rest is made up mainly of water. It may cause dryness of the skin. Rubbing alcohol is for outer use only and is flammable.

rubefacient /roo'bəfā'shənt/, something that increases the reddish color of the skin.

rubella, a contagious virus disease marked by fever, symptoms of a mild upper breathing tract infection, swollen lymph nodes, joint pain, and a fine, red rash. The virus is spread by droplets from coughs or sneezes. The dormant time is from 12 to 23 days. The symptoms usually last only 2 or 3 days except for the joint pain, which may last longer or return. One attack gives lifelong vaccination. If a woman gets rubella (German measles) in the first 3 months of pregnancy, birth defects may result, as heart disorders, eye clouding (cataracts), deafness, and mental retardation. An infant exposed to the virus in the uterus at any time during pregnancy may carry the virus for up to 30 months after birth. The illness itself is mild and needs no special treatment. A vaccine is used for all children to lower the chances of an epidemic and thus to protect pregnant women. The vaccine is not given to women already pregnant. Pregnancy should be avoided for 3 months after given rubella vaccine. Spread of the virus from a recently vaccinated person rarely occurs. Temporary joint pain is common after vaccination. Women of childbearing age working with children may be tested for vaccination to rubella and are vaccinated if not immune. The rash and discomfort of rubella look like those of other diseases, as scarlet fever, leading some people to think they have had rubella when they have not. Also called **German measles, three-day measles.** Compare **measles, scarlet fever.**

rubella and mumps virus vaccine, a live virus vaccine used for vaccination against rubella and mumps.
★CAUTION: Infection or known allergy to this drug prohibits its use. It is not given to a patient whose immune function is slowed or to a pregnant woman. Pregnancy is avoided for 3 months after vaccination.
★ADVERSE EFFECTS: Among the more serious side effects are allergic reactions.

rubella embryopathy, any birth defect in an infant caused by German measles (rubella) in the mother in the early stages of pregnancy.

rubella panencephalitis, a disease of adolescents and linked to the rubella virus. It is a long-term disease marked by motor nerve and mental breakdown. See also **panencephalitis.**

rubella virus vaccine, a live virus vaccine used to vaccinate against German measles (rubella).
★CAUTION: Fever, infection, untreated tuberculosis, or allergy to certain animal proteins prohibits its use. It is not given to pregnant women. Pregnancy should be avoided for 3 months after vaccination.
★ADVERSE EFFECTS: Among the most serious side effects are allergic reactions and pain.

rubeola. See **measles.**

rubescent /roobes'ənt/, reddening.

-rubicin, a combining form for an anticancer antibiotic (daunorubicin-type antineoplastic).

Rubin's test, a test of female infertility by checking the opening of the fallopian tubes. Carbon dioxide gas (CO_2) is sent under pressure through a tube (cannula) put into the cervix. The CO_2 is passed through from a needle connected to a pressure gauge. If the tubes are open, the gas passes from the uterus and enters the stomach space. The recorded pressure then falls. There may be shoulder pain from irritation of the diaphragm. If the tubes are blocked, gas cannot escape from the tubes into the stomach space and the pressure remains high. After the test, the patient rests for 3 hours. Crampy pain, dizziness, nausea, and vomiting may occur. A position with the pelvis higher than the head allows the gas to stay in the pelvis and gives some relief.

rubivirus /rōō′bēvī′rəs/, a member of the virus family, as rubella virus.

rubor /rōō′bôr/, redness, especially when there is swelling.

rubricyte, the marrow stage in the normal growth of a red blood cell (erythrocyte).

ructus. See **eructation.**

rudiment, an organ or tissue that is incompletely grown or does not work. **–rudimentary,** *adj.*

Ruffini's corpuscles /rōōfē′nēz/, many oval-shaped nerve endings in the tissue under the skin. They are made of strong coverings around nerve fibers with many branches that end in small knobs.

ruga /rōō′gə/, *pl.* **rugae** /rōō′jē/, a ridge or fold, as the rugae of the stomach, that form large folds in the mucous membrane of that organ.

rule of co-occurrence, a rule that a person must use the same level of vocabulary and grammar when speaking.

rule of nines, a way of estimating the amount of body surface covered by burns. It is done by giving 9% to the head and each arm, twice 9% (18%) to each leg as well as the front and back of the body, and 1% to the space between the anus and the urethral opening (perineum). This is changed in infants and children because of the different body size.

rumination /rōō′minā′shən/, the spitting up (regurgitation) of small amounts of undigested food with little force after every feeding. It is commonly seen in infants. It may be a symptom of overfeeding, of eating too fast, or of swallowing air. It is not a problem. Forceful regurgitation may mean a more serious condition, as an allergic reaction, or a block of the intestinal tract. See also **vomit.**

rupture, 1. a tear or break in an organ or body tissue. It includes those instances when other tissues break through the opening. See also **hernia. 2.** to cause a break or tear.

ruptured intervertebral disk. See **herniated disk.**

Russell dwarf, a patient with Russell's syndrome. It is an inherited disorder in which there is short height with many defects of the head, face, and skeleton. Patients also show many degrees of mental retardation.

Russell traction, a device that combines suspension and traction to hold, position, and line up the lower legs. It is used to treat broken upper legs and to treat diseases or disorders of the hip and knee.

Russian bath, a hot steam bath followed by a cold plunge. Also called **Finnish bath.**

rutin /rōō′tin/, a substance (bioflavonoid) taken from buckwheat and used to treat weak small blood vessels (capillaries).

S

s, 1. abbreviation for **steady state. 2.** abbreviation for *sinister (left).*

S, 1. symbol for **sulfur. 2.** symbol for *saturation of hemoglobin.*

SA, 1. abbreviation for **sinoatrial. 2.** abbreviation for **surface area. 3.** abbreviation for **surgeon's assistant.**

Sabin-Feldman dye test /sā'binfeld'mən/, a test for toxoplasmosis.

Sabin vaccine. See **oral poliovirus vaccine.**

sac, a pouch or a baglike organ.

saccade, referring to something jerky, broken, or abrupt, as rapid shifts of eye movement or a staccato voice.

saccadic eye movement, an extremely fast movement of the eyes, allowing them to focus on a stationary object as the person moves or the head turns.

saccharide /sak'ərīd'/, any of a large group of carbohydrates, including all sugars and starches. Almost all carbohydrates are saccharides. See also **carbohydrate, sugar.**

saccharin /sak'ərin/, 1. a white, crystal-like artificial sweetener, sweeter than table sugar (sucrose). Saccharin is often used as a substitute for sugar. 2. having a sweet taste, almost too sweet. Also called **saccharine** /-rīn', -rin'/.

Saccharomyces /sak'ərōmī'sēz/, a genus of yeast fungi, including brewer's and baker's yeast, as well as some harmful fungi, that cause such diseases as bronchitis, moniliasis, and pharyngitis.

saccharomycosis /sak'ərōmīkō'sis/, infection with yeast fungi, as the genera *Candida* or *Cryptococcus.*

saccular, referring to a pouch, or shaped like a sac.

saccular aneurysm, a limited widening of an artery in which only a small part of the vessel wall bulges, forming a saclike swelling. It is usually caused by an injury. Also called **sacculated aneurysm, amullary aneurysm.** Compare **fusiform aneurysm.**

saccule /sak'yōōl/, a small bag or sac, as the air saccules of the lungs. See also **sacculus. –saccular,** *adj.*

sacculus /sak'yōōləs/, *pl.* **sacculi,** a little sac or bag, especially the ones found in the inner ear. See also **saccule.**

Sachs' disease. See **Tay-Sachs disease.**

sacral /sā'krəl, sak'rəl/, referring to the sacrum.

sacral foramen, one of a number of openings between the vertebrae in the pelvic area through which the nerves pass.

sacral node, a knot in one of the seven groups of lymph nodes of the midsection and the pelvis. The sacral nodes collect lymphatics from the rectum and the back of the pelvis. Compare **lumbar node.** See also **lymph, lymphatic system, lymph node.**

sacral plexus, a network of nerves that controls motion and feeling. It lies against the inner back wall of the pelvis. It becomes the sciatic nerve and serves the upper legs and pelvic area. Compare **lumbar plexus.**

sacral vertebra, one of the five parts of the vertebral column that are joined together in the adult to form the sacrum. Compare **cervical vertebra, coccygeal vertebra, lumbar vertebra, thoracic vertebra.** See also **sacrum, vertebra.**

sacro-, a combining form meaning 'of or relating to the sacrum.'

sacroiliac, relating to the part of the skeleton that includes the sacrum and the ilium bones of the pelvis.

sacroiliac articulation, a joint in the pelvis that does not move.

sacrospinalis /sak'rōspīnal'sis/, a large, meaty muscle of the back. It straightens and supports the vertebral column and the head, and it pulls the ribs downward. Also called **erector spinae.**

sacrum /sā'krəm, sak'rəm/, the large, triangle-shaped bone at the top part of the pelvis. It looks like a wedge set between the two hip bones. The sacrum is shorter and wider in women than in men. **–sacral,** *adj.*

saddle block anesthesia, a form of local anesthetic that affects the parts of the body that would touch a saddle if the patient were riding a horse. Saddle block anesthesia is common in some places for anesthesia during childbirth. See also **obstetric anesthesia.**

saddle joint, a kind of joint, as the wrist and thumb. Also called **articulatio sellaris.** Compare **condyloid joint, pivot joint.**

sadism /sā'dizəm, sad'izəm/, 1. abnormal pleasure derived from causing physical or mental pain or abuse on others; cruelty. 2. also called **active algolagnia.** (In psychiatry) a mental and sexual disorder marked by the wish to hurt or destroy the self-respect of another person, either a willing or unwilling partner, to get sexual satisfaction. The condition is usually long-term, is usually found in men, may be caused by concious or unconcious desires, and, in serious cases, can lead to rape, torture, and murder. Kinds of sadism are **anal sadism** and **oral sadism.** Compare **masochism.** See also **algolagnia, sadomasochism. –sadistic,** *adj.*

sadist, a person who suffers from or practices sadism.

sadomasochism, a personality disorder marked by traits of sadism and masochism. See also **algolagnia, masochism, sadism.**

safe period. See **natural family planning method.**

safety director, a member of a hospital staff who is concerned with safety, as fire prevention, environmental safety, and disaster planning.

sagittal /saj′ətəl/, (in anatomy) of or relating to an imaginary line running from the front to the back of the body that divides the right and left sides.

sagittal fontanel, a soft area on the top of an infant's head, halfway between the front and back fontanels. It may be found in some normal newborns and also some with Down's syndrome. See also **fontanel.**

sagittal suture, the saw-toothed line in the top of the skull that is formed where the two parietal bones of the skull come together.

SaH, SAH, abbreviation for **subarachnoid hemorrhage.**

sal-, -sal, a combining form for salicylic acid derivatives.

salbutamol. See **albuterol.**

salicylanilide /sal′isilan′ilīd/, an antifungus drug used on the skin to treat tinea capitis caused by *Microsporum audouini.*

salicylate /səlis′əlāt/, any of several widely used drugs that are made from salicylic acid.

salicylate poisoning, a poisonous condition caused by eating salicylate, most often in aspirin or oil of wintergreen. It is marked by rapid breathing, vomiting, headache, irritability, ketosis, hypoglycemia, and, in severe cases, convulsions and breathing failure. Treatment usually includes a quick cleaning out of the stomach, the use of vitamin K if there is bleeding, and proper steps to treat loss of water, hypoglycemia, and hypokalemia. Sodium bicarbonate should not be taken by mouth.

salicylazosulfapyridine. See **sulfasalazine.**

salicylic acid /sal′isil′ik/, a drug that gets rid of warts and other such growths. It is used to treat bumps and growths on the skin and to help fight infections caused by a fungus. ★CAUTION: Diabetes, poor circulation, or known allergy to this drug prohibits its use. ★ADVERSE EFFECTS: Among the more serious side effects are skin swelling and salicylism.

salicylism /sal′isil′izəm/, a syndrome of salicylate poisoning.

saline cathartic, one of a large group of laxatives used to empty the bowel. It usually takes effect withing 3 to 4 hours.

saline infusion, the healthy injection of a mild salt solution into a vein.

saline irrigation, the washing out of a body space or wound with a salt solution.

saline solution, a solution containing salt (sodium chloride).

saliva, the clear, viscous fluid secreted by glands in the mouth. Saliva contains water, mucin, organic salts, and the enzyme ptyalin that helps digest food. It keeps the mouth wet, starts to digest starches, and helps the patient to chew and swallow food.

salivary, of or relating to saliva or to the forming of saliva.

salivary duct, any one of the tubes that carry saliva. Kinds of salivary ducts are **Bartholin's duct, duct of Rivinus, parotid duct,** and **submandibular duct.**

salivary fistula, an abnormal hole between a salivary gland or duct and the mouth or the skin of the face or neck.

salivary gland, one of the three pairs of glands that make the mouth wet, thus aiding in digesting food.

salivary gland cancer, a cancer-forming disease of a salivary gland, found most often in a parotid gland. About 75% of tumors that develop in the salivary glands are harmless, slow-growing, and painless rubbery bumps. On the other hand, cancerous tumors are fast-growing, hard, lumpy, and often very sore. Pain, trismus, and facial palsy may occur. In some cases, the tumor is cut out. In others, x-ray treatment is used. Chemical treatment may also be used.

salivation, the secreting of saliva by the salivary glands.

Salk vaccine. See **poliovirus vaccine.**

salmon calcitonin. See **calcitonin.**

Salmonella /sal′mənel′ə/, a genus of moving rod-shaped bacteria that includes species causing typhoid fever, paratyphoid fever, and some forms of gastroenteritis. See also **salmonellosis.**

salmonellosis /sal′mənəlō′sis/, a form of gastroenteritis, caused by eating food contaminated with a species of *Salmonella,* marked by sudden, sharp pain in the stomach or intestines, fever, and bloody, watery diarrhea that occur 6 to 48 hours after eating the bad food. Nausea and vomiting are common. Symptoms usually last from 2 to 5 days, but diarrhea and fever may persist for up to 2 weeks. Dangerous loss of water may occur. There is no special cure. Cooking food long enough, keeping food in the refrigerator, and careful handwashing may help prevent the disease. See also **food poisoning.**

salol camphor /sal′ôl/, a clear, oily mixture of camphor and phenyl salicylate, used to kill germs on contact.

Salonica fever. See **trench fever.**

salpingectomy /sal′pinjek′təmē/, removal of one or both fallopian tubes, done to remove a cyst or tumor, cut out an abscess, or, if both tubes are removed, to sterilize a female patient. Often the operation is done with a hysterectomy or an oophorectomy. Either spinal block or general anesthesia may be used. After the operation, the patient should not flex suddenly the muscles of the thighs or knees. Continuous low back pain or urine that is bloody or less than normal shows that a ureter may have been hurt during surgery.

salpingitis /sal'pinjī'tis/, a swelling or infection of the fallopian tube. See also **pelvic inflammatory disease.**

salpingo-, a combining form meaning 'of or relating to a tube, especially a fallopian tube.'

salpingo-oophorectomy, the surgical removal of a fallopian tube and an ovary.

salpingostomy /sal'ping·gos'təmē/, the operation in which a new opening is made in a fallopian tube. This is done to clear a tube that has been closed by infection, by long-term swelling, or to drain an abscess. Either regional or general anesthesia is used. A device may be put in to keep the fallopian tube open. After the operation, the patient should not suddenly flex the thighs or knees. Low back pain or less-than-normal or bloody urine may show that a ureter has been injured and more surgery may be needed.

salpinx /sal'pingks/, pl. **salpinges** /salpin'jēz/, a tube, as the *salpinx auditiva* or the *salpinx uterina.* **–salpingian,** *adj.*

salt, 1. a substance made by mixing together an acid and a base. **2.** sodium chloride (common table salt). **3.** a substance, as magnesium sulfate (Epsom salt), used as a purgative.

saltation /saltā'shən/, (in genetics) a change in the genes that causes an important difference between the looks of a child and its parents. **–saltatorial, saltatoric, saltatory** /sal'tətôr'ē/, *adj.*

salt depletion, the loss of salt from the body through too-much sweating, diarrhea, vomiting, or urination, without replacing what was lost. See also **electrolyte balance, heat exhaustion.**

Salter fracture. See **epiphyseal fracture.**

salt-free diet. See **low-sodium diet.**

Saluron, a trademark for a drug used to treat high blood pressure and to make the patient urinate more (hydroflumethiazide).

salvage therapy, treatment used when other treatments have not worked.

salve. See **ointment.**

sand bath, putting warm, dry sand or damp sand on the body.

sand flea. See **chigoe,** def. 1.

sandfly fever. See **phlebotomus fever.**

Sandhoff's disease, a type of Tay-Sachs disease that includes defects in two enzymes (hexosaminidase A and B). It is marked by a more rapid course and is found in the general population, not restricted, as is Tay-Sachs disease. Also called **gangliosidosis type II.** See also **Tay-Sachs disease.**

Sandoz Clinical Assessment-Geriatric, a test of mental function given to elderly persons to help determine the cause of a psychological problem.

sand tumor. See **psammoma.**

sangui-, a combining form meaning 'of or relating to blood.'

sanguineous /sang·gwin'ē·əs/, relating to blood.

San Joaquin fever /san'wôkēn'/, the first stage of coccidioidomycosis.

SA node. See **sinoatrial node.**

Sanorex, a trademark for an appetite-controlling drug (mazindol).

Sansert, a trademark for a vasoconstrictor (methysergide maleate).

Santyl, a trademark for an enzyme (collagenase).

saphenous nerve /səfē'nəs/, the largest and longest branch of the femoral nerve that goes along the inner side of the leg. One branch of the saphenous nerve below the knee goes to the ankle. Another branch below the knee goes to the inner side of the foot. See also **femoral nerve.**

saphenous vein. See **great saphenous vein.**

saponin /sap'ənin/, a soapy substance found in some plants, especially soapwort (Bouncing Bet) and certain lilies. It is used to make suds in medicines that soothe sore mucous membranes. Natural saponins, which can be poisonous to the blood, are no longer used since they have been replaced by artificial substances.

saprophyte, an organism that lives on dead organic matter. **–saprophytic,** *adj.*

saralasin, a substance that is injected to test the way that the renin-angiotensin system is helping to control the blood pressure.

sarcoidosis /sär'koidō'sis/, a long-term disease of unknown origin marked by small, round bumps in the tissue around the organs of the body, usually the lungs, spleen, liver, skin, mucous membranes, and tear and salivary glands, usually along with the lymph glands. The sores usually go away after a period of some months or years, but lead to widespread grainy swelling and fibrosis. Also called **sarcoid of Boeck.**

sarcoidosis cordis, a form of sarcoidosis in which grainy growths develop in the heart. The number and the size of the growths vary. Mild cases with few growths are without symptoms. In severe cases the heart may have many growths, and heart failure may follow. See also **sarcoidosis.**

sarcoma /särkō'mə/, pl. **sarcomas, sarcomata,** a cancerous growth of the soft tissues usually appearing at first as a painless swelling. About 40% of sarcomas occur in the legs and feet, 20% in the hands and arms, 20% in the trunk, and the rest in the head or neck. The growth tends to spread very quickly. It is usually not caused by an injury, but it can grow in burn scars. It must be cut out, and then the body is usually given x-ray and chemical treatment. See specific sarcomas.

-sarcoma, a combining form meaning a cancerous growth.

sarcoma botryoides /bot′rē·oi′dēz/, a tumor that can grow in muscle cells, found most often in young children and marked by a painful, grapelike mass in the upper vagina or on the cervix or the neck of the bladder. See also **rhabdomyosarcoma.**

sarcomagenesis /särkō′məjen′əsis/, the birth and growth of a sarcoma. Compare **carcinogenesis, oncogenesis, tumorigenesis. –sarcomagenetic,** *adj.*

sarcomere /sär′kōmir/, the smallest working part of a muscle fiber.

sarcoplasmic reticulum, a network of little tubes and sacs in muscles attached to the skeleton that play an important part in tensing and relaxing the muscles.

Sarcoptes scabiei /särkop′tēz skā′bē·ī/, the genus of itch mite that causes scabies.

sartorius /särtôr′ē·əs/, the longest muscle in the body, stretching from the pelvis to the calf of the leg. It is a narrow muscle that runs across the top of the thigh at an angle from the outside of the pelvis to the inside of the knee. It causes the thigh to move up and out and causes the leg to move in. Compare **quadriceps femoris.**

S.A.S. 500, a trademark for a sulfonamide (sulfasalazine), used to treat ulcerative colitis.

satellite clinic, a clinic or hospital run by a larger hospital, but in another building far away.

satiety, the satisfied feeling of being full after eating.

saturated, having absorbed or dissolved the largest possible amount of a given substance, and unable to absorb any more. Compare **unsaturated.**

saturated fatty acid, certain fats that are found mainly in beef, lamb, pork, veal, whole-milk products, butter, most cheeses, and a few plant fats, as cocoa butter, coconut oil, and palm oil. Ordinary margarine and hydrogenated shortenings also contain saturated fatty acids. A diet high in saturated fatty acids may lead to a high level of cholesterol in the blood and, in some patients, is linked to heart disease. Compare **unsaturated fatty acid.**

saturated solution, a liquid that has absorbed as much of another substance as it can.

saturation-dependent drugs, drugs that act on many tissues rather than at the site of specific nerve endings.

satyriasis /sat′irī′əsis/, excessive or uncontrollable sexual desire in the male. Also called **satyromania.** Compare **nymphomania.**

sauna bath, a bath in which steam is used to induce sweating, followed by rubbing of the body, and ending with a cold shower. Also called **Finnish bath, Russian bath.**

Sayre's jacket /serz/, a cast used for support in treating injuries to and defects of the spinal column.

Sb, symbol for **antimony.**

SBE, 1. abbreviation for **self-breast examination. 2.** abbreviation for **subacute bacterial endocarditis.**

sc, abbreviation for *sine correctione,* a Latin phrase meaning "without correction."

Sc, symbol for **scandium.**

scab. See **eschar.**

scabicide /skab′isīd/, any one of a large group of drugs that destroy the itch mite, *Sarcoptes scabiei.* These drugs are applied to the skin as a lotion or a cream. All are possibly poisonous and may irritate the skin. They are used with caution in treating children. Kinds of scabicides include **crotamiton, lindane.**

scabies /skā′bēz/, a contagious disease caused by *Sarcoptes scabiei,* the itch mite, marked by intense itching of the skin and damage to the skin from scratching. The mite, passed by close contact with infected humans or domestic animals, burrows into the layers of the skin where the female lays eggs. Two to 4 months later, the eggs hatch and the itching begins. A rash often occurs on the fingers, wrists and thighs. This disease is treated with drugs and lotions.

scag, *slang.* heroin.

scalded skin syndrome. See **toxic epidermal necrolysis.**

scalp, the skin that covers the head. The face and ears are not included.

scalp medication, 1. a cream, ointment, lotion, or shampoo used to treat skin disorders of the scalp. **2.** a medication of the scalp. If a cream, ointment, or lotion is to be applied, a shampoo is usually used first. The hair is dried, combed, and parted in the middle, and the medication is spread with the fingertips. After treatment, the medication may need to be washed off the scalp and hair with an alkaline shampoo.

scalp vein needle, a thin-gauge needle designed for use in the veins of the scalp or other small veins.

scamping speech, abnormal speech in which consonants or whole syllables are left out of words because of the person's inability to shape the sounds. Also called **clipped speech.**

scanning, carefully looking at a part of the body, an organ, or a system of the body by making a picture of the area. Sometimes a substance is injected to make a certain area or body part stand out on the x-ray film. The liver, brain, and thyroid can be looked at, tumors can be found, and other important knowledge may be gotten by various scanning techniques. See specific scanning techniques. –**scan,** *n., v.*

scanning electron microscope (SEM), an instrument, like an electron microscope, that forms a picture that seems to be lifelike. Compare **electron microscope, transmission scanning electron microscope.**

scanning electron microscopy, the technique using a scanning electron microscope.

scanning speech, abnormal speech marked by a short, broken way of speaking in which the words are clipped and broken because the person stops between syllables.

scanography /skanog'rəfē/, a special method of making an x-ray of an organ of the body. It is used mainly for making x-ray tests of the long bones.

Scanzoni rotation /skanzō'nē/, an operation used in the delivery of a baby in which a special kind of forceps is used to turn the fetus in the womb just before birth. It is not done very much any more because cesarean section is usually safer for the mother and the baby. See also **forceps delivery, obstetric forceps.**

scaphocephaly /skaf'ōsef'əlē/, a defect of the skull present at birth in which the skull has an unusually long, narrow shape. It is often linked with mental retardation. Also called **scaphocephalis, scaphocephalism, dolichocephaly, mecocephaly.** See also **craniostenosis. –scaphocephalic, scaphocephalous,** *adj.*

scaphoid abdomen, a stomach with a sunken front wall.

scaphoid bone, either of two similar bones of the hand and the foot. Also called **navicular bone.**

scapula /skap'ələ/, one of the pair of large, flat, three-sided bones that form the back of the shoulder. Also called **shoulder blade.**

scapular line, an imaginary vertical line drawn through the lower angle of the shoulder blade.

scapulohumeral, of or relating to the muscles and the area around the scapula and humerus that make up the shoulder.

scapulohumeral muscular dystrophy, a form of muscular dystrophy that begins in the shoulder. Also called **Erb's muscular dystrophy.**

scapulohumeral reflex, a normal response to tapping the side of the scapula nearest the spine, causing the arm to jerk. If the arm does not move, it may be a sign of damage to the spine.

scar. See **cicatrix.**

scarification /sker'ifikā'shən/, a number of light scratches or cuts in the skin, as are made for the applying of a vaccine. The term does not mean "causing a scar."

scarify /sker'əfī/, to make a number of light cuts into the skin; to scratch. Vaccination for smallpox is done by scarifying the skin under a drop of vaccine. See also **scarification.**

scarlatina. See **scarlet fever.**

scarlatiniform /skär'lətē'nifôrm/, looking like the rash of **scarlet fever.**

scarlet fever, a very easily spread disease of childhood caused by a type of *Streptococcus.* The infection is marked by sore throat, fever, enlarged lymph nodes in the neck, prostration, and a widespread bright red rash. Also called **scarlatina.**

scarlet red, a red dye that is used to color medicines.

schema /skē'mə/, a naturally present knowledge structure that allows children to organize in their minds ways to behave in their environment.

Scheuermann's disease /shoi'ərmonz/, an abnormal disease of the skeleton that leaves the patient a hunchback. Its cause is not known. It occurs most often in children between 12 and 16 years of age, with the beginning at puberty, and it occurs more often in girls than in boys. It begins very slowly and is often linked with a history of unusual physical activity or participation in sports. The most common symptom is poor posture with tiredness and pain in the back. The back may also be sore and stiff. If the disease is discovered early, the posture may be cured. Otherwise, the posture becomes fixed within a period of 6 to 9 months. This disease may be treated by putting the body in a cast for 10 or 12 months. After the cast is taken off, the patient must do a special set of exercises. In adults, continuous pain in the middle and lower back may be a sign of a milder form, and an operation may be needed. Also called **adolescent vertebral epiphysitis, juvenile kyphosis.**

Schick test, a skin test to find out if the patient can catch diphtheria. In this test, a small amount of a substance that fights diphtheria germs is injected into the skin. A positive reaction, showing that the patient can have diphtheria, is marked by redness and swelling at the site of injection; a negative reaction, showing that the patient cannot catch diphtheria, is marked by absence of redness or swelling.

Schilder's disease /shil'dərz/, a group of serious nerve diseases that begin in childhood. These diseases attack parts of the brain, and many of the symptoms are like those of multiple sclerosis. There is no known treatment. The cause may be viral or genetic. Also called **Schilder's encephalitis, encephalitis periaxialis diffusa, Flatau-Schilder disease, progressive subcortical encephalopathy.** See also **adrenoleukodystrophy.**

Schiller's test, a test used to choose sections of the skin in the vagina or cervix for further tests looking for possible cancers.

Schilling's leukemia. See **monocytic leukemia.**

Schilling test, a test used to find certain blood diseases (pernicious anemia). The patient swallows a small amount of cobalt, then waits for 24 hours. The urine is then tested.

schindylesis /skin'dilē'sis/, coming together of certain bones of the skull.

Schiötz' tonometer /shē·ets'/, an instrument used to measure the pressure inside the eyeball.

Schistosoma /shis'təsō'mə/, a genus of microscopic worms that live in the blood; these worms may cause disease in the bladder, liver, or intestines in humans. It lives in freshwater snails. *Schistosoma hematobium,* found chiefly in Africa and the Middle East, affects the bladder and pelvic organs, causing painful, frequent urination and bloody urine. *S. japonicum,* found in Japan, the Philippines, and Eastern Asia, causes ulcers in the intestines and liver disease. *S. mansoni,* found in Africa, the Middle East, the Caribbean, and tropic America, causes symptoms like those caused by *S. japonicum.* See also **schistosomiasis.**

schistosomiasis /shis'təsōmī'əsis/, an infection caused by a parasite *(Schistosoma)* in humans by contact with freshwater fouled with human waste (feces). One worm may live in one part of the body, laying eggs often, for up to 20 years. The eggs attack the mucous membrane, causing it to become thick and to develop a number of little harmless growths. Symptoms depend on the part of the body infected. *Schistosoma* may be found in the bladder, rectum, liver, lungs, spleen, intestines, and some veins. It may cause pain, blockage, damage to the infected organ, and anemia. It is hard to treat, but fairly easy to prevent. This may be done by properly disposing of human waste, putting chlorine in the water, and wiping out the freshwater snail *Australorbis glabratus,* which carries the parasite. Second only to malaria in the number of people affected, schistosomiasis most often occurs in the tropics and in the Orient. Also called **bilharziasis.** See also **blood fluke,** *Schistosoma.*

schistosomicide /shis'təsō'məsīd/, a drug that kills schistosomes, blood worms carried by snails to human hosts in many parts of Africa, Brazil, and Asia. **–schistosomicidal,** *adj.*

schizo-, a combining form meaning 'divided, or related to division.'

schizoaffective disorder /skit'sō·afek'tiv/, a condition that has some of the same symptoms as schizophrenia and bipolar disorder or of other major emotional disorders.

schizoid /skit'soid, skiz'oid/, **1.** typical of or resembling schizophrenia; schizophrenic. **2.** a person, not necessarily a schizophrenic, who shows the traits of a schizoid personality.

schizoid personality, an unbalanced person, who has difficulty getting along in society, who seems to be very shy, easily angered or insulted and quiet, and who likes to be alone all of the time and who does not want to get close to others. See also **schizoid personality disorder, schizophrenia.**

schizoid personality disorder, a state marked by the lack of the ability to make friends. Other symptoms are a lack of feelings, the wish to be alone all the time, and no concern for the opinions and feelings of others. The person is not able to show anger or any hostile feelings and does not seem to react to disturbing experiences. It may lead to schizophrenia.

schizophasia /skit'səfā'zhə, skiz'ə-/, the rambling babble typical of some types of schizophrenia. See also **word salad.**

schizophrene /skit'səfrēn', skiz'ə-/, a person who suffers from schizophrenia.

schizophrenia /skit'səfrē'nē·ə, skiz'ə-/, any one of a large group of mental disorders in which the patient loses touch with reality and in which the person is no longer able to think, talk, or act normally. It can be mild or serious and the person may need to spend some time in a hospital. The cause of this disorder is not known. It is often treated with tranquilizers and drugs to ease depression. Counseling and group therapy can be helpful. Kinds of schizophrenia include **acute schizophrenia, catatonic schizophrenia, childhood schizophrenia, disorganized schizophrenia, latent schizophrenia, paranoid schizophrenia, process schizophrenia, reactive schizophrenia,** and **residual schizophrenia.** Also called **schizophrenic disorder, schizophrenic reaction.**

schizophrenic /skit'səfren'ik, skiz'ə-/, **1.** of or relating to schizophrenia. **2.** a person with schizophrenia.

schizophrenic disorder, schizophrenic reaction. See **schizophrenia.**

schizophreniform disorder, a condition exhibiting the same symptoms as schizophrenia but marked by a sudden beginning with resolution in 2 weeks to 6 months.

schizophrenogenic /skit'səfren'əjen'ik, skiz'ə-/, tending to cause or produce schizophrenia.

Schizotrypanum cruzi. See **Chagas' disease.**

schizotypal personality disorder /skit'sōtī'pəl/, a condition marked by odd thinking, talking, and acting that is not serious enough to be schizophrenia. See also **schizoid personality disorder, schizophrenia.**

Schlatter-Osgood disease, Schlatter's disease. See **Osgood-Schlatter disease.**

Schlemm's canal. See **canal of Schlemm.**

Schneiderian carcinoma /shnīdir'ē·ən/, a skin cancer of the mucous membranes in the nose and sinuses.

Schönlein-Henoch purpura. See **Henoch-Schönlein purpura.**

school phobia, a strong continuing fear of going to school, usually found in young children. It usually goes away as the child grows older; if it does not go away, counseling may be needed.

Schultz-Charlton phenomenon, a skin reaction to the injection into the skin of scarlatina antiserum in a person who has a scarletiniform rash. The rash turns white.

Schultze's mechanism, the delivery of an afterbirth (placenta) with the side closest to the baby emerging first.

schwannoma /shwänō'mə/, *pl.* **schwannomas, schwannomata,** a harmless, single, self-contained tumor arising in the coverings of certain nerves. Also called **Schwann cell tumor, neurilemoma.**

Schwann's sheath. See **neurilemma.**

Schwartz bed. See **hyperextension bed.**

sciatic /sī·at′ik/, near the hip, as the sciatic nerve or the sciatic vein.

sciatica /sī·at′ikə/, a swelling of the sciatic nerve, usually marked by pain and soreness along the thigh and leg. It may lead to a wasting of the muscles of the lower leg.

sciatic nerve, a long nerve stretching through the muscles of the thigh, leg, and foot, with many branches.

SCID, abbreviation for **severe combined immunodeficiency disease.**

science, a system that attempts to organize facts learned by study and to explain how the world and everything in it works; also, the knowledge learned in this study. **Pure science** is concerned with learning new facts only for the sake of gaining new knowledge. **Applied science** is the practical use of scientific theory and laws. See also **hypothesis, law, scientific method, theory.**

scientific method, a logical, orderly way to study and solve a problem. Simply put, the method is first to state the problem, then to suggest a possible answer. Some experiment is made up that tests the suggested answer. Depending on the way the experiment turns out, the suggested answer is found either to be right or wrong.

scientific rationale, a reason, based on supporting scientific evidence, why a particular action is chosen.

scirrhous carcinoma, a hard, fiberlike, very fast-spreading tumor in which the cancer cells are found one at a time or in groups. It is the most common form of breast cancer. Also called **carcinoma fibrosum.** See also **breast cancer.**

SCL, abbreviation for **soft contact lens.**

sclera /sklir′ə/, the tough, hard, dense membrane covering most of the back of the eyeball. It helps the eyeball hold its shape. The muscles that move the eyeball are attached to the sclera. It is the white visible portion of the eyeball.

scleredema /sklir′ədē′mə/, a skin disease that arises mysteriously. It is marked by a number of hard growths that spread from the face or neck to the rest of the body, except for the hands and feet. It will go away by itself, but often comes back. There is no specific treatment. Compare **scleroderma.**

sclerodactyly /skler′ōdak′tilē/, a deforming of the muscles and skeleton affecting the hands of patients with scleroderma. The fingers are frozen in a half-bent position, and the fingertips are pointed and have sores.

scleroderma /sklerʹōdur′mə/, a fairly rare disease affecting the blood vessels and connecting tissue. It is marked by the skin of the face and hands becoming hard. Scleroderma is most common in middle-aged women. Also called **progressive systemic sclerosis (PSS).**

scleromalacia perforans, a condition of the eyes in which the sclera is attacked as a complication of rheumatoid arthritis, causing parts of the eye to be exposed. Glaucoma, cataracts, and a detached retina may result.

sclerose /sklerōz′/, to harden or to cause hardening. **–sclerotic,** adj.

sclerosing hemangioma, a solid, tumorlike small growth of the skin.

sclerosing solution, a liquid that causes swelling in tissues. It may be used in burning out ulcers, in stopping bleeding, and in treating hemangiomas.

sclerosis /sklerō′sis/, a condition marked by hardening of tissue resulting from any of several causes, including swelling, the deposit of mineral salts, and damaged connective tissue fibers. **–sclerotic,** adj.

scolex /skō′leks/, pl. **scoleces** /skō′ləsēz/, the head of an adult tapeworm that has hooks, grooves, or suckers by which it attaches itself to the wall of the intestine.

scoliosis /skō′lē·ō′sis/, a sideways curve of the spine that results in an S shape of the back, a common defect in childhood. Early discovery and treatment may prevent it from getting worse. Treatment includes braces, casts, exercises, and corrective surgery. See also **congenital scoliosis, kyphoscoliosis, kyphosis, lordosis, spinal curvature.**

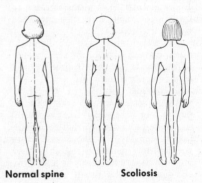

Normal spine   **Scoliosis**

scopolamine /skōpol′əmēn/, a drug used to prevent sea sickness, to prevent vomiting, and as a sedative. Also called **hyoscine.**

scopolamine hydrobromide, a drug used to treat nausea and vomiting, as a sedative, and in eye operations.

★CAUTION: Some kinds of glaucoma, asthma, blocking of the intestines, severe ulcerative colitis, or known allergy to this drug prohibits its use.

★ADVERSE EFFECTS: Among the more serious side effects are blurred vision, central nervous system effects, a fast heart beat, dry mouth, decreased sweating, and allergic reactions.

scopophilia /skō′pəfil′ē·ə, skop′-/, **1.** sexual pleasure gotten by looking at sexually exciting scenes or at another person's genitals; voyeurism. **2.** an unhealthy desire to be seen; exhibitionism. Also called **scotophilia. –scopophiliac, scopophilic, scoptophiliac, scoptophic.** *adj., n.*

scopophobia /skō′pə-/, an unhealthy fear of being seen or stared at by others. The condition is common in schizophrenia. See also **phobia.**

scorbutic gingivitis /skôrbyōō′tik/, an abnormal condition marked by swollen or bleeding gums and caused by a lack of vitamin C.

scorbutic pose, the typical posture of a child with scurvy, with thighs and legs half-bent and hips turned outward. The child usually lies still without moving the hands or feet because of the pain that any movement causes. See also **scurvy.**

scorbutus. See **scurvy.**

scorpion sting, a painful wound of a scorpion, a member of the spider family with a hollow stinger in its tail. The stings of many species are only slightly poisonous, but the sting of certain scorpions may lead to death, especially in small children. The first pain is followed within several hours by numbness, nausea, muscle spasm, shortness of breath, and convulsion. It is treated by putting ice on the wound. Severe cases require a doctor's care. An antivenin is available in some areas.

scotoma, a defect in vision in a specific area in one or both eyes. A common early symptom is a shimmering film appearing as an island in the field of vision.

scratch test, a skin test for finding an allergy, made by placing a small amount of liquid containing a suspected substance on a lightly scratched area of the skin. If a bump on the skin forms within 15 minutes, the patient is allergic to that substance.

screamer's nodule. See **vocal cord nodule.**

screening, 1. a beginning step, as a test or examination, to detect the most obvious sign of illness before further testing. **2.** testing a very large number of patients to find a certain disease, as high blood pressure.

Scribner shunt, a type of artificial vein bypass, used in clearing the blood, consisting of a special tube connection outside the body.

scripting, a technique of family therapy involving the development of new ways for family members to deal with one another.

scrofula /skrof′yələ/, an old name for tuberculosis of the lymph glands in the neck.

scrotal cancer, a cancer of the scrotum, marked at first by a small sore that may become an open sore. The sore occurs most often in elderly men who have been exposed to soot, pitch, crude oil, mineral oils, or arsenic fumes

from copper smelting. Treatment involves cutting out the tumor. In the 18th century, Sir Percival Pott linked scrotal cancer in chimney sweeps with exposure to soot. It is the first cancer shown to be caused by a cancer-causing substance in the air. Also called **chimneysweeps' cancer, soot wart.**

scrotal raphe, a line where the two halves of the scrotum join together. It is generally darker in color than the tissue around it.

scrotum /skrō′təm/, the bag of skin that holds the testicles. In older men, sick men, and in warm weather, the scrotum becomes long and floppy. The left side of the scrotum usually hangs lower than the right. See also **testis. –scrotal,** *adj.*

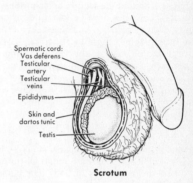

Spermatic cord:
Vas deferens
Testicular artery
Testicular veins
Epididymus
Skin and dartos tunic
Testis

Scrotum

scrubbed team members, the surgeons and physicians, nurses, and technicians who are scrubbed for surgical procedures in a sterile environment.

scrub typhus, a serious fever disease of Asia, India, northern Australia, and the western Pacific islands, caused by *Rickettsia tsutsugamushi* and carried from sick rats and mice to humans by mites. It can be prevented by staying away from places where the mites live, killing off the rats and mice, destroying scrub vegetation, and using insect repellents. Also called **Japanese flood fever, Japanese river fever, mite typhus, tsutsugamushi disease.** Compare **Q fever, Rocky Mountain spotted fever, typhus.**

sculpting, a technique of family therapy in which a live family portrait is constructed to show family alliances and conflicts.

scurvy, a disease that is caused by a lack of vitamin C in the diet. It is marked by weakness, anemia, edema, spongy gums, often with open sores in the mouth and loosening of the teeth, bleeding in the mucous membranes, and hard bumps of the muscles of the legs. It is treated and prevented by taking vitamin C and eating fresh vegetables and fruits. Also called **scorbutus.** See also **ascorbic acid, citric acid, infantile scurvy, scorbutic pose.**

seal limbs. See **phocomelia.**

seasickness. See **motion sickness.**

seasonal affective disorder (SAD), a mood disorder associated with the shorter days and longer nights of autumn and winter. Symptoms include sluggishness, depression, social withdrawal, and work difficulties. Patients also eat too many carbohydrates, gaining weight. Symptoms disappear in the spring when the days become longer. The condition is linked to the effect of light on the skin and is treated with bright light for 3 to 6 hours per day.

seatworm. See *Enterobius vermicularis.*

sea urchin sting, an injury inflicted by any sea urchin, in which the skin is pierced and, in some species, venom released. A poisonous sting is marked by pain, muscular weakness, numbness around the mouth, and shortness of breath. The spines must be taken out at once and a doctor's care may be needed. In all cases the broken spines cause local pain and irritation. Infection may result. See also **stingray.**

seawater bath, a bath taken in warm seawater or in saline solution.

sebaceous /siba'shəs/, fatty, oily, or greasy, usually referring to the oil-secreting glands of the skin or to their secretions.

sebaceous cyst, a wrong name for epidermoid cyst or pilar cyst.

sebaceous gland, one of the many small saclike organs in the skin. They are found all through the body near all types of body hair but are especially in the scalp, the face, the anus, the nose, the mouth, and the external ear. They are not found in the palms of the hands and the soles of the feet. Compare **sudoriferous gland.**

seborrhea /seb′ərē′ə/, any of several common skin conditions in which there is too much grease (sebum) made that causes very oily skin or dry scales. See also **seborrheic blepharitis, seborrheic dermatitis. –seborrheic** /seb′-ərē′ik/, *adj.*

seborrheic blepharitis, a form of seborrheic dermatitis in which the eyelids are abnormally red and the edges are covered with a grainy crust.

seborrheic dermatitis, a common, long-term, inflammatory skin disease marked by dry or moist greasy scales and yellowish crusts. Common sites are the scalp, eyelids, face, outer surfaces of the ears, armpits, breasts, groin, and gluteal folds. It is treated with special shampoos, creams, lotions, and drugs. Kinds of seborrheic dermatitis include **cradle cap, dandruff,** and **seborrheic blepharitis.**

seborrheic keratosis, a harmless, well-defined, slightly raised, tan to black, wartlike bump of the skin of the face, neck, chest, or upper back. Itching is common. It is usually taken off by a doctor. Also called **seborrheic wart.**

sebum /sē'bəm/, the oily secretion of the sebaceous glands of the skin, composed of keratin, fat, and cellular debris. Mixed with sweat, sebum forms a moist, oily, acidic film that is mildly harmful to bacteria and fungus and protects the skin against drying.

Seckel's syndrome. See **bird-headed dwarf.**

secobarbital, a drug that is used to calm and put a patient to sleep.

Seconal, a trademark for a drug used to calm and put a patient to sleep (secobarbital).

secondary, less important, second in order, or less well-developed.

secondary amenorrhea. See **amenorrhea.**

secondary amputation, amputation done after draining has begun after an injury. A place is left open for drainage, and antibiotics are given. Compare **primary amputation.**

secondary amyloidosis. See **amyloidosis.**

secondary apnea, an abnormal condition in which breathing has stopped and will not start again. Artificial breathing is needed at once. Secondary apnea may be caused by any event that does not allow oxygen to be absorbed into the blood. Compare **primary apnea.**

secondary areola, a second ring appearing around the areola of the breast during pregnancy that is darker in color than the areola before pregnancy.

secondary biliary cirrhosis, an abnormal liver disease marked by the blocking of the bile duct, which may or may not be infected. Compare **primary biliary cirrhosis.**

secondary dementia, madness caused by another form of insanity that the patient has at the same time. See also **dementia.**

secondary dental caries, cavities that form in teeth that are already decayed; often a new cavity forms next to or beneath the filling of an old cavity.

secondary dentition. See **permanent dentition.**

secondary diabetes. See **other types of diabetes.**

secondary dysmenorrhea. See **dysmenorrhea.**

secondary fracture. See **neoplastic fracture.**

secondary host. See **intermediate host.**

secondary hypertension, high blood pressure linked to diseases of the kidneys, lungs, glands, and vessels. See also **hypertension.**

secondary hypertrophic osteoarthropathy. See **clubbing.**

secondary infection, an infection by a microorganism that comes after another kind of organism.

secondary nutrient, a substance that helps to digest food in the intestines.

secondary occlusal traumatism, a strain caused by biting down so hard that it injures an already weak part of the gums that holds the teeth. The strain may not be too much for normal tissues but can be harmful to weakened areas.

secondary prevention, a level of preventive medicine that aims to detect disease early, send the patient to the right doctor, and to start the right treatment as soon as possible.

secondary proximal renal tubular acidosis. See **proximal renal tubular acidosis.**

secondary sequestrum, a piece of dead bone that partly comes apart from healthy bone in the course of some diseases, but can be pushed back into place. Compare **primary sequestrum.**

secondary sex characteristic, any of the visible bodily features of sexual maturity that develop as the patient grows older. These features include the growth of body hair and the development of the penis or breasts and the labia.

secondary shock, a state of bodily collapse and weakness caused by many types of serious injury or disease. It occurs some time after the injury has happened. The main symptoms are weakness, restlessness, low body temperature, low blood pressure, cold sweat, and a smaller amount of urine. Blood pressure drops steadily and death may occur in a fairly short time unless proper treatment is given. Secondary shock is often linked with heat stroke, crushing injuries, heart attacks, poisoning, very serious infections, burns, and other life-threatening conditions. Compare **hemorrhagic shock, primary shock.**

secondary thrombocytosis. See **thrombocytosis.**

second cuneiform bone. See **intermediate cuneiform bone.**

second nerve. See **optic nerve.**

second opinion, the patient's right to ask to be seen by another doctor so that the patient will get more knowledge about his or her health. It is most often used when the first doctor wants to operate on the patient's body.

second-order change, a change that changes the system itself.

second sight. See **senopia.**

secrete, to release a substance into a cavity, vessel, or organ or onto the surface of the skin, as a gland. **–secretion,** *n.*

secretin /sikrē′tin/, a hormone made by the lining of the intestines that helps digest food. It also helps to make bile. See also **pancreas.**

secretin test, a test of the pancreas using the hormone, secretin. It is used to test for certain cancers and diseases of the pancreas.

secretory duct, (of a gland) a small tube that has a releasing function and joins with an excretory duct.

secretory phase, the part of the cycle of menstruation that follows the release of the egg (ovum) from the ovaries. Also called **luteal phase, progestational phase.** Compare **menstrual phase, proliferative phase.**

sectional arch wire, a wire fixed to only a few teeth used to straighten teeth.

Sectral, a trademark for a beta-adrenergic blocking agent (acebutolol).

secundigravida /səkund′dəgrav′idə/, a woman who is pregnant for the second time. Also called **gravida 2.** –secundigravid, *adj.*

secundines /səkun′dīnz/, the placenta, umbilical cord, and membranes of afterbirth.

secundipara /sek′əndip′ərə/, a woman who has borne two live children in separate pregnancies.

security operations, (in psychology) mechanisms, as indifference and ignoring certain things, that may appear logical but are actually defenses against recognizing or feeling anxiety.

sedation, a drug-caused state of quiet, calmness, or sleep, as by means of a sedative or sleeping pill.

sedative, 1. of or relating to a substance or action that has a calming effect. **2.** a drug that slows down or calms the patient. Some sedatives affect the whole body and some affect one or two parts at a time. Barbiturates and nonbarbiturate sedatives, as chloral hydrate, ethinamate, furazepam, glutethimide, and various minor tranquilizers, are used to bring sleep, ease pain, aid the giving of anesthesia, and treat convulsions, nervous attacks, and irritable bowel syndrome. See also **sedative-hypnotic.**

sedative bath, putting the body in water for a very long time, used especially to calm excited patients.

sedative-hypnotic, a drug that temporarily slows down the central nervous system, used mostly to bring sleep and to calm nervousness. It is used to treat a lack of sleep, nervous attacks, convulsions, and to help activate anesthesia. These drugs should be used carefully because they can become habit-forming. See also **barbiturate.**

sedimentation rate. See **erythrocyte sedimentation rate.**

segmental fracture, a bone break in which several large pieces of bone break away from the broken bone. If the ends of these pieces come through the skin, it is called an open fracture; if they stay inside of the skin, it is called a closed fracture.

segmental resection, an operation in which a part of an organ, gland, or other part of the body is cut out.

segmentation cavity. See **blastocoele.**

segmentation cell. See **blastomere.**

segmentation method, a method for filling tooth root canals in which a cone is cut into sections and the tip section sealed into the tip of a root. The other sections are usually warmed and pressed against the first piece with a plugger. More cone segments are then added until the canal is filled.

segmented hyalinizing vasculitis, a long-term, recurring swelling disease of the blood vessels of the lower legs linked with bumpy or purple-colored skin sores that may become open sores and leave scars. Also called **livedo vasculitis**.

seizure.   See **convulsion**.

seizure threshold,   the amount of stimulus necessary to cause a seizure. All humans can have seizures if the stimulus is strong enough. Those who have sudden seizures for no seeming reason are said to have a "low seizure threshold."

selective abstraction,   a type of abnormal thought process in which the person focuses on one aspect of an event and ignores all other aspects.

selective angiography,   a method of taking x-ray films of the heart.

selective grinding,   any change made by grinding the teeth to improve the bite.

selective inattention,   ignoring something unpleasant on purpose.

selenium (Se),   a metal-like element related to sulfur. It is found in very small amounts in food. Eating a very large amount over a long period of time may be harmful. It is used, in small amounts and mixed with other drugs, to treat dandruff and some other scalp diseases.

selenium sulfide,   a drug used to kill fungus and to treat certain scalp diseases. See also **selenium**. ★CAUTION: Sudden inflammation of the scalp or known allergy to this drug prohibits its use. ★ADVERSE EFFECTS: Among the more serious side effects are dermatitis after long skin contact or keratitis after getting it in the eyes accidentally.

self-alien.   See **ego-dystonic**.

self-alienation.   See **depersonalization**.

self-breast examination (SBE),   a way for a woman to examine her breasts for any changes that might be early signs of cancer. It is usually done 1 week to 10 days after the first day of menstruation, when the breasts are smallest. It should be done throughout the woman's life. Doing this test regularly and carefully gives a much better chance to find any cancer early, when treatment is possible. Also called **breast self-examination (BSE)**. See also **breast examination**.

self-catheterization,   a method done by a person to empty the bladder and prevent it from becoming overfilled with urine. The person who cannot empty the bladder completely but can retain urine for 2 to 4 hours at a time can be taught self-catheterization if the person is willing to learn and has good hand movements and the ability to feel the bladder.

self-destructive behavior,   any behavior, direct or indirect, that if uninterrupted, will ultimately lead to the death of the individual.

self-diagnosis,   forming an opinion about one's own health or sickness without asking a doctor.

self-help group,   a group of people who meet to talk about health matters. Usually these groups are not led by a doctor or nurse. Compare **group therapy**.

self-ideal,   an idea of how one should behave based on certain personal standards. The standard may be either an image of the kind of person one would like to be or simply a number of goals one would like to achieve.

self-imposed guilt,   a restrictive type of guilt that the individual is aware of and from which he or she is unable to break free.

self-limited,   (of a disease or condition) tending to resolve without treatment.

self-management approach,   a treatment approach in which patients take responsibility for their behavior, changing their environment, and planning their future.

self-other,   an idea that prescribes persons believing that sources of power come from within as opposed to those who believe the source of power is in others.

self-responsibility,   a concept of holistic health by which individuals take responsibility for their own health.

self-retaining catheter,   an indwelling urinary catheter that has two channels. One channel allows urine to drain from the bladder into a collecting bag. The other channel has a balloon at the bladder end and a diaphragm at the other end. Several centimeters of air or sterile water are injected through the diaphragm to fill the balloon in the bladder and hold the catheter in place. To remove the catheter, the air or water is withdrawn through the diaphragm or allowed to escape by cutting the diaphragm off the tube.

self-threading pin,   a threaded pin screwed into a hole drilled in a tooth to help hold a filling.

sella turcica /sel′ə tur′sikə/,   a sideways furrow crossing the middle of the back of the skull where the pituitary gland is found.

Selsun,   a trademark for a drug used to kill fungus and to treat certain scalp diseases (selenium sulfide), used as a shampoo.

SEM.   See **scanning electron microscope**.

semen /sē′mən/,   the thick, whitish fluid released by the male sex organs, it carries the sperm. Also called **seminal fluid, sperm**. –**seminal**, *adj*.

semicircular canal,   any of three bony, fluid-filled loops inside the inner ear; involved in the sense of balance.

semicircular duct,   one of three tubes that make up the membranes of the inner ear. See also **membranous labyrinth**.

semicoma.   See **coma**.

semifixed feature space,   (in psychology) objects in the environment, as furniture, that can be moved.

semi-Fowler's position,   placing the patient in a leaning position, with the upper half of the body raised by elevating the head of the bed.

semilente insulin.   See **intermediate-acting insulin**.

semilunar bone.   See **lunate bone**.

semilunar valve,   **1.** a valve with half-moon-shaped cusps, as the aortic valve and the pulmonary valve. **2.** any one of the cusps forming such a valve. See also **heart valve, mitral valve, tricuspid valve.**

semimembranosus /sem'ēmem'brənō'səs/, one of three muscles at the back and inside of the thigh. It helps to bend the leg. Compare **biceps femoris, hamstring muscle, semitendinosus.**

seminal duct, any tube through which semen passes, as the vas deferens or the ejaculatory duct.

seminal fluid. See **semen.**

seminal fluid test, any of several tests of semen to detect defects in the male sexual system and to determine fertility. Normal values in some of these tests are sperm count, 60 million to 150 million/ml of seminal fluid; pH, more than 7 (7.7 average); ejaculation volume, 1.5 to 5.0 ml; motility, 60% of sperm.

seminal vesicle, either of the paired, saclike glands that lie behind the bladder in the male and act as part of the reproductive system. The seminal vesicles release a fluid that forms part of semen.

seminal vesiculitis, swelling of a seminal vesicle.

seminarcosis. See **twilight sleep.**

semination, the introduction of semen into the female genital tract.

seminiferous /sem'inif'ərəs/, carrying or releasing semen, as the tubules of the testicles.

seminoma /sem'inō'mə/, pl. **seminomas, seminomata,** the most common cancer of the testicles. Compare **dysgerminoma.** See also **testicular tumor.**

semipermeable membrane, a membrane that allows certain substances to pass through, but does not allow others, depending on the size of the atoms.

semirecumbent, a lying-down position.

semitendinosus /sem'iten'dinō'səs/, one of three muscles on the back of the thigh that help to move the leg. Compare **biceps femoris, hamstring muscle, semimembranosus.**

semustine /səmus'tēn/, a drug used to treat cancer. It is used to treat Lewis lung carcinoma, brain tumors, malignant melanoma, and Hodgkin's disease.

★CAUTION: Acute myelosuppression or known allergy to this drug prohibits its use. It is not given during pregnancy or to breast-feeding mothers.

★ADVERSE EFFECTS: Among the more serious side effects are delayed bone marrow depression and thrombocytopenia.

senescent /sines'ənt/, aging or growing old. See also **senile. −senescence,** n.

Sengstaken-Blakemore tube, a thick catheter having a triple bore and two balloons, used to stop bleeding in the throat. Attached to a tube, one balloon is blown up in the stomach and exerts pressure against the upper opening. Similarly attached, another longer and nar-

rower balloon exerts pressure on the walls of the throat. The third tube is used for removing the contents of the stomach. Also called **Blakemore-Sengstaken tube.** See also **tube.**

senile, relating to or characteristic of old age or the process of aging, especially the wasting of the mind and body that come with aging. See also **aging, senescent, senility,** n.

senile angioma. See **cherry angioma.**

senile cataract, a kind of cataract, linked with aging.

senile delirium, weakness of the mind linked with very old age and marked by restlessness, insomnia, aimless wandering, and, less commonly, hallucination. See also **delirium, senile psychosis.**

senile dementia. See **senile psychosis.**

senile dental caries, tooth decay occurring in old age. Senile dental caries is usually marked by cavities that form near or below the gums. See also **dental caries.**

senile involution, a pattern of steady shrinking and breakdowns in tissues and organs that come in old age.

senile keratosis. See **actinic keratosis.**

senile memory. See **anterograde memory.**

senile nanism, stunted growth linked with premature old age.

senile psychosis, a mental disorder of the aged that is caused by a shrinking of the brain. It is not known why this happens. Symptoms include loss of memory, not being able to think clearly, and periods of confusion and irritability, all of which may be serious. It is more common in women than men. There is no known cure. Also called **primary degenerative dementia, senile onset.** See also **multiinfarct dementia.**

senile wart. See **actinic keratosis.**

senna, the dried leaflets or pods of Cassia acutifolia or Cassia augustifolia, used as a cathartic.

senopia /senō'pē-ə/, an eye condition in which the hardening of the lenses causes the eyes to focus better on things nearby. It is linked with increasing lenticular nuclear sclerosis. This type of sclerosis commonly leads to the development of cataracts. Also called **genontopia, second sight.**

sensate focus technique, a kind of treatment of the inability to obtain or maintain an erection (erectile dysfunction).

sensation, 1. a feeling, impression, or awareness of a bodily state or condition that occurs whenever a nerve is excited and sends a signal to the brain. Kinds of sensation include **delayed sensation, epigastric sensation, primary sensation, referred sensation,** and **subjective sensation. 2.** a feeling of a mental or emotional state, which may or may not be caused by something outside of the body.

sense, 1. the ability or structure that allows events both inside and outside of the body to be felt and understood. The major senses are sight, hearing, smell, taste, touch, and pressure. Other senses include hunger, thirst, pain, temperature, ability to feel the muscles move, space, time, and to be able to tell when the stomach, bladder, and bowel are full or empty. **2.** the ability to feel; a sensation. **3.** normal mental ability. **4.** to perceive through a sense organ.

sensible perspiration, sweating enough to see it. Compare **insensible perspiration.**

sensitivity, 1. able to feel, transmit, or react to a stimulus. **2.** allergy to a substance, as a drug or an antigen. See also **allergy, hypersensitivity.** –**sensitive,** *adj.*

sensitization, 1. an acquired reaction in which specific antibodies develop in response to an antigen. This is done on purpose in vaccination. It is done by injecting a disease-causing organism that has been changed in such a way that it is no longer infectious. It remains able to cause the making of antibodies to fight the disease. Allergic reactions are sensitization reactions that result from excess sensitization to a foreign protein. **2.** a method of destroying microorganisms by inserting into a solution substances, as fluorescing dyes, that absorb visible light and emit energy at wavelengths that will kill the organism. **3.** *nontechnical.* anaphylaxis. –**sensitize,** *v.*

sensitized, referring to tissues that have been made susceptible to antigenic substances. See also **allergy.**

sensorimotor therapy, therapy designed to improve the relationship between reflex actions and voluntary physical movements concerned with posture and locomotion.

sensorineural hearing loss, a form of hearing loss in which sound passes properly through the outer and middle ear but is distorted by a defect in the inner ear. Use of a hearing aid helps in some, but not all, cases. Compare **conductive hearing loss.**

sensorium, (in psychology) the part of the conscious mind that includes the special powers of sensory awareness and their relationship in the brain. A clear sensorium provides a reasonably accurate memory along with a correct awareness of time, place, and identity.

sensory apraxia. See **ideational apraxia.**

sensory-based language, the use of behavior rather than words in communication. Examples include puzzled expressions, scowling, and fingerpointing.

sensory deficit, a defect in the function of one or more of the senses.

sensory deprivation, an unwilling loss of bodily awareness caused by being shut off from outside for a very long time. It can cause panic, confusion, depression, and hallucinations. It may be linked with various handicaps and conditions, as blindness, heavy sedation, and prolonged isolation.

sensory discrimination, the ability to tell the difference between specific characteristics of a sensation, as one versus two points of pressure on the skin.

sensory integration, the processing and organization of sensory input, a perception of the body or environment, an adaptive response, or the development of some neural function.

sensory integrative dysfunction, a disorder in brain function that makes it difficult to process and organize sensations. Many, but not all, learning disorders are caused by sensory integrative dysfunctions.

sensory integrative therapy, therapy that involves sensory stimulation and appropriate (adaptive) responses to it according to a child's nervous system needs. Treatment usually involves full body movements. It usually does not include desk activities, speech training, reading lessons, or training in specific mental or physical skills. The goal is to improve the brain's ability to process and organize sensations.

sensory nerve, a nerve that carries sense signals from the parts of the body to the brain or spinal chord. Compare **motor nerve.**

sensory-perceptual overload, a state in which the loudness and strength of numerous sensations go beyond the ability of the patient to sort them out.

sentinel node. See **Virchow's node.**

SEP, abbreviation for **somatosensory evoked potential.**

separation anxiety, fear and nervousness caused by being away from home and friends. It happens most often when a child is taken away from its mother. See also **anxiety, anxiety neurosis.**

separator, a tool used to hold teeth apart when the dentist needs to work between two teeth.

sepsis /sep′sis/, infection. Compare **asepsis.** –**septic,** *adj.*

septal defect, an abnormal defect usually present at birth in the wall separating two chambers of the heart. Kinds of septal defects are **atrial septal defect** and **ventricular septal defect.**

septate, relating to a structure divided by a septum.

septic abortion, an abortion that is needed when the womb becomes infected and threatens the life of the mother. It may happen by itself or it may be done by a doctor. Compare **infected abortion.** See also **criminal abortion, induced abortion.**

septic arthritis, a serious form of arthritis, marked by joint swelling caused by the spread of bacteria through the bloodstream from an infection elsewhere in the body or by infection of a joint during injury or surgery. The joint is stiff, painful, tender, warm, and swollen. Physical therapy as the joint heals is helpful to restore it to full motion. Also called **acute bacterial arthritis.**

septicemia /sep'tisē'mē·ə/, an infection of the whole body caused by germs that spread from an infected part of the body through the bloodstream. It is treated with antibiotic drugs. Usually septicemia causes fever, chill, prostration, pain, headache, nausea, or diarrhea. Also called **blood poisoning.** Compare **bacteremia.** See also **septic shock.** –**septicemic,** *adj.*

septicemic plague, a form of bubonic plague that kills very quickly in which septicemia with meningitis occurs before the lymph nodes have had time to become swollen. Compare **bubonic plague, pneumonic plague.** See also **plague,** *Yersinia pestis.*

septic fever, a rise of body temperature linked with infection by disease-causing germs.

septic shock, a form of shock that occurs in septicemia. Fever, rapid heart beat, fast breathing, and confusion or coma may also occur. Septic shock usually follows signs of severe infection, often in the urinary system or in the intestines. Kinds of septic shock include **toxic shock syndrome** and **bacteremic shock.** See also **shock.**

septostomy /septos'təmē/, an operation to make a hole in a septum.

Septra, a trademark for a drug used to kill bacteria.

septum /sep'təm/, *pl.* **septa,** a dividing wall, as found separating the chambers of the heart.

sequester, to keep apart, or away from others, as a patient sequestered to prevent the spread of an infection.

sequestered edema, the collection of fluid in the tissues surrounding a newly created surgical wound.

sequestrum /sikwes'trəm/, *pl.* **sequestra,** a fragment of dead bone that is partly or totally broken free from the nearby healthy bone.

sequoiasis /sikwoi'əsis/, a type of allergic swelling of the lungs common among workers in sawmills where redwood is sawn. Symptoms of the disease include chills, fever, cough, shortness of breath, loss of appetite, nausea, and vomiting. Long-term symptoms include a cough that brings up matter from the lungs, shortness of breath when exercising, and weight loss.

Ser, abbreviation for **serine.**

Ser-Ap-Es, a trademark for drug used to treat high blood pressure.

Serax, a trademark for a tranquilizer (oxazepam).

Serentil, a trademark for a phenothiazine tranquilizer (mesoridazine).

serial extraction, the pulling out of certain baby teeth over a number of years, to prevent crowding when the permanent teeth grow in.

serial processing, digital computer processing in which programs are run one after another rather than all at one time.

serial speech, learned speech involving a series of words, as counting numbers or reciting the days of the week.

series /sir'ēs/, *pl.* **series** / sir'ēs/, a chain of objects or events arranged in a set order, as the series of stages through which a mature blood cell grows.

serine (Ser) /ser'ēn/, an amino acid found in many proteins in the body. See also **amino acid, protein.**

Sernylan, a trademark for an anesthetic (phencyclidine hydrochloride), used to treat animals. It is also used illegally as a euphoric called **PCP.**

Seromycin, a trademark for a tuberculostatic (cycloserine).

serosa /sirō'sə/, any serous membrane, as the tunica serosa that lines the walls of body cavities and releases a watery fluid.

serosanguineous /sir'ōsang·gwin'ē·əs/, thin and red; a mixture of serum and blood. Also **serosanguinous** /sir'ōsang'gwinəs/.

serotonin /ser'ətō'nin, sir'-/, a substance found naturally in the brain and intestines. Serotonin is released from certain cells when the blood vessel walls are damaged. It acts as a strong vessel-narrowing substance. Also called **5-hydroxytryptamine.**

serous fluid /sir'əs/, a thin, watery liquid.

serous membrane, one of the many thin sheets of tissue that line certain areas inside the body, as the sac that surrounds the heart. Between the inner layer of serous membrane covering various organs and the outer layer of the organ itself is a space kept wet by serous fluid. The fluid allows the covered organ to move easily, as the lungs, which move in breathing. Compare **mucous membrane, skin, synovial membrane.**

Serpasil, a trademark for a high blood pressure drug (reserpine).

Serpasil-Apresoline, a trademark for a drug containing two high blood pressure medicines (reserpine and hydralazine hydrochloride).

Serpasil-Esidrix, a trademark for a high blood pressure drug containing a diuretic (hydrochlorothiazide) and an antihypertensive (reserpine).

serpent ulcer, an open sore of the skin that heals in one place while growing in another. Also called **serpiginous ulcer.**

Serratia /serā'shə/, a genus of bacilli that are capable of causing infection in humans, including bacteremia, pneumonia, and urinary tract infections. *Serratia* infections often happen in hospitals. See also **nosocomial infection.**

serratus anterior /serā'təs/, a thin muscle of the chest wall stretching from the ribs under the arm to the shoulder blade. It moves to raise the shoulder and arm. Compare **pectoralis major, pectoralis minor, subclavius.**

Sertoli-Leydig cell tumor. See **arrhenoblastoma.**

serum /sir'əm/, **1.** also called **blood serum.** any thin, watery fluid, especially one that keeps serous membranes wet. **2.** any clear, watery fluid that has been separated from its more solid elements, as the exudate from a blister. **3.** the clear, thin, and sticky liquid part of the blood that remains after clotting. **4.** a vaccine made from the serum of a patient who has had some disease and used to protect another patient against that same infection or poison.

serum albumin, an important substance found in the blood. It is needed to help control blood pressure.

serum C-reactive protein. See **C-reactive protein.**

serum creatinine level, the level of creatinine in the blood serum, used in diagnosing possible kidney problems.

serum glutamic oxaloacetic transaminase (SGOT), an enzyme found in various parts of the body, especially the heart, liver, and muscle tissue. The body makes more of it when there has been some cell damage. See also **transaminase.**

serum glutamic pyruvic transaminase (SGPT), an enzyme normally found in large amounts in the liver. Having much more of it than normal in the blood is a sign of liver damage. See also **transaminase.**

serum hepatitis. See **hepatitis B.**

serum sickness, a sickness that may occur 2 to 3 weeks after being given an antiserum. It is caused by a reaction to serum and is marked by fever, a swollen spleen, swollen lymph nodes, skin rash, and joint pain. Treatment may include the use of steroids. See also **angioneurotic edema, antigen-antibody reaction, Arthus reaction.**

sesamoid bone, any one of numerous small, round bones buried in certain tendons that go through much stress and strain. The largest is the kneecap.

sessile /ses'əl/, permanently attached.

set, a habit of behaving a certain way.

seventh cranial nerve. See **facial nerve.**

severe combined immunodeficiency disease (SCID), an illness marked by the total or partial lack of certain cells in the body fluids that fight infection. It is a disease of the genes, usually fatal. Its cause is not yet known.

Sever's disease. See **calcaneal epephysitis.**

Sevin, a trademark for carbaryl, a widely used insect poison that can harm humans if it is spilled directly on the skin. Besides irritating the skin, it may cause nausea, vomiting, cramps, diarrhea, heavy sweating, drooling, shortness of breath, weakness, loss of coordination, and slurred speech; large doses may cause coma and death. Carbaryl on the skin should be immediately washed off with water. Poisoning requires the attention of a doctor.

sex, 1. a division of male or female based on many features, as body parts and genetic differences. Compare **gender. 2.** sexual intercourse.

sex-linked disorder, any disease or abnormal condition that is caused by a defect in the genes on the sex chromosomes.

sex-linked ichthyosis, a skin disorder present at birth and marked by large, thick, dry scales that are dark in color and that cover the neck, scalp, ears, face, trunk, and the folds of the arms and the backs of the knees. It is carried by females and appears only in males. The condition is treated with several kinds of lotions and creams. Also called **X-linked ichthyosis.** See also **ichthyosis.**

sexual, of or relating to sex.

sexual abuse, taking advantage of another person by fondling, rape, or forcing another to take part in unnatural sex acts or other perverted behavior. When children are victims, they tend to get a harmful feeling of loss of control of themselves.

sexual assault, the act of forcing sexual contact with another person, male or female, without his or her consent. Legal definitions vary in different communities.

sexual aversion disorder, a persistent or extreme dislike or avoidance of all or nearly all genital sexual contact with a partner.

sexual dwarf, an adult dwarf whose genitals are normally developed.

sexual dysfunction, a sex-related difficulty. It may be a bodily or mental problem. See also **female sexual dysfunction, male sexual dysfunction, nursing diagnosis.**

sexual fantasy, mental images of an erotic nature that can lead to sexual arousal.

sexual harassment, any bothersome act of a sexual nature, including sexual talk, committed by someone in power, as a boss or supervisor. Sexual harassment on the job is against the law. Sexual harassment may involve a man and a woman, two men, or two women.

sexual history, (in a patient record) the part of the patient's personal history concerned with sexual activity. A sexual history is very important for deciding on the proper treatment of a patient who has a disease of the reproduction system, who has sexual difficulties, or who asks for contraception, abortion, or sterilization. The extent of the history varies with the patient's age and condition and the reason for securing the history. A short sexual history is recommended as part of every complete physical examination. It may include the age when the patient first had sexual intercourse, the kind and frequency of sexual activity, and the satisfaction gained from it.

sexual hormones, chemical substances produced in the body that control the activity of organs of the reproductive system.

sexual intercourse. See **coitus.**

sexuality, 1. all of the physical, functional, and mental traits that are shown by one's sex identity and sex behavior, whether related to the sex organs or to procreation. **2.** the genital organs that tell apart males from females.

sexually deviant personality, a sexual behavior that differs significantly from what is considered normal for a society.

sexually transmitted disease (STD), a contagious disease usually caught by sexual intercourse or genital contact. These diseases are quite common. Kinds of venereal diseases are gonorrhea, syphilis, chancroid, granuloma inguinale, lymphogranuloma venereum, scabies, herpes genitalis and anorectal herpes and warts, pediculosis, trichomoniasis, genital candidiasis, molluscum contagiosum, nonspecific urethritis, chlamydial infections, cytomegalovirus, and AIDS. Also called **venereal disease.** See also specific diseases.

sexual mores, socially acceptable sexual behavior, usually based on moral customs regarding sexual behaviors that are harmful to others, as rape, incest, and sexual abuse of children.

sexual orientation, the clear, persistent desire of a person for association with one sex rather than the other.

sexual psychopath, an individual whose sexual behavior is openly perverted, antisocial, and criminal. See also **antisocial personality disorder.**

sexual reassignment, a sex change.

sexual response cycle, the four phases of biological sexual response: excitement, plateau, orgasm, and resolution.

sexual tasks, specific skills learned in various stages of development to allow an adult to function normally sexually.

sexual therapist, a health-care professional with specialized knowledge and skill in helping individuals with sexual difficulties.

sexual therapy, a type of counseling that aids in maintaining a healthy sexuality.

SFD, abbreviation for **small for dates.** See **small for gestational age infant.**

SGA, abbreviation for **small for gestational age.** See **small for gestational age infant.**

SGOT, abbreviation for **serum glutamic oxaloacetic transaminase.**

SGPT, abbreviation for **serum glutamic pyruvic transaminase.**

shadow, (in psychology) a concept that represents the unacceptable aspects and parts of behavior.

shake test, a test to determine how mature the fetal lungs are.

shallow breathing, a kind of breathing that is slow, shallow, and usually not very useful. It is usually caused by drugs.

shared paranoid disorder, an abnormal mental disorder in which two close or related patients have exactly the same symptoms. Also called **folie à deux** /fôlē′äd′, -dä′, -dōō′/ .

Sharpey's fiber, (in dentistry) any one of a number of certain fibers found in a tooth near the gum.

shear, force or pressure applied against the surface and layers of the skin as tissues slide in opposite but parallel directions.

shearling, a sheepskin placed on a bed to help prevent bed sores.

sheath, a tubelike structure that surrounds an organ or any other part of the body, as the sheath of the rectus abdominis muscle or the sheath of Schwann, which covers various nerve fibers.

Sheehan's syndrome, a condition occurring after giving birth in which the pituitary gland is damaged. It is caused by a lessening of blood circulation after bleeding of the womb.

sheep cell test, a method that mixes human blood cells with the red blood cells of sheep. It is used to diagnose several diseases, as DiGeorge's syndrome.

sheet bath, applying of wet sheets to the body, used mainly to treat burns.

sheet wadding, stretchable sheets of cotton padding used to cover the skin before a cast is applied. The stretching allows for some swelling of the arm or leg without the cast becoming too tight.

shellfish poisoning, an illness caused by eating clams, oysters, or mussels that are tainted with the parasite known as the "red tide." The symptoms appear within a few minutes and include nausea, lightheadedness, vomiting, and tingling or numbness around the mouth, followed by paralysis of the hands and feet and, possibly, the inability to breathe. The poison is not destroyed by cooking; however, the illness is less serious if the water used in cooking is not eaten or drunk. It is treated with drugs after breathing has been restored.

shell shock, any of a number of mental disorders, ranging from extreme fear to dementia, caused by the stress of combat. See also **combat fatigue, posttraumatic stress disorder.**

shell teeth, a type of tooth disease in which the teeth are not formed properly.

Shigella /shigel′ə/, a genus of harmful bacteria that causes gastroenteritis and bacterial dysentery, as *Shigella dysenteriae.* See also **shigellosis.**

shigellosis /shig′əlō′sis/, a serious infection of the bowel marked by diarrhea, stomach pain, and fever, that is carried by hand-to-mouth contact with the feces of infected individuals. The disease occurs only rarely in the United States but is native to underdeveloped areas of the world. It is especially common and usually most severe in children. It is treated with drugs. An infected patient must be kept apart from others, and anyone coming in contact must wash the hands very well. Shigellosis infections must be reported to the public health department. Also called **bacillary dysentery.**

shin bone. See **tibia.**

shingles. See **herpes zoster.**

shin splints, a painful condition of the lower leg caused by strain after very hard exercise, as running. Many times it is the result of a lack of proper training. Treatment usually involves rest and exercise therapy. Surgery is sometimes necessary.

Shirodkar's operation /shir'odkärz'/, an operation done to repair a damaged or defective cervix. It allows a pregnancy to develop normally.

shistocytes /shis'tōsīts/, cell fragments of red blood cells, caused by the breaking down of blood cells linked with very bad burns and internal clotting.

shock, an abnormal condition that occurs when not enough blood flows through the body, causing very low blood pressure, a lack of urine, and dangerous cell disorders. It may be caused by a heart problem, changes in the blood vessels, or an injury. It may be caused by bleeding, vomiting, diarrhea, not drinking enough liquid, or improper action of the kidneys. Kinds of shock include **anaphylactic shock, bacteremic shock, cardiogenic shock, diabetic shock, electric shock, hypovolemic shock,** and **neurogenic shock.** The signs and symptoms of different kinds of shock are very much alike. The pulse and breathing become faster. The patient may appear to be very nervous. Later, the body becomes cooler. The patient should not be given anything to drink. There may also be weakness, lethargy, pallor, and a cool, moist skin.

shock lung. See **acute respiratory distress syndrome.**

shock trousers, a pair of trousers that can be filled with air; it puts pressure on the legs to treat shock and very low blood pressure.

short-acting, referring to a drug that begins to take effect very soon after being taken by the patient.

short-acting insulin, a watery fluid of beef or pork pancreas used to treat diabetics that begins to act within 1 hour after being injected and acts most strongly in 2 to 4 hours. The acting time of regular insulin is 4 to 6 hours and of crystalline zinc insulin 5 to 8 hours. Also called **rapid-acting insulin.** See also **insulin.** Compare **intermediate-acting insulin, long-acting insulin.**

short-arm cast, a cast used to keep the hand or wrist from moving. It is used to treat broken bones, to hold the hand or wrist after surgery, or to correct a defect or deformity in the hand or wrist. Compare **long-arm cast.**

short bones, bones that occur in groups and usually permit movement of the hands and feet, as the carpals and tarsals.

short gut syndrome, a disorder present at birth in which an infant's intestine is too short or not developed enough to allow normal food digestion. The child is given nutritional fluids through a vein (parenteral feeding) until the intestine grows, develops further, or is replaced by surgical transplant. When the short gut syndrome is eventually corrected, a small child may have to be taught to chew and swallow.

shorting, A type of fraud in which the patient is given a smaller amount of a prescription than he or she pays for. See also **kiting.**

short-leg cast, a cast covering the leg from the knee to the toes that does not allow the foot or ankle to move. It is used to treat a sprained or broken ankle, to secure an ankle or foot following an operation, and to correct a deformity in the ankle or foot. Compare **long-leg cast.**

short-leg cast with walker, a short-leg cast with a rubber device fixed to the bottom of the foot to help the patient walk.

Short Portable Mental Status Questionnaire, a 10-question test used to determine if older adults have difficulty thinking clearly. It tests awareness of time and place, past and recent memory, practical skills, and math ability.

short-PR-normal-QRS syndrome. See **Lown-Ganong-Levine syndrome.**

short sight. See **myopia.**

short-term memory, memory of recent events.

shoulder, the place where the collarbone and the shoulder blade meet and where the arm attaches to the trunk of the body. See also the **Color Atlas of Human Anatomy.**

shoulder blade. See **scapula.**

shoulder-hand syndrome, a condition of the nerves and bones marked by pain and stiffness in the shoulder and arm, limited joint motion, swelling of the hand, muscle wasting, and a loss of calcium from the underlying bones. The condition occurs most commonly after a heart attack but may be linked with other known or unknown causes.

shoulder joint, the ball-and-socket joint of the humerus and the shoulder blade. Also called **humeral articulation.**

shoulder spica cast, a bone cast applied to keep the body to the hips, the wrist, and the hand rigid. It uses a diagonal shoulder support between the hip and arm parts. The shoulder spica cast is used to treat shoulder dislocations and injuries. It is also used to put into place and keep rigid the shoulder after surgery.

shoulder subluxation, an injury to the tissues around the shoulder joint.

show. See **vaginal bleeding.**

shreds, very shiny little threads of mucus in the urine, showing an infection in the urinary tract. Also called **mucos shreds.**

shunt, **1.** to reroute the flow of a body fluid from one place to another. **2.** a tube or device put into the body to redirect a body fluid from one place to another.

shunt, left to right, a rerouting of blood from the left side of the heart to the right, as through a defect in the wall separating two chambers of the heart, or from the circulation of the entire body directly to the lungs, bypassing the right side of the heart.

Shy-Drager syndrome /shī'drā'gər/, a rare, gradual nerve disorder of young and middle-aged adults. It is marked by very low blood pressure, no control over bladder or bowel, narrowing of the iris of the eye, a lack of sweat, trembling, stiffness, lack of coordination, and muscle wasting. It is treated with certain drugs to control the muscles and the blood pressure. Antigravity stockings may prevent blood from settling in the legs and feet. See also **orthostatic hypotension.**

SIADH, abbreviation for **syndrome of inappropriate antidiuretic hormone secretion.**

sialogogue /sī·al'əgog'/, anything that causes saliva to be released.

sialography /sī·əlog'rəfē/, a technique in x-ray photography in which a salivary gland is filmed after a certain substance is injected into its duct. **–sialogram** /sī·al'əgram'/, *n.,* **sialographic,** *adj.*

sialolith /sī·al'əlith/, a small stone formed in a salivary gland or duct.

sialorrhea /sī·al'ərē'ə/, a flow of too much saliva that may be linked with a number of conditions, as acute swelling of the mouth, mental retardation, mercury poisoning, pregnancy, teething, alcoholism, or malnutrition. Also called **hypersalivation, ptyalism.**

Siamese twins, equally developed twin fetuses, produced from the same egg, that have not developed completely, resulting in their being joined together at some part of the body. With modern surgical methods, most Siamese twins can be successfully separated. See **conditioned twins.**

Siberian tick typhus, a mild, short fever illness seen in north, central, and east Asia, caused by *Rickettsia siberica,* carried by ticks, and marked by a widespread rash with dark, hard bumps, headache, swelling in the eyes, and a small ulcer at the tick bite. Treatment with chloramphenicol or tetracycline is usually helpful. Also called **North Asian tick-borne rickettsiosis.** See also **rickettsia, typhus.**

sibilant rale, an abnormal whistling sound that may be made by a patient with a lung or breathing disease. It is caused by air passing through a lumen that is partly clogged with mucus.

Siblin, a trademark for a bulk laxative containing psyllium seed.

sickle cell, an abnormal, crescent-shaped red blood cell typical of sickle cell anemia.

sickle cell anemia, a serious, long-term, incurable blood disease. It attacks the red blood cells. Sickle cell anemia results in joint pain, blood clots, fever, and long-term anemia, with enlargement of the spleen, lack of energy, and weakness. See also **congenital nonspherocytic hemolytic anemia, elliptocytosis, hemoglobin S, sickle cell crisis.**

sickle cell crisis, a serious, short attack that occurs in children with sickle cell anemia. See also **hemoglobin S, sickle cell anemia.** The most common form is a painful closing of the blood vessels. It is linked with an infection in the lungs or throat or in the intestines. Typical of this kind of crisis are acute stomach pain, painful swelling of the soft tissue of the hands and feet (hand-foot syndrome), and joint pain, often so severe that movement of the joint is limited. Persistent headache, dizziness, convulsions, visual or auditory disturbances, facial nerve palsies, coughing, shortness of breath, and rapid breathing may occur if the central nervous system or lungs are affected. A common problem of young children with sickle cell anemia is the high risk of infection that may be greatly increased during periods of crisis.

sickle cell thalassemia, a blood disorder in which the genes for sickle cell and for thalassemia are both inherited. See also **hemoglobinopathy, hemoglobin S, hemoglobin S-C disease, hemoglobin variant.**

sickle cell trait, a form of sickle cell anemia. People who have the trait are told of it and advised of the possibility of having an infant with sickle cell disease if both parents have the trait. See **hemoglobin S.**

sick sinus syndrome, a complex of syndromes linked with sinus node disorders. The condition may be caused by several types of heart disease. The most common symptoms are lethargy, weakness, lightheadedness, dizziness, and episodes of near fainting to actual loss of consciousness. At present the only treatment is by implanting a permanent demand pacemaker.

side effect, any reaction that results from a medication or therapy. Usually, although not necessarily, the effect is not wanted, and may manifest itself as nausea, dry mouth, dizziness, blood disorders, blurred vision, discolored urine, or a ringing or roaring in the ears.

sideroblastic anemia /sid'ərōblas'tik/, any one of a group of long-term blood disorders. It affects the red blood cells. The cause of the disease is not known. Treatment may include extract of liver, pyridoxine, folic acid, and blood transfusion. Compare **iron deficiency anemia, siderosis.**

sideropenic dysphagia. See **Plummer-Vinson syndrome.**

siderosis /sid'ərō'sis/, a type of lung disease caused by the inhalation of iron dust or particles. An increase in the amounts of iron in the blood. See also **hemochromatosis, hemosiderosis, sideroblastic anemia.**

SIDS, abbreviation for **sudden infant death syndrome.**

sigh. See **periodic deep inspiration.**

sight, 1. the sense of vision. It is the major junction of the eye. 2. that which is seen.

sigmoid /sig'moid/, 1. of or relating to an S shape. 2. the sigmoid colon.

sigmoid colon, the part of the colon that extends from the end of the colon in the pelvis to the beginning of the rectum.

sigmoidectomy /sig'moidek'təmē/, cutting out the sigmoid bend of the colon, most commonly performed to remove a cancerous tumor. Most cancers of the lower bowel occur in the sigmoid colon.

sigmoid flexure. See **sigmoid colon.**

sigmoid mesocolon /mez'ōkō'lən/, a fold of membrane that connects the sigmoid colon to the pelvic wall. Compare **mesentery proper, transverse mesocolon.**

sigmoid notch, a furrow on the top of the jaw bone where it is joined to the skull.

sigmoidoscope /sigmoi'dəskōp/, an instrument used to examine the lumen of the sigmoid colon. It consists of a tube and a light, allowing the mucous membrane lining the colon to be looked at. Compare **proctoscope.**

sigmoidoscopy /sig'moidos'kəpē/, the examination of the rectum and the sigmoid colon with the aid of a special instrument (sigmoidoscope).

sign, something seen by an examiner, as a fever, a rash, the whisper heard over the chest in lung disease, or the light band of hair seen in children after recovery from faulty diet (kwashiorkor). Many signs go along with symptoms, as bumps and rashes are often seen when a patient complains of itching. Compare **symptom.**

signal molecule, a hormone, neurotransmitter, or other agent that transfers information from one cell or organ to another. Examples include steroid hormones, insulin, and growth factors.

signal node. See **Virchow's node.**

signal symptom. See **symptom.**

silent heart attack. See **silent ischemia.**

silent ischemia, reduction of blood flow to the heart muscle that causes no symptoms but can result in severe damage or sudden death. Studies indicate that nearly 75% of all instances of reduced blood flow to the heart (cardiac ischemia) are painless; episodes may last up to 40 minutes, compared with ischemia with chest pains (angina pectoris), which usually lasts no longer than 3 minutes. Silent ischemia is most likely to occur during the first 6 hours after awakening in the morning. In more than three-fourths of the cases studied, episodes are triggered by mental activity, while cardiac ischemia with chest pains usually follows physical activity.

silicate dental cement, a relatively hard, clear material used mostly to repair front teeth.

silicosis /sil'ikō'sis/, a lung disorder caused by inhaling silicon dioxide continuously over a long period of time. Silicon dioxide is found in sands, quartzes, flints, and many other stones. Silicosis is marked by the development of small fiberlike growths in the lungs. In advanced cases, severe shortness of breath may develop. The incidence of silicosis is highest among industrial workers exposed to silica powder in manufacturing processes, in those who work with ceramics, sand, or stone, and in those who mine silica. Also called **grinder's disease, quartz silicosis.** See also **chronic obstructive pulmonary disease, inorganic dust.**

silk suture, a braided, fine, black thread, usually used to close deep cuts, wounds, and cuts in the skin. It is not absorbed by the body and is removed after about 7 days.

silo filler's disease, a rare, acute respiratory condition seen in agricultural workers who have inhaled nitrogen oxide as they work with fermented fodder in closed silos. Typically, symptoms of respiratory distress and pulmonary edema occur several hours after exposure. Loss of consciousness may occur. A stay in the hospital and help in breathing are often required. The condition is rarely fatal.

Silvadene, a trademark for a drug that kills bacteria (sulfadiazine silver).

silver (Ag), a whitish precious metal used in certain medications and, blended together with other metals, to fill teeth.

silver cone method, a method for filling tooth root canals. A small silver cone is sealed into the tip of a root canal, and any canal space that is left is filled with gutta-percha or a sealer.

Silver dwarf, a person who has Silver's syndrome, a disorder present at birth in which short stature is linked with each side of the body being a different size, numerous deformities of the head, face, and skeleton, and early puberty.

silver-fork fracture. See **Colles' fracture.**

Silverman-Anderson score, a system for rating the amount of difficulty in breathing.

silver nitrate, a drug applied to the skin to treat infection.

★CAUTION: Known allergy to this drug prohibits its use. It should not be used with bacitracin, which does not allow silver nitrate to work properly.

★ADVERSE EFFECTS: Among the more serious

side effects are severe limited swelling, burns, and argyria.

silver salts poisoning, a poisonous condition caused by the eating of silver nitrate, marked by discoloration of the lips, vomiting, stomach pain, dizziness, and convulsions. Treatment includes rinsing the stomach with salt water, followed by soothing fluids. Treatment of convulsions and low blood pressure may also be needed.

Silver's syndrome. See **Silver dwarf.**

silver sulfadiazine, a drug used on the skin to prevent or treat infection in second- and third-degree burns.

★CAUTION: Known allergy to this drug, to silver, or to sulfonamides prohibits its use. It is not given in the last weeks of pregnancy or to newborn or premature infants.

★ADVERSE EFFECTS: Among the most serious side effects are rashes, fungal infections, and certain blood disorders.

simethicone, a drug used to prevent the patient from passing gas. It is used to reduce excess gas in the stomach and intestines. Side effects include belching and rectal flatus.

simian crease, a single crease across the palm from the joining of the front and back creases of the palm, seen in birth defects, as Down's syndrome. Also called **simian line.**

Similac preparations, a trademark for a group of commercial milk products that are prepared especially for infant feeding. The formulas are packaged in both powder and liquid form.

Simmond's disease. See **postpubertal panhypopituitarism.**

simple angioma, a tumor consisting of a network of small vessels or bulging capillaries surrounded by connecting tissue.

simple cavity, a cavity that involves only one surface of a tooth.

simple fission. See **binary fission.**

simple fracture, a bone break in which the bone does not break the skin. Compare **compound fracture.**

simple mastectomy, an operation in which a breast is completely removed and the underlying muscles and nearby lymph nodes are left intact. It is done to treat breast cancer. Compare **modified radical mastectomy, radical mastectomy.** See also **mastectomy.**

simple phobia, an irrational fear of specific things, as animals, dirt, light, or darkness. Compare **social phobia.** See also **phobia.**

simple schizophrenia, a slow, very gradual form of schizophrenia marked by a lack of feeling, a lack of concern for others, and no energy and no desire to do anything or to be around other people. See also **schizotypal personality disorder.**

simple sugar, a basic form of sugar.

simple tubular gland, one of the many glands with only one tube-shaped duct, as various glands in the lining of the intestine.

simple vulvectomy. See **vulvectomy.**

sinciput, the upper half of the head. See also **bregma.**

Sinemet, a trademark for a central nervous system drug.

Sinequan, a trademark for an antidepression drug (doxepin hydrochloride).

sinew, the tendon of a muscle. See also **tendon.**

singer's nodule. See **vocal cord nodule.**

single footling breech. See **footling breech.**

single monster, a fetus with a single body and head but severely deformed parts or organs.

single-parent family, a family consisting of only the mother or the father and one or more dependent children.

singultus. See **hiccup.**

sinistrality. See **left-handedness.**

sinoatrial (SA) block /sī′nō·ā′trē·əl/, a disorder in the heart in which a nerve signal is blocked. Causes include excessive vagal stimulation, acute infections, and atherosclerosis. SA block may also be a side effect to quinidine or digitalis. Treatment for symptomatic SA block includes the use of atropine, isoproterenol, and, if these are not effective, the use of a pacemaker. See also **atrioventricular block, heart block, intraarterial block, intraventricular block.**

sinoatrial (SA) node, a cluster of hundreds of cells in the heart. It generates nerve signals that cause the heart to beat. Implanting an artificial pacemaker is a common operation for individuals suffering from a defective sinoatrial node, and more than 150,000 persons are leading active lives with permanently implanted devices. Also called **Keith-Flack node, pacemaker.** Compare **atrioventricular node, Purkinje's network.**

sinus arrhythmia, an irregular heart rhythm caused by interference in the nerve signals that cause the heart to beat.

sinus bradycardia. See **bradycardia.**

sinusitis /sīnəsī′tis/, a swelling of one or more nasal sinuses. It may be a complication of an upper respiratory infection, dental infection, allergy, a change in atmosphere, as in air travel or underwater swimming, or a defect of the nose. With swelling of nasal mucous membranes the openings from sinuses to the nose may be blocked, causing pressure, pain, headache, fever, and local tenderness. Complications include spread of infection to bone, brain, or meninges. Treatment includes steam inhalations, nasal decongestants, analgesics, and, if infection is present, antibiotics. Surgery to improve drainage may be done to treat chronic sinusitis.

sinus node, an area of special heart tissue that generates the cardiac electric impulse and is in turn controlled by the autonomic nervous system. Also called **sinus pacemaker.**

sinusoid, a blood vessel, somewhat larger than a capillary.

sinus pacemaker. See **sinus node.**

sinus rhythm, an expected, natural regular heart rhythm.

sinus tachycardia. See **tachycardia.**

sinus venosus defect. See **atrial septal defect.**

sippy diet, a very limited diet for peptic ulcer patients. It consists of hourly servings of milk and cream for several days, with the gradual addition of eggs, refined cereals, pureéd vegetables, crackers, and other simple foods until the regular bland diet is reached. Because the diet limits all fresh vegetables and fruits, additional iron and vitamins should be used to prevent deficiency. See also **bland diet.**

sireniform fetus. See **sirenomelus.**

sirenomelia /sī′rənəmē′lē·ə/, a birth defect in which both legs have grown together and there are no feet. Also called **apodial symmelia.**

sirenomelus /sī′rənom′ələs/, an infant who has sirenomelia. Also called **sireniform fetus, sympus apus.**

siriasis /siri′əsis/, sunstroke. See also **heat hyperpyrexia.**

Sister Kenny's treatment, a polio treatment in which the patient's limbs and back are wrapped in warm, moist woolen cloths and, after the pain goes away, the patient is taught to exercise affected muscles, especially by swimming. Equally important is passive movement of affected limbs while massaging the muscles at the same time, carried out after hot packs.

site, 1. location. See also **situs.** 2. an area of space occupied by a group of people.

sitosterol /sītos′tərôl/, a mixture of sterols made from plants, as wheat germ, used for treating hyperbetalipoproteinemia and hypercholesterolemia. Its use is controversial. Use in pregnancy is not recommended.

situational anxiety, a state of nervousness or fear caused by new experiences. It is not abnormal and requires no treatment; it usually disappears as the person adjusts to the new experiences. See also **anxiety, anxiety neurosis.**

situational depression, an episode of emotional and mental depression that is caused by something outside of the patient.

situational loss, the loss of a person, thing, or quality, resulting from a change in a life situation, including changes related to illness, body image, environment, and death.

situational supports, persons who are available and can be depended on to help a patient solve problems.

situational theory, a leadership theory in which the manager chooses a leadership style to match the particular situation.

situs /sī′təs/, the normal position or location of an organ or part of the body.

sitz bath /sits, zits/, literally *(German)* "seat" bath, a bath in which only the hips and buttocks are soaked in water or saline solution. The procedure is used for patients who have had surgery in the area of the rectum. Also called **hip bath.**

sixth disease. See **roseola infantum.**

sixth nerve. See **abducens nerve.**

Sjögren-Larsson syndrome /shō′grenlär′sən/, a condition present at birth, marked by dry, scaly skin, mental deficiency, and spastic paralysis.

SK-Ampicillin, a trademark for an antibacterial drug (ampicillin).

SK-Bamate, a trademark for a sedative (meprobamate).

skeletal enchondromatosis. See **enchondromatosis.**

skeletal fixation, any method of holding together the fragments of a broken bone by the attaching of wires, screws, plates, or nails. See also **external pin fixation.**

skeletal muscle. See **striated muscle.**

skeletal system, all of the bones and cartilage of the body that provide the framework for the muscles and organs. See also the **Color Atlas of Human Anatomy.**

skeletal traction, one of the two basic kinds of traction used to treat broken bones and to correct deformities of the skeleton. It is applied to the affected structure by a metal pin or wire put into the tissue of the structure and attached to traction ropes. It is often used when continuous traction is needed to allow a broken bone to heal properly. Infection of the pin may develop with skeletal traction, and a careful watch of pin sites is an important precaution. Compare **skin traction.** See also **Dunlop skeletal traction.**

skeleton, the supporting frame for the body, it has 206 bones that protect delicate structures, provide attachments for muscles, allow body movement, serve as major reservoirs of blood, and produce red blood cells. See also **bone,** and see the **Color Atlas of Human Anatomy. –skeletal,** *adj.*

Skene's duct. See **paraurethral duct.**

Skene's glands /skēnz/, the largest of the glands that open into the urethra of women.

skew, a deviation from a line or symmetric pattern, as data in a research study that do not follow the expected statistic curve of distribution because of the unwitting introduction of another variable.

skia-, scia-, a combining form meaning 'of or related to shadows, especially of internal structures as produced by roentgen rays.'

skilled nursing facility (SNF), an institution or part of an institution that meets guidelines for accreditation set by the sections of the Social Security Act that determine the basis for Medicaid and Medicare payments for skilled nursing care, including rehabilitation and various medical and nursing procedures. Written policies and protocols are made with appropriate professional consultation. It is required by law that these policies include a designation of which level of caregiver is responsible for carrying out each policy, that the care of every patient be under the supervision of a physician, that a physician be available on an emergency basis, that records be kept regarding the condition and care of every patient, that nursing service be available 24 hours a day, and that at least one full-time registered nurse be employed. Other criteria demand that the facility have proper facilities for storing and dispensing drugs and biologics, that it maintain and use a review plan, that all licensing requirements of the state in which it is located be met, and that an overall budget be maintained.

Skillern's fracture /skil′ərnz/, an open fracture of the thumb (distal radius) linked with a greenstick break.

skill play, a form of play in which a child continuously repeats an action or activity until it has been mastered, as throwing or catching a ball.

skills training, the teaching of specific behaviors and the practicing of these behaviors by the patient.

skimmed milk, milk from which the fat has been removed. Most of the vitamin A is removed with the cream, although all other nutrients remain. It appears as fluid skimmed milk, fortified skimmed milk, nonfat dry milk, and a form of buttermilk. Also called **nonfat milk, skim milk.**

skimming, a practice, sometimes used by health programs that receive their income on a prepaid basis, of seeking to enroll only relatively healthy individuals as a means of raising profits by lowering costs. See also **skimping.**

skimping, a practice, sometimes used by health programs, that receive their income on a prepaid basis, of delaying or denying services to enrolled members of the program as a means of raising profits by lowering costs. See also **skimming.**

skin, the tough, supple membrane that covers the entire surface of the body. It is the largest organ of the body and is composed of five layers of cells. Each layer is named for its unique function, texture, or position. The deepest layer is the stratum basale. It anchors the more superficial layers to the underlying tissues, and it provides new cells to replace the cells lost by abrasion from the outermost layer. The cells of each layer move upward as they mature. Above the stratum basale lies the stratum spinosum. The cells in this layer have tiny spines on their surfaces. As the cells move to the next layer, the stratum granulosum, they become flat, lying parallel with the surface of the skin. Over this layer lies a clear, thin band of tissue called the stratum lucidum. The boundaries of the cells are not visible in this layer. The outermost layer, the stratum corneum, is made up of scaly, squamous plaques of dead cells that contain keratin. This horny layer is thick over areas of the body subject to abrasion, as the palms of the hands, and thin over other more protected areas. The color of the skin varies according to the amount of melanin in the epidermis. Genetic differences determine the amount of melanin. The ultraviolet rays of the sun stimulate the production of melanin, which absorbs the rays and at the same time darkens the skin. Altered skin continues into various parts of the body as mucous membrane, as in the lining of the vagina, the bladder, the lungs, the intestines, the nose, and the mouth. Mucous membrane lacks the heavily keratinized layer of the outside skin. It releases the mucus that lubricates and protects nearby structures. The skin helps to cool the body when the temperature rises by radiating the heat flow in widened blood vessels and by providing a surface for the evaporation of sweat. When the temperature drops, the blood vessels narrow and the production of sweat lessens. Also called **cutaneous membrane, integument.**

skin barrier, an artificial layer of skin, usually made of plastic, applied to skin before the application of tape or ostomy drainage bags. It protects the real skin from chronic irritation.

skin button, a plastic and fabric device that covers the drive lines of an artificial heart at their exit point from the skin. Its purpose is to get rid of pumping pressure to the surrounding tissues.

skin cancer, a cancer of the skin caused by contact with various chemical substances or by too much exposure to the sun or other sources of ultraviolet light. Skin cancers, the most common and most curable cancers, are also the most frequent secondary lesions in patients with cancer in other sites. Risk factors are a fair complexion, xeroderma pigmentosa, vitiligo, senile and seborrheic keratitis, Bowen's disease, radiation dermatitis, and hereditary basal cell nevus syndrome. The most common skin cancers are basal cell carcinomas and squamous cell carcinomas. Tumors of the sebaceous glands or sweat glands occur rarely. Basal cell carcinomas — typically raised, hard, reddish sores with a pearly surface — do not spread to other places in contrast to scaly, slightly raised squamous cell tumors that may become exophytic, friable growths with widespread open sores and a nonhealing scab. A certain diagnosis may be made by cutting the cancer out, which may be the only treatment needed for small lesions. Surgery is usually used if the lesion is large, if bone or cartilage is invaded, or if lymph nodes are involved. Radiotherapy may be better for some smaller facial lesions and is commonly recommended for the treatment of skin tumors without clear edges. Because of the possibility of recurrence of cancer, surgery is favored for the treatment of younger patients. Despite the curability of skin cancer, it causes many deaths because people fail to obtain treatment. Lesions caused by actinic rays may be prevented by applying a sunscreen containing paraaminobenzoic acid (PABA).

skinfold calipers, an instrument used to measure the width of a fold of skin, usually on the back of the upper arm or over the lower ribs of the chest.

skin graft, a portion of skin implanted to cover areas where skin has been lost through burns or injury or by surgical removal of diseased tissue. To prevent tissue rejection of permanent grafts, the graft is taken from the patient's own body or from the body of an identical twin. Skin from another person or animal can be used as a temporary cover for large burned areas to lessen fluid loss. The area from which the graft is taken is called the donor site, that on which it is placed is called the recipient site. Various techniques are used including pinch, split-thickness, full-thickness, pedicle, and mesh grafts. In pinch grafting, quarter-inch pieces of skin are placed as small islands on the donor site that they will grow to cover. These will grow even in areas of poor blood supply and resist infection. The split-thickness graft consists of sheets of superficial and some deep layers of skin. Grafts of up to 4 inches wide and 10 to 12 inches long are removed from a flat surface—abdomen, thigh, or back—with an instrument called a dermatome. The grafts are sewed into place; compression dressings may be applied for firm contact, or the area may be left exposed to the air. A split-thickness graft cannot be used for weight-bearing parts of the body or to cover those subject to friction, as the hand or foot. A full-thickness graft contains all of the layers of skin and is more durable and effective for weight-bearing and friction-prone areas. A pedicle graft is one in which a portion remains attached to the donor site whereas the remainder is moved to the recipient site. Its own blood supply remains intact, and it is not cut loose until the new blood supply has fully developed. This type is often used on the face, neck, or hand. A mesh graft is made up of multiple slices of new skin. A successful new graft of any type is well established in about 72 hours and can be expected to survive unless a severe infection or trauma occurs. The procedure may be done with local anesthesia. Before the operation, both the donor and the recipient site must be free of infection and the recipient site must have a good blood supply. After the operation, stretching or moving the recipient site is avoided. Strict sterile technique is used for handling dressings, and antibiotics may be given to prevent infection. Good nutrition with a high-protein, high-caloric diet is essential.

Skinner box, a boxlike laboratory apparatus used in operant conditioning in animals, usually containing a lever or other device that when pressed produces reinforcement by either giving a reward, as food, or an escape outlet, or avoiding a punishment, as an electric shock. Also called **standard environmental chamber.** See also **operant conditioning.**

skin prep, a method of cleaning the skin with an antiseptic before surgery or injecting a fluid into a vein. Skin preps are done to kill bacteria and germs and to reduce the risk of infection. Various skin prep devices may be used. Such devices are commonly made of plastic, filled with a specific antiseptic, and equipped with an applicator. The antiseptic is applied by rubbing the device in a circular motion over the skin.

skin tag. See **cutaneous papilloma.**

skin test, a test to determine the reaction of the body to a substance by watching what happens when a certain substance is injected into the skin or is wiped on the skin. Skin tests are used to detect allergies and to diagnose disease. Kinds of skin tests include **patch test, Schick test,** and **tuberculin test.**

skin traction, one of the two basic types of traction used to treat broken bones and to correct deformities of the skeleton. Skin traction applies pull to an affected body structure by straps attached to the skin surrounding the structure. Kinds of skin traction are **adhesive skin traction** and **nonadhesive skin traction.** Compare **skeletal traction.** See also **Dunlop skin traction.**

SK-Penicillin VK, a trademark for an antibacterial drug (penicillin V potassium).

SK-Pramine, a trademark for an antidepression drug (imipramine hydrochloride).

SK-65 Compound, a trademark for a drug containing painkillers (propoxyphene hydrochloride, aspirin, and phenacetin) and a stimulant (caffeine).

SK-Tetracycline, a trademark for an antibiotic (tetracycline).

skull, the bony structure of the head, consisting of the skull (cranium) and the skeleton of the face. The cranium, which holds and protects the brain, consists of eight bones. The skeleton of the face has 14 bones.

SL, abbreviation for **soda lime.**

slander, any words spoken with malice that are untrue and prejudicial to the reputation, professional practice, commercial trade, office, or business of another person. Formerly, slander included published defamation, but at present it is limited to spoken accusation. To bring legal action in slander, the slandered person must be able to demonstrate real temporal damages—except for cases in which the defamation relates to the person's business or profession or in which the malicious words question the person's chastity or accuse the person of being a criminal or of having a loathsome disease. Compare **libel.**

slant of occlusal plane, (in dentistry) the inclination measured by the angle between the extended occlusal plane and the axis-orbital plane.

SLE, abbreviation for **systemic lupus erythematosus.**

sleep, a state marked by lessened consciousness, lessened movement of the skeletal muscles, and slowed-down metabolism. People normally sleep in patterns that follow four definite, gradual stages. These four stages make up three-fourths of a period of typical sleep and are called, as a group, **nonrapid eye movement (NREM)** sleep. The remaining time is usually occupied with **rapid eye movement (REM)** sleep. The REM sleep periods, lasting from a few minutes to half an hour, alternate with the NREM periods. Dreaming occurs during REM time. Individual sleep patterns change throughout life because daily needs for sleep gradually diminish from as much as 20 hours a day in infancy to as little as 6 hours a day in old age. Infants tend to begin a sleep period with REM sleep, whereas REM activity usually follows the four stages of NREM sleep in adults.

sleeping pill, 1. a sedative taken for insomnia or for sedation after an operation. **2.** an over-the-counter pill, sold as an aid to sleeping. Any drugs that slow down the central nervous system should not be used by pregnant or breast-feeding women or by patients with asthma, glaucoma, or prostatic hypertrophy.

sleeping sickness. See **African trypanosomiasis.**

sleep terror disorder, a condition occurring during sleep, it is marked by repeated episodes of waking up suddenly, usually with a panicky scream, accompanied by intense fear, confusion, agitation, jerking arms or legs, and total amnesia concerning the event. The disorder is usually seen in children, is more common in boys than in girls, and is not at all regular but is more likely to occur if the individual is very tired or under stress or has been given a tricyclic antidepressant or neuroleptic at bedtime. Compare **nightmare.** See also **pavor nocturnus.**

sleepwalking. See **somnambulism.**

sling, a bandage or device used to hold an injured part of the body.

sling restraint, a bone device, usually made to keep patients rigid in traction. Compare **diaper restraint, jacket restraint.**

slipped disk. See **herniated intervertebral disk.**

slipped femoral epiphysis, a displacement of the growth plate at the end of the thigh bone (femur) that happens most often in overweight teenagers as a result of hormonal changes. Symptoms include hip stiffness and pain, with difficulty in walking. There may also be knee pain, and the leg may turn outward. The condition is treated by orthopedic surgery.

slipping rib, a chest pain caused by a loose ligament that allows one of the lower five ribs to slip. The rib may slip inside or outside an adjoining rib, causing pain like that caused by a disorder of the pancreas, gallbladder, or other organ of the upper stomach.

Slo-Phyllin, a trademark for a bronchodilator (theophylline).

slough /sluf/, **1.** to shed or cast off dead tissue cells of the uterus, which are shed during menstruation. **2.** the tissue that has been shed.

slow-acting insulin. See **long-acting insulin.**

Slow-K, a trademark for a slow-release tablet of an electrolyte replacement (potassium chloride).

slow virus, a virus that remains inactive in the body after first infection. Years may go by before symptoms occur. Several wasting diseases of the central nervous system are believed to be caused by slow viruses.

slurred speech, abnormal speech in which words are not spoken clearly or completely but are run together or only partly said. The condition may be caused by weakness of the muscles of the lips, tongue, and mouth, damage to a motor nerve, brain disease, drug usage, or carelessness.

Sm, symbol for **samarium.**

SMA, a trademark for a food supplement for infants.

smack, *slang.* heroin.

small calorie. See **calorie.**

small cardiac vein, one of five tiny veins within the heart. Also called **right coronary vein.** Compare **great cardiac vein, middle cardiac vein, oblique vein of left atrium, posterior vein of left ventricle.**

small cell carcinoma. See **oat cell carcinoma.**

smallest cardiac vein, one of the tiny vessels that drain blood from within the heart. Also called **vein of Thebesius.** Compare **anterior cardiac vein.** See also **coronary vein.**

small for gestational age (SGA) infant, a baby whose weight and size at birth is smaller than 90% of all babies born. Factors linked with smallness other than hereditary include any disorder causing short stature, as dwarfism, malnutrition in the womb, and certain infections, including cytomegalovirus, rubella virus, and *Toxoplasma gondii.* Other causes linked with the smallness of an SGA infant include cigarette smoking by the mother during pregnancy, her addiction to alcohol or heroin, and her having received methadone treatment. This condition can cause complications in the birth of the baby. Given enough of the proper food, some SGA infants show phenomenal catch-up growth. Also called **small for dates (SFD) infant.** Compare **large for gestational age infant.** See also **dysmaturity.**

small intestine, the longest part of the digestive tract, extending for about 7 m (23 feet) from the top opening of the stomach to the anus. It is divided into the duodenum, jejunum, and ileum. Decreasing in width from beginning to end, it is found in the middle and back part of the lower body, surrounded by large intestine. Compare **large intestine.**

small omentum. See **lesser omentum.**

smallpox, a highly contagious virus-caused disease marked by fever, prostation, and a blister-like rash. It is caused by one of two species of poxvirus. Because human beings are the only carrier for the virus, worldwide vaccination with vaccinia, a related poxvirus, has been effective in wiping out smallpox. For several years no natural case of the disease has been known to occur. Also called **variola.**

smegma /smeg'mə/, a substance released by sebaceous glands, especially the cheesy, foul-smelling secretion often found under the foreskin of the penis and at the base of the labia minora near the glans clitoris.

smell, **1.** the special sense that allows odors to be perceived. See also **anosmia. 2.** any odor, pleasant or unpleasant.

Smith fracture, a broken wrist; a reverse Colles' fracture.

Smith-Hodge pessary. See **pessary.**

smoke inhalation, the breathing in of noxious fumes or irritating dust that may cause severe lung damage. Lung disease, suffocation, and serious injury to the lungs and throat may occur. Symptoms include irritation of the throat and lungs, singed nasal hairs, shortness of breath, a lack of oxygen, dusty gray spittle, wheezing, noisy breathing, restlessness, nervousness, cough, and hoarseness. Fluid in the lungs may develop up to 48 hours after exposure.

smooth muscle, one of two kinds of muscle, not under the patient's conscious control, as the smooth muscle of the intestines and stomach. Also called **involuntary muscle, unstriated muscle.** Compare **striated muscle, cardiac muscle.**

smooth pursuit eye movement, the tracking of the eyes of a slowly moving object at a steady coordinated speed, rather than in a jerky motion.

smooth surface cavity, a cavity formed by decay that starts on surfaces of teeth without pits, cracks, or enamel faults.

snail, an animal without a backbone, it belongs to the order Gastropoda, several species of which are carriers of the blood worms that cause schistosomiasis in humans. See also **Schistosoma, schistosomiasis.**

snakebite, a wound resulting from piercing of the flesh by the fangs of a snake. Bites by snakes known to be nonpoisonous are treated as puncture wounds; those produced by an unknown or poisonous snake need immediate attention. The person is kept still, the wound is washed with soap and water, and a partly tightened tourniquet is used to slow the spread of the poison. The skin is cut into through the bite marks and suction applied to assist bleeding and in removing the poison. To avoid cutting muscles, nerves, or blood vessels, the incision should be only skin deep. An appropriate antivenin may be given that protects against the venom of most pit vipers, including the rattlesnakes, copperheads, and cottonmouths that are responsible for 98% of the poisonous snakebites in the United States. Bites of pit vipers are marked by pain, redness, and collection of fluids, followed by weakness, dizziness, heavy sweating, nausea, vomiting, or weak pulse, bleeding under the skin, and, in severe cases, shock. Treatment includes the use of painkilling drugs and sedatives, antibiotics, and antitetanus shots to prevent infections from germs found in the mouths of snakes. Patients sensitive to horse serum in antivenin may require cortisone for the control of hives, urticaria, and other allergic reactions. Coral snakes rarely bite, but their venom contains a nerve poison that can cause lung paralysis.

sneeze, a sudden, forceful, involuntary burst of air through the nose and mouth occurring as a result of irritation to the mucous membranes of the throat, as by dust, pollen, or virus infection. Also called **sternutation.**

Snellen chart, one of several charts used in testing the vision. Letters, numbers, or symbols are arranged on the chart, large on top and getting smaller toward the bottom. See p. 715.

Snellen test, a vision test using a Snellen chart. The person being tested stands 20 feet from the chart and reads as many of the symbols as possible, reading each line and proceeding downward from the top. A score is assigned. A person who can read what the average person can read at 20 feet has 20/20 vision.

snout reflex, an abnormal response caused by tapping the nose, resulting in a marked facial grimace. It usually indicates the presence of a brain tumor.

SNP, abbreviation for **sodium nitroprusside.**

snuff dipping, the practice of sucking juices from a wad of moist, fine-cut chewing tobacco placed in the mouth between the cheek and gums. It has been associated with abnormal oral mucous membranes (leukoplakia), tooth and gum diseases, and possible mouth cancer.

LETTER CHART FOR 20 FEET
Snellen Scale

E

H N

D F N

P T X Z

U Z D T F

D F N P T H

P H U N T D Z

N P X T Z F H

Snellen chart

snuffles, a nasal discharge in infancy typical of congenital syphilis. See also **syphilis.**

SOAP /sōp, es'ō'ā'pē'/, (in a medical record) abbreviation for *subjective, objective, assessment, and plan,* the four parts of a written account of the health problem. In taking the patient history and physical examination, a SOAP statement is made for each condition, problem, symptom, or diagnosis. Charting by this is said to be "soaped" and charts made using it are called "soap charts." See also **problem-oriented medical record (POMR).**

Social Behavior Assessment Scale, an interview guide that gathers information from friends and family members about a patient's functioning.

social breakdwon syndrome, the progressive breaking down of social and interpersonal skills in patients with long-term mental illness.

social deviance, behavior that violates social standards, causing anger, resentment, and a desire for punishment in many members of the society.

social learning theory, a concept that the urge to behave aggressively is influenced by learning, socialization, and experience. Social learning theorists believe aggression is learned by seeing aggressive behavior in others, and by direct experience.

social margin, the sum total of all resources (material, personal, and interpersonal) available to assist an individual in coping with stress.

social medicine, an approach to the prevention and treatment of disease that is based on the study of human heredity, environment, social structures, and cultural values.

social phobia, a nervous condition marked by a strong wish to avoid, and a continuous, unreasonable fear of, situations in which the patient may be closely watched and judged by others, as speaking, eating, or performing in public, or using public toilets or transportation. Compare **simple phobia.** See also **phobia.**

social radical therapy, a form of mental therapy that attempts to bring about change by merging treatment into a radical political movement, usually one that represents the personal views of the therapist. Its major assumption is that all therapy is characterized by numerous social and political value choices.

social readjustment scale, a checklist that can be used to measure the amount of atress in a person's life. It is thought that a person with a very stressful life is more likely to get sick. See checklist on p. 716.

Social Security Act, a U.S. federal law that provides for a national system of old-age assistance, survivors' and old-age insurance benefits, unemployment insurance and payments, and other public welfare programs, including Medicare and Medicaid.

society, a nation, community, or broad group of people who establish particular aims, beliefs, or standards of living and conduct.

sociolinguistics, the study of the relationship between language and the social context in which it occurs.

sociopath. See **psychopath.**

sociopathic. See **psychopathic.**

sociopathic personality. See **antisocial personality.**

soda, a compound of sodium, particularly sodium bicarbonate, sodium carbonate, or sodium hydroxide.

sodium (Na), a soft, grayish and metallic element, needed in small amounts for health. It is eaten in the form of salt. It is also used in many forms to make various medicines. Sodium salts, as sodium bicarbonate, are widely used in medications. Sodium bicarbonate has an immediate and rapid antacid action on the stomach, but any excess rapidly enters the intestine so that the substance has a shorter action than other antacids. Sodium bicarbonate is an ingredient in many solutions used as douches, mouthwashes, and enemas.

sodium acid glutamate. See **sodium glutamate.**

sodium arsenite poisoning, a poisonous condition caused by eating sodium arsenite, an insect poison and weed-killer. The typical symptoms of arsenite poisoning are similar to those of arsenic poisoning, as is the treatment. See also **arsenic poisoning.**

The social readjustment rating scale

Life event	Mean value
1. Death of spouse	100
2. Divorce	73
3. Marital separation	65
4. Jail term	63
5. Death of close family member	63
6. Personal injury or illness	53
7. Marriage	50
8. Fired at work	47
9. Marital reconciliation	45
10. Retirement	45
11. Change in health of family member	44
12. Pregnancy	40
13. Sex difficulties	39
14. Gain of new family member	39
15. Business readjustment	39
16. Change in financial state	38
17. Death of close friend	37
18. Change to different line of work	36
19. Change in number of arguments with spouse	35
20. Mortgage or loan major purchase (home, etc.)	31
21. Foreclosure of mortgage or loan	30
22. Change in responsibilities at work	29
23. Son or daughter leaving home	29
24. Trouble with in-laws	29
25. Outstanding personal achievement	28
26. Spouse begins or stops work	26
27. Begin or end school	26
28. Change in living conditions	25
29. Revision of personal habits	24
30. Trouble with boss	23
31. Change in work hours or conditions	20
32. Change in residence	20
33. Change in schools	20
34. Change in recreation	19
35. Change in church activities	19
36. Change in social activities	18
37. Mortgage or loan for lesser purchase (car, TV, etc.)	17
38. Change in sleeping habits	16
39. Change in number of family get-togethers	15
40. Change in eating habits	15
41. Vacation	13
42. Christmas	12
43. Minor violations of the law	11

Reprinted with permission from Holmes, T.H., and Rahe, R.H.: J. Psychosom. Res. 11:213-218, 1967, Pergamon Press, Ltd.

sodium bicarbonate, a substance used to control excess acid in the stomach and to treat stomach ulcers and indigestion.

★CAUTION: Pyloric blockage, kidney disease, heart disease, or bleeding ulcer prohibits its use.

★ADVERSE EFFECTS: Among the more serious side effects are stomach bloating, acid rebound, bicarbonate-induced alkalosis, hypernatremia, and hyperkalemia.

sodium chloride, common table salt, used for many medical procedures.

sodium chloride and dextrose. See **dextrose and sodium chloride injection.**

sodium etidronate. See **etidronate disodium.**

sodium glutamate, a salt of glutamic acid used to treat hepatitis-caused coma and to make food taste better. Also called **monosodium glutamate (MSG), sodium acid glutamate.**

sodium iodide, an iodine supplement, used to treat several diseases of the thyroid gland.

★CAUTION: Hyperkalemia or known allergy to this drug prohibits its use.

★ADVERSE EFFECTS: Among the more serious side effects are salivary gland swelling, metallic taste, rashes, and stomach disorders. Acute poisoning may result in the collection of fluids in the heart and lungs.

sodium lactate injection, an injection to replace electrolytes given for metabolic acidosis.

sodium nitroprusside (SNP), a vessel-widening drug. It is used in the emergency treatment of high blood pressure and in heart failure.

★CAUTION: Certain forms of high blood pressure or known allergy to the drug prohibits its use.

★ADVERSE EFFECTS: Among the most serious side effects are a rapid fall in blood pressure or symptoms of cyanide poisoning. Muscle spasms also may occur.

sodium perborate, an antiseptic that may be used in treating gingivitis and other kinds of swelling of the gums and for bleaching pulpless teeth. Very long or careless use of the compound may cause burns of the mucous membranes of the mouth and blacken the tongue.

sodium phosphate, a salt-based laxative. It is used to achieve prompt, thorough evacuation of the bowel and, in lower dosage, for laxative effect.

★CAUTION: Congestive heart failure, stomach pain, collection of fluids, enlargement of the colon, low blood volume, salt-restricted diet, or allergy to this drug prohibits its use. It should not be used very often.

★ADVERSE EFFECTS: Among the more severe side effects are loss of water, low blood volume, and stomach cramps.

sodium phosphate P32, a drug used to treat certain blood diseases and some cancers, as eye tumors.

★CAUTION: Polycythemia vera with leukopenia or decreased platelet count, chronic myelocytic leukemia with leukopenia or erythrocytopenia, concurrent use of other alkalating agents, or allergy to this drug prohibits its use.

★ADVERSE EFFECTS: The most serious side effect is radiation sickness.

sodium-restricted diet. See **low-sodium diet.**

sodium salicylate, a drug used to treat pain and fever.

sodium sulfate, a salt-based drug used to treat constipation by causing a bowel movement.

★CAUTION: Heart disease, low blood volume, or allergy to this drug prohibits its use. It should not be used very often.

★ADVERSE EFFECTS: Among the more severe side effects are loss of water, low blood volume, and chemical imbalances in the body.

Sodium Versenate, a trademark for a drug used to treat various kinds of metal poisoning (edetate disodium).

sodoku. See **rat-bite fever.**

sodomy, 1. anal intercourse. 2. intercourse with an animal. 3. a vague term for "unnatural" sexual intercourse. **–sodomite,** *n.,* **sodomize,** *v.*

soft diet, a diet that is soft in texture, low in residue, easily digested, and well tolerated. It provides the essential nutrients in the form of liquids and semisolid foods, as milk, fruit juices, eggs, cheese, custards, tapioca and puddings, strained soups and vegetables, rice, ground beef and lamb, fowl, fish, mashed, boiled, or baked potatoes, wheat, corn, or rice cereals, and breads. Left out are raw fruits and vegetables, coarse breads and cereals, rich desserts, strong spices, all fried foods, veal, pork, nuts, and raisins. It is commonly recommended for people who have disorders of the stomach or intestines, or serious infections, or for anyone unable to eat a normal diet.

soft fibroma, a tumor that contains many cells. Also called **fibroma molle** /mol′ē/.

soft neurologic sign, a mild or slight nervous system abnormality that is difficult to find or interpret.

soft palate, the structure composed of mucous membrane, muscular fibers, and mucous glands, hanging from the back of the hard palate forming the roof of the mouth. When the soft palate rises, as in swallowing and in sucking, it closes off the nose and sinuses from the throat and mouth. The back edge of the soft palate hangs like a curtain between the mouth and the voice box. The uvula is the small, round piece of flesh hanging from the back of the soft palate. Compare **hard palate.**

solar fever. See **dengue fever, sunstroke.**

solarium /sōler′ē·əm/, a large, sunny room in a hospital serving as a lounge for patients who are able to leave their beds.

solar keratosis. See **actinic keratosis.**

solar plexus, a compact knot of nerves found behind the stomach in the middle of the body. It is one of the most important nerve centers in the body. It is sometimes called "the pit of the stomach." Also called **celiac plexus.**

solar radiation, the emission and diffusion of ultraviolet rays from the sun. Overexposure may result in sunburn, scaly skin, skin cancer, or sores linked with a sensitivity to light.

Solatene, a trademark for a sunscreen (beta-carotene), used to treat certain skin diseases.

soleus /sō′lē·əs/, one of three muscles found at the back of the calf. It is a broad flat muscle that moves the foot. Compare **gastrocnemius, plantaris.**

Solfoton, a trademark for a drug used to prevent convulsions and as a sleeping pill (phenobarbital).

Solganal, a trademark for a drug used to treat rheumatism (aurothioglucose).

solitary coin lesion, a small, rounded mass identified on a chest x-ray film by clear normal lung tissue surrounding it. A coin lesion is usually between 1 and 6 cm in size and often cancerous.

Solu-Cortef, a trademark for a steroid (hydrocortisone sodium succinate).

Solu-Medrol, a trademark for a steroid (methylprednisolone sodium succinate).

solute /sol′yo͞ot, sō′lo͞ot/, a substance dissolved in a solution.

solution, a mixture of one or more substances dissolved in another substance. A solution may be a gas, a liquid, or a solid. Compare **colloid, suspension.** See also **solute, solvent.**

solvent, 1. any liquid in which another substance can be dissolved. 2. a liquid, as benzene, carbon tetrachloride, and certain oil-based liquids that when breathed in can be poisonous, and can do damage to mucous membranes of the nose and throat and the tissues of the kidney, liver, and brain. Repeated exposure over a long time can result in addiction, brain damage, blindness, and other serious results, some of them fatal. See also **benzene poisoning, carbon tetrachloride, glue sniffing, petroleum distillate poisoning.**

som-, a combining form for growth hormone derivatives.

Soma, a trademark for a skeletal muscle relaxing drug (carisoprodol).

somatic cavity. See **coelom.**

somatic therapy, a form of treatment that affects the functioning of one's body.

somatization disorder, a disorder marked by numerous recurring physical complaints and symptoms that do not seem to have a medical cause. The condition typically occurs in adolescence or in the early adult years and is rarely seen in men. The symptoms vary according to the patient and the hidden emotional cause. Some common symptoms are stomach disorders, paralysis, temporary blindness, lung and heart problems, painful or irregular menstruation, lack of interest in sex, and pain during intercourse. Hypochondriasis may develop if the condition is untreated. Also called **Briquet's syndrome.**

somatoform disorder, any of a group of nervous disorders marked by symptoms that look like a physical illness or disease, for which there is no real disease. The symptoms are usually caused by some mental conflict within the patient's mind. Kinds of somatoform disorders are **conversion disorder, hypo chondriasis, psychogenic pain disorder, somatization disorder.**

somatoliberin. See **growth hormone-releasing factor.**

somatomedin. See **growth hormone.**

somatomegaly /sō′matōmeg′əlē/, a condition in which the body is abnormally large because of hormonal imbalance within the body.

somatosplanchnic /sōmat′ōsplangk′nik/, of or relating to the trunk of the body and the internal organs of the lower body, as the stomach and intestines.

somatostatin /sō′matōstat′in/, a hormone that controls growth and helps to control the release of certain other hormones. Also called **growth hormone release inhibiting hormone.**

somatotropic hormone, somatotropin. See **growth hormone.**

somatotype, **1.** body build or physique. **2.** the classification of body types based on certain physical traits. The primary types are **ectomorph, endomorph,** and **mesomorph.**

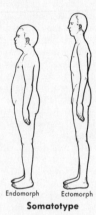

Endomorph   Ectomorph

Somatotype

Somnafac, a trademark for a sleeping pill (methaqualone hydrochloride).

somnambulism /somnam′byəliz′əm/, **1.** also called **noctambulation, sleepwalking;** a condition occurring during sleep that is marked by moving parts of the body, usually ending up by leaving the bed and walking about, with no memory of the event upon waking up. The episodes, which usually last from several minutes to half an hour or longer, are seen mostly in children, more commonly in boys than in girls, and are more likely to occur if the individual is very tired or under stress, or has taken a sedative at bedtime. Seizure disorders, central nervous system infections, and injury may be part of the cause, but the condition is more commonly related to fear and nervousness. In adults, the condition is less common. **2.** a hypnotic state in which the person has full possession of the senses but no memory of the episode.

somnolent, **1.** sleepy or drowsy. **2.** tending to cause sleepiness. **–somnolence,** *n.*

somnolent detachment, (in psychology) a term introduced by Sullivan for a type of reaction in which a person falls asleep when facing anxiety-producing experience. The mechanism originates in infancy.

Somophyllin, a trademark for a bronchodilator (theophylline).

sonogram, sonography. See **ultrasonography.**

sonorous rale, a snoring sound that may be made by the vibration of a mass of thick released matter lodged in tube leading from the lung to the throat. This sound is linked with various lung or breathing disorders.

soot wart. See **scrotal cancer.**

soporific /sop′ərif′ik/, **1.** of or relating to a substance, condition, or method that causes sleep. **2.** a soporific drug. See also **hypnotic, sedative.**

sorbic acid /sôr′bik/, a compound occurring naturally in berries of the mountain ash. Some forms are sorbic acid used in fungus-killing drugs, food preservatives, and lubricants.

Sorbitrate, a trademark for a drug used to treat angina (isosorbide dinitrate).

sordes /sôr′dēz/, *pl.* **sordes,** dirt or waste matter, especially the crusts consisting of food, germs, and cells that collect on teeth and lips during a fever illness or one in which the patient takes nothing by mouth. Sordes gastricae is undigested food and mucus in the stomach.

sore, **1.** a wound, ulcer, or lesion. **2.** tender or painful.

Sorrin's operation, an operation to treat an abscess of the gums.

s.o.s., (in prescriptions) abbreviation for *si opus sit,* a Latin phrase meaning "if necessary."

sound, an instrument used to find the opening of a space (cavity) or canal, to test the workings of a canal, to find the depth of a cavity, or to show the contents of a canal or cavity. A sound is used to find the depth of the uterus, to detect stones in the bladder, and, less commonly, to aid in correctly inserting a urinary catheter in the urethra through the urinary meatus.

South African genetic porphyria. See **variegate porphyria.**

South American blastomycosis. See **paracoccidioidomycosis.**

South American trypanosomiasis. See **Chagas' disease.**

Southern blot test, a gene analysis method used to identify specific DNA fragments and in the diagnosis of cancers and inherited blood disorders (hemoglobulinopathies). The DNA fragments are analyzed for changes in the order of antibodies (immunoglobulins) or cell receptor genes, movement of chromosomes, increases in potentially cancer-causing genes (oncogenes), and changes (point mutations) in these genes. Immunoglobulins and T cell receptor genes have marks that identify various diseases of the white blood cells (leukemias) and cancers of the lymph nodes (lymphomas). See also **Northern blot test.**

sp. *pl.* **sp., spp,** abbreviation for **species.**

space maintainer, a fixed or movable device for holding open the space formed by the early loss of one or more teeth.

space obtainer, a device for widening the space between two teeth next to one another.

space regainer, a fixed or removable device for moving a displaced permanent tooth into its normal position.

Spanish fly. See **cantharis.**

sparganosis /spär′gənō′sis/, an infection with larvae of the fish tapeworm, marked by painful swellings under the skin or swelling and destruction of the eye. It is caught by drinking contaminated water or in undercooked, infected frog flesh. Treatment includes surgery and local injection of ethyl alcohol to kill the larvae.

Sparine, a trademark for a phenothiazine antipsychotic and antivomiting drug (promazine hydrochloride).

sparteine sulfate, an alkaloid salt used to treat heart disorders.

spasm, 1. a sudden unconscious muscle tightening, as habit spasms, hiccups, stuttering, or a tic. **2.** a convulsion or seizure. **3.** a sudden, brief tightening of a blood vessel, bronchus, esophagus, pylorus, ureter, or other hollow organ. Compare **stricture.** See also **bronchospasm, pylorospasm.**

spasmodic dysphonia, a speech disorder in which vocalization is irregularly blocked by spasms of the voicebox. The cause is unknown. Also called **spastic dysphonia.**

spasmodic torticollis, a form of torticollis (also called "wryneck") marked by attacks of spasms of the neck muscles. The condition often only lasts a brief while, and examination rarely reveals a physical cause. In some cases, severe stress and muscular spasm may be the cause.

spasmogen /spas′məjən/, any substance that produces smooth muscle contractions, as in the small airways of the lungs. Examples are histamines, bradykinin, and serotonin.

spastic, of or relating to spasms or other uncontrolled tightenings of the skeletal muscles. See also **cerebral palsy. –spasticity,** *n.*

spastic aphonia, a condition in which a person is unable to speak because of spasmodic tightening of the muscles of the throat.

spastic bladder, a form of a nerve-related disorder caused by a tumor of the spinal cord. It is marked by loss of bladder control and feeling, incontinence, and automatic, interrupted, incomplete emptying. It is most often caused by injury, but may be a result of a tumor or multiple sclerosis. Also called **reflex bladder, automatic bladder.** Compare **flaccid bladder.**

spastic colon. See **irritable bowel syndrome.**

spastic dysphonia. See **spasmodic dysphonia.**

spastic entropion. See **ectropion, entropion.**

spastic hemiplegia, paralysis of one side of the body with increased tendon reflexes and uncontrolled spasms occurring in the affected muscles.

spastic paralysis, an abnormal condition marked by the uncontrolled tightening of one or more muscles with related loss of muscular function. Compare **flaccid paralysis.**

spastic pseudoparalysis. See **Creutzfeldt-Jakob disease.**

spatial dance, body shifts or movements used by individuals as they try to adjust the distance between them. See also **spatial zones.**

spatial zones, the areas of personal space in which most people function. Four basic spatial zones are the intimate zone, in which distance between individuals is less than 18 inches; the personal zone, between 18 inches and 4 feet; the social zone, extending between 4 and 12 feet; and the public zone, beyond 12 feet.

SPE, abbreviation for **sucrose polyester.**

special care unit, a hospital unit with the necessary special equipment and personnel for handling critically ill or injured patients, as an intensive care unit, burn unit, or cardiac care unit.

specialist, a health-care professional who makes a detailed study of one part of the body and the related diseases, or of a particular type of disease. A specialist usually has advanced training.

special sense, the sense of sight, smell, taste, touch, or hearing.

specialty, a branch of medicine or nursing in which the professional is specially able to practice by having had advanced study, by having passed an examination given by an organization of the members of the specialty, or by having gained experience by long practice in the specialty.

specialty care, specialized medical services provided by a physician specialist.

species (Sp) /spē′sēz, spē′shēz/, *pl.* **species (sp., spp)** /spē′sēz, spē′shēz/, the category of living things below genus in rank. A species includes individuals of the same genus who are similar in structure and chemical composition and who can interbreed. See also **genus.**

species immunity, a form of natural immunity shared by all members of a species. Compare **individual immunity, racial immunity.**

specific immune globulin, a special substance made from human blood, it is used to protect against a specific disease, as varicella zoster immune globulin.

specific treatment. See **treatment.**

specimen /spes′imən/, a small sample of something, tested to show the nature of the whole, as a urine specimen.

Spectazole, a trademark for a fungus-killing drug (econazole nitrate).

spectinomycin hydrochloride, an antibiotic. It is used to treat gonorrhea and certain infections in patients who are allergic to penicillin.
★CAUTION: Known allergy to this drug prohibits its use.
★ADVERSE EFFECTS: Among the more serious side effects are lessened urine, rash, chills, fever, dizziness, and nausea.

Spectrobid, a trademark for a certain kind of penicillin (bacampicillin).

Spectrocin, a trademark for a drug used to kill bacteria infections on the skin (neomycin sulfate and gramicidin).

speculum /spek′yo͞oləm/, a tool used to hold open a body space to make examination possible, as an ear speculum, an eye speculum, or a vaginal speculum.

speech, 1. the making of definite vocal sounds that form words to express one's thoughts or ideas. 2. communication by means of spoken words. 3. the faculty of language production, which involves the complex coordination of the muscles and nerves of the organs of articulation. Any nerve or muscle injury or defect involving these organs results in various speech defects or disorders. Kinds of disorders include **ataxic speech, explosive speech, mirror speech, scamping speech, scanning speech, slurred speech,** and **staccato speech.** See also **speech dysfunction.**

speech dysfunction, any defect or abnormality of speech, including aphasia, alexia, stammering, stuttering, aphonia, and slurring. Speech problems may develop from any of a number of causes, among them nerve injury in the brain, muscular paralysis because of injury, disease, structural defect of the organs of speech, emotional or mental tension, strain, depression, hysteria, and severe mental retardation. See also **speech.**

speech-language pathologist, an individual with graduate professional training in human communication, its development, and disorders. The person specializes in the measurement and evaluation of language abilities and speech production, clinical treatment of children and adults with speech and language disorders, and research methods in the study of communication process. See also **speech therapist.**

speech pathologist. See **speech therapist.**

speech pathology, 1. the study of defects of speech or of the organs of speech. 2. the diagnosis and treatment of defects of speech as practiced by a speech pathologist or a speech therapist.

speech therapist, a person trained in speech pathology who treats people with disorders affecting normal speech.

speed, 1. the rate of change of position with time. Compare **velocity.** 2. *slang.* any stimulating drug, as amphetamine.

speed shock, a sudden side effect of a patient to shots or drugs that are given too quickly. Some signs of speed shock are a flushed face, headache, a tight feeling in the chest, uneven pulse, loss of consciousness, and heart attack.

sperm. See **semen, spermatozoon.**

spermatic cord, a structure by which each testicle is attached to the body. The left spermatic cord is usually longer than the right, thus the left testis usually hangs lower than the right. Each cord is made up of arteries, veins, lymphatics, nerves, and the excretory duct of the testicles.

spermatic duct. See **vas deferens.**

spermatic fistula, an abnormal passage leading to or away from a testicle or a seminal duct.

spermatocele /spərmat′əsēl′, spur′-/, a cystlike swelling that contains sperm. It lies above, behind, and separate from the testis; it is usually painless and requires no therapy.

spermatocide /spərmat′əsīd, spur′-/, a chemical substance that kills spermatozoa. Also called **spermicide.**

spermatozoon /spur′mətəzō′ən, spərmat′-/, *pl.* **spermatozoa** /-zō′ə/, the male seed, contained in semen, that fertilizes the female egg in the womb in order to create a fetus. Looking like a tadpole, it is about 50 micrograms (1/500 inch) long and has a head, a neck, and a tail that propels it. See **spermatogenesis.**

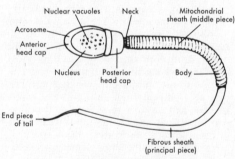

Spermatozoon

spermicidal /spur′misī′dəl/, a substance that kills sperm.

spermicide. See **spermatocide.**

S-phase, the stage of cell reproduction in which DNA is produced before the cell goes through the process of cell division (mitosis).

sphenoid bone, the bone at the base of the skull. It looks like a bat with its wings spread.

sphenoid fontanel, the area of the skull between the bone of the forehead and the two bones above the ears. In the infant this area contains cartilage, but in the adult the bones are meshed together. It cannot be felt with the fingers. See also **fontanel.**

sphenomandibular ligament /sfē'nōmandib'yələr/, one of a pair of flat, thin ligaments that connect the top of the jaw bone to the skull.

spherocytic anemia, a blood disorder marked by misshaped red blood cells. Attacks of stomach pain, fever, jaundice, and enlargement of the spleen occur. Because repeated transfusions are often needed to treat the anemia, too-much iron in the blood may develop. Removal of the spleen may then be necessary. The condition is inherited. Compare **congenital nonspherocytic hemolytic anemia.** See also **elliptocytosis.**

spherocytosis /sfir'ōsītō'sis/, the abnormal presence of diseased red blood cells in the blood. Compare **elliptocytosis.**

spheroidea. See **ball and socket joint.**

sphincter /sfingk'tər/, a circular band of muscle fibers that narrows a passage or closes a natural opening in the body, as the outer anal sphincter, which closes the anus.

sphincter pupillae, a muscle that widens the iris, narrowing the pupil of the eye. Compare **dilatator pupillae.**

sphingolipid, a certain substance found in large amounts in the brain and other tissues of the nervous system, especially membranes.

sphingomyelin /sfing'gōmī'əlin/, any of a group of sphingolipids containing phosphorus. It occurs mainly in the tissue of the nervous system, generally in membranes, and in the lipids in the blood.

sphingomyelin lipidosis, any of a group of diseases marked by an abnormality in the ability of the body to store sphingolipids. Kinds of sphingomyelin lipidosis include **Gaucher's disease, Niemann-Pick disease,** and **Tay-Sachs disease.** See also **Fabry's disease.**

sphingosine /sfing'gōsēn/, an amino alcohol, a major constituent of sphingolipids and sphingomyelin.

sphygmogram /sfig'məgram/, a graph made by a sphygmograph. It may be useful in determining the health of the heart.

sphygmograph /sfig'məgraf/, an instrument that records the force of the arterial pulse on a graph called a sphygmogram. –**sphygmographic,** *adj.*

sphygmomanometer /sfig'mōmənom'ətər/, a device for measuring the blood pressure. It consists of an arm or leg cuff with an air bag attached to a tube and a bulb for pumping air into the bag, and a gauge for showing the amount of air pressure being pressed against the artery. See also **blood pressure, manometer.**

spica bandage /spī'kə/, a figure-of-eight bandage in which each turn usually overlaps the next to form a succession of V-like designs. It may be used to give support, to apply pressure, or to hold a dressing in place on the chest, limbs, thighs, or pelvis.

spica cast, a cast applied to hold in place part or all of the trunk of the body and part or all of one or more arms or legs. It is used to treat various fractures, as of the hip and the thigh, and in correcting hip deformities. Kinds of spica casts are **bilateral long-leg spica cast, one-and-a-half spica cast, shoulder spica cast, and unilateral long-leg spica cast.**

spicule /spik'yōol/, a sharp body with a needle-like point.

spider angioma, a form of blood vessel disorder marked by a central, raised red dot the size of a pinhead from which small blood vessels radiate. Spider angiomas are often linked with high estrogen levels as occur in pregnancy or when the liver is diseased and unable to detoxify estrogens. Also called **spider nevus.** See also **telangiectasia.**

spider antivenin. See **black widow spider antivenin.**

spider bite, a puncture wound made by the bite of a spider. Fewer than 100 of some 30,000 species of spiders are known to bite. Two of them, the black widow spider and the brown recluse spider, found in the United States, are poisonous.

spider nevus. See **spider angioma.**

spina /spī'nə/, *pl.* **spinae, 1.** the spinal column. **2.** a spine or a thornlike point.

spina bifida /spī'nə bif'ədə, bī'fədə/, a nerve tube defect present at birth that results in a gap in the bone that surrounds the spinal cord. Spina bifida is relatively common, occurring about 10 to 20 times per 1,000 births. The gap may be very small, a condition that only rarely needs treatment, or it may be large enough to allow parts of the spinal cord to stick through, in which case surgery may be needed. Direct symptoms are rarely noted in spina bifida, which is often diagnosed accidentally during x-ray examinations needed for other reasons. Also called **spinal dysrhaphis.**

spina bifida anterior, a gap along the front surface of the spinal column. The defect is often linked with growth defects of the organs of the lower body.

spina bifida cystica, a growth defect of the central nervous system in which a cyst containing meninges (meningocele), spinal cord (myelocele), or both (myelomeningocele) sticks out through a gap in the vertebral column present at birth. The sac can easily break, causing the leakage of fluid and a higher risk of infection. Compare **spina bifida occulta.** See also **myelomeningocele, neural tube defect.**

spina bifida occulta, a gap in the vertebral column in the lower back without hernia of the spinal cord. The defect, which is quite common, occurs in about 5% of the population and is identified from outside by a dimple, dark tufts of hair, certain blood vessel disorders, or soft tumors beneath the skin. There is usually no nerve damage linked with the defect. However, certain disorders may occur, as problems with gait and foot weakness and with the bowel and bladder sphincters. Compare **spina bifida cystica.**

spinal, **1.** of or relating to a spine, especially the spinal column. **2.** *informal.* spinal anesthesia, as saddle block or caudal anesthesia.

spinal accessory nerve. See **accessory nerve.**

spinal arachnoid. See **arachnoidea spinalis.**

spinal canal, the space within the vertebral column.

spinal caries. See **tuberculous spondylitis.**

spinal column. See **vertebral column.**

spinal cord, a long, almost round structure found in the vertebral canal and reaching from the base of the skull to the upper part of the lower back. A major part of the central nervous system, the adult cord is about 1 cm in diameter with an average length of 42 to 45 cm and a weight of 30 g. The cord carries sense and movement signals to and from the brain and controls many reflexes. Also called **chorda spinalis, medulla spinalis.** See also **spinal nerves.**

spinal cord compression, an abnormal and often serious condition caused by pressure on the spinal cord. The symptoms range from temporary numbness of an extremity to permanent quadriplegia, depending on the cause, severity, and location of the pressure. Causes include spinal fracture, vertebral dislocation, tumor, bleeding, and edema linked with a crushing or bruising injury with contusion. See also **herniated disk, spondylolisthesis.**

spinal cord injury, any one of the traumatic injuries to the spinal cord, often linked with widespread effects on the muscles and skeleton. Common spinal cord injuries are spinal fractures and dislocations, as those commonly suffered by individuals involved in car accidents, airplane crashes, or other violent impacts. Such injuries may cause varying degrees of paralysis. Spinal cord injuries produce a state of spinal shock, marked by placid paralysis, and complete loss of skin feeling at the time of the injury. Within a few weeks the muscles affected may become spastic, and the skin feeling may return to a slight degree. The motor and the sensory losses that prevail a few weeks after the injury are usually permanent. Treatment of spinal cord injuries varies a great deal and involves many different methods, as certain exercises and techniques, and special physical and psychological treatment.

spinal cord tumor, a cancerous growth on the spinal cord. Symptoms usually develop slowly and may progress from prickling skin on one side of the body to stabbing pain, weakness in one or both legs, abnormal deep tendon reflexes, and, in advanced cases, some type of paralysis. Function of the nervous system is sometimes disturbed, causing areas of dry, cold, bluish-pink skin or profuse sweating of the legs and feet. Tumors of the spinal cord may arise at any age but appear most often in the third decade of life and are one-fourth as common as brain cancers.

spinal curvature, any continuous, abnormal change of shape of the vertebral column from its normal position. Kinds of spinal curvature are **kyphoscoliosis, kyphosis, lordosis,** and **scoliosis.**

spinal dysrhaphis. See **spina bifida.**

spinal fasciculi. See **spinal tract.**

spinal fluid. See **cerebrospinal fluid.**

spinal fusion, the joining of an unstable part of the spine, done by skeletal traction or keeping the patient rigid in a body cast but most often by surgery. Also called **spondylosyndesis.**

spinal headache, a headache occurring after spinal anesthesia or a lumbar puncture. It is caused by a loss of spinal fluid from the subarachnoid space, resulting in pressure on the fibers of the spine and skull.

spinal manipulation, the forced passive movement of spinal bones. It may be done to treat sprains, breaks, and dislocations.

spinal nerves, the 31 pairs of nerves without special names that are connected to the spinal cord. See also **spinal cord.**

spinal puncture. See **lumbar puncture.**

spinal shock, a form of shock linked with serious injury to the spinal cord. See also **shock.**

spinal tract, any one of the pathways for nerve signals that are found in the white matter of the spinal cord.

spindle, any one of the special sensing organs found throughout the body. These spindles detect the degree of stretch in a muscle or at the meeting of a muscle with its tendon and are needed to maintain muscle tone.

spindle cell carcinoma, a rapidly growing tumor.

spindle cell nevus. See **benign juvenile melanoma.**

spine, the vertebral column, or backbone.

spin-lattice relaxation time. See **relaxation time.**

spinnbarkeit /spin'bärkīt, shpin'-/, the clear, slippery, elastic consistency typical of cervical mucus during ovulation. It has the texture of an uncooked egg white, and it is a valuable sign of the most fertile period in a woman's menstrual cycle. Observation of spinnbarkeit is useful in natural methods of family planning, in the clinical evaluation of infertility, and in finding the best time for artificial insemination. Spinnbarkeit may be tested by the length to which a string of mucus can be drawn between the fingers before breaking. (The literal meaning of this German word is "weavability.") See also **ovulation method of family planning.**

spinocerebellar /spī'nōser'əbel'ər/, of or relating to the spinal cord and the cerebellum.

spinocerebellar disorder, an inherited disorder marked by a gradual wasting of the spinal cord and brain, often involving other parts of the nervous system as well. These disorders tend to occur within families. It usually attacks early, during childhood or adolescence. No treatment is known. Some kinds of spinocerebellar wasting are **ataxia telangiectasia, Charcot-Marie-Tooth atrophy, Dejerine-Sottas disease, Friedreich's ataxia, olivopontocerebellar atrophy,** and **Refsum's syndrome.**

spinofallopian tube shunt. See **ventriculofallopian tube shunt.**

spin-spin relaxation time. See **relaxation time.**

spiral fracture, a bone break in which the break of bone tissue is in a corkscrew fashion following the long axis of the broken bone.

spiral organ of Corti. See **organ of Corti.**

spirillary rat-bite fever, spirillum fever. See **rat-bite fever.**

spirochete /spī'rəkēt/, a bacterium (*Spirochaeta*) that causes leptospirosis, relapsing fever, syphilis, and yaws. Compare **bacillus, coccus, vibrio.** –**spirochetal,** *adj.*

spirogram /spī'rōgram/, a chart of breathing movements made by a spirometer, used in judging the health of the lungs.

spirograph /spī'rəgraf/, a device for recording breathing movements. See also **spirometer.** –**spirographic,** *adj.*

spirometer /spīrom'ətər/, a machine that measures and records the amount of inhaled and exhaled air, used to test the health of the lungs. Information is recorded on a chart, called a spirogram. –**spirometric,** *adj.*

spirometry /spīrom'ətrē/, laboratory test of the lungs by means of a spirometer. Compare **blood gas determination.** –**spirometric,** *adj.*

spironolactone, a drug that controls a certain hormone (aldosterone). It is used to treat primary hyperaldosteronism, edema of heart failure, cirrhosis of the liver with edema, kidney damage, high blood pressure, and a lack of potassium in the blood.

★CAUTION: Certain kinds of kidney disorder or too much potassium in the blood prohibits its use.

★ADVERSE EFFECTS: Among the most serious side effects are too much potassium in the blood, the growth of male breasts, mental confusion, loss of coordination, impotence, lack of menstruation, hairiness, and a patchy rash.

Spitz nevus. See **benign juvenile melanoma.**

SPL. See **Staphage Lysate.**

splanchnic engorgement, the overfilling or pooling of blood within the blood vessels of the stomach cavity following the removal of pressure from the stomach area, as in the removal of a large tumor, birth of a child, or drainage of a large amount of urine from the bladder.

splanchnocele, hernia of any internal organ of the lower body.

spleen, a soft, vessel-filled, egg-shaped organ found between the stomach and the diaphragm on the left half of the body. It contains lymphatic nodules. It has a dark purple color and varies in shape in different individuals and within the same individual at different times. The exact function of the spleen is not known, but the most recent research shows that it helps keep the blood healthy. The size of the spleen becomes larger during and after digestion and often during illness. It can weigh as much as 9 kg in a victim of malarial fever. Compare **thymus.** –**splenic** /splen'ik/, *adj.*

spleen scan, an x-ray test of the spleen done to find a tumor, damage, or other problem.

splenectomy /splənek'təmē/, the removal by surgery of the spleen.

splenic. See **spleen.**

splenic flexure syndrome, a pain coming back time after time and a bloating in the area of the stomach caused by a pocket of gas trapped in the large intestine below the spleen. The symptoms are eased by a bowel movement or by breaking wind.

splenic gland. See **pancreaticolienal node.**

splenic vein. See **lienal vein.**

splenius capitis, one of a pair of deep muscles of the back. It acts to turn and bend the head.

splenius cervicis, one of a pair of deep muscles of the back. It acts to turn, bend, and extend the head and neck. Also called **splenius colli.**

splenomedullary leukemia. See **acute myelocytic leukemia, chronic myelocytic leukemia.**

splenomegaly /splē'nōmeg'əlē, splen'-/, an abnormal enlargement of the spleen, as linked with certain types of high blood pressure and anemia, Niemann-Pick disease, or malaria.

splenomyelogenous leukemia. See **acute myelocytic leukemia, chronic myelocytic leukemia.**

splint, 1. a device for holding in place any part of the body. It may be stiff (of metal, plaster, or wood) or flexible (of felt or leather). 2. (in dentistry) a device for anchoring the teeth or changing the bite. Compare **brace, cast.**

splinter fracture, a crushing break resulting in thin, sharp bone chips.

splinter hemorrhage, bleeding under a finger- or toenail, looking like a splinter. It is seen after injury and in patients with bacterial endocarditis.

splinting, the process of restraining, supporting, or fixing a body part so that it cannot move.

split personality. See **multiple personality.**

split Russell traction, a kind of traction used to treat injuries and deformities of the hip and knee. Compare **Russell traction.**

splitting, a primitive defense mechanism with failure to bring together and deal with both positive and negative experiences and ideas of oneself, other people, situations, and institutions. Overuse shows a lack of emotional development.

spondylitis /spon'dəlī'tis/, a swelling of any of the spinal vertebrae, usually marked by stiffness and pain. The condition may follow injury to the spine, or it may be the result of infection or rheumatoid disease. See also **ankylosing spondylitis.**

spondylolisthesis /spon'dilōlisthē'sis/, the partial dislocation of one vertebra over the one below it. See also **spinal cord compression.**

spondylosis /spon'dilō'sis/, a condition of the spine marked by stiffness of a vertebral joint. See also **ankylosing spondylitis, spondylitis.**

spondylosyndesis. See **spinal fusion.**

sponge bath, the method of washing the patient with a damp washcloth or sponge, used when a full bath is not needed or as a method of reducing body temperature.

sponge contraceptive. See **vaginal sponge.**

sponge gold. See **mat gold.**

spongioblastoma /spun'jē·ōblastō'mə/, pl. **spongioblastomas, spongioblastomata,** a tumor made up of early fetal cells that develop around the neural tube and change into cells of the supporting connective tissue of nerve cells or cells of lining membranes of the ventricles and the spinal cord canal. A kind of spongioblastoma is **spongioblastoma unipolare.** Spongioblastoma is also called **glioblastoma, gliosarcoma, spongiocytoma.**

spongioblastoma multiforme. See **glioblastoma multiforme.**

spongioblastoma unipolare, a rare growth occurring in the spinal cord or brain.

spongiocytoma. See **spongioblastoma.**

spontaneous abortion, an end of pregnancy before the 20th week and occurring by itself because of defects of the fetus or womb. More than 10% of pregnancies end as spontaneous abortions, almost all caused by defective eggs. Compare **induced abortion.**

spontaneous delivery, a normal birth occurring without any mechanical help.

spontaneous evolution, the unassisted birth of a fetus in the crosswise (transverse) position. See also **Denman's spontaneous evolution.**

spontaneous fracture. See **neoplastic fracture.**

spontaneous ventilation, normal breathing, unassisted, in which the patient creates the range of pressure through muscle and chest wall movements that moves air into and out of the lungs.

sporadic, (of a number of events) occurring at scattered, interrupted, and seemingly random intervals.

spore, a form taken by some bacteria that is resistant to heat, drying, and chemicals. Under proper conditions the spore may change back into the active form of the bacterium. Diseases caused by spore-forming bacteria include anthrax, botulism, gas gangrene, and tetanus.

sporicide /spôr'isīd/, any substance used to kill spores.

sporiferous /spôrif'ərəs/, making or carrying spores.

sporogenous /spôroj'ənəs/, describing an animal or plant that reproduces by spores.

sporophore /spôr'əfôr/, the part of an animal or plant that makes spores.

sporotrichosis /spôr'ōtrikō'sis/, a common, long-term, fungus-caused infection usually marked by skin ulcers and little bumps under the skin. It rarely spreads to bones, lungs, joints, or muscles. The fungus is found in soil and rotting vegetation and usually enters the skin by accidental injury. Treatment may include amphotericin B.

sports medicine, a branch of medicine that specializes in the prevention and treatment of injuries resulting from training and participation in athletic events. More than 1 million persons are treated for sports injuries each year in the United States alone. Most sports injuries are injuries to the muscles (sprains) from overuse and too much effort, injuries to the joints (strains), and tears, which frequently result from not doing enough "warm-up" exercises. Among the most common sports injuries are shin splints, runner's knee, pulled hamstring muscles, Achilles' tendonitis, ankle sprain, arch sprain, charley horse, tennis elbow, baseball finger, dislocations, muscle cramps, inflammation of joint connective tissue (bursitis), inflammation of muscles and membranes enclosing them (myofascitis), inflammation of the rib cage muscles (costochondritis), hernia, and "Little League elbow."

sprain, an injury to the tendons, muscles, or ligaments around a joint, marked by pain, swelling, and discoloration of the skin over the joint. The length of time and seriousness of the symptoms vary with the amount of damage to the tissues. Treatment requires support, rest, and alternating cold and heat. Ultrasound therapy may speed recovery. X-ray pictures are often used to be certain that no break has occurred.

sprain fracture, a break that results from the separation of a tendon or ligament linked with the separation of a bone.

spreader bar, a metal bar with curved hoop areas for attaching hooks or pins for traction.

sprinter's fracture, a break of a certain part of the pelvis caused by a fragment of bone being pulled by a very strong muscle spasm.

sprue, a long-term disorder caused by poor absorption of digested food in the small intestine and marked by numerous symptoms, including diarrhea, weakness, weight loss, poor appetite, pallor, muscle cramps, bone pain, ulceration of the mucous membrane lin ing the digestive tract, and a smooth, shiny tongue. It occurs in both tropic and nontropic forms and affects both children and adults. Also called **catarrhal dysentery.** See also **malabsorption syndrome, nontropical sprue, tropical sprue.**

SPRX, a trademark for a drug used to lessen appetite (phendimetrazine tartrate).

spurious pregnancy. See **pseudocyesis.**

sputum /spyo͞o′təm/, material coughed up from the lungs and spit out through the mouth. It contains mucus, cellular debris, or microorganisms, and it may also contain blood or pus. The amount, color, and contents of the sputum are important in the diagnosis of many illnesses, including tuberculosis, pneumonia, cancer of the lung, and the pneumoconioses.

squamous cell /skwā′məs/, a flat, scaly cell.

squamous cell carcinoma, a slow-growing, cancerous tumor often found in the lungs and skin and occurring also in the anus, cervix, larynx, nose, bladder, and other sites. The typical skin sore—a firm, red, horny, painless little bump, ranging from less than 1 to several centimeters in size—is often the result of overexposure to the sun. The cancer cells typically resemble prickle cells. Also called **epidermoid carcinoma.**

squeeze dynamometer, an instrument for measuring the strength of the grip of the hand.

squint. See **strabismus.**

squinting eye, the abnormal eye in a person with strabismus that cannot be focused with the fixated eye. See also **strabismus.**

ss, abbreviation for **steady state.**

SSKI, a trademark for a drug used to clear mucus and other matter from the mouth and throat (potassium iodide).

SSSS, abbreviation for **staphylococcal scalded skin syndrome.**

S's test. See **Sulkowitch's test.**

ST, abbreviation for *slow-twitch.* See **slow-twitch fiber.**

stab form. See **band.**

stabile diabetes. See **non-insulin-dependent diabetes.**

stabilization, 1. the physical process of becoming stable. 2. the seating of a fixed or removable denture so that it will not tilt or be moved under pressure. 3. the control of induced stress loads and the development of measures to counteract such forces so that the movement of the teeth or of a device does not irritate nearby tissues.

staccato speech, abnormal speech in which the person pauses between words, breaking the rhythm of the phrase or sentence. The condition is sometimes seen linked with multiple sclerosis.

Stadol, a trademark for a painkilling drug (butorphanol tartrate) used as an aid to anesthesia.

stages of dying, the five emotional and behavioral stages that often occur after a patient first learns of approaching death. The stages, identified and described by Elizabeth Kübler-Ross, are denial and shock, anger, bargaining, depression, and acceptance. See also **emotional care of the dying patient, hospice.**

stagnant anoxia, a condition in which there is not enough blood flowing through the body. This state is linked with shock, cardiac standstill, and thrombosis.

stain, 1. a pigment, dye, or substance used to give color to very tiny objects or tissues to make easier their examination and identification. Kinds of stains include **acid-fast stain, Gram's stain,** and **Wright's stain. 2.** to apply color to a substance or tissue to examine it under a microscope.

stammering, a speech disorder marked by sudden starts and stops in the middle of words. The term is often used to mean stuttering.

stanozolol /stənō′zəlol, -ōl/, a male hormone steroid. It is used to treat aplastic anemia and osteoporosis.

★CAUTION: Cancer of the breast or prostate, nephrosis, pregnancy, or known allergy to this drug prohibits its use.

★ADVERSE EFFECTS: Among the most serious side effects are various hormone disorders in males and females, and allergic reactions. Disorders of the stomach and intestines also may occur.

stapedectomy /stā′pədek′təmē/, removal of the stapes of the middle ear and replacing it with a small plastic tube of stainless steel wire, done to restore hearing in the treatment of otosclerosis. Headache and dizziness are normal soon after the operation. The patient's hearing does not improve until the edema subsides and the packing is removed. Possible complications include infection of the outer, middle, or inner ear, rejection of the replacement, and leaking of fluid into the middle ear, with ringing in the ear and dizziness. Compare **incudectomy.**

stapes /stā′pēz/, one of the three little bones in the middle ear, resembling a tiny stirrup. It carries sound vibrations to the inner ear. Compare **incus, malleus.** See also **middle ear.**

Staphage Lysat (SPL), a trademark for an active immunizing drug (staphylococcal antigen phage lysed) used in staphylococcal infection.

Staphcillin, a trademark for a bacteria-killing drug (methicillin sodium).

staphylococcal antigen phage lysed. See **Staphage Lysate.**

staphylococcal infection /staf′ilōkok′əl/, an infection caused by any one of several disease-causing types of *Staphylococcus,* commonly marked by the formation of abscesses on the skin or other organs. Staphylococcal infections of the skin include carbuncles, folliculitis, furuncles, and hidradenitis suppurativa. Bacteremia is common and may result in endocarditis, meningitis, or osteomyelitis. Staphylococcal pneumonia often follows influenza or other viral disease and may be linked with long-term or weakening illness. Acute gastroenteritis may result from a poison made by certain species of staphylococci in tainted food. Treatment usually includes bed rest, and pain-killing and other drugs. Surgical drainage, especially of deep abscesses, is often necessary.

staphylococcal scalded skin syndrome (SSSS), an abnormal skin condition, marked by reddening of the skin, peeling, and scabs, that gives the skin a scalded look. This disorder mainly affects infants 1 to 3 months of age and other children, but it may also affect adults. It is caused by infections. SSSS is more common in the newborn infant because of undeveloped immunity and kidney systems. It is treated with antibiotics.

Staphylococcus /staf′ilōkok′əs/, a type of bacteria. Some kinds are normally found on the skin and in the throat; certain kinds cause severe, pus-forming infections or produce a poison, which may cause nausea, vomiting, and diarrhea. Life-threatening staphylococcal infections may arise in hospitals. *Staphylococcus aureus* is a species that often causes abscesses, endocarditis, impetigo, osteomyelitis, pneumonia, and septicemia. *S. epidermidis,* formerly called *S. albus,* sometimes causes endocarditis in the presence of intracardiac prostheses. See also **staphylococcal infection.** –staphylococcal, *adj.*

staple, a piece of stainless steel wire used to close certain surgical wounds.

Starr-Edwards prosthesis, an artificial heart valve. A caged-ball form of device, it blocks the valve opening and prevents the backward flow of blood. See also **prosthesis.**

startle reflex. See **Moro reflex.**

starvation, 1. a condition caused by the lack of proper food over a long period of time and marked by numerous disorders of the body and metabolism. 2. the act or state of starving or being starved. See also **malnutrition.**

stasis /stā′sis, stas′is/, 1. a disorder in which the normal flow of a fluid through a vessel of the body is slowed or stopped. 2. stillness.

stasis dermatitis, a condition, caused by too little circulation in the legs, beginning with a swelling of the ankles and progressing to a tan-colored skin, patchy reddening, tiny, round, purplish-red spots, and hardening of the skin. It can lead to shrinking of the skin and tissues. The skin is very easily irritated or sensitized to topical medications. The underlying vein problem must be treated. The dermatitis is often treated by bed rest, Burow's solution for oozing sores, antibiotics for infection, and ste roids to reduce swelling. Also called **venous stasis dermatitis.** See also **stasis ulcer.**

stasis ulcer, a scaly, craterlike sore on the skin of the lower leg caused by long-term clogging of veins. The sore is often linked with stasis

dermatitis and varicose veins. Healing is slow, and care to prevent irritation and infection is essential. Bed rest, raising the legs, and pressure bandages are usually used. Appropriate antibiotics, Burow's solution compresses, Unna's paste boot, pinch grafts, and surgery to improve vein flow are useful in treatment. Also called **varicose ulcer.** See also **stasis dermatitis.**

static, without motion, at rest, in balance. Compare **dynamic.**

static equilibrium, the ability of an individual to adjust to changes in the position of his or her center of gravity while maintaining a constant base of support.

stationary lingual arch, a wire that is shaped to fit the side of the teeth facing the tongue and is soldered to the connecting anchor bands.

statistic, a number that describes a property of a set of data or other numbers.

statotonic reflex. See **attitudinal reflex.**

status, 1. a specified state or condition, as emotional status. 2. a continuing state or condition, as status asthmaticus.

status asthmaticus, an acute, severe, and long-lasting asthma attack. A lack of oxygen in the blood, blue skin, and unconsciousness may follow. Treatment includes the giving of certain drugs and the use of artificial breathing methods. A bronchodilator may be given by aerosol inhalation from a ventilator. See also **allergic asthma, asthma.**

status dysraphicus. See **dysraphia.**

status epilepticus, a medical emergency marked by continual attacks of convulsive seizures occurring without intervals of consciousness. Unless convulsions are stopped, permanent brain damage results. Status epilepticus can be brought on by the sudden withdrawal of anticonvulsant drugs, low blood sugar, a brain tumor, a head injury, a high fever, or poisoning. Therapy includes intravenous administration of anticonvulsant drugs, nutrients, and electrolytes, preferably given in an intensive care unit. An adequate airway is usually kept open with an oral pharyngeal or endotracheal tube.

status spongiosus, a condition of poisonous and decaying change in the brain, usually linked with the death of the brain substance.

statutory rape, (in law) sexual intercourse with a female below the age of consent, which varies from state to state. See also **rape.**

STD, abbreviation for **sexually transmitted disease.**

Stearns' alcoholic amentia, a form of insanity brought on by alcohol, marked by an emotional disturbance of a less severe nature than that of delirium tremens but longer lasting and with greater mental clouding and amnesia.

stearyl alcohol, a solid substance, made from stearic acid, used in various ointments.

steatorrhea /stē′ətərē′ə/, greater-than-normal

amounts of fat in the feces, marked by frothy, foul-smelling fecal matter that floats, as in celiac disease, some malabsorption syndromes, and any condition in which fats are poorly absorbed by the small intestine.

Steele-Richardson-Olszewski syndrome, a rare, gradual, nerve disorder of unknown cause, occurring in middle age, more often in men. It is marked by paralysis of eye muscles, loss of coordination, neck and trunk rigidity, pseudobulbar palsy, and parkinsonian face. Madness and inappropriate emotional responses are also common. Treatment usually includes the antiparkinsonian drug levodopa for control of symptoms. Also called **progressive supranuclear palsy.** See also **Parkinson's disease.**

steeple head. See **oxycephaly.**

Steinert's disease. See **myotonic muscular dystrophy.**

Stein-Leventhal syndrome. See **polycystic ovary syndrome.**

Stelazine, a trademark for a tranquilizer (trifluoperazine).

stellate /stel'it, -āt/, star-shaped or arranged in the pattern of a star.

stellate fracture, a bone break in the form of a star.

stem cell, a cell that may give rise to other cell types when it divides. A **pluripotential stem cell** is one that has the potential to develop into several different types of mature cells, including white blood cells (lymphocytes), white blood cells with granules (granulocytes), platelets (thrombocytes), and red blood cells (erythrocytes).

stem cell leukemia, a cancerous growth on a blood-making organ. The disease is extremely acute and has a rapid, relentless course. Also called **embryonal leukemia, hemoblastic leukemia, hemocytoblastic leukemia, lymphoidocytic leukemia, undifferentiated cell leukemia.**

stem cell lymphoma. See **undifferentiated malignant lymphoma.**

stem pessary. See **pessary.**

stenosis /stinō'sis/, an abnormal condition marked by the tightening or narrowing of an opening or passageway in a body structure. Kinds of stenosis include **aortic stenosis** and **pyloric stenosis. –stenotic,** *adj.*

Stensen's duct. See **parotid duct.**

stent, 1. a substance used in making dental impressions and medical molds. 2. a mold or device made of stent, used in anchoring skin grafts and for supporting body openings and cavities during grafting of vessels and tubes of the body during certain surgery.

step-care therapy, a treatment program that begins with a simple, conservative type of treatment but may advance to more complex stages as needed to achieve control of a disease or disorder. An example is step-care therapy of high blood pressure, in which the first step is

limited to nondrug treatments, as weight control, low-salt diet, and exercise for the patient. If the first step fails to produce results, the next step may be the prescription of drugs that increase urine output (diuretics), followed by the use of stronger drugs, until an effective form of treatment is found.

step reflex. See **dance reflex.**

Sterane, a trademark for a nerve-blocking drug (prednisolone).

Sterapred, a trademark for a nerve-blocking drug (prednisone).

stereognostic perception /ster'ē-ōgnos'tik/, the ability to recognize objects by the sense of touch.

stereoscopic parallax. See **binocular parallax.**

stereotypy /ster'ē-ətī'pē/, the continuous, improper repetition of actions, body postures, or speech patterns, usually occurring with a lack of variation in thought processes or ideas. It is often seen in patients with schizophrenia. **–stereotypical,** *adj.*

sterile /ster'il/, 1. barren; unable to produce children because of a physical abnormality, often the lack of sperm in a man or blockage of the fallopian tubes in a woman. Compare **impotence.** 2. aseptic. **–sterility,** *n.*

sterile field, 1. a specified area, as within a tray or on a sterile towel, that is considered free of tiny organisms. 2. an area immediately around a patient that has been prepared for a surgical procedure. The sterile field includes the scrubbed team members, who are properly clothed, and all furniture and fixtures in the area.

sterilization, 1. a process or act that makes a person unable to produce children. See also **hysterectomy, tubal ligation, vasectomy.** 2. a technique for destroying microorganisms using heat, water, chemicals, or gases. **–sterilize,** *v.*

sternal node /stur'nəl/, a bump in one of the three groups of lymph nodes in the front of the rib cage. They drain the lymph from the breast, the surface of the liver, and the deep stomach wall. Also called **internal mammary node.** Compare **diaphragmatic node, intercostal node.** See also **lymphatic system, lymph node.**

sternoclavicular articulation, the double joint between the breastbone (sternum) and the collar bone (clavicle). It is at the center and top of the rib cage.

sternocostal articulation, the flexible joint of the cartilage of each true rib and the sternum. Each sternocostal articulation also has five ligaments.

sternohyoideus /stur'nōhī·oi'dē·əs/, one of the four muscles in the front of the neck that stretch from near the collarbone up to the voicebox (larynx). It is used in swallowing and speaking. Also called **sternohyoid muscle.** Compare **omohyoideus, sternothyroideus, thyrohyoideus.**

sternothyroideus /stur'nōthīroi'dē·əs/, one of the

four muscles in the front of the throat that stretch from near the collarbone up to the voicebox (larynx). It is used in swallowing and speaking. Also called **sternothyroid muscle.** Compare **omohyoideus, sternohyoideus, thyrohyoideus.**

sternum, the long, flat bone in the middle of the front of the rib cage. It is sometimes called the breastbone. The sternum is longer in men than in women.

sternutation. See **sneeze.**

sterognosis /ster´ŏgnō´sis/, **1.** the sense of feeling and understanding the form and nature of objects by the sense of touch. **2.** perception by the senses of the solidity of objects. −**sterognostic,** *adj.*

steroid, any of a large number of hormonelike substances.

stertorous /stur´tərəs/, relating to an act of breathing that is labored or struggling; having a snoring sound.

stethomimetic /steth´ōmimet´ik/, referring to any condition causing or linked with a decrease in chest volume below its normal value. The condition may be present at birth, temporary, or permanent.

stethoscope /steth´əskōp/, an instrument consisting of two earpieces connected by means of flexible tubing to a diaphragm, which is placed against the skin of the patient's chest or back to hear heart and lung sounds.

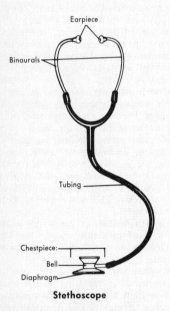

Earpiece

Binaurals

Tubing

Chestpiece

Bell

Diaphragm

Stethoscope

Stevens-Johnson syndrome, a serious, sometimes fatal inflammatory disease affecting children and young adults. It is marked by the rapid attack of fever, blisters on the skin, and open sores on the mucous membranes of the lips, eyes, mouth, nasal passage, and genitals. Pneumonia, pain in the joints, and prostration are common. The syndrome may be an allergic reaction to certain drugs, or it may follow pregnancy, herpesvirus I, or other infection. It is rarely seen linked with cancer or with radiation therapy. Treatment includes bed rest, antibiotics for pneumonia, glucocorticoids, painkilling drugs, mouthwashes, and sedatives.

sthenic fever /sthen´ik/, high body temperature linked with thirst, dry skin, and, often, madness.

stibogluconate sodium, a drug used to fight leishmaniasis available from the Centers for Disease Control.

stibophen /stib´əfin/, a drug used to treat schistosomiasis.

★CAUTION: Severe liver, kidney, or heart disorders or known allergy to this drug prohibits its use.

★ADVERSE EFFECTS: Among the more serious side effects are pain at the site of injection, disorders of the stomach and intestines, fever, and blood disorders.

sticky ends. See **cohesive termini.**

Stieda's fracture /stē´dəz/, a fracture of the end of the thighbone (femur).

stiff lung. See **congestive atelectasis.**

stigma, *pl.* **stigmata, stigmas, 1.** a moral or physical blemish. **2.** a physical trait that serves to identify a disease or a condition.

stilbestrol. See **diethylstilbestrol.**

stillbirth, the birth of a fetus that died before or during delivery.

stillborn, 1. an infant that was born dead. **2.** of or relating to an infant that was born dead.

Still's disease. See **juvenile rheumatoid arthritis.**

Stilphostrol, a trademark for a female hormone (diethylstilbestrol diphosphate).

stimulant, any substance that speeds up a body system.

stimulant cathartic, a laxative that acts by helping the motion of the bowel, especially the longitudinal peristalsis of the colon. Kinds of stimulant cathartics are **cascara** and **senna.**

stimulating bath, a bath taken in water that contains an aromatic substance, a pore-closing substance, or a tonic.

stimulus, *pl.* **stimuli,** anything that excites an organism or part to function, become active, or respond. −**stimulate,** *v.*

sting, an injury caused by a sharp, painful puncture of the skin, often accompanied by irritating chemicals or the poison of an insect or other animal. In cases of allergy, a highly poisonous sting, or numerous stings, shock may occur. Kinds of stings include bee, jellyfish, scorpion, sea urchin, and shellfish stings. See also **stingray, wasp.**

stingray, a flat, long-tailed fish that has barbed spines on its back; these spines are connected to sacs of venom. Spasm of the skeletal muscles, severe local pain, seizures, and shortness of breath may occur if the skin is broken by the spines. The wound is washed with cold saltwater, and the injured limb is placed in very hot water for 30 to 60 minutes; an antiseptic is applied and tetanus protection is given. See also **sea urchin sting.**

St. Louis encephalitis, an infection of the brain carried from birds to humans by the bite of an infected mosquito. It occurs most commonly in the central and southern portions of the United States and is marked by headache, malaise, fever, stiff neck, delirium, and convulsions. Resulting conditions may include sight and speech disorders, difficulty in walking, and personality changes. Recovery may be slow and take a long time, and death may result. Compare **California encephalitis, equine encephalitis.** See also **encephalitis.**

stoker's cramp. See **heat cramp.**

Stokes-Adams syndrome. See **Adams-Stokes syndrome.**

stoma, *pl.* **stomas, stomata, 1.** a pore or opening on a surface. **2.** an artificial opening from an internal organ to the surface of the body, created surgically, as for a colostomy, ileostomy, or tracheostomy. **3.** a new opening created surgically, between two body structures, as for a gastroenterostomy, pancreaticogastrostomy, pancreatoduodenostomy, or pyeloureterostomy.

stomach, the main organ of digestion, which is divided into a body and a pylorus. It receives and partly digests food and drink funneled from the mouth through the throat and moves material into the intestines. The shape of the stomach is changed by the amount of contents, stage of digestion, development of the muscles, and condition of the intestines. It is lined with mucous membranes that contain many blood vessels and nerves, and contains several important glands. Also called **gaster.**

stomach pump, a pump for removing the contents of the stomach through a tube passed through the mouth or nose into the stomach.

stomal peptic ulcer, a marginal peptic ulcer. See also **peptic ulcer.**

stomatitis /stō′mətī′tis/, any inflammatory condition of the mouth. It may result from infection by bacteria, viruses, or fungi, from exposure to certain chemicals or drugs, from vitamin deficiency, or from a swelling disease. Kinds of stomatitis include **aphthous stomatitis, pseudomembranous stomatitis, thrush,** and **Vincent's infection.**

stomatognathic system /stō′mətōnath′ik/, the combination of organs, structures, and nerves involved in speech and reception, mastication, and deglutition of food. This system is composed of the teeth, the jaws, the masticatory muscles, the tongue, the lips, and surrounding tissues and the nerves that control these structures.

stomatology, the study of the morphology, structure, function, and diseases of the oral cavity. **–stomatologist,** *n.,* **stomatologic, stomatological,** *adj.*

stomion, the median point of the oral slit when the mouth is closed.

-stomy, a combining form meaning 'surgical opening.'

stone. See **calculus.**

-stone, a combining form meaning a 'stone in a human organ or duct.'

stool. See **feces.**

stool softener. See **fecal softener.**

stopcock, a valve that controls the flow of fluid or air through a tube.

storage capacity, the amount of data that can be stored on a computer disk or tape, usually expressed in kilobytes or megabytes.

storing fermentation, the rapid, gaseous clotting of milk caused by *Clostridium perfringens.*

stork bite. See **telangiectatic nevus.**

Stoxil, a trademark for an antivirus drug (idoxuridine).

STP, *slang.* a psychedelic agent, dimethoxy-4-methylampetamine (DOM). STP is an abbreviation for *serenity, tranquillity,and peace.*

STPD, abbreviation for *standard temperature, standard pressure, dry.*

strabismus, an abnormal condition in which the eyes are crossed. There are two kinds of strabismus—paralytic and nonparalytic. Paralytic strabismus results from the inability of the muscles to move the eye because of nerve defects or muscle failure. Because this kind of strabismus may be caused by tumor, infection, or injury to the brain or the eye, an ophthalmological examination is recommended. Nonparalytic strabismus is a defect in the position of the two eyes in relation to each other. The condition is inherited. The person cannot use the two eyes together but has to focus with one or the other. Some people have alternating strabismus, using one eye and then the other; some have monocular strabismus affecting only one eye. Nonparalytic strabismus is treated most successfully in early childhood. Treatment consists mainly of covering the strong eye, forcing the child to use the weak eye. The earlier it is begun the more rapid and effective the treatment. By 6 years of age, a weak eye has usually become so weakened that treatment is not effective and permanent sight loss has occurred. The eyes might be straightened by surgery, but certain cases cannot be corrected. Also called **squint. –strabismal, strabismic, strabismical,** *adj.*

straight sinus, one of the six vein passages on the top and front of the brain, draining blood from the brain into the jugular vein. It has no valves. Compare **inferior sagittal sinus, superior sagittal sinus, transverse sagittal sinus.**

straight wire fixed orthodontic appliance, a device used for correcting and improving a crooked bite.

strain, 1. to use physical force in a manner that may result in injury, usually of a muscle. **2.** damage, usually muscular, that results from excessive physical effort. **3.** an emotional state reflecting mental pressure or fatigue.

straitjacket, a coat of canvas with long sleeves that can be tied behind the wearer's back to prevent movement of the arms. It is used to restrain violent or uncontrollable people.

strangulation, the tightening or closing of a tubular structure of the body, as the throat, a section of bowel, or the blood vessels of a limb, that prevents function or slows circulation. See also **intestinal strangulation. –strangulate,** *v.,* **strangulated,** *adj.*

strap, 1. a band, as that made of adhesive plaster, that is used to hold dressings in place or to attach one thing to another. **2.** to bind securely.

strapping, putting overlapping strips of adhesive tape to an arm, leg, or other parts of the body or body area to exert pressure and hold a structure in place, done to treat strains, sprains, dislocations, and certain fractures.

stratiform cartilage. See **fibrocartilage.**

stratiform fibrocartilage, a structure made of fiberlike cartilage that forms a thin coating of bony grooves through which tendons of certain muscles glide. Compare **circumferential fibrocartilage, connecting fibrocartilage, interarticular fibrocartilage.**

stratum /strā′təm, strat′əm/, *pl.* **strata,** an even, thick sheet or layer, usually linked with other layers, as the stratum basale of the skin.

stratum basale, 1. also called **stratum germinativum;** the deepest of the five layers of the skin. This layer provides new cells. Compare **stratum corneum, stratum granulosum, stratum lucidum, stratum spinosum.** See also **skin. 2.** the deepest layers of the mucous membranes of the womb.

stratum corneum, the horny, outermost layer of the skin, composed of dead cells converted to keratin that continually flakes away. The thickness of the layer is controlled with the normal wear of the area it covers. The stratum corneum is thick on the palms of the hands and the soles of the feet but thin over more protected areas. Also called **horny layer.** Compare **stratum basale, stratum granulosum, stratum lucidum, stratum spinosum.** See also **skin.**

stratum germinativum. See **stratum basale.**

stratum granulosum, one of the layers of the skin lying just below the stratum corneum except in the palms of the hands and the soles of the feet, where it lies just under the stratum

lucidum. Compare **stratum basale, stratum corneum, stratum lucidum, stratum spinosum.** See also **skin.**

stratum lucidum, one of the layers of the skin, lying just beneath the stratum corneum and present only in the thick skin of the palms of the hands and the soles of the feet. Also called **clear cell layer.** Compare **stratum basale, stratum corneum, stratum granulosum, stratum spinosum.** See also **skin.**

stratum spinosum, one of the layers of the skin. It lies on top of the stratum basale and beneath the stratum granulosum. Also called **prickle cell layer.** Compare **stratum basale, stratum corneum, stratum granulosum, stratum lucidum.** See also **skin.**

stratum spongiosum, one of the three layers of the lining of the womb, containing twisting, widened glands and a small amount of tissue. With the stratum compactum it forms the functional part of the lining during pregnancy. Compare **stratum basale.** See also **decidua, placenta.**

strawberry gallbladder, a tiny, yellow gallbladder spotted with deposits on the red mucous membrane, typical of cholesterolosis.

strawberry hemangioma, strawberry mark. See **capillary hemangioma.**

strawberry tongue, a symptom of scarlet fever, marked by a strawberrylike coloration of the swollen tongue.

strength, the ability of a muscle to produce or resist physical force.

strep throat, *informal.* an infection of the throat and tonsils caused by a bacterium *(Streptococcus).* The infection is marked by sore throat, chills, fever, swollen lymph nodes in the neck, and, sometimes, nausea and vomiting. The symptoms usually begin suddenly a few days after exposure to the germs in airborne droplets or after direct contact with an infected person. Also called **streptococcal sore throat.**

streptobacillary rat-bite fever. See **Haverhill fever.**

Streptobacillus moniliformis, a species of bacteria that can cause rat-bite fever in humans.

streptococcal angina /strep′təkok′əl/, a condition in which feelings of choking, suffocation, and pain occur as the result of a streptococcal infection.

streptococcal infection, an infection caused by disease-causing bacteria of one of several types of *Streptococcus* or their poisons. Almost any organ of the body may be involved. The infections occur in many forms, including cellulitis, endocarditis, erysipelas, impetigo, meningitis, pneumonia, scarlet fever, tonsillitis, and urinary tract infection. See also **strep throat.**

streptococcal sore throat. See **strep throat.**

Streptococcus /strep′təkok′əs/, a bacterium, causing disease in humans. *Streptococcus fecalis,* a type that normally lives in the intestines, may cause infection of the urinary tract or endocardium. *S. pneumoniae* causes 90% of the cases of bacterial pneumonia in the United States. *S. pyogenes* may cause tonsillitis, respiratory, urinary, or skin infections. Some types may lead to rheumatic fever or to glomerulonephritis. *S. viridans,* a type normally found in the mouth, is the most common cause of bacterial endocarditis, especially when introduced into the bloodstream during dental procedures.

streptokinase /strep′təkī′nās/, an enzyme made by streptococci.

streptokinase-streptodornase /-strep′tōdôr′nās/, two enzymes derived from a type of *Streptococcus hemolyticus.* It is used in removing pus, clotted blood, x-ray burns or certain deposits caused by injury or infection.

★CAUTION: Active bleeding, swelling of certain tissue, or danger of reopening bronchopleural fistulas prohibits its use.

★ADVERSE EFFECTS: Among the more serious side effects are fever and irritation.

streptolysin /streptol′isis/, a substance, made by various streptococci, that frees hemoglobin from red blood cells.

streptomycin sulfate /strep′təmī′sin/, an antibiotic. It is used to treat tuberculosis, endocarditis, and certain other infections.

★CAUTION: Labyrinthine disease or known allergy to this drug prohibits its use. It must be used with caution in damaged kidney function and in the elderly.

★ADVERSE EFFECTS: Among the most serious side effects are damage to the ears and hearing, kidney damage, muscle weakness, and allergic reactions.

streptozocin /strep′təzō′sin/, an experimental antitumor drug used to treat many tumors, including tumors of the pancreas. It is an antibiotic substance from *Streptomyces acromogenes.*

stress, any emotional, physical, social, economic, or other factor that requires a response or change, as severe loss of fluid, which can cause a rise in body temperature, or a separation from parents, which can cause a young child to cry. See also **general adaptation syndrome.**

stress-adaption theory, a concept that stress lessens an individual's ability to adjust (reserve capacity) and increases chances for health problems.

stress behavior, a change from a person's normal behavior in response to something that causes wear and tear on the body's physical or mental resources (stressor).

stress fracture, a bone break, especially of one or more of the foot bones, caused by repeated, long-term, or abnormal stress.

stress inoculation, a procedure useful in helping patients control anxiety by substituting positive coping statements for statements that bring about anxiety.

stress management, methods of controlling factors that require a response or change within a person by identifying the causes of stress, eliminating negative stresses, and developing coping mechanisms. Examples include progressive relaxation, guided imagery, biofeedback, and active problem solving.

stressor, anything that causes wear and tear on the body's physical or mental resources. See also **general adaptation syndrome.**

stress reaction. See **general adaptation syndrome, posttraumatic stress disorder.**

stress response syndrome. See **posttraumatic stress disorder.**

stress test, a test that measures a system of the body when subjected to carefully controlled stress. It allows the doctor to know the condition of the system being tested. This kind of test is often used to test the heart and lungs, and the health of the fetus in pregnant women. See also **exercise electrocardiogram, oxytocin challenge test.**

stress ulcer, a stomach ulcer that develops in patients who are under heavy stress, as when badly burned. See also **Curling's ulcer.**

stria /strī′ə/, *pl.* **striae,** a streak or a narrow furrow in the skin that often results from a stretching of the skin, as seen on the stomach after pregnancy. Purplish striae are one of the classic findings in hyperadrenocorticism. Also called **stretch mark.**

striae atrophica. See **linea albicantes.**

striae gravidarum, uneven furrows, red to purple in color, that appear in the skin of the stomach, thighs, and buttocks of pregnant women.

striated muscle, muscle tissue, including all the muscles of the skeleton, that are made up of bundles of parallel, streaklike fibers under conscious control; the heart, a striated involuntary muscle, is an exception. Also called **skeletal muscle, voluntary muscle.** Compare **cardiac muscle, smooth muscle.**

stricture, an abnormal short-term or permanent narrowing of the tube of a hollow organ, as the throat, pylorus of the stomach, ureter, or urethra, because of inflammation, pressure from outside the body, or scarring. Treatment varies depending on the cause. Compare **spasm.**

stridor /strī′dôr/, an abnormal, high-pitched, musical breathing sound, caused by a blockage in the throat or larynx. It is usually heard when breathing in. Stridor may indicate several cancerous or swelling conditions, including glottic edema, asthma, diphtheria, laryngospasm, or papilloma. Compare **pleuropericardial rub, rales, rhonchi, wheeze.**

string carcinoma, a cancer of the large intestine, usually of the colon that, in an x-ray photo, causes the intestine to appear to be tied in segments like a string of large beads.

stripping, 1. an operation for the removal of the long and the short saphenous veins of the legs. See also **milking, varicose veins. 2.** the removal of a very small amount of enamel from the top and sides of teeth to ease crowding.

stroboscopic illusion. See **phi phenomenon.**

stroke. See **cerebrovascular accident.**

stroke prone profile, a list of risk factors that show whether a patient may be likely to have a stroke. The factors include advanced age, high blood pressure, previous attacks of poor circulation, cigarette smoking, heart disorders, embolism, family history of strokes, use of birth-control pills, diabetes mellitus, lack of exercise, overweight, high cholesterol, and hyperlipidemia.

stroma /strō'mə/, *pl.* **stromata,** the supporting tissue for an organ. Some kinds of stromata are the vitreous stroma, which encloses the vitreous humor of the eye, and Rollet's stroma, which contains the hemoglobin of a red blood cell. **–stromatic,** *adj.*

Strongyloides /stron'jiloi'dēz/, a group of worms that are parasites of the intestines. One type of *Strongyloides, S. stercoralis,* causes strongyloidiasis.

strongyloidiasis /stron'jəloidī'əsis/, infection of the small intestine by the worm *Strongyloides stercoralis,* acquired when larvae from the soil penetrate intact skin, causing an itching rash. The larvae pass to the lungs by way of the bloodstream, sometimes causing pneumonia. Larvae then move up the air passages to the throat, are swallowed, and develop into adult worms in the small intestine. Bloody diarrhea and disorders of the intestines may result. Rarely, fatal disseminated strongyloidiasis occurs. Diagnosis depends on finding larvae in freshly passed feces. Treatment often includes giving thiabendazole. Proper sanitary methods for the disposal of excrement could prevent the disease. Wearing shoes prevents catching the disease from contaminated soil. Also called **threadworm infection.**

structural integration, a technique of deep massage intended to help by realigning the body by changing the length and tone of certain tissues. It is believed by some that improper posture and mental and bodily injuries may have a bad effect on a person's energy level, self-image, muscular efficiency, perceptions, and general health. Also called **Rolfing.**

structural model, a model of family therapy that views the family as an open system and identifies groups within the family that have specific functions. When faced with demands for change, individual family members, parts of the family, or the whole family respond with growth behaviors or with poor adaption behaviors. The goal of family therapy is to help family members learn new ways to behave.

structure, a part of the body, as the heart, a bone, a gland, a cell, or a limb.

struma lymphomatosa. See **Hashimoto's disease.**

Stryker wedge frame, a special bed that allows the patient to be turned onto his or her back or front as needed. It is used to treat patients with certain disorders of the spine or with very bad burns. Compare **Circolectric bed, Foster bed, hyperextension bed.**

Stuartnatal 1+1, a trademark for a drug given by mouth to pregnant women, containing vitamins and minerals.

Stuart-Power factor. See **factor X.**

stump, the part of a limb that is left after amputation.

stump hallucination, the feeling of the continued presence of an amputated limb. See also **hallucination, phantom limb syndrome.**

stupor, a state, marked by a lack of energy and an uncaring attitude, in which a person seems unaware of the surroundings. The condition occurs in nerve and mental disorders. Kinds of stupor are **anergic stupor, benign stupor, delusion stupor,** and **epileptic stupor.**

Sturge-Weber syndrome /sturj'web'ər/, a disease of the nerves of the skin marked by a port-wine-colored noncancerous tumor on the face. It may be linked with certain kinds of brain damage, certain eye disorders, and seizures. There is no known cure. Drugs may be given to control convulsions. Also called **Dimitri's disease, encephalotrigeminal angiomatosis.**

stuttering, a speech defect marked by halting speech, involving many hesitations, stumbling, repeating the same syllables, and holding some sounds for a long time. The condition may result from a brain or nerve disorder or an injury to the organs of speech, but in most cases the cause is emotional and mental. Hesitancy in speech are normal traits of language development during the preschool years when a child's mental ability and level of understanding are beyond muscle coordination and vocabulary. However, if too much emphasis or stress is placed on this pattern, the child becomes conscious of the difficulties and may develop a fear of speaking. Stuttering can usually be cured until about 7 years of age. Prevention must begin early in childhood. If stuttering continues, treatment by a speech therapist may be necessary. See also **stammering.**

sty, a pus-forming infection of a gland of the eyelid, often caused by a staphylococcal organism. Also spelled **stye.** Also called **hordeolum.**

stylohyoideus /stī'lōhī·oi'dē·əs/, one of the neck muscles. Also called **stylohyoid bone.** Compare **digastricus, geniohyoideus, mylohyoideus.**

stylohyoid ligament /stī'lōhī'oid/, the ligament attached to the side of the head that runs to the throat.

stylomandibular ligament /stī'lōmandib'yələr/,

one of a pair of special bands of neck muscles. It extends from the side of the head to the top of the jaw in front of the ear. Compare **sphenomandibular ligament.**

styptic /stip'tik/, **1.** a substance used to control bleeding. **2.** acting as an agent to control bleeding.

sub-, suf-, sup-, a combining form meaning 'under, near, almost, or moderately.'

subacromial bursa, the small fluid-filled sac in the shoulder joint.

subacute, of or relating to a disease or other abnormal condition present in a patient who appears to be well. The condition may be identified or discovered by means of a laboratory test or by x-ray test.

subacute bacterial endocarditis (SBE), a long-term infection caused by a bacteria of the valves of the heart, marked by a slow, quiet onset with fever, heart murmur, enlargement of the spleen, and the development of clumps of abnormal tissue, called vegetations, around an artificial heart valve or on the cusps of a valve. Various types of *Streptococcus* or *Staphylococcus* are commonly the cause of SBE. Dental procedures are linked with infection by *Streptococcus viridans,* surgical procedures with *Streptococcus facalis,* and self-infection (especially by drug abusers) with *Staphylococcus aureus.* See also **bacterial endocarditis, endocarditis, Janeway lesions.** It is treated with antibiotics. If an artificial heart valve has become infected, it is usually removed. Before surgery or a dental procedure, antibiotics are given. During the most serious phase of illness, the fever is treated with antifever drugs and bed rest; adequate high-protein diet and fluids are encouraged.

subacute glomerulonephritis, an uncommon disease of the kidney marked by blood and protein in the blood, lessened production of urine, and edema. Of unknown cause, the disease may grow rapidly, and kidney failure may occur. Kidney transplantation and dialysis are the only treatments available. See also **chronic glomerulonephritis, postinfectious glomerulonephritis, uremia.**

subacute myelooptic neuropathy (SMON), a condition of pain and weakness in the muscles, usually below the 12th vertebra in the chest region; numbness and burning feelings in the arms and legs; and, in some cases, decaying of the eyes. The patient usually has a significant change in his or her walking pattern.

subacute sclerosing panencephalitis, an uncommon, slow infection caused by the measles virus and marked by widespread swelling of brain tissue, personality change, seizures, blindness, madness, fever, and death. The condition occurs in children and in adolescents who have had measles at a very early age. No useful treatment is known. See also **slow virus.**

subacute thyroiditis. See **de Quervain's thyroiditis.**

subarachnoid block anesthesia, a form of spinal anesthesia involving the injection of an anesthetic into the space at the base of the brain. See also **obstetric anesthesia.**

subarachnoid hemorrhage (SaH, SAH), a bleeding into a fluid-filled space between the layers of membranes at the base of the brain near the spine. It may bleed into the brain under certain conditions. The cause may be an injury or breaking of a berry aneurysm or an arteriovenous anomaly. The first symptom of a subarachnoid hemorrhage is a sudden very painful headache that begins in one area and then spreads, becoming dull and throbbing. Other symptoms include dizziness, stiffness of the neck, vomiting, drowsiness, sweating and chills, stupor, and loss of consciousness. It may result in continued unconsciousness, coma, and death. Madness and confusion often continue through the first weeks of recovery, and permanent brain damage is common.

subcapital fracture, a break just below the head of a bone that pivots in a ball-and-socket joint, as the head of the femur.

subcapsular cataract, a condition marked by cloudiness beneath the capsule of the lens of the eye.

subclavian /səbklā'vē·ən/, situated under the clavicle, or collarbone, as the subclavian vein.

subclavian artery, one of a pair of arteries that rise in the neck and supply blood to the vertebral column, spinal cord, ear, and brain. See also **left subclavian artery, right subclavian artery.**

subclavian steal syndrome, a vessel condition caused by a blockage in the subclavian artery near the beginning of the vertebral artery. The block causes a change in blood pressure and blood flow. This condition is marked by attacks of paralysis of the arm and pain behind the ear and in the back of the skull. Very different blood pressure readings from the arms are sometimes symptoms of the condition.

subclavian vein, the continuation of the axillary vein in the upper body.

subclavius /səbklā'vē·əs/, a short muscle of the chest wall. It moves the shoulder down and forward. Compare **pectoralis major, pectoralis minor, serratus anterior.**

subclinical, of or relating to a disease or abnormal condition that is so mild it produces no symptoms.

subclinical diabetes. See **impaired glucose tolerance.**

subcutaneous /sub'kyo͞otā'nē·əs/, beneath the skin.

subcutaneous emphysema, the presence of free air or gas in the tissues under the skin. The air or gas may come from the bursting of an airway or small pocket in the lung and move through the chest between the lungs (mediastinum) up into the neck. The face, neck, and chest appear swollen. Skin tissues can be painful and may produce a "crackling" sound as air moves under them. The patient may experience shortness of breath (dyspnea) and have a bluish color in the skin (cyanosis) if the air leak is severe. Treatment may require a cut to release the trapped air. Also called **aerodermectasia.**

subcutaneous fascia, a continuous layer of connecting tissue over the entire body between the skin and the muscles. It is made up of an outer, normally fatty layer, and an inner, thin elastic layer. Between the two layers lie blood vessels, nerves, lymphatics, the mammary glands, most of the facial muscles, and the platysma. Compare **deep fascia, subserous fascia.**

subcutaneous fat necrosis. See **adiponecrosis subcutanea neonatorum.**

subcutaneous infusion. See **hypodermoclysis.**

subcutaneous injection, the puncturing by a hypodermic needle into the subcutaneous tissue beneath the skin, usually on the upper arm, thigh, or abdomen.

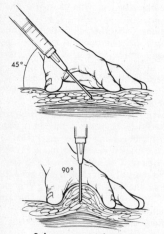

Subcutaneous injection

subcutaneous mastectomy, an operation in which all the breast tissue of one or both breasts is removed leaving the skin, areola, and nipple intact. The nearby lymph nodes and the underlying muscles are not removed. It may be done on women who are at great risk of getting breast cancer. Reconstruction of the breasts is done by a plastic surgeon, through inserting prostheses to return the normal shape to the breasts.

subcutaneous nodule, a small, solid bump beneath the skin that can be detected by touch.

Certain kinds are found in patients with rheumatic fever. Very tiny subcutaneous nodules are linked with typhus fever.

subcutaneous test. See **intradermal test.**

subcutaneous tunnel, a tunnel under the skin between the exit site of a small tube (catheter) and the entrance site into the vein through which the catheter is threaded to an atrium in the heart.

subdural hygroma, a collection of fluid between certain membranes covering the brain, caused by a spinal fluid leak.

subendocardial infarction, death of cells in the innermost layer of the heart (myocardium) from lack of blood. In some cases, portions of the middle layer of tissue are affected but not the outer region of the heart (epicardium).

suberosis. See **cork worker's lung.**

subgerminal cavity. See **blastocoele.**

subgingival calculus, a small stone, made up of collected minerals, bits of food, and other matter found in the mouth, which occurs on the teeth or in the gum next to the teeth.

subgingival curettage, a method of removing certain growths on or within the gums. It is used to reduce swelling and to restore the health of the gums.

subintentional suicide. See **benign suicide.**

subintimal, the area beneath the membrane lining a blood vessel, usually a large artery.

subinvolution, a condition that occurs when the womb does not return to normal after the birth of a child. It is marked by longer and heavier bleeding after childbirth and, on pelvic examination, a larger and softer uterus than would be expected at that time. Treatment includes ergonovine given by mouth for 2 or 3 days, and, if an infection is present, an antibiotic. The blood is also tested, and iron is given if necessary. A follow-up examination is performed 2 weeks later.

subjective sensation, a feeling that is not linked with or is not directly caused by something outside of the body. See also **sensation,** def. 1.

subjects, people, animals or events selected for study, as the effects of a new medication or therapy.

subleukemic leukemia. See **aleukemic leukemia.**

Sublimaze Citrate, a trademark for a powerful painkilling drug (fentanyl citrate).

sublingual /səbling′gwəl/, beneath the tongue.

sublingual administration of a medication, the giving of a drug, as nitroglycerin, usually in tablet form, by placing it beneath the tongue until the tablet dissolves.

sublingual duct. See **Bartholin's duct, duct of Rivinus.**

sublingual gland, one of a pair of small salivary glands found under the mucous membrane of the floor of the mouth beneath the tongue. It is a narrow, almond-shaped structure, and weighs about 2 g. The sublingual gland releases mucus. Compare **parotid gland, submandibular gland.**

subluxation /sub′luksā′shən/, a partial dislocation.

submandibular duct, a tube through which a submandibular gland releases saliva. Also called **submaxillary duct.**

submandibular gland, one of a pair of round, walnut-sized salivary glands found below the jaw in the front of the neck. The gland releases both mucus and a thinner fluid, which aid the digestive process. Compare **sublingual gland, parotid gland.** See also **salivary gland.**

submaxillary duct. See **submandibular duct.**

submucous, beneath a mucous membrane.

subperiosteal fracture /sub′perē·os′tē·əl/, a break in a bone beneath the membrane that covers each bone.

subphrenic, referring to the area beneath or under the diaphragm.

subserous fascia, one of three kinds of connecting tissue, lying between the membranes lining the body spaces in much the same manner as the subcutaneous connecting tissue lies between the skin and the deep fascia. It is thin in some areas, as between the pleura and the chest wall, and thick in other areas, where it forms a pad of fat-storing tissue. Compare **deep fascia, subcutaneous fascia.**

substance, 1. any drug, chemical, or biological object. **2.** any material that can be taken or abused because of its effects on the body and mind.

substance abuse, the overuse of and addiction to a stimulant, depressant, or other chemical substance, leading to effects that are harmful to the patient's health, or the welfare of others.

substance P, a nerve-carrying substance made by the body and used to help the widening of the vessels and tightening of the intestines and other smooth muscles. It also plays a part in the release of saliva and urine, and it affects the function of the nervous systems.

substantivity, the ability of some substances to continue to have a therapeutic effect even after they are removed, as some shampoos.

substernal goiter, an enlargement of the thyroid gland, a portion of which is beneath the sternum.

substitution, a mental mechanism, operating in the unconscious, by which an unreachable or unacceptable goal, emotion, or object is replaced by one that is more reachable and acceptable.

substratum, any underlying layer; a foundation.

subsystem, a smaller part of a large system.

subthalamus, a portion of the brain that serves as a center for signals from the eye and eye spaces. Compare **epithalamus, hypothalamus, metathalamus, thalamus.** –**subthalamic,** *adj.*

subtle, not severe and having no serious results,

as a mild infection or swelling.

subungual /səbung′gwəl/, under a fingernail or toenail.

subungual hematoma, a collection of blood beneath a nail, usually resulting from injury. The pain accompanying this condition may be quickly eased by burning or drilling a small hole through the nail to release the blood.

succus /suk′əs/, *pl.* **succi** /suk′sī/, a juice or fluid, usually one released by an organ, as succus prostaticus of the prostate.

succussion splash /səkush′ən/, the sound gotten by shaking the body of a patient who has free fluid and air or gas in a hollow organ or body space. This sound may be heard over a normal stomach but may also be heard with hernias or blockages.

sucking blisters, the pale, soft pads on the upper and lower lips of a baby that look like blisters but are not. They form as soon as the baby begins to suck well, at the breast or on a bottle. They seem to improve the seal of the lips around the nipple or breast. Some babies are born with them, having sucked on their own fingers, hand, or arm before birth.

suckle, 1. to provide nourishment, specifically to breast feed. **2.** to take in as nourishment, especially by feeding from the breast.

suckling, an infant who has not been weaned.

Sucostrin, a trademark for a drug used in anesthesia (succinylcholine).

sucrose, sugar derived from sugar cane, sugar beets, and sorghum.

sucrose polyester (SPE), an artificial fat that, when added to the diet, lowers blood cholesterol levels by increasing the excretion of cholesterol in the feces. It is made to have the texture, taste, and consistency of regular margarine or vegetable oil and adds no calories to the diet.

suction, the removal of gas or fluid by lowering air pressure over its surface, usually by mechanical means.

suction curettage, a method of removing material from the womb by suction. Using local or light general anesthesia, the cervix is widened, a tube is inserted into the womb, and suction is applied. Also called **vacuum aspiration.** Compare **dilatation and curettage.**

suction drainage. See **drainage.**

suction lipectomy. See **liposuction.**

Sudafed, a trademark for a vessel-narrowing drug (pseudoephedrine hydrochloride), used as a decongestant and bronchodilator.

sudden infant death syndrome (SIDS), the unexpected and sudden death of a seemingly normal and healthy infant that occurs during sleep and with no physical evidence of disease. It is the most common cause of death in children between 2 weeks and 1 year of age, with an incidence rate of 1 in every 300 to 350 live births. The origin is unknown. Also called **cot**

Characteristics of SIDS

Factors	Occurrence
Incidence	1.5 to 2/1,000 live births
Peak age	2 to 4 months; 90% occur by 6 months
Sex	Higher percentage of males affected
Time of death	Usually during nighttime
Time of year	Increased incidence in winter
Birth	Higher incidence in: Premature infants Multiple births Neonates with low Apgar scores Infants with central nervous system disturbances
Feeding habits	Not significant; breast feeding does not prevent SIDS
Siblings	Ten times greater incidence
Possible causes	CNS anomaly Cardiovascular anomaly Airway anomaly Infection Chronic hypoxia

death, crib death. See also **parental grief.**

sudoriferous duct /sōō′dərif′ərəs/, a tube leading from a sweat gland to the surface of the skin. Also called **sweat duct.**

sudoriferous gland, one of about 3 million tiny structures within the skin that make sweat. The average quantity of sweat secreted in 24 hours varies from 700 to 900 g. The number of glands per square centimeter of skin varies in different parts of the body, the sudoriferous glands being very plentiful on the palms of the hands and on the soles of the feet and fewest in the neck and the back. They are completely absent in the deeper portions of the external auditory meatus, the prepuce, and the glans penis, and are more numerous in the fingers of Filipinos, Hindus, and black Americans than in the fingers of white Americans. Also called **sweat gland.** Compare **sebaceous gland.**

sudorific /sōō′dərif′ik/, 1. referring to a substance or condition, as heat or emotional tension, that causes sweating. 2. a sudorific drug. Also called **diaphoretic.**

suf-. See **sub-.**

Sufenta, a trademark for a pain-relieving drug (sufentanil citrate) given in the bloodstream.

sufentanil citrate, a pain-relieving drug given by injection into the bloodstream and used with general anesthetics.
★CAUTION: It can cause breathing problems and muscle stiffness. Drugs and equipment to reduce these effects should be available.
★ADVERSE EFFECTS: Among the more serious side effects are low blood pressure, high blood pressure, slowing of the heart beat, and stiffness of the chest wall.

suffocative goiter, an enlargement of the thyroid gland causing a feeling of suffocation on pressure.

suggestibility, referring to the likeliness of a person having his or her ideas or actions changed by the influence of others

suicidal, relating to tending toward killing one self.

suicide, 1. the intentional taking of one's own life. 2. a person who kills or tries to kill himself or herself. Early signs of suicidal intent include depression; expressions of guilt, tension, and nervousness; insomnia; loss of weight and appetite; neglect of personal appearance; and direct or indirect threats to commit suicide.

Suladyne, a trademark for an anti-infection drug containing antibacterials (sulfamethizole and sulfadiazine) and a urinary antiseptic (phenazopyridine hydrochloride).

sulcus centralis cerebri. See **fissure of Rolando.**

sulcus pulmonalis, a depression on each side of the spine that holds up part of the lung.

sulfa-, a combining form for sulfur-containing antibiotics (sulfonamide antimicrobials).

sulfacetamide /sul′fəset′əmīd/, an antibacteria drug used to protect against infection after injury to the eye and to treat certain eye diseases. It is also used to treat infections of the urinary system.
★CAUTION: Known allergy to the drug or to other sulfonamides, or kidney damage prohibits its use.
★ADVERSE EFFECTS: Among known side effects are local pain, growth of other bacteria, and an allergic reaction to the drug.

Sulfacet-R, a trademark for a drug containing a substance to prevent scabies (sulfur), an antibacteria drug (sulfacetamide sodium), and an antiseptic and cell-tightening substance (zinc oxide).

sulfachlorpyridazine /sul′fəklôr′pirid′əzēn/, an antibacteria drug. It is used to treat infection, particularly of the urinary tract.
★CAUTION: Porphyria, urinary tract blockage, or known allergy to this or to other sulfonamides prohibits its use.
★ADVERSE EFFECTS: Among the more serious side effects are crystalluria, severe allergic reactions, sensitivity to light, and blood disorders.

sulfacytine, an antibacteria drug. It is used to treat infection, particularly primary pyelonephritis and cystitis.
★CAUTION: Porphyria, urinary tract blockages, or known allergy to sulfonamides prohibits its use.
★ADVERSE EFFECTS: Among the more serious side effects are crystalluria, sensitivity to light, severe allergic reactions, and blood disorders.

sulfadiazine /sul′fədī′əzēn/, an antibacteria drug used to treat infections, mainly of the urinary tract, and to protect against rheumatic fever.
★CAUTION: Porphyria, urinary tract blockages, or known allergy to sulfonamides prohibits its use.

★ADVERSE EFFECTS: Among the more serious side effects are crystalluria, sensitivity to light, severe allergic reactions, and blood disorders.

sulfamethizole, an antibacteria drug. It is used to treat infection, particularly pyelonephritis, pyelitis, and cystitis.

★CAUTION: Porphyria, urinary tract blockages, or known allergy to sulfonamides prohibits its use.

★ADVERSE EFFECTS: Among the more serious side effects are crystalluria, sensitivity to light, blood disorders, and severe allergic reactions.

sulfamethoxazole, an antibacteria drug used to treat otitis media, bronchitis, and certain urinary tract infections.

★CAUTION: It is not given during the last 3 months of pregnancy, during breast feeding, or to children under 2 months of age. Known allergy to this drug or to other sulfonamides prohibits its use.

★ADVERSE EFFECTS: Among the more serious side effects are crystalluria and rash, fever, and other allergic reactions.

sulfamethoxazole and trimethoprim, an antibacteria drug. It is used to treat urinary tract infections, otitis media, and shigellosis.

★CAUTION: It is used with caution in patients with kidney and liver damage, or with known allergy to either drug or to sulfonamides. It is not for use in infants under 2 months of age or in the last 3 months of pregnancy.

★ADVERSE EFFECTS: Among the more serious side effects are crystalluria and rashes, fever, and other allergic reactions.

Sulfamylon, a trademark for an anti-infection drug (mafenide acetate).

sulfasalazine, a sulfonamide drug used to treat mild to moderate ulcerative colitis and as therapy in severe cases.

★CAUTION: Urinary blockage or known allergy to this drug, to other sulfonamide drugs, or to salicylates prohibits its use. It is not given during the last 3 months of pregnancy.

★ADVERSE EFFECTS: Among the more serious side effects are urine problems, blood diseases, and severe allergic reactions. Stomach symptoms and loss of appetite commonly occur.

sulfate lipidosis, an inherited fat metabolism disorder of childhood caused by a lack of an enzyme (cerebroside sulfatase). It results in an increase of fats in the tissues of the central nervous system, kidney, spleen, and other organs, leading to loss of mental abilities (dementia), paralysis, and death by the age of 10. Also called **metachromatic leukodystrophy.** See also **lipidosis.**

sulfhemoglobin, a form of hemoglobin containing a bound sulfur molecule that stops normal oxygen binding. It is present in the blood in small amounts.

sulfhemoglobinemia, the presence of abnormal sulfur-containing hemoglobin circulating in the blood.

sulfinpyrazone /sul'finpir'əzōn/, a drug used to aid in excreting uric acid in the urine. It is used to treat long-term gout and intermittent gouty arthritis.

★CAUTION: Peptic ulcer, ulcerative colitis, kidney failure, or known allergy to this drug or to phenylbutazone prohibits its use. It is not usually given during an acute attack of gout.

★ADVERSE EFFECTS: Among the more serious side effects are ulcers in the stomach and intestines, blood disorders, and dermatitis.

sulfisoxazole, an antibacteria drug. It is used to treat conjunctivitis and urinary tract infections, including vaginitis, cystitis, and pyelonephritis.

★CAUTION: Porphyria, urinary tract blockage, or known allergy to this drug or to sulfonamide drugs prohibits its use. It is not given during the last 3 months of pregnancy or to children under 2 months of age.

★ADVERSE EFFECTS: Among the more serious side effects are crystalluria, blood disorders, and severe allergy reactions.

sulfiting agents, food preservatives used in processing of beer, wine, baked goods, soup mixes, and some imported seafoods and by restaurants to impart a "fresh" appearance to salad fruits and vegetables. The chemicals can cause a severe reaction in persons who are allergic to sulfites. The reactions are marked by flushing, faintness, hives, headache, distress in the stomach and intestines, breathing difficulty, and, in extreme cases, loss of consciousness and death.

sulfobromophthalein /sul'fəbrō'məfthal'ēn,-ē·in/, a substance used in testing the function of the liver. See also **Bromsulphalein test.**

sulfonamide /səlfon'əmīd/, one of a large group of artificial drugs that are effective in treating infections.

sulfonates, a class of drugs (anticholinesterase compounds) affecting the nervous system and used as insect poisons.

sulfonylurea /sul'fənilyŏŏr'ē·ə/, an antidiabetes drug that causes the pancreas to make insulin. Allergy to sulfonamides prevents it from being used. Alcoholic drinks should not be taken while using this drug.

sulfoxone sodium, an antibiotic used to treat leprosy and dermatitis herpetiformis.

★CAUTION: Advanced kidney disease or known allergy to this drug prohibits its use.

★ADVERSE EFFECTS: Among the most serious side effects are anemia, skin disorders, and many blood diseases.

Sulfoxyl, a trademark for a drug containing a disinfectant (benzoyl peroxide) and a substance to prevent scabies (sulfur).

sulfur (S), a tasteless, odorless chemical element that is used to make sulfuric acid and used commercially in many industrial processes. Sulfur has been used to treat gout, rheumatism, and bronchitis and as a mild laxative. The sulfonamides, or sulfa drugs, are used to treat various bacteria infections. Also spelled **sulphur.**

sulfuric acid, a clear, colorless, oily, highly dangerous liquid that creates great heat when mixed with water. A very poisonous substance, sulfuric acid causes severe skin burns, blindness on contact with the eyes, serious lung damage if the vapors are breathed in, and death if it is eaten or drunk. In industry, sulfuric acid is used in the making of fertilizers, dyes, glue, and other acids, in the purifying of petroleum, and in the pickling of metals. Weak solutions of sulfuric acid are used to treat gastric hypoacidity and serious diarrhea. It was formerly called **oil of vitriol.**

sulindac, an antiswelling drug. It is used to treat osteoarthritis, rheumatoid arthritis, and ankylosing spondylitis.

Sulkowitch's test /sul′kəwichs/, a test of the urine for calcium. Also called **S's test.** See also **hypercalciuria.**

Sultrin, a trademark for a vaginal drug containing antibacterials (sulfathiazole, sulfacetamide, and sulfabenzamide).

Sumycin, a trademark for an antibiotic (tetracycline hydrochloride).

sunbath, the exposure of the naked body to the sun.

sunDare, a trademark for a sunscreen (cinoxate).

sundowning, a condition in which elderly patients tend to become confused at the end of the day. Many of them have trouble seeing and varying degrees of hearing loss. With less light, they lose visual cues that help them to make up for their sensory impairments.

sunrise syndrome, a condition of unstable mental ability on arising in the morning. Compare **sundowning.**

sunstroke, a condition caused by overexposure to the sun and marked by a high fever, convulsions, and coma. See also **heat hyperpyrexia.**

sup-. See **sub-.**

Supen, a trademark for an antibacteria drug (ampicillin).

super-, a combining form meaning 'above, or implying excess.'

superfecundation, the fertilization of two or more eggs released during one menstrual cycle by sperm from the same or different males during separate acts of sexual intercourse.

superfetation, the fertilization of a second egg after the onset of pregnancy, resulting in the presence of two fetuses of different degrees of maturity developing within the uterus at the same time. Also called **superimpregnation.**

superficial, 1. of or relating to the skin or another surface. 2. not grave or dangerous.

superficial fading infantile hemangioma, a superficial, short-term, salmon-colored patch in the center of the forehead, face, or back of the head of many newborns. It fades during the first 2 years of life, but it may temporarily deepen in color if the child becomes flushed or angry.

superficial inguinal node, a bump in one of the two groups of lymph glands in the upper thigh that supply the skin of the penis, scrotum, perineum, buttocks, and abdominal wall below the level of the navel. Compare **anterior tibial node, popliteal node.**

superficial reflex, any nerve reflex begun by stimulation of the skin. Kinds of superficial reflexes are **abdominal reflex, anal reflex,** and **cremasteric reflex.** Compare **deep tendon reflex.**

superficial sensation, the awareness of feelings in the superficial layers of the skin of touch, pressure, temperature, and pain. Compare **deep sensation.**

superficial spreading melanoma, a cancerous tumor that grows outward, spreading over the surface of the affected organ or tissue, most often on the lower legs of women and the torso of men. Occurring in late middle age, it is raised and easily felt, is usually unevenly colored, and has an irregular shape and unclear border. It is the most common of the three types of melanoma, occurring in nearly 70% of melanoma patients. See also **lentigo-maligna melanoma, nodular melanoma.**

superficial temporal artery, an artery at each side of the head that can be easily felt in front of the ear and is often used for taking the pulse. Compare **deep temporal artery, middle temporal artery.**

superficial vein, one of the many veins between the layers of tissue just under the skin. Compare **deep vein.**

superimpregnation. See **superfetation.**

superinfection, an infection occurring while treating another infection. It is often a result of change in the normal tissue favoring growth of some organisms by lowering the vitality and then the number of competing organisms, as yeast microbes flourish during penicillin therapy used to cure a bacterial infection.

superior, found above or higher, as the head is superior to the torso. Compare **inferior.**

superior conjunctival fornix, the space in the fold of the conjunctiva of the eye created by the reflection of the conjunctiva covering the eyeball and the lining of the upper lid. Compare **inferior conjuctival fornix.**

superior costotransverse ligament, one of five ligaments that help connect each rib to the spine. Compare **posterior costotransverse ligament.**

superior gastric node, a bump in one of two sets of stomach lymph glands. Compare **inferior gastric node.**

superior hemorrhagic polioencephalitis. See **Wernicke's encephalopathy.**

superior mediastinum, the top part of the space (mediastinum) in the middle of the chest, containing the windpipe, the throat, and the largest vein and artery of the heart. Compare **anterior mediastinum, middle mediastinum, posterior mediastinum.**

superior mesenteric artery, a large artery in the lower body that supplies blood to the small intestine and parts of the colon.

superior mesenteric node, a bump in one of the three groups of lymph nodes that serve the abdomen and the pelvis. Compare **gastric node, inferior mesenteric node.**

superior mesenteric vein, a branch of the vein that drains the blood from the small intestine, the cecum, and the colon. See also **portal vein.**

superior profunda artery. See **deep brachial artery.**

superior radioulnar joint. See **proximal radioulnar articulation.**

superior sagittal sinus, one of the six vein paths in the front of the membrane lining the skull (dura mater), draining blood from the brain. Compare **inferior sagittal sinus, straight sinus, transverse sinus.**

superior subscapular nerve /səbskap′yələr/, one of two small nerves on opposite sides of the body that supplies the top part of the muscle in the front of the shoulder. Compare **inferior subscapular nerve.**

superior thyroid artery, one of a pair of arteries in the neck that supplies the thyroid gland and several muscles in the head.

superior ulnar collateral artery, a long, slender division of the main artery of the upper arm.

superior vena cava, the second largest vein of the body, returning blood from the upper half of the body to the right chamber of the heart. It is about 2 cm in diameter and 7 cm long. Compare **inferior vena cava.**

supernumerary nipples, a larger than normal number of nipples, which are usually not linked with underlying glands. They may vary in size from small pink dots to that of normal nipples.

superoxide, a common reactive form of oxygen formed when an oxygen molecule gains a single electron. Superoxide molecules (radicals) can attack susceptible biological targets, including fats, proteins, and nucleic acids.

superoxide dismutase (SOD), an enzyme composed of metal-containing proteins that convert superoxide molecules (radicals) into less poisonous agents. It is the main enzyme for clearing superoxide radicals from the body.

supervision, (in psychology) a process whereby a therapist is helped to become more effective through the direction of a supervisor who provides theoretical knowledge, practical techniques, and support in working through problems.

supinate /soo′pənāt/, referring to lying flat on the back or turning the palm upward.

supination /soo′pinā′shən/, **1.** one of the kinds of turning allowed by certain joints, as the elbow and the wrist joints, which allow the palm of the hand to turn up. **2.** the position of lying on the back, face up. See also **supine.** Compare **pronation.** –**supinate,** v.

supinator longus. See **brachioradialis.**

supine /səpīn′, soo′pīn/, lying flat on the back. Compare **prone.** See also **body position.**

supine hypotension, a fall in blood pressure that occurs when a pregnant woman is lying on her back. It is caused by lessened vein flow that results from pressure of the heavy womb and fetus on the vena cava. Also called **vena caval syndrome.**

supporting area, any of the areas of the upper or lower jaw that are considered best able to bear the force of chewing with false teeth.

supportive treatment. See **treatment.**

suppository, an easily melted cone or cylinder of material mixed with a drug for placing in the rectum, urethra, or vagina. Drugs given in this way are absorbed into the system, and this route is especially useful in babies, in uncooperative patients, and in cases of vomiting or certain digestive disorders.

suppression amblyopia, a partial loss of sight, usually in one eye. It occurs commonly when the eyes are crossed (strabismus) and the weaker eye does not focus properly. Early detection is absolutely necessary because early treatment can improve the child's sight. It is useless after 6 years of age, and near blindness in the affected eye may result.

suppressor T cell. See **T cell.**

suppurate /sup′yərāt/, to make pus. –**suppuration,** n., **suppurative** /sup′yərā′tiv/, adj.

supra-, a combining form meaning 'above or over.'

supraclavicular, the area of the body above the clavicle, or collarbone.

supraclavicular nerve, one of a pair of nerves that run along the collarbone from the neck to the shoulder.

supracondylar fracture /soo′prəkon′dilər/, a certain kind of break at the big end of an arm or thigh bone.

supragingival calculus, a stony deposit, made up of various minerals, bits of food, and other matter found in the mouth, that forms on the teeth.

suprainfection, an unrelated infection usually caused in a patient weakened by another illness.

suprapubic, located above the pubic bone.

suprarenal, situated above the kidney.

suprascapular nerve /soo′prəskap′yələr/, one of a pair of nerves that run from the neck to the shoulder and shoulderblade.

suprasellar cyst. See **craniopharyngioma.**

suprasternal, referring to the area above the breastbone (sternum), next to the neck.

Surfacaine, a trademark for a local anesthetic (cyclomethycaine sulfate).

surface anesthesia. See **topical anesthesia.**

surface biopsy, the removal of living tissue for testing by scraping the surface of a sore or tumor. The method is used mainly to detect cancer of the cervix. See also **exfoliative cytology.**

surface therapy, a form of x-ray treatment given by placing a certain substance on or near a part of the skin.

surface thermometer, a device that takes and shows the temperature of the skin of any part of the body.

Surfadil, a trademark for a drug containing a substance to treat an allergy or a cold (methapyrilene hydrochloride) and an anesthetic (cyclomethycaine sulfate).

Surfak, a trademark for a drug used to soften feces (docusate calcium).

surfer's nodules, little bumps on the skin of the knees, ankles, feet, or toes of a surfer caused by repeated contact of the skin with a gritty, sandy surfboard. They will slowly get smaller and go away if surfing is stopped. When treatment is necessary, injection of steroids is usually helpful.

surgery, a branch of medicine concerned with diseases and injury needing an operation. –surgical, *adj.*

surgical abdomen. See **acute abdomen.**

surgical diathermy. See **electrocoagulation.**

surgical induction of labor. See **induction of labor.**

surgical ligature, an operation in which the gum is opened to allow a metal band to be placed around a tooth and then tiny chains fastened to the band are attached to a device that will help the tooth grow properly.

surgical microscope. See **operating microscope.**

surgical sectioning, a dental operation in which a tooth is broken into several pieces in order to make it easier to remove.

surgical treatment. See **treatment.**

Surital Sodium, a trademark for a barbiturate (thiamylal sodium), used as a general anesthetic.

Surmontil, a trademark for an antidepression drug (trimipramine maleate).

susceptibility, the condition of being more-than-normally likely to fall ill to a disease or disorder. –susceptible, *adj.*

suspension, a treatment, used mainly in disorders of the spine, consisting of hanging the patient by the chin and shoulders.

suspensory ligament of the lens. See **zonula ciliaris.**

sustained release. See **prolonged release.**

susto /sōō'tō/, a culture-bound syndrome found in Central American populations. It is related to stress from a person feeling that he or she has failed to fulfill sex-role expectations.

sutilains /sōō'tilānz/, an enzyme. It is used to treat certain wounds, ulcers, and second- and third-degree burns.

★CAUTION: Wounds opening into major body spaces, wounds containing exposed major nerves or nervous tissue, or certain types of ulcer prohibits its use. It is not given during pregnancy.

★ADVERSE EFFECTS: Among the more serious side effects are bleeding, paresthesias, and dermatitis.

sutura /sōōtōōr'ə/, *pl.* **suturae,** an immovable, fiberlike joint in which certain bones of the skull are connected by a thin layer of tissue. Compare **gomphosis, syndesmosis.**

sutura dentata, an immovable fiberlike joint that is one kind of true suture in which toothlike processes interlock along the margins of connecting bones of the skull. Compare **sutura limbosa, sutura serrata.**

sutura limbosa, an immovable fiberlike joint that is one kind of true suture in which curved and jagged edges of certain connecting bones of the skull, as the parietal and temporal bones, overlap and interlock. Compare **sutura dentata, sutura serrata.**

sutura plana, a fibrous joint that is one kind of false suture in which rough, contiguous edges of certain bones of the skull, as the maxillae, form a connection. Compare **sutura squamosa.**

sutura serrata, an immovable fibrous joint that is one kind of true suture in which connecting bones interlock along serrated edges that resemble fine-toothed saws. Compare **sutura dentata, sutura limbosa.**

sutura squamosa, an immovable fibrous joint that is one kind of false suture in which overlapping, beveled edges unite certain bones of the skull, as the temporal and the parietal bone. Compare **sutura plana.**

suture /sōō'chər/, **1.** a border or a joint, as between the bones of the cranium. **2.** to stitch together cut or torn edges of tissue with suture material. **3.** a surgical stitch taken to repair a cut, tear, or wound. **4.** material used for surgical stitches, as absorbable or nonabsorbable silk, catgut, wire, or synthetic material.

Sv, abbreviation for **sievert.**

swab, a stick or clamp for holding absorbent gauze or cotton, used for washing, cleansing, or drying a body surface, for collecting a specimen for laboratory tests, or for applying a topical medication.

swamp fever. See **leptospirosis, malaria.**

swanneck deformity, a defect of the kidney tubules linked with rickets.

sweat. See **perspiration.**

sweat bath, a bath given to induce sweating.

sweat duct, any one of the tiny little tubes carrying sweat to the surface of the skin from about 2 million sweat glands throughout the body. The sweat ducts in the armpits and in the groin are larger than in other parts of the body.

Ducts and sweat glands are found in great numbers on the palms of the hands and the soles of the feet.

sweat gland. See **sudoriferous gland.**

sweating. See **diaphoresis.**

sweat test, a method for measuring sodium and chloride released from the sweat glands, often the first test performed to detect cystic fibrosis. The sweat glands are made to work with a drug, and the sweat that results is tested. The test is very trustworthy and although it may be useful at any age, it is usually done on infants from 2 weeks to 1 year of age. See also **cystic fibrosis.**

Sweet localization method, a type of x-ray test used to find a foreign body in the eye by making two x-ray films of the eye while the patient's head is held still.

Swift's disease. See **acrodynia.**

swimmer's ear, infection of the ear carried in the water of a swimming pool.

swimmer's itch, an allergic skin condition caused by sensitivity to schistosome cercarias that die under the skin, leading to reddening of the skin, the appearance of wheals, and a rash lasting 1 or 2 days. Treatment usually includes antihistamines by mouth and antipruritic lotions. See also **schistosomiasis.**

swimming pool conjunctivitis. See **pharyngoconjunctival fever.**

sy-. See **syn-.**

sycosis barbae /sikō′sis/, a swelling of hair follicles of skin that has been shaved. Treatment includes light and infrequent shaving, antibiotics, and daily plucking of infected hairs. Also called **barber's itch, sycosis vulgaris.**

Sydenham's chorea /sid′ənhamz/, a form of chorea, a disorder marked by uncontrolled jerking of the arm and face muscles, linked with rheumatic fever, usually occurring during childhood. The cause is a streptococcal infection of the tissues of the brain. The choreic movements increase over the first 2 weeks, reach a plateau, and then diminish. The child is usually well within 10 weeks. With undue exertion or emotional strain, the condition may recur. Also called **chorea minor, rheumatic chorea.**

syl-. See **syn-.**

sylvatic plague, a native disease of wild rodents caused by *Yersinia pestis* and may be carried to humans by the bite of an infected flea. It is found on every continent except Australia. See also **bubonic plague.**

sym-. See **syn-.**

symbiotic phase, in Mahler's system of development, the stage between 1 and 5 months when the infant participates in a close association ("symbiotic orbit") with the mother. All parts of the mother, including voice, gestures, clothing, and space in which she moves, are joined with the infant.

symelus. See **symmelus.**

symmelia, a defect of the fetus marked by the growing together of the lower limbs with or without feet. Kinds of symmelia are **apodial symmelia, dipodial symmelia, monopodial symmelia,** and **tripodial symmelia.**

symmelus /sim′ələs/, a deformed fetus marked by symmelia. Also spelled **symelus.**

Symmer's disease. See **giant follicular lymphoma.**

Symmetrel, a trademark for an antivirus drug (amantadine hydrochloride).

symmetric, (of the body or parts of the body) equal in size or shape; very similar in placement about an axis. Also **symmetrical. Compare asymmetric. −symmetry,** *n.*

symmetric lipomatosis. See **nodular circumscribed lipomatosis.**

symmetric tonic neck reflex, a normal response in infants to get into the crawl position by pushing with the arms and bending the knees when the head and neck are raised. The reflex disappears when the development of the nerves and muscles allow real crawling. Also called **crawling reflex.** See also **tonic neck reflex.**

sympathectomy /sim′pəthek′təmē/, an operation, done using local anesthetic, to ease long-term pain in certain vessel diseases, as arteriosclerosis, claudication, Buerger's disease, and Raynaud's phenomenon. The sheath around an artery carries the sympathetic nerve fibers that control tightening of the vessel. Removing part of the sheath causes the vessel to relax and expand and allows more blood to pass through it. The operation may also be done with a graft, to increase the blood flow through the graft area.

sympathetic amine, a drug that causes effects that look like those made normally by the sympathetic nervous system.

sympathetic nervous system. See **autonomic nervous system.**

sympathetic ophthalmia, a swelling of parts of the eye that causes grainy, fiberlike bumps to form. It occurs in one eye after the other has already been infected by an injury. Steroids may be helpful in treatment, but it may be necessary to remove the eye that was injured to save the other eye. Also called **metastatic ophthalmia, migratory ophthalmia.**

sympathetic trunk, one of a pair of chains of nerve bunches that lie along the side of the vertebral column from the base of the skull to the tailbone. Each trunk is part of the sympathetic nervous system and consists of a series of ganglia connected by cords containing various types of fibers.

sympathizing eye, (in sympathetic ophthalmia) the uninfected eye that becomes infected by the spread of harmful germs.

sympatholytic, sympatholytic agent. See **antiadrenergic.**

sympathomimetic /sim'pəthōmimet'ik/, a drug that causes effects that look like those caused by the sympathetic nervous system. Various sympathomimetic drugs are used as decongestants of the mucous membranes of the nose and eyes. It is also used to treat asthma and other lung diseases and to treat low blood pressure and shock. Side effects may be nervousness, severe headache, anxiety, vertigo, nausea, vomiting, widened pupils, and certain urine disorders. Also called **adrenergic.**

sympathomimetic bronchodilator, a medication that reduces bronchial muscle spasms because of action like that of the sympathetic nervous system in relaxing smooth muscle.

symphalangia /sim'fəlan'jē·ə/, **1.** a condition, usually inherited, marked by the fingers or toes being stiff and joined together. **2.** a birth defect in which webbing of the fingers or toes occurs in varying degrees, often along with other defects of the hands or feet. Also called **symphalangism.** See also **syndactyly.**

symphocephalus, twin fetuses joined at the head. The term is often used as a general term for fetuses with varying degrees of the defect. See also **cephalothoracopagus, craniopagus, syncephalus.**

symphyseal angle /simfiz'ē·əl/, (in dentistry) the angle of the chin, which may be striking out, straight, or receding, according to type.

symphysic teratism, a birth defect in which there is a fusion of normally separated parts or organs, as a horseshoe kidney, or in which parts close prematurely, as the skull bones in craniostenosis.

symphysis /sim'fəsis/, pl. **symphyses** /-ēz/, **1.** also called **fibrocartilaginous joint;** a joint made of cartilage in which bony surfaces lying next to one another are firmly united by fiber-like cartilage. **2.** pubic symphysis. **–symphysic,** adj.

symphysis pubis. See **pubic symphysis.**

sympodia /simpō'dē·ə/, a birth defect marked by fusion of the lower extremities. See also **sirenomelus, sympus.**

symptom, something felt or noticed by the patient that can help to detect a disease or disorder. Compare **sign.**

symptomatic esophageal peristalsis, a condition in which the series of contractions (peristalsis) in the body of the throat (esophagus) is normal, but contractions near the stomach are increased in strength and length. Also called **esophageal spasm, nutcracker esophagus.**

symptomatic nanism, dwarfism linked with defects in bone growth, tooth formation, and sexual development.

symptomatic treatment. See **treatment.**

symptom-bearer, (in psychology) a family member frequently seen as the patient who functions poorly because family behavior interferes with functioning at a higher level.

symptothermal method of family planning, a natural method of family planning that incorporates the ovulation and basal body temperature methods of family planning. It is safer than either method used alone and requires fewer days of avoiding sexual intercourse, because it enables the fertile period of the menstrual cycle to be more exactly determined.

sympus /sim'pəs/, a deformed fetus in which the legs are completely grown together or twisted and the pelvis and genitals are defective. Kinds of sympuses are **sirenomelus, sympus dipus,** and **sympus monopus.** See also **symmelus.**

sympus apus. See **sirenomelus.**

sympus dipus /dē'pəs/, a deformed fetus in which the legs are grown together and both feet are formed.

sympus monopus /mon'əpəs/, a deformed fetus in which the legs are grown together and one foot is formed. Also called **monopodial symmelia, uromelus.**

syn-, sy-, syl-, sym-, a combining form meaning 'with, together, or at the same time.'

synadelphus /sin'ədel'fəs/, pl. **synadelphi,** a conjoined twin fetal monster with a single head and trunk and eight limbs. Also called **syndelphus, cephalothoracoiliopagus.**

Synalar, a trademark for a nerve-blocking drug (fluocinolone acetonide).

Synanon, a residential center that provides a therapeutic community approach to rehabilitation for drug abusers.

synapse /sin'aps/, **1.** the point where one nerve signal jumps from one nerve cell to another. Normally, nerve signals only travel in one direction; they are also subject to fatigue, oxygen deficiency, anesthetics, and other chemical agents. Kinds of synapses include **axoaxonic synapse, axodendritic synapse, axodendrosomatic synapse, axosomatic synapse,** and **dendrodendritic synapse.** Compare **ephapse. 2.** to form a synapse or connection between nerve cells. **–synaptic,** adj.

synarthrosis. See **fibrous joint.**

syncephalus /sinsef'ələs/, a conjoined twin monster having a single head and two bodies. Also called **monocephalus.**

synchilia /singkē'lē·ə/, a birth defect in which the lips are partly or totally grown together. Also spelled **syncheilia.**

synchronized intermittent mandatory ventilation (SIMV), periodic assisted mechanical breaths occurring at preset intervals when the patient makes an effort to inhale that is sensed by the breathing machine (ventilator). The patient breathes on his or her own between the assisted breaths. The machine will provide a mechanical breath if the patient fails to breathe within a set time.

syncopal attack /sing'kəpəl/, any period of un-

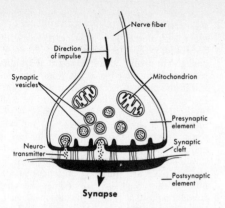

Synapse

consciousness or fainting, especially one linked with fear or pain. Many patients, especially men, suffer such attacks during violent coughing spells because of rapid changes in blood pressure. Syncopal attacks also occur as the result of any of a number of heart and lung disorders.

syncope /sing′kəpē/, a fainting spell. It usually follows a feeling of lightheadedness and may often be prevented by lying down or by sitting with the head between the knees. It may be caused by many different factors, including emotional stress, pooling of blood in the legs, heavy sweating, or sudden change in room temperature or body position.

syndactylus, a person with webbed fingers or toes.

syndactyly /sindak′təlē/, a birth defect marked by the growing together of the fingers or toes. It varies in degree of severity from partial webbing of the skin of two digits to complete union of the fingers or toes and the growing together of the bones and nails. Also called **syndactylia, syndactylism. –syndactyl, syndactylous,** adj.

syndelphus. See **synadelphus.**

syndrome, a group of signs and symptoms that occur together and are typical of a particular disorder or disease. See also specific syndromes.

syndrome of inappropriate antidiuretic hormone secretion (SIADH), an abnormal condition marked by a release of too much of a certain hormone that creates an imbalance in the body. It is linked with certain cancers of the lung. Common signs and symptoms of SIADH are weight gain despite loss of appetite, vomiting, nausea, muscle weakness, and irritability. In some patients, SIADH may cause coma and convulsions.

synechia /sinek′ē·ə/, pl. **synechiae,** an adhesion, especially of the iris to the cornea or lens of the eye. It may develop from glaucoma, cataracts, uveitis, or keratitis or as a complication of surgery or injury to the eye. Synechiae may

soon lead to blindness. Immediate treatment consists of widening the pupils with a certain solution, followed by treatment of the underlying cause.

Synemol, a trademark for a nerve-blocking drug (fluocinolone acetonide).

synergistic agent, a substance that assists or adds to the activity of another substance or agent.

synergistic muscles, groups of muscles that act together to accomplish the same body movement.

Synkayvite, a trademark for an artificial form of vitamin K (menadiol sodium diphosphate).

synophthalmia. See **cyclopia.**

Synophylate, a trademark for a bronchodilator (theophylline sodium glycinate).

synostotic joint /sin′ostot′ik/, a joint in which bones are joined to bones and there is no movement between them, as in the large triangular bone (sacrum) at the back of the pelvis or the bones of the adult skull.

synotia /sīnō′shə/, a birth defect marked by the drawing together of the ears in front of the neck, often with the absence of the lower jaw. Compare **agnathia.** See also **otocephaly.**

synotus /sīnō′təs/, a fetus with synotia.

synovectomy, the cutting out of a synovial membrane of a joint.

synovia /sinō′vē·ə/, a clear, sticky fluid, resembling the white of an egg, released by synovial membranes and acting as a lubricant for many joints, bursae, and tendons. It contains mucin, albumin, fat, and mineral salts. Also called **synovial fluid. –synovial,** adj.

synovial bursa, one of the many closed sacs filled with synovial fluid in the connecting tissue between the muscles, the tendons, the ligaments, and the bones. The synovial bursae make the gliding of muscles and tendons over bones easier. Compare **synovial membrane, synovial tendon sheath.**

synovial crypt, a pouch in the synovial membrane of a joint.

synovial fluid. See **synovia.**

synovial joint, a freely movable joint in which touching bony surfaces are covered by cartilage and connected by ligaments lined with synovial membrane. Kinds of synovial joints are **ball-and-socket joint, condyloid joint, gliding joint, hinge joint, pivot joint, saddle joint,** and **uniaxial joint.** Also called **diarthrosis.** Compare **cartilaginous joint, fibrous joint.**

synovial membrane, the inner layer of a capsule surrounding a freely movable joint. The synovial membrane secretes into the joint a thick fluid that normally oils the joint but that may collect in painful amounts when the joint is injured. Compare **synovial bursa, synovial tendon sheath.**

synovial sarcoma, a cancerous tumor that begins as a soft swelling and often spreads through the bloodstream to the lung before it is discovered.

synovitis /sin′əvī′tis/, a swelling condition of the synovial membrane of a joint as the result of a wound or an injury, as a sprain or severe strain. The knee is most commonly affected. Fluid collects, the joint is swollen, tender, and painful, and motion is limited. In most cases, the swelling goes down, and the fluid is absorbed without medical or surgical treatment.

syntax, the rules of language governing the arrangement of words into phrases, clauses, or sentences.

synthetic, of or relating to a substance that is artificial instead of natural.

synthetic oleovitamin D. See **viosterol.**

Synthroid, a trademark for a thyroid hormone (levothyroxine sodium).

Syntocinon, a trademark for a drug used to speed up childbirth (oxytocin).

syphilis, a sexually carried disease caused by a type of bacteria *(Treponema pallidum),* marked by three clear stages over a period of years. Any organ system may become involved. The bacteria are able to pass into a fetus in the womb, causing syphilis in the newborn at birth. The first stage **(primary syphilis)** is marked by the appearance of a small, painless, red pus-forming bump on the skin or mucous membrane between 10 and 90 days after exposure. The sore may appear anywhere on the body where contact with a sore on an infected person has occurred, but is seen most often in the pelvic region. It quickly wears away, forming a painless, bloodless ulcer, called a chancre, releasing a fluid that swarms with bacteria. The chancre may not be noticed by the patient, and many people may become infected. It heals by itself within 10 to 40 days, often creating the mistaken impression that the sore was not a serious event. The second stage **(secondary syphilis)** occurs about 2 months later, after the bacteria have increased in number and spread throughout the body. This stage is marked by general malaise, loss of appetite, nausea, fever, headache, hair loss, bone and joint pain, or the appearance of a rash that does not itch, flat white sores in the mouth and throat, or pimples on the moist areas of the skin. The disease remains highly contagious at this stage and can be spread by kissing. The symptoms usually continue for from 3 weeks to 3 months but may recur over 2 years. The third stage **(tertiary syphilis)** may not develop for 3 to 15 or more years. It is marked by the appearance of soft, rubbery tumors, called gummas, that fester and heal by scarring. Gummas may develop anywhere on the surface of the body and in the eye, liver, lungs, stomach, or sexual organs. Tertiary syphilis may be painless, unnoticed except for gummas, or it may be accompanied by deep, burrowing pain. The ulceration of the gummas may result in punched-out areas of the palate, nasal septum, or larynx. Various

tissues and structures of the body, including the central nervous system, and the wall and the valves of the heart may be damaged or destroyed, leading to mental or physical disorders and premature death. **Congenital syphilis** resulting from infection in the womb may result in the birth of a deformed or blind infant. In some cases, the infant appears to be well until, at several weeks of age, snuffles, sometimes with a bloodstained discharge, and skin sores are observed, particularly on the palms and soles or in the genital region. Such children may also have visual or hearing defects, and early old age (progeria) and poor health may develop. Syphilis is sometimes detected from blood tests, but often the only evidence is the patient's report that he or she has been exposed. The disease may be treated with antibiotics in the first and second stages. It is also very important to tell the doctor about any sexual partners who have been exposed to syphilis so that they can be treated. In many states, active cases of syphilis must, by law, be reported to the Department of Health. See also **chancre, Hutchinson's teeth, Hutchinson's triad, snuffles.**

syphilitic aortitis, a swelling condition of the aorta, occurring in tertiary syphilis and marked by widespread widening with gray, wheal-like plaques containing calcium on the inner coat and scars and wrinkles on the outer coat. There may be damage to the valves, narrowing of the mouths of the arteries, and the formation of blood clots. Cerebral embolism may result. Signs of syphilitic aortitis are pain in the middle of the chest, shortness of breath, bounding pulse, and high blood pressure. Penicillin may slow the disease, but it cannot heal the damage to the vessels and the heart. Also called **Döhle-Heller disease, Heller-Döhle disease, luetic aortitis.**

syphilitic meningoencephalitis. See **general paresis.**

syphilitic periarteritis, a swelling condition of the outer coat of one or more arteries occurring in tertiary syphilis. Also called **periarteritis gummosa.** See also **syphilitic aortitis.**

syringe, a device for withdrawing, injecting, or instilling fluids. Kinds include **asepto syringe, bulb syringe, hypodermic syringe, Luer-Lok syringe, tuberculin syringe.**

syringomyelocele /siring′gōmī′əlōsēōsēl′/, a condition in which a section of the spinal cord sticks out through a hole, present at birth, in the spinal column. It forms a fluid-filled sac. See also **myelomeningocele, neural tube defect, spina bifida.**

syrup of ipecac, a preparation of ipecac fluid, glycerin, and syrup used to produce vomiting to treat certain types of poisonings and drug overdoses. See also **ipecac.**

system, a collection of parts that make a whole. Systems of the body, as the cardiovascular or reproductive systems, are made up of structures specially adapted to perform functions necessary for life.

systematic heating, the raising of the temperature of the whole body.

system documentation. See **documentation.**

systemic /sistem′ik/, of or relating to the whole body rather than to a single area or part of the body.

systemic lupus erythematosus (SLE), a long-term swelling disease affecting many systems of the body. The disease includes severe swelling of the blood vessels, kidney disorders, and tumors of the skin and nervous system. The cause of the disease is not known. Four times more women than men have SLE. Also called **disseminated lupus erythematosus, lupus erythematosus.** The first sign is often arthritis. A red rash over the nose and cheeks, weakness, fatigue, and weight loss are also often seen early in the disease. Sensitivity to light, fever, skin sores on the neck and loss of hair where the sores reach beyond the hairline may occur. The skin sores may spread to the mucous membranes and other tissues of the body. They cause wasting of the tissues affected. Depending on the organs involved, the patient may also have glomerulonephritis, pleuritis, pericarditis, peritonitis, neuritis, or anemia. Kidney failure and severe nerve dis orders are among the most serious results of the disease. In many cases SLE may be controlled with steroid medication given for the whole body. Care and treatment vary with the severity and nature of the disease and the body systems that are affected. Topical steroids may be applied to the rash; salicylates may be given to ease pain and swelling in the joints. Fatigue and stress are avoided, and all body surfaces are protected from direct sunlight. Antimalarial drugs are sometimes given to treat skin sores, but eye damage may occur with continued use.

systemic remedy, a substance that is given by mouth, or placed in the intestines or rectum to be absorbed into the bloodstream for treatment of a health problem. Drugs systemically may have various local effects, but the intent is to treat the whole body.

systemic vein, one of a number of veins that drain deoxygenated blood from most of the body. They are larger and more numerous than the arteries, have thinner walls, and collapse when they are empty. Groups of systemic veins include the heart veins.

systole /sis′tǝlē/, the tightening of the heart, driving blood into the aorta and lung arteries. The systole is heard as the first heart beat and felt as the peripheral pulse.

systolic murmur, a heart murmur occurring during systole. Systolic murmurs are generally less meaningful than diastolic murmurs and are found in many people with no sign of heart disease. Systolic murmurs include ejection murmurs often heard in pregnancy or in patients with anemia, thyroid disease, or heart and lung disease. Pansystolic murmurs are heard in patients with heart valve defects.

systolic pressure, the blood pressure measured during contraction of the heart (systole). In blood pressure readings, it is normally the higher of the two measurements.

T

T, 1. symbol for **temperature.** 2. abbreviation for *tumor.* See **cancer staging.**

T₁, T₂. See **relaxation time.**

TA, abbreviation for **transactional analysis.**

ta-. See **tono-.**

tabe-, a combining form meaning 'of or referring to wasting (away).'

tabes dorsalis, an abnormal condition marked by the slow breakdown of all or part of the body and the progressive loss of reflexes at the outer part of the body. This disease involves the spinal cord. It destroys the large joints of affected limbs in some individuals. It is often seen with the inability to control the release functions of the body (incontinence) and impotence. Severe flashing pains in the stomach and the extremities also occur. The cause of tabes dorsalis is unclear. It is believed to be an uncommon disorder. Some surveys have indicated that about 10% of individuals with late syphilis and 40% of those with clinical neurosyphilis have tabes dorsalis.

tablet, a small, solid dose form of a drug. It may be pressed or molded in its manufacture. It may be of almost any size, shape, weight, and color. Most tablets are meant to be swallowed whole. However, some may be dissolved in the mouth, chewed, or dissolved in liquid before swallowing. Some may be placed in a body cavity.

taboo, something that is forbidden by a society as unacceptable and improper. Incest is a taboo common to many societies.

tabula rasa /tä′bo̅o̅lä rä′sä, tab′yəle rä′sə/, a term used to describe a child's mind at birth as a receptive "blank slate."

Tacaryl, a trademark for an antihistamine (methdilazine).

TACE, a trademark for female hormone (chlorotrianisene).

tache noir /täshnô·är′/, a circular, open sore marking the point of infection in certain diseases, as African tick typhus and scrub typhus.

tacho-, a combining form meaning 'of or referring to speed.'

tachy-, a combining form meaning 'swift or rapid.'

tachycardia /tak′ikär′dē·ə/, an abnormal condition in which the heart (myocardium) contracts regularly but at a rate greater than 100 beats per minute. The heart rate normally speeds up in response to fever, exercise, or nervous excitement. Pathological tachycardia goes along with lack of oxygen (anoxia), as caused by anemia, congestive heart failure, bleeding, or shock. A slow heart beat (bradycardia) develops because the heart muscle gets too-little oxygen and cannot maintain the sped-up pace. Tachycardia acts to increase the amount of oxygen given to the cells of the body by increasing the amount of blood circulated through the vessels.

tachykinin. See **substance P.**

tachyphylaxis /tak′əfəlak′sis/, 1. (in pharmacology) an event in which the repeated use of some drugs results in a marked decrease in effectiveness. 2. also called **mithridatism.** (in immunology) rapidly developing resistance to a toxin because of previous exposure, as from previous injection of small amounts of the toxin.

tachypnea /tak′ipnē′ə/, an abnormally rapid rate of breathing, as seen with too-high body temperature (hyperpyrexia). See also **respiratory rate.**

tact-, a combining form meaning 'of or referring to touch.'

-tactic, -tactical, -taxic, 1. a combining form meaning 'displaying agent-controlled orientation or movement.' 2. a combining form meaning 'having an arrangement of something.'

tactile /tak′təl/, of or referring to the sense of touch.

tactile anesthesia, the absence or lack of the sense of touch in the fingers. It can possibly result from injury or disease. This condition can be inborn or psychosomatic. It may cause the patient to get severe burns, serious cuts, bruises, or scraped areas. See also **traumatic anesthesia.**

tactile corpuscle, any one of many small, oval end organs linked to the sense of touch. They are widely distributed throughout the body in outer areas, as the hand and foot, front of the forehead, skin of the lips, mucous membrane of the tongue, eyelid, and skin of the nipples of the breasts. Each corpuscle is made up of a tiny, round structure. It is surrounded by a capsule penetrated by a nerve fiber that spirals through the inside of the capsule and ends in global-shaped enlargements. Also called **Meissner's corpuscle.**

tactile corpuscle of Meissner. See **Wagner-Meissner corpuscle.**

tactile defensiveness, an abnormal reaction to touch in which some sensations cause extreme emotional reactions, hyperactivity, or other behavior problems.

tactile fremitus, a shaking vibration of the chest wall during breathing. It can be felt on physical examination. It may indicate swelling, infection, congestion, or, most commonly, hardening of a lung or a part of a lung due to fluid in the lung.

tactile image, a mental concept of an object as perceived through the sense of touch. See also **image.**

Taenia /tē'nē·ə/, a genus of large, parasitic, intestinal flatworm of the family Taeniidae, class Cestoda. Taeniae are among the most common parasites infecting humans and include *Taenia saginata,* the beef tapeworm, and *T. solium,* the pork tapeworm.

taenia-. See **tenia-.**

Taenia saginata, a species of tapeworm. It is in the tissues of cattle during its larval stage. It infects the intestine of humans in its adult form. *Taenia saginata* may grow to a length of between 12 and 25 feet. It is the tapeworm species that most often infects humans. Also called **beef tapeworm.** See also **tapeworm, tapeworm infection.**

taeniasis /tēnī'əsis/, an infection with a tapeworm of the genus *Taenia.* See also **tapeworm infection.**

Taenia solium, a species of tapeworm that most commonly inhabits the tissues of pigs during its larval stage. It infects the intestine of humans in its adult form. Humans will sometimes serve as the intermediate hosts for this tapeworm. Larval infestation of the muscle and brain tissue may occur. Also called **pork tapeworm.** See also **cysticercosis, tapeworm, tapeworm infection.**

Tagamet, a trademark for a histamine H_2 receptor antagonist (cimetidine).

taijin kyofu, a culturally patterned fear of meeting people, observed in some areas of Japan.

tail bud. See **end bud.**

tail fold, a curved ridge formed at the tail end of the early developing embryo. It is made up of the tail bud, which in lower animals gives rise to the tail appendage. In human forms it gives rise mainly to the colon.

tail of Spence, the upper outer tail of breast tissue that extends into the armpit.

tailor's bottom. See **weaver's bottom.**

tailor's bunion. See **bunionette.**

Takayasu's arteritis /tä'kəyä'sŌōz/, a disorder marked by progressive closure of several arteries having their origin in the aortic arch (carotid arteries). Signs of the disorder are absence of a pulse in both arms and in the carotid arteries. Other signs are temporary paralysis of the lower part of the body (paraplegia), temporary blindness, and wasting of facial muscles. Also called **brachiocephalic arteritis, Martorell's syndrome, pulseless disease, reversed coarctation.**

talbutal, a barbiturate sedative-hypnotic. It is given as a sleeping drug (hypnotic) to treat the inability to sleep (insomnia).

★CAUTION: Previous addiction to sedative-hypnotics, porphyria, blocked liver function, or known allergy to this drug or to other barbiturates prohibits its use.

★ADVERSE EFFECTS: Among the more serious side effects are lowered breathing, drug hangover, allergic reactions, porphyria, and physical dependence.

talip-, a combining form meaning 'clubfooted.'

talipes /tal'ipēz/, a deformity of the foot. It is usually inherited. The foot is twisted and relatively fixed in an abnormal position. Talipes refers to deformities that involve the foot and ankle. Pes refers only to a deformity of the foot. Kinds of talipes include **talipes calcaneovalgus, talipes calcaneovarus, talipes equinovarus.** See also **pes cavus, pes planus.**

talipes calcaneovalgus. See **clubfoot.**

talipes cavus. See **pes cavus.**

talipes equinovarus. See **clubfoot.**

talo-, a combining form meaning 'of or referring to the ankle.'

talus /tā'ləs/, *pl.* **tali,** the second largest bone of the ankle. It is made up of a body, neck, and head. Also called **ankle bone, astragalus.**

Talwin, a trademark for a painkiller (pentazocine).

tamoxifen /təmok'səfin/, a cancer drug that counters the effects of a female hormone (estrogen). It is used to relieve advanced breast cancer in premenopausal and postmenopausal women whose tumors are estrogen-dependent.

tampon, a pack of cotton, a sponge, or other material. Its purpose is checking bleeding or absorbing fluids in cavities or canals or holding displaced organs in position.

tamponade /tam'pənād'/, stoppage of the flow of blood to an organ or a part of the body by pressure, as by a tampon or a pressure dressing applied to stop a bleeding.

tangentiality, a disturbance in association. It is marked by a tendency to step away from an original topic of conversation. Tangentiality can destroy or seriously block the ability of people to communicate effectively.

tangible elements, objects that can be seen or touched.

Tangier disease /tanjir'/, a rare lack of high-density lipoproteins. It runs in families. It is marked by low blood cholesterol and an abnormal orange or yellow discoloration of the tonsils and throat. There may also be large lymph nodes, liver, and spleen, muscle wasting, and disturbances of the peripheral nervous system (peripheral neuropathy). No specific treatment is known.

tannin, any of a group of substances that cause contractions. It comes from plants and is used for the tanning of leather. Tannic acid, a mixture of tannins, is used in the treatment of burns.

tanning, a process in which the color of the skin deepens as a result of exposure to ultraviolet light. Skin cells with dark pigment (melanin) darken immediately. New melanin is formed within 2 to 3 days. It moves upward rapidly. This allows the darkening process to continue.

tantalum (Ta), a silvery metallic element. Its atomic number is 73; its atomic weight is 180.95. Tantalum is used in prosthetic devices, as skull plates and wire sutures.

tantrum, a sudden outburst or violent display of rage, frustration, and bad temper. It usually occurs in a poorly adjusted child and certain emotionally disturbed persons. The activity is usually not directed at anyone or anything specific but toward the environment in general. It is used mainly as an attempt to control others and the surroundings. Also called **temper tantrum.**

TAO, a trademark for an antibacterial (troleandomycin).

tapeworm, a parasitic intestinal worm. It belongs to the class Cestoda. Humans usually get tapeworms by eating the undercooked meat of intermediate hosts infected with the larval form of the tapeworm. In the human food canal, the worm develops into an adult with an attaching head and numerous segments. Each of the segments can produce eggs. Kinds of tapeworm include *Diphyllobothrium latum, Taenia saginata, Taenia solium.* Also called **cestode.**

tapeworm infection, an intestinal infection by one of several species of parasitic worms. It is caused by eating raw or undercooked meat infested with a tapeworm or its larvae. Tapeworms live as larvae in one or more vertebrate intermediate hosts. They grow to adulthood in the intestine of humans. Symptoms of intestinal infection with adult worms are usually mild or absent. However, diarrhea, stomach pain, and weight loss may occur. Diagnosis is made when eggs or portions of the adult worm are passed in the stool. The drugs niclosamide and quinacrine are used to loosen and dissolve the worm so that it may be released. Sanitary disposal of fecal material from affected patients is needed to prevent the passage of larvae or eggs to humans or other hosts. Certain species of tapeworm can infect humans during the larval stage. This causes a serious condition of larval infestation, often with lumps (cysts). Also called **cestodiasis.** See also **cysticercosis, tapeworm.**

tapho-, a combining form meaning 'of or referring to the grave.'

tapotement /täpôtmäN′/, a type of massage in which the body is tapped in a rhythmic manner with the tips of the fingers or the sides of the hands. Short, rapid, repetitive movements are used. The procedure is often used on the chest wall of patients with swelling of the bronchi (bronchitis) to help loosen the mucus in the air passages. See also **massage.**

Taractan, a trademark for a tranquilizer (chlorprothixene).

tardive dyskinesia /tär′div/, an abnormal condition with involuntary, repetitious movements of the muscles of the face, the limbs, and the trunk. This disorder most commonly affects older people who have been treated for extended periods with phenothiazine drugs to alleviate the symptoms of parkinsonism. The involuntary movements linked to the condition may slacken or disappear after weeks or months. They have been lessened in some individuals by giving large doses of choline chloride. See also **antiparkinsonian.**

tardy peroneal nerve palsy, an abnormal condition in which the peroneal nerve is excessively pressured where it crosses the head of the smaller leg bone. Such compression may occur when an individual falls asleep with the legs crossed.

tardy ulnar nerve palsy, an abnormal condition marked by wasting of the hand muscles and difficulty in the performance of fine manipulations. It may be caused by injury of the ulnar nerve at the elbow. It commonly affects individuals with a shallow elbow groove or those who persistently rest their weight on their elbows. Signs and symptoms of this disorder may include numbness of the small finger, of part of the ring finger, and of the elbow border of the hand. Treatment of this condition centers on the prevention of further injury of the ulnar nerve. Therapy may include the use of a doughnut cushion for the elbow to relieve the pressure on the ulnar nerve. Severe cases of this disorder may be corrected by surgical procedures.

target, (in radiotherapy) any object area subjected to bombardment by radioactive particles or other form of diagnostic or therapeutic radiation.

target cell, 1. also called **leptocyte.** an abnormal red blood cell marked, when stained and examined under a microscope, by a densely stained center surrounded by a pale unstained ring circled by a dark, irregular band. Target cells occur in the blood after the removal of the spleen (splenectomy) and in blood diseases (anemias, hemoglobin C disease). Compare **discocyte, spherocyte. 2.** any cell having a specific receptor that reacts with a specific hormone, antigen, antibody, antibiotic, sensitized tumor cell, or other substance.

target organ, 1. (in radiotherapy) an organ that receives a therapeutic dose of irradiation, as the kidney when high-energy x-rays or gamma rays are beamed to the kidney area for the treatment of a tumor. 2. (in nuclear medicine) an organ that receives the greatest concentration of a diagnostic radioactive tracer, as the liver, which pools 99Tc sulfur colloid when it is injected by vein to detect tumors of the liver. 3. (in endocrinology) an organ most affected by a specific hormone, as the thyroid gland, which is the target organ of thyroid-stimulating hormone released by the anterior pituitary gland.

target symptoms, symptoms of an illness that are most likely to respond to a specific treatment.

tarnishing, a tendency by patients with left-sided psychomotor epilepsy to make a harsh assessment of themselves by stressing negative qualities in their self-descriptions.

tarsal /tär'səl/, of or referring to the tarsus (ankle bone) or to the eyelid.

tarsal bone, any one of seven bones comprising the ankle of the foot, made up of the talus, calcaneus, cuboid, navicular, and the three cuneiforms.

tarsal gland, one of numerous sebum-releasing glands on the inner surfaces of the eyelids. About 30 tarsal glands, resembling tiny, parallel strings of pearls, line each upper eyelid. Somewhat fewer tarsal glands line each lower eyelid. Bacterial infection of a tarsal gland causes a swelling (sty). Also called **meibomian gland.** Compare **ciliary gland.**

tarsal tunnel syndrome, an abnormal condition marked by pain and numbness in the sole of the foot. This disorder may be caused by a broken ankle that presses the posterior tibial nerve. It may be corrected by appropriate orthopedic therapy or by surgery.

tarso-, a combining form meaning 'of or referring to the edge of the foot, or to the eyelid.'

tarsometatarsal, of or referring to the bones of the foot between toes and ankle (metatarsus) bones and the ankle of the foot.

tarsus, *pl.* **tarsi, 1.** the area between the foot and the leg (the ankle). **2.** also called **tarsal plate.** Any one of the plates of cartilage, each about 2.5 cm long, forming the eyelids. One tarsal plate shapes each eyelid. The superior tarsal plates form the upper eyelids. The inferior tarsal plates form the lower eyelids. The superior tarsal plates have the shape of a half moon. They are about 10 mm wide at the center.

tartar /tär'tär/, **1.** a hard, gritty deposit. It is made of organic matter, phosphates, and carbonates that collect on the teeth and gums. An excess of tartar may cause gum disease and other dental problems. See also **gingivitis, pyorrhea. 2.** any of several compounds with tartrate, the salt of tartaric acid. See **antimony potassium tartrate.**

tartar emetic. See **antimony potassium tartrate.**

tartaric acid /tärter'ik/, a colorless or white powder found in various plants and prepared commercially from maleic anhydride and hydrogen peroxide. It is used in baking powder, certain beverages, and a drug causing vomiting (tartar emetic).

-tas, a noun-forming combining form.

task group, a group in which structured verbal and nonverbal exercises are used to help a person gain emotional, physical, and other personal awareness.

task-oriented behavior, actions involving a person's mental abilities in an attempt to solve problems, resolve conflicts, and satisfy the person's needs for reducing or avoiding distress.

taste, the sense of perceiving different flavors in soluble substances that contact the tongue and send nerve impulses to special taste centers in the cortex and the thalamus of the brain. The four basic traditional tastes are sweet, salty, sour, and bitter. The front of the tongue is most sensitive to salty and sweet substances. The sides of the tongue are most sensitive to sour substances. The back of the tongue is most sensitive to bitter substances. The middle of the tongue produces virtually no taste sensation. Chemoreceptor cells in the taste buds of the tongue detect different substances. Adults have about 9,000 taste buds. Most of the taste buds are on the upper surface of the tongue. The sense of taste is linked with the sense of smell. Taste discrimination is very complex. Many experts believe the capacity to perceive different tastes involves a synthesis of chemoreactive nerve impulses and coordinating brain processes, still not completely understood.

taste bud, any one of many outer taste organs distributed over the tongue and the roof of the mouth. The four basic taste sensations of the taste buds are sweet, sour, bitter, and salty. All other tastes are combinations of these four basic flavors. Each taste bud rests in a spheric pocket. Taste (gustatory) cells and supporting cells form each bud. It has a surface opening and an opening in the basement membrane. Also called **gustatory organ.**

TAT, abbreviation for **tetanus antitoxin.**

tattoo, a permanent coloration of the skin by the introduction of foreign color. A tattoo may accidentally occur when a bit of graphite from a broken pencil point is embedded in the skin. Small tattoos can be removed by surgery. Mechanical abrasion (dermabrasion) of the skin is preferred for removal of extensive areas of pigment. **–tattoo,** *v.*

tauto-, a combining form meaning 'same.'

Tavist, a trademark for an antihistamine (clemastine).

tax-, a combining form meaning 'order or arrangement.'

-taxia, -taxis, -taxy, 1. a combining form meaning '(condition of) blocked mental or physical control.' **2.** a combining form meaning '(condition of) inner ordering or arrangement.' See also **-taxis.**

-taxic. See **-tactic.**

-taxis, -taxia, -taxy, 1. a combining form meaning a '(specified) arrangement.' **2.** a combining form meaning a 'movement of an organism in response to a stimulus.' See also **-taxia.**

taxonomy /takson'əmē/, a system for classifying organisms on the basis of natural relationships and giving them appropriate names. **–taxonomic,** *adj.*

-taxy. See **-taxia, -taxis.**

Taylor brace, a padded steel brace used to support the spine. Also called **Taylor splint.**

Tay-Sachs disease /tā'saks'/, an inherited nerve breakdown disorder of lipid metabolism. It is caused by a lack of the enzyme hexosaminidase A. This results in the pooling of sphingolipids in the brain. The condition is carried as a non-sex-related (autosomal) recessive trait. It occurs foremost in families of Eastern European Jewish origin, specifically Ashkenazic Jews. It is marked by progressive mental and physical retardation and early death. Symptoms first appear by 6 months of age. After this age no new skills are learned, and there is progressive loss of those skills already learned. Convulsions and washing of the optic nerve head occur after 1 year. It is followed by blindness, with a cherry-red spot on each retina, spasticity, dementia, and paralysis. Most children die between 2 and 4 years of age. There is no specific therapy for the condition. Intervention is merely to take care of symptoms and to offer some relief. The disease can be diagnosed before birth through amniocentesis. Also called **amaurotic familial idiocy, gangliosidosis type I, infantile cerebral sphingolipidosis, Sachs' disease.** See also **Sandhoff's disease.**

Tay's spot. See **cherry-red spot.**

TB, abbreviation for **tuberculosis.**

T bandage, a bandage in the shape of the letter T. It is used for the pelvic floor (perineum) and sometimes for the head. Also called **crucial bandage, Heliodorus' bandage.**

TBP, 1. abbreviation for **bithionol. 2.** abbreviation for *total bypass.*

TBT, abbreviation for **tracheobronchial tree.**

TBW, abbreviation for **total body water.**

TBZ, abbreviation for *tetrabenazine,* an anesthetic aid.

T cell, a small, circulating lymphocyte made in the bone marrow. It matures in the thymus or as a result of exposure to thymosin released by the thymus. T cells live for years. They have several functions but mainly involve cellular immune responses, as graft rejection and delayed allergy. One kind of T cell, the **helper cell,** affects the production of antibodies by B cells; a **suppressor T cell** suppresses B cell activity. Compare **B cell.** See also **antibody, immune response.**

Td, abbreviation for **tetanus and diptheria toxoids.**

TD, abbreviation for **toxic dose.**

TD50. See **median toxic dose.**

tDNA, abbreviation for **transfer DNA.**

tea. See **cannabis.**

teacher's nodule. See **vocal cord nodule.**

teaching hospital, a hospital with recognized programs in medical, nursing, or related health personnel education.

teaching rounds, the somewhat informal conferences held often at the beginning of the day. Various members of the department and staff may attend, including nurses, residents, interns, students, attending physicians, and faculty. Specific problems in the care of current patients are discussed. See also **nursing rounds.**

team nursing, a system in which the care of a patient is distributed among the members of a team. The nurse in charge gives authority to a team leader who must be a professional nurse. This nurse leads the team—usually of four to six members—in the care of between 15 and 25 patients. The team leader gives tasks, schedules care, and instructs team members in details of care. A conference is held at the beginning and at the end of each shift to allow team members to exchange information. It also gives the team leader the chance to make changes in the nursing care plan for any patient. Compare **primary nursing.**

team practice, professional practice by a group of professionals that may include physicians, nurses, and others, as a social worker, nutritionist, or physical therapist. They organize the care of a specified number of patients as a team, usually in an outpatient setting.

teardrop fracture, a break of one of the short bones, as a vertebra, causing a tear-shaped disruption of bone tissue.

tear duct, any duct that carries tears, including the tear ducts, nose ducts, and the ducts of the tear glands.

tearing /tir'ing/, watering of the eye. It it usually caused by excess tear production, as by strong emotion, infection, or mechanic irritation by a foreign body. Tearing occurs when more tears are made than are drained by the ducts and sacs of the eyes. Also called **epiphora.**

technetium (Tc), a radioactive, metallic element. Its atomic number is 43; its atomic weight is 99. The first synthetic element, technetium also occurs in nature. Isotopes of technetium are used in radioisotope scanning procedures of internal organs, as the liver and spleen. Formerly called **masurium.**

technetium 99, the radionuclide most commonly used to image the body in nuclear medicine scans. It is preferred because of its short half-life and because the emitted photon has an appropriate energy for normal imaging techniques.

technic. See **technique.**

-technics, -technology, -techny, a combining form meaning 'the art or mechanics of.'

technique, the method and details followed in performing a procedure, as those used in conducting a laboratory test, a physical examination, a psychiatric interview, or a surgical operation. It is used to refer to any process needing certain skills or an ordered sequence of actions. Also spelled **technic.**

-technique, -technic, a combining form meaning 'the skillful way in which something is done.'

techno-, a combining form meaning 'art.'

-techny, -technics, -technology, a combining form meaning 'the art or mechanics of' a specified area.

tecto-, a combining form meaning 'rooflike.'

Tedral, a trademark for a breathing drug. It is made up of a bronchi widener (theophylline), a stimulation (adrenergic) drug (ephedrine hydrochloride), and a sleeping and relaxation (sedative-hypnotic) drug (phenobarbital).

teenager. See **adolescent.**

teether, an object, as a teething ring, on which an infant can bite or chew during the teething process.

teething, the physiological process of the eruption of the first teeth (which will eventually fall out) through the gums. It normally begins between the sixth and eighth months of life. It occurs periodically until the complete set of 20 teeth has appeared at about 30 months. Discomfort and swelling result from the pressure against the tissue supporting the teeth as the crown of the tooth breaks through the membranes. General signs of teething include excess drooling, biting on hard objects, irritability, difficulty in sleeping, and refusal of food. Fever or diarrhea often occurs during teething. However, it points to illness rather than to teething. The pain and swelling may usually be softened by cold, as with a frozen teething ring, cold metal spoon, or ice wrapped in a washcloth. Use of teething powders and procedures, as rubbing or cutting the gums, are discouraged because of the possibility of infection or problems from swallowing the drug. –**teethe,** *v.*

teething ring, a circular device, usually made of plastic or rubber, on which an infant may chew or bite during the teething process.

Teflon, a trademark for a substance (polytetrafluorethylene) used for the construction of surgical implants in restorative surgery.

teg-, a combining form meaning 'of or referring to a cover.'

Tegopen, a trademark for an antibacterial (cloxacillin sodium).

Tegretol, a trademark for a painkiller and a drug that prevents convulsions (carbamazepine).

TEIB, abbreviation for *triethylene-immunobenzoquinone.*

tela-, a combining form meaning 'a web or weblike structure.'

-tela, a combining form meaning a 'weblike membrane.'

telangiectasia /təlan'jē·ektā'zhə/, permanent widening of groups of superficial capillaries and small vessels (venules). Common causes are damage due to excess sunlight, some skin diseases, as rosacea, too-high levels of female hormone, and collagen blood vessel diseases. See also **Osler-Weber-Rendu syndrome, spider angioma.**

telangiectatic epulis /təlan'jē·ektat'ik/, a harmless, red tumor of the gum. It contains visible blood vessels. Low-grade or long-term irritation usually occurs. The tumor is easily injured.

telangiectatic fibroma. See **angiofibroma.**

telangiectatic glioma, a tumor made up of nerve (glial) cells and a network of blood vessels. This gives the mass a vivid pink appearance.

telangiectatic granuloma. See **pyogenic granuloma.**

telangiectatic lipoma. See **angiolipoma.**

telangiectatic nevus, a common skin condition of newborn infants. It is marked by flat, deep-pink localized areas of capillary widening. They occur foremost on the back of the neck, lower back part of the head, upper eyelids, upper lip, and bridge of the nose. The areas go away for good by about 2 years of age. Also called **capillary flames, stork bite.**

telangiectatic sarcoma, a cancerous tumor of embryo (mesodermal) cells with an unusually rich blood vessel network.

tele-, 1. a combining form meaning 'of or related to the end.' 2. a combining form meaning 'operating at a distance, or far away.'

telegraphic speech, a type of language dysfunction commonly experienced by persons with brain damage, as organic brain syndrome or some forms of aphasia. It is characterized by replies that are relevant but carry very little information.

telepathist /təlep'əthist/, 1. a person who believes in telepathy. 2. a person who claims to have telepathic powers.

telepathy /təlep'əthē/, the unproved communication of thought from one person to another by means other than the physical senses. Also called **thought transference.** See also **extrasensory perception, parapsychology.** –**telepathic,** *adj.,* **telepathize,** *v.*

telereceptive, referring to the nerve endings for hearing, sight, and smell that detect stimuli outside and distant from the body (exteroceptors).

teletherapy, radiation therapy given by a machine that is positioned at some distance from the patient. Typically, a teletherapy unit can turn around a patient and thus allow use of beams that intersect at the tumor. This lowers the dose to surrounding normal tissue.

tellurium (Te), an element with metallic and nonmetallic chemical properties. Its atomic number is 52; its atomic weight is 127.60. Breathing vapors of tellurium results in a breath that smells like garlic.

telo-, a combining form meaning 'of or referring to the end.'

telocentric /tel'əsen'trik/,   referring to a chromosome in which the centromere is located at the end. Thus the chromatids appear as straight fibers. Compare **acrocentric, metacentric, submetacentric.**

telogen.   See **hair.**

telophase /tel'əfāz/,   the final of the four stages of nuclear division in certain cell divisions (mitosis and meiosis). See also **anaphase, interphase, meiosis, metaphase, mitosis, prophase.**

Temaril,   a trademark for an antihistamine (trimeprazine tartrate).

temazepam,   a sleeping drug. It is given for the occasional sleeping problems (insomnia).
★CAUTION: Pregnancy or breast feeding prohibits its use. It is not advised for patients under 18 years of age. Patients should avoid use of alcohol while using tenazepam.
★ADVERSE EFFECTS: The most serious side effects are confusion, abnormal sense of well-being, loss of appetite, lack of muscular coordination (ataxia), palpitations, hallucinations, horizontal involuntary rapid movements of the eyeball (nystagmus), and paradoxic reactions.

temperate phage,   a virus whose hereditary factors (genome) are incorporated into the host bacterium. It lasts through many cell divisions of the bacterium without destroying the host, in contrast to a virulent phage that destroys and kills its host.

temperature,   **1.** a relative measure of sensible heat or cold. **2.** (in physiology) a measure of sensible heat linked to the processing of the human body, normally maintained at a constant level of 98.6° F (37° C) by the thermotaxic nerve mechanism that balances heat gains and heat losses. **3.** *informal.* a fever.

temper tantrum.   See **tantrum.**

template /tem'plit/,   (in genetics) the strand of DNA that acts as a mold for the synthesis of messenger RNA. This messenger RNA has the same sequence of nucleic acids as the DNA strand. It carries the code to the ribosomes for the synthesis of proteins.

tempo-,   **1.** a combining form meaning 'of or referring to time.' **2.** a combining form meaning 'of or referring to the temples, in the side regions of the head.'

temporal arteritis,   a progressive, swellinglike disorder of head blood vessels, principally the temporal artery. It occurs most often in women over 70 years of age. Symptoms are headache that cannot be relieved, difficulty in chewing, weakness, rheumatic pains, and loss of vision if the central retinal artery becomes closed. Also called **cranial arteritis, giant cell arteritis, Horton's arteritis.**

temporal artery,   any one of three arteries on each side of the head: the superficial temporal artery, the middle temporal artery, and the deep temporal artery.

temporal bone,   one of a pair of large bones forming part of the lower head. It has many cavities and small empty spaces linked to the ear, as the tympanic cavity and the auditory tube. Each temporal bone consists of four portions: the mastoid, the squama, the petrous, and the tympanic.

temporal bone fracture,   a break of the temporal bone of the skull. It is sometimes marked by bleeding from the ear. Diminished hearing, facial paralysis, or infection of the tympanic cavity of the ear leading to swelling of the brain and spinal membranes (meningitis) may occur.

temporalis /tem'pəral'is/,   one of the four muscles of food chewing. The temporalis closes the jaws. Also called **temporal muscle.** Compare **masseter, pterygoideus lateralis, pterygoideus medialis.**

temporal lobe,   the outer lower region of the brain. The center for smell is located within the temporal lobe of the brain. It also has some association areas for memory and learning, and a region where thoughts are selected. Compare **frontal lobe, occipital lobe, parietal lobe.**

temporal lobe epilepsy.   See **psychomotor seizure.**

temporal muscle.   See **temporalis.**

temporal summation.   See **summation,** def. 2.

temporary stopping,   a mixture of gutta-percha, zinc oxide, white wax, and coloring. It is used for temporarily sealing covering materials (dressings) in tooth cavities. It softens on heating. It rehardens at room temperature. However, it is not hard enough to be used effectively in tooth areas under stress from closing the mouth.

temporary tooth.   See **deciduous tooth.**

temporomandibular joint,   one of two joints connecting the lower jaw bone to the temporal bone of the skull. It is a combined hinge and gliding joint.

temporomandibular joint pain dysfunction syndrome (TMJ),   an abnormal condition with facial pain and dysfunction of the lower jaw. It is apparently caused by a defective or dislocated temporomandibular joint. Some common indications of this syndrome are the clicking of the joint when the jaws move, limitation of jaw movement, partial dislocation, and temporomandibular dislocation. Also called **myofacial pain dysfunction syndrome.**

temporoparietalis /tem'pərōpərī'ətal'is/,   one of a pair of broad, thin muscles of the scalp, divided into three parts, which fan out over the forehead. The temporoparietalis acts in combination with the occipitofrontal muscle to wrinkle the forehead, to widen the eyes, and to raise the ears. Compare **occipitofrontalis.**

TEN,   abbreviation for **toxic epidermal necrolysis.**

tenacious, referring to fluids that are sticky or adhesive or otherwise tend to hold together, as mucus and sputum.

tenaculum /tənak′yələm/, *pl.* **tenacula,** a clip or clamp with long handles used to grasp and hold an organ or a piece of tissue. Kinds of tenacula include the **abdominal tenaculum,** which has long arms and small hooks, the **forceps tenaculum,** which has long hooks and is used in gynecological surgery, and the **uterine** or **cervical tenaculum,** which has short hooks or open, eye-shaped clamps used to hold the the lower narrow end of the uterus (cervix).

tendinitis /ten′dəni′tis/, a swelling condition of a tendon. It usually results from strain. Treatment may include rest, corticosteroid injections, and support. Also spelled **tendonitis.**

tendinous cords. See **chordae tendineae.**

tendo calcaneus, the common tendon of the sole and back leg. It is the thickest and strongest tendon in the body. It begins near the middle of the back part of the leg. In an adult it is about 15 cm long. The tendon becomes contracted about 4 cm above the heel and flares out again to insert into the heel bone (calcaneus). Also called **Achilles tendon, tendon of Achilles.**

tendon, one of many white, glistening fibrous bands of tissue that attach muscle to bone. Except at points of attachment, tendons are tubular shaped in delicate fibroelastic connective tissue. Larger tendons have a thin inner dividing wall (septum), a few blood vessels, and specialized sterognostic nerves. Tendons are extremely strong and flexible, inelastic, and occur in various lengths and thicknesses. Compare **ligament.** **–tendinous,** *adj.*

tendonitis. See **tendinitis.**

tendon of Achilles. See **tendo calcaneus.**

tendon reflex. See **deep tendon reflex.**

tenesmus /tənez′məs/, persistent, ineffectual spasms of the rectum or bladder. It goes along with the desire to empty the bowel or bladder. Intestinal tenesmus is a common complaint in swelling bowel disease and irritable bowel syndrome.

tenia-, taenia-, a combining form meaning 'ribbon, band.'

tennis elbow. See **lateral humeral epicondylitis.**

teno-, tenonto-, a combining form meaning 'of or referring to a tendon.'

tenofibril. See **tonofibril.**

Tenon's capsule. See **fascia bulbi.**

tenonto-. See **teno-.**

Tenormin, a trademark for a beta-blocker (atenolol).

tenosynovitis /ten′ōsin′əvi′tis/, swelling of a tendon sheath caused by calcium deposits, repeated strain, or trauma. High levels of blood cholesterol, rheumatoid arthritis, gout, or gonorrhea are other causes. In some instances, movement yields a crackling noise over the

tendon. Most cases not linked to systemic disease respond to rest. Local injections of adrenocorticosteroids may provide relief. Surgery is needed if the condition lasts.

tenotomy /tənot′əmē/, the total or partial severing of a tendon. It is done to correct a muscle imbalance, as in the correction of squint (strabismus) of the eye or in clubfoot.

TENS, abbreviation for **transcutaneous electric nerve stimulation.**

Tensilon, a trademark for a cholinesterase reactivator (edrophonium). It is used as an antitoxic drug and as a diagnostic aid in muscle weakness (myasthenia gravis).

tension, 1. the act of pulling or straining until strained. 2. the condition of being strained, tense, or under pressure. 3. a state or condition resulting from the psychological and physiological reaction to a stressful situation. It is marked physically by a general increase in muscle tonus, heart rate, breathing rate, and alertness. Psychologically, it is marked by feelings of strain, uneasiness, irritability, and anxiety. See also **stress.**

-tension. See **-tention.**

tension headache, a pain that affects the back (occipital) region of the body as the result of overwork or emotional strain. It tenses the body and blocks rest and relaxation.

tensor, any one of the muscles of the body that tenses a structure, as the tensor fasciae latae of the thigh. Compare **abductor, adductor, depressor, sphincter.**

tensor fasciae latae, one of the 10 muscles of the buttocks region. It functions to flex the thigh and to rotate it slightly toward the middle. Also called **tensor fasciae femoris.**

tent, 1. a transparent cover, usually of plastic, supported over the upper part of a patient by a frame. It is used to treat breathing conditions. It gives a controlled environment into which steam, oxygen, vaporized drugs, or droplets of cool water may be sprayed, as an oxygen tent. 2. a cone made of various materials put into a cavity (or its entrance or outlet) of the body to widen its opening, as a laminaria tent. 3. a pack placed in a wound to hold it open. This ensures that healing goes from the base of the wound upward to the skin.

tenth nerve. See **vagus nerve.**

tenth-value layer (TVL), the thickness of material needed to lessen a beam of radiation to one tenth of its original intensity. See also **half-value layer.**

-tention, a combining form meaning the 'condition of being held.'

-tention, -tension, a combining form meaning 'condition of being stretched.'

tentorial herniation, a protrusion of brain tissue. It is caused by increased pressure in the brain. It results from edema, bleeding, or a tumor. Characteristic signs are severe headache, fever, flushing, sweating, abnormal reflex of the pupils, drowsiness, low blood pressure, and loss of consciousness. Also called **transtentorial herniation.**

tentorium /tentôr′ē·əm/, *pl.* **tentoria,** any part of the body that looks like a tent, as the tentorium of the pituitary gland that covers the gland's hollow area (hypophyseal fossa).

tentorium cerebelli, one of the three extensions of the dura mater that separates the back brain (cerebellum) from the occipital lobe of the brain. Compare **falx cerebelli, falx cerebri.**

Tenuate, a trademark for a drug that lessens the appetite (diethylpropion hydrochloride).

tenure, (in a university) a faculty appointment without a limit on the number of years it may be held. It is a permanent appointment usually awarded to a person who has advanced to the rank of professor and who shows scholarship and excellence in a specific field of study.

-tepa, a combining form for anticancer derivatives of thiotepa.

Tepanil, a trademark for a drug that lessens appetite (diethylpropion hydrochloride).

tephr-, a combining form meaning 'ash-colored.'

tepid, moderately warm to the touch.

teramorphous, of the nature of or characteristic of a monster.

teras /ter′əs/, *pl.* **terata,** a severely deformed fetus; a monster. **–teratic,** *adj.*

teratism, any inborn or developmental anomaly that is produced by inherited or environmental factors, or by a combination of the two. It can be any condition in which a severely defected fetus is produced. Kinds of teratism include **atresic teratism, ceasmic teratism, ectopic teratism, ectrogenic teratism, hypergenetic teratism,** and **symphysic teratism.** Also called **teratosis.**

terato-, a combining form meaning 'of or related to a monster.'

teratogen /ter′ətəjen′/, any substance, agent, or process that blocks normal growth of the fetus, causing one or more developmental abnormalities in the fetus. Teratogens act directly on the developing organism or indirectly, affecting such supplemental structures as the placenta or some maternal system. The type and extent of the defect are determined by the specific kind of teratogen and its mode of action. It also depends on the embryonic process affected, genetic predisposition, and the stage of development at the time the exposure occurred. The period of highest vulnerability in the growing embryo is from about the third through the 12th week of gestation. The reason is that differentiation of the major organs and systems occurs at this period. Susceptibility to teratogenic influence decreases quickly in the later periods of growth. Among the known teratogens are chemical agents, including drugs, as thalidomide, alkylating agents,

and alcohol. Infectious agents, especially the rubella virus and cytomegalovirus, have the same effect. Other teratogens include ionizing radiation, particularly x-rays, and environmental factors, as the general health of the mother or any trauma in the uterus that may affect the fetus, especially during the later stages of pregnancy. Compare **mutagen. –teratogenic,** *adj.*

teratogenesis /ter′ətōjen′əsis/, the development of physical defects in the embryo. Also called **teratogeny** /ter′ətoj′ənē/ . **–teratogenetic,** *adj.*

teratogenic agent. See **teratogen.**

teratogeny. See **teratogenesis.**

teratoid /ter′ətoid/, of or referring to abnormal physical development; looking like a monster.

teratoid tumor. See **dermoid cyst.**

teratologist, one who specializes in the science of teratology.

teratology, the study of the causes and effects of inborn malformations and developmental abnormalities. **–teratologic, teratological,** *adj.*

teratoma, *pl.* **teratomas, teratomata,** a tumor made up of different kinds of tissue, none of which normally occur together or at the site of the tumor. Teratomas are most common in the ovaries or testes.

teratosis. See **teratism.**

terbium (Tr), a rare earth metallic element. Its atomic number is 65; its atomic weight is 158.294.

terbutaline sulfate, a beta-adrenergic stimulant. It is given as a bronchial widener to treat asthma, bronchitis, and emphysema and as a uterine relaxant to treat premature labor.

★CAUTION: Irregular heart beat (cardiac arrhythmias) or known allergy to this drug prohibits its use.

★ADVERSE EFFECTS: Among the most serious side effects are dizziness and irregular heart rate. Nervousness and trembling are common side effects.

teres /tir′ēz, ter′ēz/, *pl.* **teretes** /ter′ətēz/, a long, cylindrical muscle, as the teres minor or the teres major. **–teres,** *adj.*

teres major, a thick, flat muscle of the shoulder. It functions to pull forward, extend, and rotate the arm to the middle. Compare **teres minor.**

teres minor, a cylindrical, long muscle of the shoulder. It functions to rotate the arm outward, weakly pull up the arm, and to strengthen the shoulder joint. Compare **teres major.**

terminal, (of a structure or process) near or approaching its end, as a terminal bronchiole or a terminal disease. **–terminate,** *v.,* **terminus,** *n.*

terminal bronchiole. See **bronchiole.**

terminal disinfection, the process of cleaning equipment and airing a room after the release of a patient who has been treated for an infectious disease.

terminal drop, a rapid decline in cognitive function and coping ability that occurs 1 to 5 years before death.

terminal nerve, a small nerve originating in the cerebral hemisphere near the roots of the olfactory tract. Most anatomists see it as part of the olfactory, or first cranial, nerve.

terminal stance, one of the five stages in the stance phase of a walking gait. It is directly linked to the continuation of single limb support or the period during which the body moves forward on the supporting foot. Double limb support is started during the latter part of terminal stance. It is often a factor in the analysis of many abnormal orthopedic conditions and the diagnosis of weaknesses that may develop in certain muscles used in walking, as the quadriceps femoris and the gluteus maximus. Compare **initial contact stance stage, loading response stance stage, midstance, preswing stance stage.** See also **swing phase of gait.**

terminal sulcus of right atrium, a shallow channel on the outer surface of the right heart chamber (atrium) between the upper and lower venae cavae veins.

termination phase, the last phase of a therapy in which attained goals are evaluated and outcomes achieved. During this stage, therapists may also help patients establish networks of support, other than the therapist-patient relationship, that may help in coping with future problems.

termination sequence, (in molecular genetics) a DNA segment at the end of a unit that is transcribed to messenger RNA from the DNA template.

term infant, any newborn, regardless of birth weight, born after the end of the 37th and before the beginning of the 43rd week of gestation. Infants born at term usually measure from 48 to 53 cm from head to heel. They weigh between 2,700 and 4,000 g.

terpin hydrate and codeine elixir, a preparation of the drug terpin hydrate. It promotes coughing up (expectorant). It is made of sweet orange peel tincture, benzaldehyde, glycerin, alcohol, syrup, water, and the coughing suppressing narcotic codeine. Terpin hydrate reduces secretions and promotes healing of the mucous membrane. Codeine depresses the cough center in the medulla oblongata. Prolonged use may lead to addiction.

Terra-Cortril, a trademark for a drug with a glucocorticoid (hydrocortisone) and an antibiotic (oxytetracycline).

Terramycin, a trademark for an antibiotic (oxytetracycline).

territorial, a type of body movement that aids in communication. A territorial will frame an interaction and define an individual's "territory." See also **territoriality.**

territoriality, an emotional attachment to and defense of certain areas related to one's existence. Humans and animals generally make a claim to or occupy a defined or undefined area over which they can keep some degree of control.

terti-, a combining form meaning 'third.'

tertian /tur'shən/, occurring every 48 hours or 3 days, including the first day of occurrence, as tertian malaria, in which fever occurs every third day. Compare **quartan.** See also **malaria.**

tertian malaria, a form of malaria. It is caused by the protozoon *Plasmodium vivax* or *Plasmodium ovale.* It is marked by chill, fever, and sweat attacks that occur every 48 hours. **Vivax malaria,** the most common form of malaria, caused by *Plasmodium vivax.* It is rarely fatal. However, it is the most difficult form to cure. Relapses are common. **Ovale malaria,** caused by *Plasmodium ovale,* is usually milder and causes only a few, short attacks. Both types of tertian malaria are treated with chloroquine. Compare **falciparum malaria, quartan malaria.** See also **malaria.**

tertiary /tur'shē·ərē, tursh'ərē/, third in frequency or in order of use; belonging to the third level of sophistication of development, as a tertiary health-care facility.

tertiary health care, a specialized, highly technical level of health care. It includes diagnosis and treatment of disease and disability in sophisticated, large research and teaching hospitals. Specialized intensive care units, advanced diagnostic support services, and highly specialized personnel are usually characteristic of tertiary health care. It offers a highly centralized care to the population of a large region; in some cases, to the world.

tertiary prevention, a highly technical level of health care. It deals with the return of a patient to a status of maximum usefulness with a minimum risk of renewed physical or mental disorders.

Teslac, a trademark for a drug that blocks the growth of tumors (testolactone).

Tessalon, a trademark for a local anesthetic agent (benzonatate).

test, 1. an examination or trial intended to establish a principle or determine a value. 2. a chemical reaction or reagent that has clinical importance. 3. to detect, identify, or conduct a trial. See also **laboratory test.**

test-, a combining form meaning 'of or referring to the testicles.'

testamentary capacity, a person's ability to make a will, including the requirement that he or she be aware that the will is being made, the kind and amount of the property covered by the will, and the identities of those who will benefit from the will.

testcross, 1. (in genetics) the cross of a dominant phenotype with a recessive phenotype to determine either the degree of genetic linkage or whether the dominant phenotype is homozygous or heterozygous. **2.** the subject undergoing such a test.

testes determining factor (TDF), a Y-chromosome gene that is believed to determine male sexual development. Studies show that individuals with the normal female (XX) sex chromosome pair may develop as males if the TDF gene has moved to one of the X chromosomes. Also, an individual with the normal (XY) chromosome pair may develop as female if the TDF gene is missing from the Y chromosome.

testicle. See **testis.**

testicular /testik′yələr/, of or referring to the testicle.

testicular artery, one of a pair of long, slender branches of the stomach aorta, arising backward to the kidney arteries and supplying the testicles.

testicular cancer, a cancerous disease of the testicles. It occurs most often in men between 20 and 35 years of age. An undescended testicle is often involved. In many cases the tumor is detected after an injury. However, injury is not thought to be a cause. Patients with early testicular cancer often have no symptoms. Cancerous tumors may have moved to the lymph nodes, the lungs, and liver before the original tumor can be felt. In the later stages there may be lung symptoms, urethral obstruction, excess growth of the male mammary glands (gynecomastia), and a stomach mass. Diagnostic measures include transillumination of the scrotum, radiography of the lymph and urine tracts, and a urine or serum test to evaluate circulating levels of luteinizing hormone. Tumors develop more often in the right than in the left testicle. Seminomas are the most curable lesions and the most common. They represent 40% of all testicular tumors. Embryonal carcinomas are more highly cancerous and represent 15% to 20% of these tumors. Teratocarcinomas and choricarcinomas also occur. Radiotherapy and surgical removal are usually recommended to treat seminoma. Chemotherapy using combinations of drugs is recommended for nonseminomatous tumors. Chemotherapeutic agents, used in various combinations, are increasing the survival of patients with testicular cancer. Some of these drugs are actinomycin D, bleomycin, cis-platinum, cyclophosphamide, methotrexate, and vincristine.

testicular duct. See **vas deferens.**

testicular feminization. See **feminization.**

testicular self-examination (TSE), a recommended (National Health Institute) procedure for detecting tumors or other abnormalities in the males testes. TSE should be performed once a month, usually after a warm bath or shower because the heat causes scrotal skin to relax, thereby increasing the chances of detecting any tissue abnormality. The TSE is conducted in four simple steps. The first is to stand in front of a mirror and look for any swelling on the skin of the scrotum. One testicle may appear larger than the other and one may hang lower, which is usually normal. Next, each testicle is examined with both hands, placing the fingers under the testicle while the thumbs are placed on top. The testicle is then rolled gently between the thumbs and fingers. In the next step, the epididymis, a normal cordlike structure on the top and back of each testicle, should be found. A small pea-sized lump is felt for on the front or side of a testicle. The lump is usually painless. Testicular cancer almost always occurs in only one testicle. It is curable when detected at an early stage.

testicular vein, one of a pair of blood veins that arises from networks of veins (venous plexuses), forming the greater mass of the spermatic cords. Veins from each plexus start from small veins at the back of the testes, go up along the spermatic cords, and pass through the deep groin ring and unite to form a single vein. The right testicular vein opens into the lower vena cava. The left testicular vein opens into the left kidney vein. Both testicular veins contain valves. Compare **ovarian vein.**

testimony, the statement of a witness, usually made orally and given under oath, as at a court trial.

testis /tes′tis/, *pl.* **testes,** one of the pair of male gonads that produce semen. The adult testes are suspended in the scrotum by the spermatic cords. In early fetal life they are within the abdominal cavity behind the lining (peritoneum). Before birth they normally lower into the scrotum. Each testis is an oval body about 4 cm long, 2.5 cm wide. It weighs about 12 g. The ducts in which the sperm is stored (epididymic) are located on the back of the testis. They are about 20 feet long and connect with the vas deferens through which sperm pass during ejaculation. Each testis consists of several hundred conical lobules with the tiny coiled seminiferous tubules, each about 75 mm long, in which spermatozoa develop. A man with both testes undescended is sterile but may not be impotent. The testes are supplied with blood by the two internal spermatic arteries that arise from the aorta. Compare **ovary.** See also **scrotum.**

test method, a method chosen for experimental testing or study by means of method evaluation.

testolactone, a drug that counteracts tumor growth. It is given to treat postmenopausal breast cancer and in premenopausal women whose ovarian function has been ended.

★CAUTION: Pregnancy, breast feeding, or

known allergy to this drug prohibits its use. It is not given to men.

★ADVERSE EFFECTS: Among the more serious side effects are excess calcium in the blood (hypercalcemia) and nerve disturbances at the outer part of the body with numbness or tingling.

testosterone /testos'tərōn/, a naturally occurring hormone that stimulates the growth of male characteristics (androgen). It is given for androgen lack, female breast cancer, and for stimulation of growth, weight gain, and red blood cell production.

★CAUTION: Cancer of the male breast or prostate, liver disease, pregnancy or suspected pregnancy, or known allergy to this drug prohibits its use.

★ADVERSE EFFECTS: Among the more serious side effects are fluid buildup, masculinization, swelling of the skin (acne), and a blood disease (erythrocythemia).

testosterone propionate, a drug, given intramuscularly, which stimulates the growth of male characteristics. See also **testosterone.**

test tube, a tube made of transparent material having one open end. It is used in the growth of bacteriological specimens. It is also used in the analysis of some chemical functions, and in many other common laboratory functions. See also **tube.**

-tetanic, a combining form meaning 'relating to or producing tetanus or tetany.'

tetano-, a combining form meaning 'of or referring to tetanus.'

tetanus /tet'ənəs/, a sudden, potentially deadly infection of the central nervous system. It is caused by a bacteria-formed toxin (exotoxin), tetanospasmin, elaborated by an anaerobic bacillus, *Clostridium tetani.* More than 50,000 people a year die of tetanus infection worldwide. The toxin is a neurotoxin and is one of the most lethal poisons known. *C. tetani* infects only wounds that contain dead tissue. The bacillus is a common resident of the superficial layers of the soil. It is a normal inhabitant of the intestinal tracts of cows and horses. Therefore, barnyards and fields fertilized with manure are heavily contaminated. The bacillus may come into the body through a puncture wound, abrasion, cut, or burn. It also may come into the body via the uterus, into the bloodstream in abortion or afterbirth contamination (sepsis), or through the stump of the umbilical cord of the newborn. The dead tissue of the area is low in oxygen. This is the environment essential for the replication of *C. tetani.* The infection occurs in two clinical forms. The first one shows a sudden beginning, high mortality, and a short incubation period (3 to 21 days); the second one shows less severe symptoms, a lower mortality, and a longer incubation period (4 to 5 weeks). Wounds of the face, head, and neck are the ones most likely to result in fatal infection, because the bacillus may travel rapidly to the brain. The disease is marked by irritability, headache, fever, and painful spasms of the muscles resulting in lockjaw, spasms of the face muscles (risus sardonicus), spasm with the body forward and the head and heels backward (opisthotonos), and throat spasm. Eventually every muscle of the body is in continuous spasm. The motor nerves carry the impulses from the infected central nervous system to the muscles. There is no injury. Even at autopsy no organic injury is seen, and the fluid of the brain and spine is clear and normal. Prompt and thorough cleansing and removal of foreign bodies from the wound are necessary for prevention. A booster shot of tetanus toxoid is given to previously vaccinated people. Tetanus immune globulin and a series of three injections of tetanus toxoid are given to those not vaccinated. People who are known to have been adequately immunized within 5 years do not usually need vaccination. Treating people who have the infection includes maintenance of an airway, giving an antitoxin as soon as possible, sedation, control of the muscle spasms, and assuring a normal fluid balance. The room is kept quiet. Benzodiazepines may be given to lessen excess tension of the muscles (hypertonicity). Penicillin G is given for infection. An incision in the windpipe is made and oxygen given for ventilation.

tetanus and diphtheria toxoids (Td), an active vaccination drug with detoxified tetanus and diphtheria toxoids that slowly makes antibodies to the diseases. It is a vaccination against tetanus and diphtheria in children under 7 years of age when whooping cough vaccine present in the usual diphtheria, pertussis, and tetanus trivalent vaccine is prohibited.

★CAUTION: Lessened resistance (immunosuppression), simultaneous use of corticosteroids, or serious infection prohibits its use.

★ADVERSE EFFECTS: Among the most serious side effects are allergic reactions and stinging at the site of injection.

tetanus antitoxin (TAT), a tetanus immune serum that neutralizes exotoxins in tetanus infection. It is given for short-term vaccination against tetanus after possible exposure to the organism and in tetanus treatment.

★CAUTION: It is not given if the more effective tetanus immune globulin is available or if there is a known allergy to equine serum.

★ADVERSE EFFECTS: Among the most serious side effects are allergic reactions and pain and swelling at the site of injection.

tetanus immune globulin (TIG), an injectable solution prepared from the globulin of an immune human. It is effective and much safer than tetanus antitoxin. It is given for short-term vaccination against tetanus after possible exposure to the organism and tetanus treatment.

★CAUTION: Known allergy to this drug prohibits its use. It should not be substituted for tetanus toxoid.

★ADVERSE EFFECTS: The most serious side effect is an overreaction (anaphylaxis). Fever and pain and swelling at the site of injection may occur.

tetanus toxoid, an active immunizing agent prepared from detoxified tetanus toxin that makes antibodies in the body. This gives permanent immunity to tetanus infection. It is given for primary active immunization against tetanus.

★CAUTION: Lessened resistance (immunosuppression) or immunoglobulin abnormalities, serious infection, or illness prohibits its use.

★ADVERSE EFFECTS: The most serious side effect is an allergic reaction. Pain and swelling at the site of injection may occur.

tetany /tet′ənē/, a condition with cramps, convulsions, twitching of the muscles, and sharp bending of the wrist and ankle joints. These symptoms are sometimes linked with attacks of harsh breathing sounds (stridor). Tetany is a manifestation of an abnormality in calcium processing, which can be linked to a lack of vitamin D, lessened function of the parathyroid glands (hypoparathyroidism), too-much base (alkalosis) in the body, or the ingestion of alkaline salts. Kinds of tetany are **duration tetany, grass tetany, hyperventilation tetany,** and **lactation tetany.** Compare **tetanus.**

tetart-, a combining form meaning 'fourth.'

tetra-, tetro-, a combining form meaning 'four.'

tetrachlormethane. See **carbon tetrachloride.**

tetracycline /tet′rəsī′klēn/, an antibiotic with many uses. It is given to treat many bacterial and rickettsial infections.

★CAUTION: Significantly blocked liver or kidney functions or known allergy to this drug prohibits its use. Because it may cause permanent discoloration of the teeth, its use is prohibited in the last half of pregnancy and during a child's first 8 years of life.

★ADVERSE EFFECTS: Among the more serious side effects are poisoning of the kidneys and liver, disturbances of the stomach and intestines, swelling of the small intestine and colon (enterocolitis), swelling tumors with bacterial overgrowth in the anogenital area, blood diseases (hemolytic anemia, thrombocytopenia, eosinophilia), and rashes.

tetracycline hydrochloride, a tetracycline antibiotic. It is given to treat a variety of infections.

★CAUTION: Known allergy to this drug or to other tetracyclines prohibits its use. Use during pregnancy or in children under 8 years of age may result in discoloration of the child's teeth. It is to be given carefully with kidney or liver problems.

★ADVERSE EFFECTS: Among the most common side effects are potentially serious suprainfections, various allergic reactions, toxic reactions due to light exposure (phototoxicity), and disturbances of the stomach and intestines.

tetrahydrocannabinol (THC), the active substance of marijuana, hashish, bhang, and ganja. THC increases pulse rate, causes eye reddening, a feeling of great excitement, and has variable effects on blood pressure, breathing rate, and pupil size. The drug affects memory, cognition, and the senses. It decreases motor coordination, and increases appetite. Overdoses of THC may be treated by "talking down" the patient and by giving sedative barbiturates or diazepam by injection. Nonintoxicating doses of THC are used experimentally to treat glaucoma and to relieve nausea and increase the appetite in patients receiving cancer chemotherapy. See also **cannabis.**

tetrahydrozoline hydrochloride, an adrenergic constrictor of vessels. It is given to treat nose and nose-throat (nasopharangeal) congestion and as an eye vasoconstrictor.

★CAUTION: Glaucoma or known allergy to this drug or to other vasoconstrictors prohibits its use. It is used carefully in patients who have heart disease.

★ADVERSE EFFECTS: Among the more serious side effects are irritation to mucosa, rebound nasal congestion, and effects linked with systemic absorption, including sedation and alterations in heart function.

tetraiodothyronine. See **thyroxine.**

tetralogy of Fallot /falō′/, an inborn heart problem that is made up of four defects: lung narrowing (pulmonic stenosis), a defect in the dividing wall of the lower chamber of the heart (ventricular septal defect), malposition of the aorta so that it arises from the septal defect or the right ventricle. The main symptoms in the infant are bluish skin due to too-little hemoglobin (cyanosis) and lack of oxygen (hypoxia), usually during crying, difficulty in feeding, failure to gain weight, and poor development. In older children a typical squatting position and clubbing of the fingers and toes are evident. A heart (pansystolic) murmur is usually heard, and the second heart sound is faint or absent. Diagnosis of the condition is mainly based on the history and physical symptoms. However, cardiac catheterization is done to evaluate the severity of the defects. Treatment includes supportive measures and surgery. It is mainly done to open up the lungs (pulmonary anastomoses), to lessen tissue hypoxia, and to prevent complications until the child is old enough to tolerate total corrective surgery. The optimal age for surgical repair is about 4 or 5 years. Also called **Fallot's syndrome.** See also **blue baby, trilogy of Fallot.**

tetramer /tet′rəmer/, something that is made up of four parts, as a protein composed of four polypeptide subunits.

tetraploid (4n), **1.** also **tetraploidic**, of or referring to an individual, organism, strain, or cell that has four complete sets of chromosomes. It is extremely rare in humans, found only occasionally in abortuses and stillborn fetuses. **2.** such an individual, organism, strain, or cell. Compare **diploid, haploid, triploid.** See also **polyploid.**

tetraploidy /tet′rəploi′dē/, the state or condition of having four complete sets of chromosomes.

Tetrex, a trademark for an antibiotic (tetracycline phosphate complex).

tetro-. See **tetra-.**

T fracture, a break in the rounded end of a bone (condyle) in which the fracture lines are T-shaped.

TGF, abbreviation for **transforming growth factor.**

T group. See **sensitivity training group.**

Th, symbol for **thorium.**

thalamus /thal′əməs/, *pl.* **thalami**, one of a pair of large, oval organs forming most of the outer walls of the third ventricle of the brain and part of the back part of the front brain (diencephalon). It measures about 4 cm long and 1.5 cm wide and is made up of numerous nuclei arranged in groups. It is made up mainly of gray substance. It translates impulses from appropriate receptors into crude sensations of pain, temperature, and touch. It also joins in associating sensory impulses with pleasant and unpleasant feelings, in the arousal mechanisms of the body, and in the mechanisms that produce complex reflex movements. Compare **epithalamus, hypothalamus, subthalamus.** **–thalamic,** *adj.*

thalassemia /thal′əsē′mē·ə/, a disease marked by microcytic, hypochromic, and short-lived red blood cells caused by insufficient hemoglobin synthesis. People of Mediterranean origin are more often affected than others. It is a non-sex-related (autosomal) recessive, genetically carried disease occurring in two forms. **Thalassemia major (Cooley's anemia)**, the homozygous form, evident in infancy, is recognized by anemia, fever, failure to thrive, and too-large spleen (splenomegaly). It is confirmed by characteristic changes in the red blood cells. Frequent transfusions are needed to keep up the oxygen-carrying capacity of the blood. Red cells are rapidly destroyed, freeing large amounts of iron to be deposited in the skin, which becomes bronzed and freckled. The iron is also deposited in the heart, liver, and pancreas, which become fibrotic and dysfunctional. The spleen may become so large that breathing movement is blocked, and the stomach organs are crowded. Headache, stomach pain, weakness, and loss of appetite often

occur. There is no cure. The child is uncomfortable. Growth and sexual development are usually slowed. Rarely, a child with thalassemia major is able to function without transfusions, thereby avoiding the massive ill effects of accumulated iron deposits. **Thalassemia minor,** the heterozygous form, is marked only by a mild anemia and minimal red blood cell changes. Thalassemia minima is a form that lacks clinical symptoms although patients show hematological evidence of the disease. Education and counseling about the disease, and referral for genetic counseling are needed. See also **hemochromatosis, hemosiderosis.**

thalasso-, a combining form meaning 'of or referring to the sea.'

thalidomide /thalid′əmīd/, a sleeping pill. It was withdrawn from general use because of its potential for creating defects in the growing fetus, particularly defects of limbs, hands, and feet (phocomelia), when taken during pregnancy. It is sometimes given to treat leprosy.

thallium (Tl), a soft, bluish-white metal element with some nonmetallic chemical properties. Its atomic number is 81; its atomic weight is 204.37. Many of its compounds are highly toxic. Thallium sulfate is widely used as a rat poison.

thallium poisoning, a toxic condition caused by the ingestion or the absorption through the skin of thallium salts, especially thallium sulfate. Characteristic of the condition are stomach pain, vomiting, bloody diarrhea, trembling, delirium, and baldness (alopecia). Treatment may include gastric lavage, binding the toxic with Prussian blue, and a laxative. Anticonvulsant and anti-low-blood-pressure drugs may be necessary. Thallium has been used in insect and rodent poisons, fireworks, and in some cosmetic hair removers. However, this very toxic and cumulative poison was banned for use in household products in 1965.

thanato-, a combining form meaning 'of or referring to death.'

thanatology /than′ətol′əjē/, the study of death and dying. **–thanatologist,** *n.*

thanatophoric dwarf /than′ətōfôr′ik/, an infant with severe shortness or smallness of the limbs (micromelia). The limbs usually extend straight out from the trunk. An extremely narrow chest and flattened vertebral bodies with wide intervertebral spaces also occur. Death usually occurs from breathing problems shortly after birth.

Thanatos /than′ətəs/, a Freudian term for the death instinct.

thanatopsy. See **autopsy.**

THC, abbreviation for **tetrahydrocannabinol.**

the Blues, *informal.* Referring to Blue Cross (an insurance system that pays the costs of treatment by a hospital or clinic) and Blue Shield (an insurance system that pays the cost of treatment by a professional).

thec-, a combining form meaning 'of or referring to a sheath, as of a tendon.'

theca /thē′kə/, *pl.* **thecae** /thē′sē/, a sheath or capsule, as the theca cordis or pericardium.

theca cell tumor, an uncommon, harmless fibroid tumor of the ovary. It is made up of theca cells and usually contains granulosa (follicular) cells. The tumors are typically solid masses with yellow, fatty streaks. They are often linked to excess female hormone production and tend to develop breakdown with lumps. Also called **fibroma thecocellulare xanthomatodes, thecoma.**

-thecium, a combining form meaning 'sack or container.'

thecoma. See **theca cell tumor.**

Theden's bandage /tā′dənz/, a roller bandage applied below the injury and continued upward over a compress. It is used to stop bleeding. Also called **Genga's bandage.**

thel-, a combining form meaning 'of or referring to the nipple.'

thelarche /thilär′kē/, the beginning of female pubertal breast growth that normally occurs before puberty at the beginning of the phase of fast growth between 9 and 13 years of age. **Premature thelarche** is breast growth in a female without other evidence of sexual maturation. Compare **menarche.**

-thelia, a combining form meaning '(condition of the) nipples.'

-thelioma, a combining form meaning a 'tumor in a cellular tissue.'

-thelium, a combining form meaning a 'layer of (specified kind of) cellular tissue.'

thely-, a combining form meaning 'female.'

thenar /thē′när/, 1. the ball of the thumb. 2. of or referring to the thumb side of the palm.

theo-, a combining form meaning 'of or referring to a god.'

Theobid, a trademark for a smooth muscle relaxant (theophylline).

theobromine, a substance (methylxanthine) that is related chemically to caffeine and theophylline. Theobromine occurs naturally in cocoa, cola nuts, and tea. It acts to increase urine output, to widen the blood vessels, to stimulate the heart, and to relax smooth muscle.

Theo-Dur, a trademark for a bronchial widener (theophylline).

Theolair, a trademark for a bronchial widener (theophylline). It is used for the relief of sudden bronchial asthma.

theophylline, a bronchial widener. It is given to relax the smooth muscle of the bronchial passages in the treatment of bronchospasm in bronchial asthma, bronchitis, and emphysema. ★CAUTION: High blood pressure, heart disease, liver disease, kidney disease, or simultaneous treatment with other xanthines prohibits its use.

★ADVERSE EFFECTS: Among the most serious side effects are allergy, bleeding in the stomach and intestines, palpitations, and seizures.

theoretic effectiveness, (of a contraceptive method) the effectiveness of a drug, device, or method in preventing pregnancy if used consistently and exactly as intended, without error. Compare **use effectiveness.**

theotherapy /thē′ōther′əpē/, a therapeutic approach to the prevention, diagnosis, and treatment of disease and dysfunction based on religious or spiritual beliefs.

Theovent, a trademark for a smooth muscle relaxant (theophylline).

therapeutic, 1. beneficial. 2. referring to a treatment.

-therapeutic, a combining form meaning 'referring to medical treatment by (specified) techniques.'

therapeutic abortion, 1. the ending of pregnancy thought necessary by a physician. 2. *informal.* any legal, induced abortion. Compare **elective abortion.** See also **induced abortion.**

therapeutic communication, (in psychiatric nursing) a process in which the nurse consciously influences a client or helps the client to a better understanding through spoken or unspoken communication.

therapeutic community (TC), (in mental health) a treatment facility in which the entire environment is part of the treatment. The physical environment, the other clients, the staff, and the policies of the facility influence the function of the patient in the activities of daily living in the community. The concept of a therapeutic community is an intrinsic part of milieu therapy.

therapeutic equivalent, a drug that has in essence the same effect in the treatment of a disease or condition as one or more other drugs. A drug that is a therapeutic equivalent may or may not be chemically equivalent or bioequivalent. See also **bioequivalent, chemical equivalent, generic equivalent.**

therapeutic exercise, any exercise planned and done to get a specific physical benefit, as maintenance of the range of motion, strengthening of weakened muscles, increased flexibility of a joint, or improved heart and breathing function.

therapeutic gain, the ratio of the biological effect of a therapy on a tumor compared with the effect on surrounding normal tissue. Higher therapeutic gains mean fewer problems of therapy.

therapeutic index, the difference between the lowest therapeutic and lowest poisonous amounts of a drug.

therapeutic radiopharmaceutic, a radioactive drug given to a patient to get radiation to the inner body tissues, as iodide 131 or cesium 137.

therapeutic recreation specialist, a person who helps patients in their recovery or rehabilitation after physical or emotional illness or disability. This specialist plans and supervises recreation programs.

-therapeutics, a combining form meaning 'medical treatment by (specified) techniques.'

therapeutic temperature, in treatment through increased body temperature (hyperthermia), temperatures between 42° and 45° (107° and 113° F).

-therapin, -therapy, a combining form meaning 'medical care.' See also **-therapy.**

therapist, a person with special skills, gotten through education and experience, in one or more areas of health care.

therapy, the treatment of any disease or abnormal condition. For example, breathing therapy, which gives some drugs for patients suffering from diseases of the breathing tract.

-therapy, -therapia, 1. a combining form meaning 'medical treatment of disease' by specified means. 2. a combining form meaning 'medical treatment of a (specified) disorder or body area.' See also **-therapia.**

therio-, a combining form meaning 'of or referring to beasts.'

therm-. See **thermo-.**

-therm, a combining form meaning an 'animal with a (specified) body temperature.'

thermal, of or referring to the production, application, or upkeep of heat. Also **thermic.**

thermal burn, tissue injury, usually of the skin. It is caused by exposure to extreme heat. See also **burn.**

thermal dilution, a method of heart output determination.

-thermia, -thermy, 1. a combining form meaning a 'state of body temperature.' 2. a combining form meaning 'making of body heat.'

thermic fever. See **heat hyperpyrexia.**

thermistor /thərmis′tər/, a kind of thermometer for measuring very small changes in temperature. See also **temperature, thermometer.**

thermo-, therm-, a combining form meaning 'of or referring to heat.'

thermocautery /thur′mōkô′tərē/, the use of a hot needle or loop wire in the destruction of tissue. See also **Paquelin's cautery.**

thermocouple, a temperature measuring.

thermodilution, a heart output testing method in which a small amount of a cold liquid, as a salt solution, is injected into the bloodstream. The temperature change is recorded by a special thermometer (thermistor) at a point farther along the bloodstream. Heart output is calculated as a function of the flow rate of the salt solution multiplied by a factor derived from the temperature differences.

thermogenesis /thur′mōjen′əsis/, making of heat, especially by the cells of the body. **–thermogenetic,** adj.

thermography /thərmpg′rəfē/, a technique for sensing and recording on film hot and cold areas of the body by means of an infrared detector that reacts to blood flow. Disease states that manifest increased or decreased blood flow present thermographic patterns that can be distinguished from those of normal areas. **–thermographic,** adj.

thermolabile /thur′mōlā′bəl/, easily destroyed or changed by heat. Also called **heat labile.** Compare **thermostable.**

thermoluminescent dosimetry, a method of measuring the ionizing radiation to which a person is exposed. It is done by a device that stores the radient energy and releases it later as ultraviolet or visible light. The device contains a crystalline material that is changed in structure by the radiation. It stores the radiation's energy, which is later released by heating the material. The light emitted reflects the amount of ionizing radiation originally received.

thermometer, an instrument for measuring temperature. It is usually made of a sealed glass tube, marked in degrees of Celsius or Fahrenheit. It has a liquid, as mercury or alcohol. The liquid rises or falls as it expands or contracts according to changes in temperature. Some kinds of thermometers are **clinical thermometer, digital thermometer,** and **electronic thermometer.**

thermoneutral environment, 1. an environment that keeps body temperature at an optimum point at which the least amount of oxygen is consumed for processing. 2. an environment that enables a newborn to keep a body temperature of 36.5° C (97.7° F) with a minimal requirement of energy and oxygen.

thermopenetration, the use of heating techniques to make warmth within the body tissues for therapeutic purposes. Also called **transthermia.**

thermoradiotherapy, a therapeutic process that applies ionizing radiation to any part of the body in which the temperature has been raised by artificial means. Thermoradiography seeks to increase the radiosensitivity of the body part being treated.

thermoregulation, the control of heat production and heat loss, specifically keeping the body temperature normal through physical mechanisms set off by the hypothalamus.

thermostable, unaffected by or resistant to change by an increase in temperature. Compare **thermolabile.**

thermostat, a device for the automatic control of a heating or cooling system. **–thermostatic,** adj.

thermotaxis, 1. the normal adjustment and control of body temperature. 2. the movement of an organism in response to heat, either toward the stimulus (positive thermotaxis) or away from the stimulus (negative thermotaxis). Also called **thermotropism.**

thermotherapeutic penetration, the depth to which heating to therapeutic temperatures is likely to go.

thermotherapy, the treatment of disease by the application of heat. Thermotherapy may be given as dry heat with heat lamps, heating (diathermy) machines, or electric pads. Hot water bottles or moist heat with warm compresses or immersion in warm water are other methods. Warm soaks or compresses may be used to treat local infections to relax muscles and to relieve pain in patients with motor problems. It also helps to promote circulation in outer blood vessel (peripheral vascular) disorders, as thrombophlebitis. –**thermotherapeutic,** *adj.*

thermotropism. See **thermotaxis.**

-thermy. See **-thermia.**

theta wave, one of the several types of brain waves. They are marked by a relatively low frequency of 4 to 7 Hz and a low amplitude of 10 μV. Theta waves are the "drowsy waves" of the temporal lobes of the brain. They are recordings of electrical changes in the brain (electroencephalograms) when the patient is awake but relaxed and sleepy. Also called **theta rhythm.** Compare **alpha wave, beta wave, delta wave.**

-thetic, -thetical, a combining form meaning 'to put, place, set.'

thiabendazole, a drug that destroys worms (anthelmintic). It is given to treat a variety of worm infestations, including hookworms, roundworms, and pinworms.

★CAUTION: Skin diseases (erythema multiforme, Stevens-Johnson syndrome) or known allergy to this drug prohibits its use.

★ADVERSE EFFECTS: Among the more serious side effects are loss of appetite, central nervous system effects, severe disturbances of the stomach and intestines, dizziness, and low blood pressure.

thiamine /thī'əmin/, a water-soluble, crystalline compound of the B complex vitamin group. It is necessary for normal processing and for the health of the heart and nervous systems. Thiamine joins with pyruvic acid to form a coenzyme necessary for the breakdown of carbohydrates into glucose. Rich sources of thiamine are pork, organ meats, green leafy vegetables, legumes, sweet corn, egg yolk, and corn meal. Brown rice, yeast, the germ and husks of grains, berries, and nuts are other rich sources. It is not stored in the body and must be supplied daily. A lack of thiamine affects chiefly the nervous system, the circulation, and the stomach and intestines. Symptoms include irritability, emotional disturbances, loss of appetite, swelling of nerves, increased pulse rate,

difficult breathing (dyspnea), lessened intestinal ability to move spontaneously (mobility), and heart irregularities. Severe lack causes beriberi. Thiamine is not known to cause any toxic effects. Also spelled **thiamin. Also called antiberiberi factor, antineuritic vitamin, vitamin B₁.**

thiazide diuretic. See **diuretic.**

thiethylperazine, a drug that relieves nausea and vomiting (antiemetic).

★CAUTION: Parkinson's disease, central nervous system disorders, liver or kidney dysfunction, severe low blood pressure, or known allergy to this type of drug prohibits its use.

★ADVERSE EFFECTS: Among the more serious side effects are low blood pressure, liver toxicity, a variety of extraabnormal involuntary movement (pyramidal) reactions, blood disease, and allergic reactions.

thigh, the section of the lower limb between the hip and the knee.

thigh bone. See **femur.**

thigm-, a combining form meaning 'of or referring to touch.'

thinking, **1.** the cognitive process of forming mental images or concepts. **2.** the process of cognitive problem solving through the sorting, organizing, and classification of facts. Kinds of thinking include **abstract thinking, concrete thinking,** and **syncretic thinking.** See also **imagination.**

thio-, a combining form designating the presence of sulfur.

thioamide derivative /thī'ō·am'īd/, one of a group of antithyroid drugs given to treat excess thyroid gland activity (hyperthyroidism). Thioamide drugs act by blocking the making of thyroid hormone. The main thioamides are propylthiouricil, methimazole, methylthiouricil, and carbamizole. Side effects increase in cells with granules (agranulocytosis), allergy, and a mild temporary itching (pruritus). Because agranulocytosis may occur very rapidly, serial white blood cell counts are not useful in diagnosing that problem of treatment. Instead, the patient is asked to report immediately instances of sore throat and fever, which often arise with the beginning of agranulocytosis. Prompt discontinuation of the drug, before serious lack of granulocytic white cells develops, usually results in complete recovery. Use of antithyroid drugs in pregnancy may result in fetal hypothyroidism, a large thyroid gland, and arrested physical and mental growth (cretinism).

thioctic acid /thī·ok'tik/, a pyruvate oxidation factor found in liver and yeast. It is used in bacterial culture media.

thioester /thī'ō·es'tər/, an important group of biological chemicals. They are formed by the hydrosulfides and carboxylic acids. Examples include the coenzyme A thioesters.

thioguanine /thī'ōgwä'nēn/, an antitumor drug. It is given to treat some cancerous tumor diseases, including the serious leukemias.
★CAUTION: Known allergy or resistance to this drug prohibits its use. It is not given to pregnant women.
★ADVERSE EFFECTS: Among the most serious side effects are bone marrow depression, distress of the stomach and intestines, and swelling of the mouth (stomatitis).

thiopental sodium, a potent, short-acting drug to aid sleep and relaxation. It is used as a general anesthetic for surgical procedures that are expected to require 15 minutes or less. It is also used as an induction agent for other general anesthetics, as a sleeping component in balanced anesthesia, and as an aid to effectiveness of local anesthesia. It is given by vein in adults. In children it is occasionally given rectally. By depressing the central nervous system, thiopental sodium induces hypnotic sleep in less than 1 minute. It has no painkilling properties and therefore must be supplemented by painkillers. It is a powerful breathing and heart depressant. It may be habit-forming. See also **barbiturate.**

thioridazine hydrochloride, an antipsychotic. It is given for childhood behavioral disorders, mental disorders of the elderly, depression, and alcohol withdrawal.
★CAUTION: Parkinson's disease, simultaneous administration of central nervous system depressants, liver or kidney dysfunction, severe low blood pressure, or known allergy to this drug or to other similar drugs prohibits its use.
★ADVERSE EFFECTS: Among the more serious side effects are low blood pressure, poisoning of the liver, a variety of abnormal involuntary movement (pyramidal) reactions, blood disease, and allergic reactions.

Thiosulfil, a trademark for a sulfonamide antibacterial (sulfamethizole).

thiotepa /thī'ōtep'ə/, an antitumor alkylating drug. It is given to treat some cancerous diseases, including cancer of the breast and ovary, and urinary bladder cancers.
★CAUTION: Bone marrow depression, pregnancy, liver or kidney dysfunction, or known allergy to this drug prohibits its use.
★ADVERSE EFFECTS: Among the most serious side effects are bone marrow depression, loss of appetite, nausea, and headache.

thiothixene, a thioxanthene antipsychotic. It is given to treat sudden agitation and mild to severe psychotic disorders.
★CAUTION: Parkinson's disease, simultaneous use of central nervous system depressants, liver and kidney dysfunction, severe low blood pressure, known allergy to this drug or to phenothiazine drugs prohibits its use. It is not advised for children under 12 years of age.
★ADVERSE EFFECTS: Among the more serious side effects are low blood pressure, poisoning of the liver, many involuntary movement (extrapyramidal) reactions, blood diseases, and allergic reactions.

thioxanthine derivative, any one of a group of antipsychotic drugs, each of which is similar to the phenothiazenes in indication, action, and side effects.

third cranial nerve. See **oculomotor nerve.**

third cuneiform bone. See **lateral cuneiform bone.**

third-party reimbursement, reimbursement for services given to a person in which someone other than the giver or receiver of the service is responsible for the payment. Third-party reimbursement for the cost of a subscriber's health care is commonly paid by insurance plans, as Blue Shield or Blue Cross.

third ventriculostomy /ventrik'yəlos'təmē/, a surgical procedure for draining fluid of the brain and spine into the cisterna chiasmatis of the subarachnoid space in excess fluid in the brain (hydrocephalus), usually in the newborn. The procedure is not commonly done. It is used chiefly when the cisterna magna is not available for Torkildsen's operation. The third ventriculostomy makes an opening on the front wall of the floor of the third ventricle into the interpeduncular cistern. It is done to correct a blocking type of hydrocephalus.

thirst, a perceived desire for water or other fluid. The sensation of thirst is usually referred to the mouth and throat.

Thiry-Vella fistula /thī'rēvel'ə/, an artificial passage from the stomach surface of an experimental animal to an isolated intestinal loop. It is created by surgery for the study of intestinal fluids.

thixo-, a combining form meaning 'of or referring to touch.'

Thomas' splint, 1. a rigid splint made of steel bars that are curved to fit the involved limb and held in place by a cast or a rigid bandage. It is used to treat long-term joint diseases. **2.** also called **Thomas' ring splint.** A rigid metal splint that extends from a ring at the hip to beyond the foot. It is used to treat a broken leg. It is used together with many traction and suspension devices to immobilize and position a fractured thigh of the patient after and before surgery.

Thomsen's disease. See **myotonia congenita.**

thoracentesis. See **thoracocentesis.**

thoracic /thôras'ik/, of or referring to the chest (thorax).

-thoracic, a combining form meaning 'of, referring, or relating to the chest.'

thoracic actinomycocis. See **actinomycosis.**

thoracic aorta, the large, upper portion of the descending aorta, starting at the caudal border of the fourth chest bone. It divides into seven branches. It supplies many parts of the body, as the heart, ribs, chest muscles, and stomach. Its seven branches are the pericardial, bronchial, esophageal, mediastinal, posterior intercostal, subcostal, and superior phrenic. See also **descending aorta**. Compare **abdominal aorta**.

thoracic duct, the common trunk of all the lymphatic vessels in the body, except those on the right side of the head, the neck, the chest, the right upper limb, the right lung, the right side of the heart, and the diaphragmatic surface of the liver. In the adult, it is 38 to 45 cm long and 3 to 5 mm in diameter. It begins high in the stomach at the cisterna chyli, directed toward the second lumbar backbone, enters the chest through the aortic hiatus of the diaphragm, and goes up into the neck through the back mediastinum, between the aorta and the azygous vein. In the neck it arches over the shoulder bone and opens into the junction of the left internal jugular and the left subclavian veins. The thoracic duct has many valves, including two at the entrance that prevent venous blood from flowing into the lymphatic system. Compare **right lymphatic duct**. See also **lymphatic system**.

thoracic fistula, an abnormal opening in the chest wall that ends blindly or that communicates with the chest cavity.

thoracic medicine, the branch of medicine concerned with the diagnosis and treatment of disorders of the structures and organs of the chest, especially the lungs.

thoracic nerves, the 12 spinal nerves on each side of the thorax, including 11 intercostal nerves and one subcostal nerve. They are distributed mainly to the walls of the chest and stomach. The thoracic nerves do not enter a network (plexus) but follow independent courses, making them different from other spinal nerves. The first two intercostal nerves stimulate the upper limb and the chest. The next four supply only the thorax. The lower five supply the walls of the chest and stomach. Each subcostal thoracic nerve supplies the stomach wall and the skin of a buttock. See also **autonomic nervous system**.

thoracic outlet syndrome, an abnormal condition and a type of nerve disorder. It is marked by a morbid sensation of the fingers. It may be caused by nerve root pressure by a neck disk or by pressure of the middle nerve in the carpal tunnel (carpal tunnel syndrome).

thoracic parietal node, one of the lymph glands in the chest. It is linked to various lymphatic vessels and divided into sternal nodes, intercostal nodes, and diaphragmatic nodes. See also **lymphatic system, lymph node**.

thoracic vertebra, one of the 12 bony segments of the spinal column of the upper back. They are named T1 to T12. T1 is just below the seventh cervical backbone (C7). T12 is just above the first lumbar backbone (L1). The chest portion of the spine is flexible and has a rounded and somewhat hollowed-out ventral curvature. Each vertebra has a broad, thick plate (lamina). It also has long, obliquely directed spinous processes, and thick, strong articular facets. The vertebrae are separated from each other by intervertebral disks. The vertebrae become thicker and heavier in descending order from T1 to T12. Compare **cervical vertebra, lumbar vertebra, sacral vertebra**.

thoracic visceral node, a node in the three groups of lymph nodes connected to the part of the lymphatic system that serves certain structures within the chest, as the thymus, heart sac, esophagus, windpipe, lungs, and bronchi. The thoracic visceral nodes include the anterior mediastinal nodes, the posterior mediastinal nodes, and the tracheobronchial nodes. Compare **thoracic parietal node**. See also **lymph, lymphatic system, lymph node**.

thoraco-, a combining form meaning 'of or referring to the chest.'

thoracocentesis /thôr′əkōsentē′sis/, surgery to break into the chest wall and long membrane space with a needle for the removal of fluid for diagnostic or therapeutic purposes. It may also be done for the removal of a specimen for biopsy. The procedure is usually done using local anesthesia. The patient is seated leaning forward over a table that is chest high. Puncture of a cavity of the chest wall may be used to treat pleural effusion, as may occur in cancer of the lung (bronchogenic carcinoma). Fluid samples may be examined for erythrocyte, leukocyte, and differential white cell counts, protein, glucose, and amylase concentrations. They may be cultured for studies of microorganisms that may be present. Also called **thoracentesis**.

thoracodorsal nerve /thôr′əkōdôr′səl/, a branch of the nerve network of the arm (brachial plexus), usually arising between the two subscapular nerves. It courses along the back wall of the armpit. It ends in branches that supply the latissimus dorsi.

thoracostomy /thôr′əkos′təmē/, a cut made into the chest wall to provide an opening for draining.

thoracotomy /thôr′əkot′əmē/, a surgical opening into the chest cavity.

thorax, *pl.* **thoraces, thoraxes,** the chest area, with the bone and cartilage containing the principal organs of respiration and circulation and covering part of the abdominal organs. The chest (thorax) of women has less capacity, a flat bone forming the front wall of the chest (sternum), and more movable upper ribs than that of men. Also called **chest**.

Thorazine, a trademark for a phenothiazine (chlorpromazine). It is used as a drug that prevents or relieves nausea and vomiting, and as a tranquilizer.

thorium (Th), a heavy, grayish, radioactive, metallic element. Its atomic number is 90; its atomic weight is 232.04. Thorium is used in radiographic procedures and in radiation therapy.

thought broadcasting, a symptom of mental disorder (psychosis) in which the patient believes that his or her thoughts are "broadcast" beyond the head so that other persons can hear them.

thought insertion, a belief by some mentally ill patients that thoughts of other persons can be put into their own minds.

threadworm, See *Enterobius vermicularis.*

threadworm infection. See **strongyloidiasis.**

thready pulse, an abnormal pulse that is weak and often fairly rapid. The artery does not feel full, and the rate may be difficult to count. It is characteristic of abnormal decrease of circulating fluid (hypovolemia), as occurs with severe bleeding.

threatened abortion, a condition in pregnancy before the 20th week of pregnancy. It is marked by bleeding of the uterus and cramping sufficient to suggest that miscarriage may result. A threatened abortion is generally managed with rest and observation. Compare **incomplete abortion, inevitable abortion, imminent abortion.**

three-day fever. See **phlebotomus fever.**

three-day measles. See **rubella.**

thronine (Thr), an essential amino acid needed for proper growth in infants and for keeping the nitrogen balance in adults. See also **amino acid, protein.**

threp-, a combining form meaning 'of or referring to nutrition.'

threshold, the point at which a stimulus is great enough to make an effect. For example, a pain threshold is the point at which a person becomes aware of pain.

threshold limit values, the maximum concentration of a chemical to which workers can be exposed for a fixed period, as 8 hours per day, without developing a physical problem.

thrill, a fine vibration, felt by an examiner's hand on the body of a patient over the site of a bulging of an artery wall (aneurysm) or on the region over the heart and lower chest (precordium). Compare **bruit, murmur.**

throat. See **pharynx.**

throb, a deep, pulsating kind of discomfort or pain. –**throbbing,** *adj., n.*

thrombapheresis. See **plateletpheresis.**

thrombasthenia /throm'basthē'nē·ə/, a rare bleeding disease. It is marked by a defect in the stopping of bleeding. The cause is that abnormal platelets prevent clotting. Bleeding

is the result. Transfusion with platelets is usually effective in stopping the bleeding. The condition is an inherited non-sex-determined (autosomal) recessive trait.

thrombectomy /thrombek'təmē/, the removal of a solid mass (thrombus) from a blood vessel. It is done as emergency surgery to restore circulation to the affected part. Before surgery, anticlotting therapy is begun. A radiography of the arteries is done to locate the clot. Using general anesthesia, a lengthwise incision is made into the blood vessel, and the clot is removed. After the operation, the blood pressure is maintained close to its level before the operation. The reason is that a decrease may lead to further clotting. Compare **embolectomy.**

thrombin /throm'bin/, an enzyme formed in plasma during the clotting process from prothrombin, calcium, and thromboplastin. Thrombin causes fibrinogen to change to fibrin, essential in the formation of a clot. See also **blood clot.**

thrombo-, a combining form meaning 'of or referring to a clot, or thrombosis.'

thromboangiitis obliterans /throm'bō·an'jē·ī'tis/, a condition in which the veins close. It happens usually in a leg or a foot. The small and medium-sized arteries are swollen and clotted. Early signs of the condition are burning, numbness, and tingling of the foot or leg. Swelling (phlebitis) and dead tissue (gangrene) may develop as the disease progresses. Pulsation in the limb below the damaged blood vessels is often absent. The goal of therapy is to avoid all factors that lessen the blood supply to the extremity, as cigarette smoking, and to use all means possible to increase the supply. Amputation may be necessary if the condition progresses to dead tissue (gangrene) with long-term infection and extensive tissue destruction. Men are affected 75 times more often than women. Most of the affected men smoke and are between 20 and 40 years of age. Also called **Buerger's disease.**

thrombocytapheresis. See **plateletpheresis.**

thrombocyte. See **platelet.**

thrombocytopathy /throm'bōsītop'əthē/, any disorder of the blood-clotting mechanism caused by an abnormality or dysfunction of platelets. Kinds of thrombocytopathies include **thrombocytopenia and thrombocytosis.** –**thrombocytopathic,** *adj.*

thrombocytopenia /throm'bōsī'təpē'nē·ə/, an abnormal blood condition in which the number of platelets is reduced. It is usually caused by breakdown of erythroid tissue in bone marrow linked to certain tumor diseases or an immune response to a drug. There may be decreased production or survival of platelets. There also may be increased consumption of platelets, and a large spleen. Thrombocytopenia is the most common cause of bleeding disorders. Bleeding is usually from many small capillaries. Treatment requires a specific diagnosis of the cause. All drugs are stopped because nearly any drug may cause the condition. Adrenal corticosteroids may be given. Transfusion may be necessary.

thrombocytopenic purpura, a bleeding disorder marked by a decrease in the number of platelets. This results in many bruises, red blood spots (petechiae), and bleeding into the tissues. It may occur secondary to a number of causes, including infection and drug allergy and poisoning. Until recently it was called idiopathic thrombocytopenic purpura (ITP), a diagnosis reached only by the exclusion of other causes. Today it is considered to be a manifestation of an immune response against one's own body tissues (autoimmunity). Two distinct entities, sudden and long-term thrombocytopenia, can be kept apart from clinical manifestations alone. The acute form usually but not always occurs in children between 2 and 6 years of age. It is harmless. Complete recovery usually is apparent within 6 weeks. The long-term form usually occurs in adults between 20 and 50 years of age. Recovery is rarely spontaneous. It often requires adrenocortical steroids, or, possibly, removal of the spleen (splenectomy). Compare **disseminated intravascular coagulation.** See also **hemophilia, hemorrhagic diathesis, thrombasthenia.**

thrombocytosis /throm'bōsītō'sis/, an abnormal increase in the number of platelets in the blood. **Benign thrombocytosis,** or **secondary thrombocytosis,** has no specific symptoms. It usually occurs after removal of the spleen (splenectomy), a swelling disease, a blood disease (hemolytic anemia), bleeding, or a lack of iron, as a response to exercise, or after treatment with an antitumor drug (vincristine). It may also occur in advanced cancer or Hodgkin's disease or in other cancers of the lymphs. **Essential thrombocythemia** is marked by periods of spontaneous bleeding alternating with thrombotic episodes. The platelets may reach levels exceeding 1,000,000/μL. Compare **thrombocytopenia.** See also **polycythemia.**

thromboembolism, a condition in which a blood vessel is blocked by a clot (embolus) carried in the bloodstream from the site of formation of the clot. The area supplied by an obstructed artery may tingle and become cold, numb, and bluish-colored (cyanotic). Treatment includes quiet bed rest, warm wet packs, and anticlotting drugs to prevent the formation of additional clots. Removal of clots by surgery (embolectomy) may be needed especially if the aorta or common iliac artery is blocked. A clot in the lungs causes a sudden, sharp, chest or upper stomach pain, breathing difficulty (dys-

pnea), a violent cough, fever, and spitting of blood (hemoptysis). Blockage of the lung artery or one of its branches may rapidly cause death. Clots in smaller lung arteries may be diagnosed by x-ray films and other radiological techniques, including lung scans and x-ray tests of the blood vessels.

thrombolytic, referring to the dissolution of blood clots.

thrombophlebitis, swelling of a vein, often along with the formation of a clot. It occurs most commonly as the result of injury to the vessel wall, abnormal increased clotting capacity of the blood (hypercoagulability), infection, and chemical irritation. Less blood flow after surgery, prolonged sitting, standing, or immobilization, or a long period of vein catheterization are other causes. Also called **phlebitis.** Thrombophlebitis of a superficial vein is generally evident. The vessel feels hard and thready or cordlike and is extremely sensitive to pressure. The surrounding area may be red (erythematous) and warm to the touch. The entire limb may be pale, cold, and swollen. Deep vein thrombophlebitis is marked by aching or cramping pain, especially in the calf when the patient walks or bends the foot backward (Homan's sign). Thrombophlebitis of a vein of the arm or hand caused by the irritation of a vein catheter is usually treated by removing the catheter, lifting up the arm, and applying moist heat. When the condition occurs in a vein of the leg, the patient is kept on complete bed rest in a comfortable position that does not limit blood return. The legs are lifted, if ordered, but pillows are not used and the knees are never bent unless the foot of the bed is raised. Anticlotting therapy and streptokinase may be given. Moist heat is applied to the affected area. Intense heat, which may burn bloated (edematous) skin, is avoided. Every 4 hours the blood pressure, temperature, pulse, breathing, circulation of the affected extremity, skin condition, and pulses in all the extremities are checked. A Doppler ultrasonic sensing device may be used. The patient is kept warm and dry. He or she is helped to turn, cough, and deep breathe every 2 hours. The chest is listened to for breath sounds every 4 hours. Observation for signs of lung clots, heart disease, or decreased kidney function is constant. The affected limb is covered with a bed cradle. It is not washed or massaged. It is measured daily, with the size recorded. Active and passive range-of-motion exercises are done with the unaffected extremities. Constipation is avoided. During the acute phase, the patient is lifted on and off the bedpan. When radiography of the vein is done, the patient is told how the contrast medium will be injected before an x-ray study of the affected vein. As swelling becomes less, the use of support or anticlotting stockings is demonstrated. An exercise program is started. The patient is told to alternate exercise with bed rest, never to dangle the legs, and to walk 10 minutes every hour. He or she is also told to avoid long standing, to avoid becoming overweight, and, when sitting, to lift the legs, flex the calf muscles, and contract the quadriceps 10 minutes per hour. The patient is also told to avoid narrowing circulation in the groin or crossing the legs at the knees.

thrombophlebitis migrans. See **migratory thrombophlebitis.**

thrombophlebitis purulenta, a swelling of a vein. It is linked to the formation of a soft, pus-forming mass that infiltrates the wall of the vessel.

thromboplastin, a complex substance that starts the clotting process by changing prothrombin to thrombin in the presence of calcium ion. It is found in most tissue cells and, in somewhat different form, in red blood cells and leukocytes. Both substances function as factor III in the series of blood-clotting steps. See also **blood clotting.**

thrombosis /thrombō'sis/, *pl.* **thromboses,** an abnormal blood condition in which a clot develops within a blood vessel of the body. See also **blood clotting.**

thrombotic phlegmasia. See **phlegmasia alba dolens.**

thrombotic thrombocytopenic purpura (TTP), a disorder marked by blood and nerve abnormalities. It goes together with bleeding and small clotting within the capillaries and smaller arterioles. It is seen in a long-term form and in a sudden intense form that may lead to death in weeks. Therapy includes steroids and removal of the spleen. Compare **disseminated intravascular coagulation.** See also **thrombocytopenic purpura.**

thrombus /throm'bəs/, *pl.* **thrombi,** a cluster of platelets, fibrin, clotting factors, and the cellular elements of the blood attached to the interior wall of a vein or artery. It sometimes closes the vessel. Kinds of thrombi include **agonal thrombus, hyaline thrombus, laminated thrombus, marasmic thrombus, parasitic thrombus, and white thrombus.** Also called **bloot clot.** Compare **embolus.**

thrush, fungi infection of the tissues of the mouth.

thulium (Tm), a rare earth metallic element. Its atomic number is 69; its atomic weight is 168.93. Thulium that has been irradiated in a nuclear reactor gives off x-rays. It has been used in portable x-ray devices.

thumb, the first and shortest finger (digit) of the hand. It is classified by some anatomists as one of the fingers because its metacarpal bone hardens in the same manner as the finger bones. Other anatomists classify the thumb separately, regarding it as composed of one metacarpal bone and only two phalanges, while the fingers have three phalanges. Shaping of the metacarpal bone begins in the middle of the eighth or ninth week of fetal life. About the third year of life, the base extremity of the metacarpal of the thumb starts to harden, uniting with the body of the metacarpal about the 20th year of life. The phalanges of the thumb harden from centers in the bodies of the phalanges and from centers at their nearest extremities. Formation of the phalangeal body begins about the eighth week of fetal life.

thumb forceps, a surgical instrument used to grasp soft tissue, especially while making stitches.

thumbsucking, a habit of sucking the thumb for oral satisfaction. It is normal in infants and young children as a pleasure-seeking or comforting device, especially when the child is hungry or tired. The habit reaches its peak when the child is between 18 and 20 months of age. It normally goes away as the child grows and becomes older. Thumbsucking beyond 4 to 6 years of age may lead to teeth that do not properly close. It may also lead to an abnormality of the bony tissue of the thumb. Excess thumbsucking, especially in older children, may be caused by some emotional problem.

-thymia, a combining form meaning '(condition of the) mind or will.'

thymic /thī'mik/, of or referring to the thymus gland.

thymic hypoplasia, thymic parathyroid aplasia. See **DiGeorge's syndrome.**

thymo-, 1. a combining form meaning 'of or referring to the thymus gland.' 2. a combining form meaning 'of or referring to the spirit or mind.'

thymol /thī'mol/, a synthetic or natural thyme oil. It is used as an antibacterial and antifungal. It is a part of some over-the-counter drugs used to treat hemorrhoids, a skin disease (acne), and athlete's foot (tinea pedis). It is also used as a stabilizer in various pharmaceutical preparations.

thymoma /thīmō'mə/, *pl.* **thymomas, thymomata,** a usually benign tumor of the thymus gland. It may be linked to muscle disease (myasthenia gravis) or an immune deficiency disorder.

thymosin /thī'məsin/, 1. a naturally occurring immunological hormone released by the thymus gland. It is present in greatest amounts in young children and lessens in amount throughout life. 2. an experimental drug derived from bovine thymus extracts. It is given as a drug that changes resistance to certain diseases.

thymus /thī'məs/, *pl.* **thymuses, thymi,** a single, unpaired gland located in the upper chest cavity extending upward into the neck to the lower edge of the thyroid gland and downward as far as the fourth costal cartilage. Research has established that the thymus is the primary central gland of the lymphatic system. The endocrine activity of the thymus is believed to depend on the hormone thymosin. This hormone is made up of biologically active peptides critical to the maturation and growth of the immune system. The gland is made up of two lateral lobes closely bound by connective tissue, which also encloses the entire organ in a capsule. The two lobes of the gland differ in size, and, in many individuals, the right lobe overlaps the left lobe. The thymus is about 5 cm long, 4 cm wide, and 6 mm thick. The lobes are composed of numerous segments (lobules) that vary from 0.5 to 2 mm in diameter. The lobules are separated by a delicate connective tissue. Each lobule has small lymphocytes and reticular cells. The thymus grows in the embryo from the third branchial pouch. It increases in size until attaining a weight of 12 to 14 g before birth. The size of the organ relative to the rest of the body is largest when the individual is about 2 years of age. The thymus usually attains its greatest absolute size at puberty, when it weighs about 35 g. After puberty, the organ shrivels as the small lymphocytes disappear and the reticular tissue is compressed. Fatty tissue often replaces the receding thymic tissue. With aging, the gland may change in color from pinkish-gray to yellow. In the elderly individual it may appear as small islands of thymic tissue covered with fat and surrounded by the yellowish capsule. The normal shriveling of the thymus may be displaced by rapid accidental shriveling caused by starvation or by serious disease. Compare **spleen.**

Thypinone, a trademark for the synthetic thyrotropin-releasing hormone (protirelin). It is used to help in the diagnostic assessment of thyroid function. Thyrotropin is naturally released by the pituitary gland and stimulates the thyroid gland.

Thyrar, a trademark for thyroid hormone.

-thyrea, -thyreosis, -thyroidism, a combining form meaning a 'condition of the thyroid gland.'

thyro-, a combining form meaning 'of or referring to the thyroid gland.'

thyrocalcitonin. See **calcitonin.**

thyrocervical trunk, one of a pair of short, thick, arterial branches, arising from the first portion of the subclavian arteries. It supplies many muscles and bones in the head, neck, and back. Each is divided into three branches: the inferior thyroid, supracapsular, and transverse cervical.

thyroglobulin, a purified extract of porcine thyroid. See also **thyroid hormone.** It is given to treat slowed growth (cretinism), swelling

(myxedema), and large thyroid gland (goiter), and other diseases caused by a lack of thyroid release.

★CAUTION: Heart disease, abnormal pituitary gland functioning, or known allergy to this drug prohibits its use.

★ADVERSE EFFECTS: Among the more serious side effects are trembling, nervousness, irregular and too-rapid heart rate (tachycardia), and abnormal heart beats (arrythmias) when given in excess doses.

thyroid. See **thyroid gland, thyroid hormone.**

thyroid acropathy /thī'roid/, swelling beneath the skin of the extremities and excess soft tissue at the ends of the fingers and toes (clubbing). It occurs seldom in patients with thyroid disease. It is usually linked to swelling of the legs (pretibial myxedema) or abnormal thrusting outward of the eye (exophthalmos).

thyroid cancer, a cancer of the thyroid gland. It is usually marked by slow growth and a slower and longer clinical course than that of other cancers. A significant cancerous effect of exposure to ionizing radiation is demonstrated by the high rate of thyroid cancer in survivors of exposure to atomic bomb explosions and in patients who have been treated with radiotherapy for a large thymus in infancy or for acne or other skin disorders in adolescence. Large soft thyroid glands and tumors in the sacs of the thyroid gland (follicular adenomas) may be a beginning of cancerous thyroid tumors. The first sign of cancer may be an increase in size of the thyroid gland, a lump that can be felt by hand, hoarseness, difficulty swallowing (dysphagia), breathing problems (dyspnea), or pain on pressure. Diagnostic measures include x-ray examination, inspection with a strong light (transillumination) of the gland, radioisotope scanning, needle biopsy, and ultrasonic examination. More than one-half of thyroid cancers are papillary cancers; about one-third are cancers of the sacs of the gland (follicular carcinomas). The rest is made up of cancer spreading to other body parts. Total or partial removal of the thyroid gland and related lymph nodes is usually recommended. Radioactive iodine may be given after the operation. High doses of thyroid are often used to suppress thyroid stimulating hormone (TSH) in an effort to cause the disappearance of remaining tumor dependent on TSH. Various chemotherapeutic drugs, especially adriamycin, may be effective in patients with metastatic thyroid cancer that is unresponsive to conventional treatment. Cancer of the thyroid is twice as common in women as in men. Although it is diagnosed most frequently in patients between 30 and 50 years of age, it may occur in children and the elderly.

thyroid cartilage, the largest cartilage of the larynx. It is made up of two thin flat plates fused together at an acute angle in the middle line of the neck to form the Adam's apple. Immediately above this area the laminae are separated by the upper thyroid notch. Compare **cricoid.**

thyroid dermoid cyst, a tumor derived from embryonal tissues that are believed to have developed in the thyroid gland or in the thyrolingual duct.

thyroidectomy /thī'roidek'təmē/, the surgical removal of the thyroid gland. It is done for large, soft thyroid glands, tumors, or excess thyroid gland activity (hyperthyroidism) that does not respond to iodine therapy and antithyroid drugs. All but 5% to 10% of the gland is removed. Regrowth usually begins shortly after surgery. The thyroid function may return to normal. For cancer of the thyroid, the entire gland is removed, along with surrounding structures from neck to collarbone, in a radial neck dissection. Before surgery, the body's activity rate (basal metabolic rate) is lowered to normal by giving iodine and antithyroid drugs. If a tumor is present, a frozen section of the affected tissue is examined by a pathologist. If cancerous cells are found, most or all of the gland is removed. After surgery, the patient is most comfortable with the head raised (semi-Fowler's position) with continuous mist inhalation given to change mouth secretions into liquid. Mouth suctioning may be necessary. An emergency set for making a cut in the windpipe is kept in the room. Oxygen is also available. After the operation the patient is observed for signs of bleeding, breathing problems caused by fluid pooling in the vocal apparatus (edema of the glottis), muscular twitching from accidental removal of a parathyroid gland, and uncontrolled excess activity of the thyroid gland.

thyroid function test, any of several laboratory tests done to evaluate the function of the thyroid gland. Often several of the tests are done at the same time.

thyroid gland, an organ with many veins. It is at the front of the neck. It usually weighs about 30 g. It is made up of bilateral lobes connected in the middle by a narrow connection. Each lobe is about 5 cm long, a maximum of 3 cm wide, and usually about 2 cm thick. The thyroid gland is slightly heavier in women than in men. It becomes bigger during pregnancy. The thyroid gland releases the hormone thyroxin directly into the blood and is part of the endocrine system of ductless glands. It is essential to normal body growth in infancy and childhood. Its removal greatly lessens the oxidative processes of the body. This causes a lower metabolic rate characteristic of hypothyroidism. The thyroid is activated by the pituitary thyrotrophic hormone. It needs iodine to make thyroxine. Compare **parathyroid gland.**

thyroid hormone, an iodine-containing compound released by the thyroid gland, mainly as thyroxine (T_4) and in smaller amounts as four times more potent triiodothyronine (T_3). These hormones increase the rate of processing, affect body temperature, regulate protein, fat, and carbohydrate catabolism in all cells. They keep up growth hormone release, skeletal maturation, and the heart rate, force, and output. They promote central nervous system growth, stimulate the making of many enzymes, and are necessary for muscle tone and vigor. All phases of the making and the release of T_4 and T_3 are regulated by the thyroid-stimulating hormone (TSH) released by the front pituitary gland. The production of thyroid hormones is too-great in excess thyroid gland activity (hyperthyroidism) and related diseases. The production is too-small in swelling of the face (myxedema), and absent in blocked development (cretinism). T_4's normal 6 to 7-day half-life in blood is reduced to 3 or 4 days in hyperthyroidism and extended to 9 or 10 days in myxedema. T_3 has a normal half-life of 2 days or less and, like T_4, is used most actively in the liver. Pharmaceutical preparations of thyroid hormones gotten from animal glands and the synthetic compounds levothyroxine sodium and liothyronine sodium are used as replacement therapy in patients with hypothyroidism. The dosage is initially low. It is slowly increased to the optimal level based on the patient's clinical response. Overdosage or a rapid increase in the dosage may result in signs of excess thyroid gland activity, as nervousness, tremor, rapid heart beat (tachycardia), irregular heartbeat (cardiac arrhythmia), and menstrual irregularity.

-thyroidism. See **-thyrea.**

thyroiditis /thī'roidī'tis/, inflammation of the thyroid gland. Sudden thyroiditis is caused by infections. It is marked by pus and abscess formation. It may progress to the less sudden (subacute) disease of the gland. Subacute thyroiditis is marked by fever, weakness, sore throat, and a painfully large gland with tumorlike lumps of tissue (granulomas). Long-term lymphocytic thyroiditis (Hashimoto's disease) is marked by lymphocyte and plasma cell infiltration of the gland and by a larger gland. It seems to be carried as a dominant trait. It may be linked to some autoimmune disorders. Another long-term form of thyroiditis is Riedel's struma, a rare progressive formation of fibers (fibrosis) usually of one lobe of the gland but sometimes involving both lobes, the windpipe, and surrounding muscles, nerves, and blood vessels. Radiation thyroiditis occasionally occurs 7 to 10 days after the treatment of hyperthyroidism with radioactive iodine 131.

thyroid releasing hormone. See **thyrotropin releasing hormone.**

thyroid stimulating hormone (TSH), a substance released by the front lobe of the pituitary gland. It controls the release of thyroid hormone and is necessary for the growth and function of the thyroid gland. Also called **thyrotropin.** See also **thyroid hormone.**

thyroid storm, a crisis in uncontrolled excess thyroid gland activity (hyperthyroidism). It is caused by the release into the bloodstream of increased amounts of thyroid hormones. The storm may occur spontaneously. It may also follow after infection, stress, or a surgical removal of the thyroid gland done on a patient who is inadequately prepared with antithyroid drugs. Characteristic signs are fever that may reach 106° F, a rapid pulse, sudden breathing problems, fear, restlessness, irritability, and extreme exhaustion. The patient may become delirious, fall into a coma, and die of heart failure.

Thyrolar, a trademark for a thyroid hormone (liotrix).

thyronine. See **thyroid hormone.**

thyrotoxicosis. See **Graves' disease.**

thyrotropin. See **thyroid stimulating hormone.**

thyrotropin (systemic) /thīrot′rəpin, thī′rətrō′pin/, a preparation of bovine thyroid-stimulating hormone. It increases the uptake of radioactive iodine in the thyroid and the release of thyroxine by the thyroid. It is given in diagnostic tests and to enhance uptake of ^{131}I in the treatment of thyroid cancer.

★CAUTION: Clotting of the heart arteries or known allergy to this drug prohibits its use. It should not be given in untreated low adrenal function (Addison's disease) or after heart attack.

★ADVERSE EFFECTS: Among the most serious side effects are symptoms of excess thyroid gland activity, allergic reactions, low blood pressure, and irregular heart beats.

thyrotropin releasing hormone, a substance of the hypothalamus that stimulates the release of thyrotropin (thyroid stimulating hormone) from the front pituitary gland. Also called **thyrotropin releasing factor (TRF), TSH releasing factor.**

thyroxine (T₄), a hormone of the thyroid gland. It comes from tyrosine. It influences the processing rate. Also called **tetraiodothyronine.**

thyroxine-binding globulin, a plasma protein that binds with and transports thyroxine in the blood.

Thytropar, a trademark for bovine thyroid-stimulating hormone (thyrotropin).

TIA, abbreviation for **transient ischemic attack.**

tibia, the second longest bone of the skeleton. It is located in the middle of the lower leg located at the medial side of the leg. It joins with the fibula, the talus, and the femur, forming part of the knee joint. It attaches to the ligament of the kneecap and to various muscles. Also called **shin bone.**

tibialis anterior, one of the outside muscles of the leg, situated on the outside of the tibia. Also called **tibialis anticus.** Compare **extensor digitorum longus.**

tibial torsion, a twisting rotation of the tibia on its longitudinal axis. Compare **femoral torsion.**

tic. See **mimic spasm.**

Ticar, a trademark for an antibiotic (ticarcillin).

ticarcillin, an antibiotic. It is given to treat bacterial blood poisoning (septicemia), and skin, soft tissue, and breathing infections caused by both gram-negative and gram-positive organisms.

★CAUTION: A history of allergic reactions to any of the penicillins prohibits its use.

★ADVERSE EFFECTS: Among the most serious side effects are allergic (anaphylactic) reactions, decrease in platelets in the blood (thrombocytopenia), decrease of leukocytes in the blood (leukopenia), fewer neutrophils in the blood (neutropenia), vein irritation, and swelling of the vein (phlebitis).

tic douloureux. See **trigeminal neuralgia.**

tick bite, a puncture wound produced by the toothed beak of a bloodsucking tick. Ticks carry several diseases to humans. A few species carry a neurotoxin in their saliva that may cause ascending paralysis beginning in the legs. Nervousness, loss of appetite, and tingling and headache followed by muscle pain may occur. In extreme cases, breathing failure may occur. Symptoms often disappear when the attached tick is carefully removed with forceps. Placing a drop of alcohol or ether on the tick or coating it with petrolatum or nail polish makes removal easier. See also **Lyme arthritis, Q fever, relapsing fever, Rocky Mountain spotted fever, tularemia.**

tick fever. See **relapsing fever.**

tick paralysis, a rare, progressive, changeable disorder. It is caused by several species of ticks that release a neurotoxin that causes weakness, incoordination, and paralysis. The tick must feed on the host for several days before the symptoms appear. The removal of the tick leads to rapid recovery. Because breathing, lip, tongue, throat, and vocal cord paralysis can cause death, it is important to search for ticks. They are hidden in scalp hair on a patient with the symptoms.

t.i.d., (in prescriptions) abbreviation for *ter in die* /dē′ā/, a Latin phrase meaning "three times a day."

tidal drainage. See **drainage.**

tidal volume (TV), the amount of air inhaled and exhaled during normal breathing. Inspiratory reserve volume, expiratory reserve volume, and tidal volume make up vital capacity. See also **pulmonary function test.**

tide, a change, increase or decrease, in the concentration of a particular component of body fluids, as acid tide, fat tide. **–tidal,** *adj.*

Tietze's syndrome /tēt'sēz/, **1.** a disorder marked by swellings without pus of one or more rib cartilages causing pain that may radiate to the neck, shoulder, or arm and feel like the pain of heart artery disease. The syndrome may go along with breathing infections. If the costal swellings are extremely painful, infiltration with procaine and hydrocortisone may give relief. **2.** albinism, except for normal eye pigment, accompanied by deafness, inability to speak (mutism), and incomplete growth (hypoplasia) of the eyebrows.

TIG, abbreviation for **tetanus immune globulin.**

Tigan, a trademark for a drug used against nausea and vomiting (trimethobenzamide hydrochloride).

timed collection, the collection of the specimen, as a urine or stool sample, for a specific period of time.

timed release. See **prolonged release.**

timesharing, performing two or more tasks with a computer at the same time. The computer actually processes a small portion of each task at one time, switching from one to another, but it can handle so many data in brief time segments that the operator or operators are not aware of the computer switching.

timolol maleate, a beta-adrenergic receptor blocking drug. It is given for lessening eye pressure in long-term open-angle and secondary glaucoma.
★CAUTION: Bronchial asthma, COPD, slow heart beat (sinus bradycardia), or known allergy to this drug prohibits its use. It is used carefully in patients who are sensitive to beta-adrenergic receptor blocking drugs.
★ADVERSE EFFECTS: The most serious side effect is blurring of vision. Mild eye irritation also may occur.

Timoptic, a trademark for a beta-adrenergic receptor blocking agent (timolol maleate).

tin (Sn), a whitish metallic element. Its atomic number is 50; its atomic weight is 118.69. Tin oxide is used in dentistry as a polishing agent for teeth. It is also used in some restorative procedures.

Tinactin, a trademark for an antifungal (tolnaftate).

tincture, a substance in a solution that is mixed with alcohol.

Tindal, a trademark for a phenothiazine (acetophenazine maleate), used as a tranquilizer.

tinea /tin'ē·ə/, a group of fungal skin diseases. They are caused by several kinds of parasitical fungi. They are marked by itching, scaling, and, sometimes, painful sores. Tinea is a general term that refers to infections of various causes, which are seen on several sites. The specific type is usually designated by a modifying term. Diagnosis is made by demonstrating fungus on smear or by culture. Also called, loosely, **ringworm.**

tinea capitis, a contagious fungal disease. It is marked by circular, bald patches of from 1 to 6 cm in diameter with slight redness of the skin (erythema), scaling, and crusting. Diagnosis is made by bright fluorescence of infected hairs under Wood's light. Microscopic examination of infected hairs and culture of the fungus are other diagnosis techniques. Treatment consists of 3 to 6 weeks of griseofulvin given by mouth. Also called **ringworm.**

tinea corporis, a fungal infection of the nonhairy skin of the body. It occurs most often in hot, humid climates. It is usually caused by species of *Trichophyton* or *Microsporum.* Fungi killers, as miconazole, are used for moderate cases. Severe infection calls for the antibiotic griseofulvin.

tinea cruris /krōō'ris/, a fungal infection of the groin. It is caused by species of *Trichophyton* or *Epidermophyton floccosum.* It is most common in the tropics and among males. Topical antifungals, as miconazole and clotrimazole, are often given. The antibiotic griseofulvin is used only for severe, resistant cases. Also called **jock itch.**

tinea pedis, a long-term fungal infection of the foot. It occurs especially on the skin between the toes and on the soles. It is common worldwide. It is usually caused by *Trichophyton mentagrophytes, T. rubrum,* and *Epidermophyton floccosum.* Adults are most susceptible. The wearing of constricting footwear, as sneakers, seems to induce the infection. Drying the feet well after bathing and applying powder between the toes help prevent it. The antibiotic griseofulvin is the most effective treatment. However, miconazole and tolnaftate are also used. Recurrence is common. Also called **athlete's foot.**

tinea unguium, a fungal infection of the nails. It is caused by some species of *Trichophyton* and, occasionally, by *Candida albicans.* It is more common on the toes than the fingers. It can cause complete crumbling and destruction of the nails. The antibiotic griseofulvin is the drug of choice. It must be continued until the nail has regrown completely.

tinea versicolor, a fungus infection of the skin. It is marked by finely shedding, pale tan patches on the upper trunk and upper arms that may itch and do not tan. It is caused by *Malassezia furfur.* In dark-skinned persons the injury may be depigmented. The fungus fluoresces under Wood's light. The fungus also may be easily identified in scrapings viewed under a microscope. Treatment usually includes a single application of selenium sulfide left on overnight.

It is rinsed off by thorough showering in the morning. The pale patches may last for up to 1 year after successful treatment.

Tinel's sign /tinelz'/, an indication of irritability of a nerve. It results in a remote tingling sensation on percussion of a damaged nerve. The sign is often present in the abnormal tingling sensation in the fingers and the hand (carpal tunnel syndrome). It is produced by tapping over the median nerve on the flexing surface of the wrist.

tine test, a tuberculin skin test. A small disposable disk with multiple prongs bearing tuberculin antigen is used to puncture the skin. The method is widely used to test for sensitivity to the tuberculin antigen. Hardening around the puncture site indicates previous exposure or active disease, requiring further testing. See also **tuberculin test.**

tingling, a prickly sensation in the skin or a part of the body. It goes along with less sensitivity to stimulation of the sensory nerves. It is felt by a patient as the area is numbed by local anesthetic or by exposure to the cold, or as it "goes to sleep" from pressure on a nerve.

tinnitus /tini'təs/, tinkling or ringing heard in one or both ears. It may be a sign of acoustic injury.

tinted denture base, a denture base that simulates the coloring of natural oral tissue.

tissue, a collection of similar cells that act together in doing a particular function.

tissue activator. See **fibrinokinase.**

tissue-base relationship, (in dentistry) the relationship of the base of a removable prosthesis to nearby structures.

tissue committee, a group that evaluates all surgery done in a hospital or other health care facility. See also **tissue review.**

tissue dextrin. See **glycogen.**

tissue dose, (in radiotherapy) the amount of radiation absorbed by tissue in the region of treatment, expressed in rad.

tissue fixation, a process in which a tissue sample is placed in a fluid that keeps the cells as nearly as is possible in their natural state.

tissue fixative, a fluid that keeps cells in their natural state, so that they may be identified and examined.

tissue kinase. See **fibrinokinase.**

tissue plasminogen activator (TPA), a clot-dissolving substance produced naturally by cells in the walls of blood vessels. It is also manufactured synthetically by genetic engineering techniques. TPA activates plasminogen to dissolve clots. It has been used to remove blood clots blocking heart arteries.

tissue response, any reaction or change in living cell tissue when it is acted on by disease, toxin, or other outer stimulus. Some kinds of tissue responses are **immune response, inflammation,** and **necrosis.**

tissue review, a review of the surgery done in a hospital or other health-care facility. See also **tissue committee.**

tissue typing, a series of tests to evaluate whether tissues of a donor and a recipient fit with each other. It is done before transplantation. It is done by identifying and comparing a large series of human leukocyte antigens (HLA) in the cells of the body. See also **HLA, immune system, transplant.**

titanium (Ti), a grayish, brittle metallic element. Its atomic number is 22; its atomic weight is 47.9. An alloy of titanium is used in the manufacture of orthopedic prostheses. Titanium dioxide is the active part in a number of skin ointments and lotions.

titer, **1.** a measurement of the concentration of a substance in a solution. **2.** the quantity of a substance needed to get a reaction with another substance. **3.** the smallest amount of a certain substance that shows the presence of a colon bacillus under standard conditions. **4.** the highest dilution of a serum that causes joining in irregular masses (clumping) of bacteria.

title, a section of the Social Security Act that provides for the establishment, funding, and regulation of a service to a specific part of the population, as Title XIX. This title includes medical coverage. Medicaid Title X awards lump-sum grants for family planning programs.

titubation /tich'ōōbā'shən/, unsteady posture. It is marked by a staggering or stumbling style of walking. It is also marked by a swaying head or trunk while sitting. It may be caused by a disease of the back brain (cerebellum). Compare **ataxia.**

TLC, **1.** abbreviation for **total lung capacity.** **2.** *informal.* abbreviation for *tender loving care.*

T lymphocyte. See **lymphocyte, T cell.**

TMJ, abbreviation for **temporomandibular joint.**

TMP/SMX, abbreviation for **trimethoprim sulfamethoxazole.**

TNM, a system for staging cancerous tumor disease. See also **cancer staging.**

toadstool poisoning, a toxic condition. It is caused by ingestion of certain varieties of poisonous mushrooms. See **mushroom poisoning.**

tobacco, a plant whose leaves are dried and used for smoking and chewing, and in snuff. See also **nicotine.**

tobacco withdrawal syndrome, a change in mood or performance linked to stopped or lessened exposure to nicotine. Symptoms may range from lack of concentration to anxiety and temper outbursts.

TOBEC, abbreviation for **total body electrical conductivity.**

tobramycin sulfate, an aminoglycoside antibiotic. It is used to treat outer eye infections, blood poisoning (septicemia), and lower breathing tract and central nervous system infections.

★CAUTION: Kidney dysfunction, use of strong drugs that stimulate urine release, or known allergy to this or other aminoglycosides prohibits its use.

★ADVERSE EFFECTS: Among the more serious side effects are harm to nerves, hearing, and balance (ototoxicity), and harm to the kidney cells (nephrotoxicity).

Tobruk plaster /tō'brŏŏk/, a plaster cast splint with tapes for skin traction coming through openings in the plaster and connected with Thomas' splint. It covers and immobilizes the leg from foot to groin. Also called **Tobruk splint.**

tocanide hydrochloride, a drug taken by mouth to treat irregular heart beats (cardiac arrhythmias).

-tocia, 1. a combining form meaning 'conditions of labor.' **2.** a combining form meaning the 'product of giving birth.'

-tocin, a combining form for oxytocin derivatives.

toco-, toko-, a combining form meaning 'referring to childbirth or labor.'

tocodynamometer /tō'kōdī'nəmom'ətər/, an electronic device for monitoring and recording contractions of the uterus in labor. It is made up of an electronic device (tocotransducer) that is connected to the lower stomach with a belt, and a machine that records the duration of the contractions and the interval between them on graph paper. The relative intensity of the contractions is also indicated but cannot be quantified. The tocodynamometer is a component of outer monitoring in childbirth. Also spelled **tokodynamometer. See also electronic fetal monitor.**

tocolytic drug, any drug used to suppress premature labor.

tocopherol. See vitamin E.

tocotransducer, an electronic device used to measure contractions of the uterus. See also **tocodynamometer.**

toddler, a child between 12 and 36 months of age. During this period of development the child gets a sense of autonomy and independence through the mastery of various specialized tasks. Some of these tasks are control of bodily functions, refinement of motor and language skills, and learning socially acceptable behavior, especially toleration of delayed satisfaction of needs and acceptance of separation from the mother or parents. The period is marked by exploration of the environment and by rapid cognitive growth. The child strives for self-assertion and personal interaction with others while struggling with parental discipline and sibling rivalry.

toddlerhood, the state or condition of being a toddler.

toe, any one of the digits of the feet.

toeing in. See metatarsus varus.

toeing out. See metatarsus valgus.

toenail, one of the heavy nail structures covering the end bones of the toes. Also called **unguis** /ung'gwis/.

Tofranil, a trademark for a tricyclic antidepressant (imipramine hydrochloride).

togaviruses /tō'gəvī'rəsəs/, a family of arboviruses. They include the organisms causing swelling of the brain (encephalitis), tropic diseases (dengue, yellow fever), and rubella.

toilet training, the process of teaching a child to control the functions of the bladder and bowel. Training programs differ. However, all stress a positive, consistent approach without punishment and great pressure. Each program is individualized. The specific training depends on the mental and physical age and state of the child, the parent-child relationship, and readiness of the child to learn. Training often begins between 18 and 24 months of age. At this time, voluntary control of the anus and urine tract muscles is achieved by most children. When the child has mastered some motor skills, is aware of his or her ability to control the body, and can communicate adequately, training is likely to be easy. Resistance occurs if the parents try to train the child before the child is physically and mentally ready. Bowel training is usually successful before bladder training because the urge to empty the bowel is stronger than the urge to empty the bladder. Also, the need is less frequent and more regular. Nighttime bladder control may not be achieved until the child is 4 or 5 years of age or older. Behavior changing, using a system of rewards for each of the many phases of the training, has been successful with both normal and mentally slow children.

-toin, a combining form for derivatives of hydantoin used in treatment of epilepsy.

token economy, a technique of strengthening behavior used in behavior therapy in the management of a group of people, as in hospitals, institutions, or classrooms. Individuals are rewarded for specific activities or behavior with tokens they can exchange for desired objects or privileges.

toko-. See toco-.

tokodynamometer. See tocodynamometer.

tolazamide, a sulfonylurea drug used against diabetes. Taken by mouth, it is given to treat stable or non-insulin-dependent diabetes mellitus and for some patients sensitive to other types of sulfonylureas or who have failed to respond to other similar drugs.

★CAUTION: Unstable diabetes, serious blockage of kidneys, liver, or thyroid function, pregnancy, or known allergy to this drug or to other sulfonylurea drugs prohibits its use.

★ADVERSE EFFECTS: Among the more serious

side effects are lack of glucose in the blood (hypoglycemia) and skin reactions. Blood disorders may occur.

tolazoline hydrochloride, a drug for widening the veins in the outer part of the body (peripheral vasodilator). It is given to treat spastic peripheral vascular disorders, including Buerger's disease, Raynaud's disease, and scleroderma.

★CAUTION: Heart artery disease, brain vessel (cerebrovascular) accident, or known allergy to this drug prohibits its use.

★ADVERSE EFFECTS: Among the more serious side effects are irregular heart beat (cardiac arrhythmia), high blood pressure, increase of peptic ulcer, and a contradictory response in seriously damaged limbs.

tolbutamide, a sulfonylurea drug used against diabetes. Taken by mouth, it is given to treat stable non-insulin-dependent diabetes mellitus uncontrolled by diet alone and for some patients changing from injected insulin to therapy by mouth.

★CAUTION: Unstable diabetes, serious blockage of kidney, liver, or thyroid function, pregnancy, or known allergy to this drug or to other sulfonylurea drugs prohibits its use.

★ADVERSE EFFECTS: Among the more serious side effects are lack of glucose in the blood (hypoglycemia) and skin reactions. Blood diseases may occur.

Tolectin, a trademark for a nonsteroid antiswelling drug (tolmetin sodium).

tolerance, the ability to live through hardship, pain, or ordinarily injurious substances, as drugs, without apparent physiological or psychological injury. A kind of tolerance is **work tolerance.**

tolerance dose. See **maximum permissible dose.**

Tolinase, a trademark for a drug used against diabetes (tolazamide).

tolmetin sodium /tol′mətin/, a nonsteroid antiinflammatory drug. It is mainly given to treat different forms of joint swelling (arthritis and osteoarthritis).

★CAUTION: Blocked kidney function, stomach and intestinal disease, or known allergy to this drug, to aspirin, or to nonsteroid antiswelling drugs prohibits its use.

★ADVERSE EFFECTS: Among the more serious side effects are peptic ulcer and distress of the stomach and intestines. Dizziness, skin rash, and ringing in the ears (tinnitus) commonly occur. This drug interacts with many other drugs.

tolnaftate /tolnaf′tāt/, an antifungal. It is given to treat fungus infections of the skin, including athlete's foot, infection of the thighs (tinea pedis), tinea cruris, and infection with patches (tinea versicolor).

★CAUTION: Known allergy to this drug prohibits its use.

★ADVERSE EFFECTS: Among the more common side effects are allergic reactions and mild irritation of the skin.

-tome, 1. a combining form meaning a 'cutting instrument.' **2.** a combining form meaning a '(specified) segment or region.'

-tomic, -tomical, a combining form meaning 'related to incisions or sections of tissue.'

tomographic DSA, seeing blood vessels in the body in three dimensions. See also **digital subtraction angiography (DSA).**

tomography /təmog′rəfē/, an x-ray technique that makes a film representing a detailed cross section of tissue structure at a predetermined depth. It is a valuable diagnostic tool for the discovery and identification of space-occupying tumors, as might be found in the brain, liver, pancreas, and gallbladder.

-tomy, a combining form meaning a 'surgical incision.'

tone. See **tonus.**

tongue, the main organ for the sense of taste. It also assists in the chewing and swallowing of food. It is located in the floor of the mouth within the curve of the mandible. The front two-thirds of the tongue are covered with small, nipple-shaped elevations. The back third is smoother and has numerous mucous glands and lymph follicles. The use of the tongue as an organ of speech is not anatomic but a learned characteristic. Also called **lingua.**

tongue-thrust swallow, an immature form of swallowing in which the tongue is pushed forward instead of backward during the act of swallowing. It may cause the upper jaw to move too far forward, so that the upper and lower teeth do not meet properly.

tongue-tie. See **ankyloglossia.**

-tonia, -tony, a combining form meaning '(condition or degree of) muscle contraction of a sort or in a region of the body.'

-tonic, 1. a combining form meaning the 'quality of muscle contraction or tonus.' **2.** a combining form meaning a 'solution with a comparative concentration.'

tonicity /tōnis′itē/, the quality of possessing muscle contraction (tone or tonus).

tonic labyrinthine reflex, a normal body reflex in animals. It is abnormally accentuated in patients with brain defects (decerebrate patients). It is marked by extension of all four limbs when the head is positioned in space at an angle above the horizontal in four-footed animals or in the neutral, erect position in humans. Also called **decerebrate rigidity.**

tonic neck reflex, a normal response in newborns to extend the arm and the leg on the side of the body to which the head is quickly turned while the infant is lying with the face upward and to flex the limbs of the opposite side. The reflex prevents the infant from rolling over until adequate neurological and motor development occurs. It disappears by 3 to 4 months of age to be replaced by symmetric positioning of both sides of the body. Absence or continuation of the reflex may indicate central nervous system damage. Also called **asymmetric tonic neck reflex.** See also **symmetric tonic neck reflex.**

tono-, a combining form meaning 'referring to muscle contraction (tone) or tension.'

Tonocard, a trademark for a numbing (lidocaine-type) drug (tocainide hydrochloride) given by mouth that prevents, relieves, or corrects abnormal heart rhythm.

tonofibril, a bundle of fine fibers found in the cytoplasm of epithelial cells. Also called **epitheliofibril, tenofibril.** See also **keratohyalin.**

tonometer /tōnom'ətər/, an instrument used in measuring tension or pressure, especially within the eye.

tonometry /tōnom'ətrē/, the measuring of pressure in the eyes. It is done by determining the resistance of the eyeball to flattening by an applied force. Several kinds of tonometers are used. The air-puff tonometer, which does not touch the eye, records turning aside of the cornea from a puff of pressurized air. The Schiötz impression and the aplanation tonometers record the pressure needed to flatten the corneal surface.

tonsil, a small, rounded mass of tissue, especially lymphoid tissue, as that comprising the palatine tonsils in the oropharynx. Compare **intestinal tonsil, lingual tonsil, palatine tonsil, pharyngeal tonsil.**

tonsillectomy, the surgical removal of the palatine tonsils. It is done to prevent returning swelling of the tonsil (streptococcal tonsillitis). Before surgery, several laboratory tests, including a bleeding and clotting time, complete blood count, and an analysis of the urine, are done. Tonsillar tissue is cut apart and removed. General anesthesia is usually used. Bleeding areas are stitched or destroyed by heat (cauterized). An airway remains in place until swallowing returns. An increase in pulse rate, falling blood pressure, restlessness, or frequent swallowing warns of possible bleeding. On recovery from anesthesia, ice chips or clear liquids without a drinking straw may be offered. Tonsillectomy is often combined with surgical removal of the adenoids.

tonsillitis, an infection or inflammation of a tonsil. Sudden tonsillitis is often caused by a streptococcus infection. It is marked by severe sore throat, fever, headache, malaise, difficulty in swallowing, earache, and large, tender lymph nodes in the neck. Sudden tonsillitis may go along with scarlet fever. Treatment includes systemic antibiotics, painkillers, and warm irrigations of the throat. Soft foods and enough fluids are given. Tonsillectomy is sometimes done for returning tonsillitis or tonsillar abscess. See also **peritonsillar abscess, scarlet fever, strep throat.**

tonus /tō'nəs/, **1.** the normal state of balanced tension in the tissues of the body, especially the muscles. Partial contraction or alternate contraction and relaxation of nearby fibers of a group of muscles hold the organ or the part of the body in a neutral, functional position without weakness. Tone is essential for many normal body functions. For example, holding the spine erect, the eyes open, and the jaw closed. **2.** the state of the tissues of the body being strong and fit. Also called **tone.**

-tony, -tonia, a combining form meaning a 'condition of motor control.'

tooth, *pl.* **teeth,** one of numerous dental structures that develop in the jaws as part of the digestive system. They are used to cut, grind, and process food in the mouth for ingestion. Each tooth is made up of a crown above the gum; two to four roots in the sockets; and a neck, stretching between the crown and the root. Each tooth also has a cavity filled with pulp, richly supplied with blood vessels and nerves that enter the cavity through a small opening at the base of each root. The solid portion of the tooth consists of dentin, enamel, and a thin layer of bone on the surface of the root. The dentin comprises the bulk of the tooth. The enamel covers the exposed portion of the crown. Two sets of teeth appear at different periods of life. The 20 temporary teeth appear during infancy. The 32 permanent teeth appear during childhood and early adulthood. See also **deciduous tooth, permanent tooth.**

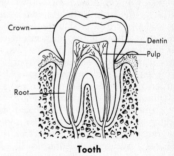

Tooth

tooth alignment, the arrangement of the teeth in relation to their supporting bone, adjacent teeth, and opposing teeth.

tooth-borne, describing a dental prosthesis or part of a prosthesis that depends entirely on real teeth for support.

tooth-borne base, a denture base restoring an area without teeth that has real teeth at each end for support. The tissue that it covers is not used for support of the base.

tooth form, the identifying curves, lines, angles, and contours of a tooth that differentiate it from other teeth.

tooth germ, a primitive cell in the embryo that is the precursor of a tooth.

tophaceous /təfā'shəs/, referring to the presence of abnormal stones of mineral salts (tophi).

tophus /tō'fəs/, *pl.* **tophi,** urate deposits around the joint. It is seen in patients with swelling of the joints (gout).

-topia, -topy, a combining form meaning '(condition of) placement of organs in the body.'

topical, **1.** of or referring to the surface of a part of the body. **2.** of or referring to a drug or treatment applied topically.

topical anesthesia, surface painkilling produced by application of a anesthetic in the form of a solution, gel, or ointment to the skin, mucous membrane, or cornea. Also called **surface anesthesia.** Compare **general anesthesia, local anesthesia, regional anesthesia.**

Topicort, a trademark for a topical drug that raises the concentration of liver glycogen and blood sugar (desoximetasone).

topo-, a combining form meaning 'place.'

topognosis, the ability to recognize stimuli through the sense of touch.

TORCH /tôrch/, an abbreviation for *toxoplasmosis, other, rubella virus, cytomegalovirus, and herpes simplex viruses.* This is a group of agents that can infect the fetus or the newborn infant causing a set of morbid effects called the TORCH syndrome.

TORCH syndrome, infection of the fetus or newborn by one of the TORCH agents. A pregnancy with a TORCH agent may lead to abortion or stillbirth, slowed growth within the uterus, or too-early childbirth. At birth and during the first days after birth, an infant infected with any one of the organisms may demonstrate various clinical manifestations, as fever, weakness, poor feeding, red spots (petechiae) on the skin, purplish-brownish skin (purpura), pneumonia, large liver and spleen (hepatosplenomegaly), liver disease (jaundice), and anemias. Other manifestations are swelling of the brain (encephalitis), too-small head (microcephaly), fluid in the brain (hydrocephalus), calcium formation in the head, hearing deficits, eye swellings (chorioretinitis), and too-small eyes (microophthalmia). In addition, each of the agents is linked to several other abnormal clinical findings involving abnormal immune response, cataracts, glaucoma, blisters (vesicles), ulcers, and inborn heart defects. Before pregnancy, women may be tested for susceptibility to the rubella virus. They may be vaccinated against it if not immune. There are currently no vaccines that confer immunity to the other TORCH agents. However, the mother may be tested for antibody levels to them. During pregnancy a nerve disorder (toxoplasmosis) does not show symptoms in about 90% of cases, making diagnosis unlikely. If infection is suspected, serial paired antibody tests are done. A high, rising titer indicates recent infection. Transplacental infection occurs in 35% of mothers infected during pregnancy. If it is contracted in the first 3 months, before the placenta is fully developed, the infant may not become infected. If the infection is contracted, severe inborn manifestations of the syndrome usually occur. If the fetus is infected after the first 3 months, the baby is usually born without symptoms or with mild disease. The infection may be spread from the baby during the newborn period. Sulfadiazone, pyrimethamine, and folinic acid are sometimes given to treat the infection. Primary cytomegalovirus infection during pregnancy is usually without symptoms. If the infection is suspected, antibody testing may be done to demonstrate primary infection. The reason is that infants born to mothers infected for the first time during pregnancy are much more likely to develop severe inborn abnormalities than if the infection is a reactivation of previous cytomegalovirus infection. There is no specific treatment. The child is thought to be infectious. However, getting an infection among newborns from an infected infant has not been proven. Transplacental rubella virus infection in pregnancy during the first 8 weeks is likely to cause infection in 50% of fetuses. It results in demonstrable defects in 85% of those infected. The risk becomes less as the pregnancy increases to 24 weeks, after which time infection has not been known to result in defects. Rubella is the only TORCH virus that is usually symptomatic. It is, therefore, often recognized. Many mothers infected during the first 3 months choose to abort the pregnancy. Screening and immunization before pregnancy could prevent virtually all cases of inborn rubella. Herpesvirus infection (HSV) in pregnancy is rarely carried to the fetus through the placenta. Primary infection during pregnancy sometimes results in spontaneous abortion or too-early childbirth. In the newborn the infection is usually life-threatening. The fetus is most likely to become infected by the virus shed from an active genital blister during vaginal birth. Infection can also be the result of vaginal examination or the placement of an intrauterine catheter or a fetal scalp electrode during labor. There is no treatment: If the mother has an active, genital herpesvirus tumor, intrapartal internal monitoring is prohibited. Vaginal examinations are often not done. Regional anesthetic techniques are avoided, and the infant is delivered by cesarean section. The TORCH infections caused by other agents are without symptoms in pregnancy. They reveal themselves by the syndrome after birth. The inborn effects are not subject to change or to improvement by any known treatment.

Torecan, a trademark for a phenothiazine drug used against nausea and vomiting (thiethylperazine maleate).

Torkildsen's procedure. See **ventriculocisternostomy.**

torque /tôrk/, **1.** a twisting force produced by contraction of the thigh muscles that tend to rotate the thigh inwards. **2.** (in dentistry) a force applied to a tooth to rotate it. **3.** a rotary force applied to a denture base. Compare **torsion.**

tors-, a combining form meaning 'twisted.'

torsades de pointes /tôrsäd′ depô·aNt′, tôrsäd dəpoint′/, an abnormal fast beat of the lower heart chambers. It shows a spiral-like look ("twisting of the points") and complexes that at first look positive and then negative on an electrocardiogram. It is begun by a long duration of electric activity in the lower heart chambers (QT interval), which often is drug induced (quinidine, procainamide, disopyramide, or amiodarone), but which may be the result of low potassium levels in the blood (hypokalemia) or profound slow heart beat (bradycardia). The abnormal rapid beat may be sudden. The patient may be conscious. Thus the diagnosis may be missed. The treatment is a temporary electronic pacemaker until the offending drug can be processed and released. Drugs that shorten the QT interval (atropine, isoproterenol) may be given.

torsion, 1. the process of twisting in a positive (clockwise) or negative (counterclockwise) direction. **2.** the state of being turned. **3.** (in dentistry) the twisting of a tooth on its long axis.

torsion dystonia. See **dystonia musculorum deformans.**

torsion fracture, a spiral broken bone. It is usually caused by a torsion injury.

torsion of the testis, the axial rotation of the sperm cord that cuts off the blood supply to the testicle, epididymis, and other structures. Complete ischemia for 6 hours may result in dying off (gangrene) of the testis. Partial loss of circulation may result in wasting away (atrophy). Certain testes are more likely to get torsion because of inadequate connective tissue. However, the condition may be caused by injury with severe swelling. Torsion of the testis occurs more often on the left than on the right side. It happens most often in the first year of life and during puberty. Surgical correction is needed in most cases. If surgery is done within 5 hours of the beginning of symptoms, the testis can usually be saved.

torsion spasm. See **dystonia musculorum deformans.**

torticollis /tôr′tikol′is/, an abnormal condition in which the head is inclined to one side as a result of the contraction of the muscles on that side of the neck. It may be inborn or gotten later in life. Treatment may include surgery, heat, support, or immobilization depending on the cause and the severity of the condition. Also called **wryneck.** See also **spasmodic torticollis.**

Torula histolytica. See **Cryptococcus neoformans.**

torulopsosis /tôr′yōōlop′səsis/, an infection with the yeast *Torulopsis glabrata.* This yeast is normally found in the throat, the intestinal and stomach tract, and the skin. However, it causes disease in severely weakened patients or in those with blocked immune function. It sometimes causes disease in patients with a long catheterization of the urine tract. General infection is usually treated with amphotericin B.

torulosis. See **cryptococcosis.**

torus fracture. See **lead pipe fracture.**

total anomalous venous return, a rare, inborn heart problem. The pulmonary veins attach directly to the right upper chamber of the heart (atrium) or to various veins draining into the right atrium rather than directing flow to the left atrium. Clinical manifestations include bluish skin (cyanosis), congestion of the lungs, and heart failure. Other heart defects may also be present. Corrective surgery is needed, usually after 1 year of age. However, it may be necessary at an earlier age if pulmonary venous obstruction or severe congestive heart failure is present. See also **congenital cardiac anomaly.**

total body electrical conductivity (TOBEC), a method of measuring body composition by the difference in the movement of electricity through fat, bone, and muscle. It is used for tracking the fitness of athletes; in clinical studies of weight control in which physicians want to determine if weight loss is due to fat, water, or other tissues; and in measurement of fat content of dietary meats. See also **bioelectric impedance analysis (BIA).**

total body radiation, radiation that exposes the entire body so that, theoretically, all cells in the body receive the same radiation.

total body water (TBW), all the water within the body, including intracellular and extracellular water plus the water in the stomach and intestines and urinary tract.

total cleavage, cell (mitotic) division of the fertilized egg (ovum) into blastomeres. Compare **partial cleavage.**

total communication, the combined use of spoken language and sign language by a person with hearing loss.

total iron, the total iron concentration in the blood. The normal concentrations in serum are 50 to 150 micrograms/dl.

total lung capacity (TLC), the volume of gas in the lungs at the end of a maximum breathing in. It equals the vital capacity plus the residual capacity.

total macroglobulins, the heavy serum macroglobulins that are raised in various diseases, as cancer, and infections. The normal concentrations in serum are 70 to 430 mg/dl.

total nitrogen, the nitrogen content of the stool. It is measured to detect various disorders, improper functioning of the pancreas, and blocked protein digestion. The normal amount in a 24-hour fecal specimen is 10% of intake, or 1 to 2 g.

total parenteral nutrition (TPN), the giving of a nutritionally adequate solution with glucose, protein hydrolysates, minerals, and vitamins through an indwelling catheter into the vein that drains into the right upper chamber of the heart (superior vena cava). The high rate of blood flow results in rapid dilution of the solution. Full nutritional requirements can be met indefinitely. The procedure is used in a long coma, severe uncontrolled malabsorption, extensive burns, stomach and intestinal fistulas, and other conditions in which feeding by mouth cannot give adequate amounts of the essential nutrients. In infants and children it is used when feeding by way of the stomach and intestinal tract is impossible, inadequate, or hazardous, as in long-term intestinal obstruction, inadequate intestinal length, or long-term severe diarrhea. The nutritional solution is put through normal tubing with a filter attached to remove any contaminants. A strict infection-free environment must be kept because infection is a grave and ever-present danger of this therapy. Also called **hyperalimentation, intravenous alimentation, parenteral hyperalimentation, total parenteral alimentation.**

total peripheral resistance, the maximum degree of resistance to blood flow caused by narrowing of the body blood vessels.

total renal blood flow (TRBF), the total volume of blood that flows into the kidney arteries. The average TRBF in a normal adult is 1,200 ml per minute.

touch, 1. the ability to feel objects and to keep their various traits apart; the tactile sense. **2.** the ability to note pressure when it is put on the skin or the mucosa of the body. **3.** to examine with the hand.

touch deprivation, a lack of touch stimulation. It happens especially in early infancy. If it is continued for some length of time, it may lead to serious developmental and emotional disturbances, as slow growth, personality disorders, and social regression. In severe cases, a child

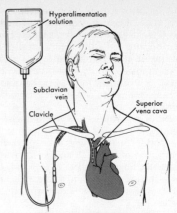

Total parenteral nutrition

who lacks adequate physical handling and emotional stimulation may not survive infancy. See also **hospitalism.**

Tourette's syndrome. See **Gilles de la Tourette's syndrome.**

tourniquet /tur′nikit, toŏr′-/, a device used in controlling bleeding. It is made up of a wide constricting band applied to the limb immediate to the site of bleeding. The use of a tourniquet is a drastic measure. It is to be used only if the bleeding is life-threatening and if other, safer measures have proved ineffective. See also **hemorrhage.**

tourniquet infusion method, a technique of intraarterial regional chemotherapy. It is used to treat a bone tumor (osteogenic sarcoma). The technique uses one or two external tourniquets, depending on the location of the tumor, which slow or interrupt the blood flow to a limb temporarily while an anticancer drug, as adriamycin, is infused into the area. The method increases the concentration of the anticancer drug by as much as 100 times as compared with an alternative technique of injecting the drug into the circulation.

tourniquet test, a test of capillary fragility. A blood pressure cuff is applied for 5 minutes to a person's arm. It is inflated to a pressure halfway between the diastolic and systolic blood pressure. The number of small red spots (petechiae) within a certain area of the skin may be counted. Alternatively, the results may be reported in a range from negative (no petechiae) to +4 positive (confluent petechiae).

tower head, tower skull. See **oxycephaly.**

toxemia /toksē′mē·ə/, the presence of bacterial poison in the bloodstream. Also called **blood poisoning.** See also **preeclampsia. –toxemic,** adj.

-toxemia, -toxaemia, a combining form meaning a '(specified) toxic substance in the blood.'

toxemia of pregnancy. See **preeclampsia.**

-toxia, a combining form meaning 'condition resulting from a poison in a (specified) region of the body.'

toxic, 1. of or referring to a poison. **2.** (of a disease or condition) severe and progressive.

-toxic, -toxical, a combining form meaning 'referring to poison.'

toxic amblyopia, partial loss of vision because of swelling of the part behind the eyeball (retrooptic bulbar neuritis). It is caused by poisoning with quinine, lead, wood alcohol, nicotine, arsenic, or certain other poisons.

toxic dementia, loss of intellectual function (dementia) resulting from excess use of or exposure to a poisonous substance. See also **dementia.**

toxic dose (TD), (in toxicology) the amount of a substance that may be expected to produce a poisonous effect. See also **median toxic dose.**

toxic epidermal necrolysis (TEN), a rare skin disease. It is marked by redness of the outer skin (epidermal erythema), death of skin cells (superficial necrosis), and skin erosion. This condition, which affects mainly adults, makes the skin appear scalded, often leaving scars. The cause of TEN is unknown. It may result from poisonous or allergic reactions. It is commonly linked to drug reactions, as those linked to butazones, sulfonamides, penicillins, barbiturates, and hydantoins. Other drugs may be involved. The disease has also been linked to airborne poisons, as carbon monoxide. TEN may also indicate an immune response, or it may be linked to severe physiological stress. Early signs of the condition include swelling of the mucous membranes, fever, malaise, a burning sensation in the membranes of the eyes (conjunctivae), and tenderness of the skin. The first phase of TEN is manifested by diffuse redness of the skin (erythema). The second phase involves blistering. The third phase is marked by extensive dropping off of dead skin tissue and general shedding (epidermal necrolysis, desquamation). As the disease progresses, large, soft blisters develop and rupture, exposing wide expanses of denuded skin. Tissue fluids and electrolytes are consequently lost. This results in extensive body complications, as fluid pooling in the lungs, swelling of the lungs, bleeding in the stomach, intestines, and esophagus, poison in the blood (sepsis), shock, kidney failure, and disseminated intravascular clotting. These extreme conditions contribute to the high mortality linked to TEN—about 30%—especially among the infirm and the elderly. Confirming diagnosis is based on symptoms in the third phase of the disease, as skin is denuded by even slight friction, affecting the areas of red skin. Diagnosis is commonly supported by bacteriological culture and Gram's stains of blisters to determine if infection exists. The presence of leukocytosis, fluid and electrolyte imbalances, albuminuria, and high transaminase levels are characteristic and help confirm the diagnosis. Treatment of TEN commonly involves giving fluids in the veins to replace body fluids and to maintain electrolyte balance. Laboratory analyses are necessary to monitor hematocrit and hemoglobin, serum proteins, electrolytes, and blood gases.

toxic erythema of the newborn. See **erythema toxicum neonatorum.**

toxic gastritis. See **corrosive gastritis.**

toxic goiter, a large thyroid gland linked to abnormal bulging of the eye (exophthalmia) and disease of the whole body. See also **Graves' disease.**

toxic hemoglobinuria. See **hemoglobinuria.**

toxicity /toksis'itē/, **1.** the degree to which something is poisonous. **2.** a condition that results from exposure to a poison or to poisonous amounts of a substance that does not cause side effects in smaller amounts.

toxic nodular goiter, an enlarged thyroid gland. It is marked by many injured nodules and excess release of thyroid hormones. It occurs most often in elderly individuals. Typical signs of thyrotoxicosis, as nervousness, trembling, weakness, weight loss, and irritability, are usually present. Bulging of the eyes (exophthalmia) may also occur. Loss of appetite is more common than excess eating (hyperphagia). Irregular heart rate (cardiac arrhythmia) or congestive heart failure may be a dominant manifestation. When clinical findings suggest thyrotoxicosis, a trial of antithyroid drugs, as propylthiouracil or methimazole, is advised. However, once the diagnosis is established, radioactive iodine is thought to be the best treatment. Large doses are usually required.

toxico-, toxo-, a combining form meaning 'referring to poison, poisonous.'

toxicokinetics, the passage through the body system of a poisonous substance or its products.

toxicologist, a specialist in the scientific study of poisons and the diseases they bring about (toxicology).

toxicology, the scientific study of poisons, their detection, their effects, and methods of treatment for conditions they produce. **–toxicologic, toxicological,** adj.

toxic psychosis, a severe mental disorder that results from the effects of chemicals or drugs, including those produced by the body itself.

toxic shock syndrome (TSS), a severe sudden disease. It is caused by infection with strains of *Staphylococcus aureus,* phage group I. These strains make a unique poison, enterotoxin F. It is most common in menstruating women using high absorbency tampons. However, it has been seen in newborn infants, children, and men. The beginning of the syndrome is marked by sudden high fever, headache, sore throat with swelling of the mucous membranes, diarrhea, nausea, and red spots on the skin (erythroderma). Acute kidney failure, abnormal liver function, confusion, and hard-to-treat low blood pressure usually follow. Death may occur. It is probable that mild forms of the syndrome are not reported and, therefore, are not diagnosed. There does not appear to be any seasonal or geographical factor in the cause of the disease. There is no evidence of contagion among household members or through sexual contacts of people who have TSS. Bacteremia, or discernible local infection, is absent in most cases. *Staphylococcus aureus* may be cultured from many sites, including the throat, the nostrils, and the lower narrow end of the uterus (cervix). However, the drastic effects of infection are the result of the toxin released from the organism rather than from the infection itself. Aggressive volume expansion by giving large amounts of fluid in the vein, help with ventilation, and giving drugs that contract the muscle tissue of blood veins (vasopressors) may be necessary in treating severe TSS. Early recognition and active supportive treatment greatly improve the survival rates. They also lessen both long occurrences of the disease and its returning.

toxin, a poison, usually one produced by or occurring in a plant or microorganism. See also **endotoxin, exotoxin.**

-toxin, a combining form meaning 'poison.'

toxo-. See **toxico-.**

toxocariasis /tok'sōkərī'əsis/, infection with the larvae of *Toxocara canis,* the common roundworm of dogs and cats. Ingestion of viable eggs, commonly found in soil, leads to the spread of tiny larvae throughout the body. This results in breathing symptoms, large liver, skin rashes, pooling of leukocytes in the blood (eosinophilia), and delayed eye injury. Children who eat dirt are particularly subject to this disease. Specific drug therapy is not very useful. The outcome is usually good without therapy. Regular worming of pets helps prevent infection. Also called **visceral larva migrans.**

toxoid, a toxin that has been treated with chemicals or with heat to lessen its poisonous effect but keeps its power to stimulate antibody formation. It is given to make immunity by stimulating the creation of antibodies. See also **toxin, vaccine.**

Toxoplasma /tok'sōplaz'mə/, a genus of protozoa with only one known species, *Toxoplasma gondii.* It is an intracellular parasite of cats and other hosts that causes a nerve disease (toxoplasmosis) in humans.

toxoplasmosis /tok'sōplazmō'sis/, a common infection with the protozoan intracellular parasite *Toxoplasma gondii.* It is marked in its in-

born form by liver and brain involvement with calcium in the brain (cerebral calcification), convulsions, blindness, too-small head and fluid on the brain (microcephaly and hydrocephaly), and mental retardation. The acquired form is marked by rash, disease of the lymph nodes (lymphadenopathy), fever, malaise, central nervous system disorders, swelling of the heart wall (myocarditis), and swelling of lung tissue (pneumonitis). Cats acquire the organism by eating infected birds and mice. Lumps (cysts) of the organism are carried from cat feces to humans or by human ingestion of inadequately cooked meat containing the lumps. Carrying through the placenta occurs only during acute infection of the mother. The disease is very serious in the fetus and in those with a blocked immune system. Diagnosis is made by demonstrating rising antibody titers or by immunofluorescent antibody tests. Infection confers immunity. Combinations of sulfonamides with pyrimethamine are advised as treatment. This may lessen the severity of the illness in the fetus.

TPA, abbreviation for **tissue plasminogen activator.**

TPAL. See **parity.**

TPN, abbreviation for **total parenteral nutrition.**

trabecula carnea /trəbek'yələ/, *pl.* **trabeculae carneae,** any one of the irregular bands and bundles of muscle that project from the inner surfaces of the lower heart chambers (ventricles), except in the arterial cone of the right lower heart chamber. Some of these trabeculae are ridges of muscle along the lower heart chamber walls. Others are short projections into the ventricular cavities. Still others form the ventricular papillary muscles. Compare **chordae tendineae.** See also **heart, left ventricle, right ventricle.**

trabeculae, the part of the eye in front of the canal of Schlemm and in the angle created by the iris and the cornea.

trabecula septomarginalis. See **moderator band.**

trabeculectomy, the removal by surgery of a section of corneoscleral tissue to increase the outflow of eye fluid (aqueous humor) in patients with severe glaucoma. The procedure usually involves removal of the canal of Schlemm and the trabecular meshwork.

trabeculotomy, an opening by surgery in an orbital trabecula to increase the outflow of eye fluid (aqueous humor).

trace element, an element needed for nutrition or mental processes, found in such small amounts that analysis shows almost none of it.

trace gas, a gas or vapor that escapes into the atmosphere during an anesthetic procedure. The substances may have negative effects on the health of personnel exposed to them.

Equipment is often installed in operating rooms to clean the air. See also **gas scavenging system.**

tracer, 1. see also **radioisotope scan.** a radioactive isotope used in diagnostic x-ray techniques to allow a biological process to be seen. The tracer, which is put into the body, binds with a specific substance and is followed with a scanner or fluoroscope as it passes through many organs or systems in the body. Kinds of tracers include **radioactive iodine** (^{131}I) and **radioactive carbon**(^{14}C). 2. a mechanical device that records on a graph the outline or movements of an object, or part of the body. 3. a cutting instrument used to isolate vessels and nerves. –**trace,** v.

tracer depot method, (in nuclear medicine) a technique used to determine local skin or muscle blood flow. It is based on the rate at which a radioactive tracer put in a tissue is removed by spreading into the capillaries and washed out by the local blood supply. If blood flow is less or absent, as in dead skin, the deposited tracer does not wash out.

trachea /trā′kē·ə/, a nearly cylindrical tube in the neck. Consisting of cartilage and membrane, it extends from the voicebox (larynx) at the level of the sixth cervical vertebra to the fifth thoracic vertebra, where it divides into two bronchi. The trachea leads air to the lungs. It is about 11 cm long and 2 cm wide. It is covered in the neck by the isthmus of the thyroid gland and various other structures. The trachea is in contact with the esophagus. Also called **windpipe.** See also **primary bronchus.** –**tracheal,** adj.

tracheal breath sound, a normal breath sound heard in the windpipe. Breathing in and out are equally loud. Compare **vesicular breath sound.**

tracheitis /trā′kē·ī′tis/, any swelling condition of the windpipe. It may be sudden or long-term. It may result from infection, allergy, or physical irritation.

trachelo-, a combining form meaning 'referring to the neck or a necklike structure.'

trachelodynia. See **cervicodynia.**

tracheo-, a combining form meaning 'referring to the trachea.'

tracheobronchial tree (TBT), an anatomic complex that includes the windpipe, the bronchi, and the bronchial tubes. It brings air to and from the lungs. It is the main structure in breathing. See also **bronchial tree.**

tracheobronchitis /trā′kē·ōbrongkī′tis/, swelling of the windpipe and bronchi. It is a common form of breathing infection.

tracheobronchomegaly, an abnormally large upper airway, in which the windpipe may be as wide as the spinal column.

tracheoesophageal fistula, an inborn abnormality. There is an abnormal tubelike passage between the windpipe and the esophagus.

tracheoesophageal shunt, a surgical procedure that makes a passageway between the windpipe and the throat, allowing a person without a voicebox to speak. The operation results in an ability to produce throat speech with normal breathing as a source of air and without the need to belch to produce voice sounds.

tracheomalacia /trā′kē·ōmälā′shə/, a decaying of the windpipe, usually caused by too-much pressure from a cuffed tube inside the windpipe.

tracheostomy /trā′kē·os′təmē/, an opening through the neck into the windpipe through which an indwelling tube may be inserted. After tracheostomy, the patient's chest is listened to for breath sounds indicative of pulmonary congestion. Mucous membranes and fingertips are observed for bluish coloring (cyanosis). Humidified oxygen is given via tent or directly into the tracheostomy tube. The patient is reassured that the tube is open and that air can

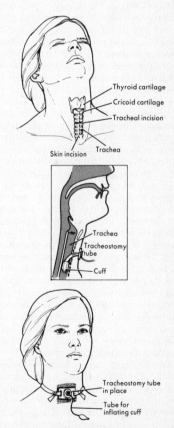

Thyroid cartilage
Cricoid cartilage
Tracheal incision
Skin incision
Trachea

Trachea
Tracheostomy tube
Cuff

Tracheostomy tube in place
Tube for inflating cuff

Tracheostomy

pass through it. The tube is suctioned frequently to keep it free from tracheobronchial fluids using a suction catheter attached to a Y-connector. The catheter is inserted 6 to 8 inches into the tube. The catheter is rotated. Intermittent suction is applied for no longer than 5 seconds. The patient is taught to cough to move fluids up and out of the bronchi. The nurse holds the tube stable during intense coughing to prevent its moving. Should the outer tube be moved out, the nurse uses an instrument to hold the windpipe open until another tube can be inserted. A fluid intake of 3,000 ml per day is recommended. The dressing is changed as necessary. The area is kept dry and clean. Frequent mouth care is given. Pen and paper or a magic slate is kept available for communication because the patient cannot speak. Complications of tracheostomy include air or gas in the lung space (pneumothorax), breathing insufficiency, obstruction of the tracheostomy tube or its displacement from the windpipe, and lung infection. Other problems are lung collapse, an abnormal passage between the windpipe and esophagus (tracheoesophageal fistula), and bleeding. If the procedure was done as an emergency, the tracheostomy is closed once normal breathing is restored. If the tracheostomy is permanent, as with a removed voicebox (larynx), the patient is taught self-care. Compare **tracheotomy.**

tracheotomy /trāˈkē·otʼəmē/, an incision made into the windpipe through the neck below the voice box (larynx). It is done to get access to the airway below a blockage with a foreign body, tumor, or fluid pooling in the vocal apparatus (edema of the glottis). The opening may be made as an emergency measure at an accident site, at a hospitalized patient's bedside, or in the operating room. Local or general anesthesia may be used, if available. The patient's neck is stretched out. An incision is made through the skin through the second, third, or fourth windpipe ring. A small hole is made in the fibrous tissue of the windpipe. The opening is then widened to allow the intake of air. In an emergency any available instrument may be used as a widener, even the barrel of a ballpoint pen with the inner portion removed. If the blockage lasts, a tracheostomy tube is inserted. If the blockage does not last, the incision is closed once normal breathing is established. After surgery the patient is observed for renewed breathing problems or bluish skin (cyanosis). Compare **tracheostomy.**

trachoma /trəkōˈmə/, a long-term, infectious disease of the eye. It is caused by the bacterium *Chlamydia trachomatis.* It is marked initially by swelling, pain, abnormal intolerance to light (photophobia), and release of tears (lacrimation). If untreated, sacs form on the upper eyelids and grow larger until the granulations invade the cornea, eventually causing blindness. Tetracycline, erythromycin, and topical sulfonamides usually give effective treatment. Scarred eyelids may be surgically repaired. Trachoma is a significant cause of blindness. It is present in hot, dry, poverty-ridden areas. In the United States, it is found on Native American reservations in the Southwest. Teaching an affected population about the spread of trachoma and having an adequate water supply for washing hands, towels, and handkerchiefs are important factors in getting rid of the disease. Also called **Egyptian ophthalmia, granular conjunctivitis.**

trackball, a ball-like mechanism nested in a box used to control cursor movements on a computer screen. See also **joystick, mouse.**

tract, 1. a long group of tissues and structures that function together as a pathway, as the digestive tract or the breathing tract. 2. (in neurology) the neuronal axons that are grouped together to form a pathway.

traction, 1. (in orthopedics) the process of putting a limb, bone, or group of muscles under tension by means of weights and pulleys to align or to keep rigid the part or to relieve pressure on it. See also **orthopedic traction. 2.** the process of pulling a part of the body along, through, or out of its socket or cavity, as axis traction with obstetric forceps in giving birth to an infant. Kinds of traction include **Bryant's traction, Buck's traction, Russell traction, skeletal traction, skin traction, and split Russell traction.**

traction frame, a bone apparatus that supports the pulleys, the ropes, and the weights by which traction is applied to many parts of the body or by which many parts of the body are hung. Traction frames are used to treat bone fractures and dislocations, disease processes of the muscle and skeleton system, to correct many bone defects, and to keep rigid specific areas of the body. The main parts of a traction frame are metal uprights that attach to the bed and support an overhead metal bar. In addition to traction equipment, traction frames are often rigged with trapeze bars that the patient can grasp to help in changing position and to exercise the muscles of the arms and the trunk. The parts of a traction frame are securely clamped together when in use. However, they can be easily taken apart and put back together. Compare **IV-type traction frame, claw-type traction frame, Balkan traction frame.**

traction, 90-90, a bone mechanism that combines skeletal traction and suspension with a short-leg cast or a splint to keep still and position the leg in the treatment of a displaced broken thigh. It is especially used for children. The pin used in this kind of skeletal traction is inserted into bone in the knee area. It is attached to a riser running through a pulley on an overhead traction frame to a pulley and weight system fitted over the foot of the bed. The pulley and weight system at the foot of the bed also accommodates additional attachments to the short-leg cast or splint of the involved lower limb. Use of 90-90 traction may also have a jacket restraint to help keep the patient rigid. One type of this traction is often used with adults to treat low back pain.

trademark, a word, symbol, or device given to a product by its manufacturer. It is registered as a part of its identity. See also **generic name.**

tragus /trā′gəs/, *pl.* **tragi** /trā′jī/, an area of cartilage on the flap of the ear at the opening of the outer ear passage.

trained reflex. See **conditioned response.**

trait, **1.** a mode of behavior or any mannerism or physical feature that separates one individual or culture from another. **2.** any quality or condition that is inborn. A trait is shown as one that appears often and strongly (dominant) or appears seldom and weakly (recessive) for the particular trait. See also **dominance, gene, Mendel's laws, recessive.**

Tral, a trademark for a nerve-blocking drug (hexocyclium methylsulfate).

trance, **1.** a sleeplike state marked by the complete or partial loss of consciousness and the loss or lack of muscle movement, as seen in hypnosis. **2.** a dazed or confused condition; stupor. **3.** a state of being removed from the things and people around one, as in deep concentration or daydreaming. Kinds of trances are **alcoholic trance, death trance, hypnotic trance, hysteric trance, induced trance.**

Trancopal, a trademark for a tranquilizer (chlormezanone).

Trandate, a trademark for a drug that relieves high blood pressure (labetalol hydrochloride).

tranquilizer, a drug to calm people who are nervous, excited, or worried about the future. Major tranquilizers are generally used to treat mental conditions. Minor tranquilizers are given to treat anxiety, irritability, tension, or failure to deal with unsolved problems. Tranquilizers often bring on drowsiness and can cause physical or mental addiction to the drug. See also **antipsychotic.**

trans-, a combining form meaning 'across, through, over.'

transactional analysis (TA), a form of mental treatment that focuses on three stages of ways to deal with differences between animal desires and inner rules that keep one from following up on those desires (ego). These stages represent the child, the adult, and the parent. Every time someone deals with another person (transaction) it is out of need for support or contact. Each transaction starts by a person in one of these stages dealing with another person who may or may not be in that same stage.

Treatment using TA tries to help the adult to control signals that come from the child stage and the parent stage.

transcendence, the rising above limits or restrictions one had set for oneself earlier.

transcondylar fracture /transkon′dilər/, a broken bone near the end of a long bone, as the elbow or ankle.

transcortical apraxia. See **ideomotor apraxia.**

transcutaneous, referring to a procedure that is performed through the skin.

transcutaneous electric nerve stimulation (TENS), a method of pain control using electric signals sent to the nerve endings. Electrodes are placed on the skin and joined to a machine by wires. The electric signals are like those of the body. They are different enough to block pain signals sent to the brain. It is a fairly safe method with no known side effects. It is not done with patients who have pacemakers.

transcutaneous nerve stimulation. See **transcutaneous electric nerve stimulation.**

transdermal delivery system, to apply a drug to unbroken skin. The drug is absorbed through the skin and enters the blood system. It is used mainly to give a heart drug and a nerve-blocking drug (nitroglycerin and scopolamine).

transect, to sever or cut across, as in doing a cross section of tissue.

transference, **1.** shifting symptoms from one part of the body to another, as occurs in conversion disorder. **2.** a way of defending oneself by shifting feelings that are linked to earlier events on people in one's life to others that are currently in one's life. This is often done without knowing it. **3.** the feelings of a patient for the physician working on mental treatment with the patient, to whom the patient has given or assigned the qualities, attitudes, and feelings of a person or persons, usually from childhood. See also **countertransference, parataxic distortion.**

transfer factor, a substance made from white blood cells (leukocytes) that transfers a delayed allergy from one person to another. Transfer factor may be used to treat a long-term infection (mucocutaneous candidiasis) and an immune system disease (Wiskott-Aldrich syndrome). It is also used to give immunity against tumors in patients with many types of cancer.

transferrin /transfer′in/, a protein in the blood that is needed to move iron from one place in the body to another. It moves iron from the intestine into the blood. The bone marrow can then use it. It may also take part in a slower transfer with iron forms in the tissues. See also **hemosiderin, iron transport.**

transfusion, the placing into the bloodstream of whole blood or blood components, as plasma, platelets, or packed red cells. Whole blood may be given to a patient by transfusion directly from a donor, but more often the donor's blood is collected and stored by a blood bank. See also **blood transfusion.**

transfusion reaction, a response by the patient's body to being given blood that has a different blood group than his or her own. The causes include red blood cells that are different than each other, allergy to the white blood cells (leukocytes) or other parts of the blood, or to a substance used to preserve the blood in the blood bank. Symptoms are fever and itching. Other symptoms are asthma, blood vessel collapse, and kidney failure. An allergic hemoglobin (hemolytic) reaction from red blood cells that do not match is serious and must be diagnosed and treated promptly. Symptoms start shortly after beginning the transfusion, before 50 ml have been given, and include a throbbing headache, sudden, deep, and severe lumbar pain in the loins, upper chest pain, difficult breathing, and restlessness. Signs include a red face followed by bluish skin and neck veins that stick out, rapid, thready pulse, heavy sweating, and cold, clammy skin. Deep shock may occur within 1 hour. Antihistamines relieve itching but do not help bring down fever. If a red blood cell reaction occurs, the transfusion is stopped at once. The tube in the vein is kept open with a normal saltwater solution. Blood must be checked, typed, and crossmatched carefully. The patient is always watched during the transfusion to check for fever and transfusion reaction.

transient, referring to a condition that is temporary, as a transient ischemic attack.

transient ischemic attack (TIA), an episode of brain blood vessel breakdown (stroke). It is caused by a blockage of a vessel, by a blood clot, or a buildup of fats. The symptoms depend on where the blockage is and how much of the vessel is blocked. Normal vision in one or in both eyes may be disturbed, and dizziness, weakness, difficulty in swallowing, numbness, or unconsciousness may occur. The attack is most often brief, lasting a few minutes; rarely, symptoms continue for several hours.

transillumination, shining a light through body tissue to look at its structure.

transition, the last phase of the first stage of labor, sometimes shown by the cervix dilating 8 to 10 cm.

transitional cell carcinoma, a malignant, nipplelike tumor. It is caused by a form of manylayered linings (mucous membranes) of tissues. It occurs most often in the bladder, urinary tubes, and the kidneys. Most tumors in the collecting system of the kidney are this kind. Patients with this disease have a better chance of recovery than squamous cell carcinomas in the same site.

transitional dentition. See **mixed dentition.**

transitional object, an object used by a child to provide comfort and security while he or she is away from a secure base, as mother or home.

transitory mania, a mood disorder marked by the sudden onset of excessive excitement (manic) reactions that only last a short time, usually from 1 hour to a few days. See also **mania.**

transmission, the transfer or carrying of a thing or condition, as a signal from the brain, infectious or inborn disease, or an inborn trait, from one person or place to another. **–transmissible,** adj.

transmission electron microscopy. See **electron microscopy.**

transmitter substance. See **neurotransmitter.**

transmural, referring to the entire thickness of the wall of an organ, as in a blockage of blood to the whole heart wall (transmural myocardial infarction).

transmural infarction, the death of heart muscle tissue that extends from the inner layer (endocardium) to the outer tissue layer (epicardium) as a result of a heart attack (myocardial infarction).

transneuronal degeneration, breakdown of permanently damaged nerve cells that may move near or far to involve nerve cells (neurons) more than one nerve junction (synapse) away.

transovarial transmission, the transfer of germs to the following generations through germs getting into the ovary and infecting the egg, as occurs in ticks and mites.

transplacental /trans′pləsen′təl/, across or through the placenta, especially referring to the exchange of nutrients, waste products, and other material between the growing fetus and the mother.

transplant, 1. to transfer an organ or tissue from one person to another or from one body part to another in order to replace a diseased structure, to restore function, or to change appearance. Skin and kidneys are the structures most often transplanted. Others include cartilage, bone, corneal tissue, portions of blood vessels and tendons, and recently, but seldom, hearts and livers. The best donors are identical twins or persons having the same blood type and immune features. Success of the transplant depends on overcoming the rejection of the donor tissue by the immune system of the patient receiving the transplant. Signs of rejection reaction include fever, pain, and loss of function, usually occuring in the first 4 to 10 days after transplantation. A forming of pus (abscess) may occur if the reaction is not treated quickly. The transplanted structure may need several weeks to become established. Late rejection may occur several months or even 1 year later. 2. any tissue or organ that is transplanted. 3. of or referring to a tissue or organ that is transplanted, or to the patient who receives donated tissue or an organ or to something linked to the procedure. Also called **graft, transplantation.**

transposition, 1. an abnormality occuring during growth in the womb in which a part of the body normally on the left is found on the right or vice versa. **2.** the shifting of genetic material from one chromosome to another at some point in the reproductive process, often resulting in a birth defect. **–transpose,** *v.*

transposition of the great vessels, a heart birth defect in which the lung blood vessel (pulmonary artery) arises from the left lower heart chamber (ventricle) and the main heart vessel (aorta) from the right ventricle so that there is no linkage between the two circulations. Life is impossible without defects that allow the mixing of blood with and without oxygen. The severity of the condition depends on the type and size of the associated defect. The primary symptoms are bluish skin and lack of oxygen, especially in infants with small defects, although a swollen heart is usually evident a few weeks after birth. Signs of congestive heart failure develop rapidly, especially in infants with large ventricle defects. The diagnosis is based on running a tube through the vessels into the heart. Surgical correction of the defect is put off, if possible, until after 6 months of age when the infant can better tolerate the procedure. Surgery, as by putting a tube in the heart and filling it with air (balloon septostomy), may be done to decrease lung vessel problems and to prevent congestive heart failure. See also **blue baby.**

transsexual, a person whose gender identity is opposite his or her biological sex.

transtentorial herniation /trans′tentôr′ē·əl/, a bulge of brain tissue out of the skull through a hole (tentorial notch), caused by pressure in the brain. See also **tentorial herniation.**

transthermia. See **thermopenetration.**

transudate /tran′so͞odāt′/, a fluid passed through a membrane or squeezed through a tissue or into the space between the cells of a tissue. It is thin and watery and contains few blood cells or other large proteins. See also **edema.**

transudative ascites /transyo͞o′dətiv/, an abnormal collecting in the bowel space of a fluid that usually has very small amounts of protein and cells. Fluids (ascites) with protein counts of less than 2.5 g/ml are labelled transudates. Transudative ascites is a sign of cirrhosis or congestive heart failure rather than infection, swelling, or the presence of a tumor.

transurethral resection (TUR) /trans′yo͞orē′thrəl/, a surgical process through the urethra, as in transurethral prostatectomy. Compare **suprapubic.**

transverse, at right angles to the long part of any common part, as the planes that cut the long part of the body into upper and lower portions and are at right angles to the back and front.

transverse colon, the segment of the colon that goes from the end of the ascending colon at the liver on the right side across the middle intestinal area to the beginning of the descending colon at the spleen on the left side.

transverse fissure, a crack dividing two surfaces of the brain. Also called **fissure of Bichat.**

transverse fracture, a broken bone that occurs at right angles to the long part of the bone involved.

transverse lie, abnormal position of a fetus just before childbirth. Here, the baby's body lies crossways in the uterus, with the length of its body at a right angle to the up and down channel through the mother's pelvic bone. Unless the baby turns by itself or is turned by means of inside or outside turning of the fetus, childbirth through the vagina is impossible.

transverse mesocolon /mez′ōkō′lən/, a broad fold of the bowel connecting the large intestine (transverse colon) to the wall of the abdomen. Compare **mesentery proper, sigmoid mesocolon.**

transverse palatine suture, the joining line between the jawbones and the side-lying parts of the bones that form the hard palate.

transverse plane, any one of the planes that cut across the body at right angles to the front and the back. It divides the body into upper and lower parts. Also called **cardinal horizontal plane.** Compare **frontal plane, median plane, sagittal plane.**

transverse relaxation time. See **relaxation time.**

transvestism, a tendency to achieve psychic and sexual relief by dressing in the clothing of the opposite sex.

Tranxene, a trademark for a tranquilizer (chlorazepate dipotassium).

tranylcypromine sulfate /tran′əlsip′rəmēn/, a monoamine oxidase (MAO) inhibitor that acts as an antidepressant. It is given to treat severe mental depression.

★CAUTION: Diseases of the heart or brain vessels, paranoid schizophrenia, liver problems, alcoholism, adrenal gland tumors, or known allergy to this drug prohibits its use. It is not given to children under 16 years of age.

★ADVERSE EFFECTS: Among the most serious side effects are severe periods of high blood pressure that can be brought on by eating foods high in tyramine or by being given at the same time many nervous system drugs. Common side effects include headache, dizziness, dry mouth, blurred vision, and fainting when standing up.

trapezium /trəpē′zē·əm/, *pl.* **trapeziums, trapezia,** a wrist bone. Also called **greater multangular, os trapezium.**

trapezius /trəpē′zē·əs/, a large flat triangular muscle of the shoulder and upper back. It raises the shoulder, and flexes the arm.

trapezoidal arch, a dental arch that has slightly less convergence than that of a tapering arch. The front teeth in the arch are somewhat square or sharply rounded from tip to tip of the canines, which are at the corners of the arch.

trapezoid bone, the smallest wrist bone. Also called **lesser multangular bone, or trapezoideum.**

trauma /trou′mə, trô′mə/, **1.** physical injury caused by violent or disruptive action, or by a poisonous substance getting into the body. **2.** mental or emotional injury caused by a severe emotional shock. **–traumatic,** *adj.,* **traumatize,** *v.*

-trauma, a combining form meaning a 'wound or injury, psychic or physical.'

trauma center, a service that gives emergency and specialized intensive care to very ill and injured patients.

traumatic anesthesia, a total lack of normal feeling in a part of the body, caused by injury, destruction of nerves, or blocking of nerve pathways. See also **tactile anesthesia.**

traumatic delirium, mental confusion or excitement (delirium) after severe head injury, marked by alertness and conciousness with disorientation, talking about imagined things (confabulation), and amnesia. See also **delirium.**

traumatic fever, a rise in body temperature following physical injury, particularly a crushing injury. Such fevers may last 1 or 2 days. The higher body temperature may help provide resistance to infection that may follow, and increased wound temperature may speed local healing.

traumatic myositis, inflammation of the muscles caused by a wound or other trauma.

traumatic neuroma, a tangled mass of nerve elements and fibrous tissue produced by the increase of nerve and connective tissue cells (Schwann cells and fibroblasts) after severe injury to a nerve. A kind of traumatic neuroma is **amputation neuroma.**

traumatic occlusion, a closure of the teeth that injures the teeth, the periodontal tissues, the residual ridge, or other mouth structures.

traumato-, a combining form meaning 'referring to trauma, or to an injury or wound.'

traumatology /trô′mətol′əjē/, **1.** the study of wounds and injuries. **2.** a surgical specialty dealing with the treatment of wounds, injuries, and resulting problems. **–traumatologic, traumatological,** *adj.*

traumatopathy /trô′mətop′əthē/, a disease condition resulting from a wound or injury. **–traumatopathic,** *adj.*

traumatophilia /trô′mətōfil′ē·ə/, a mental condition in which the patient gets unknowing plea-

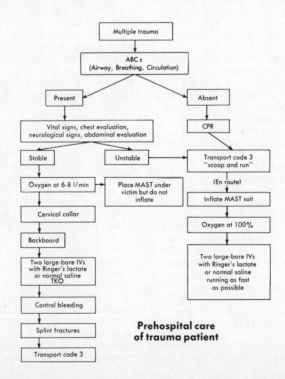

Prehospital care of trauma patient

sure from injuries and surgical operations. **–traumatophiliac,** *n.,* **traumatophilic,** *adj.*

traumatopnea /trô'mətop'nē·ə/, partial suffocation with collapse of the patient, caused by a wound that cuts through the chest allowing air to enter the chest space and collapse the lungs.

traumatopyra /trô'mətōpī'rə/, a high temperature caused by a wound or injury.

traumatotherapy, the medical, surgical, and mental treatment of wounds, injuries, and disorders caused by trauma. **–traumatotherapeutic,** *adj.*

traumatropism /trômat'rəpiz'əm/, the tendency of damaged tissue to attract bacteria and to help their growth, often causing infections after injuries, especially burns.

travail /trəvāl'/, 1. physical or mental effort, especially when it causes distress. 2. the effort of labor and childbirth.

Travase, a trademark for an enzyme that splits proteins (sutilains).

traveler's diarrhea, any of several diarrheal disorders commonly seen in people visiting regions of the world other than their own. Some strains of *Escherichia coli,* which produce a powerful poison enzyme (exotoxin), are the common cause. Other organisms that cause the condition include *Giardia lamblia* and species of *Salmonella* and *Shigella.* Symptoms last for a few days and include stomach and intestinal cramps, nausea, vomiting, slight fever, and watery stools. Having the condition return is rare. Treatment depends on knowing the cause and includes restoring the body's water level with drinks that have electrolytes. Preventive measures include using pure or boiled water and beverages for drinking and brushing the teeth and eating only fruits and vegetables that have a skin or peel. Also called **Montezuma's revenge, turista.**

TRBF, abbreviation for **total renal blood flow.**

Treacher Collins' syndrome, an inborn disorder, marked by an incomplete form of a head and face birth defect (mandibulofacial dysostosis). See also **Pierre Robin's syndrome.**

treatment, 1. the care and overseeing of a patient to fight, reduce, or prevent a disease, disorder, or injury. 2. a method of fighting, reducing, ameliorating, or preventing a disease, disorder, or injury. Active or curative treatment is designed to cure; palliative treatment is directed to ease pain and distress; prophylactic treatment is for the prevention of a disease or disorder; causal treatment focuses on the cause of a disorder; conservative treatment avoids drastic measures and procedures; empiric treatment employs methods shown to work by experience; rational treatment is based on a knowledge of a disease process and the action of the measures used. Treatment may be pharmacological, using drugs; surgical, involving surgery; or supportive, building the patient's strength. It may focus on finding a cure for the disorder, or just try to relieve symptoms without bringing about a cure.

treatment guardian, a person appointed by the court for the purpose of agreeing to or refusing medical treatment for a patient.

treatment room, a room in a patient care unit, usually in a hospital, in which various treatments or procedures that need special equipment are done, as removing stitches, draining a blood blister, packing a wound, or doing a diagnostic test.

Trecator-SC, a trademark for a tuberculosis drug (ethionamide).

Trechona /trikon'ə/, a genus of spiders, family Dipluridae, the bite of which is poisonous and irritating to humans.

-trema, 1. a combining form meaning a 'hole, orifice, opening.' 2. a combining form meaning 'creatures possessing an opening.'

trematode /trem'ətōd/, any species of flatworm of the class Trematoda, some of which live in humans, infecting the liver, the lungs, and the intestines. Kinds of trematodes include the organisms causing **clonorchiasis, fascioliasis, paragonimiasis,** and **schistosomiasis.** Also called **fluke.**

tremor, rhythmic, quivering movements with no purpose caused by the uncontrolled tightening and relaxing of groups of muscles attached to the skeleton. This disorder occurs in some older patients, in certain families, and in patients with different nerve disorders that get worse and worse. Senile tremor is marked by fine, quick movements, especially of the hands, rhythmic head nodding, and increased trembling during useful movements. Familial tremor, which may be inborn, and the tremor occurring in multiple sclerosis also get worse during normal, controlled muscle movement and may be made worse by worry, excitement, and being worried about how one looks or acts to others. The tremors of Graves' disease, alcoholism, mercury poisoning, and other disorders caused by poisons are usually less rhythmic, and the tremor in lead poisoning often affects the lips. The fine, quick, unbroken tremor in Parkinson's disease sometimes goes away during useful muscle movements. Kinds of tremors are **continuous tremor** and **intention tremor.**

tremulous, referring to tremors, or uncontrolled muscular contractions.

trench fever, an infection that goes away by itself, caused by *Rochalimaea quintana,* an organism in the Rickettsia group of microorganisms, carried by body lice, marked by weakness, fever, rash, and leg pains. It was common during World War I but is now rare. Also called **quintana fever.**

trench mouth. See **acute necrotizing gingivitis.**

Trendelenburg gait /trendel'ənbərg/, an abnormal way of walking (gait) linked to weakness of the thigh muscle (gluteus medius). The Trendelenburg gait is marked by the dropping of the pelvis on the unaffected side of the body at the moment of heelstrike on the affected side. In this condition, the pelvic drop during the walking cycle lasts until heelstrike on the unaffected side and has with it the sideways jutting out of the affected hip. The person with a Trendelenburg gait also shortens the step on the unaffected side and has a sideways movement of the entire trunk and the affected side during the stance phase of the affected lower limb. The Trendelenburg gait is one of the more common walking abnormalities. Also called **uncompensated gluteal gait.** Compare **compensated gluteal gait.**

Trendelenburg's operation, tying off varicose veins whose valves no longer work, done to take out weak parts of veins and pockets in which clots might lodge. After surgery, the patient should walk but should not stand or sit. Bluish-colored toes shows possible cutting off of blood supply by the bandages. Elastic bandages remain in place until the seventh day after surgery, when the stitches are usually removed. Possible new problems include bleeding, infection, nerve damage, and blood clots.

Trendelenburg's position, a position in which the head is low and the body and legs are on an upward angle. It is sometimes used in pelvic surgery to move the stomach and intestinal organs upward, out of the pelvis.

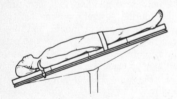

Trendelenburg's position

Trendelenburg's test, a simple test for nonworking valves in a person who has varicose veins. The person lies down and raises the leg to empty the vein, then stands, and the vein is looked at as it fills. If the valves are not working correctly, the vein fills from above; if the valves are normal, they do not allow backflow of blood, and the vein fills from below.

Trental, a trademark for a drug (pentoxyfylline) given by mouth. The drug thins the blood and improves its flow.

trephine /trifīn', trifēn'/, a circular, sawlike instrument used in removing pieces of bone or tissue, usually from the skull. Also called

trepan /trē'pan, tripan'/.

Treponema /trep'ənē'mə/, a genus of slender, spiral microorganisms (spirochetes), including some harmful to humans, as the organisms causing bejel, pinta, syphilis, and yaws.

Treponema pallidum, a self-moving slender spirochetal organism that causes syphilis.

treponematosis /trep'ənē'mətō'sis/, pl. **treponematoses,** any disease caused by slender, spiral microorganisms (spirochetes) of the genus *Treponema.* All of these infections are effectively treated with penicillin; often one dose, given in the muscle, results in cure. Kinds of treponematoses are **bejel, pinta, syphilis, yaws.**

-tresia, a combining form meaning 'perforation.'

tretinoin, a drug used to treat acne.

★CAUTION: Known allergy to this drug prohibits its use.

★ADVERSE EFFECTS: Among the more serious side effects are red, fluid-filled, blistered, or crusted skin.

Trexan, a trademark for a drug (naltexone hydrochloride) given by mouth which is used to block the effects of drugs, as heroin, morphine, and methadone in patients recovering from addiction.

TRF, abbreviation for **thyrotropin releasing factor.** See **thyrotropin releasing hormone.**

tri-, a combining form meaning 'three or thrice.'

triacetin /trī·as'itin/, an antifungus drug used to treat surface fungus infections of the skin, including athlete's foot.

triacetyloleandomycin. See **troleandomycin.**

triad, a combination of three, as two parents and a child.

triage /trē·äzh'/, **1.** a sorting of casualties of war and other disasters according to the severity of injuries, urgency of treatment, and place for treatment. **2.** a process in which a group of patients is sorted according to their need for care. The kind of illness or injury, the severity of the problem, and the facilities available are the factors used to sort the patients. **3.** a process in which a large group of patients is sorted so that care can be focused on those who are likely to survive.

trial forceps, an operation consisting of an attempt to bring on childbirth with obstetric forceps. The forceps grasp the baby's head, and moderate pulling is done. The childbirth is continued only if the trial shows that childbirth can be done safely. The procedure is given up if proper use of the forceps or rotation of the baby's head is not possible or if the trial shows that completing the childbirth will mean using unusually strong pulling that will cause more injury to the mother or baby than would cesarean section. Trial forceps is usually done with a double setup so that cesarean section can be carried out immediately if necessary. Compare **failed forceps.** See also **double setup.**

triamcinolone /trī'amsin'əlōn/, a steroid drug

used to bring down swelling. It is given to treat many skin diseases.

★CAUTION: Fungus infections or known allergy to this drug prohibits its systemic use. Viral or fungus infections of the skin, slowed circulation, or known allergy to this drug prohibits its local use.

★ADVERSE EFFECTS: Among the more serious side effects to the systemic use of the drug are stomach and intestinal, endocrine, nervous system, fluid, and electrolyte disturbances. A variety of skin reactions may occur from local use of this drug.

triamterene /trī·am'tərēn/, a fluid-releasing drug (diuretic) that keeps potassium from being excreted. It is given alone or with another diuretic to treat fluid buildup, high blood pressure, and congestive heart failure.

★CAUTION: Absence of urine (anuria), severe liver or kidney problems, high levels of potassium in the blood, or known allergy to this drug prohibits its use.

★ADVERSE EFFECTS: Among the most serious side effects are electrolyte disturbances, especially high levels of potassium in the blood. Stomach and intestinal problems may also occur.

triangle, an emotional process that takes place when there is difficulty in a relationship. Triangles represent dysfunctional efforts to keep distance or lower conflict in a relationship. The three corners of the triangle can be composed of three people or of two people and an object or group or issue.

triangular bandage, a square of cloth folded or cut into the shape of a triangle. It may be used as a sling, a cover, or a thick pad to control bleeding.

triangular bone, a wrist bone. Also called **cuneiform bone,** or **triquetrum.**

Triavil, a trademark for a nervous system drug that has a calming drug (perphenazine) and a drug to control depression (amitriptyline hydrochloride).

triazolam, a sleeping pill. It is given in the short term to treat insomnia.

★CAUTION: Known allergy to this drug or other drugs like it prohibits its use. It is not given to pregnant women, nursing mothers, or patients younger than 18 years of age.

★ADVERSE EFFECTS: Among the most serious side effects are loss of memory, reactions conflicting with the expected, rapid heart beat, depression, confusion or reduced memory, and vision problems.

-tribe, a combining form meaning a 'surgical instrument used to crush a body part.'

TRIC /trik/, abbreviation for *trachoma inclusion conjunctivitis* agent, which refers to *Chlamydia trachomatis,* the organism that causes two eye diseases (inclusion conjunctivitis and trachoma). See also *Chlamydia.*

triceps brachii /trī'seps brak'ē·ī/, a large muscle that runs along the entire length of the back of the upper arm. It extends the forearm and moves the arm toward the body. Also called **triceps, triceps extensor cubiti.** Compare **biceps brachii.**

triceps reflex, a deep tendon reflex brought on by tapping sharply the triceps tendon next to the elbow with the forearm in a relaxed position. The response is a clear extension movement of the forearm. The reflex is made stronger by injury to the pyramidal tract of the spinal cord above the level of the seventh or eighth backbones. Also called **triceps jerk.** See also **deep tendon reflex.**

triceps skinfold, the thickness of a fold of skin around the muscle along the back of the upper arm (triceps muscle). It is measured primarily to estimate the amount of fat under the skin.

triceps surae limp, an abnormal action in the walking cycle, linked to a weakness in the raising and forward motion muscles in the elevating muscles on the affected side of the body, especially a weakness of the knee muscle (triceps surae). Such a weakness keeps the triceps surae from raising the pelvis and carrying it forward during the walking cycle. As a result, the pelvis sags below its normal level and lags behind in the walking movement.

-trichia, -trichosis, 1. a combining form meaning a 'disease condition of the hair.' 2. a combining form meaning a '(specified) hairiness.'

trichiasis /trikī'əsis/, an abnormal turning inward of the eyelashes that irritates the eyeball. It usually follows infection or swelling. Compare **ectropion.**

trichinosis /trik'inō'sis/, a condition of having the parasitic roundworm *Trichinella spiralis,* gotten by eating raw or undercooked pork or bear meat. Early symptoms of infection include stomach or intestinal pain, nausea, fever, and diarrhea; later, muscle pain, tenderness, fatigue, and a buildup of white blood cells (eosinophilia) are observed. Light infections may have no symptoms. Also called **trichinellosis, trichiniasis.** Larvae surrounded by membrane in improperly cooked pork develop in the intestines of the patient, with mature worms depositing their larvae in the intestinal wall. The larvae get through the mucous lining of the intestine and move to other parts of the body through the blood and lymphatic systems. They finally get into skeletal muscles, especially the diaphragm and the chest muscles, where they form new lumps. Larvae getting into the brain or the heart may cause death. Blood serum tests, skin sensitivity tests, and microscopic examination of samples of muscles that have larvae, gotten by surgically removing a part of the tissue, often help in the diagnosis. There is no specific treatment. Painkillers or steroid drugs may relieve symptoms. Bed rest is best to prevent relapse and possible death. After 2 or 3 months, the organisms are completely surrounded by membrane and cause no further symptoms. Prevention requires cooking pork or wild game at 350° F (176° C) for 35 minutes a pound. Freezing at 10° F (– 12° C) for 20 days also kills the larvae. Pork or pork products should never be eaten raw, and even smoked or salted meat may still have living larvae. Routine inspection of carcasses for trichinella organisms is not done in the United States, where the disease is on the decline.

trichlormethiazide /trī′klôrməthī′əzīd/, a fluid releasing and high blood pressure drug. It is given to treat high blood pressure and fluid buildup.
★CAUTION: Urine buildup (anuria) or known allergy to this drug or to other drugs like it prohibits its use.
★ADVERSE EFFECTS: Among the more serious side effects are too-little potassium in the blood, high blood sugar levels, high uric acid blood levels, and many allergic reactions.

trichloroethylene /trīklôr′ō·eth′ilēn/, a general anesthetic, given by mask with N_2O, for dentistry, minor surgery, and the first stages of labor. It is too harmful to the heart for deep anesthesia; even low levels may cause irregular heart rates but may be reversed by giving oxygen and stopping use of the anesthesia. Trichloroethylene must not be given by rebreathing devices using soda lime, because highly poisonous gases may result. Its safety for use in early pregnancy has not been proven. It should not be used in severe heart disease of any kind, diseases of pregnancy (eclampsia or preeclampsia), and should not be combined with epinephrine.

tricho-, a combining form meaning 'referring to hair.'

trichobasalioma hyalinicum. See **cylindroma,** def. 2.

trichoepithelioma /trik′ō·ep′ithē′lē·ō′mə/, pl. **trichoepitheliomas, trichoepitheliomata,** a skin tumor that comes from the cells of the sacs (follicles) of fine body hair. One form of trichoepithelioma is an inborn condition and usually occurs as multiple growths. Also called **acanthoma adenoides cysticum, epithelioma adenoides cysticum.**

trichoid /trik′oid/, looking like a hair.

trichologia /trik′əlō′jē·ə/, an abnormal condition in which a person pulls out his or her own hair, usually seen only in a state of confusion (delirium).

trichomonacide, a drug that destroys *Trichomonas vaginalis,* a microorganism that causes a stubborn form of irritation of the outer urinary tract and vagina. Metronidazole is given for this disorder and for other similar disorders with no symptoms. **–trichomonacidal,** adj.

Trichomonas vaginalis /trik′əmon′əs/, a self-

moving microorganism that causes irritation of the vagina with large amounts of bad smelling discharge and severe itching. See also **trichomoniasis.**

trichomoniasis /trik′əmənī′əsis/, a vaginal infection caused by the microorganism *Trichomonas vaginalis,* marked by itching, burning, and frothy, pale yellow to green, bad-smelling vaginal discharge. With long-term infection all symptoms may disappear, although the organisms are still present. In men, infection is usually without symptoms but may be shown by a continuing or recurrent irritation of the urethra. Infection is carried by sexual intercourse, rarely by moist washcloths, or, in newborns, by passage through the birth canal. Diagnosis is by microscopic examination of fresh substances released through the vagina. Treatment is by metronidazole given by mouth. Reinfection is common if sexual partners are not treated at the same time.

trichophytic granuloma. See **Majocchi's granuloma.**

Trichophyton /trikof′iton/, a genus of fungi that infects skin, hair, and nails. See also **dermatomycosis, dermatophyte.**

-trichosis. See **-trichia.**

trichostrongyliasis /trik′ōstron′jəlī′əsis/, a condition of being infested with *Trichostrongylus,* a genus of nematode worm. Also called **trichostrongylosis.** See also **nematode.**

Trichostrongylus /trik′ōstron′jiləs/, a genus of roundworm, some species of which live in humans, as *Trichostrongylus orientalis.* See also **trichostrongyliasis.**

trichotillomania /trik′ōtil′ōmā′nē·ə/, an abnormal impulse or desire to pull out one's hair, often seen in cases of severe mental retardation and conditions of severe confusion (delirium). Also called **trichomania, hair pulling.** See also **trichologia. –trichotillomanic, trichomanic,** adj.

trichuriasis /trik′yŏŏrī′əsis/, a condition of being infested with the roundworm *Trichuris trichiura.* The condition usually has no symptoms, but heavy infestation may cause nausea, stomach and intestinal pain, diarrhea, and, occasionally, low red blood cell levels (anemia), and the dropping down of the rectum. It is common in tropic areas with poor sanitation. Eggs are passed in feces. Contamination of the hands, food, and water results in taking the eggs into the body that hatch in the intestines, where the adult worms embed two-thirds of their length in the mucous lining of the intestines. The worms may live 15 to 20 years. Treatment is with mebendazole. Prevention includes proper disposal of feces and good personal hygiene. Also called **trichiuriasis** /trik′ē-/.

Trichuris /trikyŏŏr′is/, a genus of roundworms that live in the body of which the species *Tri-*

churis trichiura infects the intestinal tract. Adult worms, which are 30 to 50 mm long, resemble a whip, with a threadlike front and a thicker rear. Also called **whipworm.** See also **trichuriasis.**

tricuspid /trīkus′pid/, **1.** of or referring to three points or points of the crowns of teeth (cusps). **2.** of or referring to the tricuspid valve of the heart.

tricuspid atresia, a heart birth defect marked by not having the tricuspid valve so that there is no opening between the right upper heart chamber (atrium) and right lower heart chamber (ventricle). Other cardiac defects are usually present, allowing some flow of blood into the lungs. Clinical symptoms include bluish skin from lack of oxygen, difficulty in breathing, lack of oxygen to tissues, and signs of right-sided heart failure. Definitive diagnosis is made by running a tube into the heart, although x-ray studies usually show a small, underdeveloped right ventricle and large atria, giving the heart a round shape, and decreased lung vessel blood flow. Immediate treatment includes grafting blood vessels to the lung to increase blood flow to the lungs, and a surgical opening of the wall between the atria if the defect in that wall is small. Total corrective surgery has been successful in a limited number of older children.

tricuspid stenosis. See **valvular heart disease.**

tricuspid valve, a valve with three main divisions in the heart valves (cusps) located between the right upper chamber (atrium) and the right lower chamber (ventricle) of the heart. The cusps of the tricuspid valve include the ventral, dorsal, and medial cusps. The ventral cusp is the largest, the posterior cusp the smallest. The cusps are made of strong fibrous tissue and are attached to the papillary muscles of the right ventricle by several tendons. As the right and the left ventricles relax during the relaxation (diastole) phase of the heart beat, the tricuspid valve opens, allowing blood to flow into the ventricle. In the contraction (systole) phase of the heart beat both blood-filled ventricles contract, pumping out their contents, while the tricuspid and mitral valves close to prevent any backflow. Also called **right atrioventricular valve.** Compare **aortic valve, mitral valve, pulmonary, valve, semilunar valve.** See also **atrioventricular valve, heart valve.**

tricyclic antidepressant. See **antidepressant.**

Tridesilon, a trademark for a steroid drug (desonide).

tridihexethyl chloride, a nerve-blocking drug. It is given to treat stomach and intestinal muscle spasm and to lower the level of liquids being released by the gastric gland of the stomach and movement by the stomach and intestines. ★CAUTION: Narrow-angle eye cataracts (glau-

coma), asthma, blockage of the genitals, urinary tract, or of the stomach and intestinal tract, severe open-sore irritation of the colon, or known allergy to this drug prohibits its use. ★ADVERSE EFFECTS: Among the more serious side effects are blurred vision, rapid heartbeat, dry mouth, decreased sweating, and allergic reactions. It may cause a wasting of the prostate gland in elderly men.

Tridione, a trademark for an antiseizure drug (trimethadione).

triethanolamine polypeptide oleate-condensate, a drug given to reduce a buildup of too-much earwax. It is used as a solution in propylene glycol. A possible serious side effect is a severe skin rash (contact dermatitis).

trifacial nerve. See **trigeminal nerve.**

trifluoperazine hydrochloride /trī′floo·ōper′əzēn/, a tranquilizer. It is given to treat anxiety, delusions (schizophrenia), and other mental disorders, and as an antinausea and antivomiting drug. ★CAUTION: Parkinson's disease, use of central nervous system depressants at the same time, liver or kidney disorders, severe low blood pressure, or known allergy to this drug prohibits its use. ★ADVERSE EFFECTS: Among the more serious side effects are low blood pressure, liver disease, many motor disorders, a variety of blood diseases, and allergic reactions.

trifluorothymidine /trīfloōr′ōthī′mədēn/, an antivirus drug. Also called **trifluridine.** It is given to treat eye diseases caused by herpes simplex virus. ★CAUTION: Known allergy to this drug prohibits its use. Poisoning of the eyes may result from being given this drug for more than 21 days. ★ADVERSE EFFECTS: Among the more serious side effects are allergic reactions, fluid buildup, and increased eye pressure.

triflupromazine hydrochloride, a tranquilizer. It is given to treat severe agitation and other mental disorders and for the control of severe vomiting. ★CAUTION: Parkinson's disease, use of central nervous system depressants at the same time, liver or kidney disease, severe low blood pressure, or known allergy to this drug or to other similar drugs prohibits its use. ★ADVERSE EFFECTS: Among the more serious side effects are low blood pressure, many motor problems, blood diseases, and allergic reactions.

trifluridine. See **trifluorothymidine.**

trigeminal nerve /trījem′inəl/, either of the largest pair of skull nerves, necessary for the act of chewing and general control of the face. The trigeminal nerves have sensory, motor, and intermediate roots and connect to three areas in the brain. Also called **fifth nerve, nervus trigeminus, trifacial nerve.**

trigeminal neuralgia, a nerve condition of the trigeminal facial nerve, marked by sudden spasms of flashing, stablike pain moving along the course of a branch of the nerve from the angle of the jaw. It is caused by breakdown of the nerve or by pressure on it. Any of the three branches of the nerve may be affected. Severe, sharp pain (neuralgia) of the first branch results in pain around the eyes and over the forehead; of the second branch, in pain in the upper lip, nose, and cheek; of the third branch, in pain on the side of the tongue and the lower lip. The quick bursts of pain happen again in clusters lasting many seconds; periods of sharp painful spasms may last for hours. Also called **prosopalgia, tic douloureux** /tik´do͞olo͞oroe´/.

trigeminal pulse, an abnormal pulse in which every third beat is absent. See also **bigeminal pulse, trigeminy.**

trigeminy /trījem´inē/, **1.** a grouping in threes. **2.** an irregular heart beat marked by three heart beats, a normal beat followed by two irregular beats that follow each other quickly. **–trigeminal,** *adj.*

triglyceride /trīglis´ərīd/, a compound made up of a fatty acid (oleic, palmitic, or stearic) and glycerol. Triglycerides make up most animal and vegetable fats and are the basic substances that cannot be dissolved in water (lipids) that appear in the blood where they circulate. Here they are bound to a protein, forming high- and low-density lipoproteins. The total amount of triglyceride, and the amount and level of the kinds of lipoproteins are important in the diagnosis and treatment of many diseases and conditions including diabetes, high blood pressure, and heart disease. Normally the total amount of triglyceride in the blood does not exceed 200 mg to 300 mg/dl.

trigone /trī´gōn/, **1.** a triangle. **2.** the first three main high points of a crown (cusps), taken together, of an upper molar.

trigone of the bladder. See **trigonum vesicae.**

trigonitis /trī´gənī´tis/, swelling of the triangular area of the bladder, which often occurs with a swollen bladder tube (urethritis).

trigonum vesicae, a triangular area of the bladder between the opening of the bladder tubes (ureters) and the opening of the urethra. Also called **trigone of the bladder.**

trihexyphenidyl hydrochloride, a nerve-blocking drug. It is given to treat Parkinson's disease and to control motor problems brought on by the giving of drugs.
★CAUTION: Narrow-angle eye disease (glaucoma), asthma, blockage of the genitals or urinary tract, or of the stomach and intestinal tract, severe swelling of the colon with open sores, or known allergy to this drug prohibits its use.

★ADVERSE EFFECTS: Among the more serious side effects are blurred vision, central nervous system problems, rapid heart beat, dry mouth, decreased sweating, and allergic reactions.

triiodothyronine (T₃) /trī´ī·ō´dōthī´rənēn/, a hormone that helps control growth and development, the body's chemical processes, and body temperature. It also acts to prevent, as needed, the release of a hormone (thyrotropin) by the pituitary. It is used to treat an underactive thyroid gland (hypothyroidism) and simple enlargement of the thyroid gland (goiter). See also **thyroid hormone.**

Trilafon, a trademark for a tranquilizer (perphenazine).

trilaminar blastoderm, the stage of growth in the embryo in which all three of the primary germ layers, the ectoderm, mesoderm, and entoderm, have formed. Compare **bilaminar blastoderm.**

trilogy of Fallot /falō´/, a heart birth defect made up of the combination of narrowing of lung vessels, a heart vessel defect, and a wasting of a heart chamber. For discussion of diagnosis and treatment, see **tetralogy of Fallot.**

trimalleolar fracture. See **Cotton's fracture.**

trimeprazine tartrate /trīmep´rəzēn/, an anti-itching drug. It is given to treat itching and allergic reactions of the skin.
★CAUTION: Coma, decrease of the function of bone marrow, producing breast milk, or known allergy to this drug prohibits its use. It is not given to children under 6 months of age or to patients receiving large amounts of central nervous system depressants.
★ADVERSE EFFECTS: Among the more serious side effects are confused excitement, parkinsonlike problems, a swelling condition of the liver (hepatitis), and disorders of the stomach and intestines.

trimester /trīmes´tər, trī´-/, one of the three periods of roughly 3 months into which pregnancy is divided. The first trimester includes the time from the first day of the last menstrual period to the end of 12 weeks. The second trimester, closer to 4 months in length than 3, extends from the 12th to the 28th week of pregnancy. The third trimester begins at the 28th week and extends to the time of childbirth.

trimethadione /trī´methədī´ōn/, an anticonvulsing drug. It is given to prevent seizures in petit mal epilepsy, especially seizures that do not respond to other treatments.
★CAUTION: Severe kidney or liver conditions, blood diseases, or known allergy to this drug prohibits its use.
★ADVERSE EFFECTS: Among the more serious side effects are skin disorders, blood diseases, and low red blood cell levels. Sleepiness and poor vision in bright light (hemeralopia) may occur.

trimethaphan camsylate, a nerve-blocking agent. It is given to produce an even, low blood pressure during surgery and to lower blood pressure in high blood pressure emergencies.
★CAUTION: It is not used where low blood pressure places a patient in undue risk or when allergy to this drug prohibits its use.
★ADVERSE EFFECTS: The most serious side effect is severe low blood pressure.

trimethobenzamide hydrochloride, an antivomiting drug. It is given to relieve nausea and vomiting.
★CAUTION: Disease of the brain and spinal cord (Reye's syndrome) or known allergy to this drug prohibits its use.
★ADVERSE EFFECTS: Among the most serious side effects with high doses are drowsiness, diarrhea, allergic reactions, and motor problems. Side effects are rare at usual dosages.

trimethoprim /trīmeth'əprim/, an antibacteria drug. It is given to treat many infections, especially of the urinary tract, middle ear, and breathing tubes.
★CAUTION: Known allergy to this drug prohibits its use. It should not be used to treat strep throat.
★ADVERSE EFFECTS: Among the more serious side effects are blood diseases and allergic reactions, stomach and intestinal problems, and central nervous system disorders.

trimethoprim and sulfamethoxazole. See **sulfamethoxazole and trimethoprim.**

trimethylene. See **cyclopropane.**

trimipramine maleate /trimip'rəmēn/, an antidepressant. It is given to treat anxiety, depression, and insomnia.
★CAUTION: Use at the same time of an MAO antidepressant (monoamine oxidase) within 14 days or known allergy to this drug prohibits its use. It is not given during recovery from heart attack or to patients with a mental disorder (schizophrenia). It should not be given to children.
★ADVERSE EFFECTS: Among the more serious side effects are rapid heart rate, seizures, parkinsonlike disorders, blurred vision, low blood pressure, and making glaucoma worse.

Trimox, a trademark for an antibiotic drug (amoxicillin trihydrate).

Trimpex, a trademark for an antibacterial drug (trimethoprim).

trioxsalen, a skin-coloring drug. It is given to increase skin color (pigmentation), for repigmentation of the skin in idiopathic vitiligo, and to increase the body's ability to deal with sunlight.
★CAUTION: Diseases linked to sensitivity to light, as porphyria, a long-term swelling disorder of the joints (acute lupus erythematosus), or a shortage of skin pigment (leukoderma) gotten by infection, or the simultaneous use of drugs having any light sensitizing activity prohibits its use.
★ADVERSE EFFECTS: Among the most serious side effects are severe burns from too-much exposure to ultraviolet light. Stomach irritation and nausea also may occur.

tripelennamine citrate. See **tripelennamine hydrochloride.**

tripelennamine hydrochloride, an antihistamine. It is given to treat stuffy nose and allergic reactions of the skin.
★CAUTION: Asthma, glaucoma, difficulty in urination, simultaneous use of an antidepressant (monoamine oxidase inhibitor), or known allergy to this drug prohibits its use. It is not given to premature or newborn infants or to mothers producing breast milk.
★ADVERSE EFFECTS: Among the more serious side effects are sleepiness, high heart rate, and stomach and intestinal upset.

triple-dye treatment, a treatment for burns in which three dyes, 6% gentian violet, 1% brilliant green, and 0.1% acriflavin base, are applied.

triple point, a situation in which a given substance may exist in solid, liquid, and vapor forms at the same time.

triple response, a three-part response to injection of histamine in the skin. First, a red spot develops, spreading outward for a few millimeters, reaching its largest size within 1 minute and then turning bluish. Next, a brighter red flush of color spreads slowly in an irregular flare around the original red spot. Finally, a bump, filled with fluid, forms over the original spot. Also called **triple response of Lewis.**

triple sugar iron reaction, any one of several reactions seen in certain kinds of bacteria growing on triple sugar iron agar, a substance used to aid in the identification of *Escherichia coli, Proteus, Salmonella, Shigella,* and other disease-causing bacteria of the small intestine.

triplet, any one of three offspring born of the same gestation period during a single pregnancy. See also **Hellin's law.**

triple X syndrome. See **XXX syndrome.**

tripodial symmelia /trīpō'dē·əl/, an abnormal fetus marked by the joining of the legs and the presence of three feet.

triprolidine hydrochloride, an antihistamine. It is given to treat many allergic reactions, including stuffy nose, skin rash, and itching.
★CAUTION: Asthma or known allergy to this drug prohibits its use. It is not given to newborn infants or mothers producing breast milk. Side effects may occur in elderly patients.
★ADVERSE EFFECTS: Drowsiness, skin rash, allergic reactions, dry mouth, and fast heart rate may occur.

-tripsy, a combining form meaning a 'crushing of a body part by a surgical instrument or other device.'

trismus /triz'məs/, a long-term spasm of the muscles of the jaw. Also called (informal) **lockjaw.** See also **tetanus.**

Trisoralen, a trademark for a skin-coloring drug (trioxsalen).

Trobicin, a trademark for an antibacteria drug (spectinomycin hydrochloride).

trocar /trō'kär/, a sharp, pointed rod that fits inside a tube. It is used to pierce the skin and the wall of a cavity or canal in the body to suck in or out fluids, to put in a drug or solution, or to guide the placement of a soft tube (catheter). The trocar is usually removed and the catheter, tube, or instrument is left in place. See also **cannula.**

trochanter /trōkan'tər/, one of the two bony structures that stick out on the end of the thigh. It serves for the attachment of various muscles. The two structures are the greater trochanter and the lesser trochanter.

troche /trō'kē/, a small oval, round, or oblong tablet that has a drug mixed in a flavored, sweetened vegetable or fruit base that dissolves in the mouth, releasing the drug. Also called **lozenge, rotula, trochiscus.**

trochlea /trok'lē·ə/, a pulley-shaped part or structure. **–trochlear,** adj.

trochlear nerve, either of the smallest pair of skull nerves, necessary for eye movement and eye muscle sensibility. The trochlear nerves branch to supply the superior oblique muscle and link to the eye (ophthalmic) division of the trigeminal nerve, connecting with two areas in the brain. Also called **fourth nerve, nervus trochlearis.**

trochoid joint. See **pivot joint.**

trolamine, a short form for **triethanolamine.**

troleandomycin, an antibiotic. It is given to treat certain infections, including pneumococcal pneumonia and Group A streptococcal infections of the upper breathing tract.
★CAUTION: Known allergy to this drug prohibits its use.
★ADVERSE EFFECTS: Among the more serious side effects are stomach and intestinal disturbances, mild to severe allergic reactions (including anaphylaxis), and poisoning of the liver.

trombiculosis /trombik'yo͞olō'sis/, a condition of being infested with mites of the genus *Trombicula,* some species of which carry scrub typhus.

Tronothane Hydrochloride, a trademark for a local anesthetic (pramoxine hydrochloride).

-tropal. See **-tropic.**

troph-. See **tropho-.**

-troph, 1. a combining form meaning 'that which nourishes an embryo.' **2.** a combining form meaning an 'organism that gets nourishment from a (specified) source.'

trophectoderm. See **trophoblast.**

-trophic, a combining form meaning 'referring to a type of nutrition or nutritional requirement.'

trophic action, the starting of cell reproduction and enlargement by nurturing and causing growth.

trophic fracture, a break in a bone caused by the weakening of bone tissue caused by nutritional disturbances.

trophic ulcer, a pressure sore (decubitus ulcer) caused by outer injury to a part of the body that is in poor condition caused by disease, low levels of blood flow, or loss of nerve fibers that carry signals to the brain. Trophic ulcers may be painless or linked to severe burning pain (causalgia). See also **decubitus ulcer.**

tropho-, troph-, a combining form meaning 'referring to food or nourishment.'

trophoblast, the layer of tissue that forms the wall of the early embryo (blastocyst) of mammals with placentas in the early stages of the growth of the embryo. It functions in the placing of the blastocyst in the uterine wall and in supplying nutrients to the embryo. Also called **trophectoderm. –trophoblastic,** adj.

trophoblastic cancer, a cancerous abnormal tissue-forming disease of the uterus gotten from early fetal skin cells, marked by the production of high levels of a hormone (human chorionic gonadotropin, HCG). This type of cancer forms a dark red, bleeding, nodular tumor on or in the uterine wall and spreads early in its course to the lungs, brain, liver, bones, vagina, or vulva. Initial symptoms are vaginal bleeding and a heavy, foul-smelling discharge; a persistent cough or coughing up of blood signals lung involvement. As the disease spreads, there may be frequent bleeding, weakness, and extreme thinness. Diagnostic measures include a series of tests over time to see if the HCG level in the blood is high and microscopic examination of specimens obtained by scraping of the lining of the uterus. Removal of the uterus (hysterectomy) should be done in most cases, but does not end the chance of the disease coming back. Chemotherapy is effective in curing a large percentage of patients with trophoblastic tumors. Also called **trophoblastic disease.** See also **choriocarcinoma, hydatid mole.**

trophotropic, referring to a state, as resting or sleeping, in which the parasympathetic nervous system maintains the vital involuntary functions of the body, as breathing and heart rate, while skeletal muscles relax, and beta waves from the outer regions of the brain are synchronized.

-trophy, -trophia, a combining form meaning a 'condition of nutrition or growth.'

-tropia, a combining form meaning '(condition of) change in the visual axis.'

-tropic, -tropal, -tropous, 1. a combining form meaning a 'turn or change in the visual axis.' **2.** a combining form meaning a 'tendency to have an influence on, or be influenced by.'

tropic medicine, the branch of medicine that deals with the diagnosis and treatment of diseases commonly occurring in tropic and subtropic regions of the world, generally between 30 degrees north and south of the equator.

tropic sore. See **oriental sore.**

tropic sprue, a disorder of not absorbing enough nutrients through the intestine (malabsorption syndrome) of unknown cause that occurs continuously in the tropics and subtropics. It is marked by abnormalities in the mucous lining of the small intestine that cause protein malnutrition and multiple nutritional shortages, often made worse by severe infection. Symptoms include diarrhea, loss of appetite, and weight loss. Megaloblastic anemia may result from folic acid and vitamin B_{12} deficiency. Treatment includes use of antibiotics, especially tetracycline, folic acid, iron, calcium, and vitamins A, D, K, and the B complex group, as well as a balanced diet high in protein and normal in fat content. See also **nontropic sprue.**

tropic typhus. See **scrub typhus.**

-tropous. See **-tropic.**

-tropy, -tropism, a combining form meaning 'influenced by or having a closeness for' something specified.

Trousseau's sign /trōosōz'/, a test for muscle cramps in which a wrist spasm is brought about by inflating a blood pressure cuff on the upper arm to a higher-than-normal systolic blood pressure for 3 minutes. A positive test may be seen in results that show abnormally low calcium (hypocalcemia) and magnesium (hypomagnesemia) in the blood.

Trp, abbreviation for **tryptophan.**

true birth rate, the ratio of total births to the total female population of childbearing age, between 15 and 45 years of age. Compare **birth rate, crude birth rate, refined birth rate.**

true chondroma. See **enchondroma.**

true denticle, a calcified mass, composed of irregular dentin, found in the pulp chamber of a tooth.

true dwarf. See **primordial dwarf.**

true glottis. See **glottis.**

true labor, contractions of the uterus that cause a change in the cervix leading to childbirth.

true neuroma, any new, abnormal tissue formation (neoplasm) made up of nerve tissue.

true pelvis. See **pelvis.**

true rib. See **rib.**

true twins. See **monozygotic twins.**

true vocal cord. See **vocal cord.**

truncal ataxia, a loss of coordinated muscle movements for maintaining normal posture of the body from the chest to the pelvis.

truncus arteriosus, the main artery in the embryo that initially opens from both lower heart chambers (ventricles) and later divides into the aorta and the main lung artery (pulmonary trunk), the two portions separated by the bulbar septum.

trunk incurvation reflex. See **Galant reflex.**

truss, a device worn to prevent or slow the pushing through of the intestines or other organ through an opening in the abdominal wall.

Trypanosoma /trip'ənōsō'mə/, a genus of organisms that live in the body. Several species can cause serious diseases in humans. Most *Trypanosoma* organisms live part of their life-cycle in insects and enter humans by insect bites. See also **trypanosome, trypanosomiasis.**

Trypanosoma brucei gambiense. See **Gambian trypanosomiasis.**

Trypanosoma brucei rhodesiense. See **Rhodesian trypanosomiasis.**

Trypanosoma cruzi. See **Chagas' disease.**

trypanosomal infection. See **trypanosomiasis.**

trypanosome /trip'ənōsōm', tripan'-/, any organism of the genus *Trypanosoma.* See also **trypanosomiasis. –trypanosomal,** *adj.*

trypanosomiasis /trip'ənōsōmī'əsis/, an infection by an organism of the *Trypanosoma* genus. Kinds of trypanosomiasis are **African trypanosomiasis** and **Chagas' disease.**

trypanosomicide /trip'ənōsō'misīd/, a drug that destroys trypanosomes, especially the species of the protozoon parasite given to humans by various insect carriers common in Africa, Central America and South America. Various arsenic drugs are used to treat African sleeping sickness, caused by *Trypanosoma gambiense* and *T. rhodesiense,* and Chagas' disease, caused by *T. cruzi,* in the Americas. **–trypanosomicidal,** *adj.*

Tryptacin, a trademark for an amino acid (L-tryptophan), used as an antidepressant and to bring on sleep.

tryptophan (Trp) /trip'təfan/, an amino acid necessary for normal growth in infants and for nitrogen balance in adults. Tryptophan is the basis of several substances, including serotonin and niacin. About 50% of the daily requirement of tryptophan is gotten by the body's processing of niacin. The rest is gotten from protein in foods, especially legumes, grains, and seeds. See also **amino acid, protein.**

tsetse fly /tset'sē, tsē'tsē/, an insect of the genus *Glossina,* found in Africa, that carries the organisms of trypanosomiasis.

TSH, abbreviation for **thyroid stimulating hormone.**

TSH releasing factor. See **thyrotropin releasing hormone.**

TSS, abbreviation for **toxic shock syndrome.**

tsutsugamushi disease. See **scrub typhus.**

TTP, abbreviation for **thrombotic thrombocytopenic purpura.**

T tube, a tubed-shaped device in the shape of a T, inserted through the skin into a cavity or a wound and used for drainage.

T tubule cholangiography, a type of x-ray test of the bilary tract in which iodine dissolved in water is injected into the bile duct through a T-tube. The T-shaped rubber tube is inserted in the common bile duct as a routine process after operations to allow drainage.

tubal abortion, a condition of pregnancy in which an embryo, implanted outside of the uterus, is forced out from the uterine tube into the peritoneal cavity. Tubal abortion often has with it significant internal bleeding that causes severe intestinal and pelvic pain, but may have no symptoms, the products of conception being absorbed again. Rarely, the products of conception reimplant on the peritoneum and continue growing to become an abdominal pregnancy. See also **abdominal pregnancy, ectopic pregnancy, tubal pregnancy.**

tubal dermoid cyst, a tumor that comes from embryonal tissues that grows in an oviduct.

tubal ligation, one of several sterilization processes in which both fallopian tubes are blocked to prevent conception from occurring. Spinal or local anesthesia is used unless the procedure goes along with major surgery. Through a small incision in the intestinal area, the fallopian tubes are tied off in two places with suture. The segment between the two tied places is then burnt, crushed, or cut out. The procedure is less commonly done through the vagina. Problems that result from the procedure, which are rare but serious, include blockage of the pulmonary artery, bleeding, infection, and tubal pregnancy. The requirements for giving one's legal permission to have sterilization operations are different among states and institutions.

tubal pregnancy, a pregnancy where the embryo is implanted outside of the uterus (ectopic), in which the products of conception implant in the fallopian tube. Roughly 2% of all pregnancies are ectopic; of these, roughly 90% occur in the fallopian tube. Tubal pregnancy seldom occurs in first pregnancies. The most important factor that might bring on tubal pregnancy is prior tubal injury. Pelvic infection, scarring and healing tissue from surgery, or problems from using an IUD birth-control device may cause damage that decreases the self-movement of the tube. Transport of the ovum through the tube after fertilization is slowed, and implantation takes place before the products of conception (conceptus) reach the uterine cavity. Most often the tube, which cannot hold the growing fetus for very long, breaks. This causes bleeding in the peritoneal cavity that, if not stopped, can lead rapidly to shock and, often, death. Occasionally, the conceptus does not firmly implant in the tube and is pushed out from the fringed end of the tube as a tubal abortion. Some conceptuses seem to die and are absorbed back into the tube. Diagnosis of tubal pregnancy is often difficult. With breaking open of the fallopian tube, women often feel sudden sharp pain in one side of the lower intestinal area, but signs and symptoms of tubal pregnancy are different with each patient, and the classic three symptoms of absence of menstruation, pelvic pain, and a tender adnexal mass are present only 50% of the time. Drawing out blood from the rear vaginal sac (cul-de-sac) usually means a ruptured fallopian tube and tubal pregnancy; it requires immediate surgical examination of the lower intestinal area. Absence of blood in this process does not rule out the presence of an unruptured tubal pregnancy. Use of an exploration device used in the lower intestinal area, or surgical exploration may be required, especially if a woman's pregnancy test is positive, the pelvic findings show a possible tubal pregnancy, and ultrasound tests (sonography) of the pelvis cannot show a normal pregnancy. Because of the deadly consequences of an undiagnosed tubal pregnancy, women who report any of these symptoms early in their pregnancies, especially during the time before a normal pregnancy can be confirmed, must be considered at risk. In women who have had prior pelvic disease and in those who have symptoms or signs that are of tubal pregnancy, emergency treatment requires an immediate infusion by vein of blood, type and cross match of blood for blood replacement, and treatment of shock as necessary. Treatment is surgical and involves opening the lower intestinal area for examination (laparotomy), taking out the conceptus and any blood in the peritoneal cavity, and removing or repairing the involved tube. Conditions that help bring on a first tubal pregnancy also help bring on a second; a woman who has had one tubal pregnancy has one chance in five of having another in a following pregnancy. Depending on the location of the developing embryo, the condition is classified as an ampullary, fimbrial, or interstitial tubal pregnancy.

tube, a hollow, cylinder-shaped piece of equipment or structure of the body.

tube feeding, the giving of nutritionally balanced liquefied foods through a tube inserted into the stomach or first part of the small intestine (duodenum). The process is used after mouth or stomach surgery, in severe burns, in paralysis or blockage of the food pipe (esophagus), in severe cases of a mental disorder causing severe weight loss (anorexia nervosa), and for unconscious patients or those unable to chew or swallow. Also called **gavage feeding, nasogastric feeding.** See also **parenteral nutrition.**

tube feeding care, the nursing care and management of a patient receiving nourishment through a nose tube that goes into the stomach (nasogastric).

tubercle /tōō'bərkəl/, **1.** a small group of cells or a bump (nodule), as that on a bone. **2.** a nodule, especially an elevation of the skin that is larger than a pimple, as Morgagni's tubercles of the dark circles around the nipples (areolae) of the breasts. **3.** a small, rounded nodule caused by infection with *Mycobacterium tuberculosis,* made up of a gray translucent mass of small round cells surrounded by connective cells.

tubercles of Montgomery, small pimples (papillae) on the surface of nipples and dark circles around the nipples (areolae) that release a fatty lubricating substance.

tuberculin. See **tuberculin test, tuberculosis.**

tuberculin purified protein derivative /tōōbur'-kyōolin/, a solution that has a pure protein fraction gotten from substances grown in laboratories that are taken from strains of *Mycobacterium tuberculosis.* It is used as an aid in the diagnosis of tuberculosis, in the Mantoux test, and in multiple puncture skin test devices. See also **Mantoux test, Tine test.**

tuberculin test, a test to find past or present tuberculosis infection based on a positive skin reaction, using one of several methods. A purified protein derivative (PPD) of tubercle bacilli, called **tuberculin,** is placed into the skin by scratch, puncture, or skin injection. If a raised, red, or hard zone forms around the tuberculin test site, the person is said to be sensitive to tuberculin, and the test is read as positive. However, a negative tuberculin reaction does not rule out a diagnosis of earlier or active tuberculosis. Bacteria grown from samples taken from saliva and from stomach material, acid-fast staining, and x-ray studies are often needed to make a sure diagnosis of tuberculosis. Kinds of tuberculin tests include **Heaf test, Mantoux test, Pirquet's test,** and **tine test.**

tuberculoid leprosy. See **leprosy.**

tuberculoma /tōōbur'kyōolō'mə/, a tumorlike growth of tuberculous tissue in the central nervous system, marked by symptoms of an expanding brain, or spinal mass. Treatment consists of the use of antibacteria drugs to take away the primary growth and to prevent swelling of the membranes of the brain or spinal cord (meningitis).

tuberculosis (TB), a long-term grainy tumorous infection caused by an acid-fast bacillus, *Mycobacterium tuberculosis.* Generally exposure is by breathing in or eating infected droplets, and it usually affects the lungs, although infection of other organ systems by other ways of getting the disease occurs. Listlessness, vague chest pain, swelling of the membranes around the lungs (pleurisy), loss of appetite, fever, and weight loss are early symptoms of lung (pulmonary) tuberculosis. Night sweats, bleeding in the lungs, coughing up of sputum with pus, and shortness of breath (dypsnea) develop as the disease progresses. The lung tissues react to the bacterium by making protective cells that go around the disease organism, forming small groups of cells or bumps (tubercles). Untreated, the tubercles enlarge and merge to form larger tubercles that undergo a change into a grainy mass of tissue (caseation). Eventually the separated dead tissue ends up in the cavities of the lungs. Coughing up of blood occurs as a result of cavitary spread. Physical examination reveals sounds from the highest part of the lungs (apical rales), resonating breathing tube sounds, lower breathing movement, and, in advanced cases, bluish skin. The infecting organism does not produce bacterial poisons (endotoxins) or substances that disrupt red blood cells (hemolysins), but **tuberculin,** a poisonous substance, is released as the bacillus breaks apart. Tuberculin has no effect in people who have never been infected but produces a typical skin reaction when injected in the skin in people who have or have had tuberculosis. Purified protein derivative (PPD) is a stable, purified active drug used to test for current or past infection. X-ray films of the lungs show various signs of tubercular activity. Tuberculosis may spread from the lungs via the lymphatics and blood vessels. Such seedlike infection is marked by tiny, seedlike tubercles in the liver, spleen, and other organs. The bacillus is generally sensitive to isoniazid (INH), paraaminosalicylic acid, streptomycin, rifampin, dihydrostreptomycin, ultraviolet radiation, and heat. A combination of drugs is given, with regular tests of the function of the kidneys, liver, eyes, and ears done to find early signs of drug poisoning. This is especially important because drug treatment will usually continue for more than 1 year. The person is usually hospitalized for the first weeks of treatment to limit the possible spread of infection, to encourage rest and excellent nutrition, to ensure the patient follows the drug schedule, and to watch for drug side effects. Samples of sputum are regularly looked at. The disease cannot be spread once the bacillus is no longer present in the sputum. Care of an outpatient includes continued use of drugs, checking for drug side effects, sputum analyses, and support to complete the long course of treatment. All contacts are tested periodically with PPD. People who are at increased risk of infection may be treated under the likelihood they may have the disease without a positive diagnosis having been made. Before discharge, the patient is taught the following: how to prevent the spread of the disease, the elements of good nutrition, the name, dose, action, and side effects of all drugs given, the need to take the drugs regularly, and how and where to get the next supply of drugs. Plans for follow-up are discussed; they include date, time, and place of the next laboratory tests, and a reminder that a cough, weight loss, fever, night sweats, and coughing up blood are danger signals that are to be reported immediately. See also **miliary tuberculosis, tuberculin test.**

tuberculosis vaccine. See **BCG vaccine.**

tuberculous spondylitis /tōobur′kyələs/, a rare, serious form of tuberculosis caused by the invasion of *Mycobacterium tuberculosis* into the spinal backbones. The disks between the backbones may be destroyed, causing the collapse and wedging of affected backbones and the shortening and angling of the spine. Upper backbones are more often involved than the lower parts of the spine. More than one area of the spine may be affected, and normal backbones may be seen between affected and unaffected sections. The infection usually cuts into backbones in front and to one side and produces pus-filled sores (abscesses). The pressure of the abscess may cause blockage of blood to the nearby spinal cord, and abscesses in the cervical area may put out of place or block the windpipe (trachea) and the food pipe (esophagus). Also called **Pott's disease, spinal caries.** See also **tuberculosis.**

tuberosity /tōo′bəros′itē/, a raising or bump, especially of a bone.

tuberosity of the tibia, a large, oblong elevation at the end of the large leg bone (tibia) that attaches to the ligament of the kneecap.

tuberous carcinoma, a hard, cancerous tumor of the skin, marked by bumps. Also called **carcinoma tuberosum.**

tuberous sclerosis, a familial, nervous system and skin (neurocutaneous) disease marked by epilepsy, mental breakdown, tumorlike growths on the face (adenoma sebaceum), nodules and hardened patches on the outer brain (cerebral cortex), tumors on the eyes, discolored patches on the skin, tumors of the heart or kidneys, and calcium deposits on the brain. There is no effective treatment. Also called **epiloia.** See also **adenoma sebaceum.**

tuberous xanthoma. See **xanthoma tuberosum.**

tuboplasty, a surgical procedure in which cut or damaged fallopian tubes are repaired.

tubular necrosis, the death of cells in the small tubes of the kidneys as a result of disease or injury.

tubule /tōo′byōol/, a small tube, as one of the collecting tubules in the kidneys, the semen-producing tubules of the testicles, or Henle's tubules between the distal and proximal convoluted tubules of the kidney. **–tubular,** *adj.*

tuft fracture, fracture of any one of the distal phalanges.

tularemia /tōo′lərē′mē·ə/, an infectious disease of animals caused by the bacillus *Francisella (Pasteurella) tularensis,* which may be gotten by insect carriers or direct contact. It is marked in humans by fever, headache, and an open skin sore with localized lymph node enlargement, or by eye infection, stomach and intestinal sores, or pneumonia, depending on the site of entry and the response of the patient. Treatment includes antibiotics. Recovery produces lifelong immunity. A vaccine is available. Also called **deerfly fever, rabbit fever.**

-tumescence, a combining form meaning a 'swelling.'

tumor, 1. a growth or enlargement occurring in conditions that produce swelling. 2. also called **neoplasm.** a new growth of tissue marked by continuing, uncontrolled growth of cells. The tumor may be localized or spreading, harmless or cancerous. A tumor may be named for its location, for its cellular makeup, or for the person who first identified it.

tumor albus, a white swelling occurring in a tuberculous bone or joint.

tumoricide /tōomōr′isīd/, a substance that can destroy a tumor. **–tumoricidal,** *adj.*

tumorigenesis /tōo′mərijen′əsis/, the process of starting and helping the growth of a tumor. Compare **carcinogenesis, oncogenesis, sarcomagenesis. –tumorigenic,** *adj.*

tumor marker, a substance in the body that is linked to the presence of a cancer. Some doctors feel the term is misleading because the marker molecules found in blood or other tissue samples do not mean the presence only of cancer.

tumor necrosis factor (TNF), a natural body protein, also produced by artificial means, with anticancer effects. It is produced in the body in response to the presence of poisonous substances, as poisons of bacteria. Side effects are shock from poisonous levels of TNF and ill health and poor nutrition.

tumor volume, a part of an organ or tissue that includes both the tumor and affected areas next to it.

tungsten (W), a metallic element. Its atomic number is 74; its atomic weight is 183.85. It has the highest melting point of all metals.

tunica, a surrounding coat or covering membrane.

tunica adventitia, the outer layer or coat of an artery or other tube-shaped structure.

tunica intima, the membrane lining an artery.

tunica media, a muscular middle coat of an artery.

tunica vaginalis testis, the serumlike membrane surrounding the testicle and an attached tube (epididymis).

tunica vasculosa bulbi. See **uvea.**

tuning fork, a small metal instrument consisting of a stem and two prongs that makes a constant pitch when either prong is struck. It is used in sound tests of nerve function and of air and bone carrying signals.

tunnel vision, a defect in sight in which there is a great loss of side vision, as if looking through a hollow tube or tunnel. The condition occurs in advanced long-term glaucoma.

TUR, abbreviation for **transurethral resection.**

turban tumor, a noncancerous tumor made up of many pink or maroon bumps that may cover the entire scalp and may also occur on the trunk and arms and legs. The growth seems to occur often within single families and often recurs after being removed.

turgid /tur'jid/, swollen, hard, and blocked, usually as a result of a gathering of fluid.

turgor /tur'gər/, the normal strength and tension of the skin caused by the outward pressure of the cells and the fluid that surrounds them. Loss of body water causes decreased skin turgor, which appears as loose skin that, when grasped and raised between two fingers, slowly returns to a position level with the tissue next to it. Marked fluid gain or too-much fluid in the peritoneal cavity (ascites) causes increased turgor that appears as smooth, taut, shiny skin that cannot be grasped and raised. An evaluation of the turgor of the skin is an important part of physical examination.

turista. See **traveler's diarrhea.**

turnbuckle cast, a deformity correcting (orthopedic) device used to encase and immobilize the entire trunk, one arm to the elbow, and the opposite leg to the knee. It is made of plaster of Paris or fiberglass and uses hinges as part of its design in the treatment of curvature of the spine (scoliosis). The hinges are placed at the level of the top of the curvature. Used for preoperative and postoperative positioning, it is used less frequently than the Risser cast. A version of the turnbuckle cast is used sometimes as a extreme stretching-out (hyperextension) cast for the treatment of spinal curvature disorders (kyphosis or kyphoscoliosis). Compare **Risser cast.**

Turner's sign. See **Grey Turner's sign.**

Turner's syndrome, a chromosome disorder seen in about 1 in 3,000 live female births, marked by the absence of one X chromosome, inborn ovarian failure, genital tissue defects, heart and circulation problems, dwarfism, short metacarpals, "shield chest," bone growths on the larger bone of the leg, and underdeveloped breasts, uterus, and vagina. Confusion about space and distances and some learning disorders are common. Treatment includes hormone treatment (estrogens, androgens, pituitary growth hormone) and, often, surgical correction of heart and circulation problems and the webbing of the neck skin. Also called **Bonnevie-Ullrich syndrome, monosomy X.** See also **Noonan's syndrome.**

turricephaly. See **oxycephaly.**

-tuse, **1.** a combining form meaning 'dull or blunt.' **2.** a combining form meaning 'to beat or thrust.'

Tussionex, a trademark for a drug containing an antitussive (hydrocodone bitartrate) and an antihistamine (phenyltoloxamine citrate).

TV, abbreviation for **tidal volume.**

TVL, abbreviation for **tenth value layer.**

twelfth cranial nerve. See **hypoglossal nerve.**

twin, either of two offspring born of the same pregnancy and developed from either a single egg or from two eggs that were released from the ovary and fertilized at the same time. Twin births occur approximately 1 in 80 pregnancies. Kinds of twins include **conjoined twins, dizygotic twins, interlocked twins, monozygotic twins, Siamese twins, unequal twins.** See also **Hellin's law.**

twin monster. See **double monster.**

twinning, **1.** the development of two or more fetuses during the same pregnancy, either by itself or through outside control for experimental purposes in animals. **2.** the making of two like structures or parts by division.

two-way catheter, a catheter that has two tubes within it, one for injection of drugs or fluids and the other for taking out fluid or specimens.

Tylenol, a trademark for a painkiller and fever-reducing drug (acetaminophen).

tyloxapol /tīlok'səpôl/, a breathing tract detergent given for bronchitis, emphysema, pus-filled sores in the lungs, long-term enlargement of the breathing tubes (bronchiectasis), or unexpanded lungs in the fetus (atelectasis).

tympanic /timpan'ik/, of or referring to a structure that sounds when struck; drumlike, as a **tympanic abdomen** that sounds on percussion because the intestines are enlarged with gas. **–tympanum** /tim'pənəm/, n. (pl. **tympana**).

tympanic antrum, a relatively large, irregular opening in the upper front part of the mastoid process of the temporal bone at the base of the skull. It is linked to the mastoid air cells and lined by the extension of the mucous membrane of the tympanic cavity. The bony tegmen tympani separates the tympanic antrum from the middle fossa of the cranial cavity, and the sideways semicircular canal of the inner ear sticks out into the antrum. See also **mastoid process.**

tympanic cavity. See **middle ear.**

tympanic membrane, a thin, semitransparent membrane in the middle ear that carries sound vibrations to the inner ear by means of the bones of the middle ear (auditory ossicles). It is nearly oval in form, with an up and down diameter of about 10 mm, and separates the tympanic cavity from the bottom of the outer acoustic meatus. Also called **eardrum, membrana tympani.**

tympanic reflex, the reflection of a beam of light shining on the eardrum. In a normal ear a bright, wedge-shaped reflection is seen; its highpoint is at the end of the malleus, and its base is at the front lower edge of the eardrum. In disorders of the middle ear or eardrum, this shape may be distorted. Also called **light reflex.**

tympanoplasty /timpan'əplas'tē/, any of several operations on the eardrum or small bones of the middle ear, to restore or improve hearing in patients with conductive deafness. These operations may be used to repair a broken eardrum, for increasing deafness (otosclerosis), or dislocation or death of one of the small bones of the middle ear. See also **myringoplasty.**

tympanotomy. See **myringotomy.**

tympanum. See **tympanic.**

-type, a combining form meaning a 'representative form or class.'

Type A personality, a behavior pattern described by Meyer Friedman and Ray Rosenman as linked to individuals who are highly competitive and work compulsively to meet deadlines. The behavior also goes with a higher-than-usual rate of coronary heart disease.

Type B personality, a form of behavior Friedman and Rosenman argue goes with persons who seem to be passive and who lack an inner need to meet deadlines, are not highly competitive at work and play, and have a lower risk of heart attack.

Type E personality, a term introduced by Harriet Braiker to describe professional women who fit neither Type A or Type B personality categories, but who have a high sense of insecurity and try to convince themselves that they are worthwhile. Type E women try to be "all things to all people," according to Braiker, and tend to suffer mental strain.

Type I diabetes mellitus. See **insulin-dependent diabetes mellitus.**

Type II diabetes mellitus. See **non-insulin-dependent diabetes mellitus.**

type I hyperlipidemia, a familial form of primary lipoproteinemia. A rare disease carried as a recessive genetic trait, it is marked by the gathering of triglycerides in the bloodstream, causing recurring bouts of swelling of the pancreas (acute pancreatitis). The symptoms begin in childhood. The disease is caused by a low level of activity of an enzyme, lipoprotein lipase, that normally removes triglycerides from the blood. The accumulation of triglycerides is basically in proportion to the amount of fat in the diet. Treatment is mainly dietary; both saturated and unsaturated fats are limited to amounts that produce less than 500 mg/dl of blood, checked after not eating overnight. Also called **exogenous hyperlipemia.**

type II hyperlipoproteinemia. See **familial hypercholesterolemia.**

type I hypersensitivity. See **anaphylactic hypersensitivity.**

type II hypersensitivity. See **cytotoxic hypersensitivity.**

type III hypersensitivity. See **immune complex hypersensitivity.**

type IV hypersensitivity. See **cell-mediated immune response.**

typhlo-, **1.** a combining form meaning 'referring to the cecum.' **2.** a combining form meaning 'referring to blindness.'

-typhoid, **1.** a combining form meaning a '(specified) form of typus.' **2.** a combining form meaning 'of or resembling typhus.'

typhoid fever, a bacterial infection usually caused by *Salmonella typhi,* carried by contaminated milk, water, or food. It is marked by headache, mental confusion and excitement, cough, watery diarrhea, rash, and a high fever. Also called **enteric fever.** Compare **cholera, paratyphoid fever, salmonellosis.** The period between first being exposed to the bacteria and getting the first symptoms may be as long as 60 days. Patches of rosy spots and pimples are scattered over the skin of the intestinal area. Enlargement of the spleen and a decrease in the number of white corpuscles develop first. The diagnosis is made by growing bacterial cultures from samples of blood and stool and by rising concentrations of antibodies (agglutinins) in Widal's test. The disease is serious and may be fatal. Further problems are bleeding or holes in the intestines and swelling and blood clotting in veins (thrombophlebitis). Some people who recover from the disease continue to be carriers and release the organism, spreading the disease. Antibiotics as chloramphenicol, ampicillin, amoxicillin, and trimethoprin-sulfamethoxazole are all useful in treatment. Prolonged use of antibiotics or removal of the gallbladder may stop the patient from carrying the disease. Typhoid vaccine gives some protection but requires annual booster doses for best effect. To lower the temperature, sponge baths are preferred to temperature-reducing drugs (salicylates) because they may cause extreme loss of body temperature or low blood pressure. Laxatives and enemas should not be used because of the danger of holes being made in the bowel. Proper disposal of human wastes is essential to prevent epidemics, and carriers should not be allowed to prepare food.

typhoid pellagra, a form of food shortage disease (pellagra) in which the symptoms also include continued high temperatures.

typhoid vaccine, a bacterial vaccine prepared from an inactivated, dried strain of *Salmonella typhi.* It is given for primary immunization against typhoid fever for adults and children.

★CAUTION: Acute infection or use of steroids at the same time prohibits its use.

★ADVERSE EFFECTS: Among the more serious side effects are allergic reaction, and pain and swelling at the site of injection.

typhus, any of a group of acute infectious diseases caused by various species of *Rickettsia* and usually carried from infected rodents to humans by the bites of lice, fleas, mites, or ticks. These diseases are all marked by headache, chills, fever, malaise, and red patches and pimples. Kinds of typhus are **epidemic typhus, murine typhus,** and **scrub typhus.** See also **Brill-Zinsser disease, Rocky Mountain spotted fever.**

typhus vaccine, any one of three vaccines, each of which is made to deal with the different rickettsial organisms that cause epidemic typhus, murine typhus, or Brill-Zinsser disease. Each of the vaccines is given for immunization against a form of typhus.

★CAUTION: Acute infection, diseases that cause weakness, use of corticosteriods at the same time, or allergy to eggs prohibits its use.

★ADVERSE EFFECTS: Among the most serious side effects are allergic reactions. Pain at the site of injection also may occur.

-typia, a combining form meaning '(condition of) conformity to type.'

typing, the process of finding out the classification of a specimen of blood, tissue, or other substance. See also **blood typing, tissue typing.**

Tyr, abbreviation for **tyrosine.**

tyramine, an amino acid made in the body from the essential acid tyrosine. Tyramine starts the release of the catecholamines epinephrine and norepinephrine. It is important that people taking MAO (monoamine oxidase) inhibitors avoid eating foods and drinks that have tyramine, especially aged cheeses and meats, bananas, yeast-containing products, and alcoholic beverages. See also **adrenergic drug, amine, catecholamine, epinephrine, norepinephrine, vasoconstriction.**

tyro-, a combining form meaning 'referring to cheese.'

tyroma /tīrō′mə/, *pl.* **tyromas, tyromata,** a new growth or nodule with a caseous or cheesy texture.

tyrosinemia /tī′rōsinē′mē·ə/, **1.** also called **neonatal tyrosinemia.** a harmless, temporary condition of the newborn, especially premature infants, in which too much of the amino acid tyrosine is found in the blood and urine. The disorder is caused by a problem in amino acid processing, usually late development of the enzymes necessary to process tyrosine, and is controlled by dietary measures and vitamin C treatment. The defect goes away with treatment, or it may disappear by itself. **2.** also called **hereditary tyrosinemia.** an inborn disorder that involves an inborn problem of processing the amino acid tyrosine. The condition, which is carried as a non-sex-related chromosome (autosomal) recessive trait, is caused by an enzyme shortage and causes liver failure or cirrhosis of the liver. It can also cause defects in the kidney tubes that can lead to renal rickets and sugar in the urine of the kidney, generalized excess amino acids in the urine, and mental retardation. Treatment consists of a diet low in tyrosine and phenylalanine and high in doses of vitamin C. In severe cases the outlook is extremely poor, and a liver transplantation may be the only lifesaving measure.

tyrosinosis /tī′rōsinō′sis/, a condition caused by a defect in amino acid processing and carried as a non-sex-related chromosome (autosomal) recessive trait. It is marked by the release of an excessive amount of parahydroxyphenylpyruvic acid and a moderate product of tyrosine, in the urine. There is no known treatment. See also **tyrosinemia.**

tyrosinurea /tī′rōsinŏŏr′ē·ə/, tyrosine in the urine.

Tyzine, a trademark for an alpha-adrenergic drug (tetrahydrozoline hydrochloride).

Tzanck test /tsangk/, a microscopic examination of material from skin sores to help diagnose certain small blister diseases. The tissue is scraped from the base of a blister, placed on a slide, and stained with Wright's or Giemsa's stain. Giant cells with many nuclei show the presence of herpesvirus or varicella. Typical pemphigus and other cells can also be identified.

U

ulcer, a craterlike skin lesion or mucous membrane caused by some inflammatory, infectious, or malignant process. Some kinds of ulcer are **decubitus ulcer, peptic ulcer,** and **serpent ulcer. –ulcerate,** *v.,* **ulcerative** /ul'sərā'tiv/, *adj.*

ulcerative blepharitis, an inflammation of the edges of the eyelids in which a staphylococcal infection of the follicles of the eyelashes and eyelids causes sticky crusts on the lid margins. If the crusts are pulled off, the skin bleeds. Tiny pustules develop in the follicles and form ulcers. Other signs include burning, itching, swelling, and redness of the eyelids; loss of eyelashes; irritation of the conjunctiva with tearing; photophobia; and gluing together of the eyelids during sleep by the dried secretions. Compare **nonulcerative blepharitis.**

ulcerative colitis, a chronic, episodic, inflammatory disease of the large intestine and rectum, marked by profuse watery diarrhea containing varying amounts of blood, mucus, and pus. See also **Crohn's disease.** The diarrhea is accompanied by tenesmus, severe intestinal pain, fever, chills, anemia, and weight loss. Children with the disease may have retarded physical growth. Patients with ulcerative colitis often cannot perform the normal activities of daily living. Diagnosis of the disease is based on clinical signs, the results of barium x-ray films of the colon, and colonoscopy with biopsy. It is often hard to distinguish between ulcerative colitis and Crohn's disease. Treatment with steroids or other anti-inflammatory drugs may help to control the symptoms. Those with severe disease or life-threatening problems often need surgery. Total proctocolectomy with ileostomy is a permanent cure for ulcerative colitis.

ulocarcinoma /yōō'lōkär'sinō'mə/, *pl.* **ulocarcinomas, ulocarcinomata,** cancer of the gums.

ulterior transactions, (in psychiatry) communication between two people with two levels of meaning. The first level is usually of relevant verbal statements. The second level is usually nonverbal and has hidden psychological meaning.

Ultracef, a trademark for an antibiotic (cefadroxil monohydrate).

Ultralente, a trademark for an insulin zinc suspension.

ultralente insulin. See **long-acting insulin.**

ultramicroscopy. See **darkfield microscopy.**

ultrasonic cardiography. See **echocardiography.**

ultrasonography, the process of imaging deep structures of the body by recording the reflection of high-frequency sound waves. It is used to diagnose fetal abnormalities, gallstones, heart defects, and tumors. Also called **sonography.**

ultrasound imaging, the use of high-frequency sound to image internal structures. Ultrasound diagnosis differs from radiological diagnosis in that there is no ionizing radiation involved. Also called **ultrasound diagnosing.**

ultraviolet (UV), light beyond the range of human vision. It occurs in sunlight; it burns and tans the skin and converts in the skin to vitamin D. Ultraviolet lamps are used to control infectious airborne bacteria, and viruses and to treat psoriasis and other skin conditions. Black light is ultraviolet light used in fluoroscopy. See also **angstrom, light, radiation, spectrum.**

ultraviolet microscopy. See **fluorescent microscopy.**

ultraviolet radiation, a range of electromagnetic waves. Ultraviolet radiation is used to treat rickets and certain skin conditions. Milk and some other foods become activated with vitamin D when exposed to this type of energy.

umbilical /umbil'ikəl/, **1.** of or referring to the umbilicus. **2.** of or referring to the umbilical cord.

umbilical catheterization, a procedure in which a catheter is passed through an umbilical artery to give a newborn parenteral fluids, to take blood samples, or through the umbilical vein for a transfusion or for giving emergency amounts of drugs, fluids, or volume expanders.

umbilical cord, a flexible structure connecting the umbilicus with the placenta in the pregnant uterus, and giving passage to the umbilical arteries and vein. In the newborn it is about 2 feet long and one-half inch in diameter. First formed during the fifth week of pregnancy, it contains the yolk sac and the body stalk. Also called the **chorda umbilicalis, funiculus umbilicalis.** See also **allantois.**

umbilical duct. See **vitelline duct.**

umbilical fistula, an abnormal passage from the umbilicus to the intestine or to the remnant of the canal in the median umbilical ligament that connects the fetal bladder with the allantois.

umbilical hernia, a soft, skin-covered protrusion of intestine through a weakness in the abdominal wall around the umbilicus. It often closes on its own within 1 to 2 years, but large hernias may need surgery.

umbilical region, the part of the abdomen around the umbilicus. See also **abdominal regions.**

umbilical vasculitis, an inflammation of the umbilical cord and its blood vessels.

umbo, a landmark on the eardrum created by the attachment of the eardrum to the first small bone in the middle ear.

uncal herniation, a state in which part of the temporal lobe protrudes over the tentorial edge because of increased intracranial pressure. If uncorrected, the disorder causes pressure on the brain stem after first impinging on the third cranial nerve. A dilated pupil on the side of the herniation is a sign of the disorder.

unciform bone. See **hamate bone.**

Uncinaria, a genus of nematode causing hookworm in dogs, cats, and other carnivores.

uncompensated gluteal gait. See **Trendelenburg gait.**

unconditioned response, a normal, instinctive, unlearned reaction to a stimulus. It is one occurring naturally, not acquired by association and training. Also called **inborn reflex, instinctive reflex, unconditioned reflex.** Compare **conditioned response.**

unconscious, 1. being unaware of the environment; insensible; unable to respond to sensory stimuli. **2.** (in psychiatry) the part of mental function in which thoughts, ideas, emotions, or memories are beyond awareness and not subject to ready recall. It contains data that have never been conscious or were conscious at one time, usually for a brief period, and later repressed. Compare **preconscious.** See also **collective unconscious, personal unconscious.**

unconsciousness, a state of unawareness or lack of response to sense stimuli as a result of a lack of oxygen caused by breathing difficulties or shock. It can also be caused by depressants, as drugs, poisons, ketones or electrolyte imbalance. Other causes are from a brain pathological condition, as injury, seizures, stroke, or brain tumor or infection. Many kinds of unconsciousness can occur during hypnotic and dream states. See also **coma.**

unction. See **ointment.**

undecylenic acid, an antifungus drug. It is given to treat athlete's foot and ringworm.

★CAUTION: Known allergy to this drug prohibits its use. It is not used in the eyes or on mucous membranes. Caution is advised when the patient is diabetic.

★ADVERSE EFFECTS: Among the more serious side effects are skin irritation and allergic reactions.

underdriving, a state in artificial heart functioning in which there is too-little compressed air during systole to eject the entire end diastolic volume of the ventricle.

underlying assumption, a set of rules one holds about oneself, others, and the world. These rules are regarded as unquestionably true.

underwater exercise, any physical activity in a pool or large tub where the buoyancy of the water aids movement of weak or injured muscles. See also **exercise.**

underwater seal, a seal over one end of a tube made by water, the other end of the tube is in the chest cavity of a patient. The water acts as a one-way valve. It lets air flow in but not out. Also called **water trap.**

underweight, less-than-normal body weight given height, body build, and age.

undescended testis. See **cryptorchidism, monorchism.**

undifferentiated cell leukemia. See **stem cell leukemia.**

undifferentiated family ego mass, an emotional connectedness in a family in which all members express emotions in the same way.

undifferentiated malignant lymphoma, a lymphoid neoplasm with many large cells with large nuclei, small amounts of pale cytoplasm, and poorly defined borders. Also called **reticulosarcoma, stem cell lymphoma.**

undifferentiated schizophrenia. See **acute schizophrenia.**

undifferentiation, the lack or absence of normal cell differences creating an identifiable cell type.

undisplaced fracture, a bone break in which cracks in the tissue may radiate in several directions without the separation of fragmented sections.

undulant fever. See **brucellosis.**

unengaged head, the head of a fetus before it moves down into the mother's pelvic area. See **engagement.** See also **ballottement.**

unequal twins, two nonjoined fetuses born of the same pregnancy in which only one of the pair is fully formed, with the other showing developmental defects.

unfinished business, the concerns of a dying patient that need resolution before death can be accepted by the patient. Unfinished business may range from money matters to personal relations.

ungual phalanx. See **distal phalanx.**

unguent. See **ointment.**

unguis. See **nail.**

UNICEF /yōo′nisef′/, abbreviation for **United Nations International Children's Emergency Fund.**

unicentric blastoma. See **blastoma.**

unidirectional block, a pathological failure of cardiac impulse conduction in one direction while conduction is possible in the other direction.

unidisciplinary health care team, a group of health-care workers who have similar training.

unidose. See **unit dose.**

unilateral hypertrophy, enlargement of one side or part of one side of the body.

unilateral long-leg spica cast, a cast used to immobilize one leg and the trunk of the body cranially as far as the nipple line. It is used to treat a broken thigh or to correct or maintain a correction of a hip deformity. Compare **bilateral long-leg spica cast, one-and-a-half spica cast.**

unilateral paralysis. See **hemiplegia.**

uniovular /yōō′nē·ov′yələr/, developing from a single ovum as in monozygotic twins as contrasted with dizygotic twins. Also **monovular.** Compare **binovular.**

uniovular twins. See **monozygotic twins.**

Unipen, a trademark for an antibacterial (nafcillin sodium).

unipolar depressive response, an affective disorder marked by symptoms of depression only.

unique radiolytic product, a product, as a food substance, that has undergone chemical changes as a result of exposure to ionizing radiation, as x-rays.

unit dose, a method of preparing medications in which single doses are prepared by the pharmacy and delivered in individual labeled packages to the patient's unit to be given by the nurses on the ordered schedule. Also called **unidose.**

unit dose system, a system of drug distribution in which a movable cart containing a drawer for each patient's medication is prepared by the hospital pharmacy with a 24-hour supply of the medications.

United Nations International Children's Emergency Fund (UNICEF) /yōō′nisef′/, a fund established by the United Nations in 1946 to aid children of the world. It is funded by member nations. It acts to prevent disease, including tuberculosis, whooping cough, and diphtheria, and gives food and clothing to needy children in more than 50 countries.

United States Pharmacopeia (USP), a compendium, recognized officially by the Federal Food, Drug, and Cosmetic Act, with descriptions, uses, strengths, and standards of purity for certain drugs and their dosage.

United States Public Health Service (USPHS), an agency of the federal government responsible for the control of any people, goods, or substances from abroad that may affect the health of U.S. citizens. The agency sets standards for domestic handling and processing of food and the manufacture of serums, vaccines, cosmetics, and drugs. It supports and does research, aids localities in times of disaster and epidemics, and provides medical care for certain groups of Americans.

univalent antiserum. See **antiserum.**

universal antidote, a mixture of 50% activated charcoal, 25% magnesium oxide, and 25% tannic acid, formerly thought useful as an antidote for most types of acid, heavy metal, alkaloid, and glycoside poisons. It is now thought that the mixture is no more effective than activated charcoal given with water.

universal cuff, a device worn on the hand to help hold items, as utensils, shaver, or pencil, allowing a patient with a weak grasp to increase participation in self-care activities.

universal donor, a person with blood of type O, Rh factor negative. Such blood may be used for emergency transfusion with little risk of incompatibility. See also **blood donor, blood group, transfusion.**

universalizability principle, a principle that an act is good if everyone should, in similar circumstances, do the same act without exception.

universal qualifiers, (in neurolinguistical programing) the use of terms that give general impressions of limitations, as all, common, every, only, and never.

Unna's paste boot /ōō′nəz/, a dressing for varicose ulcers made by putting gelatin-glycerin-zinc oxide paste on the leg and then a spiral bandage that is covered with coats of paste to make a rigid boot.

unresolved grief, a severe, continuous grief reaction in which a person does not come to terms with his or her grief within a reasonable time.

unsaturated, describing a solution that is capable of dissolving more of the solute; not saturated.

unsaturated fatty acid, any glyceryl esters of certain organic acids in which some of the atoms are joined by double or triple valence bonds. Monounsaturated fatty acids have only one double or triple bond per molecule and are found in such foods as fowl, almonds, pecans, cashew nuts, peanuts, and olive oil. Polyunsaturated fatty acids have more than one double or triple bond per molecule and are found in fish, corn, walnuts, sunflower seeds, soybeans, cottonseeds, and safflower oil. Diets high in polyunsaturated fatty acids and low in saturated fatty acids have been correlated with low serum cholesterol levels in some study populations. Compare **saturated fatty acid.**

unsaturated hydrocarbon. See **unsaturated.**

unscrubbed team members, the members of a surgical team, including the anesthetist and circulating nurse, who wear surgical attire but do not wear a gown or gloves and do not enter the sterile field.

unsocialized aggressive reaction, a behavior disorder of childhood marked by hostility, disobedience, aggression, vengefulness, quarreling, and destructiveness. It includes lying, stealing, temper tantrums, vandalism, and violence. It is more prevalent in boys than in girls. Typically it is caused by an unstable home with harsh and inconsistent discipline, general frustration, rejection, marital discord, or divorce. Punitive treatment is ineffective. Recommended techniques reinforce desirable behavioral patterns and try to change unfavorable environmental conditions. If untreated, the condition may lead to antisocial personality disorder.

unstable, 1. in an excited or active state, as an atom with a nucleus possessing excess energy. 2. easily broken down.

unstriated muscle. See **smooth muscle.**

upper extremity suspension, an orthopedic process used to treat bone fractures and correct orthopedic abnormalities of the upper limbs. The procedure uses traction equipment, with metal frames, ropes, and pulleys to relieve the weight of the upper limb involved rather than to exert traction. Compare **balanced suspension, hyperextension suspension, lower extremity suspension.**

upper motor neuron paralysis, an injury to or lesion in the brain or spinal cord that damages cell bodies or axons of the upper motor neurons. Clinical signs include increased muscle tone and spasticity of the muscles involved, hyperactive deep tendon reflexes, diminished or absent superficial reflexes, the presence of pathological reflexes, and no local twitching of muscle groups. Compare **lower motor neuron paralysis.**

upper respiratory infection. See **respiratory tract infection.**

upper respiratory tract, one of the two divisions of the respiratory system. The upper respiratory tract consists of the nose, the nasal cavity, the ethmoidal air cells, the frontal sinuses, the sphenoidal sinuses, the maxillary sinus, the larynx, and the trachea. The upper respiratory tract moves air to and from the lungs and filters, moistens, and warms the air. Infection and irritation of the upper tract are common and often spread to the lower respiratory tract, where they may cause serious complications. See also **larynx, nose, trachea.** Compare **lower respiratory tract.**

–uracil, a combining form for uracil derivatives used as anticancer drugs and to counteract the effect of thyroid hormone.

urate /yŏor'āt/, any salt of uric acid, as sodium urate. Urates are found in the urine, blood, and tophi or calcareous deposits in tissues. They may also be deposited as crystals in body joints. See also **gout, uric acid.**

urban typhus. See **murine typhus.**

urea /yŏorē'ə/, the main nitrogen part of urine made from protein breakdown.

urea, a diuretic given to reduce intracranial and intraocular fluid pressure, it is used topically as a keratolytic agent.

★CAUTION: Severely impaired kidney function, active intracranial bleeding, marked dehydration, or liver damage prohibits its systemic use.

★ADVERSE EFFECTS: Among the more serious side effects are pain and necrosis at the site of injection, headache, stomach and intestinal disturbances, and dizziness. There are no known severe effects of topical use.

Ureaplasma urealyticum, a sexually spread microorganism often found in the urogenital systems of men and women in whom infection is asymptomatic. Neonatal death, prematurity, and perinatal morbidity are statistically associated with colonization of the surface of the placenta by *Ureaplasma urealyticum.* How the negative effects on pregnancy occur is not known. There is no characteristic lesion in the fetus or newborn.

Urecholine, a trademark for a cholinergic (bethanechol chloride).

uremia /yŏorē'mē·ə/, the presence of excessive amounts of urea and other nitrogenous waste products in the blood, as occurs in renal failure. Also called **azotemia.** See also **chronic glomerulonephritis, subacute glomerulonephritis.**

uremic frost, a pale, frostlike deposit of white crystals on the skin caused by kidney failure and uremia. Urea compounds and other waste products of metabolism that cannot be excreted by the kidneys into the urine are excreted through capillaries into the skin, where they collect on the surface.

uremic gingivitis. See **nephritic gingivitis.**

ureter /yŏorē'tər/, one of a pair of tubes that carry the urine from the kidney into the bladder. The ureter enters the bladder through an oblique tunnel that works as a valve to stop the backflow of urine into the ureter when the bladder contracts. **–ureteral** /yŏorē'tərəl/, *adj.*

ureteral dysfunction, a disturbance of the normal flow of urine through a ureter, caused by dysfunction of ureteral motor nerves. See also **megaloureter.**

ureteritis /yŏorē'tərī'tis/, an inflammatory condition of a ureter caused by infection or by irritation of a stone.

ureterocele /yŏorē'tərōsēl'/, a prolapse of the terminal portion of the ureter into the bladder. The condition may block the flow of urine and lead to hydronephrosis and loss of renal function. Cystoscopy and pyelography reveal the prolapsed ureter. Surgery is done to prevent permanent damage to the kidney. Compare **cystocele.**

ureterography, the radiological imaging of a ureter. The examination may involve injection of a radiopaque medium through a urinary catheter or by injection of a contrast medium that permits the filtering of the substance through the kidneys to the ureters.

ureterosigmoidostomy, surgery in which a ureter is implanted in the sigmoid flexure of the intestinal tract.

ureterotomy, a cut into a ureter.

urethra /yŏorē'thrə/, a small, tubular structure

that drains urine from the bladder. In men, the urethra serves as a passage for semen during ejaculation, as well as a canal for urine during voiding. See also **ureter.**

urethral /yōōrē′thrəl/, of or pertaining to the urethra.

urethral papilla. See **papilla.**

urethral sphincter, the voluntary muscle at the neck of the bladder that relaxes to allow urination.

urethritis /yōōr′ithrī′tis/, an inflammatory state of the urethra, often caused by infection in the bladder or kidneys. Drugs, as a sulfonamide or other antibacterial, a urinary antiseptic, and an analgesic, are often given once the causative organism is identified by culture of a urine specimen. See also **nongonococcal urethritis.**

urethrocele /yōōrē′thrəsēl′/, (in women) a herniation of the urethra. It is marked by a protrusion of a segment of the urethra and the connective tissue surrounding it into the anterior wall of the vagina. The herniation may be slight and high in the vagina and only palpable on digital examination when the patient strains downward. But it may be large and low in the anterior wall with visible bulging at the vaginal entrance. A large cystocele may cause voiding difficulty, and cause some incontinence, urinary tract infection, and dyspareunia. The condition may be congenital or acquired, secondary to obesity and poor muscle tone. Surgery is often done.

urethrography, the radiological examination of the urethra after the injection of a radiopaque agent into the urethra, usually through a catheter. It may be done as a part of a radiological examination of the lower urinary tract.

urethroplasty /yōōrē′thrəplas′tē/, a surgical procedure for the repair of a urethra, as to correct an abnormal exit of urine.

Urex, a trademark for an antibacterial (methenamine hippurate).

urgency, feeling the need to urinate immediately.

uric acid, a product of the metabolism of protein present in the blood and excreted in the urine. See also **gout, kidney, liver, purine, urine.**

uricaciduria /yōōr′ikas′idōōr′ē·ə/, a more-than-normal amount of uric acid in the urine, often linked to urinary calculi or gout.

uricosuric drugs, drugs given to relieve the pain of gout or to increase the elimination of uric acid.

–uridine, a combining form for uridine derivatives used as agents against viruses and cancer.

urinal, a plastic or metal receptacle for collecting urine.

urinalysis, a physical, microscopic, or chemical examination of urine. The specimen is physically examined for color, turbidity, specific-gravity, and pH. Then it is spun in a centrifuge to allow collection of a small amount of sediment that is examined microscopically for blood cells, casts, crystals, pus, and bacteria. Chemical analysis may be done to identify and quantify any of a large number of substances, most often for ketones, sugar, protein, and blood.

urinary, of or referring to urine or to the formation of urine.

urinary bladder, the muscular membranous sac in the pelvis that stores urine for discharge through the urethra. Urine reaches this reservoir from the kidneys via the ureters.

urinary calculus, a calculus formed in the urinary tract. Calculi may be large enough to block the flow of urine or small enough to be passed with the urine. Kinds of urinary calculi are **renal calculus and vesicle calculus.** See also **calculus.**

urinary frequency, a greater-than-normal frequency of the urge to void without an increase in the total daily volume of urine. The state is a sign of inflammation in the bladder or urethra or of diminished bladder capacity or other structural abnormalities. Burning and urgency with increased frequency often mark an infection of the urinary tract. Infection needs precise diagnosis and specific antibacterial drugs; structural abnormality may require surgery. See also **cystitis, cystocele.**

urinary hesitancy, a decrease in the force of the stream of urine, often with difficulty in starting the flow. Hesitancy is usually the result of a blockage or stricture between the bladder and the urethral opening; in men it may indicate a swelling of the prostate gland, in women, stenosis of the urethral opening. Cold, stress, dehydration, and various neurogenic and psychogenic factors are common causes of this condition.

urinary incontinence, involuntary passage of urine, with the failure of voluntary control over bladder and urethral sphincters. Some causes are neurogenic bladder dysfunction stemming from lesions of the brain and spinal cord, a neoplasm of calculus in the bladder, multiple sclerosis, obstruction of the lower urinary tract, trauma, aging, and multiparity in women. In children, incontinence may be psychogenic or the result of allergy. Treatment with drugs, surgery, or psychotherapy (depending on the underlying cause) is often effective.

urinary infection. See **urinary tract infection.**

urinary output, the total volume of urine excreted daily. Various metabolic and renal diseases may change the normal urinary output. See also **anuria, oliguria, polyuria.**

urinary retention, the retention of urine in the bladder. It is often caused by a temporary loss of muscle function.

urinary system assessment, an examination in which the kidneys, bladder, ureters, and urethra are evaluated. A check is made of disorders in the urinary system. The patient is asked about frequency or burning on urination, dribbling, a decreased urinary stream, nocturia, stress incontinence, headache, back pain, or if increased thirst has occurred. The color, odor, and amount of urine voided are checked. The patient's vital signs, any distention of the bladder, state of the skin, neurological changes, and the location, duration, and nature of pain, and the presence of bladder spasms are recorded. It is determined whether the patient has hypertension, diabetes, venereal disease, vaginal or urethral drainage or discharge, or a history of cystitis, pyelonephritis, kidney stones, prostatectomy, renal surgery, a kidney transplant, or a venereal infection. The patient's sexual activity, use of coffee, tea, cola beverages, alcohol, perfumed soaps, feminine hygiene sprays, drugs, and habit of bathing in a tub or shower are ascertained. A family history of polycystic kidney disease, hypertension, diabetes, or cancer is noted, with laboratory tests of the patient's urine and serum creatinine. Diagnostic tests may include cystoscopy, excretory and intravenous urography, renal angiography, and x-ray films of the kidneys, ureters, and bladder.

urinary tract, all organs and ducts involved in the release and elimination of urine.

urinary tract infection (UTI), an infection of the urinary tract. Most of these infections are caused by gram-negative bacteria, most commonly *Escherichia coli* or species of *Klebsiella, Proteus, Pseudomonas,* or *Enterobacter.* The state is more common in women than in men and may lack symptoms. Urinary tract infection is often marked by urinary frequency, burning, pain with voiding, and, if the infection is severe, visible blood and pus in the urine. Diagnosis of the cause and the location of the infection is made by microscopic examination of a urine specimen, by physical examination of the patient, by bacteriological culture of a specimen of urine, and, if necessary, by various radiological techniques or by cystoscopy. Treatment includes antibacterial, analgesic, and urinary antiseptic drugs. Kinds of urinary tract infections include **cystitis, pyelonephritis, and urethritis.**

urination, the act of passing urine. Also called **micturition.**

urine, the fluid secreted by the kidneys, transported by the ureters, stored in the bladder, and voided through the urethra. Normal urine is clear, straw-colored, slightly acid, and is odorless. It contains water, urea, sodium chloride and potassium chloride, phosphates, uric acid, organic salts, and the pigment uro bilin. Abnormal constituents indicating disease include ketone bodies, protein, bacteria, blood, glucose, pus, and certain crystals. See also **bacteriuria, glycosuria, hematuria, ketoaciduria, proteinuria.**

urinoma /yŏŏr'inō'mə/, *pl.* **urinoma, urinomatas,** a cyst filled with urine.

Urised, a trademark for a urinary fixed-combination drug with an antibacterial (methenamine), an analgesic (phenyl salicylate), anticholinergics (atropine sulfate and hyoscyamine), an antifungal (benzoic acid), and an antiseptic (methylene blue).

Urispas, a trademark for a smooth muscle relaxant (flavoxate hydrochloride).

Urobiotic, a trademark for a urinary drug with antibacterials (oxytetracycline hydrochloride and sulfamethizole) and an analgesic (phenazopyridine hydrochloride).

urogenital /yŏŏr'ōjen'itəl/, of or referring to the urinary and the reproductive systems. Also called **genitourinary.**

urogenital system, the urinary and genital organs and the structures that develop in the fetus to form the kidneys, the ureters, the bladder, the urethra, and the genital structures of the male and female. In women these are the ovaries, the uterine tubes, the uterus, the clitoris, and the vagina. In men these are the testes, the seminal vesicles, the seminal ducts, the prostate, and the penis. Also called **genitourinary system.** See also the **Color Atlas of Human Anatomy.**

urogram /yŏŏr'əgram'/, an x-ray film of the urinary tract. See also **pyelogram.**

urography /yŏŏrog'rəfē/, x-ray techniques used to check the urinary system. A radiopaque substance is injected, and x-ray films are taken as the substance is passed through or excreted from the system. Some kinds of urography are **cystoscopic urography, intravenous pyelography, and retrograde pyelography.**

urokinase /yŏŏr'əkī'nās/, an enzyme, produced in the kidney and found in urine, that is a potent plasminogen activator of the fibrinolytic system. A pharmaceutical preparation of urokinase is given in the veins to treat pulmonary embolism.

urolagnia /yŏŏr'əlag'nē·ə/, sexual stimulation gained from acts involving urine, as watching people urinate or a desire to be urinated on.

urolithiasis. See **urinary calculus.**

urologist, a licensed physician who has completed an approved residency program, who specializes in urology.

urology, the branch of medicine concerned with the anatomy and physiology, disorders, and the care of the urinary tract in men and women and of the male genital tract.

uromelus. See **sympus monopus.**

uropathy /yŏŏrop'əthē/, any disease or abnormal state of the urinary tract. **–uropathic,** *adj.*

uroporphyria /yŏŏr'ōpôrfir'ē·ə/, a rare, genetic disease marked by too-much release of uroporphyrin in the urine, blistering dermatitis, photosensitivity, splenomegaly, and hemolytic anemia. Steroid ointments may help the skin lesions; splenomegaly may be needed to aid the hemolytic anemia. Most patients die from hematological complications before middle age. See also **porphyria.**

uroporphyrin /yo͞or′ōpôr′firin/, a porphyrin normally excreted in the urine in small amounts. See also **uroporphyria.**

uroradiology, the study of the urinary tract using x-rays.

urostomy /yo͞oros′təmē/, the diversion of urine away from a diseased or defective bladder through a surgically created opening (stoma) in the skin.

ursodeoxycholic acid, a secondary bile salt. It is used to dissolve gallstones. See also **chenodeoxycholic acid.**

urticaria /ur′tiker′ē·ə/, a skin eruption marked by transient wheals of varying shapes and sizes with clear margins and pale centers, caused by capillary dilation. The capillary dilation is caused by vasoactive mediators, including histamine, kinin, and the reactive substance of anaphylaxis found with antigen-antibody reaction. Treatment includes antihistamines and removal of the stimulus or allergen. Cholinergic urticaria appears as wheals surrounded by a large axon flare. It may be caused by drugs, food, insect bites, inhalants, emotional stress, exposure to heat or cold, and exercise. Also called **hives.** See also **angioneurotic edema.** –**urticarial,** *adj.*

urticaria pigmentosa, a rare form of mastocytosis marked by pigmented skin lesions that often begin in infancy and become urticarial on irritation. Duration of the state is unpredictable. Prognosis is good. Treatment is symptomatic and often includes antihistamines to stop itching.

urushiol /əro͞o′shē·ôl/, a toxic resin in the sap of certain plants of the genus *Rhus,* as poison ivy, poison oak, and poison sumac, that produces allergic contact dermatitis in many people.

USAN /yo͞o′san, yo͞o′es′ā′en′/, abbreviation for *United States Adopted Names,* a list of approved drugs.

use effectiveness, (of a contraceptive method) the actual effectiveness of a drug, device, or method to prevent pregnancy. Inconsistent use and human error often reduce the theoretical effectiveness of a method of contraception. Compare **theoretical effectiveness.**

useful radiation, the portion of direct radiation that is permitted to pass from an x-ray tube housing through the tube head port, aperture, or collimator. Also called **useful beam.**

user documentation. See **documentation.**

use test, a way to find offending allergens in foods, cosmetics, or fabrics by cutting out and adding specific items of the life-style of the patient. Allergic reactions to the use test may be right away or spread over a long time. Some patients having the test become frustrated and

discouraged, needing encouragement to keep looking for the sources of their allergies by this method. See also **allergy testing.**

USPHS, abbreviation for **United States Public Health Service.**

uta /yo͞o′tə/, a mild form of American leishmaniasis, found in the Andes of Peru and Argentina, caused by *Leishmania peruana.* The lesions are small and tend to be on the exposed surfaces of the skin. They often heal on their own within 1 year. The disease has been slowly disappearing because of the increased use of insecticides.

uterine anteflexion, an abnormal position of the uterus in which the uterine body is bent forward on itself at the juncture of the isthmus of the uterine cervix and the lower uterine segment.

uterine anteversion, a position of the uterus in which the body of the uterus is directed ventrally. Mild degrees of anteversion are of no significance. On speculum examination of the vagina, acute anteversion of the uterus may be deduced from the location of the cervix in the posterior of the vaginal vault. Slight anteversion is the most common position of the uterus; on speculum examination the cervix is in the middle of the top of the vaginal vault, and it protrudes directly downward toward the vaginal orifice.

uterine bruit, a sound made by blood passing through the vessels of the pregnant uterus. The sounds are in rhythm with the fetal heart beat.

uterine cancer, any cancer of the uterus. It may be cervical cancer affecting the cervix or endometrial cancer affecting the lining of the body of the uterus. See also **cervical cancer, endometrial cancer.**

uterine inertia, abnormal relaxation of the uterus during labor, stopping the progress of the baby, or after childbirth, causing bleeding in the uterus.

uterine ischemia, a decreasing or ineffective blood supply to the uterus.

uterine prolapse, the falling, sinking, or sliding of the uterus from its normal location in the body.

uterine retroflexion, a position of the uterus in which the body of the uterus is bent backward on itself at the isthmus of the cervix and the lower uterine segment. It has no significance. It does not prevent conception or adversely affect pregnancy. On speculum examination of the vagina, the condition may be deduced by the location of the cervix in the anterior of the vaginal vault.

uterine retroversion, a position of the uterus in which the body of the uterus is directed away from the midline, toward the back. Mild degrees of retroversion are common and have no significance. Severe retroversion may be found with vague persistent pelvic discomfort and dyspareunia and may prevent the fitting of a contraceptive diaphragm. Compare **uterine anteversion.** See also **uterine retroflexion.**

uterine souffle, a soft, blowing sound made by the blood in the arteries of a pregnant uterus. The sound is in rhythm with the woman's pulse.

uterine tenaculum. See **tenaculum.**

uterine tetany, a condition in which contractions of the uterus last longer than normal.

uterine tube. See **fallopian tube.**

uteritis. See **metritis.**

uteroglobulin. See **blastokinin.**

uteroovarian varicocele, a swelling of the veins of the female pelvis. Compare **ovarian varicocele, varicocele.**

uteroplacental apoplexy. See **Couvelaire uterus.**

uterovesical. See **vesicouterine.**

uterus /yōō'tərəs/, the hollow, pear-shaped inner female organ of reproduction in which the fertilized ovum is implanted and the fetus develops, and from which the decidua of menses flows. The uterus is composed of three layers: the endometrium, the myometrium, and the parametrium. The endometrium lines the uterus and becomes thicker and more vascular in pregnancy and during the second half of the menstrual cycle under the influence of the hormone progesterone. The myometrium is the muscular layer of the organ. Its muscle fibers wrap around the uterus. After childbirth the fibers contract, creating natural ligatures that stop the flow of blood from the large blood vessels supplying the placenta. The parame-

trium is the outermost layer of the uterus. During pregnancy it becomes many times its usual size, almost entirely by cellular hypertrophy. Few new cells develop. The uterus has two parts: a body and a cervix. The walls of the body touch, unless the woman is pregnant. The cervix has a vaginal portion protruding into the vagina, and a supravaginal portion at the juncture of the lower uterine segment.

uterus masculinis. See **prostatic utricle.**

utilization review (UR), an assessment of the need for and economy of an admission to a health-care facility or a continued hospitalization. The length of the hospital stay is compared with the average length of stay for similar diagnoses.

uvea /yōō'vē·ə/, the fiberlike place under the sclera that includes the iris, the ciliary body, and the choroid of the eye. Also called **tunica vasculosa bulbi, uveal tract.** –**uveal,** *adj.*

uveitis /yōō'vē·ī'tis/, swelling of the uveal tract of the eye. It may be marked by an irregularly shaped pupil, inflammation around the cornea, pus in the anterior chamber, opaque deposits on the cornea, pain, and tearing. Causes include allergy, infection, trauma, diabetes, collagen disease, and skin diseases. A major complication may be glaucoma. See also **chorioretinitis, choroiditis, iritis.**

uvula /yōō'vyōōlə/, *pl.* **uvulae,** the small, coneshaped process suspended in the mouth from the middle of the back edge of the soft palate. –**uvular,** *adj.*

uvulitis /yōō'vyəlī'tis/, inflammation of the uvula. Common causes are allergy and infection.

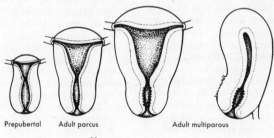

Prepubertal   Adult parcus   Adult multiparous

Uterus

V

v, abbreviation for *vein.*

V, symbol for **vanadium.**

VAC, an anticancer drug combination of vincristine, dactinomycin, and cyclophosphamide.

vaccination, any injection of weakened bacteria given to protect against or to reduce the effects of related infectious diseases. The first vaccinations in history were given to protect against smallpox. Vaccinations are now available to protect against many diseases, as typhoid, measles, and mumps. **–vaccinate,** *v.*

vaccine /vaksēn', vak'sēn, -sin/, a liquid of weakened or dead germs given either by mouth, by injection into the muscle or under the skin, or into a muscle to protect against infectious disease. Some vaccines are grown in bird eggs, rabbit brains, or monkey kidneys, and the germs are killed or weakened with chemicals. Vaccines may be used one at a time or in combinations. Compare **antiserum.**

-vaccine, a combining form meaning a 'liquid containing germs for protection against disease.'

vaccinia /vaksin'ē·ə/, an infectious disease of cattle caused by a virus that may be given to humans by direct contact or by deliberate injection as a protection against smallpox. A small bump develops at the place of infection. This is followed by a sick feeling and a fever that lasts for several days. After 2 weeks, the small bump forms a scab that drops off after a while, leaving a scar. The virus may be spread by scratching. Persons with eczema or other preexisting skin disease may develop widespread vaccinia. Rarely, a severe encephalitis follows vaccinia. Also called **cowpox.** Compare **smallpox.** See also **vaccination.**

vacuole /vak'yōō·ōl/, **1.** a clear or fluid-filled space within a cell, as when a drop of water is taken into the cell. **2.** a small space in the body enclosed by a membrane, usually containing fat or other matter. **–vacuolar, vacuolated,** *adj.*

Vacu-tainer tube, a glass tube with a rubber stopper in which air can be removed to create a vacuum.

vacuum aspiration, a method of abortion in which the fetus and placenta are removed by suction to end pregnancy, up to the 14th week. Using local or light general anesthesia, the cervix is widened and the uterus is emptied with suction. After the operation, temperature and blood pressure should be checked for signs of blood loss. Also called **suction curettage.** Compare **dilatation and curettage.** See also **therapeutic abortion.**

vagal /vā'gəl/, of or concerning the vagus nerve.

vagina, the part of the female genitals that forms a canal from the opening through the passageway to the cervix. It is behind the bladder and in front of the rectum. In the adult woman the front wall of the vagina is about 7 cm long and the back wall is about 9 cm long. The vagina is a canal in which the walls usually touch. The vagina widens from the entrance upward and narrows toward the top, forming a curved vault around the protruding cervix. The vagina is lined with mucous membranes covering a layer of tissue and muscle. The muscles of the vagina consist of a strong, lengthwise layer and an inner circular layer.

vagina bulbi. See **fascia bulbi.**

vaginal bleeding, a problem in which blood flows from the vagina at other times than during menstruation. It may be caused by problems of the uterus or cervix; by an abnormal pregnancy; by glandular problems; by abnormalities of one or both ovaries or one or both fallopian tubes; or by an abnormality of the vagina. The following terms are commonly used in approximating the amount of vaginal bleeding: **heavy vaginal bleeding,** which is greater than heaviest normal menstrual flow; **moderate vaginal bleeding,** which is equal to heaviest normal menstrual flow; **light vaginal bleeding,** which is less than heaviest normal menstrual flow; **vaginal staining,** which is a very light flow of blood barely requiring the use of a sanitary napkin or tampon; **vaginal spotting,** which is the passage of a few drops of blood; **bloody show,** which is an episode of light vaginal bleeding as often occurs in early labor, during labor, and, particularly, at the time of complete widening of the cervix at the end of the first stage of labor.

vaginal cancer, a cancer of the vagina occurring rarely as a first new growth. More often it accompanies vulvar, cervical, endometrial, or ovarian cancer. This cancer occurs in young women exposed in the uterus to diethylstilbestrol, given their mothers to prevent abortion, but most primary vaginal cancers arise in white women over 50 years of age. Symptoms are vaginal bleeding in women over 50 years of age, the discharge of pus, pain, and painful or difficult urination. Depending on the patient's age and condition and place and size of the tumor, treatment may be by radiation or by removal of the vagina or the uterus. Various drugs may be used, but chemotherapy is not usually effective.

vaginal discharge, any discharge from the vagina. A clear or pearly-white discharge is normal. During the fertile reproductive years the amount varies greatly from woman to woman, and the amount and nature vary in each woman at different times in her cycle. Before menarche and after menopause, the quantity of discharge is usually less than during the reproductive years. The discharge is largely made of fluids from the endocervical glands. Infections of the vagina and cervix often cause an increase in the discharge, which may then have a foul odor and cause itching of the pelvic area and genitals.

vaginal fornix, a recess in the upper part of the vagina caused by the protrusion of the cervix into the vagina.

vaginal instillation of medication, the application of a medicated cream, a suppository, or a gel into the vagina, usually done to treat a local infection of the vagina or cervix. The woman voids before the treatment. She then lies back. The nurse, physician, or patient sometimes, wearing gloves, separates the labia majora, exposing the vaginal opening. The medication is instilled gently. A cream or gel is squeezed into an applicator from a tube and is then placed in the vagina by depressing the plunger of the applicator while withdrawing the device from the vagina. A tablet or suppository is usually placed in the vagina near the cervix with another style of applicator that holds the medication in a slotted receptacle at its tip. The woman remains lying down after the instillation to prevent escape of the medication from the vagina. Most applicators may be washed after each instillation and reused for the same woman for the next dose. They are thrown away after a course of treatment.

vaginal jelly, a jellylike product that prevents conception by killing sperm on contact. It is usually used along with a contraceptive diaphragm or cervical cap. Some drugs are also supplied in the form of a vaginal jelly.

vaginal sponge, a plastic sponge that contains a sperm-killing chemical. The sponge is shaped like a mushroom and fits into the upper vagina. It is believed to work in three ways: by killing sperm, by absorbing semen, and by blocking the cervical opening. The sponge can be kept in place to provide protection for 24 hours. The vaginal sponge is believed to be about as effective as other vaginal methods.

vaginal spotting, vaginal staining. See also **vaginal bleeding.**

vaginismus /vaj′iniz′məs/, a mental and physical reaction of women, marked by a strong tightening of the muscles in the pelvic area and the vagina. It is caused by fear of a painful entry before intercourse or a pelvic examination. Vaginismus is considered abnormal if it occurs in the absence of genital sores and if it conflicts with a woman's desire to participate in intercourse or to permit examination, but it may be a normal response if painful genital conditions exist or if forcible or premature intercourse is expected. Abnormal vaginismus is not common. This condition can be eased through education and counseling that improve sexual self-awareness. In some cases, the condition is a symptom of serious mental illness and requires formal psychiatric testing and treatment. Gender identity conflict, a history of rape or incest, or strong denial of sexuality in childhood and adolescence are factors that are often linked to vaginismus. See also **dyspareunia.**

vaginitis /vaj′inī′tis/, a swelling of the vaginal tissues, as trichomonas vaginitis.

vagino-, a combining form meaning 'referring to the vagina.'

vaginography /vaj′inog′rəfē/, the examination of the vagina by means of x-ray tests after the injection of substances that show up well on x-ray films after injection of a radiopaque contrast medium.

Vagisec, a trademark for a vaginal douche used to treat trichomoniasis.

vagotomy /văgot′əmē/, the cutting of certain branches of the vagus nerve, done with stomach surgery, to reduce the amount of gastric acid released and to lessen the chance of a return of a gastric ulcer. With the patient under general anesthesia, a gastrectomy is done and the branches of the vagus nerve are cut out. Because the movement of the stomach will be lessened, the opening into the intestines from the stomach is enlarged or a new passage between the stomach and small intestine is made to assure proper emptying of the stomach. See also **anastomosis, gastrectomy, gastric ulcer, pyloroplasty, vagus nerve.**

vagotonus /vā′gətō′nəs/, an abnormal increase in the activity of the vagus nerve, especially abnormal slowness of the heart beat, causing faintness and a sudden loss of strength. Vagotonus may occur in clearing out the throat of a newborn infant as an instrument is accidently pressed on the back of the throat, stimulating the nerve. It also occurs in some women after surgery or simple manipulation of the cervix.

vagovagal reflex /vā′gōvā′gəl/, a stimulation of the vagus nerve by reflex in which irritation of the throat (larynx or the trachea) results in slowing of the pulse rate.

vagueness, a communication pattern in which pronouns are too general and relationships between ideas are not clear, leading to confusion and misunderstanding.

vagus nerve /vā′gəs/, either of the longest pair of cranial nerves essential for speech, swallowing, and the sensibilities and functions of many parts of the body. The vagus nerves have 13 main branches, connecting to four areas in the brain. Also called **nervus vagus, pneumogastric nerve, tenth cranial nerve.**

valeric acid /vəler′ik/, an acid with a disagreeable odor found in the roots of the garden heliotrope *(Valeriana officinalis)*. Commercially prepared, it is used to make perfumes, flavors, lubricants, and certain drugs.

valgus /val'gəs/, an abnormal position in which a part of a limb is bent or twisted outward, away from the middle of the body, as the heel of the foot in **talipes valgus.** Compare **varus.** See also **hallux valgus.**

validation, an agreement of the listener with certain points of the patient's communication.

validity, (in research) the extent to which a test measurement or other device measures what it is intended to measure. Kinds of validity include **content validity, current validity, construct validity, face validity,** and **predictive validity.**

valine (Val), an essential amino acid needed for optimal growth in infants and for nitrogen balance in adults. See also **amino acid, maple syrup urine disease, protein.**

Valisone, a trademark for a drug that raises the blood sugar (betamethasone valerate).

Valium, a trademark for a tranquilizer (diazepam), used to assist in achieving anesthesia.

vallecula /vəlek'yōōlə/, **1.** any groove or furrow on the surface of an organ or structure. **2.** *See* **vallecula epiglottica. –vallecular,** *adj.*

vallecula epiglottica, a furrow between the three folds of tissue at the base of the tongue on each side of the back of the throat. Also called *(informal)* **vallecula.**

vallecular dysphagia, difficulty or pain on swallowing caused by swelling of the vallecula epiglottica. Compare **contractile ring dysphagia, dysphagia lusoria.**

valley fever. See **coccidioidomycosis.**

Valmid, a trademark for a sedative (ethinamate).

Valpin, a trademark for an anticholinergic (anisotropine).

valproic acid, a drug used to stop or prevent convulsions. It is given to prevent certain types of seizure activity, particularly complex absence and petit mal seizures.

★CAUTION: It is not recommended for use during pregnancy or lactation. Known allergy to this drug prohibits its use.

★ADVERSE EFFECTS: Among the more severe side effects are harm to the blood and liver. Stomach and intestinal upset are common, and hair loss, rash, headache, and insomnia may also occur.

Valsalva's maneuver /valsal'vəs/, any forced effort of the breath against a closed throat as when a person holds the breath and tightens the muscles while making a strong effort to move a heavy object or to change position in bed. Most healthy people perform Valsalva's maneuvers during normal daily activities without any ill effects; but such efforts are dangerous for many patients with diseases of the heart and blood vessels. Constipation increases the risk of heart attack in such patients, especially if they perform Valsalva's maneuver in trying to bear down while moving their bowels. Orthopedic patients often use Valsalva's maneuver in changing their position in bed with the aid of an overhead trapeze bar. Patients who may be harmed by performing Valsalva's maneuver are commonly instructed to exhale instead of holding their breath when they move. The exhalation decreases the risk of heart attack.

Valsalva's test, a method for proving that the eustachian tubes are wide open. With mouth and nose kept tightly closed, the patient breathes out very forcefully; if the eustachian tubes are open, air will enter into the middle ear cavities and the patient will hear a popping sound. See also **Valsalva's maneuver.**

value, a personal belief about the worth of a given idea or behavior.

value clarification, a method for discovering one's own values by assessing, exploring, and determining what those personal values are and how they affect one's decisions.

valve, a structure, either natural or artificial, in a passage that opens to allow fluid to flow in one direction, but closes to prevent it from flowing back in the other direction. Valves in veins are membranous folds that prevent the backflow of blood. **–valvular,** *adj.*

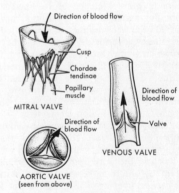

Direction of blood flow

Cusp

Chordae tendinae

Papillary muscle

MITRAL VALVE

Direction of blood flow

AORTIC VALVE (seen from above)

Direction of blood flow

Valve

VENOUS VALVE

Valves

-valve, a combining form meaning 'a thing that controls the flow of.'

valve of Kerkring. See **circular fold.**

valve of lymphatics, one of the tiny half-moon-shaped structures in the vessels and trunks of the lymphatic system that help regulate the flow of lymph and prevent venous blood from entering the system. Usually, two valves of equal size are found opposite each other. Most are found near the lymph nodes, and there are more in the neck and arms than in the legs. See also **lymphatic system.**

valvotomy /valvot'əmē/, the cutting into a valve, especially one in the heart, to correct a defect and allow the valve to open and close properly. Before surgery a catheter is inserted into the heart through a vein in the arm. With the patient under general anesthesia, the damaged valve is repaired, if possible, or removed and an artificial valve put in its place. Special problems of valve replacement include broken stitches, blockages, leaking within the heart, infection, and blood clots.

valvular heart disease, a flaw in a heart valve, either present from birth or acquired later, marked by a narrowing of the vessels and blocked blood flow or by damage to the valve and a backward blood flow. This may be caused by defects present at birth, bacterial endocarditis, syphilis, or, most frequently, rheumatic fever. Episodes of rheumatic fever often affect heart valves, causing them to remain open or causing the valves to become stiff and constricted. Lessened action of the valves can result in changes in blood pressure and circulation. It may lead to unsteady heart-beat, heart failure, and heart attack. Weakness, loss of appetite, blood clots and fluid in the lungs often accompany valvular heart disease. In moderate or severe **aortic stenosis,** the pulse is weakened. The patient may experience pain or choking that comes and goes as well as weakness. Other symptoms are difficult breathing, profuse sweating, flushed skin, a pounding pulse in the neck. The patient with **mitral stenosis** tires easily, is short of breath on exertion, may have attacks of difficult breathing at night, and may spit up blood and develop blood clots. Mitral regurgitation is typified by difficult breathing, fatigue, intolerance of exercise, and heart palpitation. **Tricuspid stenosis** is relatively uncommon, is usually linked to damage in other valves resulting from rheumatic fever, and in rare cases is caused by tumor-related heart disease or by diseases of the heart muscles. Typical signs include engorged neck veins, enlargement of the liver and retention of fluids. The valve in the artery leading to the lungs is affected by rheumatic fever much less frequently than other heart valves. **Pulmonic stenosis** may cause some problems, but usually will not lead to a heart attack. Valvular heart disease is usually treated with a variety of drugs, but surgery may be necessary in very serious cases. The patient having heart valve repair or replacement may be hospitalized for from 4 to 6 weeks and requires the care, both before and after the operation, typical of any open-heart surgery.

valvular stenosis, a narrowing of the valves of the heart. The condition may be present at birth, or it may be caused by some disease. See also **aortic stenosis, congenital cardiac anomaly, mitral valve stenosis, pulmonic stenosis.**

valvulitis /val'vyŏŏlī'tis/, a swelling of a valve, especially a heart valve. Changes caused by swelling in the valves of the heart are caused most commonly by rheumatic fever and less often by bacterial endocarditis and syphilis. Infected valves wear out, or they become stiff and hard, resulting in stenosis and blocked blood flow.

VAMP /vamp/, abbreviation for a combination drug program, used in the treatment of cancer, containing three drugs to prevent new cancer cells from forming (vincristine sulfate, methotrexate, and mercaptopurine) and a drug to raise the blood sugar (prednisone).

vanadium (V), a grayish, metallic element. Absorption of vanadium results in a condition called **vanadiumism,** marked by anemia, conjunctivitis, pneumonitis, and irritation of the throat and lungs.

van Bogaert's disease /vanbō'gərts/, a rare disorder of lipid metabolism occurring in members of the same family in which the substance cholestanol is deposited in the nervous system, blood, and connective tissue. Patients with it suffer many physical and mental problems. No effective treatment has been found. Also called **cerebrotendinous xanthomatosis.**

Vanceril, a trademark for a drug to raise blood sugar (beclomethasone dipropionate), used for mouth-breathing therapy in asthma.

Vancocin Hydrochloride, a trademark for a drug that kills bacteria (vancomycin hydrochloride).

vancomycin, an antibiotic used to treat infections, particularly staphylococcal infections resistant to other antibiotics.
★CAUTION: Use at the same time as neurotoxical, nephrotoxical, or ototoxical drugs or known allergy to this drug prohibits its use.
★ADVERSE EFFECTS: Among the more serious side effects are allergic reactions, dizziness, and a ringing or roaring in the ears (tinnitus).

van den Bergh's test /van'dənburgs'/, a test for the presence of bilirubin in the blood serum. Blood is obtained from a patient who has fasted overnight.

vanillylmandelic acid (VMA) /va'nililmandel'ik/, a substance normally found in the urine. A greater-than-normal amount of VMA is a sign of a pheochromocytoma and neuroblastomas.

Vanoxide, a trademark for a drug with an antibacterial (benzoyl peroxide) and a keratolytic drying agent (chlorhydroxyquinoline).

Vaponefrin, a trademark for an adrenalinelike substance (epinephrine hydrochloride), used to aid in clearing the lungs.

vapor bath, the exposure of the body to vapor, as steam.

variable interval (VI) reinforcement, reinforcement that is provided after a varying amount of time has passed. By varying the amount of time between reinforcements, the recipient does not know when it will arrive and is more likely to respond in the desired manner at all times.

variable ratio (VR) reinforcement, reinforcement that is provided after a varying number of responses. By varying the number of required responses, the recipient does not know when reinforcement will be provided and is more likely to respond in the desired manner at all times.

varicella.   See **chickenpox.**

varicella zoster virus (VZV), a member of the herpesvirus family, which causes chickenpox (varicella) and shingles (herpes zoster). The virus is very contagious and may be spread by direct contact or droplets. Dried crusts of skin sores do not contain active virus. Herpes zoster is made by latent varicella virus, usually several years after the first infection. There is no simple test for measuring antibodies to this virus; however, zoster immune globulin taken from recovering zoster patients, if injected within 3 days of exposure, will prevent varicella in at-risk children. See also **chickenpox, herpesvirus hominus, herpes zoster.**

varicelliform /ver'isel'ifôrm/, resembling the rash of chickenpox.

varicocele /ver'əkōsēl'/, a widening of the pampiniform venous complex of the spermatic cord. The varicocele forms a soft, elastic swelling that can cause pain. It is most common in men between 15 and 25 years of age and affects the left sperm cord more often than the right. It is usually more noticeable and painful in the standing position. Compare **ovarian varicocele, uteroovarian varicocele.**

varicose /ver'əkōs/, **1.** (of a vein) showing varicosis, or a varicosity. **2.** abnormally and permanently distended, as the bulging veins in some individuals.

varicose aneurysm, a blood-filled, saclike projection that connects an artery and one or several veins and that is formed from a limited widening of the adjoining vessels.

varicose ulcer.   See **stasis ulcer.**

varicose vein, a twisted, widened vein with incompetent valves. Causes include congenitally defective valves, thrombophlebitis, pregnancy, and obesity. Varicose veins are common, especially in women. The veins of the legs are most often affected. Raising the legs and use of elastic stockings are frequently sufficient therapy for simple cases. Surgery (ligation and stripping) may be required in severe cases. Injection of sclerosing solutions helps prevent or treat postphlebitic syndrome.

varicosis /ver'ikō'sis/, a common condition marked by one or more twisted, abnormally widened, or varicose veins, usually in the legs or the lower trunk, occurring between 30 and 60 years of age. Varicosis may be caused by congenital defects of the valves or walls of the veins or by congestion and increased pressure

in the vessels resulting from prolonged standing, poor posture, pregnancy, abdominal tumor, or long-term disease of the system. Symptoms include pain and muscle cramps with a feeling of fullness and heaviness in the legs. Widening of less important veins is often evident before the condition causes discomfort. Varicose veins may be treated conservatively by elevating the affected limb at times or by wearing an elastic bandage or stocking. Tying off the vein above the varicosity and removal of the affected portion of the vessel may be necessary for more severe cases if deeper vessels can continue the normal flow of venous blood.

varicosity, **1.** an abnormal condition, usually of a vein, marked by swelling and twisting. **2.** a vein in this condition.

variegate porphyria, a rare form of hepatic porphyria, marked by skin tumors and sensitivity to light. The condition may be present at birth or acquired. The first form is more serious, resulting in attacks of sharp pain in the stomach and intestines and in certain complications in the nervous system. See also **porphyria.**

variola, variola major.   See **smallpox.**

variola minor.   See **alastrim.**

varioloid /ver'ē-əloid'/, **1.** resembling smallpox. **2.** a mild form of smallpox in a vaccinated person or one who has previously had the disease.

varix /ver'iks/, *pl.* **varices** /ver'əsēz/, **1.** a twisted, widened vein. **2.** an enlarged, twisting artery or an enlarged, twisting lymphatic.

varus /ver'əs/, an abnormal position in which a part of a limb is turned inward toward the midline, as the heel and foot in **talipes varus.** Compare **valgus.**

vas /vas/, *pl.* **vasa** /vā'sə/, any one of the many vessels of the body, especially those that carry blood, lymph, or sperm.

vascular /vas'kyŏŏlər/, of or relating to a blood vessel.

vascular access device (VAD), a catheter, flexible tube (cannula) or other device designed to be left in place for a period of time to allow access to a vein or artery.

vascular hemophilia.   See **Von Willebrand's disease.**

vascular insufficiency, poor circulation caused by blockage of vessels. Signs of vascular insufficiency include pale, bluish, or mottled skin over the affected area, swelling of a hand or foot, absent or lessened sense of touch, tingling, lessened sense of temperature, muscle pain, as pain in the calf when walking, and, in advanced disease, wasting of muscles of the involved extremity. Treatment of vascular insufficiency may include a diet low in saturated fats, moderate exercise, sleeping on a firm mattress, avoidance of smoking, proper standing or sitting posture, the use of vessel-widening drugs, and, if indicated, surgical repair of an arteriovenous fistula or aneurysm. See also **arterial insufficiency.**

vascularization, the process by which body tissue becomes vascular and develops small blood vessels (capillaries). It may be natural or may be caused by surgical techniques. **–vascularize,** *v.*

vascular leiomyoma, a new growth (as a tumor) that has developed from smooth muscle fibers of a blood vessel.

vascular spider. See **spider angioma.**

vasculitis /vas′kyo̅o̅li′tis/, a swelling condition of the blood vessels that is the mark of certain systemic diseases or that is caused by an allergic reaction. Kinds of vasculitis are **allergic vasculitis, necrotizing vasculitis,** and **segmented hyalinizing vasculitis.** See also **angiitis.**

vas deferens /def′ərənz/, *pl.* **vasa deferentia** /def′ərən′shē-ə/, a tube passing from the testicles through the scrotum and joining the seminal vesicle. A vasectomy severs the vas deferens and makes a man sterile by interrupting the route sperm must take to the exterior from the testicles. Also called **deferent duct, ductus deferens, spermatic duct, testicular duct.** See also **testis.**

vasectomy /vasek′təmē/, an operation that makes a man sterile by cutting out a section of the vas deferens. Vasectomy is most commonly done in the doctor's office using local anesthesia. It is also done routinely before removal of the prostate gland to prevent swelling of the testicles. Potency is not affected. A signed and witnessed form indicating informed consent is usually required before doing it.

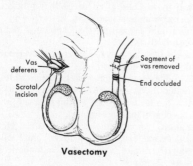

Vas deferens

Scrotal incision

Segment of vas removed

End occluded

Vasectomy

vaso-, a combining form meaning 'relating to a vessel or duct.'

vasoactive /vā′zō-ak′tiv/, (of a drug) tending to cause the widening or narrowing of a vessel.

vasoactive intestinal polypeptide (VIP), a blood vessel-widening substance secreted by pancreatic islet cancer cells. VIP causes blood vessels throughout the body to widen and in the intestinal tract causes secretion of fluid and salt, resulting in diarrhea. Its effects are like the symptoms of Asiatic cholera and can result in death from dehydration and kidney failure if either surgery or chemotherapy is not applied at an early stage of tumor development.

vasoconstriction, a narrowing of any blood vessel, especially the arterioles and the veins in the blood reservoirs of the skin and the abdominal viscera. It is done by many means that together control blood pressure and the distribution of blood throughout the body. Compare **vasodilatation.**

vasoconstrictor, **1.** of or relating to a process, condition, or substance that causes the narrowing of blood vessels. **2.** an agent that promotes vasoconstriction. Cold, fear, stress, and nicotine are common external vasoconstrictors. Epinephrine and norepinephrine produced by the body cause blood vessels to contract. Also called **vasopressor.**

vasodilatation /vā′zōdil′ətā′shən, -dī′lətā′shən/, widening or enlarging of blood vessels, particularly arterioles, usually caused by nerve impulses or certain drugs that relax smooth muscle in the walls of the blood vessels. Also called **vasodilation** /vā′zōdilā′shən/. Compare **vasoconstriction.**

vasodilator /vā′zōdī′lātər/, **1.** a nerve or agent that causes widening of blood vessels. **2.** relating to the relaxation of the smooth muscle of the vascular system. **3.** producing widening of blood vessels. Vasodilators are a recent, important addition to the treatment of heart failure. Included are hydralazine, nitroglycerin, nitroprusside, and trimethaphan. They have been used to treat severe heart failure in heart attack, in cases linked to severe mitral insufficiency, and in failure resulting from heart disease.

vasogenic shock, shock resulting from outer blood vessel-widening produced by factors, as poisons, that directly affect the blood vessels.

vasomotor, of or relating to the nerves and muscles that control the width of the blood vessels. Fibers (arranged in circles) of the muscles of arteries can contract, causing constriction, or they can relax, causing dilation.

vasomotor center, a vital collection of cell bodies in the brain stem that regulates blood pressure and heart function.

vasomotor rhinitis, rhinitis and nasal blockage without allergy or infection, marked by sneezing, rhinorrhea, nasal blockage, and vascular engorgement of the mucous membranes of the nose. A vaporizer or humidifier and systemic vasoconstrictive agents are used to ease discomfort. Nose drops and nasal sprays are avoided, because continued use may cause further vasodilatation of the mucous membrane and aggravation of the condition. Vasomotor rhinitis is common in pregnancy.

vasomotor system, the part of the nervous system that controls the narrowing and widening of the blood vessels. See also **vasoconstriction, vasodilatation.**

vasopressin. See **antidiuretic hormone.**

vasopressor. See **vasoconstrictor.**

vasospasm, a former term for **angiospasm.**

vasospastic, 1. relating to irregular narrowing of a blood vessel. **2.** any agent that produces spasms of the blood vessels.

vasospastic angina, a chest pain caused by reduced blood flow to the heart resulting from spasms of the arteries that supply blood to the heart. The pain is different from that with exertional angina. See also **Prinzmetal's angina.**

Vasotec, a trademark for a drug used to lower blood pressure (enalapril malcate).

vasovagal syncope, a sudden loss of consciousness caused by a lack of blood flow to the brain, as a result of less blood being released by the heart, widening of the blood vessels around the heart, and reduced heart rate. The condition may be caused by pain, fright, or trauma, and be accompanied by nausea, paleness, and perspiration. Also called **vasodepressor syncope, vasovagal attack.**

vasovasostomy /vā'zōvəsos'təmē/, an operation in which the function of the vas deferens on each side of the testes is restored, having been cut and tied in a preceding vasectomy. It is done if a man wants to regain his fertility. In most cases, the ability to work the canals is achieved, but in many cases fertility does not result, probably caused by flowing autoantibodies that disrupt normal sperm activity. The antibodies seem to develop after vasectomy because the growing sperm cannot be excreted through the urogenital tract.

Vasoxyl, a trademark for an alpha-adrenergic drug (methoxamine hydrochloride).

vastus intermedius, one of the four muscles of the quadriceps femoris, situated in the center of the thigh. It functions with the other three muscles of the quadriceps to extend the leg. Also called **crureus.** Compare **rectus femoris, vastus lateralis, vastus medialis.**

vastus internus. See **vastus medialis.**

vastus lateralis, the largest of the four muscles of the quadriceps femoris, situated on the outside of the thigh. It functions to help extend the leg. Compare **rectus femoris, vastus intermedius, vastus medialis.**

vastus medialis, one of the four muscles of the quadriceps femoris, situated in the inside of the thigh. It functions together with other parts of the quadriceps femoris to extend the leg. Also called **vastus internus.** Compare **rectus femoris, vastus intermedius, vastus lateralis.**

Vater-Pacini corpuscles /fä'tərpäsē'nē/, movement sensors located in the membranes covering the joints (capsules) and joint ligaments.

They may send nerve impulses faster and faster as a joint approaches the point where it can no longer bend or extend without being damaged. They are believed to protect the joints by signalling this information to the brain.

VBP, an anticancer drug combination of vinblastine, bleomycin, and cisplatin. Also called **PVB.**

VC, abbreviation for **vital capacity.**

VD, abbreviation for **venereal disease.**

VDRL test, abbreviation for *Venereal Disease Research Laboratory test,* a test for syphilis. It is also positive in other diseases, as yaws. False positive and false negative results may occur. A positive test must be confirmed by further, more precise testing.

vector, a carrier, especially one that transmits disease. A **biologic vector** is usually a parasite in which the infecting animal completes part of its life cycle. A **mechanic vector** carries the infecting organism from one host to another but is not essential to the life cycle of the parasite. Kinds of vectors include dogs, which carry rabies; mosquitoes, which transmit malaria; and ticks, which carry Rocky Mountain spotted fever. **–vector,** *v.,* **vectorial,** *adj.*

vecuronium bromide, a drug given via the vein (intravenously) to relax the muscles. It is used in conjunction with general anesthesia to allow insertion of a large tube through the mouth or nose into the windpipe, and to relax muscles during surgery or when a mechanical device is used to control a patient's breathing.

★CAUTION: The drug should be used cautiously in patients with myasthenia gravis or other disorders of the nerves and muscles, or who have been given drugs that produce or increase muscle relaxation. Effects of vecuronium may last longer than normal in patients with liver disease.

★ADVERSE EFFECTS: No serious adverse reactions have been reported.

VEE, abbreviation for **Venezuelan equine encephalitis.** See **equine encephalitis.**

Veetids, a trademark for a drug that kills bacteria (penicillin V potassium).

vegetation, an abnormal growth of tissue around a valve, made of protein, platelets, and bacteria.

vegetative nervous system. See **autonomic nervous system.**

Veillonella /vā'yənel'ə/, a bacterium. The species *Veillonella parvula* is normally present in the mouth.

vein, one of the many vessels that convey blood without oxygen back to the heart from all parts of the body. Compare **artery.** See also **portal vein, pulmonary vein, systemic vein.**

vein ligation and stripping, an operation consisting of the tying off of the saphenous vein and its removal (from groin to ankle). It is done to treat recurrent thrombophlebitis or severe varicosities or for getting a blood vessel to graft in another site, as in a coronary bypass operation.

vein lumen, the central opening through which blood flows in a vein.

vein of Thebesius. See **smallest cardiac vein.**

veins of the vertebral column, the veins that drain the blood from the spinal column, the nearby muscles, and the meninges of the spinal cord.

Velban, a trademark for a drug that prevents new growths, as tumors (vinblastine sulfate).

vellus hair. See **lanugo.**

velocity of growth, the rate of growth or change in growth measurements over a period of time.

velocity spectrum rehabilitation, a rehabilitation program that uses strength training at various speeds of movement, from slow to fast.

velopharyngeal closure /vē′lōfərin′jē·əl/, the blocking of any escape of air by the raising of the soft palate and the closing of the throat. Compare **closure, flask closure.**

velopharyngeal insufficiency, an abnormal condition resulting from a birth defect in the structure of a throat opening (velopharyngeal sphincter). Closure of the mouth beneath the nasal passages is not complete, as seen in cleft palate. Food may be spit up through the nose, and speech is impaired. Surgical repair is usually successful.

Velosef, a trademark for an antibiotic (cephradine).

Velpeau's bandage /velpōz′/, a roller bandage that stabilizes the elbow and shoulder by holding the arm against the side and the flexed forearm on the chest. The palm of the hand rests on the clavicle of the opposite side.

vena cava /vē′nə kā′və/, pl. **venae cavae,** one of two large veins returning blood from outer parts of the body to the right chamber of the heart. See also **inferior vena cava, superior vena cava. –vena caval,** adj.

vena caval syndrome. See **supine hypotension.**

vena comes /kō′mēz/, pl. **venae comites** /kom′itēz/, one of the deep paired veins that go along with the smaller arteries, one on each side of the artery. The three vessels are wrapped together.

venereal /vənir′ē·əl/, relating to or caused by sexual intercourse or genital contact.

venereal disease. See **sexually transmitted disease.**

venereal sore. See **chancre.**

venereal wart. See **condyloma acuminatum.**

venereology /vənir′ē·ol′əjē/, the study of venereal diseases. **–venereologic, venereological,** adj., **venereologist,** n.

venerupin poisoning /ven′ərōō·pin/, a form of shellfish poisoning that may cause death, resulting from eating oysters or clams contaminated with venerupin, a poison that causes reduced liver function, vomiting or diarrhea, and increased white cell production. The shellfish poison occurs in waters around Japan. About

one-third of the cases are fatal. See also **shellfish poisoning.**

venesection. See **phlebotomy.**

Venezuelan equine encephalitis. See **equine encephalitis.**

venipuncture /ven′ipungk′chər/, a technique in which a vein is punctured by a sharp instrument carrying a flexible plastic catheter or by a steel needle attached to a syringe or catheter. The purpose of the procedure is to withdraw a specimen of blood, to instill a medication, to start a feeding, or to inject a substance to aid in the x-ray examination of a part or system of the body. Antiseptics are used to avoid infection. A quick, skillful insertion is nearly painless for the patient. See also **intravenous infusion, phlebotomy.**

venogram. See **phlebogram.**

venography. See **phlebography.**

venom, a poisonous fluid substance secreted by some snakes, insects, spiders, and other animals and transmitted by their stings or bites.

venom extract therapy, the giving of antivenin as protection against the poisonous effects of the bite of a specific poisonous snake or spider, or other poisonous animal.

venom immunotherapy, the reduction of sensitivity to the bite of a poisonous insect or animal by giving a series of gradually increasing amounts of the specific substance secreted by the insect or animal.

venotomy /vēnot′əmē/, the surgical opening of a vein.

venous /vē′nəs/, of or relating to a vein.

venous blood gas, the oxygen and carbon dioxide in venous blood measured in order to test the health of a part of the body.

venous hum, a continuous musical murmur heard through a stethoscope placed over major veins at the base of the neck, especially when the patient is anemic, upright, and looking away from the side of the neck where the stethoscope is placed. It is also heard in some healthy, young individuals.

venous insufficiency, an abnormal circulatory condition marked by decreased return of vein blood from the legs to the trunk of the body. Fluid buildup (edema) is usually the first sign of the condition; pain, varicosities, and ulceration may follow. Treatment usually consists of raising the legs, using elastic hose, and correcting the cause.

venous pressure, the pressure of circulating blood on the walls of veins, normally 60 to 120 mm of water in peripheral veins but higher in congestive heart failure, in acute or chronic constrictive pericarditis, and in the blockage of a vein caused by a clot or external pressure against a vein. Symptoms of increased pressure are continued distention of veins on the back of the hand when it is raised above the top of the rib cage and enlarging of the neck veins when the individual is sitting with the head raised 30 to 45 degrees.

venous pulse, the pulse of a vein usually felt over the inner or outer or jugular veins in the neck. The pulse in the jugular vein is taken to read the pressure of the pulse and the form of the pressure wave, especially in a patient with a cardiac conduction defect or cardiac arrhythmia.

venous sinus, one of many sinuses that collect blood from the brain and drain it into the inner jugular vein.

venous stasis, a disorder in which the normal flow of blood through a vein is slowed or halted.

venous stasis dermatitis. See **stasis dermatitis.**

venous thrombosis, a condition marked by the presence of a clot in a vein in which the wall of the vessel is not swollen. Pain and swelling may follow if the vein is closed. Also called **phlebothrombosis.** Compare **thrombophlebitis.**

ventilate, **1.** to provide with fresh air. **2.** to provide the lungs with air from the atmosphere and to get air or oxygen into the blood for the lungs. **3.** (in psychiatry) to open discussion of something, as to ventilate feelings.

ventilation, the process by which gases are moved into and out of the lungs. Compare **respiration.** –**ventilatory,** *adj.*

ventilation lung scan, an x-ray examination of the lungs, done while the patient inhales a radioactive gas and the lungs are scanned to detect nonworking or damaged lung areas or other abnormalities.

ventilation perfusion defect, a disorder in which one or more areas of the lung receive oxygen but no blood, or blood but no oxygen.

ventilator, any of several devices used in respiratory therapy to provide assisted breathing and intensive positive pressure breathing. Kinds of ventilators are **pressure limited ventilator** and **volume ventilator.** See also **IPPB unit.**

Ventolin a trademark for a bronchodilator (albuterol).

ventral, of or relating to a position toward the belly of the body; frontward; anterior. Compare **dorsal.**

ventral hernia. See **abdominal hernia.**

ventricle /ven'trikəl/, a small cavity, as one of the cavities filled with cerebrospinal fluid in the brain, or the right and the left ventricles of the heart.

ventricular /ventrik'yōōlər/, of or relating to a ventricle.

ventricular aneurysm, a limited widening or saclike bulge in the wall of the left ventricle, occurring most often after a myocardial infarction. Scar tissue may be formed as a result of swelling caused by the infarction. This tissue weakens the myocardium, allowing its walls to bulge outward when the ventricle contracts.

Diagnosis may be made with the use of x-ray studies and cardiac catheterization. Treatment may consist of giving propranolol, digoxin, or procainamide but usually involves surgical removal of the scar tissue. Also called **cardiac aneurysm.**

ventricular dysfunction, abnormal functioning of the wall within the heart cavities (ventricles) that is related to abnormalities in contraction and wall motion.

ventricular extrasystole, an extra heart beat arising from the ventricle.

ventricular fibrillation, a very fast, very uneven heart beat. The condition is marked by a complete lack of a regular heart beat. Blood pressure falls to zero, resulting in unconsciousness. Death may occur within 4 minutes. Defibrillation and ventilation must be initiated immediately.

ventricular gallop, an abnormal heart beat in which a low-pitched, extra heart sound (S_3) is heard. When it is heard in an older patient with heart disease, it means heart failure. The same sound heard in a healthy child or young adult is not a problem and goes away with age. See also **gallop.**

ventricular septal defect (VSD), an abnormal opening in the wall (septum) separating the ventricles, permitting blood to flow from the left ventricle to the right ventricle and to recirculate through the pulmonary artery and lungs. It is the most common heart defect, present at birth, with openings that may be single or multiple and may range in size from 1 to 2 mm to several centimeters. Children with small defects usually have no symptoms, whereas those with large defects may have congestive heart failure linked with lower respiratory tract infections, rapid breathing, poor weight gain, restlessness, and irritability. Small defects may close on their own; larger ones may lead to bacterial endocarditis, pulmonary vascular obstructive disease, aortic regurgitation, or congestive heart failure. Diagnosis is proved by electrocardiography, cardiac catheterization, and angiography. Treatment consists of surgical repair of the defect, preferably in early childhood.

ventricular tachycardia, a fast heart beat that usually begins in the ventricular Purkinje system.

ventriculo-, a combining form meaning 'relating to a ventricle of the heart or brain.'

ventriculoatrial shunt /ventrik'yōōlō·ā'trē·əl/, a surgically created passageway, consisting of plastic tubing and one-way valves, implanted between a cerebral ventricle and the right atrium of the heart to drain excess cerebrospinal fluid from the brain in hydrocephalus.

ventriculocisternostomy, an operation done to treat water on the brain (hydrocephalus). An opening is created that allows spinal fluid to drain through a shunt from the ventricles of the brain into the cisterna magna. Also called **Torkildsen procedure, ventriculostomy.**

ventriculofallopian tube shunt, an operation with limited effectiveness for diverting spinal fluid into the abdomen. This procedure is used to correct both the blocking and the communicating types of hydrocephalus. Also called **spinofallopian tube shunt.**

ventriculogram /ventrik′yəlōgram′/, **1.** a diagnostic test in which air is inserted into the cavities (ventricles) of the brain through surgical openings in the scalp. **2.** x-ray examination of the cavities (ventricles) of the heart in which a dye is injected through a long tube inserted through the blood vessels (cardiac catheterization).

ventriculography /ventrik′yōolog′rəfē/, **1.** an x-ray examination of the head, after air or some other substance has been injected into the head. **2.** an x-ray examination of a ventricle of the heart, after injection of a substance that allows x-ray films to be made.

ventriculoperitoneal shunt, a surgically created passageway, consisting of plastic tubing and one-way valves, between a cerebral ventricle and the abdomen for the draining of excess spinal fluid from the brain in water on the brain (hydrocephalus).

ventriculoperitoneostomy /ventrik′yōolōper′itōnē-os′təmē/, an operation for temporarily diverting spinal fluid in water on the brain (hydrocephalus), usually in the newborn. This procedure is used to correct both the communicating and the blocking types of hydrocephalus.

ventriculopleural shunt, an operation for diverting spinal fluid from enlarged ventricles in water on the brain (hydrocephalus), usually in the newborn. Spinal fluid is diverted from the vessel into the chest.

ventriculostomy. See **ventriculocisternostomy.**

ventriculoureterostomy /ventrik′yōolōyōorē′tər-os′təmē/, an operation for directing cerebrospinal fluid into the general circulation done to treat hydrocephalus, usually in the newborn. Rarely used, the method is an alternative to auriculoventriculostomy. The procedure is used to correct a blocking type of hydrocephalus.

Venturi mask, a face mask used in respiratory therapy, designed to allow the air the patient inhales to mix with oxygen, which is supplied through a jet in fixed amounts.

venule /ven′yōol/, any one of the small blood vessels that gather blood from the capillary plexuses and join together to form the veins. **–venular,** *adj.*

verapamil, a drug given to treat spastic and exercise-related heart diseases.

★CAUTION: Severe heart problems, low blood

pressure, shock, sick sinus syndrome, or heart block prohibits its use.

★ADVERSE EFFECTS: Among the more serious side effects are low blood pressure, fluid buildup, heart block, heart failure, fluid in the lungs, and dizziness.

verbal aphasia. See **motor aphasia.**

vergence, movement of the two eyes in opposite directions.

vermicide, an agent that kills worms, particularly those in the intestine. Compare **anthelmintic, vermifuge.**

vermiform appendix, a wormlike, blunt tube closed at one end extending from the large intestine. Its length varies from 3 to 6 inches, and its diameter is about one-thrid of an inch. Also called **appendix vermiformis, cecal appendix.** See also **appendicitis.**

vermifuge, an agent that causes parasitic worms to be flushed from the body.

vermilion border, the pinkish to red area of the upper and lower lip.

vermis /vur′mis/, *pl.* **vermes, 1.** a worm. **2.** a structure resembling a worm. **–vermiform,** *adj.*

Vermox, a trademark for a drug used to kill parasitic worms in the intestine (mebendazole).

vernal conjunctivitis, a long-term form of conjunctivitis that affects both eyes, thought to be caused by allergies, that occurs most often in young men under 20 years of age during the spring and summer months. Most common symptoms include strong itching and crusting discharge. Topical corticosteroids may be applied, and treatment for pollen allergies may be helpful. Compare **allergic conjunctivitis.**

Vernet's syndrome /vernāz′/, a disorder of the nervous system caused by an injury to certain cranial nerves near the base of the skull. Symptoms include paralysis on the right or left side of the muscles of the roof of the mouth, throat, voicebox, and side and back of the neck (sternocleidomastoid and trapezius muscles). The patient also experiences difficulty swallowing, the voice is nasal and hoarse, and there may be some loss of taste sensations. Also called **jugular foramen syndrome.**

Verneuil's neuroma. See **plexiform neuroma.**

vernix caseosa /vur′niks kas′ē·ō′sə/, a grayish-white, cheeselike substance consisting of fatty gland secretions, a kind of woolly down (lanugo), and scaly cells. It covers the skin of the fetus and newborn. It acts as a protection for the fetus while it is in the uterus and is thought to help keep it warm.

verruca /vurōō′kə/, a harmless, warty sore on the skin caused by a virus. It has a rough surface. It is caused by a common, contagious virus. Methods of treatment include drugs, surgery, and mental suggestion. Also called **verruca vulgaris, wart. –verrucose, verrucous,** *adj.*

verruca plana, a small, slightly raised, smooth, tan or flesh-colored wart, sometimes occurring in large numbers on the face, neck, back of the hands, wrists, and knees, especially in children. Also called **flat wart.**

verruca senillis. See **basal cell papilloma.**

verruca vulgaris. See **verruca.**

verrucous carcinoma, a very distinct scaly growth of soft tissue of the mouth, larynx, or genitals. A slow-growing tumor, it does not usually spread.

verrucous dermatitis, any skin rash with wartlike sores.

verruga peruana. See **bartonellosis.**

version, the changing of the position of the fetus in the uterus, usually done to ease delivery. Version may occur by itself as a result of contractions of the uterus or be caused by action taken by the physician.

version and extraction, an operation in the delivery of a baby in which a fetus being born headfirst is turned and delivered feet-first. It is done by reaching deeply into the uterus, grasping the feet and pulling them down, and pulling out the infant. The procedure is considered out-of-date and unsafe and has been replaced by cesarean section, although it may still be done to deliver a second twin. Also called **internal podalic version and total breech extraction.** Compare **external version.** See also **breech birth.**

vertebra, *pl.* **vertebrae,** any one of the 33 bones of the spinal column. There are 7 in the neck, 12 in the back, 5 in the lower back, 5 in the pelvic area, and 4 in the tailbone.

-vertebral, a combining form referring to the spinal column.

vertebral artery, each of two arteries that carry blood to the deep neck muscles, the spine, and parts of the brain.

vertebral body, the solid central portion of a vertebra that supports the weight of the body.

vertebral column, the backbone. It is made up of 33 vertebrae that are separated by spongy disks. The average length in men is about 71 cm; in women, the average length is about 61 cm. The spine is made stronger by several curves. The spinal column also protects the spinal cord that runs inside of it. Also called **spinal column, spine.** See also **vertebra.**

vertex, **1.** the top of the head; crown. **2.** the highest point of any structure.

vertex presentation, (in the delivery of a baby) a birth in which the fetus is lying in the womb with its head downward. The head will be born first. Compare **breech presentation.**

vertical angulation, (in dentistry) an up-and-down angle used in taking x-ray films of the teeth and jaw.

vertical-integrated health care, a health delivery system in which all care, including financial services, is provided within a single organization, as a health-maintenance organization (HMO).

vertical plane. See **cardinal frontal plane.**

vertical resorption, a kind of bone loss in which the part of the jaw where the teeth grow that is next to an affected tooth is destroyed without loss of a crest. See also **resorption.**

vertical transmission, the transfer of a disease, condition, or trait from a mother to her child, either in the genes or at the time of birth, as the spread of an infection through breast milk or through the placenta.

verticosubmental, a part of the skull used as a focus for x-ray tests. It permits the central ray to pass from the vertex of the skull to its base.

vertigo. See **dizziness.**

very-low-density lipoprotein (VLDL), a blood protein that is made mainly of triglycerides with small amounts of cholesterol, phospholipid, and protein. It transports triglycerides mainly from the liver to sites in the tissues for use or storage. The triglycerides are quickly changed to smaller, more easily dissolved lipoproteins and in time to low-density lipoproteins. See also **high-density lipoprotein (HDL).**

vesical fistula, an abnormal passage leading to the bladder. Vesical fistulae may travel to the skin, vagina, uterus, or rectum.

vesicant /ves'ikənt/, a drug capable of causing tissue death when it enters the tissues.

vesicle /ves'ikəl/, a small sac or blister, as a small, thin-walled, raised bump on the skin containing clear fluid. Compare **bulla.** **–vesicular,** *adj.*

vesicle calculus, a stone formed in the bladder. Also called **bladder stone, cystolith.**

vesicle reflex, the sensation of a need to urinate when the bladder is partly full. See also **micturition reflex.**

vesico-, a combining form meaning 'relating to the bladder or to a blister.'

vesicoureteral reflux, an abnormal backflow of urine from the bladder to the ureter, resulting from a defect present at birth blocking the outlet of the bladder, or infection of the lower urinary tract. Backflow increases the water pressure in the ureters and kidneys. The condition is marked by pain in the stomach, intestines, or sides, uncontrolled urination and pus or blood in the urine, with frequent urinary infections. Surgery may be necessary to fix the damage. Drugs are used to treat any infection that occurs with this state.

vesicular /vesik'yələr/, referring to a blisterlike condition.

vesicular appendix, a closed sac near the entrance of each of the fallopian tubes.

vesicular breath sound, a normal sound of rustling or swishing heard with a stethoscope over the lung, marked by higher pitch when breathing in and fading rapidly while breathing out. Compare **tracheal breath sound.**

vesicular mole. See **hydatid mole.**

vesiculitis /vəsik'yŏolī'tis/, swelling of any vesicle, particularly the seminal vesicles. This is rarely seen by itself. It is usually linked with prostatitis.

vesiculography, the x-ray examination of the seminal vesicles and nearby structures, with a substance that shows up well on x-ray films after being injected into the area. It is used to examine the vesicles, vas deferens, and ejaculatory duct for possible tumors, cysts, or other disorders.

vessel, any one of the many small tubes throughout the body that convey fluids, as blood and lymph. The main kinds of vessels are the arteries, the veins, and the lymphatic vessels.

vestibular /vestib'yŏolər/, of or relating to a vestibule, as the vestibular part of the mouth, which lies between the cheeks and the teeth.

vestibular apparatus, the inner ear structures that are associated with balance and position sense. It includes the vestibule and semicircular canals.

vestibular-bilateral disorder, a disorder in which information received by the body's sense is not properly processed. It is characterized by short periods during which the eyes make jerky movements (nystagmus), poor coordination between the two sides of the body and brain, and difficulty in learning reading or arithmetic. The disorder occurs when the brain does not respond adequately to information about the body's position and movement.

vestibular function, the sense of balance.

vestibular gland, any one of four small glands, two on each side of the opening of the vagina. One pair of the small glands are called the greater vestibular glands; the other pair are called the lesser vestibular glands. The vestibular glands secrete a lubricating substance. Compare **Cowper's gland.** See also **Bartholin's gland.**

vestibular toxicity, poisonous (toxic) effects (commonly of drugs) on the balance center (vestibule) of the ear, resulting in dizziness and loss of balance.

vestibule /ves'tibyŏol/, a space that serves as the entrance to a passageway, as the vestibule of the vagina or the vestibule of the ear.

vestibulocochlear nerve. See **nerve for hearing and balance.**

vestibulo-ocular reflex, a normal reflex in which eye position compensates for movement of the head. It is caused by stimulation of the inner ear structures (vestibular apparatus) that are associated with balance and position sense.

vestige, a deformed, mainly useless organ or other structure of the body that was important at an earlier stage of life or in a simpler form of life. The vermiform appendix is a vestigial organ. **–vestigial,** *adj.*

viable, capable of developing, growing, and otherwise sustaining life, as a normal human fetus at 28 weeks of pregnancy. **–viability,** *n.*

viable infant, an infant who at birth weighs at least 1,000 g or has been carried in the womb for 28 weeks or more.

vial /vī'əl/, a glass container with a metal-enclosed rubber seal.

Vibramycin Hyclate, a trademark for a tetracycline antibiotic (doxycycline hyclate).

Vibramycin Monohydrate, a trademark for a drug that kills germs (doxycycline monohydrate).

vibrating. See **cupping and vibrating.**

vibration, a type of massage done by quick tapping with the fingertips, alternating the fingers in a rhythmic way, or by a mechanic device. See also **massage.**

vibrio /vib'rē-ō/, any bacterium that is curved and able to move, as those belonging to the genus *Vibrio.* Cholera and several other epidemic forms of gastroenteritis are caused by members of the genus.

Vibrio cholerae, the species of comma-shaped, motile bacillus that is the cause of cholera.

Vibrio fetus. See *Campylobacter.*

vibrio gastroenteritis, an infectious disease caught from infected seafood and marked by nausea, vomiting, stomach pain, and diarrhea, caused by *Vibrio parahaemolyticus.* Headache, mild fever, and bloody stools may also be present. Recovery usually occurs by itself in 2 to 5 days. Compare **salmonellosis, shigellosis.**

Vibrio parahaemolyticus /per'əhē'mōlit'ikəs/, a species of microorganism of the genus *Vibrio,* the cause of food poisoning linked with the eating of uncooked or undercooked shellfish, especially crabs and shrimp. This microorganism is a common cause of gastroenteritis in Japan, aboard cruise ships, and in the eastern and southeastern coastal areas of the United States. Thorough cooking of seafood prevents the infection linked with *Vibrio parahaemolyticus,* which causes watery diarrhea, stomach cramps, vomiting, headache, chills, and fever. The symptoms of infection may appear after a time of 2 to 48 hours. The food poisoning from this agent usually goes away by itself within 2 days but may be more severe, even fatal, in disease-ridden and old persons. This is usually treated by resting in bed and drinking lots of water.

vicarious menstruation, bleeding from a site other than the uterus at the time when menstruation is normally expected. Such bleeding is caused by the small blood vessels releasing more blood during menstruation.

vidarabine, a drug that is used to kill a virus (antiviral). Also called **adenine arabinoside.** It is used to treat herpes simplex encephalitis and put on the skin to treat herpesvirus I keratoconjunctivitis and keratitis.

★CAUTION: It is used in pregnancy only when the benefits are greater than the risk of damage to the baby. Known allergy to this drug prohibits its use.

★ADVERSE EFFECTS: Among the more serious side effects when given by pill or shot are severe nausea and other symptoms of upset in the stomach and intestines, various nervous system effects, and bone marrow depression. Irritation, sensitivity to light, and corneal edema may occur when put in the eyes.

villi. See **villus.**

villoma /vilō'mə/, *pl.* **villomas, villomata,** a fiberlike harmless growth, occurring chiefly in the bladder or rectum. Also called **villioma.**

villous adenoma /vil'əs/, a slow-growing, soft, spongy, possibly cancer-causing growth of the mucous membranes of the large intestine.

villous carcinoma, a tumor with many long, velvety fingerlike growths. Also called **carcinoma villosum.**

villous papilloma, a harmless tumor with long, slender growths, usually occurring in the bladder, breast, or in a brain ventricle.

villus, *pl.* **villi,** one of the many tiny projections, barely visible to the naked eye, which cover the whole lining of the small intestine. The villi absorb and carry fluids and nutrients. They are very uneven in size and are larger in some parts of the intestine than in others, flattening out when the intestine stretches. –**villous,** *adj.*

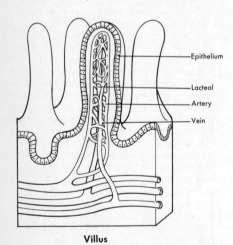

Epithelium

Lacteal

Artery

Vein

Villus

vin-, -vin, a combining form for substances that act against viruses.

vinblastine sulfate /vinblas'tēn, -tin/, a drug that prevents the growth of cancer cells. It is used to treat many cancerous diseases, as choriocar-

cinoma, testicular carcinoma, Hodgkin's disease, and non-Hodgkin's lymphoma.

★CAUTION: Leukopenia, bacterial infection, or known allergy to this drug prohibits its use. It is not given in pregnancy.

★ADVERSE EFFECTS: Among the most serious side effects are leukopenia and poisoning. Nausea, diarrhea, stomatitis, and loss of hair (alopecia) also may occur.

Vincent's angina, Vincent's infection. See **acute necrotizing gingivitis.**

vincristine sulfate /vinkris'tēn, -tin/, a drug that prevents the growth of cancer cells. It is given to treat many cancerous diseases, as leukemia, neuroblastoma, lymphomas, and sarcomas.

★CAUTION: Pregnancy, leukopenia, preexisting neuromuscular disease, or known allergy to this drug prohibits its use.

★ADVERSE EFFECTS: Among the most serious side effects are poisoning and leukopenia. Constipation, pain in the stomach and intestines, loss of hair (alopecia), and swelling at the site of injection also may occur.

vindesine sulfate, a drug that prevents the growth of cancer cells. It is used to treat acute lymphoblastic leukemia, breast cancer, cancerous melanoma, lymphosarcoma, and non-small-cell lung carcinoma.

★CAUTION: Leukopenia, bacterial infections, or known allergy to this drug prohibits its use.

★ADVERSE EFFECTS: Among the most serious side effects are neurotoxicity, leukopenia, thrombocytopenia, phlebitis, and loss of hair (alopecia).

Vioform, a trademark for a drug that kills amebas (antiamebic) and used to treat skin infections (iodochlorhydroxyquin).

Viokase, a trademark for an enzyme (pancreatin).

viosterol /vī·os'tərôl/, artificial vitamin D_2 in an oil base. Also called **synthetic oleovitamin D.** See also **calciferol, ergosterol.**

VIP, abbreviation for **vasoactive intestinal polypeptide.**

vipoma /vipō'mə/, a type of tumor of the pancreas that causes changes in the release of vasoactive intestinal polypeptide (VIP). VIP causes widening of blood vessels throughout the body and release of fluid and salt in the intestinal tract, resulting in diarrhea. The VIP effects are identical to the symptoms of Asiatic cholera and can result in kidney failure and death from dehydration if either surgery or chemotherapy is not administered at an early stage of tumor development. See also **vasoactive intestinal polypeptide.**

vir-, -vir, a combining form for substances that act against viruses.

Vira-A, a trademark for a drug used to fight a virus (vidarabine).

viral disease. See **viral infection.**

viral gastroenteritis, an inflammation of the intestine caused by a virus. The symptoms usually include stomach cramps, diarrhea, nausea, and vomiting.

viral hepatitis, a virus-caused, swelling disease of the liver, caused by one of the hepatitis viruses, A, B, or non-A, non-B. How the disease is caught, how fast it shows, and the results of the illness vary with the kind of virus, but the symptoms of the disease and its treatment are the same. See also **hepatitis A, hepatitis B, non-A, non-B hepatitis.** Symptoms of viral hepatitis are loss of appetite (anorexia), a sick feeling, headache, pain over the liver, fever, jaundice, clay-colored stools, dark urine, nausea and vomiting, and diarrhea. Severe infection, especially with hepatitis B virus, may last a long time and result in tissue destruction, liver disease (cirrhosis), and chronic hepatitis or in hepatic coma and death. The patient should not donate blood, and should not take over-the-counter drugs without asking a doctor.

viral infection, any of the diseases caused by one of about 200 viruses dangerous to humans. Some are the most dangerous diseases known; some are harmless. Disease exists when the virus damages any cells. Viruses enter the body through breaks in the skin, by being breathed into the lungs, or by entering the stomach when eaten. The disease develops as the virus goes through its life cycle. In many diseases of this type, the body makes its own protection against ever catching it again. In others, this protection lasts only a short time.

viral pneumonia, infection of the lungs caused by a virus.

Virchow's node /fēr′shōz/, a firm lymph node located above the collarbone, particularly on the left side, that is so enlarged it can be felt by examination with the fingers. Also called **sentinel node, signal node.**

viremia /vīrē′mē·ə/, viruses in the blood. Compare **bacteremia, fungemia, parasitemia.**

virile /vir′əl/, **1.** of, relating to, or typical of an adult male; masculine; manly. **2.** having masculine strength, vigor, force, or energy. **3.** of or relating to the male sexual functions; capable of making a woman pregnant. Compare **virilism, –virility,** n.

virilism, 1. See **virilization. 2.** a state in which a woman seems to have secondary male sex characteristics. **3.** early development of masculine traits in the male. Kinds of virilism are **adrenal virilism,** and **prosopopilary virilism.**

virilization, a process in which secondary male sexual traits are acquired by a female, usually as the result of adrenal gland dysfunction or hormone drugs. Also called **masculinization.** See also **adrenal virilism.**

virion /vī′rē·on/, a simple virus particle. See also **capsid.**

virologist /vīrol′əjist, vir-/, a specialist who studies viruses and diseases caused by viruses.

virology /vīrol′əjē, vir-/, the study of viruses and viral diseases. **–virologic, virological,** adj.

Viroptic, a trademark for a drug that fights viruses in the eyes (trifluridine).

virucidal, referring to the destruction of viruses.

virucide, any drug that destroys or makes harmless a virus. **–virucidal,** adj.

virulence /vir′yooləns/, the power of a microbe to cause disease.

virulent /vir′yoolənt/, of or relating to a very deadly condition.

virus, a tiny organism that can only grow in the cells of another animal. More than 200 viruses have been found to cause disease in humans. Some kinds of viruses are **adenovirus, arenavirus, enterovirus, herpesvirus,** and **rhinovirus.** See also **viral infection. –viral,** adj.

virustatic, referring to the prevention of the growth and development of viruses, rather than their destruction.

viscera /vis′ərə/, sing. **viscus** /vis′kəs/, the internal organs held within a space in the body, mainly the stomach and intestines.

visceral /vis′ərəl/, of or relating to the viscera, or internal organs in the body cavity. Also **splanchnic.**

visceral afferent fibers, the nerve fibers in the nervous system of the viscera. Some of the parts of the body with visceral afferents are the face, scalp, nose, mouth, descending colon, lungs, abdomen, and rectum. See also **autonomic nervous system.**

visceral larva migrans, infestation with parasitic larvae or *Toxocara* or, occasionally, *Ascaris, Strongyloides,* or other nematodes. See **toxocariasis.**

visceral leishmaniasis. See **kala-azar.**

visceral lymph node, a small, oval, bumpy gland that filters lymph circulating in the lymphatic vessels of the viscera of the chest, lower body, and the pelvis. Compare **parietal lymph node.** See also **lymph, lymphatic system, lymph node.**

visceral nervous system, the visceral part of the nervous system that is made up of the whole complex of nerves, fibers, ganglia, and plexuses by which signals travel from the central nervous system to the viscera and from the viscera to the central nervous system. Also called **involuntary nervous system.** See also **autonomic nervous system, visceral afferent fibers.**

visceral pain, pain in the stomach and intestines caused by any abnormal condition of the viscera. It is usually strong, scattered, and hard to point to.

visceral peritoneum, one of two parts of the largest membrane in the body that covers the viscera. Compare **parietal peritoneum.** See also **peritoneal cavity.**

visceral pleura, the inner layer of the membrane surrounding the lung that is next to the outer lung tissue.

visceral protein status, the amount of protein that is contained in the internal organs.

viscid /vis'id/, sticky or gluelike. Also **viscous** /vis'kəs/.

viscosity, relating to the quality of a sticky or gummy fluid.

viscus. See **viscera.**

vision, the ability to see.

Visken, a trademark for a heart drug (pindolol).

Vistaril, a trademark for a sedative (hydroxyzine hydrochloride).

visual, referring to the sense of sight.

visual accommodation, the way the eye is able to change its focus while seeing things either close up or far away. As the person grows older, the lens of the eye gets harder, and there may be a loss of the ability to focus on nearby things. Compare **presbyopia.**

visual field defect, one or more spots or defects in the vision that move with the eye, unlike a floater. This fixed defect may be caused by injuries to the eye, by disease, or by damage to the brain. Sudden loss of part of a person's sight is a signal to get an eye test.

visual-motor coordination, the ability to coordinate vision with the movements of the body or parts of the body.

visual-motor function, the ability to draw or copy forms or to perform constructive tasks.

visual pathway, a pathway over which a visual sensation is carried from the retina to the brain. A pathway consists of an optic nerve and other optic structures.

visual purple. See **rhodopsin.**

vital capacity (VC), a measurement of the amount of air that can be breathed out slowly after the largest possible breath has been taken. This shows the most air that the lungs can hold. The average normal values of 4,000 to 5,000 ml are affected by age, the size of the chest cage, physical fitness, posture, and sex. The vital capacity may be limited by disease, injury, or pregnancy. Compare **forced expiratory volume, residual volume.**

vital signs, the measurements of pulse rate, the rate of breathing, and body temperature. Although not strictly a vital sign, blood pressure is also usually included. Abnormalities of vital signs are often clues to diseases, and changes in vital signs are used to measure a patient's progress. See also **blood pressure, pulse, respiration, temperature.**

vital statistics, data relating to births, deaths, marriages, health, and disease.

vitamin, a natural compound needed in small quantities for normal bodily functions. With few exceptions, vitamins cannot be made by the body and must be gotten from the diet or dietary supplements. No one food contains all the vitamins. Vitamin deficiency diseases produce specific symptoms usually eased by making the appropriate vitamin. See also **avitaminosis, hypervitaminosis, oleovitamin, provitamin,** and see the specific vitamins.

vitamin A, a vitamin needed for the growth of the skeleton, maintaining the mucous membranes, and keen sight. It is present in leafy green vegetables, yellow fruits and vegetables, the liver oils of the cod and other fish, liver, milk, cheese, butter, and egg yolk. Lack of this vitamin causes diseases of the mucous membranes and the eyes. Symptoms of getting too much vitamin A are irritability, fatigue, lethargy, stomach pain, painful joints, severe throbbing headache, insomnia and restlessness, night sweats, loss of body hair, brittle nails, and a bug-eyed expression (exophthalmus). Also called **antiinfection vitamin, antixerophthalmic vitamin.** See also **oleovitamin A.**

vitamin B₁. See **thiamine.**

vitamin B₂. See **riboflavin.**

vitamin B₆. See **pyridoxine.**

vitamin B₁₂. See **cyanocobalamin.**

vitamin B₁₇. See **Laetrile.**

vitamin B complex, a group of vitamins differing from each other in structure and their effect on the human body. All of the B vitamins are found in large quantities in liver and yeast, and they are present one at a time or several together in many foods. Heat and prolonged cooking, especially cooking with water, can destroy B vitamins. See also **folic acid, and see vitamins B₁ through B₁₂.**

vitamin C. See **ascorbic acid.**

vitamin D, a vitamin related to the steroids and needed for the normal growth of bones and teeth and for absorbing calcium and phosphorus from the intestines. The vitamin is present in natural foods in small amounts, and the needed amounts are usually gotten from vitamins added to various foods, especially milk and dairy products, and exposure to sunlight. The natural foods containing vitamin D are of animal origin and include saltwater fish, especially salmon, sardines, and herring, organ meats, fish-liver oils, and egg yolk. A lack of the vitamin results in rickets in children, and other bone diseases in adults. Too-much vitamin D results in poisoning that causes a loss of appetite, vomiting, headache, drowsiness, diarrhea, and hardening of the soft tissues of the heart, blood vessels, renal tubules, and lungs. Treatment consists of stopping the vitamin dosage and beginning a low-calcium diet until symptoms stop. See also **calciferol, vitamin D₃.**

vitamin D₂. See **calciferol.**

vitamin D₃, a vitamin that is needed for calcium and phosphorus metabolism. It is found in most fish-liver oils, butter, brain, and egg yolk and is formed in the skin, fur, and feathers of animals and birds exposed to sunlight or ultraviolet rays. Also called **activated 7-dehydrocholesterol, cholecalciferol.**

vitamin deficiency, a state or condition that is caused by the lack of or inability to use one or more vitamins. The symptoms of each deficiency vary depending on the function of the vitamin in helping the body to grow, develop, and stay healthy.

vitamin D resistant rickets, a disease that seems to be rickets but cannot be cured with large doses of vitamin D. It is caused by a defect present at birth in part of the kidney and is usually seen in men. See also **rickets.**

vitamin E, any or all of the group of vitamins that are needed for normal reproduction, muscle development, and various other bodily functions. A lack of this vitamin causes muscle damage, blood disorders (anemia), liver and kidney damage, and infertility and is linked with the aging process. The richest dietary sources are wheat germ, soybean, cottonseed, peanut, and corn oils, margarine, whole raw seeds and nuts, soybeans, eggs, butter, liver, sweet potatoes, and the leaves of many vegetables, as turnip greens. It is stored in the body for long periods of time so that severe lack is rare. It is considered harmless except in patients with high blood pressure and those with long-term rheumatic heart disease. Also called **tocopherol.**

vitamin H. See **biotin.**

vitamin K, a group of vitamins that are needed to help the liver work properly and to help the blood to clot. The vitamin is widely distributed in foods, especially leafy green vegetables, pork liver, yogurt, egg yolk, kelp, alfalfa, fish-liver oils, and blackstrap molasses and is made by bacteria in the intestines. It can also be made artificially. A lack of this vitamin is marked by blood disorders. It is used to reduce the clotting time in patients with some types of jaundice and in certain kinds of bleeding linked with some diseases of the intestines and liver. It is given to infants to protect against a bleeding disease of the newborn. A form of the vitamin is used to preserve food. Natural vitamin K is stored in the body and produces no poisons. Very large doses of artificial vitamin K may cause anemia in newborn infants and hemolysis in patients with glucose-6-phosphate deficiency. See also **vitamin K_1, vitamin K_2, menadione.**

vitamin K_1, a vitamin occurring naturally, especially in alfalfa, and synthetically. It is used to help in the clotting of the blood. Also called **phylloquinone, phytonadione.**

vitamin K_2, a vitamin of the vitamin K group that is slightly weaker than vitamin K. It is found in fish meal and made by various bacteria in the intestines. See also **vitamin K.**

vitamin K_3. See **menadione.**

vitaminology /vī'təminol'əjē/, the study of vitamins, including their structures, the way they work, and the way they keep the body healthy.

vitamin P. See **bioflavonoid.**

vitellin /vitel'in/, a phosphoprotein containing lecithin, found in the yolk of eggs. Also called **ovovitellin. –vitelline** /-ēn/,*adj.*

vitelline artery, any of the simple arteries that carry blood from the primitive aorta of the early developing egg to the yolk sac. Also called **omphalomesenteric artery.**

vitelline circulation, the flow of blood and nutrients between the developing embryo and the yolk sac by way of the vitelline arteries and veins. Also called **omphalomesenteric circulation.** See also **fetal circulation.**

vitelline duct, (in embryology) the narrow channel connecting the yolk sac with the intestine. Also called **umbilical duct.**

vitelline membrane, the delicate membrane surrounding the egg (ovum). Also called **yolk membrane.** See also **zona pellucida.**

vitelline sac. See **yolk sac.**

vitelline sphere. See **morula.**

vitelline vein, any of the simple veins that return blood from the yolk sac to the primitive heart of the early developing embryo. Also called **omphalomesenteric vein.**

vitellogenesis /vitel'ōjen'əsis/, the formation of yolk. **–vitellogenetic,** *adj.*

vitellus /vitel'əs, vī-/, the yolk of an egg (ovum).

vitiligo /vit'ilē'gō/, a harmless skin disease of unknown cause, having uneven patches of various sizes totally lacking in color and often having very colorful borders. Exposed areas of skin are most often affected. Waterproof makeup is often used to cover the patches. Compare **albinism, piebald. –vitiliginous,** *adj.*

vitreous body. See **vitreous humor.**

vitreous cavity, the space behind the lens of the eyes that contains the vitreous body and vitreous membrane.

vitreous hemorrhage, bleeding into the vitreous humor of the eye.

vitreous humor, a clear, jellylike substance contained in a thin membrane filling the space behind the crystal-like lens of the eye. Also called **corpus vitreum, vitreous body.**

vitreous membrane, a membrane that lines the rear space of the eye and surrounds the vitreous body.

vitriol, oil of. See **sulfuric acid.**

Vivactil, a trademark for a drug used to relieve depression (protriptyline hydrochloride).

vivax malaria. See **tertian malaria.**

viviparous /vivip'ərəs/, bearing live babies rather than laying eggs, as most mammals and some fishes and reptiles. Compare **oviparous, ovoviviparous.**

Vivonex, a trademark for a food supplement containing protein, carbohydrate, and fat.

VLDL, abbreviation for **very-low-density-lipoprotein.**

VMA, abbreviation for **vanillylmandelic acid.**

vocal cord, either of two strong bands of yellow stretchy tissue in the larynx held by membranes called vocal folds. Also called **true vocal cord, vocal ligament.** Compare **false vocal cord.**

vocal cord nodule, a small, swelling or fiber-like growth that develops on the vocal cords of people who always strain their voices. Also called **screamer's nodule, singer's nodule, teacher's nodule.** See also **chorditis.**

vocal cues, a category of communication that includes noises and sounds but not words. Also called **paralinguistic cues.**

voice, the sounds of speech that are normally produced by vibration of the vocal folds of the voicebox (larynx).

voicebox. See **larynx.**

void, to empty, as urine from the bladder.

volar /vō'lər/, of or relating to the palm of the hand or the sole of the foot.

volar ligament. See **retinaculum flexorum manus.**

Volkmann's canal /fōlk'munz/, any one of the small blood vessel canals connecting haversian canals in bone tissue. Compare **haversian canaliculus.** See also **haversian system.**

Volkmann's contracture, a serious, continuous flexing of the forearm and hand caused by ischemia. A pressure or crushing injury in the region of the elbow usually causes this condition, and pressure from a cast or tight bandage about the elbow is also a common cause. Permanent fibrosis, muscle degeneration, and a clawlike hand may result. Also called **ischemic contracture.**

Volkmann's splint, a splint that supports and prevents movement of the lower leg. It has a footpiece attached to two sides that extends from the foot to the knee, allowing the patient to walk.

volsella forceps /volsel'ə/, a kind of forceps having a small, sharp-pointed hook at the end of each blade. Also called **volsella, volsellum forceps, vulsella forceps.**

volume, the amount of space taken up by a body, given in cubic units.

volume dose. See **integral dose.**

volumetric flow rate, the rate at which a volume of fluid flows past a designated point, usually measured in liters per second.

voluntary, referring to an action or thought that is under the patient's control.

voluntary abortion. See **elective abortion.**

voluntary muscle. See **striated muscle.**

volvulus /vol'vyŏōləs/, a twisting of the bowel on itself, causing intestinal blockage. If it is not corrected, the blocked bowel becomes damaged and death may follow. Severe, gripping pain, nausea and vomiting, a lack of bowel sounds, and tense, bloated intestines are symptoms. X-ray tests are used to find the problem. Compare **intussusception.**

volvulus neonatorum, a blocking of the intestines in a newborn baby resulting from a twisting of the bowel caused by a twisting or other complication of the colon. Typical symptoms include bloating of the intestines, continuous vomiting, and constipation. The condition needs immediate surgery to fix the problem.

vomer /vō'mər/, the bone forming the front and lower part of the nasal septum and having two surfaces and four borders.

vomit, 1. to force out the contents of the stomach through the esophagus and out of the mouth. **2.** also called **emesis, vomitus. the material expelled.**

von Economo's encephalitis. See **epidemic encephalitis.**

von Gierke's disease /fôngir'kəz/, a disease in which very large amounts of glycogen are stored in the liver and kidneys. The disorder is marked by hypoglycemia, ketoacidosis, and hyperlipemia. There is no cure for the disorder. It is treated by preventing hypoglycemia and ketoacidosis. Also called **glycogen storage disease, type I.** See also **glycogen storage disease.**

von Hippel-Lindau disease. See **cerebroretinal angiomatosis.**

von Pirquet test. See **Pirquet test.**

von Recklinghausen's disease. See **neurofibromatosis.**

von Willebrand's disease, an inherited disorder marked by abnormally slow clotting of the blood and sudden nose bleeds and bleeding gums. Excessive bleeding is common after giving birth, during menstruation, and after injury or surgery. Also called **angiohemophilia.** See also **hemophilia, thrombasthenia.**

vox /voks/, voice, as **vox cholerica,** the hard-to-hear, hoarse voice of a patient in an advanced and severe case of cholera.

voyeur /voiyur', vô·äyœr'/, one whose sexual satisfaction is obtained by the practice of voyeurism. Also called **Peeping Tom.**

voyeurism /voi'yəriz'əm, voiyur'izəm/, a mental and sexual disorder in which a person gets sexual excitement and satisfaction from looking at the naked bodies and genitals or seeing the sexual acts of others, especially from a hiding place.

VP-L-asparaginase, an anticancer drug combination of vincristine, prednisone, and asparaginase.

VSD, abbreviation for **ventricular septal defect.**

vulnerable, being in a dangerous position or condition and thereby susceptible to being infected or injured.

vulnerable period, a short period in the heart cycle during which action may result in irregular heartbeat.

vulsella forceps. See **volsella forceps.**

vulva. See **pudendum.**

vulvar /vul′vər/,   of or relating to the vulva.

vulvectomy /vəlvek′təmē/,   removing by surgery of part or all of the tissues of the vulva, done most often in treating cancerous or precancerous disease. **Simple vulvectomy** includes the removal of the skin of the labia minora, the labia majora, and the clitoris. **Radical vulvectomy** involves removing the labia majora, labia minora, clitoris, surrounding tissues, and pelvic lymph nodes.

vulvocrural /vul′vōkrŏŏr′əl/,   of or relating to the vulva and the thigh.

vulvovaginal /vul′vōvaj′inəl/,   of or relating to the vulva and the vagina.

vulvovaginitis /vul′vōvaj′inī′tis/,   a swelling of the vulva and vagina, or of the vulvovaginal glands.

VZV,   abbreviation for **varicella zoster virus.**

W

Wagner-Meissner corpuscle /wag′nərmīs′nər/, one of a number of small sensory end organs. It is sensitive to pressure. It can be found on the hand and foot, the front of the forearm, the skin of the lips, and the mucous membrane of the tongue. Also called **tactile corpuscle of Meissner.** Compare **Golgi-Mazzoni corpuscles, Krause's corpuscles.**

Wagstaffe's fracture /wag′stafs/, a fracture marked by separation of the inner malleolus.

waking imagined analgesia (WIA), the pain relief felt by a patient who uses this psychological technique. The technique is made up of concentrating on previous pleasant experiences that gave tranquillity, as lying on a summer beach beside cooling ocean water or drifting down a quiet river in a canoe. The technique is usually done with the help of a nurse or hospital aide. The patient using the WIA technique is encouraged to talk about experiences. This strengthens remembering the pleasant experiences, resulting in relaxation. This technique is often effective in reducing mild to moderate pain, especially when used with a mild pain reliever. See also **pain evaluation, pain intervention, pain mechanism.**

Waldenström's disease. See **Perthes' disease.**

Waldeyer's ring, the tonsils that surround the throat.

walker, a very light, movable apparatus, about waist high, made of metal tubing, used to help a patient in walking. It has four widely placed, sturdy legs. The patient holds onto the walker. He or she takes a step, then moves the walker forward and takes another step. Compare **crutch.**

walking belt, a leather or nylon device with handles that allows a health-care provider to help a patient walk.

walking heel, a plastic or rubber heel placed in the sole of a leg cast to allow weight to be put on it.

walking pneumonia. See **mycoplasma pneumonia.**

walking rounds, rounds in which the doctor responsible leads a group of interns and medical students on a tour to visit the patients for whom they are all responsible. In some hospitals, nurses may join in walking rounds.

wall, a structure within the body that closes a space, as the wall of the stomach or the wall of a cell.

wallerian degeneration, the fatty breakdown of a nerve fiber after it has been cut off from its cell body.

wander, 1. to move about without purpose. **2.** to cause to move back and forth in a searching manner. For example, in inserting a catheter in the uterus, the tip of the inserter must usually be wandered around the fetal head in the narrow lower end of the uterus (cervix) to find a space through which the catheter may be passed upward into the uterus.

wandering goiter. See **diving goiter.**

Wangensteen apparatus /wang′ənsten/, a catheter and a suction apparatus. It is used for constant, gentle drainage and pressure relief of the stomach or first part of the small intestines (duodenum). It may be used to relieve stomach bloating that often occurs after an operation or that may complicate a stomach and intestinal disorder, especially a blocked intestine. See also **Wangensteen tube.**

Wangensteen tube, the catheter portion of a Wangensteen apparatus.

ward, a hospital room made and equipped to house more than four patients.

warfarin poisoning, a toxic condition caused by swallowing warfarin. The poison results in nosebleed, bruising, blood in the urine, stools with blood (melena), and inner bleeding. Treatment may include gastric lavage, a cathartic, vitamin K, and blood transfusion. The goal of therapy is to destroy the poison and to restore normal clot formation.

warfarin sodium, a drug that acts to prevent clot formation. It is given to prevent and treat thrombosis and embolism.

★CAUTION: Bleeding or known allergy to this drug prohibits its use.

★ADVERSE EFFECTS: The most serious side effect is bleeding. Many other drugs interact with this drug to increase or decrease its effects.

warm-blooded, having a high and constant body temperature, as the temperatures kept by humans, other mammals, and birds, despite changes in outside temperatures. Heat is made in the warm-blooded human body by the breakdown of foods. About 80%of the body heat that is lost in humans is lost through the skin. The rest is lost through the mucous membranes of the breathing, the digestive, and the urinary systems. The average temperature of the healthy human is 98.6° F (37° C). The human body's acceptance of change in its temperature is very small. Important changes can have drastic, even deadly results. The control mechanism for temperature in the human body is made up of heat receptive neurons in the front part of the hypothalamus, more than 2 million sweat glands, and the vast network of blood vessels in the skin. Fever, which raises internal body temperature, temporarily changes the control of the hypothalamus by the action of bacteria and viruses. The temperature control mechanisms of the body serve to restore normal heat levels during fever. Also called **homoiothermal, homothermal.** Compare **cold-blooded.**

war neurosis. See **combat fatigue, shell shock.**

wart. See **verruca.**

Warthin's tumor. See **papillary adenocystoma lymphomatosum.**

washout, the destruction or removal of one gas or volatile anesthetic drug by giving another.

wasp, a slender, narrow-waisted insect with two pairs of wings that are folded lengthwise when at rest like parts of a fan. Many species of wasps may give painful stings. They may have severe results in allergic persons. Treatment is as for bee stings.

Wassermann test /was'ərmən, vos'ərmun/, a diagnostic blood test for syphilis.

wasted ventilation, the amount of air provided to the parts of the breathing system that are not involved in the exchange of oxygen and carbon dioxide.

wasting, a process of breakdown marked by weight loss and decreased physical vigor, appetite, and mental activity.

watchfulness, continuous supervision provided either openly or secretly as the situation requires.

water (H₂O), a chemical compound. A molecule of water has one atom of oxygen and two atoms of hydrogen. Almost three-quarters of the earth's surface is covered by water. Water is essential to life as it exists on this planet. It comprises more than 70% of living things. Pure water freezes at 0° C (32° F). It boils at 100° C (212° F) at sea level.

waterborne, carried by water, as a waterborne epidemic of typhoid fever.

water-hammer pulse, a pulse associated with blood forced back out of the aorta. It is characterized by a full, forcible impulse and immediate collapse, causing a jerking sensation.

Waterhouse-Friderichsen syndrome /wô'tərhous'frid'ərik'sən/,a large amount of bacteria in the blood (bacteremia). It is marked by the sudden beginning of fever, bluish discoloring of the skin (cyanosis), small red spots (petechiae), and collapse from massive bleeding. The syndrome requires immediate emergency treatment, hospitalization, and intensive care. Emergency treatment includes drugs that contract the muscular tissue of the capillaries and arteries (vasopressor drugs), fluids given in the vein, plasma, and oxygen. No sedatives or narcotics are given. Specific treatment for bacteremia is intensive antibiotic therapy, given after symptoms lessen.

water intoxication, an increase in the volume of free water in the body. This results in a lack of salt.

water moccasin. See **cottonmouth.**

water pollution, the contamination of lakes, rivers, and streams by industrial or community sources of pollutants.

waters. See **amniotic fluid.**

water trap. See **underwater seal.**

wax. See **cerumen.**

wax bath. See **paraffin bath.**

waxy flexibility. See **cerea flexibilitas.**

WBC, abbreviation for **white blood cell.** See **leukocyte.**

W/D, abbreviation for *well developed.* It is often used in the patient record to describe the patient's physical appearance.

wean, 1. to make a child give up breast-feeding and to accept other food. Many children are ready for weaning during the second half of the first year. Some wean themselves. **2.** to take from a patient something on which he or she is dependent.

weanling, a child who has just been weaned.

wear-and-tear theory, a concept of the aging process in which changes in the body's structure and function that are associated with growing old are accelerated by abuse of the body and slowed down with health care.

weaver's bottom, a form of swelling of the bursae in the hip. It is found among patients whose work involves sitting for a long time in one position. Also called *(obsolete)* **tailor's bottom.**

web, a network of fibers forming a tissue or a membrane, as the laryngeal web that spreads between the vocal cords.

webbing, skinfolds connecting structures next to each other as fingers or toes, associated with genetic abnormalities.

Weber's tuning fork test, a method of testing hearing. The test is done by placing the stem of a vibrating 256 Hz tuning fork in the center of the person's forehead or on the jaw. The loudness of the sound is equal in both ears if hearing is normal. If the person has a sensory mechanism loss in one ear, the good ear hears the sound as louder. When hearing loss caused by a defect in the sound-conducting apparatus is present, the sound is louder in the affected ear.

web of causation, an interrelationship of many factors that cause a disease.

webril, trademark for a stretchable cotton material applied over the skin to protect from plaster irritation.

Wechsler intelligence scales, a series of standardized tests made to measure the intelligence at several age levels. It is done by means of questions that examine general information, arrangement of pictures and objects, vocabulary, memory, reasoning, and other abilities.

wedge fracture, a fracture of vertebral structures with frontal pressure.

wedge pressure, the capillary pressure in the left upper heart chamber (atrium). It is determined by measuring the pressure in a cardiac catheter wedged in the most remote segment of the pulmonary artery.

wedge resection, the surgical removal of part of an organ. The segment taken away may be wedge-shaped.

WEE, abbreviation for **western equine encephalitis.** See **equine encephalitis.**

weed. See **cannabis.**

weeping, **1.** crying. **2.** slow flowing fluid, as a sore or rash.

Wegener's granulomatosis /wā'gənərz/, an uncommon, long-term swelling process leading to tumorlike masses in the air passages, the death of vessels (necrotizing vasculitis), and serious kidney disease (glomerulonephritis). Symptoms depend on the organs involved. They may include sinus pain, a bloody nasal discharge with pus, saddle-nose deformity, chest discomfort and cough, weakness, loss of appetite, weight loss, and skin injury. Glomerulonephritis, as a problem, used to lead to death within a few months. However, with the use of cytotoxic drugs, especially cyclophosphamide, a high percentage of patients achieve long-term remissions.

weight holder, a metal, T-shaped bar that holds weights for traction.

Weil's disease. See **leptospirosis.**

weismannism /vīs'muniz'əm/, the basic concepts of heredity and development as proposed by the German biologist August Weismann. Also called **weismann's theory, germ plasm theory.** Compare **pangenesis.** –**weismannian,** *adj., n.*

Weiss' sign. See **Chvostek's sign.**

well baby care, regular health care for infants and children to promote the best possible physical, emotional, and intellectual growth and development. Such health-care measures include routine vaccinations and screening procedures for early detection and treatment of illness. Parental guidance and instruction in proper nutrition, accident prevention, and specific care and rearing of the child at various stages of growth are other measures to be taken. The advised preventive health-care schedule for children who are growing normally is monthly for the first 6 months of life, every 2 months until 1 year of age, every 3 months during the second year, and every 6 months during the third year. It must be followed by yearly visits. Well baby care may be given in a clinic, a convenient local meeting place, a private doctor's office, the office of a community health nursing service, or a school. Nurses or nurse practitioners often give the care.

well baby clinic, a clinic that specializes in medical supervision and services for healthy infants.

well-being, achievement of a good existence as defined by the individual.

well-differentiated lymphocytic malignant lymphoma, a tumor of the lymph glands with a predominance of mature lymphocytes. Also called **lymphocytic lymphoma, lymphocytic lymphosarcoma, lymphocytoma.**

wellness, a dynamic state of health in which an individual grows toward a higher level of functioning, having an optimum balance between inner and outer environments.

wen. See **pilar cyst.**

Wenckebach heart block. See **Mobitz I heart block.**

Wenckebach periodicity, a form of a partial (second-degree) block at the atrioventricular junction. Also called **Mobitz I, Type I block, Wenckebach phenomenon.** See also **atrioventricular block.**

Werdnig-Hoffmann disease /verd'nighôf'mun/, a genetic disorder beginning in infancy or young childhood. It is marked by a growing wasting away of the skeletal muscles. It results from a breakdown of the cells in the front horn of the spinal cord and the motor nuclei in the brain stem. The beginning occurs within the first year of life. The condition is usually visible at birth. Symptoms include inborn lessened tone of the skeletal muscles at birth (hypotonia), absence of stretch reflexes, and paralysis, especially of the trunk and limbs. Lack of sucking ability, involuntary contractions (fasciculations) of the tongue and sometimes of other muscles, and, often, speech problems are other symptoms. Treatment depends on the symptoms. Death generally occurs in early childhood, often from breathing problems. The condition is carried as a sex-independent recessive trait. It occurs more often in siblings than in successive generations. Also called **familial spinal muscular atrophy, Hoffmann's atrophy, infantile spinal muscular atrophy, progressive spinal muscular atrophy of infants, Werdnig-Hoffmann paralysis.** See also **floppy infant syndrome.**

Werlhof's disease. See **thrombocytopenic purpura.**

Wernicke's encephalopathy /ver'nikēz/, a swelling, bleeding, degenerative condition of the brain. It is marked by tumors in several parts of the brain including the hypothalamus, mammillary bodies, and tissues surrounding ventricles and aqueducts. The condition is marked by double vision, involuntary and rapid movements of the eyes, lack of muscular coordination, and decreased mental function, which may be mild or severe. Wernicke's encephalopathy is caused by a lack of thiamine. It is linked to long-term alcoholism. It also occurs as a problem linked to stomach and intestinal disease. Excessive vomiting (hyperemesis gravidarum) linked to malabsorption and bad health is another cause.

West African sleeping sickness. See **Gambian trypanosomiasis.**

Westermark's sign, the absence of blood vessel markings beyond the location of a blockage of a lung artery as seen on an x-ray.

Western blot test, a laboratory blood test to detect the presence of antibodies to specific foreign substances (antigens). It is regarded as more accurate than the enzyme-linked immunoabsorbent assay (ELISA) and is sometimes used to check the accuracy of ELISA tests.

western equine encephalitis. See **equine encephalitis.**

West nomogram, a nomogram used in estimating the body surface area. See also **nomogram.**

wet cough. See **productive cough.**

wet dream. See **nocturnal emission.**

wet dressing, a moist dressing used to treat some skin diseases. As the moisture evaporates, it cools and dries the skin, softens dried blood and sera, and stimulates drainage. Drugs may be added if necessary.

wet lung, an abnormal condition of the lungs. It is marked by a persistent cough at the lung bases. It occurs in workers exposed to lung irritants, as ammonia, chlorine, sulfur dioxide, organic acids that evaporate, dusts, and vapors of corrosive chemicals. Treatment is made up of removing the person from expo sure to the irritant. Therapy for possible pulmonary edema is given. Compare **pulmonary edema.** See also **pleural effusion, pleurisy.**

wet nurse, a woman who cares for and breast feeds another's infant.

wetting agent, a detergent, as tyloxapol, used to dissolve mucous in breathing therapy.

W/F, symbol for *white female*. It is often used in the first identifying statement in a patient record.

Wharton's jelly, a soft, jellylike substance of the umbilical cord.

wheal /wēl/, an individual patch of itchy skin, as in hives.

wheat weevil disease, an allergic swelling of lung tissue (pneumonitis). It is caused by allergy to weevil particles found in wheat flour.

wheelchair, a mobile chair with large wheels and brakes. If long-term use of the chair is expected, a physical therapist may advise certain personalized requirements, as size, left- or right-hand propulsion, type of brakes, height of armrests, and special seat pads.

wheeze, **1.** a form of rattling in the throat. It is marked by a high-pitched musical quality. It is caused by a high velocity flow of air through a narrowed airway. It is heard both during breathing in and out. Wheezes are linked to asthma and long-term swelling of the bronchi.

Unilateral wheezes are characteristic of cancer of the bronchi, and the presence of foreign bodies. An asthmatoid wheeze is caused by blockage in the trachea or bronchus. **2.** to breathe with a wheeze. See also **rale, rhonchi.**

whiplash injury, *informal.* an injury to the cervical vertebrae or their supporting ligaments and muscles. It is marked by pain and stiffness. It usually results from sudden speeding or slowing down, as in a rear-end car collision that causes a violent back-and-forth movement of the head and neck.

Whipple's disease, a rare intestinal disease. It is marked by severe intestinal malabsorption, excess fat in feces (steatorrhea), anemia, weight loss, swelling of a joint (arthritis), and pain in a joint (arthralgia). Patients with the disease are in bad health. They also have stomach and intestinal pain, chest pain, and a long-term nonproductive cough. The diagnosis is made by a biopsy of the small intestine (jejunal biopsy). Penicillin and tetracycline may relieve the symptoms. See also **malabsorption syndrome.**

whipworm. See *Trichuris.*

whirlpool bath, putting the body or a part of the body in a tank of hot water moved by a jet of equal amounts of hot water and air.

whispered pectoriloquy, the transmission of a whisper through the breathing structures so that it is heard as normal speech through a stethoscope.

white blood cell. See **leukocyte.**

white cell, *informal.* white blood cell. See also **leukocyte.**

white corpuscle. See **leukocyte.**

white damp. See **damp.**

white fibrocartilage, a mixture of tough, white fiberlike tissue and flexible cartilaginous tissue. It is divided into four types: interarticular fibrocartilage, connecting fibrocartilage, circumferential fibrocartilage, and stratiform fibrocartilage. Compare **hyaline cartilage, yellow cartilage.**

white gold, a gold alloy with a high content of palladium or platinum. It is used in some dental restorations, as prepared tooth cavities and gold crowns. It has a higher fusion range, lower stretching range, and greater hardness than a yellow gold alloy.

whitehead. See **milia.**

white leg. See **phlegmasia alba dolens.**

white matter. See **white substance.**

white radiation, a form of radiation that results from the rapid slowdown of high-speed electrons striking a target. Most of the x-rays emitted from a diagnostic or therapeutic x-ray unit represent white radiation. Also called **braking radiation, bremsstrahlung.**

white substance, the tissue surrounding the gray substance of the spinal cord. It is made up mainly of sheathed nerve fibers, but with some unsheathed nerve fibers. It is subdivided in each half of the spinal cord into three parts (funiculi): the anterior, the posterior, and the lateral white column. Also called **white matter.** Compare **gray substance.** See also **spinal cord, spinal tract.**

white thrombus, **1.** a gathering of blood platelets, fibrin, clotting factors, and cell elements with few or no erythrocytes. **2.** a thrombus with chiefly white blood cells. **3.** a thrombus with primarily blood platelets and fibrin.

whitlow /wit'lō, hwit'lō/, a swelling of the end of a finger or toe that results in pus. See also **felon.**

WHO, abbreviation for **World Health Organization.**

whole blood, blood that is unchanged except for the presence of a drug that prevents clotting of the blood. It is used for transfusion.

whole body hyperthermia. See **systemic heating.**

whoop, a noisy spasm on inhaling after a fit of coughing in cases of whooping cough (pertussis). It is caused by a sudden, sharp increase in tension on the vocal cords.

whooping cough. See **pertussis.**

whorl /wurl, hwurl/, a spiral turn, as one of the turns of ridges that form fingerprints.

WIA, abbreviation for **waking imagined analgesia.**

wick humidifier, a respiratory-care device in which a piece of paper, sponge, or other material that absorbs water is put in the path of air flow. With the addition of heat, high levels of water vapor in the air (humidity) can be achieved over a wide range of flows and temperatures.

Widal's test /vēdäls'/, a test used to aid in the diagnosis of salmonella infections, as typhoid fever.

wide-angle glaucoma. See **glaucoma.**

Wigraine, a trademark for a drug with a substance that blocks the passage of impulses through the parasympathetic nerves (belladonna alkaloids), and a painkiller (phenacetin). It also has a substance that contracts the blood vessels (ergotamine tartrate). It is used to treat migraine.

wild-type gene, a normal or standard form of a gene, as opposed to a mutant form.

will, **1.** the mental faculty that enables one consciously to choose or decide on a course of action. **2.** the act or process of using the power of choice. **3.** a wish, desire, or conscious intention. **4.** a disposition or attitude toward another or others. **5.** determination or purpose; willfulness. **6.** (in law) an expression or declaration of a person's wishes as to the use of property, taking effect after death.

Willis' circle. See **circle of Willis.**

Willis' disease. See **diabetes mellitus.**

willow fracture. See **greenstick fracture.**

Wilms' tumor /vilms/, a cancerous tumor of the kidney. It occurs in young children, before the fifth year in 75% of the cases. The common early sign of this large cancerous tumor of childhood is high blood pressure. It is followed by the appearance of a lump that can be felt, pain, and blood in the urine (hematuria). Diagnosis usually can be established by radiography of the urinary tract (excretory urogram) and part of the body. The tumor is well enclosed in the early stage. It may later extend into lymph nodes and other sites. Prompt removal of the tumors is recommended. Radiotherapy is used before or after surgery. Chemotherapy along with surgery and irradiation is proving highly effective.

Wilson's disease, a rare, inherited disorder of copper processing. Copper comes slowly together in the liver. It is then released and taken up in other parts of the body. A blood disease (hemolytic anemia) occurs as the copper pools in the red blood cells. Pooling in the brain destroys certain tissues. It may cause tremors, muscle rigidity, speech problems (dysarthria), and dementia. Kidney function is diminished. The liver becomes swollen. Treatment of Wilson's disease includes lessening copper in the diet and giving copper-binding agents and penicillamine. Also called **hepatolenticular degeneration.**

Winckel's disease. See **hemoglobinuria.**

wind chill, the loss of heat from the body when it is exposed to wind of a given speed at a given temperature and humidity. The **wind chill index** is given in kilocalories per hour per square meter of skin surface. The **wind chill factor** is given in degrees Celsius or Fahrenheit as the real temperature felt by a person exposed to the weather.

winding sheet, a shroud for wrapping a dead body.

windkessel effect /wind'kes'əl/, the stretching of the aorta during a contraction of the heart (systole) to accommodate the volume of blood ejected. Energy that was stored pushes this volume into the peripheral artery tree during the widening of the heart (diastole).

window, a surgically created opening in the surface of a structure or an existing opening in the surface or between the chambers of a structure. **2.** a specific time period during which an event can be observed, a reaction monitored, or a procedure started.

windowed, (of an orthopedic cast) having an opening, as to relieve pressure that may irritate and swell the skin.

winged scapula, an outward projection of the shoulder blade caused by nerve damage or muscle weakness.

Winstrol, a trademark for a drug that stimulates male characteristics (stanozolol). It is used as an anabolic drug.

winter cough, *nontechnical.* a long-term condition with a persistent cough caused by cold weather. See also **cough.**

wintergreen oil. See **methyl salicylate.**

winter itch, itching occurring in cold weather in people who have dry skin, particularly in those who have long-term inflammation of the skin (atopic dermatitis). Warmer temperature, increased humidity, and soothing drugs on the skin may offer relief.

wiry pulse, an abnormal pulse that is strong but small.

wisdom tooth, either of the last teeth on each side of the upper and lower jaw. These are the last teeth to come out. This usually happens between 17 and 21 years of age. It often causes considerable pain, dental problems, and the need for pulling out the tooth. Also called **dens serotinus.** See also **molar.**

wish fulfillment, 1. the fulfillment of a desire. 2. (in psychology) the satisfaction of a desire or the release of emotional tension through dreams, daydreams, and neurotic symptoms. 3. (in psychoanalysis) one of the main motivations for dreams in which an unconscious desire or urge is expressed. The desire or urge is unacceptable to the ego and superego because of sociocultural restrictions or feelings of personal guilt.

wishful thinking, the viewing of facts or situations according to one's desires or wishes rather than as they exist in reality. It is usually used as an unconscious device to avoid painful or unpleasant feelings.

Wiskott-Aldrich syndrome /wis'kotôl'drich/, a disorder with a lack of resistance. It is inherited as a recessive, X-linked trait. It is marked by a blood disease (thrombocytopenia), a skin disease (eczema), and an increased susceptibility to viral, bacterial, and fungal infections and to cancer. Treatment includes appropriate antibiotics for specific infectious organisms. It also includes the use of transfer factor from activated lymphocytes to increase the resistance to infection and to clear the eczema. See also **transfer factor.**

witch hazel, 1. a shrub, *Hamamelis virginiana,* native to North America, from which an astringent extract is derived. 2. also called **hamamelis water.** a solution with the extract, alcohol, and water, used as a contraction drug (astringent).

witch's milk, a milklike substance released from the breast of the newborn. It is caused by circulating maternal lactating hormone. Also called **hexenmilch** /hek'-sənmilsh'/.

withdrawal, a common response to physical danger or severe stress. It is marked by a state of apathy, weakness, depression, and retreat into oneself. Catatonic schizophrenia and stupor may occur in severe cases. It is a disease if it hinders a person's view of reality and the ability to function in society, as in the various forms of schizophrenia. See also **schizophrenia.**

withdrawal behavior, the physical or mental removal of oneself from a stressful situation.

withdrawal bleeding, the passage of blood from the uterus, linked to the shedding of the lining of the uterus (endometrium) that has been stimulated and maintained by hormonal drugs. It occurs when the drug is no longer given.

withdrawal method, a birth-control technique in which the penis is withdrawn from the vagina before ejaculation. It is not reliable because small amounts of sperm may be released without sensation before full ejaculation. Also called **coitus interruptus.**

withdrawal symptoms, the unpleasant, sometimes life-threatening bodily changes that occur when some drugs are withdrawn after long-term, regular use. The effects may occur after use of a narcotic, tranquilizer, stimulant, barbiturate, alcohol, or other substance on which the person has become bodily or mentally dependent.

withdrawn behavior, a condition in which there is a blunting of the emotions and a lack of social responsiveness.

witness, a person who is present and can testify that he or she has personally observed an event, as the signing of a will or consent form.

Wittmaack-Ekbom syndrome. See **restless legs syndrome.**

W/M, symbol for *white male.* It is often used in the first identifying statement in a patient record.

W/N, symbol for *well nourished.* It is often used in the first identifying statement in a patient record to describe the patient's nutritional state.

Wolff-Chaikoff effect, the lessened formation and release of thyroid hormone in the presence of an excess of iodine.

wolffian body. See **mesonephros.**

wolffian duct. See **mesonephric duct.**

Wolff-Parkinson-White syndrome /wôlf'pär'kin-sənwit'/, a disorder of atrioventricular conduction. It is marked by two atrioventricular conduction pathways. This syndrome can be diagnosed by an electrocardiogram. See also **Lown-Ganong-Levine syndrome.**

wolfram. See **tungsten.**

Wolman's disease. See **cholesteryl ester storage disease.**

woman-year, (in statistics) 1 year in the reproductive life of a sexually active woman. A unit that represents 12 months of exposure to the risk of pregnancy. Woman-years are used in determining the pregnancy rate of the various methods of family planning. They are also used in determining the negative effect on the birth rate of many environmental factors.

womb. See **uterus.**

wood alcohol. See **methanol.**

Wood's glass, a nickel oxide filter that holds back all light except for a few violet rays of the visible spectrum and ultraviolet wavelengths of about 365 nm. It is used widely to help diagnose fungus infections of the scalp and other skin infections.

Wood's light, an ultraviolet light of about 365 nm wavelength used to diagnose certain scalp and skin diseases. The light causes hairs infected with a fungus, as *tinea capitis,* to become brilliantly fluorescent. Also called **Wood's lamp, Wood's rays.**

wool fat, a fatty substance obtained from sheep's wool, which contains lanolin. It consists primarily of cholesterol and its alcohol and organic acid groups (esters).

woolsorter's disease, anthrax of the lungs. It is so named because it is a work hazard to those who handle sheep's wool. Early symptoms look like influenza. However, the patient soon develops high fever, breathing distress, and a blood disease with bluish skin (cyanosis). If the disease is not treated at this point, it often leads to death. Also called **pulmonary anthrax.** See also **anthrax.**

word association. See **controlled association.**

word association test. See **association test.**

word length, the number of bits composing a word, or unit of computer data.

word salad, a jumble of words and phrases that lacks coherence and meaning. It is often seen in disoriented individuals and schizophrenics.

working occlusion, the closing contacts of teeth on the side of the jaw toward which the lower jaw (mandible) is moved.

working phase, (in psychology) the second stage of the nurse-patient relationship in which patients explore their experiences. Nurses assist by helping patients to describe and make clear their experiences, to plan courses of action and try out the plans, and to begin to evaluate the effectiveness of their new behavior. Should new behavior prove ineffective, nurses can assist patients in revising their courses of action.

working pressure, a recommended beginning pressure of about 50 pounds per square inch, gauge (psig) for oxygen or compressed air leaving a cylinder for use in respiratory therapy.

working through, a process by which hidden feelings are released and again made a part of the personality.

work of worrying, a coping strategy in which worrying in anticipation increases the ability to withstand threats that follow.

work therapy, an approach in which the client does a useful activity or learns a job.

work tolerance, the kind and amount of work that a physically or mentally ill person can or should do.

work-up, the process of making a complete evaluation of a patient, including history, physical examination, laboratory tests, and x-ray or other diagnostic techniques. The purpose is to get the facts on which a diagnosis and treatment plan may be established.

World Health Organization (WHO), an agency of the United Nations. It is connected to the Food and Agricultural Organization of the United Nations, the International Atomic Energy Agency, the International Labor Organization, the Pan American Health Organization, and UNESCO. The WHO is mainly concerned with worldwide or regional health problems. However, in emergencies it may give local assistance on request. Its tasks include offering technical assistance, advancing an investigation of diseases, recommending health regulations, and promoting cooperation among scientific and professional health groups. Providing information and counsel relating to health matters is one of its other tasks. Its headquarters are in Geneva, Switzerland. Its French name is **Organisation Mondiale de la Santé** /ôrgänizäsyôN′ môNdē·äl′ dələ säNtä′/ **(OMS).**

worm, any of the soft-bodied, long boneless animals of the phyla Annelida, Nemathelminthes, or Platyhelminthes. Some kinds of worms parasitic for humans are **hookworm, pinworm,** and **tapeworm.** See also **fluke, roundworm.**

wormian bone /vôr′mē·ən/, any of several tiny, smooth, segmented bones. They are soft, moist, and lukewarm to the touch. They are usually found as the sawlike borders of the joints between the skull bones. Wormian bones were named for the Danish anatomist Claus Worm.

worthlessness, feelings of uselessness and inability to contribute meaningfully to the well-being of others or to one's environment.

wound, 1. any physical injury involving a break in the skin. It is usually caused by an act or accident rather than by a disease, as a chest wound, gunshot wound, or puncture wound. 2. to cause an injury, especially one that breaks the skin.

wound irrigation, the cleansing of a wound or the cavity formed by a wound using a solution with drugs, water, or liquid substance that suppresses or kills the growth of microorganisms. The wound cover (dressing) is taken away and wrapped for disposal. The patient is helped into a position that will make the irrigation go easily. An irrigating solution is generally warmed to room temperature. An emesis or kidney basin is then fitted snugly against the patient's body beneath the wound. It may be held in place by the patient or by an assistant. A catheter is held with sterile gloves or forceps. It is then gently inserted into the wound to a certain depth and at a certain angle. A syringe filled with irrigating solution is then attached to the catheter. The solution is gently instilled. The syringe is filled again. The wound is irrigated until the returning solution runs clear. If a catheter is not used, the solution is sprayed directly on the wound from the syringe until the wound looks clean. After irrigation is completed, the body area is dried with sterile sponges working from the wound out to the area around it. A dry sterile dressing is applied. Wounds are irrigated to remove fluid and dried blood. Another purpose is to keep the wound surface open to encourage healing from the inside out. When the irrigation solution returns clear, the wound is clean.

wound repair, restoration of the normal structure after an injury, especially of the skin. See also **healing, intention.**

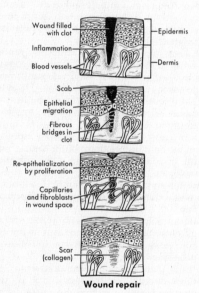

Wound repair

Wright's stain, a stain with methylene blue and eosin. It is used to color blood specimens for microscopic examination, as for complete blood count and, particularly, for malarial parasites.

wrinkle test, a test for nerve function in the hand by observing the presence of skin wrinkles after the hand has been placed in warm water for 20 to 30 minutes. Skin without a nerve supply does not wrinkle.

wrist. See **carpus.**

wrist joint. See **radiocarpal articulation.**

writer's cramp, a painful involuntary contraction of the muscles of the hand when attempting to write. It often occurs after long periods of writing. Also called **graphospasm.**

wrongful death statute, (in law) a statute existing in all states that says that the death of a person allows for legal action against the person whose willful or negligent acts caused the death. Before the existence of these statutes, a suit could be brought only if the injured person survived the injury.

wrongful life action, (in law) a civil suit usually brought against a physician or health facility on the basis of negligence that led to wrongful birth or life of an infant. The parents of the unwanted child seek to get payment from the defendant for the medical expenses of pregnancy and birth. They also seek to get payment for pain and suffering, and for the education and upbringing of the child. Wrongful life actions have been brought and won in several situations, including malpractice sterilizations (of both men and women), and abortions. Failure to diagnose pregnancy in time for abortion and incorrect medical advice leading to the birth of a defective child have also led to malpractice suits for a wrongful life.

wryneck. See **torticollis.**

Wucheria /vōō′kərē′rē·ə/, a genus of filarial worms found in warm, humid climates. *Wuchereria bancrofti* is carried by mosquitoes. It is the cause of elephantiasis. See also **filariasis.**

Wycillin, a trademark for an antibacterial (penicillin G procaine).

Wydase, a trademark for an enzyme (hyaluronidase).

Wymox, a trademark for an antibiotic (amoxicillin).

Wytensin, a trademark for drug used to fight high blood pressure (guanabenz).

Wyvac, a trademark for a rabies virus vaccine.

X

Xanax, a trademark for an antianxiety drug (alprazolam).

–xanox, a combining form for drugs of the xanoic acid group, which prevent allergic reactions in the lungs.

xanthelasma, xanthelasma palpebrarum. See **xanthoma palpebrarum.**

xanthelasmatosis /zan′thilaz′mətō′sis/, a skin disease with yellowish plaques. It is often linked to a plasma disease (multiple myeloma).

xanthemia. See **carotenemia.**

xanthine /zan′thēn/, a nitrogen byproduct of the processing of nucleoproteins. It is normally found in the muscles, liver, spleen, pancreas, and urine. **–xanthic,** *adj.*

xanthine derivative, any one of the closely linked alkaloids caffeine, theobromine, or theophylline. They are found in plants widely distributed geographically. They are consumed as components in different beverages, as coffee, tea, cocoa, and cola drinks. The xanthine derivatives or methylxanthines stimulate the central nervous system. They also promote urine release and relax smooth muscles. Theobromine has low potency. It is seldom used as a drug. Caffeine causes greater central nervous system stimulation than theophylline or theobromine. Some experiments have shown that caffeine increases the capacity for continuous intellectual effort, decreases reaction time, and improves the association of ideas. Caffeine and theophylline also affect the circulatory system. They relieve headaches caused by high blood pressure. The ability of the xanthine derivatives to relax smooth muscle is especially important in certain treatments of asthma. Theophylline is most effective in such treatments and markedly increases vital capacity. It is uncertain whether a large coffee consumption (five to six cups per day) promotes heart attack (myocardial infarction). Research continues to find out the effect of caffeine on pregnant women who use it in large amounts. Many studies show that the per capita consumption of caffeine in the United States is 200 mg daily, about 90%of which comes from coffee. One cup of coffee has about 100 mg of caffeine. One cup of tea contains about 50 mg of caffeine and 1 mg of theophylline. One cup of cocoa has about 250 mg of theobromine and 5 mg of caffeine. A 350 ml bottle of a cola beverage has about 35 mg of caffeine. Consumption of xanthine beverages may cause many problems, including restlessness and an inability to sleep, stomach and intestinal irritation, and excess heart stimulation.

xanthinuria /zan′thinyŏŏr′ē·ə/, **1.** the presence of excess quantities of xanthine in the urine. **2.** a rare disorder of purine processing. It results in the release of large amounts of xanthine in the urine because of the lack of an enzyme, xanthine oxidase, that is needed in xanthine processing. This inherited lack may cause the development of kidney stones made of xanthine precipitate.

xantho-, a combining form meaning 'yellow.'

xanthochromic /zan′thəkrō′mik/, having a yellowish color, as fluid of the brain and spine with blood or bile. Also **xanthochromatic.**

xanthochromia /zan′thəkrō′mē·ə/, a substance in the fluid of the brain and spine that accounts for its yellow color. It is caused by the presence of hemoglobin breakdown products.

xanthogranuloma /zan′thəgran′yŏŏlō′mə/, *pl.* **xanthogranulomas, xanthogranulomata,** a tumor or knot of granulated tissue with lipid deposits. A kind of xanthogranuloma is **juvenile xanthogranuloma.**

xanthoma /zanthō′mə/, *pl.* **xanthomas, xanthomata,** a harmless, fatty, fibrous, yellowish plaque, knot, or tumor that develops in the subcutaneous layer of skin, often around tendons. The plaques are marked by lipid deposits.

xanthoma disseminatum, a harmless, long-term condition in which small orange or brown knots grow on many body surfaces, especially on the mucous membrane of the throat, bronchi, and in skin folds. Also called **xanthoma multiplex.**

xanthoma eruptivum. See **eruptive xanthoma.**

xanthoma multiplex. See **xanthoma disseminatum.**

xanthoma palpebrarum, a soft, yellow spot or plaque usually occurring in groups on the eyelids. Also called **xanthelasma, xanthelasma palpebrarum.**

xanthoma planum. See **planar xanthoma.**

xanthomasarcoma /zan′thōməsärkō′mə/, *pl.* **xanthomasarcomas, xanthomasarcomata,** a tumor with xanthoma cells.

xanthoma striatum palmare, a yellow or orange flat plaque or slightly raised knot occurring in groups on the palms of the hands.

xanthoma tendinosum, a yellow or orange elevated or flat round knot occurring in groups on tendons. It is found in patients with hereditary lipid storage disease.

xanthomatosis /zan′thōmətō′sis/, an abnormal condition in which there are deposits of yellowish fatty material in the skin, internal organs, and reticuloendothelial system. It may be linked to excess lipoproteins in the blood (hyperlipoproteinemia), paraproteins in the blood (paraproteinemia), lipoid storage diseases, and other disorders of fatty tissue. Also called **xanthosis.** See also **lipemia, xanthoma, xanthoma palpebrarum.**

xanthoma tuberosum, a yellow or orange flat or elevated round knot occurring in clusters on the skin of joints, especially the elbows and knees. It occurs usually in patients who have a hereditary lipid storage disease, as excess lipoproteins in the blood (hyperlipoproteinemia). The knots may also be linked to swelling of the liver (biliary cirrhosis) and swelling of the face (myxedema). Also called **tuberous xanthoma, xanthoma tuberosum multiplex.**

xanthopsia /zanthop'sē·ə/, an abnormal visual condition in which everything appears to have a yellow hue. It is sometimes linked to liver disease (jaundice) or digitalis poisoning.

xanthosis /zanthō'sis/, **1.** a yellowish discoloration. It is sometimes seen in the wasting tissues of cancerous diseases. **2.** See **xanthomatosis. 3.** also called **carotenosis.** a changeable yellow discoloration of the skin. It is commonly caused by eating large amounts of yellow vegetables with carotene pigment. The antimalarial drug quinacrine, if taken over a long period, may produce a similar skin color. Xanthosis can be kept apart clinically from liver disease (jaundice) because the white outer coats of the eyeballs (sclerae) are colored yellow in jaundice but are not discolored in xanthosis. See also **carotenemia.**

xanthureic acid /zanth'yo͝orē'ik/, a processing product of tryptophan. It occurs in normal urine. It occurs in higher levels in patients with a lack of vitamin B_6.

X chromosome, a sex chromosome that in humans and many other species is present in both sexes. It appears singly in the cells of normal males and in duplicate in the cells of normal females. The chromosome is carried as a sex determinant by all of the female gametes and one-half of all male gametes. It has many sex-linked genes linked to important disorders, as hemophilia, Duchenne's muscular dystrophy, and Hunter's syndrome. Compare **Y chromosome.**

xeno-, a combining form meaning 'strange or referring to foreign matter.'

xenobiotic, referring to organic substances that are foreign to the body, as drugs or organic poisons.

xenogeneic, 1. (in genetics) referring to individuals or cell types from different species and different genotypes. **2.** (in transplantation biology) referring to tissues from different species. Also **heterologous.** Compare **allogenic, syngeneic.**

xenogenesis /zen'əjen'əsis/, **1.** a change of traits in successive generations; heterogene sis. **2.** the production of offspring that are totally different from both of the parents. **–xenogenetic, xenogenic,** *adj.*

xenograft /zen'əgraft'/, tissue from another species used as a temporary graft in certain cases. It is used in treating a severely burned patient when sufficient tissue from the patient or from a tissue bank is not available. It is quickly rejected. However, it gives a cover for the burn for the first few days. Thus the amount of fluid loss from the open wound is lessened. Also called **heterograft.** Compare **allograft, autograft, isograft.** See also **graft.**

xenon (Xe), an inert, gaseous, nonmetallic element; its atomic number is 54. Its atomic weight is 131.30.

xenophobia /zen'ə-, zē'nə-/, an anxiety disorder. It is marked by a strong, irrational fear or uneasiness in the presence of strangers, especially foreigners, or in new surroundings.

xero-, a combining form meaning 'referring to dryness.'

xeroderma /zir'ədur'mə/, a long-term skin condition with dryness and roughness.

xeroderma pigmentosum, a rare, inherited skin disease. It is marked by extreme sensitivity to ultraviolet light. Exposure to ultraviolet light may result in freckles, horny growths, and harmless and cancerous tumors. Horny growths and tumors developing on the eyelids and cornea may result in blindness. Exposure to sunlight must be avoided.

xerogram /zē'rəgram/, an x-ray image produced by xeroradiography.

xeromammogram, a type of breast x-ray in which x-ray thicknesses are reflected in energized atomic material released from a charged plate. The image is transferred to paper, where it is stored permanently, and the plate is used again after recharging.

xerophthalmia, a condition of dry and lusterless corneas and areas covering the eyes. It is usually the result of a lack of vitamin A and linked to night blindness.

xeroradiography, a diagnostic x-ray technique in which an image is made electrically rather than chemically. It allows lower exposure times and radiation of lower energy than that of ordinary x-rays. Xeroradiography is used mainly for radiography of the breasts.

xerosis. See **dry skin.**

xerostomia /zir'əstō'mē·ə/, dryness of the mouth. It is caused by halting normal salivary release. The condition is a symptom of many diseases, as diabetes, acute infections, and hysteria. It can be caused by paralysis of the facial nerves. It is also a common side effect of drugs.

X-inactivation theory. See **Lyon hypothesis.**

xiphi-. See **xipho-.**

xiphisternal articulation /zif'istur'nəl/, the cartilaginous connection between the xiphoid process and the body of the breastbone (sternum).

This joint usually hardens at puberty. Compare **manubriosternal articulation.**

xiphisternum. See **xiphoid process.**

xipho-, xiphi-, a combining form meaning 'referring to a sword or to the xiphoid process.'

xiphoid process /zif'oid/, the smallest of three parts of the breastbone near the seventh rib. Several muscles of the stomach wall are attached to the xiphoid process. Also called **ensiform process, xiphisternum, xiphoid appendix.** Compare **manubrium.**

X-linked, referring to genes or to the traits or conditions they transmit that are carried on the X chromosome. Most X-linked traits and conditions, as hemophilia, are recessive and therefore occur mostly in males, because they have only one X chromosome. Compare **Y-linked.** See also **sex-linked disorder.** –**X-linkage,** *n.*

X-linked dominant inheritance, a pattern of inheritance in which the carrying of a dominant gene on the X chromosome causes a trait to be manifested. Affected individuals all have an affected parent. All of the daughters of an affected male are affected but none of the sons. Half of the sons and half of the daughters of an affected female are affected. Normal children of an affected parent have normal offspring. The inheritance shows a clear positive family history. Hypophosphatemic vitamin D-resistant rickets is an example of this pattern. X-linked dominant inheritance closely looks like non-sex-linked (autosomal) inheritance. Compare **X-linked recessive inheritance.**

X-linked ichthyosis. See **sex-linked ichthyosis.**

X-linked inheritance, a pattern of inheritance in which the carrying of traits changes according to the sex of the person. The reason is that the genes on the X chromosome have no counterparts on the Y chromosome. The inheritance pattern may be recessive or dominant. The trait determined by a gene on the X chromosome is always expressed in males. Transmission from father to son does not occur. Kinds of X-linked inheritance are **X-linked dominant inheritance** and **X-linked recessive inheritance.** Compare **autosomal inheritance.** See also **sex-linked.**

X-linked mucopolysaccharidosis. See **Hunter's syndrome.**

X-linked recessive inheritance, a pattern of inheritance in which the carrying of an abnormal recessive gene on the X chromosome results in a carrier state in females and traits of the condition in males. Affected people have unaffected parents (except for the rare situation in which the father is affected and the mother is a carrier). Half of the female siblings of an affected male carry the trait. Unaffected male siblings do not carry the trait. Sons of affected males are unaffected. Daughters of affected

males are carriers. Unaffected male children of a carrier female do not carry the trait. Compare **X-linked dominant inheritance.**

XO, (in genetics) the designation for the presence of only one sex chromosome. Either the X or Y chromosome is missing so that each cell is monosomic. It has a total of 45 chromosomes. See also **Turner's syndrome.**

x-ray, 1. also called **roentgen ray.** electromagnetic radiation of shorter wavelengths than visible light. X-rays are made when electrons, traveling at high speed, strike certain materials, particularly heavy metals, as tungsten. They can go through most substances. They are used to investigate the integrity of certain structures and to destroy diseased tissue. They are also used to make photographic images for diagnostic purposes, as in radiography and fluoroscopy. **2.** also called **x-ray film.** a radiograph made by projecting x-rays through organs or structures of the body onto a photographic plate. Because some tissue, as bone, is more radiopaque (allowing fewer x-rays to pass through) than other tissue, like skin or fat, a shadow is created on the plate that is the image of a bone or of a cavity filled with a radiopaque substance. **3.** to make a radiograph. See also **contrast medium, electron, fluoroscopy, radiopaque.** –**x-ray,** *adj.*

x-ray fluoroscopy, an examination that uses an x-ray source that projects through the patient onto a fluorescent screen or image intensifier. Image-intensified fluoroscopy has replaced conventional fluoroscopy in current practice.

x-ray microscope, a microscope that makes images by x-rays and records them on fine-grain film or projects them as enlargements. Film images made by x-ray microscopes may be examined at quite large magnifications with a light microscope.

x-ray pelvimetry, a radiographic examination used to determine the dimensions of the bony pelvis of a pregnant woman. If possible, the diameter of her baby's head is also determined. It is done when there is doubt that the head can pass safely through the pelvis in labor. The method is not very precise and risky because of radiation exposure. It is rarely used. Other diagnostic tools, among them ultrasonography, often give the needed information with less apparent risk. Compare **clinical pelvimetry.** See also **cephalopelvic disproportion, contraction, dystocia.**

X-tra densities, images on x-ray film caused by the presence of foreign objects, as bullets or surgical clips, in the patient's body.

XX, (in genetics) the designation for the normal sex chromosome complement in the human female. See also **X chromosome.**

XXX syndrome, a human sex chromosomal disorder. It is marked by the presence of three X chromosomes. The condition occurs about once in every 1,000 live female births. Individuals with the syndrome show no significant symptoms. However, there is usually some degree of mental retardation. Half of the offspring of a trisomy X female will be both chromosomally and phenotypically normal. Also called **triple X syndrome.**

XXXX, XXXXX, (in genetics) an abnormal sex chromosome complement in the human female in which there are, respectively, four or five instead of the normal two X chromosomes. The risk of inborn abnormalities and mental retardation increases significantly with the increase in the number of X chromosomes.

XXXY, XXXXY, XXYY, (in genetics) an abnormal sex chromosome complement in the human male in which there are more than the normal one X chromosome. The more X chromosomes there are, the greater the number of inborn defects and the severity of mental retardation in the affected individual. See also **Klinefelter's syndrome.**

XXY syndrome. See **Klinefelter's syndrome.**

XY, (in genetics) the normal sex chromosome complement in the human male. See also **X chromosome, Y chromosome.**

xylitol /zī′litôl/, a sweet, crystal-like alcohol. It is used as an artificial sweetener.

xylo-, a combining form meaning 'referring to wood.'

Xylocaine, a trademark for a local anesthetic (lidocaine).

xylometazoline hydrochloride, a drug that is given to treat nasal congestion in colds, hay fever, sinusitis, and other upper breathing allergies.

★CAUTION: Glaucoma or known allergy to this drug or similar drugs prohibits its use. It is used carefully in patients having heart and blood vessel disease.

★ADVERSE EFFECTS: Among the more serious side effects are irritation to the mucosa, returning nasal congestion, and effects linked to systemic absorption, including sedation and changes in the function of heart and blood vessels.

XYY syndrome, having an extra Y chromosome. It tends to have a positive effect on height. It may have a negative effect on mental and psychological development. However, the extra Y chromosome also occurs in normal males. See also **trisomy.**

Y

yaws /yôs/, a nonvenereal infection caused by the spirochete *Treponema pertenue*. It is carried by direct contact. It is marked by long-term ulcerating sores anywhere on the body with eventual tissue and bone destruction. It leads to crippling if untreated. It is a disease of unsanitary tropic living conditions. It may be effectively treated with penicillin G. All blood tests for syphilis may be positive in yaws. The infection may give protection against syphilis. Also called **bouba, buba, frambesia, parangi, patek, pian.** Compare **bejel, pinta, syphilis.**

Y chromosome, a sex chromosome that in humans and many other species is present only in the male. It is present singly in the normal male. It is carried as a sex determinant by half of the male gametes and none of the female gametes. It has genes linked to triggering the development of male characteristics. There are no known medically significant traits or conditions linked to the genes on the Y chromosome. Compare **X chromosome.**

yeast, a fungus that reproduces asexually (budding). *Candida albicans* is a kind of disease-producing yeast.

yellow cartilage, the most elastic of the three kinds of cartilage. It is yellow, and made up of elastic fibers. It is in various parts of the body, as the external ear, the auditory tube, and the throat. Also called **elastic cartilage.** Compare **hyaline cartilage, white fibrocartilage.**

yellow fever, a sudden arbovirus infection. It is carried by mosquitoes. It is marked by headache, fever, liver disease (jaundice), vomiting, and bleeding. There is no specific treatment. Mortality is about 5%. Recovery is followed by lifelong immunity. Vaccination for travelers to risk areas is advised.

yellow fever vaccine, a vaccine made from live yellow fever virus grown in chick embryos. It is given for vaccination against yellow fever. Lessened immunity, pregnancy, or known allergy to chicken or egg protein prohibits its use. Among the more serious side effects are fever, discomfort, and allergic reactions.

yellow marrow. See **bone marrow.**

Yersinia arthritis /yursin′ē-ə/, a swelling of many joints. It occurs a few days to 1 month after the beginning of infection caused by *Yersinia enterocolitica* or *Y. pseudotuberculosis*. It usually lasts longer than 1 month. Knees, ankles, toes, fingers, and wrists are most often affected. Cultures of fluid of the joint (synovial fluid) yield no infectious organism. The clinical presentation may look like juvenile rheumatoid arthritis, rheumatic fever, or Reiter's syndrome. It may be linked to redness of the skin (erythema nodosum and erythema multiforme). Treatment is with antibiotics.

Yersinia pestis, a small bacillus that causes plague. The primary host is the rat. However, other small rodents also harbor the organism. A person without symptoms may be a carrier, but this happens rarely. *Yersinia pestis* is hardy, living for long periods in infected carcasses, the soil of the host's habitat, or in sputum. Also called *Pasteurella pestis*. See also **plague.**

Y fracture, a Y-shaped fracture between condyles.

Y-linked, referring to genes or to the traits or conditions they transmit that are carried on the Y chromosome. Such traits, as hypertrichosis of the pinna of the ear, can be expressed only in males. Compare **X-linked.** See also **sex-linked.** –**Y linkage,** *n.*

Yodoxin, a trademark for a drug that destroys amebas (diiodohydroxyquin).

yoga (hatha), a discipline that focuses on the body's muscles, posture, breathing mechanisms, and consciousness. The goal of yoga is to reach physical and mental well-being through mastery of the body, achieved by exercising, holding positions of the body, proper breathing, and meditation.

yogurt, a slightly acid, semisolid, curdled milk preparation. It is rich in vitamins of the B complex group and a good source of protein. It also gives a medium in the tract of the stomach and intestines that slows the growth of harmful bacteria and aids in the absorption of minerals.

yoke, a connector used to link small cylinders of medical gases, as portable oxygen tanks, to respiratory equipment.

yolk, the material, rich in fats and proteins, in the egg (ovum) to supply nourishment to the developing embryo. The amount and distribution of the yolk within the egg depends on the species of animal. In humans and most mammals, the yolk is absent or greatly diffused through the cell. The reason is that embryos absorb nutrients directly from the mother through the placenta. See also **deutoplasm.**

yolk membrane. See **vitelline membrane.**

yolk sac, a structure that develops in the inner cell mass of the embryo and expands into a sac. After supplying the nourishment for the embryo, the yolk sac usually disappears during the seventh week of pregnancy. See also **allantois, Meckel's diverticulum.**

yolk sphere. See **morula.**

yolk stalk, the narrow duct connecting the yolk sac with the midgut of the embryo during the early stages of prenatal development. Also called **omphalomesenteric duct, umbilical duct, vitelline duct.** See also **Meckel's diverticulum.**

young and middle adult, the stages of life from 22 to 65 years of age.

Young's rule, a method for the calculation of the appropriate dose of a drug for a child 2 years of age or more using the formula (age in years) ÷ (age + 12) × adult dose. See also **pediatric dosage.**

Y-plasty, a method of surgical revision of a scar. It uses a Y-shaped incision to reduce scar contractures. See also Z-plasty.

Y-set, a device made of plastic components. It is for putting fluids in the vein through a primary line connected to a combination drip chamber-filter section from which two separate plastic tubes lead to fluid sources. It is often used to transfuse packed blood cells that must be di-luted with saline solution to lessen their resistance to flow. In such a transfusion, one of the tubes is connected to the container with the packed cells. The other tube is con nected to the receptacle with the saline solution. During a long-term transfusion of packed blood cells, the tubing of the Y-set must be changed every 4 hours. Compare **component drip set, component syringe set, microaggregate recipient set, straight line blood set.**

ytterbium (Yb) /itur′bē·əm/, a rare earth metallic element. Its atomic number is 70; its atomic weight is 173.04.

yttrium (Y) /it′rē·əm/, a scaly, grayish metallic element. Its atomic number is 39; its atomic weight is 88.905. Radioactive isotopes of yttrium have been used in cancer therapy.

Yutopar, a trademark for a drug used to stop premature labor (ritodrine hydrochloride).

Z

Zahorsky's disease. See **roseola infantum.**

Zarontin, a trademark for a drug that prevents convulsions (ethosuximide).

Zaroxolyn, a trademark for a drug that lowers the blood pressure and increases urine release (metolazone).

Z chromosome. See **W chromosome and Z chromosome.**

Zenker's diverticulum, a bulging (herniation) of the mucous membrane of the throat as it joins the esophagus. Food may become trapped in the diverticulum and may be breathed into the lungs. Diagnosis is confirmed by x-ray studies. In most cases it is small, causes no dysfunction, and requires no treatment.

Zephiran Chloride, a trademark for a disinfectant (benzalkonium chloride).

zeranol, a hormonal substance used to fatten livestock. Consumption of beef from zeranol-treated cattle has been linked to too-early puberty in some boys and girls.

zero fluid balance, a state in which the amount of fluid intake is equal to the amount of fluid output.

zero population growth, a situation in which there is no population increase during a given period because the number of live births is equal to the number of deaths. In the United States this would occur at a birth rate of 2.54 children per fertile married woman.

zero-to-three infant stimulation groups, groups that provide therapeutic services for children from birth to 3 years of age, an age group not yet eligible for public school placement.

Zetar, a trademark for a drug used against eczema.

zeugmatography /zōōg'mətog'rəfē/, another name for nuclear magnetic resonance imaging.

zidovudine, a drug that acts against viruses by controlling their growth. It has been used to treat the symptoms of HIV infection, including AIDS. It was previously called azidothymidine (AZT).

Ziehl-Neelsen test /zēl'nēl'sən/, one of the most widely used methods of acid-fast staining. It is commonly used in the microscopic examination of a smear of sputum suspected of containing *Mycobacterium tuberculosis.* See also **acid-fast stain.**

Ziehl's stain. See **carbol-fuchsin stain.**

ZIG, abbreviation for **zoster immune globulin.**

Zinacef, a trademark for a cephalosporin antibiotic (cefuroxime sodium).

zinc (Zn), a bluish-white crystal-like metal. It is linked to lead ores. Its atomic number is 30; its atomic weight is 65.38. Zinc is an essential nutrient in the body. It is used in numerous drugs, as zinc acetate, zinc oxide, zinc permanganate, and zinc stearate. Zinc acetate is used as a drug that causes vomiting and stops bleeding. Zinc oxide is used as a drug that prevents spasms. It is also used as a protective in ointments. Zinc permanganate is used as a drug that causes contractions. It is also used to treat swelling of the urethra (urethritis) by injection or douche in a 1:4,000 solution. Zinc stearate is used as a water-repellent protective drug to treat acne, eczema, and other skin diseases.

zinc chill. See **metal fume fever.**

zinc deficiency, a condition resulting from a lack of zinc in the diet. It is marked by abnormal weakness, decreased alertness, a decrease in taste and odor sensitivity, poor appetite, slowed growth, delayed sexual maturity, lengthy healing of wounds, and risk of infection and injury. Other conditions that may occur with the lack include alcoholic swelling of the liver and other liver diseases, ulcers, heart attack (myocardial infarction), Hodgkin's disease, mongolism, and cystic fibrosis. Prevention and treatment are made up of a diet of foods high in protein that are also rich in zinc, including meats, eggs, liver, seafood, vegetables with pods, nuts, peanut butter, milk, and whole-grain cereals.

zinc gelatin, a protectant gel used to support varicose veins and other lesions of the lower limbs. It is available as a smooth jelly with zinc oxide (10%), gelatin (15%), glycerin (40%), and purified water (35%). It is also available put in gauze.

zinc oxide, a protectant given for a wide range of minor skin irritations.

zinc oxide eugenol dental cement, a filling material with zinc oxide and a liquid that is basically a pain and bacteria killer.

zinc phosphate dental cement, a material for cementing dental inlays, crowns, bridges, and orthodontic appliances and for some temporary restorations of teeth.

zinc salt poisoning, a poisonous condition caused by eating or breathing a zinc salt. Symptoms of ingestion include a burning sensation of the mouth and throat, vomiting, diarrhea, stomach and chest pain, and, in severe cases, shock and coma. Treatment includes gastric lavage, followed by giving an oily drug (demulcent). A drug is given that binds zinc (calcium edetate). Fluid therapy is also given. Breathing of zinc salts may cause metal fume fever. Skin contact may produce blisters. A deadly dose of 10 g of zinc sulfate has been reported.

zinc sulfate, an eye drug that causes contractions. It is given in drops for nasal congestion or irritation of the eye. It is put on the skin in deodorants. It is given by mouth in tablets to promote healing and as a diet supplement.

ZIP, abbreviation for *zoster immune plasma.* See **chickenpox.**

zirconium (Zr), a steel-gray metallic element. Its atomic number is 40; its atomic weight is 91.22. A component of zirconium dioxide was formerly used in some ointments to treat poison ivy skin rashes. However, such ointments caused skin irritation (granulomas) in some individuals. Similar skin conditions developed in individuals using deodorants with zirconium sodium lactate. The use of zirconium compounds, except for zirconyl-hydroxychloride, has been discontinued in the manufacture of skin ointments. Zirconyl hydroxychloride is still used in antiperspirants.

zoanthropy /zō·an'thrəpē/, the false belief that one has the form and characteristics of an animal. **–zoanthropic,** *adj.*

-zoite, a combining form meaning a 'simple organism' of a specified sort.

Zollinger-Ellison syndrome /zol'injərel'isən/, a condition marked by severe ulcers of the esophagus, stomach, or small intestines (duodenum), too-much release of gastric juice (gastric hypersecretion), elevated serum gastrin, and a tumor (gastrinoma) of the pancreas or of the small intestine (duodenum). The syndrome is uncommon but not rare. It may occur in early childhood. However, it is seen more often in patients between 20 and 50 years of age. Two-thirds of the tumors are cancerous. Total removal of the stomach (gastrectomy) may be necessary. However, giving cimetidine may control gastric hypersecretion and allow the ulcers to heal. See also **peptic ulcer.**

zona /zō'nə/, *pl.* **zonae,** a zone, or girdlelike segment of a rounded or spheric structure. See also **zone.**

zona ciliaris. See **ciliary zone.**

zona fasciculata, the middle portion of the adrenal cortex. It is the site of the production of glucocorticoids and sex hormones.

zona glomerulosa, the outer portion of the adrenal cortex.

zona pellucida /pəlo͞o'sidə/, the thick, transparent, noncellular membrane that encloses the egg (ovum). It is released by the ovum during its development in the ovary. It is kept until near the time of implantation. Also called **oolemma** /ō'əlem'ə/ . See also **vitelline membrane.**

zona radiata, a zona pellucida that has stripes. Also called **zona striata.**

zona reticularis, the innermost portion of the adrenal cortex. It acts together with the zona fasciculata in making many sex hormones and glucocorticoids.

zona striata. See **zona radiata.**

Zondek-Ascheim test. See **Ascheim-Zondek test.**

zone, an area with specific boundaries and traits, as the epigastric, the mesogastric, or the hypogastric zones of the stomach. See also **zona.**

zonesthesia, a painful sensation of constriction, as of a bandage bound too tightly. Also called **girdle sensation.**

zone therapy, the treatment of a disorder by mechanic stimulation and counterirritation of a body area in the same zone as the affected organ or region.

zonography, an x-ray imaging technique. It is used to produce films of body sections similar to those made by tomography.

zonula, *pl.* **zonulae,** a small zone. Also called **zonule.**

zonula ciliaris, a series of fibers connecting the ciliary body of the eye with the lens. It holds the lens in place. It relaxes by the contraction of the ciliary muscle. This relaxation allows the lens to become more rounded. Also called **zonule of Zinn.**

zoo-, zo-, a combining form meaning 'referring to an animal.'

zooerastia. See **bestiality.**

zoogenous /zō·oj'ənəs/, gotten from or originating in animals. See also **zoonosis.**

zoograft /zō'əgraft/, the tissue of an animal transplanted to a human, as a heart valve from a pig to replace a damaged heart valve in a human.

zoology, the study of animal life.

zoomania /zō·əmā'nē·ə/, a mental disorder marked by excess fondness for and attention to animals. **–zoomaniac,** *n.*

-zoon, a combining form meaning a 'living being.'

zoonosis /zō·on'əsis, zō'ənō'sis/, a disease of animals that can be carried to humans from its primary animal host. Some kinds of zoonoses are **equine encephalitis, leptospirosis, rabies,** and **yellow fever.**

zooparasite /zō·əper'əsīt/, any parasitic animal organism. Kinds of zooparasites are **arthropods, protozoa,** and **worms. –zooparasitic,** *adj.*

zoopathology, the study of the diseases of animals.

zoophilia /zō·əfil'ē·ə/ , **1.** an abnormal fondness for animals. **2.** (in psychiatry) a sexual disorder in which sexual excitement and satisfaction come from fondling animals or from the fantasy or act of having sexual activity with animals. Also called **zoophilism** /zō·of'iliz'/əm/ . See also **paraphilia. –zoophile,** *n.,* **zoophilic, zoophilous,** *adj.*

zoophobia /zō'ə-/, an anxiety disorder. It is marked by a persistent, irrational fear of animals, particularly dogs, snakes, insects, and mice. The condition is seen more often in women than in men. It always begins in childhood. It can typically be traced to some frightening or unpleasant experience involving an animal. Treatment is psychotherapy to reveal the cause of the anxiety reaction. It is followed by behavior therapy.

zoopsia /zō·op'sē·ə/, a visual hallucination of animals or insects, often occurring in mental disturbance with trembling linked to alcohol withdrawal (delirium tremens).

zootoxin /zō'ətok'sin/, a poisonous substance from an animal, as the venom of snakes, spiders, and scorpions. **–zootoxic,** *adj.*

zoster. See **herpes zoster.**

zosteriform /zoster'ifôrm/, resembling the sores with pus (pocks) seen in herpes zoster infection.

zoster immune globulin (ZIG), a passive vaccinating drug. It is now in limited experimental use for preventing or weakening herpes zoster virus infection in less resistant (immunosuppressed) individuals who are at great risk of severe herpes zoster virus infection.

Zovirax, a trademark for an antiviral drug (acyclovir).

Z-plasty, a method of surgical revision of a scar or closure of a wound using a Z-shaped cut. This lessens abnormal shortening of muscle tissue of the nearby skin. See also **Y-plasty.**

Z-track, a technique for injecting irritating preparations into muscle without tracking residual medication through sensitive tissues.

Zung Self-Rating Depression Scale, a "self-report test" of 20 negatively stated items given to determine the presence of depression.

zyg-, zygo-, a combining form meaning 'union or fusion, connected or joined, referring to a junction, or a pair.'

zygogenesis /zī'gōjen'əsis/, **1.** the formation of a zygote. **2.** reproduction by the union of gametes. **–zygogenetic, zygogenic,** *adj.*

zygoma /zīgō'mə, zig-/, **1.** a long, slender projection from the temporal bone. It arises from the lower part of the temporal bone, passing forward to join the zygomatic bone, and forming part of the zygomatic arch. **2.** the cheekbone (zygomatic bone) that forms the area of the cheek.

zygomatic bone, one of the pair of bones that forms the area of the cheek, the lower part of the orbit of the eye, and parts of the temporal and infratemporal fossae.

zygomatic head. See **zygomaticus minor.**

zygomaticus major /zī'gōmat'ikəs/, one of the 12 muscles of the mouth. It is used to smile or laugh. Also called **zygomaticus.** Compare **zygomaticus minor.**

zygomaticus minor, one of the 12 muscles of the mouth. It is used in making a sad face. Also called **quadratus labii superioris, zygomatic head.** Compare **zygomaticus major.**

zygomaxillare. See **key ridge.**

zygomycosis /zī'gōmīkō'sis/, a serious, often suddenly arising, and sometimes deadly fungal infection. It is caused by certain Phycomycetal water molds and is seen mainly in patients with long-term wasting diseases, especially uncontrolled diabetes mellitus. It often begins with fever and with pain and discharge from the nose. It soon continues to invade the eye and the lower breathing tract. The fungus may enter blood vessels and spread to the brain and other organs. It is usually carried by breathing. The diagnosis is confirmed by biopsy and the pathological examination of sputum. Treatment includes improved control of diabetes mellitus, extensive removal of tumors on the face and head, and amphotericin B given into the vein. Also called **mucormycosis.** Compare **phycomycosis.**

zygonema /zī'gənē'mə/, the synaptic chromosome formation that occurs in the zygotene stage of the first meiotic prophase of gametogenesis. **–zygonematic,** *adj.*

zygosis /zīgō'sis/, a form of sexual reproduction in one-celled organisms. It is made up of the union of the two cells and the fusion of the nuclei. **–zygotic** /zīgot'ik/,*adj.*

zygosity /zīgos'itē/, the traits or conditions of a zygote. The form occurs mainly as a suffix combining form to denote genetic makeup.

zygote /zī'gōt/, (in embryology) the developing egg (ovum) from the time it is fertilized until, as a blastocyst, it is implanted in the uterus.

zygotene /zī'gətēn/, the synaptic stage of cell division (meiosis). See also **diakinesis, diplotene, leptotene, pachytene.**

Zyloprim, a trademark for a drug that prevents xanthine oxidase (allopurinol).

-zyme, a combining form meaning a 'ferment or enzyme.'

zymo-, a combining form meaning 'referring to an enzyme or to fermentation.'

zymogenic cell. See **chief cell.**

APPENDIXES

Drugs

1-1 Commonly used medications: generic to trade name listing

The following is an alphabetical listing, by generic name, of selected prescription and over-the-counter medications.

Generic Name	Trade Name
acetaminophen	Tylenol, Datril, Anacin-3
acetazolamide	Diamox, Diamox Sequels
acetohexamide	Dymelor
acetylcysteine	Mucomyst
acetylsalicylic acid (ASA)	aspirin
acyclovir	Zovirax
albuterol	Proventil, Ventolin
allopurinol	Zyloprim
alprazolam	Xanax
aluminum hydroxide gel	Amphogel
aluminum-magnesium suspension	Maalox, Mylanta, Gelusil
amantadine	Symmetrel
ambenonium	Mytelase
amikacin	Amikin
amiloride	Midamor
aminocaproic acid	Amicar
aminoglutethimide	Cytadren
amitriptyline	Elavil, Endep
amobarbital	Amytal
amoxicillin	Amoxil, Larotid, Polymox
amoxicillin and clavulanate	Augmentin
amphotericin B	Fungizone
ampicillin	Amcil, Omnipen, Polycillin
ampicillin and sulbactam	Unasyn
ascorbic acid	Vitamin C
asparaginase	Elspar
aspirin, buffered	Bufferin
aspirin, enteric coated	Ecotrin
astemizole	Hismanal
atenolol	Tenormin
atracurium besylate	Tracrium
azatadine maleate	Trinalin, Optimine
azathioprine	Imuran
aztreonam	Azactam
baclofen	Lioresal
beclomethasone	Vanceril, Beclovent
belladonna alkaloids and phenobarbital	Donnatal
benzocaine	Americaine, Hurricaine
benzquinamide	Emeta-Con
benztropine	Cogentin
betamethasone	Celestone, Valisone
bethanechol chloride	Urecholine
biperiden	Akineton
bisacodyl	Dulcolax
bleomycin	Blenoxane
bretylium tosylate	Bretylol
bromocriptine	Parlodel
brompheniramine	Dimetane
buffered aspirin	Bufferin, Ascriptin
bumetanide	Bumex
buprenorphine	Buprenex
buspirone	Buspar
busulfan	Myleran
butabarbital	Butisol
butorphanol	Stadol
calcitonin	Calcimar
calcium carbonate	Tums, Titralac, Alka-2
camphorated tincture of opium	Paregoric
captopril	Capoten
carmiphen and phenylpropanolamine	Tuss-Ornade

From: McKenry, L. and Salerno, E. Mosby's Pharamcology in Nursing, ed. 18, 1992, Mosby–Year Book, Inc.

Continued.

Commonly used medications: generic to trade name listing—cont'd

Generic Name	Trade Name
carbamazepine	Tegretol
carbenicillin	Geocillin, Geopen, Pyopen
carbidopa	Lodosyn
carbidopa and levodopa	Sinemet
carmustine	BiCNU
cefaclor	Ceclor
cefadroxil	Duricef
cefamandol	Mandol
cefapirin	Cefatrex
cefazolin	Ancef, Kefzol
cefixime	Suprax
cefoperazone	Cefobid
cefotaxime	Claforan
cefoxitin	Mefoxin
ceftizoxime	Cefizox
ceftriaxone	Rocephin
cefuroxime	Ceftin
cephalexin	Keflex
cephalothin	Keflin
cephapirin	Cefadyl
cephazolin	Ancef, Kefzol
cephradine	Anspor, Velosef
chloral hydrate	Noctec
chlorambucil	Leukeran
chloramphenicol	Chloromycetin, Chloroptic
chlorazepate, dipotassium	Tranxene
chlorazepate, monopotassium	Azene
chlordiazepoxide	Librium, Libritab
chlordiazepoxide and amitriptyline	Limbitrol
chlordiazepoxide and clidinium	Limbrax
chloroquine	Aralen
chlorothiazide	Diuril
chlorotrianisene	Tace
chlorpheniramine	Chlortrimeton
chlorpromazine	Thorazine
chlorpropamide	Diabinese
chlorprothixene	Taractan
chlorthalidone	Hygroton
cholestyramine	Questran
cimetidine	Tagamet
cinoxacin	Cinobac
cisplatin	Platinol
clemastine	Tavist
clidinium	Quarzan
clindamycin	Cleocin-T
clofibrate	Atromid-S
clomiphene	Clomid
clonazepam	Klonopin
clonidine	Catapres
clotrimazole	Lotrimin, Myclex
colestipol	Colestid
conjugated estrogens	Premarin
corticotropin	ACTH, Acthar
cortisone acetate	Cortone
cromolyn	Intal
cyclizine	Marezine
cyclobenzaprine	Flexeril
cyclophosphamide	Cytoxan
cyproheptadine	Periactin
dactinomycin	Cosmegen
danazol	Danocrine
dantrolene sodium	Dantrium
demeclocycline	Declomycin
desipramine	Norpramin, Pertofrane
deslanoside	Cedilanid-D
dexamethasone	Decadron, Hexadrol
diazepam	Valium
diazoxide	Hyperstat, Proglycem
dibucaine	Nupercaine, Nupercainal
diclofenac	Voltaren
dicyclomine	Bentyl
diethylstilbestrol	Stilbestrol, DES
diflunisal	Dolobid

Continued.

Commonly used medications: generic to trade name listing—cont'd

Generic Name	Trade Name
digitoxin	Crystodigin
digoxin	Lanoxin
dimenhydrinate	Dramamine
diocytl calcium sulfosuccinate (DOCS)	Surfak
diocytl sodium sulfosuccinate (DSS)	Colace
diocytl sodium sulfosuccinate with casanthranol	Pericolace
diphenhydramine	Benadryl
diphenoxylate HCL with atropine	Lomotil
dipyridamole	Persantine
disopyramide	Norpace
disulfiram	Antabuse
dobutamine	Dobutrex
docusate calcium	Surfak
docusate sodium (DSS)	Colace
dopamine	Intropin
doxapram	Dopram
doxepin HCl	Adapin, Sinequan
doxorubicin HCl	Adriamycin
doxycycline	Vibramycin
dyphylline	Lufyllin
edrophonium	Tensilon
enalapril	Vasotec
encainide	Enkaid
enteric coated aspirin	Ecotrin
ephedrine	Vaponefrin
epinephrine	Adrenalin, Sus—Phrine
ergoloid mesylates	Hydergine
ergonovine	Ergotrate
ergotamine	Ergomar, Ergostat
erythromycin	Erythrocin, Ilotycin
erythromycin estolate	Ilosone
estrogens, conjugated	Premarin
ethacrynic acid	Edecrin
ethclorvynol	Placidyl
etidronate	Didronel
etoposide	Vepesid
famotidine	Pepcid
fenoprofen	Nalfon
fentanyl	Sublimaze
ferrous fumarate	Femiron
ferrous gluconate	Fergon
ferrous sulfate	Mol-iron, Feosol
flecainide	Tambocor
flucytosine	Ancobon
fludrocortisone	Florinef
fluocinolone acetonide	Synalar
fluocinonide	Lidex
fluoxetine	Prozac
fluphenazine	Prolixin
flurazepam	Dalmane
flurbiprofen	Ansaid
folic acid	Folvite
folinic acid	Leucovorin calcium
furosemide	Lasix
gemfibrozil	Lopid
gentamicin	Garamycin
glutethimide	Doriden
glyburide	Diabeta, Micronase
glycopyrrolate	Robinul
griseofulvin	Fulvicin P/G
guaifenesin (glyceryl guaiacolate)	Robitussin
guanabenz	Wytensin
guanethidine	Ismelin
guanfacine	Tenex
haloperidol	Haldol
haloprogin	Halotex
halothane	Fluothane
heparin	Lipo-Hepin, Liquaemin
hetacillin	Versapen
hyaluronidase	Wydase
hydralazine	Apresoline
hydrochlorothiazide	HydroDiuril, Esidrex
hydrochlorothiazide and spironolactone	Aldactazide

Continued.

Commonly used medications: generic to trade name listing—cont'd

Generic Name	Trade Name
hydrochlorothiazide and timolol	Timolide
hydrochlorothiazide and triamterene	Dyazide
hydrocodone	Dicodid
hydrocodone and homatropine	Hycodan
hydrocortisone	Solu-Cortef
hydromorphone	Dilaudid
hydromorphone and guaifenesin	Dilaudin cough syrup
hydroxyzine HCl	Atarax
hydroxyzine pamoate	Vistaril
ibuprofen	Advil, Motrin, Rufen
idoxuridine	Stoxil, Herplex
imipenem-cilastatin	Primaxin
imipramine	Tofranil
indomethacin	Indocin
INH (isoniazid)	Nydrazid
ipratropium	Atrovent
iron dextran	Imferon
isoetharine HCl	Bronkosol
isoproterenol	Isuprel
isosorbide dinitrate	Isordil, Sorbitrate
isotretinoin	Accutane
isoxsuprine HCl	Vasodilan
kanamycin	Kantrex
kaolin-pectin	Kaopectate
ketoconazole	Nizoral
ketoprofen	Orudis
labetalol	Normodyne, Trandate
lactulose syrup	Chronulac
lanatoside C	Cedilanid
leucovorin	Wellcovorin
levarterenol	Levophed
levodopa	Dopar, Larodopa
levorphanol	Levo-Dromoran
levothyroxine	Synthroid
lidocaine	Xylocaine
lindane	Kwell
liothyronine	Cytomel
liotrix	Euthroid, Thyrolar
lisinopril	Prinivil, Zestril
lithium carbonate	Lithane, Lithobid
lomustine	Cee Nu
loperamide	Imodium
lorazepam	Ativan
lovastatin	Mevacor
loxapine succinate	Loxitane
lypressin	Diapid
magaldrate	Riopan
magnesium sulfate	Epsom salt
maprotiline	Ludiomil
mazindol	Sanorex
mebendazole	Vermox
mecamylamine	Inversine
mechlorethamine	Mustargen, Nitrogen Mustard
meclizine	Antivert, Bonine
meclofenamate	Meclomen
medroxyprogesterone	Provera
megestrol	Megace
melphalan	Alkeran
menadiol	Synkayvite, vitamin K
meperidine	Demerol
mephenytoin	Mesantoin
mephobarbital	Mebaral
meprobamate	Miltown, Equanil
mesoridazine	Serentil
metaproterenol	Alupent
metaraminol	Aramine
methadone	Dolophine
methanodrostenolone	Dianabol
metheanime hippurate	Hiprex, Urex
methenamine mandelate	Mandelamine
methicillin	Staphcillin
methimazole	Tapazole
methocarbamol	Robaxin

Continued.

Commonly used medications: generic to trade name listing—cont'd

Generic Name	Trade Name
methoxyflurane	Penthrane
methyldopa	Aldomet
methylphenidate	Ritalin
methyprylon	Noludar
methysergide	Sansert
metoclopramide	Reglan
metolazone	Zaroxolyn
metoprolol	Lopressor
metronidazole	Flagyl
mexiletine	Mexitil
mezlocillin	Mezlin
miconazole	Monistat
milk of magnesia (MOM)	Magnesium Hydroxide
mineral oil emulsion	Kondremul
minocycline	Minocin
minoxidil	Loniten
misoprostol	Cytotec
mithramycin	Mithracin
mitotane	Lysodren
molindone	Moban
morphine sulfate	Roxanol, Duramorph
moxalactam	Moxam
nadolol	Corgard
nalbuphine	Nubain
nalidixic acid	Neg Gram
naloxone	Narcan
naproxen	Naprosyn
naproxen sodium	Anaprox
neostigmine	Prostigmin
niacin (nicotinic acid)	Nicobid, Nicolar
nicardipine	Cardene
nifedipine	Procardia
nitrofurantoin	Furadantin
nitrogen mustard	Mustargen
nitroglycerin	Nitrobid, Nitrospan, Nitrostat
nitroprusside	Nipride
nizatidine	Axid
norepinephrine	Levophed
norethindrone	Norlutin
norethindrone acetate	Norlutate
norfloxacin	Noroxin
nortriptyline	Aventyl, Pamelor
nylidrin	Arlidin
nystatin	Mycostatin, Nilstat
oprhendrine	Norflex
oxacillin	Prostaphlin
oxazepam	Serax
oxtriphylline	Choledyl
oxycodone, ASA	Percodan
oxycodone, acetaminophen	Percocet, Tylox
oxymetazoline, nasal	Afrin, Dristan Long Lasting
oxymorphone	Numorphan
oxyphenbutazone	Tandearil
oxytetracycline	Terramycin
oxytocin	Pitocin
pancrelipase	Cotazym, Viokase
pancuronium	Pavulon
papaverine	Pavabid, Cerespan
paraldehyde	Paral
pargyline	Eutonyl
pemoline	Cylert
penicillamine	Cuprimine
penicillin and benzathine	Bicillin
penicillin G potassium	Pfizepen, Pentid
penicillin procaine	Duracillin, crysticillin, Wycillin
penicillin V potassium	Pen-Vee K, V-cillin K
pentaerythritol tetranitrate	Peritrate
pentamidine isethionate	Pentam
pentazocine	Talwin
pentobarbital	Nembutal
perphenazine	Trilafon
phenzopyridine HCl	Pyridium
phenazopyridine and sulfisoxazole	Azo-Gantrisin

Continued.

Commonly used medications: generic to trade name listings—cont'd

Generic Name	Trade Name
phenelzine sulfate	Nardil
pentoxifylline	Trental
phenmetrazine	Preludin
phenobarbital	Luminal
phenolphthalein	Ex-Lax, Feen-A-Mint
phenoxymethyl penicillin	V-Cillin, Penicillin VK
phentolamine	Regitine
phenylbutazone	Butazolidin, Azolid-A
phenylephrine	Neosynephrine
phenytoin	Dilantin
phosphate enema	Fleet enema
phosphated carbohydrate solution	Emetrol
physostigmine	Antilirium
phytonadione (vitamin K_1)	Mephyton, Aquamephyton
pilocarpine	Isoptocarpine
pindolol	Visken
piperacillin	Pripracil
piroxicam	Feldene
potassium chloride	KLor, Kaon, Cl, Slow K, Micro K, Klorvess
potassium gluconate	Kaon
povidone-iodine	Betadine
prazosin	Minipress
prednisolone	Meticortelone, Delta Cortef
primidone	Mysoline
probenecid	Benemid
probucol	Lorelco
procainamide	Pronestyl
procaine	Novocain
procarbazine	Matulane
prochlorperazine	Compazine
procyclidine	Kemadrin
promazine	Sparine
promethazine	Phenergan
proprantheline	Probanthine
propoxyphene	Darvon
propoxyphene, napsylate, acetaminophen	Davocet-N
propranolol	Inderal
psyllium hydrocolloid	Effersyllium
pyridostigmine	Mestinon
pyrimethamine	Daraprim
quinacrine	Atabrine
quinidine gluconate	Quinaglute
quinidine sulfate	Quinora
quinine sulfate	Quinamm
racepinephrine	Vaponefrin, Asthmanefin
ranitidine	Zantac
rauwolfia serpentina	Raudixin
reserpine	Serpasil
ribavirin	Virazole
rifampin	Rimactane, Rifadin
ritodrine	Yutopar
salsalate	Disalcid
scopolamine	Transderm-Scop
secobarbital	Seconal
selenium sulfide	Selsun Blue, Selsun
senna	Senokot
silver sulfadiazine	Silvadene
simethicone	Mylicon
sodium polystyrene sulfonate	Kayexalate
spironolactone	Aldactone
spironolactone and hydrochlorothiazide	Aldactazide
streptokinase	Streptase
succinylcholine	Anectine
sucralfate	Carafate
sufentanil	Sufenta
sulfamethoxazole	Gantanol
sulfamethoxazole and trimethoprim	Bactrim, Septra
sulfasalzine	Azulfidine
sulfisoxazole	Gantrisin
sulfisoxazole and phenazopyridine	Azo-Gantrisin
sulindac	Clinoril
tamoxifen	Nolvadex
temazepam	Restoril
terbutaline	Brethine, Bricanyl

Continued.

Commonly used medications: generic to trade name listing — cont'd

Generic Name	Trade Name
terfenadine	Seldane
tetanus immune globulin	Hyper-tet
tetracaine	Pontocaine
tetracycline	Achromycin, Sumycin
theophylline	Elxiophyllin, Theo-Dur
thiethylperzine	Torecan
thioridazine	Mellaril
thiothixene	Navane
thyroglobulin	Proloid
ticarcillin	Ticar
ticarcillin disodium	Clavulanate-Timentin
timolol maleate	Blocadren, Timotpic
tobraymcyin	Nebcin, Tobrex
tocainide	Tonocard
tolazamide	Tolinase
tolbutamide	Orinase
t-PA	Activase
tranylcypromine sulfate	Parnate
trazodone	Desyrel
triamcinolone	Kenacort, Aristocort
trimaterene	Dyrenium
triamterene and hydrochlorothiazide	Dyazide, Maxzide
triazolam	Halcion
trifluoperazine	Stelazine
trihexphenidyl HCl	Artane, Tremin
trimeprazone	Temaril
trimethadione	Tridione
trimethaphan	Arfonad
trimethobenzamide	Tigan
trimethoprim	Proloprim, Trimpex
tripelennamine	Pyribenzamine (PBZ)
triprolidine	Actidil
triprolidine and pseudoephedrine	Actifed
undecylenic acid	Desenex
urokinase	Abbokinase
ursodiol	Actigall
valproic acid	Depakene
vancomycin	Vancocin
vasopressin	Pitressin
verapamil	Calan, Isoptin
vidarabine	Vira-A
vinblastine	Velban
vincristine	Oncovin
vitamin B_1	Thiamine
vitamin B_2	Riboflavin
vitamin B_3	Niacin, Nicotinic Acid
vitamin B_6	Pyridoxine, Hexabetalin
vitamin B_{12}	Cyanocobalamin, Redisol
vitamin C	Ascorbic acid
vitamin D	Deltalin
vitamin K_1	Phytonadione
vitamin K_2	Menadione
warfarin	Coumadin
wellbutrin	Bupropion
zidovudine	Retrovir, AZT

1-2 | Guide to common drug interactions

Drug	Interacting drug	Effect
OVER-THE-COUNTER DRUGS AND SUBSTANCES		
Antacids		
Alumina and magnesia Dihydroxyaluminum sodium carbonate	Dicumarol	Effects of dicumarol may be faster and/or increased
Magnesia	Digoxin	Effects of digoxin may be reduced
	Tetracylines Doxycycline Tetracycline	Effects of tetracyclines may be reduced Should be taken 1-3 hours apart
Painkillers		
Acetaminophen Buffered acetaminophen	Alcoholic beverages	May cause liver damage
	Blood-thinning drugs Dicumarol Warfarin sodium	High doses of acetaminophen may increase blood-thinning effects of these drugs
	Tetracycline	Buffered form may cancel the effects of tetracycline Should be taken 1 hour apart
Ibuprofen	Alcoholic beverages	May cause internal bleeding or ulcers
	Blood-thinning drugs Dicumarol Heparin Warfarin sodium	May cause internal bleeding or ulcers
	Salicylates Aspirin Aspirin and caffeine Buffered aspirin	May cause stomach upset without relieving symptoms
Salicylates Aspirin Aspirin and caffeine Buffered aspirin	Alcoholic beverages	May cause stomach ulcers or bleeding
	Antidiabetics Chlorpropamide Tolazamide	May cause blood sugar level to drop too low
	Blood-thinning drugs Dicumarol Heparin Warfarin sodium	Increases risk of internal bleeding
	Ibuprofen	May cause stomach upset without relieving symptoms
Other substances Alcoholic beverages	Tetracycline	Effects of tetracycline are reduced
	Acetaminophen	May cause liver damage
	Buffered acetaminophen	
	Antidiabetics Chlorpropamide Tolazamide	Stomach upset, vomiting, cramps, headaches, low blood sugar
	Antiseizure drugs Carbamazepine Chlordiazepoxide Diazepam Phenytoin	May cause extreme drowsiness
	Barbiturates Pentobarbital Phenobarbital Secobarbital Secobarbital and amobarbital	May cause drowsiness, increase effects of either drug, cause breathing to fail, or cause blood pressure to drop too low

This table includes only common over-the-counter and prescription drugs. Some of these drugs may interact with less common drugs and substances not described. When using any drug, always consult your doctor or pharmacist about possible interactions with other drugs, substances, or foods.

Continued.

Drug	Interacting drug	Effect
Other substances — cont'd	Ibuprofen	May cause internal bleeding or ulcers
	Narcotic analgesics Acetaminophen and codeine Meperidine Propoxyphene	May depress nervous system and breathing or cause blood pressure to drop too low
	Reserpine	May increase effects of alcohol and reserpine
	Salicylates Aspirin Aspirin and caffeine Buffered asprin	May cause stomach ulcers or internal bleeding
	Tricyclic antidepressants Amitriptyline Amoxapine Doxepin	May cause extreme drowsiness
Sodium chloride (salt)	Lithium	Low-salt diet causes lithium to build up in body and is not advised
Tobacco (smoking)	Birth control pills Norethindrone with ethinyl estradiol Norethynodrel with mestranol	May increase chances of blood clot or heart attack
Tyramine-containing foods Avocados, bananas, beer, caffeine, cheese, chicken liver, chocolate, fava beans, fermented sausages (salami, pepperoni, bologna, etc.), canned figs, pickled herring, pineapple, raisins, red wine, sauerkraut, soy sauce, yeast extract, yogurt	MAO inhibitors Isocarboxazid Phenelzine Tranylcypromine	May cause severe and sometimes fatal high blood pressure Headache, vomiting, fever, and high blood pressure are warning signals

PRESCRIPTION DRUGS

Antibiotics

Drug	Interacting drug	Effect
Erythromycins Erythromycin Erythromycin lactobionate	Penicillins Amoxicillin Ampicillin	Could interfere with the effects of penicillins
Penicillins Amoxicillin Ampicillin	Birth control pills Norethindrone with ethinyl estradiol Norethynodrel with mestranol	May interfere with and result in unplanned pregnancy or menstrual problems
	Blood-thinning drugs Dicumarol Warfarin sodium	May increase blood thinning effects of these drugs
	Erythromycins Erythromycin Erythromycin lactobionate	May interefere with effects of penicillins
	Tetracyclines Doxycycline Tetracycline	May interfere with effects of penicillins
Tetracyclines Doxcycline Tetracycline	Acetaminophen Buffered acetaminophen	
	Antacids Alumina and magnesia Dihyroxaluminum sodium carbonate Magnesia	May decrease effects of tetracyclines and should be taken 1 to 3 hours apart

Continued.

Drug	Interacting drug	Effect
	Barbiturates Pentobarbital Phenobarbital Secobarbital Secobarbital and amobarbital	May decrease effects of doxy- cycline Other tetracyclines can be used
	Penicillins Amoxicillin Ampicillin	May interfere with effects of peni- cillins
	Salicylates Aspirin Aspirin and caffeine Buffered aspirin	Effects of tetracyclines are reduced
Antidepressants Lithium	Sodium chloride (salt)	Low-salt diet causes lithium to build up in body and is not advised
	Thiazide diuretics Cyclothiazide Furosemide Methyclothiazide	May cause lithium to have toxic effect
Tricyclic antidepressants	Alcoholic beverages	May cause extreme drowsiness
Amitryptyline Amoxapine Doxepin	Antiseizure drugs Carbamazepine Chlordiazepoxide Diazepam Phenytoin	Effects of antiseizure drug may be decreased Dosage should be adjusted
	Blood-thinning drugs Dicumarol Warfarin sodium	May cause internal bleeding
	MAO inhibitors Isocarboxazid Phenelzine Tranylcypromine	Severe seizure and death could result Should be taken 14 days apart
	Narcotic analgesics Acetaminophen and codeine Meperidine Propoxyphene	May depress nervous system and breathing and cause blood pres- sure to drop too low
Antidiabetics Chlorpropamide Tolazamide	Alcoholic beverages	May cause stomach upset, vomit- ing, cramps, headaches, low blood sugar
	Beta-adrenergic blockers Metoprolol Propranolol	May increase risk of either high or low blood sugar levels May mask symptoms
	Blood-thinning drugs Dicumarol Warfarin sodium	Blood-thinning effect will be in- creased at first, later it will be decreased May also cause low blood sugar and become toxic
	MAO inhibitors Isocarboxazid Phenelzine Tranylcypromine	Can cause extreme low blood sugar level
	Salicylates Aspirin Aspirin and caffeine Buffered aspirin	May cause blood sugar level to drop too low
Isophane insulin suspension	Beta-adrenergic blockers Metoprolol Propranolol	These may mask symptoms of low blood sugar

This table includes only common over-the-counter and prescription drugs. Some of these drugs may also interact with less common drugs and substances not described. When using any drug, always consult your doctor or pharmacist about possible interactions with other drugs, substances, or foods.

Continued.

Drug	Interacting drug	Effect
	Birth control pills Norethindrone with ethinyl estradiol Norethynodrel with mestranol	May increase risk of high blood sugar levels Dosages should be adjusted
	MAO inhibitors Isocarboxazid Phenelzine Tranylcypromine	May cause extreme low blood sugar level
Antiseizure drugs Carbamazepine Chlordiazepoxide Diazepam Phenytoin	Alcoholic beverages	May cause extreme drowsiness
	Beta-adrenergic blockers Metoprolol Propranolol	Could decrease the effects of beta- blockers
	Birth control pills Norethindrone with ethinyl estradiol Norethynodrel with mestranol	Phenytoin and carbamazepine may interfere and increase risk of unplanned pregnancy May increase effect of diazepam
	Tricyclic antidepressants Amitriptyline Amoxapine Doxepin	Effects of antiseizure drug may be decreased Dosage should be adjusted
Barbiturates Pentobarbital Phenobarbital Secobarbital Secobarbital and amobarbital	Alcoholic beverages	May cause drowsiness, increase ef- fects of either drug, cause breathing to fail, or cause blood pressure to drop too low
	Birth control pills Norethindrone with ethinyl estradiol Norethynodrel with mestranol	Barbiturates may interfere with and result in unplanned preg- nancy
	Blood-thinning drugs Dicumarol Warfarin sodium	May decrease blood-thinning effects of these drugs
	Doxycycline	May decrease effects of doxy- cycline Other tetracyclines can be used
Birth control pills Norethidrone with ethinyl estradiol Norethynodrel with mestranol	Antiseizure drugs Carbamazepine Chlordiazepoxide Diazepam Phenytoin	Will increase the sedative effects of these drugs May decrease the effects of other antiseizure drugs
	Barbiturates Pentobarbital Phenobarbital Secobarbital Secobarbital and amobarbital	Barbiturates may intefere with birth control pills and result in unplanned pregnancy
	Isophane insulin suspension	May increase risk of high blood sugar levels; dosages should be adjusted
	Penicillins Amoxicillin Ampicillin	May interfere with birth control pills and result in unplanned pregnancy
	Tobacco (smoking)	May increase chances of blood clot or heart attack

This table includes only common over-the-counter and prescription drugs. Some of these drugs may also interact with less common drugs and substances not described. When using any drug, always consult your doctor or pharmacist about possible interactions with other drugs, substances, or food.

Continued.

Drug	Interacting drug	Effect
Blood pressure drugs		

Thiazide diuretics
Cyclothiazide
Furosemide
Methylchlothiazide
	Beta-adrenergic blockers
	  Metoprolol
	  Propranolol
		Can cause extremely low blood pressure

	Digitalis glycosides
	  Digitalis
	  Digoxin
		Can cause irregular heartbeat, which can be fatal
		Can cause extremely low blood pressure

	Lithium	May cause lithium to have toxic effect
	Reserpine	Can cause extremely low blood pressure
Rauwolfia alkaloids Reserpine	Alcoholic beverages	May increase effects of alcohol May increase effects of rauwolfia alkaloids

	Beta-adrenergic blockers
	  Metoprolol
	  Propranolol
		May cause extremely slow heartbeat and low blood pressure

	Digitalis glycosides
	  Digitalis
	  Digoxin
		May cause irregular heartbeat

	MAO inhibitors
	  Isocarboxazid
	  Phenelzine
	  Tranylcypromine
		May cause slight to sudden and severe high blood pressure
		May cause extreme high fever
		Either effect could be life-threatening

	Thiazide diuretics
	  Cyclothiazide
	  Furosemide
	  Methylclothiazide
		Can cause extreme low blood pressure

Blood-thinning drugs		
Dicumarol Warfarin sodium	Acetaminophen Buffered acetaminophen	High doses of acetaminophen may increase blood-thinning effects of these drugs

	Antacids
	  Alumina and magnesia
	  Dihydroxaluminum sodium
	  carbonate
	  Magnesia
		Effects of dicumarol may be faster and may also be increased

	Antidiabetics
	  Chlorpropamide
	  Tolazamide
		Blood-thinning effect will be increased at first, later it will be decreased
		May also cause low blood sugar and become toxic

	Barbiturates
	  Pentobarbital
	  Phenobarbital
	  Secobarbital
	  Secobarbital and amobarbital
		Decreases blood-thinning effect

	Heparin	May cause increased risk of internal bleeding
	Ibuprofen	May cause internal bleeding or ulcers

	Penicillins
	  Amoxicillin
	  Ampicillin
		May increase blood-thinning effects of these drugs

	Salicylates
	  Aspirin
	  Aspirin and caffeine
	  Buffered aspirin
		Blood-thinning effects will be increased
		May cause ulcers or internal bleeding

Continued.

Drug	Interacting drug	Effect
	Tricyclic antidepressants Amitryptyline Amoxapine Doxepin	May cause internal bleeding
Heparin	Blood-thinning drugs Dicumarol Warfarin sodium	May cause increased risk of internal bleeding
	Salicylates Aspirin Aspirin and caffeine Buffered aspirin	Blood-thinning effects will be increased May cause ulcers or internal bleeding
Heart drugs		
Beta-adrenergic blockers Metoprolol Propranolol	Antidiabetics Chlorpropamide Tolazamide	May increase risk of either high or low blood sugar levels May mask symptoms
	Antiseizure drugs Carbamazepine Chlordiazepoxide Diazepam Phenytoin	Could decrease the effect of beta blockers
	Digitalis glycosides Digitalis Digoxin	May cause extremely slow heartbeat with a chance of heart block
	Isophane insulin suspension	Beta blockers may mask symptoms of low blood sugar May also cause low blood sugar
	Reserpine	May cause extremely slow heartbeat and low blood pressure
	Thiazide diuretics Cyclothiazide Furosemide Methylclothiazide	Can cause extremely low blood pressure
Digitalis glycosides Digitalis Digoxin	Antacids Alumina and magnesia Dihydroaluminum sodium carbonate Magnesia	Effects of digoxin may be reduced
	Beta-adrenergic blockers Metoprolol Propranolol	May cause extremely slow heartbeat with a chance of heart block
	Reserpine	May cause irregular heartbeat
	Thiazide diuretics Cyclothiazide Furosemide Methyclothiazide	May cause extreme low blood pressure; may cause digitalis to become toxic
Monoamine oxidase inhibitors (MAO inhibitors) Isocarboxazid Phenelzine Tranylcypromine	Antidiabetics Chlorpropamide Isophane insulin suspension Tolazamide	Can cause extreme low blood sugar level
	Narcotic analgesics Acetaminophen and codeine Meperidine Propoxyphene	May cause severe and sometimes fatal reactions
	Reserpine	May cause slight to sudden and severe high blood pressure May cause extreme high fever Either effect could be life-threatening

This table includes only over-the-counter and prescription drugs. Some of these drugs may also interact with less common drugs and substances not described. When using any drug, always consult your doctor or pharmacist about possible interactions with other drugs, substances, or foods.

Continued.

Drug	Interacting drug	Effect
Monoamine oxidase inhibitors (MAO inhibitors) — cont'd	Tricyclic antidepressants Amitriptyline Amoxapine Doxepin	Severe seizure and death could result Should be taken 14 days apart
	Tyramine-containing foods Avocados, bananas, beer, caffeine, cheese, chicken liver, chocolate, fava beans, fermented sausages (salami, pepperoni, bologna, etc.), canned figs, pickled herring, pineapple, raisins, red wine, sauerkraut, soy sauce, yeast extract, yogurt	May cause severe and sometimes fatal high blood pressure. Headache, vomiting, fever, and high blood pressure are warning signals
Painkillers Narcotic analgesics Acetaminophen and codeine Meperidine Propoxyphene	Alcoholic beverages	May depress nervous system and breathing May cause blood pressure to drop too low
	MAO inhibitors Isocarboxazid Phenelzine Tranylcypromine	May cause many severe and sometimes fatal reactions
	Tricyclic antidepressants Amitriptyline Amoxapine Doxepin	May depress nervous system and breathing May cause blood pressure to drop too low

APPENDIX 2

Height and weight tables

2-1 | Height and weight tables for children

Desirable weights (pounds) for persons 5 to 19 years old

Boys

Height (in)	5 yr	6 yr	7 yr	8 yr	9 yr	10 yr	11 yr	12 yr	13 yr	14 yr	15 yr	16 yr	17 yr	18 yr	19 yr
38	34	34													
39	35	35													
40	36	36													
41	38	38	38												
42	39	39	39	39											
43	41	41	41	41											
44	44	44	44	44											
45	46	46	46	46	46										
46	47	48	48	48	48										
47	49	50	50	50	50	50									
48		52	53	53	53	53									
49		55	55	55	55	55	55								
50		57	58	58	58	58	58	58							
51			61	61	61	61	61	61	61						
52			63	64	64	64	64	64	64						
53			66	67	67	67	67	68	68						
54				70	70	70	70	71	71	72					
55				72	72	73	73	74	74	74					
56				75	76	77	77	77	78	78	80				
57					79	80	81	81	82	83	83				
58					83	84	84	85	85	86	87				
59						87	88	89	89	90	90	90			
60						91	92	92	93	94	95	96			
61							95	96	97	99	100	103	106		
62							100	101	102	103	104	107	111	116	
63							105	106	107	108	110	113	118	123	127
64								109	111	113	115	117	121	126	130
65								114	117	118	120	122	127	131	134
66									119	122	125	128	132	136	139
67									124	128	130	134	136	139	142
68										134	134	137	141	143	147
69										137	139	143	146	149	152
70										143	144	145	151	151	155
71										148	150	151	152	154	159
72											153	155	156	158	163
73											157	160	162	164	167
74											160	164	168	170	171

Girls

Height (in)	5 yr	6 yr	7 yr	8 yr	9 yr	10 yr	11 yr	12 yr	13 yr	14 yr	15 yr	16 yr	17 yr	18 yr
38	33	33												
39	34	34												
40	36	36	36											
41	37	37	37											
42	39	39	39											
43	41	41	41	41										
44	42	42	42	42										
45	45	45	45	45	45									
46	47	47	47	48	48									
47	49	50	50	50	50	50								
48		52	52	52	52	53	53							
49			54	55	55	56	56							
50			56	57	58	59	61	62						
51			59	60	61	61	63	65						
52			63	64	64	64	65	67						
53			66	67	67	68	68	69	71					
54				69	70	70	71	71	73					
55				72	74	74	74	75	77	78				
56					76	78	78	79	81	83				
57					80	82	82	82	84	88	92			
58						84	86	86	88	93	96	101		
59						87	90	90	92	96	100	103	104	
60						91	95	95	97	101	105	108	109	111
61							99	100	101	105	108	112	113	116
62							104	105	106	109	113	115	117	118
63								110	110	112	116	117	119	120
64								114	115	117	119	120	122	123
65								118	120	121	122	123	125	126
66									124	124	125	128	129	130
67									128	130	131	133	133	135
68									131	133	135	136	138	138
69										135	137	138	140	142
70										136	138	140	142	144
71										138	140	142	144	145

2-2 | Height and weight tables for adults*

Desirable weights for persons 25 to 29 years old (in indoor clothing†)

Men

Height (in shoes)‡:		Small frame:	Medium frame:	Large frame:
Ft.	In.	Pounds	Pounds	Pounds
5	2	128-134	131-141	138-150
5	3	130-136	133-143	140-153
5	4	132-138	135-145	142-156
5	5	134-140	137-148	144-160
5	6	136-142	139-151	146-164
5	7	138-145	142-154	149-168
5	8	140-148	145-157	152-172
5	9	142-151	148-160	155-176
5	10	144-154	151-163	158-180
5	11	146-157	154-166	161-184
6	0	149-160	157-170	164-188
6	1	152-164	160-174	168-192
6	2	155-168	164-178	172-197
6	3	158-172	167-182	176-202
6	4	162-176	171-187	181-207

Women

Height (in shoes)‡:		Small frame:	Medium frame:	Large frame:
Ft.	In.	Pounds	Pounds	Pounds
4	10	102-111	109-121	118-131
4	11	103-113	111-123	120-134
5	0	104-115	113-126	122-137
5	1	106-118	115-129	125-140
5	2	108-121	118-132	128-143
5	3	111-124	121-135	131-147
5	4	114-127	124-138	134-151
5	5	117-130	127-141	137-155
5	6	120-133	130-144	140-159
5	7	123-136	133-147	143-163
5	8	126-139	136-150	146-167
5	9	129-142	139-153	149-170
5	10	132-145	142-156	152-173
5	11	135-148	145-159	155-176
6	0	138-151	148-162	158-179

†Indoor clothing weighing 5 pounds for men and 3 pounds for women.
‡Shoes with 1-inch heels.
*Source of basic data *Build Study, 1979,* Society of Actuaries and Association of Life Insurance Medical Directors of America, 1980.
Copyright 1983 Metropolitan Life Insurance Company.

Nutrition

3-1 | United States Recommended Daily Allowances (U.S. RDA)*

		Weight[a]		Height[a]		Protein	Fat-soluble vitamins			
							Vita-min A	Vita-min D	Vita-min E	Vita-min K
Category	Age (years) or condition	(kg)	(lb)	(cm)	(in)	(g)	(μg RE)[b]	(μg)[c]	(mg α-TE)[d]	(μg)
Infants	0.0-0.5	6	13	60	24	13	375	7.5	3	5
	0.5-1.0	9	20	71	28	14	375	10	4	10
Children	1-3	13	29	90	35	16	400	10	6	15
	4-6	20	44	112	44	24	500	10	7	20
	7-10	28	62	132	52	28	700	10	7	30
Males	11-14	45	99	157	62	45	1,000	10	10	45
	15-18	66	145	176	69	59	1,000	10	10	65
	19-24	72	160	177	70	58	1,000	10	10	70
	25-50	79	174	176	70	63	1,000	5	10	80
	51+	77	170	173	68	63	1,000	5	10	80
Females	11-14	46	101	157	62	46	800	10	8	45
	15-18	55	120	163	64	44	800	10	8	55
	19-24	58	128	164	65	46	800	10	8	60
	25-50	63	138	163	64	50	800	5	8	65
	51+	65	143	160	63	50	800	5	8	65
Pregnant						60	800	10	10	65
Lactating	1st 6 Months					65	1,300	10	12	65
	2nd 6 Months					62	1,200	10	11	65

The allowances, expressed as average daily intakes over time, are intended to provide for individual variations among most normal persons as they live in the United States under usual environmental stresses. Diets should be based on a variety of common foods in order to provide other nutrients for which human requirements have been less well defined. See text for detailed discussion of allowances and of nutrients not tabulated.
[a]Weights and heights of Reference Adults are actual medians for the U.S. population of the designated age, as reported by NHANES II. The use of these figures does not imply that the height-to-weight ratios are ideal.

Water-Soluble Vitamins							Minerals						
Vitamin C (mg)	Thiamin (mg)	Riboflavin (mg)	Niacin (mg NE)[e]	Vitamin B^4 (mg)	Folate (µg)	Vitamin B^{12} (µg)	Calcium (mg)	Phosphorus (mg)	Magnesium (mg)	Iron (mg)	Zinc (mg)	Iodine (µg)	Selenium (µg)
30	0.3	0.4	5	0.3	25	0.3	400	300	40	6	5	40	10
35	0.4	0.5	6	0.6	35	0.5	600	500	60	10	5	50	15
40	0.7	0.8	9	1.0	50	0.7	800	800	80	10	10	70	20
45	0.9	1.1	12	1.1	75	1.0	800	800	120	10	10	90	20
45	1.0	1.2	13	1.4	100	1.4	800	800	170	10	10	120	30
50	1.3	1.5	17	1.7	150	2.0	1,200	1,200	270	12	15	150	40
60	1.5	1.8	20	2.0	200	2.0	1,200	1,200	400	12	15	150	50
60	1.5	1.7	19	2.0	200	2.0	1,200	1,200	350	10	15	150	70
60	1.5	1.7	19	2.0	200	2.0	800	800	350	10	15	150	70
60	1.2	1.4	15	2.0	200	2.0	800	800	350	10	15	150	70
50	1.1	1.3	15	1.4	150	2.0	1,200	1,200	280	15	12	150	45
60	1.1	1.3	15	1.5	180	2.0	1,200	1,200	300	15	12	150	50
60	1.1	1.3	15	1.6	180	2.0	1,200	1,200	280	15	12	150	55
60	1.1	1.3	15	1.6	180	2.0	800	800	280	15	12	150	55
60	1.0	1.2	13	1.6	180	2.0	800	800	280	10	12	150	55
70	1.5	1.6	17	2.2	400	2.2	1,200	1,200	320	30	15	175	65
95	1.6	1.8	20	2.1	280	2.6	1,200	1,200	355	15	19	200	75
90	1.6	1.7	20	2.1	260	2.6	1,200	1,200	340	15	16	200	75

[b]Retinol equivalents. 1 retinol equivalent = 1 µg retinol or 6 µg β-carotene.
[c]As cholecalciferol. 10µg cholecalciferol = 400 IU of vitamin D.

[d]α-Tocopherol equivalents. 1 mg d-α tocopherol = 1 α-TE.
[e]1 NE (niacin equivalent) is equal to 1 mg of niacin or 60 mg of dietary tryptophan.

3-2 Recommended nutrient intakes for Canadians

Summary of Examples of Recommended Nutrients Based on Energy Expressed as Daily Rates

Age	Sex	Energy kcal	Thiamin mg	Riboflavin mg	Niacin NE[b]	n-3 PUFA[a] g	n-6 PUFA g
Months							
0-4	Both	600	0.3	0.3	4	0.5	3
5-12	Both	900	0.4	0.5	7	0.5	3
Years							
1	Both	1100	0.5	0.6	8	0.6	4
2-3	Both	1300	0.6	0.7	9	0.7	4
4-6	Both	1800	0.7	0.9	13	1.0	6
7-9	M	2200	0.9	1.1	16	1.2	7
	F	1900	0.8	1.0	14	1.0	6
10-12	M	2500	1.0	1.3	18	1.4	8
	F	2200	0.9	1.1	16	1.2	7
13-15	M	2800	1.1	1.4	20	1.5	9
	F	2200	0.9	1.1	16	1.2	7
16-18	M	3200	1.3	1.6	23	1.8	11
	F	2100	0.8	1.1	15	1.2	7
19-24	M	3000	1.2	1.5	22	1.6	10
	F	2100	0.8	1.1	15	1.2	7
25-49	M	2700	1.1	1.4	19	1.5	9
	F	1900	0.8	1.0	14	1.1	7
50-74	M	2300	0.9	1.2	16	1.3	8
	F	1800	0.8[c]	1.0[c]	14[c]	1.1[c]	7[c]
75+	M	2000	0.8	1.0	14	1.1	7
	F[d]	1700	0.8[c]	1.0[c]	14[c]	1.1[c]	7[c]
Pregnancy (additional)							
1st Trimester		100	0.1	0.1	1	0.05	0.3
2nd Trimester		300	0.1	0.3	2	0.16	0.9
3rd Trimester		300	0.1	0.3	2	0.16	0.9
Lactation (additional)		450	0.2	0.4	3	0.25	1.5

[a]PUFA, polyunsaturated fatty acids
[b]Niacin Equivalents
[c]Level below which intake should not fall
[d]Assumes moderate physical activity
SOURCE: Scientific Review Committee. *Nutrition Recommendation,* Ottawa, Canada: Health and Welfare, 1990.

Summary Examples of Recommended Nutrient Intake Based on Age and Body Weight Expressed as Daily Rates

Age	Sex	Weight kg	Protein kg	Vit. A RE[a]	Vit. D µg	Vit. E mg	Vit. C mg	Folate µg	Vit. B$_{12}$ µg	Calcium mg	Phosphorus mg	Magnesium mg	Iron mg	Iodine µg	Zinc mg
Months															
0-4	Both	6.0	12[b]	400	10	3	20	25	0.3	250[c]	150	20	0.3[d]	30	2[d]
5-12	Both	9.0	12	400	10	3	20	40	0.4	400	200	32	7	40	3
Years															
1	Both	11	13	400	10	3	20	40	0.5	500	300	40	6	55	4
2-3	Both	14	16	400	5	4	20	50	0.6	550	350	50	6	65	4
4-6	Both	18	19	500	5	5	25	70	0.8	600	400	65	8	85	5
7-9	M	25	26	700	2.5	7	25	90	1.0	700	500	100	8	110	7
	F	25	26	700	2.5	6	25	90	1.0	700	500	100	8	95	7
10-12	M	34	34	800	2.5	8	25	120	1.0	900	700	130	8	125	9
	F	36	36	800	2.5	7	25	130	1.0	1100	800	135	8	110	9
13-15	M	50	49	900	2.5	9	30	175	1.0	1100	900	185	10	160	12
	F	48	46	800	2.5	7	30	170	1.0	1000	850	180	13	160	9
16-18	M	62	58	1000	2.5	10	40[e]	220	1.0	900	1000	230	10	160	12
	F	53	47	800	2.5	7	30[e]	190	1.0	700	850	200	12	160	9
19-24	M	71	61	1000	2.5	10	40[e]	220	1.0	800	1000	240	9	160	12
	F	58	50	800	2.5	7	30[e]	180	1.0	700	850	200	13	160	9
25-49	M	74	64	1000	2.5	9	40[e]	230	1.0	800	1000	250	9	160	12
	F	59	51	800	2.5	6	30[e]	185	1.0	700	850	200	13	160	9
50-74	M	73	63	1000	5	7	40[e]	230	1.0	800	1000	250	9	160	12
	F	63	54	800	5	6	30[e]	195	1.0	800	850	210	8	160	9
75+	M	69	59	1000	5	6	40[e]	215	1.0	800	1000	230	9	160	12
	F	64	55	800	5	5	30[e]	200	1.0	800	850	210	8	160	9
Pregnancy (additional)															
1st trimester			5	1000	2.5	2	0	200	0.2	500	200	15	0	25	6
2nd Trimester			20	1000	2.5	2	10	200	0.2	500	200	45	5	25	6
3rd Trimester			24	1000	2.5	2	10	200	0.2	500	200	45	10	25	6
Lactation (additional)			20	400	2.5	3	25	100	0.2	500	200	65	0	50	6

[a] Retinol Equivalents
[b] Protein is assumed to be from breast milk and must be adjusted for infant formula
[c] Infant formula with high phosphorous should contain 375 mg calcium
[d] Breast milk is assumed to be the source of the mineral.
[e] Smokers should increase vitamin C by 50%.
SOURCE: Scientific Review Committee. *Nutrition Recommendations*, Ottowa, Canada: Health and Welfare, 1990.

3-3 | The Guide to Daily Food Choices — a summary

Food Group	Serving	Major Contributions	Foods and Serving Sizes*
Milk, yogurt, and cheese	2 (adult‖) 3 (children, teens, young adults, and pregnant or lactating women)	Calcium Riboflavin Protein Potassium Zinc	1 cup milk 1½ oz cheese 2 oz processed cheese 1 cup yogurt 2 cups cottage cheese 1 cup custard/pudding 1½ cups ice cream
Meat, poultry, fish, dry beans, eggs, and nuts	2-3	Protein Niacin Iron Vitamin B-6 Zinc Thiamin Vitamin B-12†	2-3 oz cooked meat, poultry, fish 1½ cups cooked dry beans 4 T peanut butter 2 eggs ½-1 cup nuts
Fruits	2-4	Vitamin C Fiber	¼ cup dried fruit ½ cup cooked fruit ¾ cup juice 1 whole piece of fruit 1 melon wedge
Vegetables	3-5	Vitamin A Vitamin C Folate Magnesium Fiber	½ cup raw or cooked vegetables 1 cup raw leafy vegetables
Bread, cereals, rice, and pasta	6-11	Starch Thiamin Riboflavin§ Iron Niacin Folate Magnesium‡ Fiber‡ Zinc‡	1 slice of bread 1 oz ready-to-eat cereal ½-¾ cup cooked cereal, rice, or pasta
Fats, oils, and sweets		Foods from this group should not replace any from the other groups. Amounts consumed should be determined by individual energy needs.	

*May be reduced for child servings.
†Only in animal food choices.
‡Whole grains especially.
§If enriched.
‖≥ 25 years of age.

3-4   Cholesterol content of foods

Item	Amount of cholesterol in		
	100 gm edible portion[1] (mg)	Edible portion of 450 gm (1 lb) as purchased (mg)	Refuse from item as purchased (%)
Beef, raw			
with bone[2]	70	270	15
without bone[2]	70	320	0
Brains, raw	>2000	>9000	0
Butter	250	1135	0
Caviar or fish roe	>300	>1300	0
Cheese			
cheddar	100	455	0
cottage, creamed	15	70	0
cream	120	545	0
other (25% to 30% fat)	85	385	0
Cheese spread	65	295	0
Chicken, flesh only, raw	60	—	
Crab			
in shell[2]	125	270	52
meat only[2]	125	565	0
Egg, whole	550	2200	12
Egg white	0	0	0
Egg yolk			
fresh	1500	6800	0
frozen	1280	5800	0
dried	2950	13,380	0
Fish			
steak[2]	70	265	16
fillet[2]	70	320	0
Heart, raw	150	680	0
Ice cream	45	205	0
Kidney, raw	375	1700	0
Lamb, raw			
with bone[2]	70	265	16
without bone[2]	70	320	0
lard and other animal fat	95	430	0
Liver, raw	300	1360	0
Lobster			
whole[2]	200	235	74
meat only[2]	200	900	0
Margarine			
all vegetable fat	0	0	0
two-thirds animal fat, one-third vegetable fat	65	295	0
Milk			
fluid, whole	11	50	0
dried, whole	85	385	0
fluid, skim	3	15	0
Mutton			
with bone[2]	65	250	16
without bone[2]	65	295	0
Oysters			
in shell[2]	>200	>90	90
meat only[2]	>200	>900	0
Pork			
with bone[2]	70	260	18
without bone[2]	70	320	0
Shrimp			
in shell[2]	125	390	31
flesh only[2]	125	565	0
Sweetbreads (thymus)	250	1135	0
Veal			
with bone[2]	90	320	21
without bone[2]	90	410	0

[1] Data apply to 100 gm of edible portion of the item, although it may be purchased with the refuse indicated and described or implied in the first column.

[2] Designate items that have the same chemical composition for the edible portion but differ in the amount of refuse.

3-5 | Food exchange lists

STARCH/BREAD LIST

Each item in this list contains approximately 15 grams of carbohydrate, 3 grams of protein, a trace of fat, and 80 calories. Whole grain products average about 2 grams of fiber per serving. Some foods are higher in fiber. Those foods that contain 3 or more grams of fiber per serving are identified with an asterisk (*).

You can choose your starch exchanges from any of the items on this list. If you want to eat a starch food that is not on this list, the general rule is that:

- ½ cup of cereal, grain or pasta is one serving
- 1 ounce of a bread product is one serving.

Your dietitian can help you be more exact.

CEREALS/GRAINS/PASTA

*Bran cereals, concentrated (such as Bran Buds,®, All Bran®	⅓ cup
*Bran cereals, flaked	½ cup
Bulgur (cooked)	½ cup
Cooked cereals	½ cup
Cornmeal (dry)	2½ Tbsp.
Grapenuts	3 Tbsp.
Grits (cooked)	½ cup
Other ready-to-eat unsweetened cereals	¾ cup
Pasta (cooked)	½ cup
Puffed cereal	1½ cup
Rice, white or brown (cooked)	⅓ cup
Shredded wheat	½ cup
*Wheat germ	3 Tbsp.

DRIED BEANS/PEAS/LENTILS

*Beans and peas (cooked) (such as kidney, white, split, blackeye)	⅓ cup
*Lentils (cooked)	⅓ cup
*Baked beans	¼ cup

STARCHY VEGETABLES

*Corn	½ cup
*Corn on cob, 6 in. long	1
Lima beans	½ cup
*Peas, green (canned or frozen)	½ cup
*Plantain	½ cup
Potato, baked	1 small (3 oz.)
Potato, mashed	½ cup
Squash, winter (acorn, butternut)	¾ cup
Yam, sweet potato, plain	⅓ cup

BREAD

Bagel	½ (1 oz.)
Bread sticks, crisp, 4 in. long × ½ in.	2 (⅔ oz.)
Croutons, low fat	1 cup
English muffin	½
Frankfurter or hamburger bun	½ (1 oz.)
Pita, 6 in. across	½
Plain roll, small	1 (1 oz.)
Raisin, unfrosted	1 slice (1 oz.)
*Rye, pumpernickel	1 slice (1 oz.)
Tortilla, 6 in. across	1
White (including French, Italian)	1 slice (1 oz.)
Whole wheat	1 slice (1 oz.)

CRACKERS/SNACKS

Animal crackers	8
Graham crackers, 2½ in. square	3
Matzoth	¾ oz.
Melba toast	5 slices
Oyster crackers	24
Popcorn (popped, no fat added)	3 cups
Pretzels	¾ oz.
Rye crisp, 2 in. × 3½ in.	4
Saltine-type crackers	6
Whole wheat crackers, no fat added (crisp breads, such as Finn®, Kavli®, Wasa®)	

STARCH FOODS PREPARED WITH FAT

(Count as 1 starch/bread serving, plus 1 fat serving)

Biscuit, 2½ in. across	1
Chow mein noodles	½ cup
Corn bread, 2 in. cube	1 (2 oz.)
Cracker, round butter type	6
French fried potatoes, 2 in. to 3½ in. long	10 (1½ oz.)
Muffin, plain, small	1
Pancake, 4 in. across	2
Stuffing, bread (prepared)	¼ cup
Taco shell, 6 in. across	2
Waffle, 4½ in. square	1
Whole wheat crackers, fat added (such as Triscuits®)	

The exchange lists are the basis of a meal planning system designed by a committee of the American Diabetes Association and the American Dietetic Association. While designed primarily for people with diabetes and others who must follow special diets, the exchange lists are based on principles of good nutrition that apply to everyone. © 1989 American Diabetes Assocation, The American Dietetic Association.

*3 grams or more of fiber per serving.

MEAT LIST

Each serving of meat and substitutes on this list contains about 7 grams of protein. The amount of fat and number of calories varies, depending on what kind of meat or substitute you choose. The list is divided into three parts based on the amount of fat and calories: lean meat, medium-fat meat, and high-fat meat. One ounce (one meat exchange) of each of these includes:

	Carbo-hydrate (grams)	Protein (grams)	Fat (grams)	Calo-ries
Lean	0	7	3	55
Medium-fat	0	7	5	75
High-fat	0	7	8	100

You are encouraged to use more lean and medium-fat meat, poultry, and fish in your meal plan. This will help decrease your fat intake, which may help decrease your risk for heart disease. The items from the high-fat group are high in saturated fat, cholesterol, and calories. You should limit your choices from the high-fat group to three (3) times per week. Meat and substitutes do not contribute any fiber to your meal plan.

†Meats and meat substitutes that have 400 milligrams or more of sodium per exchange are indicated with this symbol.

Tips
1. Bake, roast, broil, grill, or boil these foods rather than frying them with added fat.
2. Use a nonstick pan spray or a nonstick pan to brown or fry these foods.
3. Trim off visible fat before and after cooking.
4. Do not add flour, bread crumbs, coating mixes, or fat to these foods when preparing them.
5. Weigh meat after removing bones and fat, and after cooking. Three ounces of cooked meat is about equal to 4 ounces of raw meat. Some examples of meat portions are:
2 ounces meat (2 meat exchanges) =
1 small chicken leg or thigh
½ cup cottage cheese or tuna
3 ounces meat (3 meat exchanges) =
1 medium pork chop
1 small hamburger
½ of a whole chicken breast
1 unbreaded fish fillet
cooked meat, about the size of a deck of cards
6. Restaurants usually serve prime cuts of meat, which are high in fat and calories.

LEAN MEAT AND SUBSTITUTES (One exchange is equal to any one of the following items.)

Beef	USDA Good or Choice grades of lean beef, such as round, sirloin, and flank steak; tenderloin; and chipped beef†	1 oz.
Pork	Lean pork, such as fresh ham; canned, cured or boiled ham†; Canadian bacon†, tenderloin.	1 oz.
Veal	All cuts are lean except for veal cutlets (ground or cubed). Examples of lean veal are chops and roasts.	1 oz.
Poultry	Chicken, turkey, Cornish hen (without skin)	1 oz.
Fish	All fresh and frozen fish	1 oz.
	Crab, lobster, scallops, shrimp, clams (fresh or canned in water†)	2 oz.
	Oysters	6 medium
	Tuna† (canned in water)	¼ cup
	Herring (uncreamed or smoked)	1 oz.
	Sardines (canned)	2 medium
Wild game	Venison, rabbit, squirrel	1 oz.
	Pheasant, duck, goose (without skin)	1 oz.
Cheese	Any cottage cheese	¼ cup
	Grated parmesan	2 Tbsp.
	Diet cheeses† (with less than 55 calories per ounce)	1 oz.
Other	95% fat-free luncheon meat	1 oz.
	Egg whites	3 whites
	Egg substitutes with less than 55 calories per ¼ cup	¼ cup

†400 mg or more of sodium per exchange.

MEDIUM-FAT MEAT AND SUBSTITUTES (One exchange is equal to any one of the following items.)

Beef	Most beef products fall into this category. Examples are: all ground beef, roast (rib, chuck, rump), steak (cubed, Porterhouse, T-bone), and meatloaf.	1 oz.
Pork	Most pork products fall into this category. Examples are: chops, loin roast, Boston butt, cutlets.	1 oz.
Lamb	Most lamb products fall into this category. Examples are: chops, leg, and roast.	1 oz.
Veal	Cutlet (ground or cubed, unbreaded)	1 oz.
Poultry	Chicken (with skin), domestic duck or goose (well-drained of fat), ground turkey	1 oz.
Fish	Tuna† (canned in oil and drained)	¼ cup
	Salmon† (canned)	¼ cup
Cheese	Skim or part-skim milk cheeses, such as:	
	Ricotta	¼ cup
	Mozzarella	1 oz.
	Diet cheeses† (with 56-80 calories per ounce)	1 oz.
Other	86% fat-free luncheon meat†	1 oz.
	Egg (high in cholesterol, limit to 3 per week)	1
	Egg substitutes with 56-80 calories per ¼ cup	¼ cup
	Tofu (2½ in. × 2¾ in. × 1 in.)	4 oz.
	Liver, heart, kidney, sweetbreads (high in cholesterol)	1 oz.

HIGH-FAT MEAT AND SUBSTITUTES
Remember, these items are high in saturated fat, cholesterol, and calories, and should be used only three (3) times per week. *(One exchange is equal to any one of the following items.)*

Beef	Most USDA Prime cuts of beef, such as ribs, corned beef†	1 oz.
Pork	Spareribs, ground pork, pork sausage† (patty or link)	1 oz.
Lamb	Patties (ground lamb)	1 oz.
Fish	Any fried fish product	1 oz.
Cheese	All regular cheeses†, such as American, Blue, Cheddar, Monterey, Swiss	1 oz.
Other	Luncheon meat†, such as bologna, salami, pimento loaf	1 oz.
	Sausage†, such as Polish, Italian	1 oz.
	Knockwurst, smoked	1 oz.
	Bratwurst†	1 oz.
	Frankfurter† (turkey or chicken)	1 frank (10/lb.)
	Peanut butter (contains unsaturated fat)	1 Tbsp.

Count as one high-fat meat plus one fat exchange:

Frankfurter†, (beef, pork, or combination)	1 frank (10/lb.)

VEGETABLE LIST
Each vegetable serving on this list contains about 5 grams of carbohydrate, 2 grams of protein, and 25 calories. Vegetables contain 2-3 grams of dietary fiber. Vegetables which contain 400 mg of sodium per serving are identified with a † symbol.

Vegetables are a good source of vitamins and minerals. Fresh and frozen vegetables have more vitamins and less added salt. Rinsing canned vegetables will remove much of the salt.

Unless otherwise noted, the serving size for vegetables (one vegetable exchange) is:
½ cup of cooked vegetables or vegetable juice
1 cup of raw vegetables

Artichoke (½ medium)	Mushrooms, cooked
Asparagus	Okra
Beans (green, wax, Italian)	Onions
Bean sprouts	Pea pods
Beets	Peppers (green)
Broccoli	Rutabaga
Brussels sprouts	Sauerkraut†
Cabbage, cooked	Spinach, cooked
Carrots	Summer squash (crookneck)
Cauliflower	
Eggplant	Tomato (one large)
Greens (collard, mustard, turnip)	Tomato/vegetable juice†
	Turnips
Kohlrabi	Water chestnuts
Leeks	Zucchini, cooked

Starchy vegetables such as corn, peas, and potatoes are found on the Starch/Bread List.
For free vegetables, see Free Food List.

†400 mg or more of sodium per serving

FRUIT LIST
Each item on this list contains about 15 grams of carbohydrate, and 60 calories. Fresh, frozen, and dry fruits have about 2 grams of fiber per serving. Fruits that have 3 or more grams of fiber per serving have an asterisk (*). Fruit juices contain very little dietary fiber.

The carbohydrate and calorie content for a fruit serving are based on the usual serving of the most commonly eaten fruits. Use fresh fruits or fruits frozen or canned without sugar added. Whole fruit is more filling than fruit juice and may be a better choice for those who are trying to lose weight. Unless otherwise noted, the serving size for one fruit serving is:
½ cup of fresh fruit or fruit juice
¼ cup of dried fruit

FRESH, FROZEN, AND UNSWEETENED CANNED FRUIT

Apple (raw, 2 in. across)	1 apple
Applesauce (unsweetened)	½ cup
Apricots (medium, raw) or	4 apricots
Apricots (canned)	½ cup, or 4 halves
Banana (9 in. long)	½ banana
*Blackberries (raw)	¾ cup
*Blueberries (raw)	¾ cup
Cantaloupe (5 in. across)	⅓ melon
(cubes)	1 cup
Cherries (large, raw)	12 cherries
Cherries (canned)	½ cup
Figs (raw, 2 in. across)	2 figs
Fruit cocktail (canned)	½ cup
Grapefruit (medium)	½ grapefruit
Grapefruit (segments)	¾ cup
Grapes (small)	15 grapes
Honeydew melon (medium)	⅛ melon
(cubes)	1 cup
Kiwi (large)	1 kiwi
Mandarin oranges	¾ cup
Mango (small)	½ mango
*Nectarine (1½ in. across)	1 nectarine
Orange (2½ in. across)	1 orange
Papaya	1 cup
Peach (2¾ in. across)	1 peach, or ¾ cup
Peaches (canned)	½ cup, or 2 halves
Pear	½ large, or 1 small
Pears (canned)	½ cup or 2 halves
Persimmon (medium, native)	2 persimmons
Pineapple (raw)	¾ cup
Pineapple (canned)	⅓ cup
Plum (raw, 2 in. across)	2 plums
*Pomegranate	½ pomegranate
*Raspberries (raw)	1 cup
*Strawberries (raw, whole)	1¼ cup
Tangerine (2½ in. across)	2 tangerines
Watermelon (cubes)	1¼ cup

DRIED FRUIT

*Apples	4 rings
*Apricots	7 halves
Dates	2½ medium
*Figs	1½
*Prunes	3 medium
Raisins	2 Tbsp.

*3 or more grams of fiber per serving

FRUIT JUICE

Apple juice/cider	½ cup
Cranberry juice cocktail	⅓ cup
Grapefruit juice	½ cup
Grape juice	⅓ cup
Orange juice	½ cup
Pineapple juice	½ cup
Prune juice	⅓ cup

MILK LIST

Each serving of milk or milk products on this list contains about 12 grams of carbohydrate and 8 grams of protein. The amount of fat in milk is measured in percent (%) of butterfat. The calories vary, depending on what kind of milk you choose. The list is divided into three parts based on the amount of fat and calories: skim/very lowfat milk, lowfat milk, and whole milk. One serving (one milk exchange) of each of these includes:

	Carbo- hydrate (grams)	Protein (grams)	Fat (grams)	Calories
Skim/very Lowfat	12	8	trace	90
Lowfat	12	8	5	120
Whole	12	8	8	150

Milk is the body's main source of calcium, the mineral needed for growth and repair of bones. Yogurt is also a good source of calcium. Yogurt and many dried or powdered milk products have different amounts of fat. If you have questions about a particular item, read the label to find out the fat and calorie content.

Milk is good to drink, but it can also be added to cereal, and to other foods. Many tasty dishes such as sugar-free pudding are made with milk (see the Combination Foods List). Add life to plain yogurt by adding one of your fruit servings to it.

SKIM AND VERY LOWFAT MILK

skim milk	1 cup
½% milk	1 cup
1% milk	1 cup
lowfat buttermilk	1 cup
evaporated skim milk	½ cup
dry nonfat milk	⅓ cup
plain nonfat yogurt	8 oz.

LOWFAT MILK

2% milk	1 cup
plain lowfat yogurt (with added nonfat milk solids)	8 oz.

WHOLE MILK

The whole milk group has much more fat per serving than the skim and lowfat groups. Whole milk has more than 3¼% butterfat. Try to limit your choices from the whole milk group as much as possible.

whole milk	1 cup
evaporated whole milk	½ cup
whole plain yogurt	8 oz.

FAT LIST

Each serving on the fat list contains about 5 grams of fat and 45 calories.

The foods on the fat list contain mostly fat, although some items may also contain a small amount of protein. All fats are high in calories and should be carefully measured. Everyone should modify fat intake by eating unsaturated fats instead of saturated fats. The sodium content of these foods varies widely. Check the label for sodium information.

UNSATURATED FATS

Avocado	⅛ medium
Margarine	1 tsp
‡Margarine, diet	1 Tbsp.
Mayonnaise	1 tsp
‡Mayonnaise, reduced- calorie	1 Tbsp.
Nuts and seeds:	
Almonds, dry roasted	6 whole
Cashews, dry roasted	1 Tbsp.
Pecans	2 whole
Peanuts	20 small or 10 large
Walnuts	2 whole
Other nuts	1 Tbsp.
Seeds, pine nuts, sun- flower (without shells)	1 Tbsp.
Pumpkin seeds	2 tsp.
Oil (corn, cottonseed, saf- flower, soybean, sun- flower, olive, peanut)	1 tsp.
‡Olives	10 small or 5 large
Salad dressing, mayonnaise-type	2 tsp.
Salad dressing, mayonnaise-type, reduced-calorie	1 Tbsp.
‡Salad dressing (all varieties)	1 Tbsp.
†Salad dressing, reduced- calorie	2 Tbsp.

(Two tablespoons of low-calorie salad dressing is a free food.)

SATURATED FATS

Butter	1 tsp.
‡Bacon	1 slice
Chitterlings	½ ounce
Coconut, shredded	2 Tbsp.
Coffee whitener, liquid	2 Tbsp.
Coffee whitener, powder	4 tsp.
Cream (light, coffee, table)	2 Tbsp.
Cream, sour	2 Tbsp.
Cream (heavy, whipping)	1 Tbsp.
Cream cheese	1 Tbsp.
‡Salt pork	¼ ounce

†400 mg or more of sodium per serving.
‡If more than one or two servings are eaten, these foods have 400 mg. or more of sodium.

3-6 Food exchange lists for infants

List 1: Milk/formula exchange*

	Protein/g	CHO/g	Fat/g
Whole milk	8	12	10
Similac	3.6	17.0	8.8
Enfamil	3.6	16.8	8.8
SMA	3.6	17.3	8.6
Prosobee	6.0	16.3	8.4
isomil	4.8	16.3	8.6
2% milk	8	12	5†
Advance	6.7	14.9	4.8†

List 2: Bread exchanges for diabetic infants‡

Dry baby rice cereal	5 tablespoons
Baby oatmeal cereal	5 tablespoons
High-protein cereal	9 tablespoons
"Strained" jar = 4.75 oz (135 g)	
Strained baby rice cereal with mixed fruit (also count 1 fruit exchange)	1 jar
Baby oatmeal cereal with applesauce and banana	1 jar
High-protein cereal with applesauce and banana	1 jar
Creamed corn	1 jar
Mixed vegetables	1 jar
Sweet potatoes	1 jar
"Junior" jar = 7.75 oz (200 g)	
Junior rice with mixed fruit	1 jar
Oatmeal with applesauce and banana	1 jar
Creamed corn	1 jar
Teething biscuits, arrowroot cookies, animal cookies, and pretzels	3

List 3: Fruit exchanges for diabetic infants§

Baby apple juice	¾ can (3 oz)
Mixed fruit juice	½ can (2 oz)
Prune-orange juice	⅓ can (1½ oz)
"Baby" can = 4.2 oz.	
Strained applesauce	½ jar
Bananas	⅓ jar
Peaches	⅓ jar
Plums	¼ jar
Prunes	⅓ jar
Cherry vanilla pudding	½ jar
Chocolate custard	⅓ jar
Dutch apple desert	⅓ jar
"Strained" jar = 4.75 oz (135 g)	
Junior applesauce	⅓ jar
Bananas	¼ jar
Peaches	⅕ jar (5 tbsp)
Pears	⅓ jar (5 tbsp)
Plums	⅕ jar (5 tbsp)
Prunes	⅕ jar (5 tbsp)
"Junior" jar = 7.75 oz (220 g)	

List 4: Meat exchanges for diabetic infants‖

Strained egg yolk	1 jar
Strained chicken	½ jar
Ham	½ jar
Lamb	½ jar
Beef	½ jar
Pork	½ jar
(Above also must count 1 fat)	
1 jar = 3.33 oz (94 g)	½ jar
Junior chicken	
Ham	½ jar
Lamb	½ jar
Beef	½ jar
Pork	½ jar
Meat sticks	½ jar
1 jar = 3.5 oz (99 g)	
Strained carrots	1 jar
Beets	½ jar
Creamed spinach	1 jar
Green beans	1 jar
Squash	1 jar
Peas	1 jar
"Strained" jar = 4.5 oz (128 g)	
Junior carrots	½ jar
Creamed spinach	½ jar
Green beans	½ jar
Squash	½ jar
"Junior" jar = 7.5 oz (213 g)	

List 6: Multiple exchanges for diabetic infants

Strained beef with egg noodles and vegetables	1 jar = ½ bread ½ meat
Cereal and egg yolk	1 jar = ½ bread ½ meat
Chicken and noodles	1 jar = ½ bread ½ meat
Vegetables and chicken	1 jar = ½ bread ½ meat
Macaroni and cheese	1 jar = 1 fruit ½ meat
High meat dinners	1 jar = 1 meat ½ bread
"Strained" jar = 4.5 oz (128 g)	
Junior beef with egg noodles	1 jar = 1 bread ½ meat
Cereal and egg yolk	1 jar = 1 bread 1 fat
Chicken and vegetables	1 jar = 1 bread ½ meat
Vegetables and chicken	1 jar = 1 bread ½ meat
Macaroni and cheese	1 jar = 1 bread ½ meat
"Junior" jar = 7.5 oz (213 g)	

From Kohler, E.: Baby food exchanges and feeding the diabetic infant. Diabetes Care 3:553-556, 1980. Reproduced with permission from The American Diabetes Association, Inc.

*One 8-oz cup = 160 cal.
†Add 1 fat exchange.
‡Each item is 1 bread exchange (68 cal).
‡Each item is 1 bread exchange (68 cal).
§Ech item is 1 fruit exchange (40 cal).
‖Each item is 1 meat exhcange (73 cal).
¶Each item is 1 vegetable B exchange (36 cal).

Pregnancy table for expected date of delivery

Find the date of the last menstrual period in the top line (light-face type) of the pair of lines.
The dark number (bold-face type) in the line below will be the expected day of delivery.

Jan.	1 2 3 4 5 6 7 8 9 10 11 12 13 14 15 16 17 18 19 20 21 22 23 24 25 26 27 28 29 30 31	
Oct.	**8 9 10 11 12 13 14 15 16 17 18 19 20 21 22 23 24 25 26 27 28 29 30 31 (1 2 3 4 5 6 7**	Nov.
Feb.	1 2 3 4 5 6 7 8 9 10 11 12 13 14 15 16 17 18 19 20 21 22 23 24 25 26 27 28	
Nov.	**8 9 10 11 12 13 14 15 16 17 18 19 20 21 22 23 24 25 26 27 28 29 30 (1 2 3 4 5**	Dec.
Mar.	1 2 3 4 5 6 7 8 9 10 11 12 13 14 15 16 17 18 19 20 21 22 23 24 25 26 27 28 29 30 31	
Dec.	**6 7 8 9 10 11 12 13 14 15 16 17 18 19 20 21 22 23 24 25 26 27 28 29 30 31 (1 2 3 4 5**	Jan.
April	1 2 3 4 5 6 7 8 9 10 11 12 13 14 15 16 17 18 19 20 21 22 23 24 25 26 27 28 29 30	
Jan.	**6 7 8 9 10 11 12 13 14 15 16 17 18 19 20 21 22 23 24 25 26 27 28 29 30 31 (1 2 3 4**	Feb.
May	1 2 3 4 5 6 7 8 9 10 11 12 13 14 15 16 17 18 19 20 21 22 23 24 25 26 27 28 29 30 31	
Feb.	**5 6 7 8 9 10 11 12 13 14 15 16 17 18 19 20 21 22 23 24 25 26 27 28 (1 2 3 4 5 6 7**	Mar.
June	1 2 3 4 5 6 7 8 9 10 11 12 13 14 15 16 17 18 19 20 21 22 23 24 25 26 27 28 29 30	
Mar.	**8 9 10 11 12 13 14 15 16 17 18 19 20 21 22 23 24 25 26 27 28 29 30 31 (1 2 3 4 5 6**	April
July	1 2 3 4 5 6 7 8 9 10 11 12 13 14 15 16 17 18 19 20 21 22 23 24 25 26 27 28 29 30 31	
April	**7 8 9 10 11 12 13 14 15 16 17 18 19 20 21 22 23 24 25 26 27 28 29 30 (1 2 3 4 5 6 7**	May
Aug.	1 2 3 4 5 6 7 8 9 10 11 12 13 14 15 16 17 18 19 20 21 22 23 24 25 26 27 28 29 30 31	
May	**8 9 10 11 12 13 14 15 16 17 18 19 20 21 22 23 24 25 26 27 28 29 30 31 (1 2 3 4 5 6 7**	June
Sept.	1 2 3 4 5 6 7 8 9 10 11 12 13 14 15 16 17 18 19 20 21 22 23 24 25 26 27 28 29 30	
June	**8 9 10 11 12 13 14 15 16 17 18 19 20 21 22 23 24 25 26 27 28 29 30 (1 2 3 4 5 6 7**	July
Oct.	1 2 3 4 5 6 7 8 9 10 11 12 13 14 15 16 17 18 19 20 21 22 23 24 25 26 27 28 29 30 31	
July	**8 9 10 11 12 13 14 15 16 17 18 19 20 21 22 23 24 25 26 27 28 29 30 31 (1 2 3 4 5 6 7**	Aug.
Nov.	1 2 3 4 5 6 7 8 9 10 11 12 13 14 15 16 17 18 19 20 21 22 23 24 25 26 27 28 29 30	
Aug.	**8 9 10 11 12 13 14 15 16 17 18 19 20 21 22 23 24 25 26 27 28 29 30 31 (1 2 3 4 5 6**	Sept.
Dec.	1 2 3 4 5 6 7 8 9 10 11 12 13 14 15 16 17 18 19 20 21 22 23 24 25 26 27 28 29 30 31	
Sept.	**7 8 9 10 11 12 13 14 15 16 17 18 19 20 21 22 23 24 25 26 27 28 29 30 (1 2 3 4 5 6 7**	Oct.

The Washington guide to promoting development in the young child

Motor skills

Expected tasks	Suggested activities
1 to 3 months 1. Holds head up briefly when prone 2. Head erect and bobbing when supported in sitting position 3. Head erect and steady in sitting position 4. Follows object through all planes 5. Palmar grasp 6. Moro reflex	1. Place infant in prone position 2. Support in sitting position with his head erect 3. Pull infant to sitting position 4. Provide with opportunity to observe people or activity 5. Hang bright-colored objects and mobiles within reach across crib 6. Provide with opportunity to observe objects or people while in sitting position 7. Use infant seat 8. Alternate bright shiny objects with dark and light visual patterns
4 to 8 months 1. Sits with minimal support, with stable head and back 2. Sits alone steadily 3. Plays with hands, which are open most of time 4. Grasps rattle or bottle with both hands 5. Picks up small objects, for example, cube 6. Transfers toys from one hand to other 7. Neck-righting reflex	1. Pull up to sitting position 2. Provide opportunity to sit supported or alone when head and trunk control are stabilized 3. Put bright-colored objects within reach 4. Give toys or household objects: rattles, teething ring, cloth animals or dolls, 1-inch cubes, plastic objects such as cups, rings, and balls 5. Offer small objects such as cereal to improve grasp 6. Offer a variety of patterns or textures to play with 7. Use squeak toys
9 to 12 months 1. Rises to sitting position 2. Creeps or crawls, maybe backward at first 3. Pulls to standing position 4. Stands alone 5. Cruises 6. Uses index finger to poke 7. Finger-thumb grasp 8. Parachute reflex 9. Landau reflex	1. Provide playpen, allow child to pull himself to standing 2. Give opportunity and space to practice creeping and crawling 3. Have child practice moving on knees to improve balance prior to walking 4. Have child use walker or straddle toys 5. Play airplane with child; have child practice catching himself while rolling on large ball 6. Provide with objects such as spoons, plastic bottles, cups, ball, cubes, finger foods, saucepans, and lids
13 to 18 months 1. Walks a few steps without support 2. Balanced when walking 3. Walks upstairs with help, creeps downstairs 4. Turns pages of book	1. Provide opportunity to practice walking, climbing stairs with help 2. Give toys that can be pushed around 3. Supervise activity with paper and large crayons 4. Provide toys such as cubes, cups, saucepans, lids, rag dolls, and other soft, cuddly toys 5. Begin introducing child to swing
19 to 30 months 1. Runs 2. Walks up and down stairs, one at a time (not alternating feet) 3. Imitates vertical strokes 4. Imitates building tower of four or more blocks 5. Throws ball overhand 6. Jumps in place 7. Rides tricycle	1. Provide opportunity to practice and develop activities 2. Provide pattern for child while he watches and then encourage him to try 3. Provide tricycle or similar pedal toys; secure foot on pedal if necessary
31 to 48 months 1. Walks downstairs (alternating feet) 2. Hops on one foot 3. Swings and climbs 4. Balances on one foot for 10 seconds 5. Copies circle 6. Copies cross 7. Draws person with three parts	1. Continue with blocks, combining materials, toy cars, and trains 2. Provide clay and other manipulating materials 3. Give opportunities to swing and climb 4. Provide with activities such as finger painting, chalk, and black board

Continued.

Motor skills — cont'd

Expected tasks	Suggested activities
49 to 52 months 1. Balances well 2. Skips and jumps 3. Can heel-toe walk 4. Copies square 5. Catches bounced ball	1. Provide with music and games to synchronize hand and foot, tapping with music, skipping, hopping, and dancing rhythmically to improve coordination

Feeding skills

Expected tasks	Suggested activities
1 to 3 months 1. Sucking reflex present 2. Rooting reflex present 3. Ability to swallow pureed foods 4. Coordinates sucking, swallowing, and breathing	1. Consider a change in nipple or posturing if there is difficulty in swallowing 2. Introduce solids, one kind at a time (use small spoon, place food well back on infant's tongue) 3. Hold in comfortable relaxed position while feeding 4. Pace feeding tempo to infant's needs
4 to 8 months 1. Tongue used in moving food in mouth 2. Hand-to-mouth motions 3. Recognizes bottle on sight 4. Gums or mouths solid foods 5. Feeds self cracker	1. Give finger foods to develop chewing, stimulate gums, and encourage hand-to-mouth motion (cubes of cheese, bananas, dry toast, bread crust, cookies) 2. Encourage upright supported position for feeding 3. Promote bottle holding 4. Introduce junior foods
9 to 12 months 1. Holds own bottle 2. Drinks from cup or glass with assistance 3. Finger feeds 4. Beginning to hold spoon	1. Bring child in highchair to table and include in part of or entire meal with family 2. Have child in dry comfortable position with trunk and feet supported 3. Encourage self-help in feeding; use of table foods 4. Offer spoon when interest is indicated 5. Introduce cup or glass with small amount of fluid
13 to 18 months 1. Holds cup and handle with digital grasp 2. Lifts cup and drinks well 3. Beginning to use spoon, may turn bowl down before reaching mouth 4. Difficulty in inserting spoon into mouth 5. May refuse food	1. Continue offering finger foods (wieners, sandwiches) 2. Use nontip dishes and cups; dishes should have sides to make filling of spoon easy 3. Give opportunity for self-feeding 4. Provide fluids between meals rather than having child fill up on fluids at mealtime
19 to 30 months 1. Drinks without spilling 2. Holds small glass in one hand 3. Inserts spoon in mouth correctly 4. Distinguishes between food and inedible material 5. Plays with food	1. Encourage self-feeding with spoon 2. Do not rush child 3. Serve foods plainly but in attractive servings 4. Small servings of food will encourage eating more than large servings
31 to 48 months 1. Pours well from pitcher 2. Serves self at table with little spilling 3. Rarely needs assistance 4. Interest in setting table	1. Encourage self-help 2. Give opportunity for pouring (give rice and pitcher to promote pouring skills) 3. Encourage child to help set table 4. Have well-defined rules about table manners
49 to 52 months 1. Feeds self well 2. Social and talkative during meal	1. Socialize with child at mealtime 2. Have child help with preparation, table setting, and serving 3. Include child in conversations at mealtimes by planning special times for him to tell about events, situations, or what he did during the day

Sleep

Expected tasks	Suggested activities
1 to 3 months 1. Night: 4 to 10 hour intervals 2. Naps: frequent 3. Longer periods of wakefulness without crying	1. Provide separate sleeping arrangements away from parent's room 2. Reduce noise and light stimulation when placing in bed 3. Have room at comfortable temperature with no drafts or extremes in heat 4. Reverse position of crib occasionally 5. Place child in different positions from time to time for sleep 6. Alternate from back to side to stomach 7. Keep crib sides up
4 to 8 months 1. Night: 10 to 12 hours 2. Naps: 2 to 3 (1 to 4 hours in duration) 3. Night awakenings	1. Keep crib sides up 2. Refrain from taking child into parents' room if he awakens 3. Check to determine if there is cause for awakenings: hunger, teething, pain, cold, wet, noise, or illness 4. If a baby-sitter is used, attempt to find some person with whom infant is familiar. Explain bedtime and naptime arrangements.
9 to 12 months 1. Night: 12 to 14 hours 2. Naps: one to two (1 to 4 hours in duration) 3. May begin refusing morning nap	1. Short crying periods may be source of tension release for child 2. Observe for signs of fatigue, irritability, or restlessness if naps are shorter 3. Provide familiar person to baby-sit who knows sleep routines
13 to 18 months 1. Night: 10 to 12 hours 2. Naps: one in afternoon (1 to 3 hours in duration) 3. May awaken during night crying (associated with wetting bed) 4. As he becomes more able to move about, he may uncover himself, become cold, and awaken	1. Night terrors may be terminated by awakening infant and offering reassurance 2. Check to see that child is covered 3. Avoid hazardous devices to keep child covered, including blanket clips, pins, and garments that enclose child to neck
19 to 30 months 1. Night: 10 to 12 hours 2. Naps: one (1 to 3 hours duration) 3. Doesn't go to sleep at once — keeps demanding things 4. May awaken crying if wet or soiled 5. May awaken because of environmental change of temperature, change of bed, change of sleeping room, addition of sibling to room, absence of parents from home, hospitalization, trip with family, or relatives visiting	1. Quiet period of socialization prior to bedtime — reading child book or telling story 2. Holding child — talking quietly with him 3. Ritualistic behavior may be present; allow child to carry out routine; helps him overcome fear of unexpected or fear of dark, for example, child may wish to arrange toys in certain way 4. Explain bedtime ritual to baby-sitter 5. Give more reassurance, spend more time before bedtime preparation 6. Provide familiar bedtime toys or items 7. Allow crying-out period if he is safe, comfortable, and tucked in 8. Place in bed before he reaches excessive state of fatigue, excitement, or tiredness 9. Eliminate sources of stimulation or fear 10. Maintain consistent hour of bedtime
31 to 48 months 1. Daily range: 10 to 15 hours 2. Naps: beginning to disappear 3. Prolongs process of going to bed 4. Less dependent on taking toys to bed 5. May awaken crying from dreams 6. May awaken if wet	1. Television programs may affect ability to go to sleep: avoid violent television programs 2. Anxiety about going to bed and desire to stay up with parents requires limits 3. Regularity and consistency important to promote good sleep habits 4. Reassurance — night light or leaving door ajar 5. Do not use bedtime or naptime as punishment 6. Encourage naps if signs of fatigue or irritability are evidenced
49 to 52 months 1. Daily range: 9 to 13 hours 2. Naps: rare 3. Quieter during sleep	1. Encourage napping if excessive or strenuous activity occurs and child is overly tired 2. Explain to child if baby-sitter will be there after child is asleep

Play

Expected tasks	Suggested activities
1 to 3 months	
1. Quieted when picked up	1. Encourage holding and touching of child by mother
2. Regards face of others	2. Provide with cradle gyms and mobiles, brightly colored, visually interesting objects within arm's distance
4 to 8 months	
1. Plays with own body	1. Begin patty-cake and peekaboo
2. Differentiates strangers from family	2. Provide for periods of solitary play (playpen)
3. Seeks out objects	3. Encourage holding and touching of child by mother
4. Grasps, holds, and manipulates objects	4. Provide variety of multicolored and multitextured objects that child can hold
5. Repeats activities he enjoys	5. Encourage exploration of body parts
6. Bangs toys or objects together	6. Provide floating toys for bath
9 to 12 months	
1. Puts objects in and out of containers	1. Continue mother-infant games
2. Examines objects held in hand	2. Give opportunity to place objects in containers and pour out
3. Plays interactive games (peekaboo)	3. Provide large and small objects with which to play
4. Extends toy to other person without releasing	4. Encourage interactive play
5. Works to get toy out of reach	
13 to 18 months	
1. Plays by himself — may play near others	1. Introduce to other children even though child may not play with them
2. Has preferred toys	2. Provide music, books, and magazines
3. Enjoys walking activities, pulling toys	3. Encourage imitative activities — helping with dusting, sweeping, stirring
4. Throws and picks up objects, throws again	
5. Imitates, for example, reading newspaper, sweeping	
19 to 30 months	
1. Parallel play — not interactive but plays alongside another child	1. Provide with new materials for manipulating and feeling — finger paints, clay, sand, stones, water, and soap
2. Uses both large and small toys	Wooden toys — cars and animals
3. Rough-and-tumble play	Building blocks of various sizes, crayons, and paper
4. Play periods longer than before — interested in manipulative and constructive toys	Rhythmical tunes and equipment — swing, rocking chair, rocking horse
5. Enjoys rhymes and singing (television programs)	Children's books — short, simple stories with repetition and familiar objects; enjoys simple pictures, brightly colored
	2. Guide child's hand to actively participate with specific activities, for example, using crayons, hammering
31 to 48 months	
1. In playing with others, beginning to interact, sharing toys, taking turns	1. Encourage play with small groups of children
2. Dramatizes, expresses imagination in play	2. Encourage imaginative and dramatic play activities
3. Combining playthings; more use of constructive materials	3. Music: singing and experimenting with musical instruments
4. Prefers two or three children to play with; may have special friend	4. Group participation in rhymes, dancing by hopping or jumping
	5. Drawing and painting (seldom recognizable)
49 to 52 months	
1. Dramatic play and interest in going on excursions	1. Painting and drawing (objects will be out of proportion; details that are most important to child are drawn largest)
2. Fond of cutting and pasting, creative materials	2. Encourage printing of numbers and letters
3. Completes most activities	3. Clay: making recognizable objects
	4. Cutting and pasting
	5. Provide with materials, for example, boxes, chairs, barrels, for building sturdy structures

Language

Expected tasks	Suggested activities
1 to 3 months *Receptive abilities* 1. Movement of eyes, respiration rate, or body activity changes when bell is rung close to child's head 2. Smiles when socially stimulated 3. Has facial, vocal, and generalized bodily responses to faces 4. Reacts differently to adult voices *Expressive abilities* 1. Makes prelanguage vocalizations that consist of cooing, throaty sounds, for example, gu 2. Makes "pleasure" sounds that consist of soft vowels 3. Makes "sucking" sounds 4. Crying can be differentiated for discomfort, pain, and hunger as reported by mother 5. An "A" sound as in cat is commonly heard in distress crying	1. Observe facial expressions, gestures, bodily postures, and movements when vocalizations are being produced 2. Smile and talk softly in pleasant tone while holding, touching, and handling infant 3. Hold, touch, and interact frequently with infant for pleasure 4. Refrain from letting infant engage in prolonged and incessant crying

4 to 8 months
Receptive abilities
1. Eyes locate source of sound
2. Responds to "hi, there" by looking up at face that is across and in front of him
3. Head turns to sound of cellophane held and crunched 2 feet away and at a 135-degree angle on either side of head
4. Will turn head to locate sound of "look here" when spoken at a 90-degree angle from head 2 feet away*
5. Turns head to sound of rattle
6. Responds differently to vacuum cleaner, phone, doorbell, or sound of dog barking: may cry, whimper, look toward sound, or mother may report change in body tension
7. Responds by raising arms when mother reaches toward child and says "come up"
 	
Expressive abilities
1. Uses different inflectional patterns:
  ah   ah
      uh
2. Laughs aloud when stimulated
3. Has differential patterns of crying when hungry, in pain, or angry
4. Produces vowel sounds and chained syllables (baba, gugu, didi)
5. Makes "talking sounds" in response to others talking to him
6. Babbles to produce consonant sounds: ba, da, m-m
7. Vocalizes to toys
8. Says "da-da" or "ma-ma" but not specific to presence of parents
	1. Engage in smiling eye-to-eye contact while talking to infant
	2. Vocalize in response to inflectional patterns and when infant is producing babbling sounds; echo the sounds he makes
	3. Observe for subtle communication clues such as eye aversion, struggling to move away, flushing of skin, tension of body, or movement of arms
	4. Vocalize with infant during handling, while feeding, bathing, dressing, diapering, bedtime preparation, and holding
	5. Stimulate laughing by light tickling
	6. Observe child's reactions to bells, whistles, horns, phones, laughing, singing, talking, music box, noise-making toys, and common household noises
	7. While talking to infant, hold in position so that he can see your face
	8. Have infant placed at position of eye level while talking to him throughout the day
	9. If crying or laughing sounds are not discerned at this stage, report to family physician, pediatrician, public health nurse, or well-child clinic

9 to 12 months *Receptive abilities* 1. Ceases activity when name is pronounced or "no-no" is said 2. Gives toys on request when accompanied by facial and bodily gestures 3. Attends to simple commands *Expressive abilities* 1. Imitates definite speech sounds such as tongue clicking, lip smacking, or coughing 2. Should have two words that are *specific* for parents: "mama," "dada," or equivalents	1. Gain child's attention when giving simple commands 2. Accompany oral directions with gestures 3. Vocalize with child during feeding, bathing, and playtimes 4. Provide sounds that child can reproduce such as lip smacking and tongue clicking 5. Repeat direction frequently and have child participate in action: open and close the drawer; move arms and legs up and down 6. Have child respond to verbal directions: stand up, sit down, close door, open door, turn around, come here

*Do not test for localization of sound by producing sound directly behind infant's head.

Continued.

Language — cont'd

Expected tasks	Suggested activities

13 to 18 months
Receptive abilities
1. Attends to person speaking to child
2. Finds "the baby" in picture when requested, for example, on baby food jar, in magazine, or in story-books
3. Indicates wants by gestures
4. Looks toward family members or pets when named

Expressive abilities
1. Uses three words other than mama and dada to denote *specific* objects, persons, or actions
2. Indicates wants by naming objects such as cookie

1. Incorporate repetition into daily routine of home
   a. Feeding: name baby's food and eating utensils; ask if he is enjoying his dessert; concentrate on reviewing a day's events in simple manner
   b. Household duties: mother names each item as she dusts; pronounces word while cooking and preparing foods
   c. Playing: identify toys when using them; explain their function
2. Let child see mouthing of words
3. Encourage verbalization and expression of wants.

19 to 30 months
Receptive abilities
1. Points to one named body part
2. Follows two or three verbal directions that are not accompanied by facial or body gestures, for example, put ball on table, give it to mommy, or put toy in box

Expressive abilities
1. Combines two different words, for example, "play ball," "want cookie"
2. Names object in picture, for example, cat, bird, dog, horse, man
3. Refers to self by pronoun rather than by name

1. Continue to present concrete objects with words; talk about activities child is involved with
2. Include child in conversations during mealtimes
3. Encourage speech by having child express wants
4. Incorporate games into bathing routine by having child name and point to body parts
5. As child gains confidence in remembering and using words appropriately, encourage less use of gestures
6. Count and name articles of clothing as they are placed on child
7. Count and name silverware as it is placed on table
8. Sort, match, and name glassware, laundry, cans, vegetables, and fruit with child
9. Have child keep scrapbook and add new picture every day to increase recognition of vocabulary words
10. Spend 15 to 20 minutes per day going through booklets and naming pictures; have child point to pictures as objects are named
11. Help child develop functional core vocabulary to express safety needs and information about neighborhood
12. Whenever possible, use word (for example, paper), show object, have child handle and use it, encourage him to watch your face while you say the words, and suggest that he repeat it; refrain from undue pressure

31 to 36 months
Receptive abilities
1. Takes turns when asked while playing, eating
2. Attends longer to stories and television programs
3. Demonstrates understanding of two prepositions by carrying out two commands one at a time, for example, "put the block under the chair"
4. Can follow commands asking for two objects or two actions
5. Demonstrates understanding of concepts of big and little, for example, selects larger of two balls when asked for big one
6. Points to additional body parts

Expressive abilities
1. Uses regular plurals, for example, adds "s" to apple, box, orange (does not use irregular plurals, for example, mouse to mice)
2. Gives first and last name
3. Names what he has drawn after scribbling
4. On request, tells you his sex; for example, "Are you a little boy or a little girl?"
5. Can repeat a few rhymes or songs
6. On request, tells what action is going on in picture, for example, the kitten is eating

1. Read stories with familiar content but with more detail; nonsense rhymes, humorous stories
2. Expect child to follow simple commands
3. Give child opportunity to hear and repeat his full name
4. Listen to child's explanation about pictures he draws
5. Encourage child to repeat nursery rhymes by himself and with others
6. Address child by his first name

Continued.

Language — cont'd

Expected tasks	Suggested activities
37 to 48 months	
1. Expresses appropriate responses when asked	1. Provide visual stimuli while reading stories
2. Tells stories	2. Have child repeat story
3. Common expression: I don't know	3. Arrange trips to zoo, farms, seashore, stores, and
4. Repeats sentence composed of twelve to thirteen syllables, for example, "I am going when daddy and I are finished playing"	movies and discuss with child
	4. Give simple explanations in answering questions
5. Has mastered phonetic sounds of p, k, g, v, tf, d, z, lr, hw, j, kw, l, e, w, qe, and o	
49 to 52 months	
Receptive abilities	
1. Points to penny, nickel, or dime on request	1. Play games in which child names colors
2. Carries out in order command containing three parts, for example, "pick up the block, put it on the table, and bring the book to me"	2. Encourage use of please and thank you
	3. Encourage social-verbal interactions with other children
	4. Encourage correct usage of words
Expressive abilities	5. Provide puppets or toys with movable parts that child can converse about
1. Names penny, nickel, or dime on request	6. Provide group activity for child; children may stimu-
2. Replies appropriately to questions such as, "What do you do when you are asleep?"	late each other by taking turns naming pictures
3. Counts three objects, pointing to each in turn	7. Allow child to make choices about games, stories, and activities
4. Defines simple words, for example, hat, ball	8. Have child dramatize simple stories
5. Asks questions	9. Provide child with piggy bank and encourage naming coins as they are handled or dropped into bank
6. Can identify or name four colors	

Discipline

Expected tasks	Suggested activities
1 to 3 months	
1. Draws attention by crying	1. a. Needs should be identified and met as promptly as possible
	b. Every bit of fussing should not be interpreted as emergency requiring immediate attention
	c. Infant should not be ignored and permitted to cry for exhaustive periods
2. Infant desires whatever is pleasant and wishes to avoid unpleasant situations	2. Begin to present limit of having to wait so that infant can learn that tension and discomfort are bearable for short periods
3. Beginning to "wiggle" around	3. Place infant on surfaces that have sides to protect him from falling off
4 to 8 months	
1. Begins to respond to "no-no"	1. a. Reserve "no-no" for times when it is really needed
	b. Be consistent with word "no-no" for same activity and event that requires it; be friendly and firm with verbal control of limit setting
2. Infant who is left alone for long periods of time may become bored or fretful; learns that crying and whining result in attention	2. Make special efforts to attend to infant when he is quiet and amusing himself
3. Beginning to show signs of timidity and fretfulness and may whimper and cry when mother separates from him or when strangers pick him up	3. a. Gradually introduce strangers into infant's environment
	b. Refrain from promoting frightening situations with strangers during this stage
	c. Play hiding games like peekaboo in which mother disappears and reappears
	d. Allow infant to cling to mother and get used to persons a little at a time
	e. If baby-sitter is used, find person familiar to infant or introduce for brief periods before mother leaves infant in her care
	f. Encourage gentle handling by mother, father, and siblings. Discourage rough handling, particularly by strangers

Continued.

Discipline—cont'd

Expected tasks	Suggested activities
4. Beginning to grasp objects and bring to mouth, but unable to differentiate safe from hazardous items	4. a. Provide toys that do not have small detachable parts b. Check frequently for small objects in his line of reach 5. When traveling in car, place in crib or seat with safety belts securely fastened

9 to 12 months

1. Beginning to respond to simple commands, for example, "pick up the ball, put the toy in the box"	1. a. Avoid setting unreasonable number of limits b. Give simple commands one at a time c. Once limit is set, adhere to it firmly each time and connect it immediately with misbehavior d. Respond with consistency in enforcing rule e. Allow time to conform to request f. Gain child's attention
2. Ready to go places on his own and is trying out newly developing motor capacities (not to be confused with naughtiness, "spoiled," or stubbornness)	2. a. Begin setting and enforcing limits on where child is allowed to travel and explore b. Remove tempting objects c. Remove sources of danger such as light sockets, protruding pot handles, hanging table covers, sharp objects, and hanging cords d. Keep child away from fans, heaters, and certain drawers and do not place vaporizer close to infant's crib e. Keep high chair at least 2 feet away from working and cooking surfaces in kitchen f. Use gate to keep child out of kitchen when it is being used g. Be certain that pans, basins, and tubs of hot water are never left unattended h. Remove all possible poisons or substances that are not food that can be eaten or drunk off floor, low-level cabinets, and under sink i. Keep child from objects or surfaces that he may chew, for example, porch rails, windowsills, *repainted* toys or cribs that may contain lead j. Instruct baby-sitter on all safety items
3. Has emerging desires to look at, handle, and touch objects	3. a. Experiment with diversionary measures b. Provide child with own play objects
4. Explores objects by sucking, chewing, and biting	4. a. Remove household poisons, cosmetics, pins, and buttons that he could put in his mouth b. Be certain that objects that go into mouth are hygienic c. Check toys for detachable small parts
5. Beginning to test reactions to certain parental responses during feeding and may become choosy about food	5. a. Once problem behaviors are defined, plan to work on changing only one behavior at a time until child behaves or conforms to expectations b. Be certain that child understands old rules before adding new ones c. Respond with consistency in enforcing old rules: enforce each time, do not ignore next time d. Provide regular pattern of mealtimes e. Refrain from feeding throughout day f. Allow child to decide what he will eat and how much g. Introduce new foods gradually over period of time h. Continue to offer foods that may have been rejected first time i. Do not force food j. Refrain from physically punishing child for changes in eating habits
6. Beginning to test reactions to parental responses at bedtime preparation	6. a. Provide regular time for naps and bedtime b. Avoid excessive stimulation at bedtime or naptime c. Ignore fussing and crying once safety and physical needs are satisfied and usual ritual is carried out d. Keep child in own room e. Refrain from picking up and rocking and holding if needs seem satisfied

Continued.

Discipline — cont'd

Expected tasks	Suggested activities
13 to 18 months	

1. Understands simple commands and requests	1. a. Begin with one rule; add new ones as appropriate
	   b. In selecting new rules, choose on the basis of being able to clearly define it to self and child, having it reasonable and enforceable at all times; demand no more than fulfillment of defined expectations
	   c. Plan decisive limits and plan to give consistent attention to them

2. In learning mastery over impulses and self-control, child begins testing out limit setting	2. a. Immediately correct errors in behavior as they occur
	   b. Use consistent enforcement of short-term rules (which are given as verbal commands) and long-term rules (which pertain to chores and family routines)
	   c. Ignore temper tantrums
	   d. Show child when you approve of his behavior and praise for obedience throughout day

3. With increasing fine motor control, child can manipulate objects that may be hazardous	3. a. Set limits regarding play with doorknobs and car door handles
	   b. Keep away from open windows; latch screens
	   c. Supervise around pools and ponds or drain or fence them
	   d. Lock cabinets
	   e. Keep open jars and bottles out of reach
	   c. Use gate to protect child from falling down stairs

19 to 30 months	

1. Attention span increasing	1. a. Gain attention before giving simple commands, one at a time; praise for success
	   b. Add new rules as child conforms to old ones
	   c. Refrain from expecting *immediate* obedience

2. Begins simple reasoning — asks question why; may be repetitive	2. Make special efforts to answer questions; give simple explanations; gauge need for simplicity by number of times act is repeated or question asked

3. Interested in further exploration of environment; may lack physical control	3. a. Supervise on stair rails and waxed floors
	   b. Set rules about crossing streets and carrying knives, sharp objects, or glass objects
	   c. Have outdoor play area securely fenced or supervised
	   d. When riding in car, secure child safely by seat belt or insist on his sitting in back seat; do not permit standing on car seats
	   e. Keep matches out of reach
	   f. Shield adult tools such as knives, lawnmowers, sharp tools

4. Negativistic behavior is expected; responds more frequently with word "no"; may show more resistance at bedtime preparation and during mealtime	4. a. Practice consistency in responding to behavior b. Allow more time to conform to expectation

5. Behavior may change if new sibling is introduced into family unit	5. a. Explain verbally or through play that new child is expected
	   b. Exercise more patience with child
	   c. Set special times aside for parental attention to child
	   d. Allow child to help with special care tasks of new sibling

31 to 48 months	

1. Displays more interest in conforming	1. a. Exercise consistency in parental demands; enforce each time and avoid ignoring behavior next time
	   b. Show concrete approval and give immediate recognition for acceptable behavior
	   c. Refrain from use of threats that produce fearfulness

2. Shows greater understanding when simple reasoning is communicated	2. a. Give simple explanations; allow child chance to demonstrate understanding by talking about event, situation, or rule
	   b. Eliminate unnecessary and impractical rules
	   c. Refrain from constant verbal reprimands
	   d. Denial of privileges should not be excessive or prolonged

Continued.

Discipline — cont'd

Expected tasks	Suggested activities
3. Will respond to simple commands such as putting toys away	3. a. Assign simple household tasks that child can carry out each day; show approval for performance and success b. Decide if child is capable of doing what is asked by observing him c. Determine how much time is necessary to complete a chore or activity before expecting maximum performance
4. Displays a greater independence in general activities	4. a. Be extra cautious about supervising riding tricycles in streets and watching for cars in driveways b. Do not permit dashing into street while playing c. Do not allow child to follow ball into street d. Areas under swings and slides should not be paved e. Provide an imitative model that child can copy, for example, do not jaywalk f. Provide scissors that are blunt tipped
49 to 52 months 1. Can be given two or three assignments at one time; will carry out in order 2. Complies readily with reasonable, well-defined, and consistent requirements 3. Understands reasoning	1. Give more opportunities to be independent 2. Use simple explanations and reasoning 3. Ask child to define role if he disobeys 4. Have child correct mistakes as they occur 5. Do not use punishment without warnings 6. Praise for successful performance 7. Use gold stars on chart for rewards 8. If leaving for social obligation, vacation, or visiting away from home, let child know 9. Avoid making promises that cannot be kept 10. Avoid bribing, ridicule, shaming, teasing, inflicting pain, using unfavorable comparison with other children, and exhbition of behavior in parents they are trying to stop in child 11. Remember that child may be imitating models of behavior set up by parents, brothers, sisters, a neighborhood child, or maybe a television hero 12. Recognize that there are stress periods in family or child's life that may result in changes in child's behavior including accidents, illness, moving into new neighborhood, separation from friends, death, divorce, and hopsitalization of child or parents (be more patient with child's behavior, give more time to conform, show more approval for mastery of tasks, and exercise consistency in handling problems as they occur)

Dressing

Expected tasks	Suggested activities
13 to 18 months 1. Cooperates in dressing by extending arm or leg 2. Removes socks, hats, mittens, shoes 3. Can unzip zippers 4. Tries to put shoes on	1. Encourage child to remove socks, etc., after task is initiated for him 2. Do not rush child 3. Have him practice with large buttons and with zippers
19 to 30 months 1. Can undress 2. Can remove shoes if laces are untied 3. Helps dress 4. Tries to unbutton 5. Pulls on simple clothes	1. Provide opportunities to button with extra-large—sized buttons 2. Encourage and allow opportunity for self-help in getting drink, removing clothes with help, hand washing, unbuttoning, etc. 3. Simple clothing 4. Provide mirror at height child can observe himself for brushing teeth, etc.

Continued.

Dressing — cont'd

Expected tasks	Suggested activities
31 to 48 months	
1. Greater interest and ability in dressing	1. Provide with own dresser drawer
2. Intent on lacing shoes (usually does incorrectly)	2. Simple garments encourage self-help; do not rush child
3. Does not know back from front	3. Provide large buttons, zippers, slipover clothing
4. Washes and dries hands, brushes teeth	4. Self hand washing but help with brushing teeth
5. Can button	5. Provide regular routine for dressing, either in bathroom or bedroom
49 to 52 months	
1. Dresses and undresses with care except for tying shoes and buckling belts	1. Assign regular task of placing clothes in hamper or basket
2. May learn to tie shoes	2. Continue to use simple clothing
3. Combs hair with assistance	3. Encourage self-help in dressing and undressing
	4. Allow child to select clothes he will wear

Toilet training

Expected tasks	Suggested activities
9 to 12 months	
1. Beginning to show regular patterns in bladder and bowel elimination	1. Watch for clues that indicate child is wet or soiled
2. Has one to two stools daily	2. Be sure to change diapers when wet or soiled so that child begins to experience contrast between wetness and dryness
3. Interval of dryness does not exceed 1 to 2 hours	
13 to 18 months	
1. Will have bowel movement if put on toilet at approximate time	1. Sit child on toilet or potty chair at regular intervals for short periods of time throughout day
2. Indicates wet pants	2. Praise child for success
	3. If potty chair is used, it should be located in bathroom
	4. Training should be started when social disruptions are at minimum
	5. Respond promptly to signals and clues of child by taking him to bathroom or changing pants
	6. Use training pants, once toilet training is commenced
	7. Plan to begin training when disruptions in regular routine are minimized, that is, do not begin on vacation
19 to 30 months	
1. Anticipates need to eliminate	1. Continue regular intervals of toileting
2. Same word for both functions	2. Reward success
3. Daytime control (occasional accident)	3. Dress in simple clothing that child can manage
4. Requires assistance (reminding, dressing, wiping)	4. Remind occasionally, particularly after mealtime, juicetime, naptime, and playtime
	5. Take to bathroom before bedtime
	6. Bathroom should be convenient to use, easy to open door
31 to 48 months	
1. Takes responsibility for toilet if clothes are simple	1. May still need reminding
2. Continues to verbalize need to go; apt to hold out too long	2. Dress in simple clothing that child can manage
3. May have occasional accident	3. Ignore accidents; refrain from shame or ridicule
4. Needs help with wiping	
49 to 52 months	
1. General independence (anticipates needs, undresses, goes, wipes, washes hands)	1. Praise child for his accomplishment

Immunization schedules

6-1 Current American Academy of Pediatrics immunization schedule (January 1991)

Age	Immunization(s)
2 mo	DTP, TOPV, HbOC*
4 mo	DTP, TOPV, HbOC
6 mo	DTP, HbOC
15 mo	MMR, HbCV
18 mo	DTP, TOPV†
4-6 yr	DTP, TOPV
12 yr	MMR‡
q 10 yr	dT

DTP indicates diphtheria-tetanus-pertussis; *TOPV*, trivalent oral polio vaccine; *HbOC, Haemophilus influenzae* type b conjugate vaccine (diphtheria CRM$_{197}$ protein conjugate; HibTITER); *MMR* measles-mumps-rubella; *HbCV*, Hib conjugate vaccine (ProHIBIT, Pedvax HIB, HibTITER); *dT*, diphtheria-tetanus.
*In October 1990, HbOC (HibTITER) was approved by the FDA for infants starting at 2 mo of age. Other Hib conjugate vaccines have submitted applications.
†Can be given at 15 mo of age.
‡Some states require this dose at 4-6 yr of age.
From American Academy of Pediatrics: Report of the Committee on Infectious Diseases, ed 22, Elk Grove Village, IL, 1991, The Academy.

6-2 Recommended immunization schedules for children not immunized in first year of life

Recommended time	Immunization(s)	Comments
LESS THAN 7 YEARS OLD		
First visit	DTP, OPV, MMR, HbOC	MMR if child ≥ 15 mo. old; HbOC if child between 7-11 mo; tuberculin testing may be done at same visit
Interval after first visit:		
1 mo		
2 mo	DTP, OPV, HbOC	HbOC if child between 7-11 mo
4 mo	DTP	A third dose of OPV is not indicated in the US. but is desirable in geographic areas where polio is endemic
10-16 mo	DTP, OPV, HbOC	OPV is not given if third dose was given earlier; HbOC if child between 12-14 mo, with final booster at 15 mo
4-6 yr (at or before school entry)	DTP, OPV	DTP is not necessary if the fourth dose was given after the fourth birthday; OPV is not necessary if recommended OPV dose at 10-16 mo following the first visit was given after the fourth birthday
10 yr later	Td	Repeat every 10 yr throughout life
7 YEARS OLD AND OLDER		
First visit	Td, OPV, MMR	
Interval after first visit:		
2 mo	Td, OPV	
8-14 mo	Td, OPV	
10 yr later	Td	Repeat every 10 yr throughout life

Adapted from American Academy of Pediatrics: Report of the Committee on Infectious Diseases, ed 21, Elk Grove Village, IL, 1988, The Academy.

Leading health problems and communicable diseases

Two leading health problems in the United States are cardiovascular disease and cancer. Nurses and other health care professionals encounter some form of these diseases daily. The following statistics are offered in an effort to increase understanding of the magnitude of the problem and to provide a basis for developing patient teaching strategies. In this way the health care professional becomes a tool for preventive health care, an increasingly important role in today's health-conscious society.

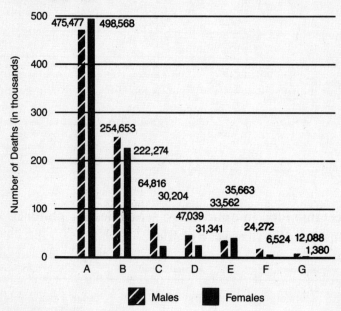

Leading Causes of Death by Sex

United States: 1987

A Cardiovascular Disease
B Cancer
C Accidents
D Chronic Obstructive Pulmonary Disease
E Pneumonia and Influenza
F Suicide
G AIDS

Source: National Center for Health Statistics, U.S. Public Health Service, DHHS and the American Heart Association.

7-1

Cardiovascular disease

VITAL STATISTICS

- 68.09 million Americans have one or more forms of cardiovascular disease (CVD).
- Stroke killed 150,300 in 1988.
- As many as 1.5 million Americans may have a heart attack this year and about 500,000 of them will die.

- High blood pressure afflicts an estimated 61.87 million Americans age six or older.
- 1.29 million Americans have rheumatic heart disease.

Reproduced with permission. © American Heart Assoiation.

HEART ATTACK — SIGNALS AND ACTION

Know the warning signs of a heart attack.

- Uncomfortable pressure, fullness, squeezing or pain in the center of your chest, lasting 2 minutes or more
- Pain may spread to shoulders, neck, or arms
- Severe pain, dizziness, fainting, sweating, nausea, or shortness of breath may also occur
- Not all these signals, however, are always present. **Don't wait.** Get help immediately.

Know what to do in case of an emergency.

- If you are having chest discomfort that lasts for 2 minutes or more, call the emergency rescue service.
- If you can get to a hospital faster by car, have someone drive you.
- Find out which hospitals in your area offer 24-hour emergency cardiac care.
- Select in advance the facility nearest your home and office and tell your family and friends to call this facility in an emergency.
- Keep a list of emergency rescue service numbers next to your telephone and in a prominent place in your pocket, wallet, or purse.

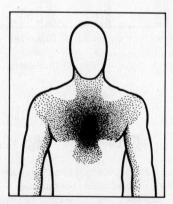

The pain of a heart attack radiates from the center of the chest to the neck and arms.

RISK FACTORS OF HEART DISEASE
Major risk factors that cannot be changed

Heredity—It appears that a tendency toward heart disease or atherosclerosis is hereditary. Race is a consideration, too. African Americans have moderate hypertension twice as often as whites and severe hypertension three times as often.

Male sex—Men have a greater risk of heart attack than women. Even after menopause when women's death rate increases, it never reaches that of men.

Age—Fifty-five percent of all heart attack victims are age 65 or older; of those who die, more than four out of five are over 65.

Major risk factors that can be changed.

Cigarette smoking—Smoker's risk of heart attack is more than twice that of nonsmokers. Smokers have two to four times the risk for sudden cardiac death as nonsmokers. For those who have given up the habit, the death rate eventu-

ally declines almost to that of people who have never smoked. Don't smoke cigarettes.

High blood pressure—A major risk factor of stroke and heart attack, high blood pressure usually has no specific symptoms but can be detected by a simple, painless test. A person with mild elevations of blood pressure often begins treatment with a program of weight reduction, if overweight, and salt (sodium) restriction before drugs are recommended.

Blood cholesterol levels—Too much cholesterol can cause buildups on the walls of arteries, narrowing the passageway through which blood flows, and leading to heart attack and stroke. A doctor can measure the amount of cholesterol in the blood by a simple test. Since the body gets cholesterol both through diet and by manufacturing it, a diet low in saturated fat and cholesterol will help lower the level of blood cholesterol if it is too high. Medications also are available to maintain cholesterol levels within the normal range.

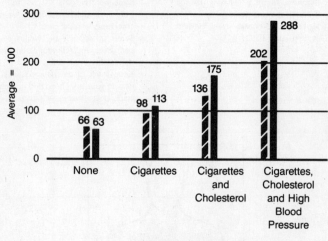

Danger of Heart Attack by Risk Factors Present

Example: 55-year-old male and female

This chart shows how a combination of three major risk factors can increase the likelihood of heart attack. For purposes of illustration, this chart uses an abnormal blood pressure level of 150 systolic and a cholesterol level of 260 in a 55-year-old male and female.

Source: Framingham Heart Study, Section 37: The Probability of Developing Certain Cardiovascular Diseases in Eight Years at Specified Values of Some Characteristics (Aug. 1987).

Other contributing factors

Diabetes — Diabetes appears most frequently during middle age, more often in people who are overweight. In its mild form, diabetes can escape detection for many years, but it can sharply increase a person's risk of heart attack, making control of other risk factors even more important. A doctor can detect diabetes and prescribe changes in eating habits, weight-control and exercise programs, and drugs, if necessary, to keep it in check.

Obesity — In most cases, obesity simply results from eating too much and exercising too little. It places a heavy burden on your heart. In addition, obesity is associated with coronary heart disease primarily because of its influence on blood pressure, blood cholesterol and precipitating diabetes. To reduce weight, doctors usually recommend a program that combines exercise with a low-calorie diet.

Lack of exercise — Lack of exercise has not been clearly established as a risk factor for heart attack. But when combined with overeating, lack of exercise may lead to excess weight, which is clearly a contributing factor. A doctor should be consulted for the physical activities that best suit the age and physical condition of the individual.

Stress — It's practically impossible to define and measure a person's emotional stress level. Moreover, each of us reacts differently to it. All human beings feel stress — life without it would be dull, indeed. But excessive stress over a long period may create health problems in some people. Most doctors agree that reduction of emotional stress will benefit the health of the average individual.

Estimated Prevalence of Major Cardiovascular Diseases

United States: 1988 Estimate

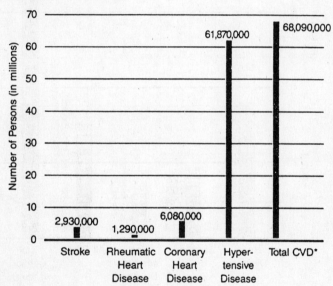

*The sum of the individual estimates exceeds 68,090,000 since many people have more than one cardiovascular disorder.

Source: National Health and Nutrition Examination Survey II, Data National Center for Health Statistics, U.S. Public Health Service, DHHS and the American Heart Association. Hypertension Prevalence and the Status of Awareness Treatment and Control in the U.S., Final Report of the Subcommittee on Detection, Evaluation, and Treatment of High Blood Pressure, 1984 and the American Heart Association.

Estimated Cost of Major Cardiovascular Diseases by Type of Expenditure: 1991

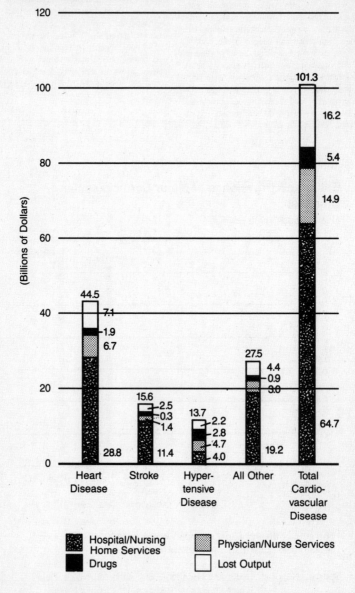

Source: American Heart Association extrapolation from Hodgson, T.A., et al., "Health Care Expenditures for Major Diseases in 1980," *Health Care Financing Review*, Vol. 5, No. 4, 1984.

WARNING SIGNALS OF STROKE

Know the warning signals of stroke.

- Sudden, temporary weakness or numbness of the face, arm, and leg on one side of the body
- Temporary loss of speech, or trouble talking or understanding speech
- Dimness or loss of vision, particularly in only one eye
- Unexplained dizziness, unsteadiness, or sudden falls.

Many major strokes are preceded by "little strokes," warning signals like the above, experienced days, weeks, or months before the more severe event.

Prompt medical or surgical attention to these symptoms may prevent a fatal or disabling stroke from occurring.

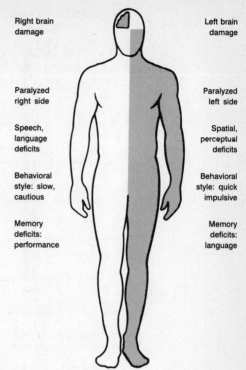

Right brain
damage

Left brain
damage

Paralyzed
right side

Paralyzed
left side

Speech,
language
deficits

Spatial,
perceptual
deficits

Behavioral
style: slow,
cautious

Behavioral
style: quick
impulsive

Memory
deficits:
performance

Memory
deficits:
language

RISK FACTORS OF STROKE

Some of the factors that increase the risk of stroke are congenital, whereas others result from the hazards of life. Some of these factors can be minimized by the individual and with a doctor's help. Other factors cannot be changed.

Risk factors that cannot be changed

Age — The incidence of stroke is strongly related to age. In fact, the incidence of stroke more than doubles in each successive decade for people over 55 years old.

Sex — The risk of stroke is greater in men than in women. However, in women who take oral contraceptives the risk of stroke is slightly increased. Women who are also heavy smokers may aggravate this risk further.

Race — The risk of death and disability from stroke is much greater among black Americans than among white Americans. This may be a result of the greater prevalence of high blood pressure among blacks.

Diabetes mellitus — Although diabetes is treatable, the fact that a person has diabetes still makes it much more likely that a stroke will occur.

Prior stroke — The risk of stroke for a person who has already suffered a stroke is many times that of a person who has never had stroke.

Heredity — The risk of stroke is greater in people who have a family history of stroke.

Asymptomatic carotid bruit — As an indication of existing atherosclerosis, a bruit is an abnormal sound heard when a stethoscope is placed over an artery (in this case, the carotid artery, which is in the neck). Carotid bruit clearly indicates an increased stroke risk, although a bruit mainly indicates that atherosclerosis is present and doesn't necessarily mean the carotid artery with the bruit will become clogged and a stroke will result.

Risk factors that can be changed

High blood pressure — The control of high blood pressure will reduce the risk of stroke.

High red blood cell count — A marked increase, as well as a moderate elevation, in the red blood cell count may be a risk factor of stroke.

Heart disease — A diseased heart increases the risk of stroke in two ways: as a failing pump and as a source of emboli, clots that form in the heart and could travel to the arteries leading to the brain and cause a blockage. Good management of heart disease reduces the risk of stroke.

Age-Adjusted Stroke Death Rates
United States: 1987

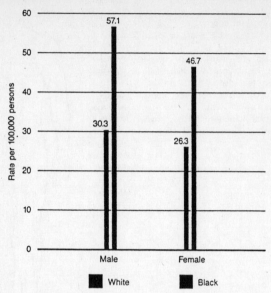

Source: National Center for Health Statistics, U.S. Public Health
Service, DHHS and the American Heart Association.

Estimated Annual Number of Americans, by Age and Sex, Experiencing First Stroke — Age 30 and Older

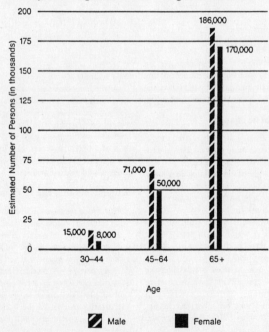

Source: Based on the Framingham Heart Study, 24-year follow-up.

Cumulative Percent Decline in Age-Adjusted Stroke Death Rates

United States: 1978–1988

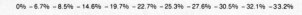

0% – 6.7% – 8.5% – 14.6% – 19.7% – 22.7% – 25.3% – 27.6% – 30.5% – 32.1% – 33.2%

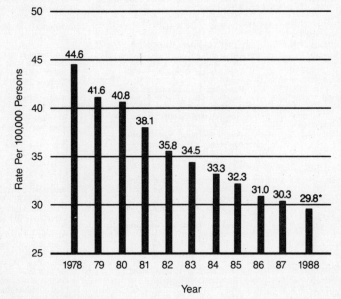

Source: National Center for Health Statistics, U.S. Public Health
Service, DHHS and the American Heart Association.

*1988 Provisional

THE AMERICAN HEART ASSOCIATION AFFILIATES

American Heart Association
Alabama Affiliate, Inc.
1449 Medical Park Dr.
Birmingham, AL 35213

American Heart Association
Alaska Affiliate, Inc.
2330 East 42nd Ave.
Anchorage, AK 99508

American Heart Association
Arizona Affiliate, Inc.
1550 East Meadowbrook
Phoenix, AZ 85014

American Heart Association
Arkansas Affiliate, Inc.
990 West Second St.
Little Rock, AR 72201

American Heart Association
California Affiliate, Inc.
805 Burlway Rd.
Burlingame, CA 94010-1795

American Heart Association of
Metropolitan Chicago, Inc.
20 N. Wacker Dr.
Chicago, IL 60606

American Heart Association of
Colorado, Inc.
1280 S. Parker Road
Denver, CO 80231

American Heart Association
Connecticut Affiliate, Inc.
5 Brookside Drive
Wallingford, CT 06492

American Heart Association
Dakota Affiliate, Inc.
1005 Twelfth Ave., S.E.
Jamestown, ND 58401

American Heart Association of
Delaware, Inc.
4C Trolley Square
Delaware Ave. and DuPont St.
Wilmington, DE 19806

American Heart Association
Florida Affiliate, Inc.
1213 16th St. North
St. Petersburg, FL 33705-1092

American Heart Association
Georgia Affiliate, Inc.
1685 Terrell Mill Rd.
Marietta, GA 30067

American Heart Association of
Hawaii, Inc.
245 North Kukui St.
Honolulu, HI 96817

American Heart Association of
Idaho, Inc.
3295 Elder St., Suite 140
Boise, ID 83705

American Heart Association
Illinois Affiliate, Inc.
1181 North Dirksen Pkwy
Springfield, IL 62708

American Heart Association
Indiana Affiliate, Inc.
8645 Guion Road, Suite H
Indianapolis, IN 46268

American Heart Association
Iowa Affiliate, Inc.
1111 Ninth St., Suite 280
West Des Moines, IA 50314

American Heart Association
Kansas Affiliate, Inc.
5375 S.W. Seventh St.
Topeka, KS 66606

American Heart Association
Kentucky Affiliate, Inc.
207 Speed Building
Louisville, KY 40202

American Heart Association
Greater Los Angeles Affiliate, Inc.
Fifth Floor
3550 Wilshire Blvd.
Los Angeles, CA 90010

American Heart Association
Louisiana, Inc.
105 Campus Drive East
Destrehan, LA 70047

American Heart Association
Maine Affiliate, Inc.
20 Winter St.
Augusta, ME 04330

American Heart Association
Maryland Affiliate, Inc.
415 N. Charles St.
Baltimore, MD 21203

American Heart Association
Massachusetts Affiliate, Inc.
33 Fourth Ave.
Needham Heights, MA 02194

American Heart Association of
Michigan, Inc.
16310 West Twelve Mile Rd.
Lathrup Village, MI 48076

American Heart Association
Minnesota Affiliate, Inc.
7401 West 77th St.
Minneapolis, MN 55435

American Heart Associaton
Mississippi Affiliate, Inc.
4830 East McWillie Circle
Jackson, MS 39236

American Heart Association
Missouri Affiliate, Inc.
105 East Ash, Suite 2
Columbia, MO 65205

American Heart Association
Montana Affiliate, Inc.
Professional Building
510 First Ave., N. #4
Great Falls, MT 59401

American Heart Association
Nation's Capital Affiliate, Inc.
2233 Wisconsin Ave., N.W.
Washington, D.C. 20007

American Heart Association
Nebraska Affiliate, Inc.
3642 Farnam
Omaha, NE 68131

American Heart Association
Nevada Affiliate, Inc.
3355 Spring Mountain Road
Suite 4
Las Vegas, NV 89102

American Heart Association
New Hampshire Affiliate, Inc.
309 Pine St.
Manchester, NH 03103

American Heart Association
New Jersey Affiliate, Inc.
2550 Rt. 1
North Brunswick, NJ 08902

American Heart Association
New Mexico Affiliate, Inc.
1330 San Pedro, N.E., Suite 105
Albuquerque, NM 87110
(505)268-3711

American Heart Association
New York State Affiliate, Inc.
100 N. Concourse
N. Syracuse, NY 13212

American Heart Association
New York City Affiliate, Inc.
205 East 42nd St.
New York, NY 10017

American Heart Association
North Carolina Affiliate, Inc.
300 Silver Cedar Court
Chapel Hill, NC 27515

American Heart Association
Northeast Ohio Affiliate, Inc.
1689 East 115th St.
Cleveland, OH 44106

American Heart Association
Ohio Affiliate, Inc.
5455 N. High St.
Columbus, OH 43214

American Heart Association
Oklahoma Affiliate, Inc.
2915 North Classen, Suite 220
Oklahoma City, OK 73136

American Heart Association
Oregon Affiliate, Inc.
1425 N.E. Irving #100
Portland, OR 97232-4201

American Heart Association
Pennsylvania Affiliate, Inc.
Pennsboro Center
1019 Mumma Rd.
P.O. Box 8835
Camp Hill, PA 17011-8835

Puerto Rico Heart
Association, Inc.
Cabo Alverio 554
Hato Rey
Puerto Rico 00918

American Heart Association
Rhode Island Affiliate, Inc.
40 Broad St.
Pawtucket, RI 02860

American Heart Association
South Carolina Affiliate, Inc.
400 Percival Rd.
Columbia, SC 29206

American Heart Association
Southeastern Pennsylvania
    Affiliate, Inc.
121 S. Broad St.
Philadelphia, PA 19107

American Heart Association
Tennessee Affiliate, Inc.
1200 Division St.
Suite 201
Nashville, TN 37203

American Heart Association
Texas Affiliate, Inc.
1700 Rutherford Ln.
Austin, TX 78754

American Heart Association
Utah Affiliate, Inc.
645E-400S
Salt Lake City, UT 84102

American Heart Association
Vermont Affiliate, Inc.
12 Hurricane Ln.
Williston, VT 05495

American Heart Association
Virginia Affiliate, Inc.
4217 Park Place Ct.
Glen Allen, VA 23060

American Heart Association
Washington Affiliate, Inc.
4414 Woodland Park Ave., N.
Seattle, WA 98103

American Heart Association
West Virginia Affiliate, Inc.
211 35th St., S.E.
Charleston, WV 25304

American Heart Association
Wisconsin Affiliate, Inc.
795 North Van Buren St.
Milwaukee, WI 53202

American Heart Association of
    Wyoming, Inc.
1320 Hugar St.
Cheyenne, WY 82001

7-2   Cancer

Cancer deaths — 1989: Estimated cancer deaths for all sites plus major sites, by state

State	All sites		Major sites									
	Number of deaths	Death rate per 100,000 population*	Female breast	Colon & rectum	Lung	Oral	Uterus	Prostate	Skin melanoma	Pancreas	Leukemia
Alabama	8,900	214	700	950	2,600	125	200	550	100	425	300
Alaska	500	221	30	50	150	10	10	20	10	25	10
Arizona	6,500	180	550	700	1,800	100	50	400	70	300	225
Arkansas	5,600	190	350	600	1,800	60	100	300	80	300	225
California	50,000	181	4,400	5,500	14,100	950	900	2,800	700	2,500	1,800
Colorado	4,700	141	450	600	1,200	60	70	275	80	250	200
Connecticut	7,200	217	650	950	1,800	125	125	375	90	400	275
Delaware	1,400	250	125	175	450	10	20	60	10	60	50
Dist. of Columbia	1,700	264	175	175	400	70	60	125	10	100	50
Florida	32,500	182	2,500	4,100	9,800	600	400	2,100	400	1,600	1,000
Georgia	11,200	202	850	1,200	3,400	250	250	700	150	500	400
Hawaii	1,700	191	150	175	375	50	80	80	20	80	50
Idaho	1,800	158	100	175	400	20	25	125	30	100	180
Illinois	24,000	201	2,100	3,100	6,600	450	600	1,300	200	1,300	900
Indiana	11,500	217	950	1,500	3,500	175	300	600	125	550	425
Iowa	6,400	190	550	850	1,600	125	125	400	70	350	300
Kansas	4,900	171	425	650	1,300	90	100	350	50	275	225
Kentucky	8,400	207	650	1,000	2,800	125	175	425	80	375	300
Louisiana	8,800	212	650	900	2,800	150	175	475	80	450	300
Maine	2,800	199	225	400	800	40	60	175	20	150	90
Maryland	9,600	244	800	1,200	2,700	175	175	500	125	425	300
Massachusetts	14,100	220	1,500	1,900	3,500	250	275	750	175	650	475
Michigan	18,600	226	1,600	2,100	5,300	275	400	1,000	200	900	650
Minnesota	8,100	181	700	1,100	2,000	125	125	550	90	450	350
Mississippi	5,100	186	325	500	1,700	80	100	350	60	300	225
Missouri	11,800	196	950	1,500	3,400	175	250	550	125	550	450
Montana	1,600	186	150	175	375	20	30	100	20	100	70
Nebraska	3,300	173	300	450	800	40	70	200	40	200	175
Nevada	2,100	216	150	200	600	40	20	100	30	80	40
New Hampshire	2,100	197	200	250	550	30	40	90	30	100	70
New Jersey	18,100	230	1,600	2,500	4,900	325	375	950	225	900	550
New Mexico	2,300	168	200	250	500	30	40	150	20	125	70
New York	38,500	200	3,800	5,400	9,800	750	950	2,200	475	2,100	1,400
North Carolina	12,200	203	1,000	1,300	3,700	225	275	750	175	550	425
North Dakota	1,300	171	125	175	300	20	20	125	10	90	60
Ohio	24,000	227	2,100	3,100	7,300	400	600	1,300	250	1,200	850
Oklahoma	7,000	163	550	800	2,300	100	100	375	100	325	275
Oregon	5,900	198	500	650	1,800	100	75	350	70	300	275
Pennsylvania	29,500	221	2,600	4,000	7,800	475	700	1,500	350	1,400	1,000

*Adjusted to the age distribution of the 1970 U.S. Census Population.

Cancer deaths — 1989: Estimated cancer deaths for all sites plus major sites, by state — cont'd

| State | All sites | | Major sites | | | | | | | | |
---	Number of deaths	Death rate per 100,000 population*	Female breast	Colon & rectum	Lung	Oral	Uterus	Prostate	Skin melanoma	Pancreas	Leukemia
Rhode Island	2,500	227	250	350	650	60	40	125	30	125	70
South Carolina	6,500	209	550	650	1,900	125	125	425	90	325	175
South Dakota	1,500	180	125	200	325	10	30	125	20	100	80
Tennessee	10,400	202	800	1,100	3,300	200	200	600	125	500	375
Texas	27,000	155	2,200	2,900	8,100	475	500	1,400	350	1,300	1,000
Utah	1,800	118	175	175	275	20	30	175	30	90	80
Vermont	1,200	196	100	150	275	20	30	70	10	60	50
Virginia	11,700	219	950	1,400	3,500	225	225	650	150	500	375
Washington	8,600	181	750	900	2,600	150	150	500	100	425	300
West Virginia	4,400	202	350	500	1,400	60	100	225	50	200	175
Wisconsin	10,000	197	950	1,300	2,500	125	175	650	90	500	425
Wyoming	700	128	70	75	175	10	10	30	10	40	30
United States	502,000	204	43,000	61,000	142,000	8,700	10,000	28,500	6,000	25,000	18,000
Puerto Rico	3,500	150	200	250	400	175	150	300	400	80	150

New cancer cases — 1989: Estimated new cancer cases for all sites plus major sites, by state

State	All sites* Number of cases	Major sites Female breast	Colon & rectum	Lung	Oral	Uterus	Prostate	Skin melanoma	Pancreas	Leukemia
Alabama	18,000	2,400	2,300	2,800	450	950	2,100	400	500	450
Alaska	1,000	150	125	150	40	20	100	50	20	10
Arizona	13,000	1,800	1,700	1,900	350	550	1,500	300	350	375
Arkansas	11,300	1,100	1,500	1,900	200	400	1,000	350	350	300
California	101,000	14,200	13,500	15,400	3,500	5,000	10,000	3,200	2,600	2,800
Colorado	9,400	1,500	1,500	1,200	225	450	1,400	400	250	250
Connecticut	14,400	2,200	2,300	2,000	450	600	1,400	400	375	375
Delaware	2,800	400	450	500	40	125	275	70	70	80
Dist. of Columbia	3,200	450	400	450	250	150	450	60	90	60
Florida	65,500	8,300	10,200	10,600	2,200	2,800	7,600	1,800	1,700	1,600
Georgia	22,500	2,800	2,900	3,700	850	1,100	2,400	600	550	600
Hawaii	3,300	350	450	450	150	150	275	90	90	80
Idaho	3,500	500	475	475	60	125	425	150	80	125
Illinois	48,000	7,000	7,800	7,400	1,400	2,400	4,700	950	1,300	1,300
Indiana	23,200	3,200	3,700	3,800	650	1,200	2,200	600	550	550
Iowa	12,700	1,800	2,100	1,800	400	550	1,500	300	375	375
Kansas	9,900	1,400	1,600	1,600	300	450	1,600	200	300	325
Kentucky	16,800	2,100	2,500	3,000	450	850	1,600	350	375	425
Louisiana	17,500	2,200	2,200	3,000	550	750	1,700	300	500	400
Maine	5,500	750	950	850	150	250	600	100	150	150
Maryland	19,300	2,700	2,900	3,000	650	800	1,900	550	400	450
Massachusetts	28,400	4,800	4,500	3,800	800	1,000	2,600	800	700	700
Michigan	37,400	5,500	5,300	5,800	1,000	1,700	3,600	900	950	1,000
Minnesota	16,400	2,300	2,600	2,100	400	650	2,000	400	450	450
Mississippi	12,000	1,100	1,400	1,800	300	600	1,200	250	325	300
Missouri	23,500	3,100	3,900	3,700	700	1,200	2,000	600	650	700
Montana	3,200	500	425	425	60	150	400	90	100	100
Nebraska	6,400	900	1,100	900	150	350	750	175	225	175

These estimates are offered as a rough guide and should not be regarded as definitive. They are calculated according to the distribution of estimated 1989 cancer deaths by state. Especially note that year-to-year changes may only represent improvements in the basic data.
*Does not include carcinoma in situ or non-melanoma skin cancer.

New cancer cases—1989: Estimated new cancer cases for all sites plus major sites, by state—cont'd

State	All sites* Number of cases	Female breast	Colon & rectum	Lung	Oral	Uterus	Prostate	Skin melanoma	Pancreas	Leukemia
Nevada	4,100	500	500	750	150	175	375	150	90	70
New Hampshire	4,000	650	650	600	80	200	400	125	125	90
New Jersey	36,500	5,500	6,200	5,300	1,200	1,800	3,500	950	1,000	850
New Mexico	4,500	600	600	550	125	175	550	80	150	150
New York	77,500	12,100	13,200	10,900	2,500	4,000	7,900	2,100	2,300	2,000
North Carolina	24,500	3,400	3,200	4,000	900	1,300	2,700	750	700	700
North Dakota	2,700	400	450	325	70	125	450	40	90	90
Ohio	49,000	6,800	7,700	7,900	1,400	2,200	4,700	1,200	1,300	1,300
Oklahoma	14,000	1,800	1,900	2,500	400	550	1,400	500	425	450
Oregon	11,800	1,700	1,600	2,000	300	425	1,200	350	325	350
Pennsylvania	59,000	8,800	10,000	8,600	1,700	2,500	5,300	1,600	1,500	1,500
Rhode Island	4,900	700	900	700	200	500	500	150	150	100
South Carolina	13,000	1,900	1,700	2,000	500	750	1,500	400	350	250
South Dakota	2,900	425	500	375	40	125	350	80	90	100
Tennessee	21,000	2,600	2,800	3,500	700	950	2,200	500	550	600
Texas	54,500	7,300	7,200	8,800	1,800	2,600	5,000	1,600	1,400	1,700
Utah	3,500	550	450	350	100	200	600	100	100	125
Vermont	2,300	350	375	350	80	150	250	50	50	90
Virginia	23,500	3,300	3,400	3,800	800	1,100	2,500	700	600	600
Washington	17,300	2,500	2,300	2,800	550	850	1,800	500	500	450
West Virginia	8,900	1,200	1,500	1,500	200	375	800	200	250	250
Wisconsin	20,200	3,100	3,200	2,700	450	900	2,300	400	550	650
Wyoming	1,300	225	200	200	30	30	150	50	30	30
United States	1,010,000	142,000	151,000	155,000	31,000	47,000	103,000	27,000	27,000	27,000
Puerto Rico	6,000	450	450	350	425	750	400	500	100	175

FIVE-YEAR CANCER SURVIVAL RATES* FOR SELECTED SITES

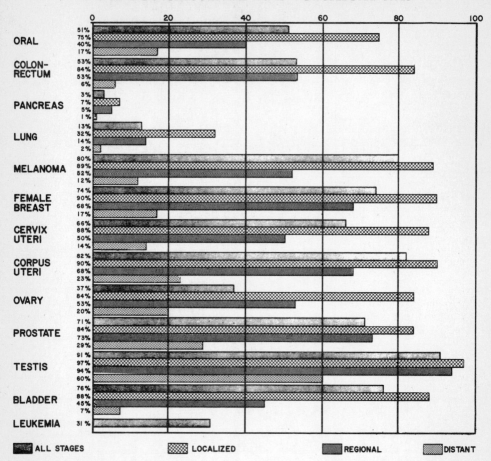

*Adjusted for normal life expectancy.
This chart is based on cases diagnosed in 1979-1984.

Source: Surveillance and Operations Research Branch,
National Cancer Institute.

How to estimate cancer statistics locally

Community population	Estimated No. who are alive, saved from cancer	Estimated No. cancer cases under medical care in 1989	Estimated No. who will die of cancer in 1989	Estimated No. of new cases in 1989	Estimated No. who will be saved from cancer in 1989	Estimated No. who will eventually develop cancer	Estimated No. who will die of cancer if present rates continue
1,000	10	5	1	3	1	280	180
2,000	20	11	4	7	3	560	360
3,000	30	16	5	10	4	840	540
4,000	40	21	7	13	5	1,120	720
5,000	50	26	9	16	6	1,400	900
10,000	100	52	18	33	12	2,800	1,800
25,000	250	131	45	79	30	7,000	4,500
50,000	500	262	90	158	59	14,000	9,000
100,000	1,000	525	180	325	122	28,000	18,000
200,000	2,000	1,050	360	650	244	56,000	36,000
500,000	5,000	2,625	900	1,575	590	140,000	90,000

NOTE: The figures can only be the roughest approximation of actual data for your community and should be used with caution. It is suggested that every effort be made to obtain actual data from a Registry source.

Estimated new cancer cases and deaths by sex for all sites — 1989*

	Estimated new cases			Estimated deaths		
	Total	Male	Female	Total	Male	Female
All sites	1,010,000*	505,000*	505,000*	502,000	266,000	236,000
Buccal cavity and Pharynx **(Oral)**	30,600	20,600	10,000	8,650	5,775	2,875
Lip	4,200	3,700	500	100	75	25
Tongue	6,000	3,900	2,100	1,950	1,300	650
Mouth	11,700	7,000	4,700	2,600	1,600	1,000
Pharynx	8,700	6,000	2,700	4,000	2,800	1,200
Digestive organs	227,800	115,200	112,600	123,000	64,400	58,600
Esophagus	10,100	7,200	2,900	9,400	6,900	2,500
Stomach	20,000	11,900	8,100	13,900	8,200	5,700
Small intestine	2,700	1,400	1,300	900	500	400
Large intestine ⎱ **(Colon-**	107,000	50,000	57,000	53,500	26,000	27,500
Rectum ⎰ **Rectum)**	44,000	23,000	21,000	7,800	4,000	3,800
Liver & Biliary passages	14,500	7,500	7,000	11,400	5,800	5,600
Pancreas	27,000	13,000	14,000	25,000	12,500	12,500
Other & Unspecified digestive	2,500	1,200	1,300	1,100	500	600
Respiratory system	171,600	114,000	57,600	147,100	96,900	50,200
Larynx	12,300	10,000	2,300	3,700	3,000	700
Lung	155,000	101,000	54,000	142,000	93,000	49,000
Other & Unspecified respiratory	4,300	3,000	1,300	1,400	900	500
Bone	2,100	1,200	900	1,300	700	600
Connective tissue	5,600	3,000	2,600	3,000	1,400	1,600
Skin	27,000†	14,500†	12,500†	8,200§	5,200	3,000
Breast	142,900‡	900‡	142,000‡	43,000	300	43,000
Genital organs	181,800‡	109,900	71,900‡	52,200	29,100	23,100
Cervix Uteri ⎱	13,000‡	—	13,000‡	6,000	—	6,000
Corpus, Endometrium ⎰ **(Uterus)**	34,000	—	34,000	4,000	—	4,000
Ovary	20,000	—	20,000	12,000	—	12,000
Other & Unspecified genital, female	4,900	—	4,900	1,100	—	1,100
Prostate	103,000	103,000	—	28,500	28,500	—
Testis	5,700	5,700	—	350	350	—
Other & Unspecified genital, male	1,200	1,200	—	250	250	—
Urinary organs	70,200	49,000	21,200	20,200	12,900	7,300
Bladder	47,100	34,500	12,600	10,200	6,900	3,300
Kidney & Other urinary	23,100	14,500	8,600	10,000	6,000	4,000
Eye	1,900	1,000	900	300	150	150
Brain & Central nervous system	15,000	8,200	6,800	11,000	6,000	5,000
Endocrine glands	12,600	3,700	8,900	1,750	775	975
Thyroid	11,300	3,000	8,300	1,025	375	650
Other endocrine	1,300	700	600	725	400	325
Leukemia	27,300	15,200	12,100	18,100	9,800	8,300
Lymphocytic leukemia	13,000	7,500	5,500	7,000	3,900	3,100
Granulocytic leukemia	13,300	7,200	6,100	10,600	5,600	5,000
Monocytic leukemia	1,000	500	500	500	300	200
Other blood & Lymph tissues	51,800	27,000	24,800	27,400	14,100	13,300
Hodgkin's disease	7,400	4,200	3,200	1,500	900	600
Non-Hodgkin's lymphomas	32,800	16,800	16,000	17,300	8,900	8,400
Multiple myeloma	11,600	6,000	5,600	8,600	4,300	4,300
All other & Unspecified sites	41,800	21,600	20,200	36,500	18,500	18,000

NOTE: The estimates of new cancer cases are offered as a rough guide and should not be regarded as definitive. Especially note that year-to-year changes may only represent improvements in the basic data. ACS six major sites appear in boldface caps. Incidence estimates are based on rates from NCI SEER program 1983-85.

*Carcinoma in situ and nonmelanoma skin cancers are not included in totals. Carcinoma in situ of the uterine cervix accounts for more than 50,000 new cases annually, and carcinoma in situ of the female breast accounts for about 10,000 new cases annually. Nonmelanoma skin cancer accounts for more than 500,000 new cases annually.

†Melanoma only.
‡Invasive cancer only.
§Melanoma 6,000; other skin 2,200.

Trends in survival by site of cancer, by race (cases diagnosed in 1960–63, 1970–73, 1974–76, 1977–78, 1979–84)

Site	White Relative 5-year survival					Black Relative 5-year survival				
	1960–63[1]	1970–73[1]	1974–76[2]	1977–78[2]	1979–84[2]	1960–63[1]	1970–73[1]	1974–76[2]	1977–78[2]	1979–84[2]
All sites	39%	43%	50%	50%	50%	27%	31%	38%	38%	37%
Oral cavity and pharynx	45	43	54	53	54	–	–	35	35	31
Esophagus	4	4	5	6	7	1	4	4	2	5
Stomach	11	13	14	15	16*	8	13	15	16	17
Colon	43	49	50	52	54*	34	37	45	44	49
Rectum	38	45	48	50	52*	27	30	40	40	34
Liver	2	3	4	3	3	–	–	1	1	5
Pancreas	1	2	3	2	3	1	2	2	3	5
Larynx	53	62	66	69	66	–	–	58	59	55
Lung and bronchus	8	10	12	13	13*	5	7	11	10	11
Melanoma of skin	60	68	78	81	80*	–	–	62‡	–	61†
Breast (females)	63	68	74	75	75*	46	51	62	62	62
Cervix uteri	58	64	69	69	67	47	61	61	63	59
Corpus uteri	73	81	89	87	83*	31	44	61	58	52*
Ovary	32	36	36	37	37*	32	32	41	40	36
Prostate gland	50	63	67	70	73*	35	55	56	64	60*
Testis	63	72	78	86	91*	–	–	77†	–	82†
Urinary bladder	53	61	73	75	77*	24	36	47	53	57†
Kidney and renal pelvis	37	46	51	50	51	38	44	49	54	53
Brain and nervous system	18	20	22	23	23	19	19	27	24	31
Thyroid gland	83	86	92	92	93	–	–	88	92	95
Hodgkin's disease	40	67	71	73	74*	–	–	67†	79†	69
Non-Hodgkin's lymphoma	31	41	47	48	49*	–	–	47	46	49
Multiple myeloma	12	19	24	24	24	–	–	28	30	29
Leukemia	14	22	34	37	32	–	–	30	31	27

Source: Surveillance and Operations Research Branch, National Cancer Institute.
[1] Rates are based on End Results Group data from a series of hospital registries and one population-based registry.
[2] Rates are from the SEER Program. They are based on data from population-based registries in Connecticut, New Mexico, Utah, Iowa, Hawaii, Atlanta, Detroit, Seattle-Puget Sound and San Francisco-Oakland. Rates are based on follow-up of patients through 1985.
*The difference in rates between 1974–75 and 1979–84 is statistically significant (p < .05).
†The standard error of the survival rate is between 5 and 10 percentage points.
‡The standard error of the survival rate is greater than 10 percentage points.
– Valid survival rate could not be calculated.

NATIONAL CANCER INSTITUTE COMPREHENSIVE CANCER CENTERS

Alabama

Comprehensive Cancer Center
University of Alabama
University Station
1824 Sixth Avenue, S.
Birmingham, AL 35294
(205) 934-5077

California

**Kenneth Norris Jr., Cancer
   Research Institute**
University of Southern California
P.O. Box 33804
1441 Eastlake Ave.
Los Angeles, CA 90033-0804
(213) 224-6416

**Jonsson Comprehensive Cancer
   Center**
University of California
UCLA Medical Center
Louis Factor Health Sciences Bldg.
10833 LeConte Ave.
Los Angeles, CA 90024
(213) 825-1532 or 5628

Connecticut

**Yale University Comprehensive
   Cancer Center**
School of Medicine
333 Cedar Street
New Haven, CT 06510
(203) 785-4095

District of Columbia

Lombardi Cancer Research Center
Georgetown University Medical
   Center
3800 Reservoir Rd, NW
Washington, DC 20007
(202) 687-2110

**Howard University
University Comprehensive
   Cancer Center**
Howard University Hospital
2041 Georgia Ave, NW
Washington, DC 20060
(202) 636-7697

Florida

**Comprehensive Cancer Center for
   the State of Florida**
University of Miami Medical School
1475 NW 12th Ave.
PO Box 016960 (D8-4)
Miami, FL 33101
(305) 548-4810

Illinois

Illinois Cancer Council
36 S. Wabash Ave., Suite 700
Chicago, IL 60603
(312) 346-9813

**University of Chicago Cancer
   Research Center**
5841 S. Maryland Avenue
Box 444
Chicago, IL 60637
(312) 702-6180

Maryland

Johns Hopkins Oncology Center
600 N. Wolfe St.
Baltimore, MD 21205
(301) 955-8822

Massachusetts

Dana-Farber Cancer Institute
44 Binney St.
Boston, MA 02115
(617) 732-3636

Michigan

**Comprehensive Cancer Center of
   Metropolitan Detroit**
Wayne State University
School of Medicine
P.O. Box 02188
Detroit, MI 48201
(313) 745-8870

Minnesota

**Mayo Comprehensive Cancer
   Center**
Mayo Clinic, East 12
200 First St, SW
Rochester, MN 55905
(507) 284-4718

New York

**Memorial-Sloane Kettering
   Cancer Center**
1275 York Ave.
New York, NY 10021
(212) 794-6561

Roswell Park Memorial Institute
666 Elm St.
Buffalo, NY 14263
(716) 845-5770

Columbia University Cancer Center
College of Physicians and
   Surgeons
701 W. 168th St.
New York, NY 10032
(212) 305-6904

Ohio

**Ohio State University
   Comprehensive Cancer Center**
410 W. 12th Ave., Suite 302
Columbus, OH 43210
(614) 292-5022

Pennsylvania

Fox Chase Cancer Center
7701 Burholme Ave.
Philadelphia, PA 19111
(215) 728-2490

**University of Pennsylvania Cancer
   Center**
7 Silverstein Pavilion
3400 Spruce St.
Philadelphia, PA 19104
(215) 662-6334

Texas

**University of Texas M. D. Anderson
Cancer Center**
1515 Holcombe Blvd.
Houston, TX 77030
(713) 792-6000

Washington

**Fred Hutchinson Cancer Research
Center**
1124 Columbia St.
Seattle, WA 98104
(206) 467-4302

Wisconsin

**University of Wisconsin Clinical
   Cancer Center**
600 Highland Ave.
Madison, WI 53792
(608) 263-8610

CHARTERED DIVISIONS OF THE AMERICAN CANCER SOCIETY. INC.*

Alabama Division, Inc.
402 Office Park Drive—Suite 300
Birmingham, Alabama 35223
(205) 879-2242

Alaska Division, Inc.
406 West Fireweed Lane
Suite 204
Anchorage, Alaska 99503
(907) 277-8696

Arizona Division, Inc.
2929 East Thomas Road
Phoenix, Arizona 85016
(602) 224-0524

Arkansas Division, Inc.
901 North University
Little Rock, Arkansas 72207
(501) 664-3480

California Division, Inc.
1710 Webster Street
Oakland, California 94612
(415) 893-7900

Colorado Division, Inc.
2255 South Oneida
Denver, Colorado 80224
(303) 758-2030

Connecticut Division, Inc.
Barnes Park South
14 Village Lane
Wallingford, Connecticut 06492
(203) 265-7161

Delaware Division, Inc.
1708 Lovering Avenue
Suite 202
Wilmington, Delaware 19806
(302) 654-6267

District of Columbia Division, Inc.
1825 Connecticut Avenue, NW
Suite 315
Washington, DC 20009
(202) 483-2600

Florida Division, Inc.
1001 South MacDill
Avenue
Tampa, Florida 33629
(813) 253-0541

Georgia Division, Inc.
46 Fifth Street, NE
Atlanta, Georgia 30308
(404) 892-0026

Hawaii-Pacific Division
Community Services Center
Building
200 North Vineyard Blvd.
Honolulu, Hawaii 96817
(808) 531-1662-3-4-5

Idaho Division, Inc.
1609 Abbs Street
Boise, Idaho 83705
(208) 343-4609

Illinois Division, Inc.
37 South Wabash Avenue
Chicago, Illinois 60603
(312) 372-0472

Indiana Division, Inc.
8730 Commerce Park Place
Indianapolis, Indiana 46268
(317) 872-4432

Iowa Division, Inc.
Suite D
8364 Hickman Road
Des Moines, Iowa 50322
(515) 253-0147

Kansas Division, Inc.
1315 SW Arrowhead Road
Topeka, Kansas 66604
(913) 273-4114
FAX: 913-267-9910

Kentucky Division, Inc.
701 West Muhammad Ali
    Boulevard
Louisville, Kentucky 40201-1807
(502) 584-6782

Long Island Division, Inc.
145 Pidgeon Hill Road
Huntington Station, New York 11746
(516) 385-9100

Louisiana Division, Inc.
Fidelity Homestead Building
837 Gravier Street
Suite 700
New Orleans, Louisiana 70112-1509
(504) 523-4188

Maine Division, Inc.
52 Federal Street
Brunswick, Maine 04011
(207) 729-3339
FAX: 207-729-0635

Maryland Division, Inc.
8219 Town Center Drive
P.O. Box 82
White Marsh, Maryland 21162-0082
(301) 529-7272

Massachusetts Division, Inc.
Carhart Memorial Building
247 Commonwealth Avenue
Boston, Massachusetts 02116
(617) 267-2650

Michigan Division, Inc.
1205 East Saginaw Street
Lansing, Michigan 48906
(517) 371-2920

Minnesota Division, Inc.
3316 West 66th Street
Minneapolis, Minnesota 55435
(612) 925-2772

Mississippi Division, Inc.
1380 Livingston Lane
Lakeover Office Park
Jackson, Mississippi 39213
(601) 362-8874

Missouri Division, Inc.
3322 American Avenue
Jefferson City, Missouri 65102
(314) 893-4800

Montana Division, Inc.
Suite #1
313 N. 32nd Street
Billings, Montana 59101
(406) 252-7111

Nebraska Division, Inc.
8502 West Center Road
Omaha, Nebraska 68124-5255
(402) 393-5800

Nevada Division, Inc.
1325 East Harmon
Las Vegas, Nevada 89119
(702) 798-6877

New Hampshire Division, Inc.
Gail Singer Memorial Building
360 Route 101
Unit 501
Bedford, New Hampshire 03102-
6821
(603) 472-8899

New Jersey Division, Inc.
CN 2201
2600 Route 1
North Brunswick, New Jersey 08902
(201) 297-8000

New Mexico Division, Inc.
5800 Lomas Boulevard, NE
Albuquerque, New Mexico 87110
(505) 586-8700

New York City Division, Inc.
19 West 56th Street
New York, New York 10019
(212) 586-8700

New York State Division, Inc.
6725 Lyons Street
East Syracuse, New York 13057
(315) 437-7025

North Carolina Division, Inc.
11 South Boylan Avenue
Suite 221
Raleigh, North Carolina 27603
(919) 834-8463

North Dakota Division, Inc.
123 Roberts Street
Fargo, North Dakota 58102
(701) 232-1385

Ohio Division, Inc.
5555 Frantz Road
Dublin, Ohio 43017
(614) 889-9565

Oklahoma Division, Inc.
3000 United Founders Boulevard
Suite 136
Oklahoma City, Oklahoma 73112
(405) 843-9888

Oregon Division, Inc.
0330 Southwest Curry
Portland, Oregon 97201
(503) 295-6422

Pennsylvania Division, Inc.
Route 422 & Sipe Avenue
Hershey, Pennsylvania 17033-0897
(717) 533-6144

*National Headquarters: American Cancer Society, Inc., 777 Third Avenue, New York, NY., 10017

CHARTERED DIVISIONS OF THE AMERICAN CANCER SOCIETY, INC.—cont'd

Philadelphia Division, Inc.
1422 Chestnut Street
Second Floor
Philadelphia, Pennsylvania 19102
(215) 665-2900

Puerto Rico Division, Inc.
Calle Alverio #577
Esquina Sargento Medina
Hato Rey, Puerto Rico 00918
(809) 764-2295

Queens Division, Inc.
112-25 Queens Boulevard
Forest Hills, New York 11375
(718) 263-2224

Rhode Island Division, Inc.
400 Main Street
Pawtucket, Rhode Island 02860
(401) 722-8480

South Carolina Division, Inc.
2214 Devine Street
Columbia, South Carolina 29205
(803) 256-0245

South Dakota Division, Inc.
4101 Carnegie Circle
Sioux Falls, South Dakota 57104-
2322

Tennessee Division, Inc.
1315 Eighth Avenue South
Nashville, Tennessee 37203
(615) 255-1ACS (1227)

Texas Division, Inc.
2433 Ridgepoint Drive
Austin, Texas 78754
(512) 928-2262
Inf. Systems: (512) 928-8921
(1-800-843-1092)

Utah Division, Inc.
610 East South Temple
Salt Lake City, Utah 84102
(801) 322-0431

Vermont Division, Inc.
13 Loomis Street
Drawer C
Montpelier, Vermont 05602
(802) 223-2348

Virginia Division, Inc.
4240 Park Place Court
Glen Allen, Virginia 23060
(804) 270-0142/800-552-7996

Washington Division, Inc.
2120 First Avenue North
Seattle, Washington 98109-1140
(206) 283-1152

Westchester Division, Inc.
30 Glenn Street
White Plains, New York 10603
(914) 949-4800

West Virginia Division, Inc.
2428 Kanawha Boulevard, East
Charleston, West Virginia 25311
(304) 344-3611

Wisconsin Division, Inc.
615 North Sherman Avenue
Madison, Wisconsin 53704
PO Box 8370
Madison, Wisconsin 53708
(608) 249-0487

Wyoming Division, Inc.
3109 Boxelder Drive
Cheyenne, Wyoming 82001
(307) 638-3331

DIVISION SERVICES, AMERICAN CANCER SOCIETY, INC.

Central
425 North Martingale Road
Suite 1130
Schaumburg, Illinois 60173
(312) 706-3280

Coastal
1599 Clifton Road, N.E.
Atlanta, Georgia 30329
(404) 329-7520

New England
World Trade Center
Commonwealth Pier, Suite 305
Boston, Massachusetts 02201
(617) 439-5260

Southern
1599 Clifton Road, N.W.
Atlanta, Georgia 30329
(404) 329-7518

East Metro
1155 Connecticut Avenue, N.W.
Suite 602
Washington, D.C. 20036
(202) 872-9220

Mid-Atlantic
1155 Connecticut Avenue, N.W.
Suite 602
Washington, D.C. 20036
(202) 872-9220

West I
4900 Southwest Meadow Drive
Meadow One
Suite 425
Lake Oswego, Oregon 97034
(503) 697-4290

West II
5660 Greenwood Plaza Boulevard
Suite 400
Englewood, Colorado 80111
(303) 773-1502

7-3 | Contagious diseases

Disease and synopsis of symptoms	Incubation period	Mode of transmission	Period of communicability
Actinomycosis Chronic disease most frequently localized in jaw, thorax, or abdomen; septicemic spread with generalized disease may occur. Lesions are firmly indurated areas of purulence and fibrosis.	Irregular; probably years after colonization in oral tissues, plus days or months after precipitating trauma and actual penetration of tissues.	Contact from person to person as part of normal oral flora.	Time and manner in which *A. israelii* becomes part of normal flora is unknown.
Amebiasis Infection with a protozoan parasite that exists in two forms: the hardy, infective cyst and the more fragile, potentially invasive trophozoite. Parasite may act as a commensal or invade tissues, giving rise to intestinal or extraintestinal disease.	Variation—from a few days to several months or years. Commonly 2 to 4 weeks.	Contaminated water or food containing cysts from feces of infected persons, often as complication of another infection such as shigellosis.	During period of cyst passing, which may continue for years.
Ascariasis (roundworm infection) Helminthic infection of small intestine. Symptoms are variable, often vague or absent, and ordinarily mild; live worms, passed in stools or regurgitated, are frequently first recognized sign of infection.	Worms reach maturity about 2 months after ingestion of embryonated eggs.	By ingestion of infective eggs from soil contaminated with human feces containing eggs, but not directly from person to person.	As long as mature female worms live in intestine. Maximum lifespan of adult worms is under 18 months; however, female produces up to 200,000 eggs a day that can remain viable in soil for months or years.
Balantidiasis Disease of colon characteristically producing diarrhea or dysentery accompanied by abdominal colic, tenesmus, nausea, and vomiting.	Unknown; may be only a few days.	By ingestion of cysts from feces of infected hosts; in epidemics, mainly by fecally contaminated water.	As long as infection persists.
Candidiasis (monoiliasis, thrush, candidosis) Mycosis usually confined to superficial layers of skin or mucous membranes with patients who have oral thrush, intertrigo, vulvovaginitis, paronychia, or onychomycosis.	Variable, 2 to 5 days in thrush of infants.	Through contact with excretions of mouth, skin, vagina, and especially from patients or carriers; from mother to infant during childbirth; and by endogenous spread.	Presumably for duration of lesions.
Carditis, Coxsackie (viral carditis, enteroviral carditis) Acute or subacute myocarditis or pericarditis, which occurs as the only manifestation, or may occasionally be associated with other manifestations.	Usually 3 to 5 days.	Fecal-oral or respiratory droplet contact with infected person.	Apparently during acute stage of disease.
Chickenpox, herpes zoster (varicella shingles) Acute generalized viral disease with sudden onset of slight fever, mild constitutional symptoms, and a skin eruption that is maculopapular for a few hours, vesicular for 3 to 4 days, and leaves a granular scab.	From 2 to 3 weeks; commonly 13 to 17 days.	From person to person by direct contact, droplet, or air-borne spread of secretion of respiratory tract of chickenpox cases or of vesicle fluid of patients with herpes zoster.	As long as 5 days but usually 1 to 2 days before onset of rash, and not more than 6 days after appearance of first crop of vesicles.

Continued.

Contagious diseases — cont'd

Disease and synopsis of symptoms	Incubation period	Mode of transmission	Period of communicability
Cholera Acute intestinal disease with sudden onset, profuse watery stools, occasional vomiting, rapid dehydration, acidosis, and circulatory collapse. Death may occur within a few hours.	From a few hours to 5 days, usually 2 to 3 days.	Through ingestion of food or water contaminated with feces or vomitus of infected persons or with feces of carriers.	Thought to be for duration of stool-positive stage, usually only a few days after recovery. Carrier stage may last for several months.
Conjunctivitis, acute bacterial Clinical syndrome beginning with lacrimation, irritation, and hyperemia of the palpebral and bulbar conjunctivae of one or both eyes, followed by edema of lids, photophobia, and mucopurulent discharge.	Usually 24 to 72 hours.	Contact with discharges from conjunctivae or upper respiratory tract of infected persons through contaminated fingers, clothing, or other articles.	During course of active infection.
Conjunctivitis, epidemic hemorrhagic (Apollo 11 disease) Virus infection with sudden onset of pain or sensation of a foreign body in eye. Disease rapidly progresses (1 to 2 days) to full case of swollen eyelids, hyperemia of the conjunctivae, often with a circumcorneal distribution, seromucous discharge, and frequent subconjunctival hemorrhages.	1 to 2 days or even shorter.	Through direct or indirect contact with discharge from infected eyes and possibly by droplet infection from those with virus in throat.	Unknown, but assumed to be for period of active disease, usually 1 to 2 weeks.
Dermatophytosis A. Ringworm of scalp and beard (tinea capitis, tinea kerion, favus) Begins as small papule and spreads peripherally, leaving scaly patches of temporary baldness. Infected hairs become brittle and break off easily. Kerions sometimes develop.	10 to 14 days	Direct or indirect contact with articles infected with hair from humans or infected animals.	As long as lesions are present and viable fungus persists on contaminated materials.
B. Ringworm of nails (tinea unguium, onychomycosis) Chronic infectious disease involving one or more nails of hands or feet. Nail thickens becoming discolored and brittle with an accumulation of caseous-appearing material beneath nail.	Unknown.	Presumably by direct extension from skin or nail lesions of infected persons. Low rate of transmission.	Possibly as long as infected lesion is present.
C. Ringworm of groin and perinanal region (dhobie itch, tinea cruris)	4 to 10 days.	Direct or indirect contact with skin and scalp lesions of infected persons or animals.	As long as lesions are present and viable fungus persists on contaminated materials.
D. Ringworm of the body (tinea corporis) Characteristically appears as flat, spreading, ring-shaped lesions. Periphery is usually reddish, vesicular, or pustular and may be dry and scaly or moist and crusted.			

Continued.

Contagious diseases — cont'd

Disease and synopsis of symptoms	Incubation period	Mode of transmission	Period of communicability
E. Ringworm of the foot (tinea pedis, athlete's foot) Scaling or cracking of skin, especially between toes, or blisters containing this watery fluid are characteristic. In severe cases vesicular lesions appear on various parts of body.	Unknown.	Direct or indirect contact with skin lesions of infected persons or contaminated floors or shower stalls.	As long as lesions are present and viable spores persist on contaminated materials.
Diphtheria Characteristic lesion marked by patch or patches of grayish membrane with surrounding dull red inflammatory zone. Throat is moderately sore in faucial diphtheria, with cervical lymph nodes enlarged and tender; occasionally swelling and edema of neck.	2 to 5 days, sometimes longer.	Contact with patient or carrier; more rarely with articles soiled with discharges from lesions of infected persons. Raw milk has been a vehicle.	Variable, until virulent bacilli have disappeared from discharge and lesions. Usual period is 2 to 4 weeks but chronic carriers may shed organisms for 6 months or more.
Gastroenteritis, viral A. Epidemic viral gastroenteritis Usually self-limited mild disease that often occurs in outbreaks with clinical symptoms of nausea, vomiting, diarrhea, abdominal pain, myalgia, headache, malaise, low-grade fever, or a combination thereof.	24 to 48 hours; in volunteer studies with Norwalk agent range was 10 to 51 hours.	Unknown; probably by fecal-oral route. Several recent outbreaks strongly suggest foodborne and waterborne transmission.	During acute stage of disease and shortly thereafter.
B. Rotavirus gastroenteritis (sporadic viral gastroenteritis of infants and children) Sporadic severe gastroenteritis of infants and young children characterized by diarrhea and vomiting, often with severe dehydration and occasional deaths.	Approximately 48 hours.	Probably fecal-oral and possibly respiratory routes.	During acute stage of disease and later while virus shedding continues. Virus is not usually detectable after eighth day of illness.
Giardiasis (*Giardia* enteritis, lambliasis) Protozoan infection principally of upper small bowel; often asymptomatic, it may also be associated with a variety of intestinal symptoms such as chronic diarrhea, steatorrhea, abdominal cramps, bloating, frequent loose and pale, greasy, malodorous stools, fatigue, and weight loss.	In a water-borne epidemic in United States, clinical illnesses occured 1 to 4 weeks after exposure; average 2 weeks.	Localized outbreaks occur from contaminated water supplies. By ingestion of cysts in fecally contaminated water and occasionally by fecally contaminated food.	Entire period of infection.
Hepatitis, viral A. Viral hepatitis A (infectious hepatitis, epidemic hepatitis, epidemic jaundice, catarrhal jaundice, Type A hepatitis) Onset is usually abrupt with fever, malaise, anorexia, nausea, and abdominal discomfort, followed within a few days by jaundice.	From 15 to 50 days, depending on dose; average 28-30 days.	Person to person by fecal-oral route. Common-vehicle outbreaks have been related to contaminated water and food.	Studies indicate maximum infectivity during latter half of incubation period, continuing for a few days, after onset of jaundice.

Continued.

Contagious diseases — cont'd

Disease and synopsis of symptoms	Incubation period	Mode of transmission	Period of communicability
B. Viral hepatitis B (Type B hepatitis, serum hepatitis) Onset is usually insidious with anorexia, vague abdominal discomfort, nausea, and vomiting, sometimes arthralgias and rash, often progressing to jaundice. Fever may be absent or mild.	Usually 45 to 160 days, average 60 to 90 days. Variation is related in part to amount of virus in inoculum, mode of transmission, and host factors.	HB$_x$Ag, the infectious agent, has been found in virtually all body secretions, but only blood, saliva, and semen have been shown to be infectious. Transmission usually by percutaneous inoculation of infected blood and blood products; contaminated needles, syringes, and IV equipment.	From several weeks before onset of symptoms through clinical course of disease; carrier state can last for years.
C. Hepatitis, non-A, non-B (non-B transfusion-associated hepatitis, hepatitis C) Chronic infection may be symptomatic or asymptomatic. Differential diagnosis depends on exclusion of hepatitis types A and B.	2 weeks to 6 months, model 6 to 8 weeks.	Most common posttransfusion hepatitis in United States and is more common when paid donors are used. Percutaneous transmission documented and other modes similar to those of hepatitis B virus are suspected.	Degree of immunity following infection is not known.
Herpangina; hand-foot-and-mouth disease, acute lymphonodular pharyngitis *Herpangina* — grayish papulovesicular pharyngeal lesions on an erythematous base. *Hand-foot-and-mouth disease* — more diffuse oral lesions on buccal surfaces of cheeks, gums, and tongue. *Acute lymphonodular pharyngitis* — lesions are firm, raised, discrete, whitish to yellow nodules.	3 to 5 days for herpangina and hand-foot-and-mouth disease. 5 days for acute lymphonodular pharyngitis.	Direct contact with nose and throat discharges and feces of infected (possibly asymptomatic) persons and by droplet spread.	During acute stage of illness and longer because virus persists in stools for as long as several weeks.
Herpes simplex Viral infection characterized by localized primary lesion, latency, and a tendency to localized recurrence. In perhaps 10% of primary infections overt disease may appear as illness of varying severity marked by fever and malaise lasting 1 week or more.	2 to 12 days.	HSV Type 1: Direct contact with virus in saliva of carriers. HSV Type 2: Sexual contact.	Secretion of virus in saliva has been reported for as long as 7 weeks after recovery from stomatitis. Patients with primary lesions are infective for about 7 to 12 days, with recurrent disease for 4 days to 1 week.
Influenza Acute viral disease of respiratory tract characterized by fever, chilliness, headache, myalgia, prostration, coryza, and mild sore throat. Cough is often severe and protracted.	Usually 24 to 72 hours.	By direct contact through droplet infection; probably airborne among crowded populations in enclosed spaces.	Probably limited to 3 days from clinical onset.

Continued.

Contagious diseases — cont'd

Disease and synopsis of symptoms	Incubation period	Mode of transmission	Period of communicability
Measles (rubeola, hard measles, red measles, morbilli) Acute, highly communicable viral disease with prodromal fever, conjunctivitis, coryza, bronchitis, and Koplik's spots on the buccal mucosa. A characteristic red blotchy rash appears on third to seventh day, beginning on face, becoming generalized, lasting 4 to 7 days and sometimes ending in branny desquamation. Leukopenia is common.	About 10 days varying from 8 to 13 days from exposure to onset of fever; about 14 days until rash appears; uncommonly longer or shorter human normal immune globulin (IG), given later than third day of incubation period for passive protection, may extend the incubation period to 21 days instead of preventing disease.	By droplet spread or direct contact with nasal or throat secretions of infected persons. Measles is one of most readily transmitted communicable diseases.	From slightly before beginning of prodromal period of 4 days after appearance of rash; communicability is minimal after second day of rash.
Meningitis, meningococcal (cerebrospinal fever, meningococcemia) Characterized by sudden onset of fever, intense headache, nausea and often vomiting, stiff neck, and frequently a petechial rash with pink macules or, very rarely, vesicles. Delirium and coma often appear; occasional fulminating cases exhibit sudden prostration.	Varies from 2 to 10 days, commonly 3 to 4 days.	By direct contact, including droplets and discharges from nose and throat of infected persons, more often carriers than cases.	Until meningococci are no longer present in discharges from nose and throat. If organisms are sensitive to sulfonamides, meningococci usually disappear from nasopharynx within 24 hours after institution of treatment. They are not fully eradicated from oronasopharynx by penicillin.
Meningitis, hemophilus (meningitis caused by *Haemophilus influenzae*) Most common bacterial meningitis in children 2 months to 3 years old in U.S. Otitis media or sinusitis may be precursor. Almost always associated with bacteremia. Onset is sudden with symptoms of fever, vomiting, lethargy, and meningeal irritation.	Probably short — within 2 to 4 days	By droplet infection and discharges from nose and throat during infectious period. May be purulent rhinitis. Portal of entry is most commonly nasopharyngeal.	As long as organisms are present, which may be for prolonged period even without nasal discharge.
Mononucleosis, infectious (glandular fever, EBV mononucleosis) Characterized by fever, sore throat (often with exudative pharyngotonsillitis), and lymphadenopathy (especially posterior cervical). Jaundice occurs in about 4% of infected young adults and splenomegaly in 50%. Duration is from 1 to several weeks.	From 4 to 6 weeks.	Person-to-person spread by oropharyngeal route via saliva. Spread may also occur via blood transfusion to susceptible recipients.	Prolonged; pharyngeal excretion may persist for 1 year after infection; 15% to 20% of healthy adults are oropharyngeal carriers.

Continued.

Contagious diseases — cont'd

Disease and synopsis of symptoms	Incubation period	Mode of transmission	Period of communicability
Mumps (infectious parotitis) Acute viral disease characterized by fever, swelling, and tenderness of one or more salivary glands, usually parotid and sometimes sublingual or submaxillary glands.	About 2 to 3 weeks, commonly 18 days.	By droplet spread and by direct contact with saliva of an infected person.	Virus has been isolated from saliva from 6 days before salivary gland involvement to as long as 9 days thereafter; but height of infectiousness occurs about 48 hours before swelling begins. Urine may be positive for as long as 14 days after onset of illness.
Paratyphoid fever Frequently generalized bacterial enteric infection, often with abrupt onset, continued fever, enlargement of spleen, sometimes rose spots on trunk, usually diarrhea, and involvement of lymphoid tissues of mesentery and intestines.	1 to 3 weeks for enteric fever; 1 to 10 days for gastroenteritis.	Direct or indirect contact with feces or urine of patient or carrier. Spread is by food, especially milk, milk products, and shellfish. Flies may be vectors.	As long as infectious agent persists in excreta, which is from appearance of prodromal symptoms, throughout illness, and for periods up to several weeks or months. Commonly 1 to 2 weeks after recovery.
Pediculosis (lousiness) Infestation of head, hairy parts of body, or clothing with adult lice, larvae, or nits (eggs), which results in severe itching and excoriation of scalp or scratch marks of body.	Under optimum conditions, eggs of lice hatch in 1 week, reach sexual maturity in approximately 2 weeks.	Direct contact with infected person and indirectly by contact with personal belongings, especially clothing and headgear. Crab lice are usually transmitted through sexual contact.	Communicable as long as lice remain alive on infested person or in clothing, and until eggs in hair and clothing have been destroyed.
The pneumonias A. Pneumococcal pneumonia Acute bacterial infection characterized by sudden onset with single shaking chill, fever, pleural pain, dyspnea, cough productive of "rusty" sputum and leukocytosis.	Not well determined; believed to be 1 to 3 days.	By droplet spread; by direct oral contact or indirectly, through articles freshly soiled with respiratory organisms is common.	Presumably until discharges of mouth and nose no longer contain virulent pneumococci in significant numbers. Penicillin will render patient noninfectious within 24 to 48 hours.
B. Mycoplasmal pneumonia (primary atypical pneumonia) Predominantly afebrile lower respiratory infection. Onset is gradual with headache, malaise, cough often paroxysmal, and usually substernal pain (not pleuritic). Sputum, scant at first, may increase later.	14 to 21 days.	Probably by droplet inhalation, direct contact with infected person or with articles freshly soiled with discharges of nose and throat from acutely ill and coughing patient.	Probably less than 10 days; occasionally longer with persisting febrile illness or persistence of the organisms in convalescence (as long as 13 weeks is known).
C. Pneumocystis pneumonia (interstitial plasmal cell pneumonia) Acute pulmonary disease occuring early in life, especially in malnourished, chronically ill, or premature infants. Characterized by progressive dyspnea, tachypnea, and cyanosis; fever may not be present.	Analysis of data from institutional outbreaks among infants indicates 1 to 2 months.	Unknown.	Unknown.

Continued.

Contagious diseases—cont'd

Disease and synopsis of symptoms	Incubation period	Mode of transmission	Period of communicability
D. Chlamydial pneumonia (pertussoid eosinophilic pneumonia) Subacute pulmonary disease occurring in early infancy, primarily in infants of mothers with infection of uterine cervix with causative organism.	Not known, but pneumonia may occur in infants from 1 to 18 weeks of age (more commonly between 4 and 12 weeks).	Presumed to be vertically transmitted from infected cervix to infant during birth, with resultant nasopharyngeal infection.	Unknown, but length of nasopharyngeal excretion can be at least 2 months.
Poliomyelitis (infantile paralysis) Acute viral infection whose symptoms include fever, malaise, headache, nausea, vomiting, and stiffness of neck and back with or without paralysis.	Commonly 7 to 14 days for paralytic cases, with a range from 3 to possibly 35 days.	Direct contact through close association. In rare instances milk, foodstuffs, and other fecally contaminated materials have been incriminated as vehicles. Fecal-oral is major route when sanitation is poor, but during epidemics and when sanitation is good, pharyngeal spread becomes relatively more important.	Not accurately known. Cases are probably most infectious during first few days after onset of symptoms.
Respiratory disease (excluding influenza) A. Acute febrile respiratory disease Viral diseases of respiratory tract are characterized by fever and one or more constitutional reactions such as chills or chilliness, headache, general aching, malaise, and anorexia; in infants by occasional gastrointestinal disturbances.	From a few days to 1 week or more.	Directly by oral contact or by droplet spread, indirectly by hands or other materials soiled by respiratory discharges of infected person.	For duration of active disease; little is known about subclinical or latent infections.
B. Common cold (acute coryza) Acute catarrhal infections of upper respiratory tract characterized by coryza, sneezing, lacrimation, irritated nasopharynx, chilliness, and malaise lasting 2 to 7 days. Fever is uncommon in children and rare in adults.		Presumably by direct oral contact or by droplet spread; indirectly by hands and articles freshly soiled by discharges of nose and throat of infected person.	
Rubella (German measles) A. Congenital rubella Mild febrile infectious disease with diffuse punctate and macular rash. Sometimes resembling that of measles, scarlet fever, or both. May be few or no constitutional symptoms in children but adults may experience 1- to 5-day prodrome characterized by low-grade fever, headache, malaise, mild coryza, and conjunctivitis. As many as 20% to 50% of infections may occur without evident rash; overall 50% are not recognized. B. Erythema infectiosum (fifth disease)	From 16 to 18 days with a range of 14 to 21 days.	Contact with nasopharyngeal secretions of infected person. Infection is by droplet spread or direct contact with patients and indirect contact.	For about 1 week before and at least 4 days after onset of rash. Highly communicable. Infants with congenital rubella syndrome may shed virus for months after birth.

Continued.

Contagious diseases—cont'd

Disease and synopsis of symptoms	Incubation period	Mode of transmission	Period of communicability
Mild nonfebrile erythematous eruption occurring as epidemics among children. Characterized by striking erythema of cheeks, reddening of skin, and lacelike serpiginous rash of body. C. Exanthema subitum (roseola infantum) Acute illness of probable viral cause characterized by high fever that suddenly appears and lasts 3 to 5 days. A maculopapular rash on trunk and later on rest of body ordinarily follows lysis of fever.			
Shigellosis (bacillary dysentery) Acute bacterial disease primarily involving large intestine, characterized by diarrhea, accompanied by fever, nausea, sometimes vomiting, cramps, and tenesmus. In severe cases stools contain blood, mucus, and pus.	1 to 7 days, usually 1 to 3 days.	By direct or indirect fecal-oral transmission from patient or carrier. Infection may occur after ingestion of very few organisms.	During acute infection and until infectious agent is no longer present in feces, usually within 4 weeks of illness.
Staphylococcal disease A. Staphylococcal disease in community, boils, carbuncles, furuncles, impetigo, cellulitis, abscesses, staphylococcal septicemia, staphylcoccal pneumonia, osteomyelitis, endocarditis Staphylococci produce variety of syndromes with clinical manifestations that range from single pustule to impetigo to septicemia to death. Lesion or lesions containing pus are primary clinical finding, abscess formation is typical.	Variable and indefinite. Commonly 4 to 10 days.	Major site of colonization is anterior nares. Autoinfection is responsible for at least one third of infections. Person with draining lesion or any purulent lesion or who is asymptomatic (usually nasal) carrier of pathogenic strain. Air-borne spread is rare.	As long as purulent lesions continue to drain or carrier state persists.
B. Staphylococcal disease in hospital nurseries, impetigo, abscess of breast Characteristic lesions develop secondary to colonization of nose or umbilicus, conjunction, circumcision site, or rectum of infants with pathogenic strain.	Commonly 4 to 10 days but may occur several months after colonization.	Spread by hands of hospital personnel is primary mode of transmission within hospitals; to a lesser extent, air-borne.	Same.
C. Staphylococcal disease in medical and surgical wards of hospitals Lesions vary from simple furuncles or stitch abscesses to extensively infected bedsores or surgical wounds, septic phlebitis, chronic osteomyelitis, fulminating pneumonia, endocarditis, or septicemia.	Variable and indefinite. Commonly 4 to 10 days.	Major site of colonization is anterior nares. Autoinfecton is responsible for at least one third of infections. Person with a draining lesion or any purulent lesion or who is an asymptomatic (usually nasal) carrier of a pathogenic strain. Air-borne spread is rare.	As long as purulent lesions continue to drain or carrier state persists.

Continued.

Contagious diseases — cont'd

Disease and synopsis of symptoms	Incubation period	Mode of transmission	Period of communicability
Streptococcal sore throat Fever, sore throat, exudative tonsillitis or pharyngitis, and tender anterior cervical lymph nodes	Short, usually 1 to 3 days, rarely longer.	Transmission results from direct or intimate contact with patient or carrier, rarely by indirect contact through objects or hands. Nasal carriers are particularly likely to transmit diseases.	In untreated uncomplicated cases 10 to 21 days; in untreated conditions with purulent discharges, weeks or months.
Syphilis, nonvenereal endemic Acute disease of limited geographical distribution, characterized clinically by eruption of skin and mucous membrane, usually without evident primary sore.	2 weeks to 3 months.	Direct or indirect contact with infectious early lesions of skin and mucous membranes. Congenital transmission does not occur.	Until moist eruptions of skin and mucous patches disappear — sometimes several weeks or months.
Trachoma Communicable keratoconjunctivitis characterized by conjunctival inflammation with papillar hyperplasia, associated with vascular invasion of cornea, and in later stages by conjunctival scarring that may eventually lead to blindness.	5 to 12 days (based on volunteer studies).	By direct contact with ocular discharges and possibly mucoid or purulent discharges of nasal mucous membranes of infected persons or materials. Flies (*Musca sorbens*) may contribute to spread of disease.	As long as active lesions are present in the conjunctivae and adnexal mucous membranes.
Tuberculosis Myocbacterial disease. Initial infection usually goes unnoticed; tuberculin sensitivity appears within a few weeks; lesions commonly heal, leaving no residual changes except pulmonary or tracheobronchial lymph node calcification. May progress to pulmonary tuberculosis or, by lympho hematogenous dissemination of bacilli, to produce miliary, meningeal, or other extrapulmonary involvement.	From infection to demonstrable primary lesion, about 4 to 12 weeks. Whereas subsequent risk of progressive pulmonary or extrapulmonary tuberculosis is greatest within 1 or 2 years after infection, it may persist for a lifetime as latent infection.	Exposure to bacilli in air-borne droplet nuclei from sputum of persons with infectious tuberculosis. Bovine tuberculosis results from exposure to tubercular cattle and ingestion of unpasteurized dairy products.	As long as infectious tubercle bacilli are being discharged.
Typhoid fever (enteric fever, typhus abdominalis) Systemic infectious disease characterized by sustained fever, headache, malaise, anorexia, relative bradycardia, enlargement of spleen, rose spots on trunk, nonproductive cough, constipation more commonly than diarrhea, and involvement of lymphoid tissues.	Depends on size of infecting dose; usual range 1 to 3 weeks.	By food or water contamined by feces or urine of patient or carrier.	As long as typhoid bacilli appear in excreta; usually first week throughout convalescence; variable thereafter. About 10% of untreated patients will discharge bacilli for 3 months after onset of symptoms; 2% to 5% become permanent carriers.

Continued.

Contagious diseases—cont'd

Disease and synopsis of symptoms	Incubation period	Mode of transmission	Period of communicability
Whooping cough (pertussis) Acute bacterial disease involving tracheobronchial tree. Initial catarrhal stage has insidious onset with irritating cough that gradually becomes paroxysmal, usually within 1 to 2 weeks, and lasts for 1 to 2 months.	Commonly 7 days; almost uniformly within 10 days, and not exceeding 21 days.	Primarily by direct contact with discharges from respiratory mucous membranes of infected persons by air-borne route, probably by droplets. Frequently brought into home by older sibling.	Highly communicable in early catarrhal stage before paroxysmal cough stage. For control purposes, communicable stage extends from 7 days after exposure to 3 weeks after onset of typical paroxysms in patients not treated with antibiotics; in patients treated with erythromycin, period of infectiousness extends only 5 to 7 days after onset of therapy.

7-4 | Sexually transmitted diseases

Disease and synopsis of symptoms	Incubation period	Mode of transmission	Period of communicability
Acquired immunodeficiency syndrome (AIDS) Acute viral infection characterized by breakdown and failure of immune system, opening body to often lethal infections and disorders such as Kaposi's sarcoma, pneumonia, and meningitis. Symptoms begin with fever, weight loss, fatigue, shortness of breath, diarrhea, and neurologic disorders.	Variable.	By direct sexual contact and transmission of semen, saliva, blood, or other body fluids. Also by blood transfusion or contaminated syringes.	For duration of infection
Chancroid (ulcus molle, soft chancre) Acute, localized, genital infection characterized by single or multiple painful necrotizing ulcers at site of inoculation, frequently accompanied by painful inflammatory swelling and suppuration of regional lymph nodes. Extragenital lesions have been reported.	From 3 to 5 days, up to 14 days.	By direct sexual contact with discharges from open lesions and pus from buboes; suggestive evidence of asymptomatic infections in women. Multiple sexual partners and uncleanliness favor transmission.	As long as infectious agent persists in original lesion or discharging regional lymph nodes; usually until healed—a matter of weeks.
Conjunctivitis, inclusion (swimming pool conjunctivitis, paratrachoma) In the newborn, acute papillary conjunctivitis with abundant mucopurulent discharge. In children and adults, acute follicular conjunctivitis with preauricular lymphadenopathy, often with superficial corneal involvement.	5 to 12 days.	During sexual intercourse; genital discharges of infected persons are infectious.	While genital infection persists; can be longer than 1 year in female.
Cytomegalovirus infections, congenital cytomegalovirus infection, cytomegalic inclusion disease Most severe form of disease occurs in perinatal period, following congenital infection, with signs and symptoms of severe generalized infection especially involving central nervous system and liver.	Information inexact. 3 to 8 weeks following transfusion with infected blood. 3 to 12 weeks after birth.	Intimate exposure to infectious secretions or excretions. Virus is excreted in urine, saliva, cervical secretions, breast milk, and semen.	Virus is excreted in urine or saliva for months and may persist for several years following primary infection.

Continued.

Sexually transmitted diseases—cont'd

Disease and synopsis of symptoms	Incubation period	Mode of transmission	Period of communicability
Gonococcal infections A. Gonococcal infection of genitourinary tract (gonorrhea, gonococcal urethritis) *Males*—purulent discharge from anterior urethra with dysuria appears 2 to 7 days after infecting exposure. *Females*—few days after exposure initial urethritis or cervicitis occurs, frequently so mild as to pass unnoticed. About 20% of patients have uterine invasion at the first, second, or later menstrual period with symptoms of endometritis, salpingitis, or pelvic peritonitis.	Usually 2 to 7 days, sometimes longer.	By contact with exudates from mucous membranes of infected persons, almost always result of sexual activity.	May extend for months if untreated, especially in females who frequently are asymptomatic. Specific therapy usually ends communicability within hours except with penicillin-resistant strains.
B. Gonococcal conjunctivitis neonatorum (gonorrheal ophthalmia neonatorum) Acute redness and swelling of conjunctiva of one or both eyes, with mucopurulent or purulent discharge in which gonococci are identifiable by microscopic and cultural methods.	Usually 1 to 5 days.	Contact with infected birth canal during childbirth.	While discharge persists if untreated; for 24 hours following initiation of specific treatment.
Granuloma inguinale (donovanosis) Mildly communicable, nonfatal, chronic and progressive, autoinoculable bacterial disease of skin and mucous membranes of external genitalia, inguinal, and anal region. Small nodule, vesicle, or papule is present.	Unknown; probably 8 to 80 days.	Presumably by direct contact with lesions during sexual activity.	Unknown and probably for duration of open lesions on skin or mucous membranes.
Herpes simplex Viral infection characterized by localized primary lesion, latency, and a tendency to localized recurrence. In perhaps 10% of primary infections overt disease may appear as illness of varying severity marked by fever and malaise lasting 1 week or more.	2 to 12 days.	HSV Type 1: Direct contact with virus in saliva of carriers. HSV Type 2: Sexual contact.	Secretion of virus in saliva has been reported for as long as 7 weeks after recovery from stomatitis. Patients with primary lesions are infective for about 7 to 12 days, with recurrent disease for 4 days to 1 week.
Lymphogranuloma venereum (lymphogranuloma inguinale, esthiomene, climactic bubo, tropical bubo) Venerally acquired infection, beginning with painless evanescent erosion, papule, nodule, or herpetiform lesion on penis or vulva, frequently unnoticed. Regional lymph nodes undergo suppuration followed by extension of inflammatory process to adjacent tissues.	Usually 7 to 12 days, with a range of 4 to 21 days to primary lesion. If bubo is first manifestation, 10 to 30 days, sometimes several months.	Direct contact with open lesions of infected persons usually during sexual intercourse.	Variable, from weeks to years, during presence of active lesions.

Continued.

Sexually transmitted diseases — cont'd

Disease and synopsis of symptoms	Incubation period	Mode of transmission	Period of communicability
Syphilis, venereal (lues) Acute and chronic treponematosis characterized clinically by primary lesion, secondary eruption involving skin and mucuous membranes, long periods of latency, and late lesions of skin, bone, viscerae, and central nervous and cardiovascular systems. Papule appears 3 weeks after exposure at site of initial invasion; after erosion, most common form is indurated chancre.	10 days to 10 weeks, usually 3 weeks.	By direct contact with infectious exudates from obvious or concealed moist early lesions of skin and mucous membrane, body fluids, and secretions of infected persons during sexual contact.	Variable and indefinite during primary and secondary stages and also in mucocutaneous recurrences; some cases may be intermittently communicable for 2 to 4 years.
Trichomoniasis Common disease of genitourinary tract, characterized in women by vaginitis, with small petechial or sometimes punctate hemorrhagic lesions and profuse, thin, foamy, yellowish discharge with foul odor; frequently asymptomatic. In men, infectious agent invades and persists in prostate, urethra, or seminal vesicles, but rarely produces symptoms or demonstrable lesions.	4 to 20 days, average 7days.	By contact with vaginal and urethral discharges of infected persons during sexual intercourse and possibly by contact with contaminated articles.	For duration of infection.

Urethritis, chlamydial
  Urethritis, nongonorrheal
  and nonspecific
Sexually transmitted urethritis of males caused by chlamydial agent. Clinical manifestations are usually indistinguishable from gonorrhea but are often milder and include opaque discharge of moderate or scanty quantity, urethral itching, and burning on urination. Infection of women results in cervicitis and salpingitis.
	5 to 7 days or longer	Sexual contact.	Unknown.

Aging

8-1 | Organizations pertaining to the elderly

AFL/CIO Social Security Department*
815 16th St., N.W.
Washington, D.C. 20006

AFSCME Retiree Program
1625 L Street, N.W.
Washington, D.C. 20036

Alzheimer's Association
551 5th Ave., Suite 601
New York, N.Y. 10176
and
70 East Lake St.
Chicago, Ill. 60601

Alzheimer's Association's board of directors is comprised of business leaders, health professionals, and family members. Additionally, there is a prestigious Medical and Scientific Advisory Board which consults on and monitors issues related to Alzheimer's Disease.

The Alzheimer's Association has five major goals: (1) Supporting *research* into causes, treatments, cures and prevention; (2) Stimulating *education and public awareness* of both laypeople and professionals on Alzheimer's Disease; (3) Encouraging *Chapter* formation for a nationwide family support network and implementation of programs at the local level; (4) *Advocacy* for improved public policy and needed legislation at federal, state and local levels; (5) *Patient and family service* to aid present and future victims and caregivers.

Those interested in help may call 800-621-0379 (Illinois residents, call 800-572-6037).

American Aging Association
University of Nebraska Medical Center
Omaha, Neb.
Made up of scientists, it seeks to promote research on aging.

American Association of Homes for the Aging*
1129 20th St. N.W., Suite 400
Washington, D.C. 20036
AAHA represents the nonprofit homes for the aging — religious, municipal, trust, fraternal.

American Association for International Aging
1511 K St., N.W., Suite 1028
Washington, D.C. 20005

American Association of Retired Persons†
1909 K St., N.W.
Washington, D.C. 20049
Age 55 or above, retired to still employed.

American Dance Therapy Association
2000 Century Plaza, Suite 108
Columbia, Md. 21044

American Foundation for the Blind, Inc.
15 West 16th St.
New York, N.Y. 10011

The American Geriatrics Society
770 Lexington, Suite 400
New York, N.Y. 10021
The American Geriatrics Society, made up of physicians, has an annual meeting.

American Nurses' Association, Inc.
Council of Nursing Home Nurses
Division on Gerontological Nursing Practice
2420 Pershing Rd.
Kansas City, Mo. 64108

American Occupational Therapy Assocation
1383 Piccard Dr.
Rockville, Md. 20850

American Osteopathic Association
142 E. Ontario
Chicago, Ill. 60611-2864

American Physical Therapy Association
200 S. Service Rd.
Roslyn Heights, N.Y. 11577
and
111 N. Fairfax St.
Alexandria, Va 22314

American Psychiatric Association
Council on Aging
1400 K St., N.W.
Washington, D.C. 20005

American Psychological Association
Division of Adult Development and Aging
1200 17th St., N.W.
Washington, D.C. 20036

American Public Health Association
Section of Gerontological Health
1015 15th St., N.W.
Washington, D.C. 20005

American Public Welfare Association
810 1st St., N.E., Suite 5
Washington, D.C. 20002

American Society on Aging
833 Market St., Room 516
San Francisco, Calif. 94103

American Speech-Language-Hearing Association
10801 Rockville Pike
Rockville, Md. 20852
8,047 audiologist members.

Asian and Pacific Coalition on Aging
1102 Crenshaw Blvd., Room 43
Los Angeles, Calif. 90019

*Denotes steering committee members of the Leadership Council.
†Denotes General Members of the Leadership Council of Aging Organizations, 1980-81.

Association for Gerontology in
Higher Education†
600 Maryland Ave., S.W.
West Wing 204
Washington, D.C. 20024

Canadian Psychiatric
Association
294 Albert St., Suite 204
Ottawa, Ontario K1P 6E6

Catholic Golden Age
1012 14th St., N.W., Suite 1003
Washington, D.C. 20005

Commission on Legal Problems
of the Elderly
American Bar Association
1800 M St., N.W.
Washington, D.C. 20036

Continental Association of
Funeral and Memorial
Societies
2001 S St., N.W., Suite 630
Washington, D.C. 20009

Council of Home Health
Agencies and Community
Health Services
National League for Nursing
10 Columbus Circle
New York, N.Y. 10019

The Gerontological Society of
America
1275 K St., N.W., Suite 350
Washington, D.C. 20005-4006
*This professional society has
an annual meeting and an
international meeting every
3 years. It is made up of
four components—biological
sciences, clinical medicine,
psychological and social
sciences and social research,
and planning and practice.*

Gray Panthers
311 S. Juniper St., Suite 601
Philadelphia, Pa. 19107
*Activistic group of older
people who resent "stereotyping."*

The Gray Panthers' National
Task Force on Older Women
6407 Maiden Lane
Bethesda, Md. 20034

Huntington's Disease Society
of America
140 W. 22nd St., 6th Floor
New York, N.Y. 10011-2420

The Institute of Retired
Professionals
The New School of Social
Research
66 W. 12th St.
New York, N.Y. 10011
*This pioneering school also led the
way in providing intellectual activi-
ties for retired professional people.*

The Institutes of Lifetime
Learning
*These are educational services of
the National Retired Teachers Associaton and the American Association of Retired Persons.*

The International Federation
on Aging
1909 K St., N.W.
Washington, D.C. 20049
*Confederation of aging organiza-
tions of various nations.*

Memorial Society Association
of Canada
Box 96
Weston, Ontario M9N 3M6

National Association of Area
Agencies on Aging
600 Maryland Ave., S.W.
Washington, D.C. 20024

National Association of Black
Social Workers, Inc.
642 Beckwith Ct., S.W.
Atlanta, Ga. 30314

National Association of Counties
Aging Program
440 First St., N.W.
Washington, D.C. 20001

National Association for
Families Caring for their
Elders, Inc.
1141 Loxford Terrace
Silver Spring, Md 20901

National Association of Foster
Grandparents Program
Directors
195 East San Fernando St.
San Jose, Calif. 95112

National Association of Meals
Programs, Inc.
204 E St., N.E.
Washington, D.C. 20002

National Association of
Nutrition and Aging
Services Programs
2663 44th St., S.W., Suite 205
Wyoming, Mich. 49509

National Association of Older
American Volunteer Program
Directors
1148 Bingham Terrace
Reston, VA 22091

National Assocation of RSVP
Directors, Inc.
RSVP of El Paso
Two Civic Center Plaza
El Paso, Tex. 79999

National Association of Retired
Federal Employees†
1533 New Hampshire Ave., N.W.
Washington, D.C. 20036
*Represents and lobbies for needs
of retired civil servants.*

National Association of Senior
Companion Project Directors
St. Landry Parish Community
Action Agency
P.O. Box 1510
Opelousas, La. 70570

National Association of Social
Workers
7981 Eastern Ave.
Silver Spring, Md. 20910

National Association of State Units
on Aging
2033 K St., S.W., Suite 304
Washington, D.C. 20006
*Information resources on state poli-
cies on aging. Represents and lobbies
for state agencies at the federal level.*

National Caucus and Center on
Black Aged
1424 K St., N.W., Suite 500
Washington, D.C. 20005
*Advocates improving the quality of
life for the black aged. Provides
comprehensive program of coordination, information, and consulta-
tive services to meet needs of black
aged.*

*Denotes steering committee members of the Leadership Council.
†Denotes General Members of the Leadership Council of Aging Organizations, 1980–1981.

**National Citizens' Coalition
for Nursing Home Reform**
1424 16th St., N.W.,
Suite L2
Washington, D.C. 20036

**National Conference of
State Legislatures**
444 N. Capital St., N.W.,
Suite 500
Washington, D.C. 20001

**National Council on the
Aging**
600 Maryland Ave., S.W.
Washington, D.C. 20024
*Research and services
regarding the elderly.*

**National Council of Senior
Citizens**
925 15th St., N.W.
Washington, D.C. 20005
*Represents and lobbies
for needs of the elderly.
Membership at any age.*

National Geriatrics Society
212 W. Wisconsin Ave.
Milwaukee, Wis. 53202

National Health Services
1200 18th St., Suite 602
Washington, D.C. 20036

**National Hispanic Council
on Aging**
2713 Ontario Road, N.W.,
Suite 200
Washington, D.C. 20009
National Hospice Organization
1901 N. Moore St., Suite 901
Arlington, Va. 22209

National Hospice Organization
1901 N. Moore St., Suite 901
Arlington, Va. 22209

**National Indian Council on
Aging, Inc.†**
P.O. Box 2088
Albuquerque, N.M. 87103

**National Institute of Senior
Centers**
National Council on Aging
600 Maryland Ave. S.W.
West Wing 100
Washington, D.C. 20024

**National Interfaith Coalition
on Aging**
P.O. Box 1924
Athens, Ga. 30605
*Coordinates the involvement
of religious groups in meeting
the needs of the elderly.*

National Organization for Women
1000 16th St., N.W., Suite 700
Washington, D.C. 20036

**National Pacific/Asian
Resource Center on Aging**
2033 6th Ave., Suite 410
Seattle, Wash. 98121

**National Retired Teachers
Association (NRTA)***
1909 K St., N.W.
Washington, D.C. 20049
*Members once active in an
educational system, public
or private.*

**National Senior Citizens Law
Center (NSCLC)**
2025 M St., N.W., Suite 400
Washington, D.C. 20036
and
1052 W. 6th St., Suite 700
Los Angeles, Calif. 90017
*The NSCLC is a national support
center, specializing in the legal
problems of the elderly poor, and is
funded by the Legal Services Cor-
poration, the Administration on Aging of the Department of Health
and Human Services; and the
Community Services Administration. Its principal function is to
provide support services to legal service attorneys, and other publicly
funded programs providing legal assistance to older persons, on the legal problems of their elderly clients.*

**National Therapeutic Recreation
Society**
National Recreation and Park
Association
3101 Park Center Dr.
Alexandria, Va. 22302

**National Voluntary Organizations
for Independent Living for the
Aging (NVOILA)**
National Council on Aging
600 Maryland Ave., S.W.
West Wing 100
Washington, D.C. 20024

**The National Women's Political
Caucus**
1275 K St., N.W., Suite 750
Washington, D.C. 20005

Retired Officers Association
201 N. Washington
Alexandria, Va. 22314
*Represents needs of retired military
officers of the United States.*

**Senior Action in a Gay Environ-
ment, Inc.**
Serving the Older Gay Community
208 W. 13th St.
New York, N.Y. 10011

**Sex Information and Education
Council of the United States
(SIECUS)**
32 Washington Place
New York, N.Y. 10003
*Part of its program is to provide
sex information to older people.*

Southern Gerontological Society
c/o Gerontology Center
Georgia State University
Atlanta, Ga. 30303

**United Auto Workers/Retired
Members Department**
8731 E. Jefferson St.
Detroit, Mich. 48214

U.S. Conference on Mayors
Task Force on Aging
1620 I St., N.W.
Washington, D.C. 20006

United Steelworkers of America
720 West Chicago Ave., Room 211
East Chicago, Ind. 46312

Villers Advocacy Associates
1334 G St., N.W.
Washington, D.C. 20005

Women's Equity Action League
1250 I St., N.W., Suite 305
Washington, D.C. 20005

**Women's Studies Program and
Policy Center**
George Washington University
2025 I St., N.W.
Washington, D.C. 20052
*Has formed a coalition with the
Congressional Women's Caucus to
draft and promote legislation to
benefit older women.*

8-2 | State agencies on aging

State agency	Telephone number
Alabama Commission on Aging	(205) 261-5743
Older Alaskans Commission	(907) 465-3250
American Samoa Territorial Administration on Aging	(684) 633-1252
Arizona Office on Aging and Adult Administration	(602) 255-4446
Arkansas Department of Human Services	(501) 371-2441
California Department of Aging	(916) 322-5290
Colorado Aging and Adult Services Division	(303) 866-5122
Connecticut Department on Aging	(203) 566-3268
Delaware Division on Aging	(302) 421-6791
District of Columbia Office of Aging	(202) 724-5622
Florida Aging and Adult Services	(904) 488-8922
Georgia Office of Aging	(404) 894-5333
Guam Public Health and Social Services	(671) 734-2942
Hawaii Executive Office on Aging	(808) 548-2593
Idaho Office on Aging	(208) 334-3833
Illinois Department on Aging	(217) 785-3356
Indiana Department on Aging and Community Services	(317) 232-7006
Iowa Commission on Aging	(515) 281-5187
Kansas Department on Aging	(913) 296-4986
Kentucky Division for Aging Services	(502) 564-6930
Louisiana Governor's Office of Elderly Affairs	(504) 925-1700
Maine Bureau of Elderly	(207) 289-2561
Maryland Office on Aging	(301) 225-1102
Massachusetts Department of Elder Affairs	(617) 727-7751
Michigan Office of Services to the Aging	(517) 373-8230
Minnesota Board on Aging	(612) 296-2270
Mississippi Council on Aging	(601) 949-2013
Missouri Division of Aging	(314) 751-3082
Montana Community Services Division	(406) 444-3865
Nebraska Department on Aging	(402) 471-2307
Nevada Division for Aging Services	(702) 885-4210
New Hampshire State Council on Aging	(603) 271-2751
New Jersey Division on Aging	(609) 292-4833
New Mexico State Agency on Aging	(505) 827-7640
New York State Office for the Aging	(518) 474-4425
North Carolina Division of Aging	(919) 733-3983
North Dakota Aging Services	(701) 224-2577
Northern Mariana Islands Departments of Community and Cultural Affairs	(670) 234-6011
Ohio Commission on Aging	(614) 466-5500
Oklahoma Services for the Aging	(405) 521-2281
Oregon Senior Services Division	(503) 378-4728
Pennsylvania Department of Aging	(717) 783-1550
Puerto Rico Gericulture Commission	(809) 724-1059
Rhode Island Department of Elderly Affairs	(401) 277-2858
South Carolina Commission on Aging	(803) 758-2576
South Dakota Office of Adult Services and Aging	(605) 773-3656
Tennessee Commission on Aging	(615) 741-2056
Texas Department on Aging	(512) 444-6890
Trust Territory of the Pacific Islands Office of Elderly Affairs	(670) 322-9328
Utah Division of Aging and Adult Services	(801) 533-6422
Vermont Office on Aging	(802) 241-2400
Virgin Islands Commission on Aging	(809) 774-5884
Virginia Department for the Aging	(804) 225-2271
Washington Bureau of Aging and Adult Services	(206) 753-2502
West Virginia Commission on Aging	(304) 348-3317
Wisconsin Office on Aging	(608) 266-2536
Wyoming Commission on Aging	(307) 777-6111

APPENDIX 9

Resources for help with disabilities and illness

800 numbers for organizations and
services for various illnesses and
disabilities

AT&T Special Needs Center; (800)
233-1222.
TDD (800) 833-3232.

AMC Cancer Information Center;
(800) 525-3777.

Alzheimer's & Related Disorders
Center; (800) 621-0379. In Illinois, (618) 985-8311.

American Association for Retarded
Citizens; (800) 433-5255.

American Cleft Palate Foundation;
(800) 232-5338; (800) 24-CLEFT.

American Council for the Blind;
(800) 424-8666.

American Diabetes Association;
(800) 232-3472.

American Foundation for the Blind;
(800) 232-5463.

American Kidney Fund
Information; (800) 638-8299.

American Liver Foundation;
(800) 223-0179.

American Paralysis Association;
(800) 225-0292.

American Parkinson's Disease Assocation, (800) 223-APDA.

Better Hearing Institute; (800) 424-
8576.

Braillegrams (Western Union);
(800) 325-6000.

Cancer Information Service;
(800) 4-CANCER.

Captioned Films for the Deaf; (800)
237-6213.

Children's Hospice International;
(800) 242-4453.

Chrysler Motors Adaptive Equipment Center; (800) 255-9877.

Clearinghouse on Adult Career and
Vocational Education;
(800) 848-4815.

Cornelia de Lange Syndrome
Foundation; (800) 223-8355.

Craniofacial Foundation; (800) 535-
3643.

Doubleday Large Print Books; (800)
343-4300.

Educators Publishing (Dyslexia);
(800) 792-5166; (800) 225-5750.

Epilepsy Foundation of America;
(301) 459-3700; (800) 332-1000.

Higher Education and Training for
People with Handicaps;
(800) 544-3284.

IBM Support Center for Persons
with Disabilities; (800) 426-2133.

Job Accomodation Network;
(800) 526-4698; (800) 526-7234.

Job Opportunities for the Blind;
(800) 638-7518.

Job Discrimination Hot Line; (800)
USA-EEOC.

Juvenile Diabetes Association; (800)
223-1138.

Library of Congress Handicapped
Hot Line; (800) 424-8567.

Lung Line (respiratory disorders);
(800) 222-LUNG.

Medicare/Medicaid Fraud, Waste
and Abuse Hot Line;
(800) 368-5779.

Multiple Sclerosis 24-Hour Information Line; (800) 624-8236.

National Adoption Center for Special Needs and Physically Disabled
Children; (800) TO-ADOPT.

National AIDS Hot Line; English,
(800) 342-AIDS. Spanish, (800)
344-SIDA.
Deaf, (800) AIDS-TTY.

National Association for Hearing
and Speech Action; (800) 638-
TALK.

National Center for Stuttering; (800)
221-2483.

National Cystic Fibrosis Foundation;
(800) 344-4823.

National Deafness Information
Center; (800) 672-6720.

National Down Syndrome Congress;
(800) 232-NDSC. In Illinois, (312)
823-7550.

National Down Syndrome Society;
(800) 221-4602.

National Easter Seal Society; (800)
221-6827.

National Health Information
Center; (800) 336-4797.

National Hearing Aid Society; (800)
521-5247.

National Organization of Social Security Claimants Representatives;
(800) 431-2804.

National Organization on Disability;
(800) 248-ABLE.

National Rehabilitation Information
Center; (800) 34-NARIC.

National Spinal Cord Injury Hot
Line; (800) 526-3456.

National Spinal Cord Injury
Association; (800) 962-9629.

National Tuberous Sclerosis
Association; (800) CAL-NTSA.

Orton Dyslexia Society; (800) 222-
3123.

Protection and Advocacy Legal
Rights Agency for Developmen-
tally and Mentally Disabled
Persons; (800) 555-1212.

Random House Audio Books; (800)
638-6460.

Recorded Books; (800) 638-1304.

Recordings for the Blind; (800) 221-
4792.

Retinitis Pigmentosa Foundation;
(800) 638-2300.

Sexually Transmitted Disease Hot
Line; (800) 227-8922.

Social Security Administration;
(800) 234-5772.

Spina Bifida Association; (800) 621-
3141.

The Living Bank—Organ
Donations; (800) 528-2971.

United Cerebral Palsy; (800) 872-
1827

From Diane B. Piastro, Living with a disability. © 1990 United Feature Syndicate, Inc. Reprinted by permission.